MOSBY'S

Canadian Textbook for the Support Worker

MOSBY'S Canadian Textbook for the Support Worker

SHEILA A. SORRENTINO
RN, PhD
Curriculum and Health Care Consultant
Normal, Illinois

CANADIAN AUTHORS
Mary J. Wilk, *RN, GNC(C), BA, BScN, MN(c)*
Fanshawe College, London, Ontario
Rosemary Newmaster, *RN*
Fleming College, Peterborough, Ontario

Second Canadian Edition

MOSBY
ELSEVIER

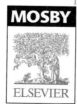

MOSBY
ELSEVIER

Library and Archives Canada Cataloguing in Publication

Sorrentino, Sheila A.
Mosby's Canadian textbook for the support worker / Sheila A. Sorrentino, Mary J. Wilk., Rosemary Newmaster – 2nd Canadian ed.

Adaptation of Mosby's textbook for nursing assistants, 7th ed., by Sheila A. Sorrentino.
Includes index.
ISBN 978-0-7796-9989-6

1. Nurses' aides–Handbooks, manuals, etc. 2. Care of the sick–Textbooks.
I. Newmaster, Rosemary II. Wilk, Mary J. III. Sorrentino, Sheila A.
Mosby's textbook for nursing assistants. IV. Title.

RT84.S67 2008 610.7306'98 C2007-902046-1

VP, Publishing: Ann Millar
Managing Developmental Editor: Martina van de Velde
Developmental Editor: Toni Chahley
Managing Production Editor: Rohini Herbert
Copy Editor: Rohini Herbert
Cover, Interior Design: Olena Sullivan/New Mediatrix
Typesetting and Assembly: Jansom
Printing and Binding: Transcontinental

Elsevier Canada
905 King Street West, 4th Floor,
Toronto, ON, Canada M6K 3G9
Phone: 1-866-896-3331
Fax: 1-866-359-9534

Printed in Canada

2 3 4 5 13 12 11 10 09 08

"To my parents.
For all that they have done for me and for so many others."

Sheila A. Sorrentino

"To my parents Michael and Natalia Wilk, who taught me everything I know about the power of love, and about growing older with dignity. I am blessed to be their daughter. I also wish to thank my husband Gord and my children Andrew and Julie for their patience, love, and support. I would also like to acknowledge my father-in-law J. Harvey Peterson for teaching me that one *can* grow as one ages."

Mary Wilk

"To my children Christopher and Stephanie, my grandson Noah, and my extended family Steve, Alaine, Madison, Andrea, and Lynn for all their love and support. I also would like to thank Susan, Taryn, and Ryan for their technical help that enabled me to meet my deadlines. Thank you to all my former students who have taught me so much over the years."

Rosemary Newmaster

CONTENTS

ABOUT THE AUTHORS

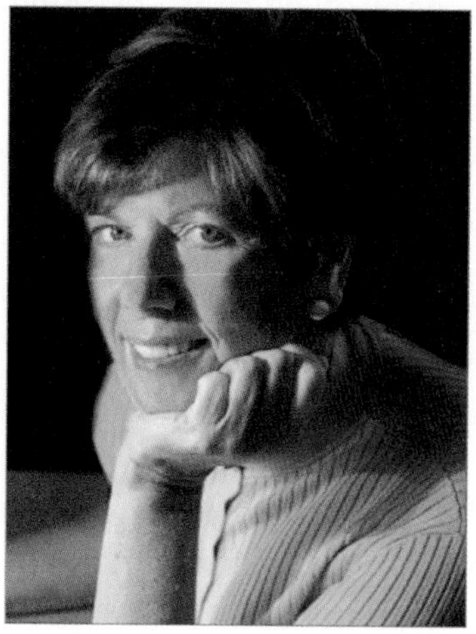

SHEILA A. SORRENTINO, RN, PhD

Sheila A. Sorrentino is currently a curriculum and health care consultant focusing on career ladder nursing programs and effective delegation and partnering with assistive personnel in hospitals, long-term care centres, and home care agencies. She also teaches part-time at Bradley University in Peoria, Illinois.

Dr. Sorrentino was instrumental in the development and approval of CAN-PA-AND programs in the Illinois Community College System and has taught in nursing assistant, practical nursing, associate degree, and baccalaureate and higher degree programs. Her career includes experience as a nursing assistant, staff nurse, charge nurse, head nurse, nursing educator, assistant dean, dean, and consultant.

A Mosby author since 1982, Dr. Sorrentino has written several textbooks for nursing assistants and other assistive personnel. She was also involved in the development of *Mosby's Nursing Assistant Skills Video* and *Mosby's Nursing Skills Videos*. An earlier version of the nursing assistant skills video won the 1992 International Medical Films Award on caregiving.

Dr. Sorrentino has a bachelor of science degree in nursing, a master of arts in education, a master of science degree in community nursing, and a PhD in higher education administration. She is a member of Sigma Theta Tau and a former member and chair of the Central Illinois Higher Education Health Care Task Force. She also served on the Iowa-Illinois Safety Council Board of Directors and the Board of Directors of Our Lady of Victory Nursing Center in Bourbonnais, Illinois. In 1998, she received an alumni achievement award from Lewis University for outstanding leadership and dedication in nursing education. Her presentations at national conferences focus on delegation and other issues relating to assistive personnel.

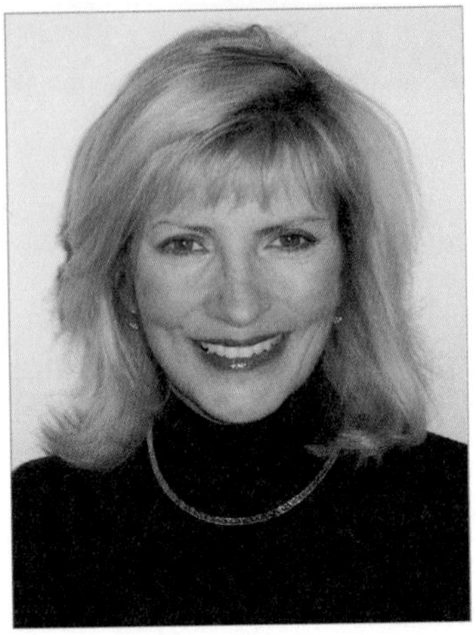

MARY J. WILK, RN, GNC(C), BA, BScN, MN(c)

Mary Wilk is currently a professor and coordinator of the personal support worker program at Fanshawe College, London, Ontario. She has taught at Fanshawe College for over 20 years in the School of Nursing, teaching pharmacology, anatomy and physiology, health promotion, communication, nursing theory, and nursing accountability, as well as clinical nursing in a variety of settings. During her teaching career, she has taught in the personal support worker, practical nurse, diploma nurse, paramedic, and recreation and leadership programs. She was also involved in curriculum development for the Collaborative Nursing Program, in affiliation with the University of Western Ontario. Her nursing career includes work experience in the emergency, coronary care, intensive care, orthopedics, gynecology, and medical-surgical nursing departments.

Mary has taught and has coordinated in the personal support worker (PSW) program at Fanshawe College since it was introduced in Ontario in 1997, and her students were the first PSW graduates in the province. She has been actively involved in PSW curriculum development at Fanshawe College and is involved in the Ontario PSW Subcommittee for the Heads of Health Sciences.

Mary has a bachelor of arts degree and a bachelor of science degree and is a candidate for the master of nursing degree from the University of Windsor. She currently holds a Gerontology Nurse Certificate through the Canadian Nurses Association, and she is on her local chapter's executive for the Gerontological Nursing Association (GNA) of Ontario. She has been a guest speaker numerous times, and her most recent topics include "Tuberculosis and the Elderly" and "The Role of PSWs in the Health Care Team."

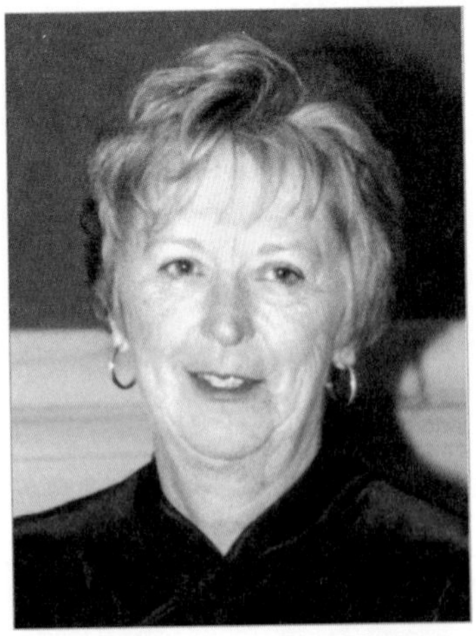

ROSEMARY NEWMASTER, RN

Rosemary Newmaster is a registered nurse currently working as a consultant, in the School of Continuing Education and Skilled Trades at Fleming College in Peterborough, Ontario. One of her areas of responsibilities is the health studies program. Rosemary started teaching and coordinating in the health care aide (HCA) program in 1987. She was involved at the provincial level as the health care aide curriculum evolved into the personal support worker program. As well as teaching HCAs, she taught the post-diploma gerontology certificate and the activation techniques in gerontology certificate programs. In 1996, she joined the School of Continuing Education and held the responsibility for the personal support worker programs at four campuses until the program was placed in the postsecondary school in 2006. She continues to be responsible for the bridging to personal support worker programs. Rosemary has been involved in the Ontario PSW Subcommittee for the Heads of Health Sciences since its beginning.

EDITORIAL ADVISORY BOARD

Elsevier Canada and the authors are grateful to our Editorial Advisory Board for sharing their knowledge and expertise; for providing their insights about support work and making many valuable content suggestions; and for their diligence in meeting very tight deadlines. Without their efforts, this textbook would not be the true representation of support work across Canada that it is. Their valuable feedback has improved the text immeasurably, and we wish to acknowledge their efforts.

CANADIAN REVIEWERS

The authors and publisher would like to acknowledge the assistance of the following reviewers:

Joanne Bailey, *RN, COHN*
Clinical Instructor
Humber College (North Campus)
Toronto, Ontario

Susan Bodis, *RN*
PSW Instructor
Georgian College
Barrie, Ontario

Mary Boivin, *RN*
Professor, PSW Program
Cambrian College
Sudbury, Ontario

Laurie Branchaud, *RN*
Clinical Instructor
St. Lawrence College
Cornwall, Ontario

Betty Buder, *BRE, RN*
Faculty and Lab Technologist, PN and PSW Program
Sheridan Institute of Technology and Advanced Learning
Oakville, Ontario

Carol Butler, *RN, BScN, MScN, MEd*
Coordinator, Clinical Learning and Simulation Nursing Labs
Fanshawe College
London, Ontario

Natalie Clark, *RN, BScN*
PSW Professor, Clinical Instructor
St. Lawrence College (Cornwall Campus and Iohahi:io Akwesasne)
Cornwall, Ontario

Stacey Copeland, *LPN*
Instructor/Supervisor, Health Care Aide Program
Horizon College
Fredericton, New Brunswick

Mary Gazel, *BA, BScN*
Professor, Personal Support Worker Program/Centre for Nursing
George Brown College
Toronto, Ontario

Helen Harrison, *BSc, BScN, BEd, MScN, PHCNP, RN(EC)*
Professor, School of Nursing, Faculty of Health Sciences
Fanshawe College
London, Ontario

Rhonda Jackson, *RN, BN*
School of Health and Human Services Faculty
Nova Scotia Community College (Cumberland Campus)
Springhill, Nova Scotia

Piera Jung, *RN, BSN, MA*
Professor, Faculty of Health and Human Services
Vancouver Island University
Nanaimo, British Columbia

Bonnie Lambkin, *RN, GCN*
Instructor, HS/RCA Program
College of New Caledonia
Prince George, British Columbia

Carole Lamothe, *RN, BA, MEd*
Coordinator, PSW Program and PN Program
College Boreal
Sudbury, Ontario

Marian MacLennan, *RN, BN*
Faculty, Continuing Care
Nova Scotia Community College (Waterfront Campus)
Dartmouth, Nova Scotia

Sally Malicki, *RN*
Professor, PSW Program
Confederation College
Thunder Bay, Ontario

Mary McDonald, *RN, BScN*
Education Director
Island Health Training Centre
Charlottetown, Prince Edward Island

Heather McGregor, *RN, BA*
Coordinator, PN and PSW Programs
School of Health and Community Services
Lambton College
Sarnia, Ontario

Jeffery Miller, *BEd*
PSW Educator, First Aid Instructor Trainer
Crisis Prevention Intervention Trainer
Medix School
London, Ontario

Glenda Montigny, *RN, OHN*
Instructor
Island Health Training Centre
Charlottetown, Prince Edward Island

Teresa Morris, *RN*
Assistant Instructor, Continuing Care,
Department of Health and Human Services
Nova Scotia Community College
Truro, Nova Scotia

Myrna O'Brien, *RN*
Faculty Head, PSW Program
triOS College of Business Technology
and Healthcare
Toronto, Ontario

Nadine Paquette, *RN, BScN*
Professor, PSW Program
Cambrian College
Sudbury, Ontario

Joanne Roberts, *RN*
Program Coordinator, PSW Program
St. Lawrence College (Cornwall Campus)
Cornwall, Ontario

Deborah Schuh, *RN, BN(P), PNC(C)*
Faculty, School of Health and Community
Services
Co-Coordinator, PSW Program
Durham College
Oshawa, Ontario

Norma Sherret, *RN, BSN, MN* (student)
College of the Rockies
Cranbrook, British Columbia

Elizabeth Sholtanuk, *RN*
Supervisor, PSW Program, and Education
Manager
Medix School (London Campus)
London, Ontario

Heather St. Jules, *RN*
Instructor, PSW Program
C/J Health Care Support College
Toronto, Ontario

Janet Szczukocki, *RN*
Manager, Education
Red Cross Community Health Services
Kingston, Ontario

Sandra Trubyk, *MSA, BN, BA, CAE*
Professor and Coordinator, School of
Community and Liberal Studies, PN, and PSW
Sheridan Institute of Technology & Advanced
Learning
Oakville, Ontario

Deborah Turner, *RN, BA, BEd*
Program Coordinator, Continuing Care
Nova Scotia Community College
(Marconi Campus)
Sydney, Nova Scotia

Debra Walker, *RN, BA, MDE*
Professor, PN Program
Confederation College
Thunder Bay, Ontario

Dorothy Wurst-Thurn, *LPN*
Instructor, Health Care Aide Program
Northern Lakes College,
Grande Prairie, Alberta

ACKNOWLEDGEMENTS

Textbooks are written and published through the combined efforts of many people. The planning, manuscript development, review, design, and production processes involve the ideas, talents, and contributions of many individuals. The authors would like to thank Ann Millar, Publisher at Elsevier, as well as Toni Chahley, Freelance Editor, for helping us stay sane and focused throughout this entire journey.

The authors and the publisher would like to acknowledge Fanshawe College, as many of the photos in this book were taken at their lab facilities.

INSTRUCTOR PREFACE

Mosby's Canadian Textbook for the Support Worker, Second Edition, is intended to prepare students to function in the role of support worker in communities and facility settings across Canada. Although the term ***support worker*** is used to describe a worker who provides personal care and support, the text also discusses programs for nursing attendants, continuing care attendants, and home care aides and other similar programs across Canada.

In keeping with the approach of the previous edition, the second edition of *Mosby's Canadian Textbook for the Support Worker,* prepared entirely *by* Canadians *for* Canadians, serves the needs of students and instructors in educational programs taught in community colleges, secondary schools, as well as private colleges. Most students in these institutions will find this an interesting textbook that is easy to read and understand.

This textbook is also designed to be an excellent resource for support workers already working in the field—whether in facilities or in community settings—who may have questions about issues they have encountered in their clinical practice. Support workers will learn many new things, experience new situations and new challenges, and even acquire new skills in the course of their work. Whatever the setting, they will find that learning is an ongoing process, and this textbook will be a valuable resource that will aid them in that process.

NEW TO THE SECOND CANADIAN EDITION

Mosby's Canadian Textbook for the Support Worker, Second Edition, has been revised, updated, and reorganized to reflect current practice across Canada. The chapter on Medical Terminology has been moved closer to the beginning of the textbook to prepare students to fully understand and appreciate the information presented in subsequent chapters. A new chapter on Caring for the Young includes a discussion of the role that support workers play when caring for children, disciplining the child as client, and caring for the challenging child. The chapter on Common Diseases and Conditions has also been moved to the earlier part of the textbook to make it easier for students and instructors to cross-reference the material with the chapters on Body Structure and Function, Growth and Development, Caring for the Young, and Caring for the Old. The chapter on Body Structure and Function has been significantly enhanced to ensure that an appropriate amount of anatomy and physiology has been covered to meet the needs of the users of this textbook. The scope of the chapter on Confusion, Delirium, and Dementia has been expanded to include an important discussion on managing disruptive behaviours.

The pedagogy of *Mosby's Canadian Textbook for the Support Worker,* Second Edition, has been brought up-to-date and enriched with the addition of new photos and figures reflecting current practice and over 30 new ***Supporting*** boxes that present real-life scenarios embodying the concepts covered in the chapters. ***Supporting*** boxes help students understand a particular client's health challenge or issue and empathize with the client. The clients discussed in each of these boxes are from different ethnic and cultural backgrounds and are described in a realistic style that is easy to understand. Instructors will find these boxes very useful to elicit discussion and dialogue from the class on various issues that students are likely to encounter in the field. Instructors who would like more information on the issues that are presented in the ***Supporting*** boxes are encouraged to refer to the Instructor's Manual that accompanies the textbook.

The new Appendix at the end of the book outlines the provincial/territorial differences in support worker titles, roles, education, and regulatory or comprehensive exams.

Also new to the Second Canadian Edition is a CD-ROM that contains Body Spectrum (with extra anatomy and physiology material, including images and a colouring book) and an Audio Glossary (the Glossary of the textbook in audio format).

Perhaps most importantly, this new edition places a stronger emphasis on understanding the role of support workers and their scope of practice.

GUIDING PRINCIPLES

This textbook is structured around several key ideas and principles:

- ***Canadian support workers need to know about Canadian issues.*** We have included chapters that discuss health care across Canada. These include Chapter 2 (The Canadian Health Care System), Chapter 3 (Workplace Settings), and Chapter 11 (Legislation: The Client's Rights and Your Rights). Relevant Canadian content on all important topics is presented throughout the textbook.
- ***Support workers provide services in a variety of community and facility settings.*** Because training programs prepare students for a variety of workplaces, multiple workplace settings—long-term care, home care, and hospital settings—are discussed throughout the text, especially in the ***Focus on Home Care*** and ***Focus on Long-Term Care*** boxes and the ***Procedures*** boxes, which highlight information and insights with regard to these settings.
- ***Each client is an individual with dignity and value.*** Throughout this textbook, students are reminded that each client is a whole person, with physical, emotional, social, intellectual, and spiritual dimensions. Students are encouraged to appreciate the client as a unique individual with a past, a present, and a future. Students are also taught to recognize a client's basic needs and protected rights.
- ***An essential part of a support worker's job is to provide compassionate care.*** The acronym DIPPS helps identify, recognize, and promote the five priorities of support work—dignity, independence, preferences, privacy, and safety—which are highlighted in ***Providing Compassionate Care*** boxes that discuss ways to promote the priorities of support work when giving the care described in the chapter.
- ***Effective communication skills are necessary to develop good working relationships.*** Chapter 13 is devoted to communication skills, and Chapter 36 discusses communication with clients who have speech and language disorders. Case studies and other boxes throughout the text also highlight the importance of communication.
- ***Support workers must respect the cultural diversity among their clients.*** Culture influences people's attitudes and beliefs. Chapter 12 discusses the role of cultural heritage in health and illness practices as well as in other aspects of life such as communication. ***Respecting Diversity*** boxes provide examples of the influence of culture on support care.
- ***Students learn best by reading about real-life examples.*** Case studies and examples that apply concepts to the real world of support work appear throughout the text. ***Support Workers Solving Problems*** boxes discuss ways to solve problems that may occur in support work in different settings. ***Supporting*** boxes help students understand a particular client's health challenge or issue and empathize with the client.
- ***Support workers need to understand their scope of practice and the delegation process.*** Because agencies and facilities across Canada vary in the way they utilize support workers, the responsibilities and limitations of support workers are emphasized throughout the text. The text presents many procedures that support workers across the country need to know and points out procedures that require extra training and supervision. Students are advised that they must understand and respect their employer's policies as well as provincial or territorial laws governing scope of practice. Chapter 5 addresses scope of practice and delegation issues; Chapter 10 focuses on ethical principles; and Chapter 11 addresses specific legislation that affects support workers in Canada.
- ***Providing safe care is at the core of support work.*** Ensuring the client's safety is one of the top priorities in support work and is therefore

emphasized throughout the text. Chapter 19 discusses the major types of accidental injuries among clients and measures to prevent them. It also discusses how support workers can take steps to ensure their own safety on the job; how to prevent the spread of infection (Chapter 20); how to recognize and report abuse (Chapter 21); and the basic principles of body mechanics and safety while moving and transferring clients (Chapter 23).

- *Following the client's care plan is critical to providing good care.* Chapter 8 describes the care planning process in both facilities and communities. Students are reminded throughout the text that support workers must follow the care plan and their supervisor's directions.

PEDAGOGICAL FEATURES AND DESIGN

Mosby's Canadian Textbook for the Support Worker, Second Edition, is presented in an attractive, four-colour, user-friendly design that makes the text easily navigable and the concepts and regulations easy to understand.

- *Objectives*—explain what is presented in the chapter and what students will learn.
- *Illustrations*—numerous full-colour photographs and illustrations.
- *Key Terms*—appear at the beginning of each chapter along with definitions and again in bold print within the body of the chapter where they are defined in the context of the subject discussed. An alphabetized list of the key terms, together with their definitions, is presented in the Glossary at the end of the book for easy reference. Key terms are set out in bold type in the chapters, and other important terms appear in italics for emphasis.
- *Boxes and tables*—list principles, guidelines, signs and symptoms, care measures, and other information.
- *Supporting boxes*—each box describes a scenario about a particular client and aims to elicit discussion about a specific concept or topic.
- *Case Study boxes*—apply some of the concepts discussed in the text to real-life examples of support workers and clients. They complement the ***Supporting*** boxes.
- *Focus on Children boxes*—provide age-specific information about the needs, considerations, and special circumstances of children.
- *Focus on Older Adults boxes*—provide age-specific information about the needs, considerations, and special circumstances of older adults.
- *Focus on Home Care boxes*—highlight information necessary for safe functioning in the home setting.
- *Focus on Long-Term Care boxes*—highlight information unique to the long-term care setting.
- *Providing Compassionate Care boxes*—remind students of the priorities of support work: respecting and promoting their client's dignity, independence, preferences, privacy, and safety. The acronym DIPPS is used to summarize these five priorities.
- *Support Workers Solving Problems boxes*—present scenarios depicting situations and problems encountered in support work on a daily basis and discuss how support workers make decisions and solve problems.
- *Respecting Diversity boxes*—help students learn to appreciate the influence of culture on health and illness practices and the importance of sensitivity to cultural diversity in support work.
- *Procedure boxes*—are usually divided into Pre-Procedure, Procedure, and Post-Procedure sections. The *Compassionate Care* section at the beginning of most of the Procedure boxes is a reminder of the priorities of support work. Asterisks are used to identify steps that are usually not applicable in community settings.
- *Review questions*—are found at the end of each chapter. Answers to the questions are presented (upside down) at the end of the section.

The authors and the publishing team at Elsevier Canada hope that this text will serve you and your students well by providing the information needed to teach and learn safe and effective care during this time of dynamic changes in Canadian health care.

AN IMPORTANT NOTE ON TERMINOLOGY

The client and his or her family who receive the services of support workers may be referred to by different terms, depending on the location and the context where these services are provided. For example, Mrs. Jones, who is receiving care in her own home (or in an assisted-living facility), would be referred to as a "client" by her caregivers. If she were to be admitted to an acute or complex care, continuing care, or subacute care facility—such as a hospital—she would then be called a "patient." If she needed to live in a continuing care (or long-term care) facility, she would then be called a "resident."

While the practice in an area or agency might be to refer to the recipient of support services as a ***patient***, ***resident***, ***consumer***, or ***customer***, for the purposes of this textbook, we have chosen to use the term ***client*** for the sake of simplicity and to make it easy for students, who are in the process of learning a large number of terms related to health care that constitute a whole new language. We discuss the issue of differences in terminology in Chapter 3: Workplace Settings.

In this text, we have also chosen to use the more generic and widely used term ***long-term care*** (referred to as **LTC** in the field) in the context of care that is ongoing and provides relatively stable assistance to people with their activities of daily living (ADLs). It also relates to any type of home or facility where clients are cared for and supported—long-term care facilities (nursing homes) or even in group homes for the developmentally delayed who are not physically or intellectually ill but are unable to care for themselves. While this term is *not* the preferred term in every province or regional area, we use "long-term care" throughout the text because it does not have different (and therefore misleading) meanings from one region to another within Canada. In contrast the term, "complex care" refers to the old terms "intermediate" and "extended" care in British Columbia, while it can mean "acute or subacute care for people with multisystem failure," a completely different meaning, in Ontario. Some provinces use the term "continuing complex care" to mean "ongoing care," while other provinces do not use the term at all. The term "continuing care" is being widely used throughout Canada in this context, but it is a relatively newer term than "long-term care" and therefore not widely used in some areas of Canada.

In summary, we suggest that instructors (and students) use the term that is the term of choice in their particular region, while being aware of the terminology differences existing within this diverse country of ours.

STUDENT PREFACE

As a support worker, you are a very important member of the health care team because you probably spend more time with your clients that any other member of the team. Team members rely on your observations, reports, and recordings, especially of any changes in your client. Your clients and their family rely on you to provide professional and safe care. You and the care you give may be the bright spots in a client's day.

This book was designed to help you learn and study using its special features that are described on the following pages. The book will continue to be a useful resource to you in the field as you gain experience and expand your knowledge.

This preface presents some study guidelines and tips to use this book effectively. Your instructor will probably assign chapters or partial chapters from the textbook to read before or after class. When given a reading assignment, do you read from the first page to the last page without stopping? How much of what you read do you remember? Using an efficient study system will help you understand and retain all the information that you read. A useful study system has these steps:

- Preview, or survey
- Question
- Read and record
- Recite and review

1 PREVIEW

Before you start a reading assignment, preview or survey the assignment to get an idea of what the assignment covers and to recall what you already know about the subject. Preview the chapter title, headings, subheadings, and terms or ideas in bold print or italics. Also, survey the objectives, key terms, introductory paragraph, boxes, and the review questions at the end of the chapter. Previewing takes only a few minutes. Remember, previewing helps you become familiar with the material.

2 QUESTION

After previewing, you need to form a list of questions to be answered as you read the material. Questions should relate to what might be asked on a test or how the information applies to giving care. Use the title, headings, and subheadings to form questions. Avoid questions that have one-word answers. Questions that begin with what, how, or why are helpful. While reading, if you find that a particular question does not help you understand and retain the assignment material, change the question to make this step more useful.

3 READ AND RECORD

Reading, which is the next step, is more productive after you have determined what you know already and what you need to learn. The purpose of reading is to:

- Gain new information
- Connect the new information to what you know already

Break the assignment into smaller parts, and as you read each part, try to find answers for the questions you had formulated earlier. Also, mark important information in the text by underlining, highlighting, or making notes, which will remind you later what you need to go back to in order to review and learn. Making notes helps you remember what you have learned. When making notes, write down important information in the text margins or in a notebook. Use words and summary statements that will jog your memory about the material.

After reading the assignment, in order to retain the information, you must organize it into a study guide—in the form of diagrams or charts that show relationships or steps in a process. Much of the information in this text is organized in this manner to help you learn. Note-taking in outline format is also very useful.

The following is a sample outline:

I. Main heading
    1. Second level
    2. Second level
        a. Third level
        b. Third level
II. Main heading

4 RECITE AND REVIEW

Finally, recite and review using your notes and the study guides and by finding the answers for the questions you formed earlier and any others that may have come up during the reading and as you answered the review questions at the end of the chapter. Answer all questions out loud (recite). If you are unsure about the answers to any of the questions, consult your instructor.

Reviewing is more about *when* to study than *what* to study. You already decided what to study during the preview, question, and reading steps. Your instructor may have emphasized key points from the reading assignment in class. The best times to review both the information in your text and your notes from class are: (1) the same day or evening of the class, (2) right after your first study session, (3) 1 week later, and (4) regularly before a quiz or test, midterm, or final exam. Studying the information many times will help you remember it.

CHAPTER 12

Caring About Culture and Diversity

OBJECTIVES

- Define the key terms listed in this chapter.
- Distinguish among race, ethnicity, and culture.
- Describe the factors that influence a person's culture.
- Summarize how culture influences a person's attitudes and behaviours in many areas.
- Describe how culture may affect communication, family organization, religious convictions, and perceptions about illness and health care.
- Analyze how your own cultural biases may affect your relationships with your clients.
- Apply the information in this chapter in your work by providing culturally sensitive care.

154

Chapter titles and subtitles tell you the subject of the chapter.

Objectives tell you what is presented in the chapter and what you will learn. As a final review of the chapter, see if you have learned all the information as listed in the Objectives.

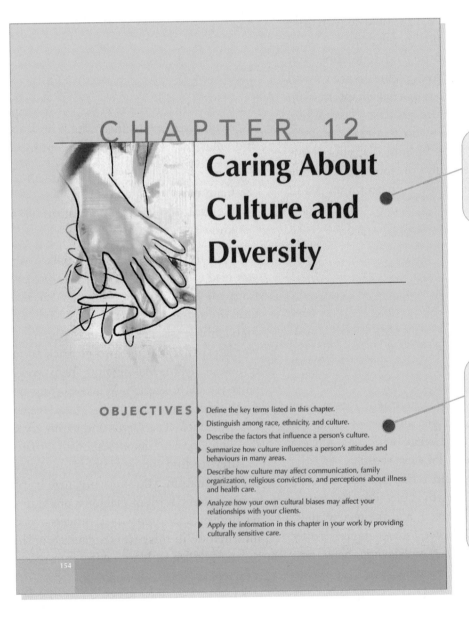

key terms

active listening A nonjudgemental communication technique that focuses not only on understanding the content of what is being said but also on the underlying emotions and feelings conveyed by the sender. This technique helps develop rapport and fosters a trusting relationship.

assertiveness A style of communication in which thoughts and feelings are expressed positively and directly without offending others.

body language Posture, appearance, facial expressions, body movements, eye contact, and gestures that send messages to others.

closed questions Questions that are structured so that the response can be restricted to one word, such as "yes" or "no," or a few words.

empathetic listening A nonjudgemental technique that requires the listener to be attentive to the sender's feelings.

focusing Limiting the conversation to a certain topic.

interpersonal communication The exchange of information between two people, usually face to face.

nonverbal communication Messages sent without words.

open-ended questions Questions that invite a person to share thoughts, feelings, or ideas.

paraphrasing Restating someone's message in one's own words.

verbal communication Messages sent through the spoken word.

Key terms are important words and phrases in the chapter. The list at the beginning of the chapter includes the definitions for all the terms. The key terms not only introduce you to the important terms in the chapter but they are also useful study guides.

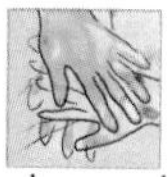

Good interpersonal communication is needed to provide safe and effective health care. Health care team members share information about what was done, what needs to be done for t[he] client, and the client's response to care and trea[t]ment. Good communication means better relatio[n]ships with clients, families, and co-workers. As [a] support worker, when you communicate wi[th] clients, you find out about their needs, feeling[s,] likes, and dislikes. You also express your though[ts] and ideas. *What* you say and *how* you say it a[re] equally important.

Successful interpersonal communication occurs when the receiver understands the meaning of the message. However, sometimes the receiver does not interpret the message in the way the sender

THE COMMUNICATION PROCESS

Interpersonal communication is the exchange [of] information between two people, usually face [to] face. A message is sent by one person (the *sende[r]*) and is received and interpreted by another pers[on] (the *receiver*). Often the receiver provides inform[a]tion in response to the message (*feedback*). Durin[g] the exchange of information, each person usual[ly] acts as both a sender and a receiver.

166

Focus on Home Care boxes highlight information necessary for providing safe care in the home setting.

260 Chapter 18 Common Diseases and Conditions

Hip Fractures. Fractured hips are common in older adults, especially in older women. They are serious because healing is slower in older people. The person is also at risk for life-threatening postoperative complications such as pneumonia, urinary tract infections, and thrombi in the leg veins, as well as pressure ulcers, constipation, and confusion.

The fractured hip is fixed in position with a pin, nail, plate, screw, or artificial hip joint. The client needs preoperative and postoperative care (see Chapter 46). Box 18–5 describes the support care required. Usually rehabilitation is needed after surgery. If home care is not possible, the client requires subacute or long-term care. Unless complications develop, the client usually returns home after successful rehabilitation (see the *Focus on Home Care: Clients Recovering From Hip Fractures* box.)

Box 18–5 Caring for Clients With Hip Fractures

- Follow the guidelines in Box 18–1 on page 251 if the client is confined to bed.
- Transfer, turn, and reposition the client, as directed. Turning and positioning depend on the type of fracture and the surgery performed. Usually the client is not positioned on the operative side.
- Keep the operated leg abducted at all times (**abduction** involves movement of a body part away from the median plane). The leg is abducted when the client is supine, being turned, or in a side-lying position (Figure 18–11, *A*). Use pillows or abductor splints, as directed (Figure 18–11, *B*).
- Prevent external rotation of the hip (turning outward). Use trochanter rolls, pillows, sandbags, or abductor splints, as directed (see Chapter 24).
- Provide range-of-motion exercises, as directed. Do not exercise the affected leg.
- Provide a straight-backed chair with armrests. The client will need a high, firm seat, so avoid placing the client in a low, soft chair.
- Position the chair on the client's unaffected side.
- Do not let the client stand on the affected leg unless allowed by the physician.
- Support and elevate the affected leg, as directed, when the client is in a chair.
- Apply elastic stockings, as directed (see Chapter 30).
- Remind the client to not cross his or her legs while seated.

focus on »HOME CARE

Clients Recovering From Hip Fractures

The artificial hip joint can dislocate (move out of place) with **adduction**, internal rotation (turning inward), and severe hip flexion. Lying on the affected side, sitting in low seats, sitting with the legs crossed, bending from the waist, and putting on shoes and socks or stockings would involve these movements and should be avoided for 6 to 8 weeks after surgery.

An occupational therapist helps the client learn to do self-care activities, and the client uses self-help devices for dressing (see Chapter 33). The client needs a raised toilet seat for elimination and a shower chair for bathing. The client uses a pillow or abductor splint between the legs when in bed. A physiotherapist helps the client learn muscle-strengthening exercises. A walker is usually needed for walking.

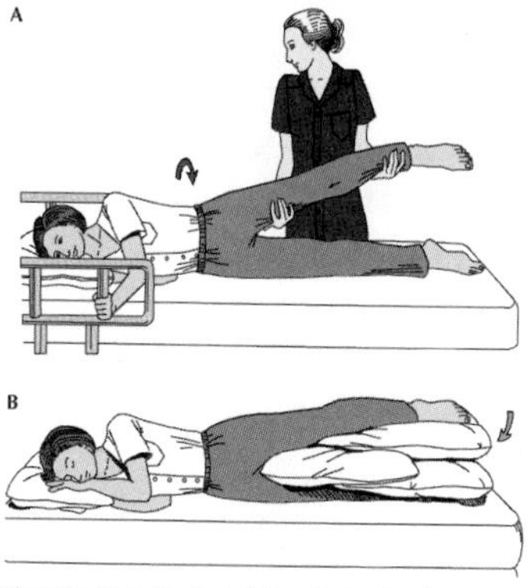

Figure 18–11 **A,** The hip is abducted when the client is turned. **B,** Pillows are used to maintain the hip in abduction.
Source: Phipps, W.J., Sands, J.K., & Marek, J.F. (1999). *Medical-surgical nursing: Concepts and clinical practice* (6th ed.). St. Louis: Mosby.

Terms in bold present the key terms and definitions again within the body of the chapter, which helps reinforce learning. The key terms and their definitions are listed alphabetically in the Glossary at the end of the book (see page 923). Whenever you come across a key term again in a later chapter, you can go to the Glossary for the definition of the term.

focus on ››CHILDREN

Hepatitis

Hepatitis A is more common among preschool and school-age children than among adults because the virus is easily spread among children. Poor hygiene practices after defecation lead to contamination of eating and drinking vessels, toys, and other surfaces. Also, young children often put their hands, toys, and other items in their mouths.

Acquired Immune Deficiency Syndrome

Acquired immune deficiency syndrome (AIDS) is a disease of the immune system caused by the *human immunodeficiency virus* (*HIV*). AIDS affects the person's ability to fight infections. Clients with AIDS may get infections such as pneumonia and tuberculosis (TB) and are also at increased risk for cancers. Sometimes they experience central nervous system damage, which may cause memory loss, loss of coordination, paralysis, mental health disorders, and dementia.

A person may be infected with HIV but not hav signs and symptoms of AIDS. This person is a carri and can transmit the virus to others. There is no cu for HIV infection; however, several medications hav been developed recently that slow its progress to ful blown AIDS. With current treatment, infected pe sons can remain AIDS-free for many years.

HIV is spread from an infected person to som one else when there is an exchange of certain bod fluids—blood, semen, vaginal secretions, or brea milk. HIV is transmitted mainly by:

- Unprotected intercourse with an infected pe son ("unprotected" means without a condom The virus enters the bloodstream through sma breaks in the mucous membranes of the re tum, vagina, penis, or mouth
- Needle-sharing among intravenous (IV) dru users
- HIV-infected mothers to their babies at birt or during breastfeeding
- ***Infection can also be spread when infecte body fluids come in direct contact with broke skin.*** Needle stick injuries can thus spread HI (see Chapter 20).

HIV is *not* spread by saliva, tears, urine, sweat, sneezing, coughing, and insects or through casual contact, including hugging, touching, or shaking hands with an infected person.

AIDS is the last stage of HIV infection. If HIV infection is not treated, AIDS develops in about 10 years after the initial infection. The following are possible warning signs of HIV infection:

- Rapid weight loss
- Dry cough
- Fever or night sweats
- Fatigue
- Swollen glands in the armpits, groin, or neck
- Diarrhea that lasts for more than a week
- White spots or unusual blemishes on the tongue, in the mouth, or in the throat
- Pneumonia
- Red, brown, pink, or purplish blotches on the skin or inside the mouth, nose, or eyelids
- Memory loss, confusion, or dementia

You may be providing support care to clients who have AIDS or who are HIV carriers. In some of the procedures, you may be in contact with the client's blood. Standard Precautions are important

Focus on Children boxes provide information about the needs, considerations, and general circumstances of children.

Terms in *italics* present other important terms and information in the text that require special attention.

Respecting Diversity boxes contain information to help you learn about the various practices of different cultures.

sive. Those living in long-term care facilities may not like the food that is served.

Loss of hearing, smell, and taste can affect appetite and social enjoyment of food, and poor vision may make shopping and meal preparation more challenging. Decreases in saliva may cause **dysphagia**—difficulty (*dys*) in swallowing (*phagia*). (See page 499.) Secretion of digestive juices also declines with age. As a result, fried and fatty foods are hard to digest and may cause indigestion, and nutrients are not absorbed as easily. Medications may have side effects, such as nausea, constipation, and loss of appetite. Loss of teeth and ill-fitting dentures can affect chewing. Decreased peristalsis, common among older adults, results in slower emptying of the stomach and colon, causing flatulence and constipation.

Energy levels are usually lower in older adults. Fewer calories are needed to sustain weight, but nutritional requirements remain high. High-protein foods are needed for tissue growth and repair. Foods high in calcium help keep bones strong; high-fibre foods, such as raw vegetables, help avoid constipation, but they can be hard to chew and can cause indigestion. Foods providing soft bulk, such as cooked fruits and vegetables, are often preferred for older clients with constipation or chewing problems. Drinking more fluids may also aid digestion, kidney function, chewing, and swallowing.

Good oral hygiene and well-fitted dentures can help prevent irritation of gums and mouth sores and improve the ability to eat and taste.

FACTORS THAT AFFECT EATING AND NUTRITION

Many factors affect nutrition and eating habits; some of them begin during infancy and continue throughout life, while others develop later:

- ***Personal choice.*** Likes and dislikes of certain foods is a matter of personal preferences that begin in childhood. They are influenced by the way foods taste, smell, and look and the way it is prepared.
- ***Allergies.*** An **allergy** is sensitivity to a substance that causes the body to react with signs and symptoms. Common allergic reactions are swelling of the lips, throat, tongue, or face; skin rash; coughing or difficulty breathing; abdominal cramps; nausea; or diarrhea. In severe cases, *anaphylactic shock*—a life-threatening sensitivity to a substance that can be fatal—can occur. For some people, food allergies are just an annoyance, while for others, avoiding certain foods is a matter of life and death. Nuts and shellfish cause the most severe reactions.
- ***Food intolerances.*** A food intolerance is a noticeable reaction to food, such as indigestion and diarrhea, but it does not involve the immune system and is not as serious as a food allergy. For example, lactose intolerance occurs in people who lack the enzyme lactase, which is needed to break down the sugar (lactose) in milk. Therefore, people who are lactose-intolerant cannot digest milk.
- ***Culture.*** Culture influences dietary practices, food choices, and food preparation (see the *Respecting Diversity: Food Practices* box). The way food is cooked—frying, baking, smoking, and roasting food—or eaten raw depends on cultural practices. The use of sauces and spices is also related to culture.
- ***Religion.*** Religious practices can often influence the selection, preparation, and eating of food. Members of a religious group may follow all, some, or none of the dietary practices of their faith. You need to be aware of and respect your clients' religious practices.

RESPECTING DIVERSITY

Food Practices

Food practices vary among cultures. For example, rice and beans are common protein sources in Mexico. Rice is also common in the Philippines, China, and Japan. A diet high in starch and fat is common in Poland. A low-fat, high-sodium diet is common in China. In some countries (such as India) beef is not eaten by most people.

Adapted from: D'Avanzo & Geissler, E.M. (2003). *Pocket guide to cultural assessment* (3rd ed.). St. Louis: Mosby.

supporting LESLIE AND MILTON

Leslie X., 17, mother of 2-week old Milton, is a single mother who is new to your community. Milton's father left Leslie during her pregnancy while they were both in drug rehab, and she does not have any contact with her family. You are the support worker assigned to Leslie to find out if she has any difficulties with her new role as a mother. She is currently breastfeeding Milton. Milton weighed 17.6 kg (8 pounds) at birth and, according to his pediatrician, has grown and gained weight well. Leslie seems to have no trouble changing him, bathing him, or bringing him to his doctor for his weekly visits.

On your visit today, Leslie greets you at the door, carrying Milton in one arm and holding a cigarette in her other hand. She looks as if she has been crying. Milton is crying, wet, and obviously needs a diaper change. Leslie says that she thinks that her decision to keep Milton was a wrong one and that she wants to spend some time with her friends. While you watch Leslie change Milton's diaper, you notice her hands are shaking. Leslie then says that she has been feeling very lonely and sad lately and asks if smoking a "joint" (i.e., marijuana cigarette) to help her relax will be harmful to Milton.

You are unsure how to answer Leslie's question. What should you do? What can you say to her? Who can she turn to for help in your community?

When assisting a new mother, you usually do one or more of the following:

- Provide physical care for the mother.
- Provide care for the newborn.
- Help with child care when other young children are in the home.
- Help with home management tasks, such as meal preparation and housekeeping.

The **postpartum**—after (*post*) childbirth (*partum*)—period starts with the birth of the baby and ends 6 weeks later. During this time, the mother begins to adjust physically and emotionally to the effects of childbirth, and her body begins to return to its normal (pre-pregnant) state. Because of the many changes experienced during the postpartum period, the mother needs to rest and recover. Encourage her to rest or nap when the baby is sleeping and to take time for herself and her partner. During this time, she also has important nutritional needs (see Chapter 27).

Lochia. In the first few weeks to months after giving birth, the mother's hormone levels will change dramatically, and her uterus will begin to contract to its pre-pregnant size. Blood and other substances will be expelled from the uterus; this vaginal discharge, called **lochia** (from the Greek word *lochos*, which means *childbirth*), is made up of blood, mucus, and placental tissue.

Lochia will typically increase with breastfeeding (*nursing*) and activity, but the amount of flow should return to normal after the mother rests. The mother wears clean sanitary pads to absorb the discharge, which eventually decreases in amount. Lochia generally has an odour similar to that of normal menstrual discharge.

Any offensive odour indicates a possible infec-

Supporting boxes present situations that have actually occurred and are intended to promote discussion in class.

SUPPORT WORKERS SOLVING PROBLEMS

Using Paraphrasing and Questioning Skills

<< Scenario >>

Sophia provides personal care to 48-year-old Mr. Dupuis. He is severely disabled by multiple sclerosis. On her first visit, she had helped Mr. Dupuis shave and dress. On this second visit, she is to assist him with bathing and preparing breakfast.

Mr. Dupuis: Oh, it's you. I was still asleep. It's awfully early.

Sophia: A 7:30 start is a little early for you. You're not ready for me. *(paraphrasing)*

Mr. Dupuis: Yes, I've asked the case manager to start the morning care at 8:00 instead.

Sophia: Perhaps she is working on the schedule change. I will check with the agency.

Mr. Dupuis: Thanks.

Sophia: The care plan calls for a bath today. Would you like to have your bath now or after breakfast? *(closed question)*

Mr. Dupuis: It doesn't matter much. I wish I didn't need to take a bath. Being bathed by someone else is not much fun.

Sophia: Can you tell me what you dislike about it? *(open-ended question)*

Mr. Dupuis: The lack of privacy really gets to me.

Sophia: We can work together on giving you privacy.

Mr. Dupuis: That would be a good idea. I don't think my last support worker cared much about my privacy.

<< Discussion >>

Paraphrasing and questioning skills can help you improve the care you provide to your clients. In this case, Sophia listens to Mr. Dupuis and uses paraphrasing, closed questions, and open-ended questions in her responses. Sophia uses paraphrasing *(A 7:30 start is a little early for you. You're not ready for me.)* to show Mr. Dupuis she has understood his concern and to prompt him to provide more information. She asks a closed question *(Would you like to have your bath now or after breakfast?)* because she needs specific information about Mr. Dupuis's preferences. She asks an open-ended question *(Can you tell me what you dislike about it?)* to encourage Mr. Dupuis to share his feelings about being given baths. Once Sophia understands Mr. Dupuis's worries about privacy, she can take steps to solve this problem.

Avoid these pat responses:

- "I know how you feel." *(Nobody can ever know how another person feels.)*
- "I feel sorry for you." *(This implies pity.)*
- "I wouldn't want to be in your shoes." *(This suggests superiority and implies pity.)*

Consider these two responses to a complaint:

Mr. Witowski: I can't believe they have made me move to this new room. I felt settled in the other room, and I liked the view of the lawn and the pond. Now, all I see when I look out the window is an asphalt parking lot.

Jane: The move can't be helped, unfortunately. The old wing was falling apart.

Carlos: Being moved can be upsetting. Your old room had a lovely view. I can see why you miss it.

Jane's response is not empathetic—she focuses on facts, not on Mr. Witowski's feelings. Carlos' response is empathetic—he paraphrases Mr. Witowski's statement, which lets Mr. Witowski know Carlos has understood his message and has acknowledged Mr. Witowski's feelings about moving.

Asking Closed Questions

Closed questions focus on specific information, so use them when you need to learn something precise. Some closed questions have "yes" or "no" answers. Others require a brief response. For example:

You: Would you like butter on your toast this morning, Mrs. Cummings?

Mrs. Cummings: Yes, please.

You: Would you like strawberry jam or marmalade?

Mrs. Cummings: Marmalade, please.

Support Workers Solving Problems boxes present scenarios depicting situations and problems that support workers may face on a typical day. The boxes discuss how support workers in these cases make decisions and solve problems. Put yourself in the same situation. What would you do?

CASE STUDY
REHABILITATION FOLLOWING A BRAIN INJURY

High school teacher Jeffery Butler, 34, was cycling to school when he was hit by a van. He sustained a severe blow to the head and broke several bones. After emergency care and surgery, he was placed in the intensive care unit (ICU). Because he had acquired a serious brain injury, he could not speak or recognize his family. After 10 days in the ICU, he was moved to the acute care unit, where he stayed for 2 months.

Eventually Mr. Butler was transferred to the hospital's rehabilitation unit, and 3 months later, he was discharged home. He received rehabilitation services at home and in the community for the next 6 months. During his long rehabilitation, Mr. Butler's rehabilitation team worked with him and his family (see the chart below). The team's main goals were helping Mr. Butler regain lost function and helping the family learn new skills for his care.

Rehabilitation Team	Role
Mr. Butler and his family	Made decisions regarding rehabilitation goals Were involved in every aspect of care Learned new skills and re-learned old skills
Neurosurgeon	Led surgical team and aspects of rehabilitation after surgery
Orthopedic surgeon	Led surgical team and aspects of rehabilitation after surgery
Nurses	Coordinated and provided care at every stage
Specialist in rehabilitation medicine	Led and coordinated rehabilitation
Neuropsychologists	Evaluated thinking, memory, emotions, behaviour, and personality Planned behaviour management treatment Headed adult day program
Case manager	Coordinated h Arranged for a
Social workers	Provided cou Headed adult
Occupational therapists	Assessed perf Conducted hc Provided treat independence
Physiotherapists (Physical therapists)	Evaluated stre Taught mobili
Speech-language pathologist	Tested speech Taught family
Family physician	Provided med
Support workers	Assisted with Assisted with Assisted with Helped with
Volunteers	Provided com Assisted with

Case Study boxes apply some of the concepts in the text to real-world examples of support workers and the clients they care for.

Box 43–2 General Guidelines for Applying Heat and Cold

These guidelines apply to application of heat or cold:

- Apply only when ordered by a professional, allowed by your employer, and assigned to do so.
- Know how to use the equipment.
- Measure the temperature of moist applications before applying, according to your employer policy.
- Follow employer policies for safe temperature ranges. See Table 43–2 for heat and cold temperature ranges.
- Do not apply hot applications above 41.1°C (106°F) because tissue damage can occur. ***Only a nurse can apply a very hot application.***
- Ask your supervisor what the temperature of the application should be (see Box 43–1).
  - Heat—are used for clients at risk, cooler temperatures.
  - Cold—for clients at risk, warmer temperatures are used.
- Know the precise site of the application. Ask your supervisor to show you the site.
- Cover dry heat or cold applications with cloth before applying them. Use a flannel or terrycloth cover, towel, or pillowcase, according to your employer policy.
- Do not leave clients at risk unattended.
- Observe the skin, at least every 5 minutes, for signs of complications (see Table 43–1 on page 821).
- Observe for changes in the client's behaviour, which may indicate the client is in pain.
- Remind the client not to change the temperature of the application.
- Prevent chills. When moist heat is applied, the increased blood flow to the affected area may cause reduced blood flow to other body parts, and the client may feel chilled. Cover the client with a blanket or robe. Eliminate room drafts.
- Ask your supervisor how long to leave the application in place. Carefully watch the time. Heat and cold are applied for no longer than 15-minute periods.
- Provide for privacy. Properly drape and screen the client. Expose only the body part on which you will apply heat or cold.
- If it is safe to leave, place the call bell within the client's reach, or remain within easy hearing distance.
- Follow Standard Practices. Wear gloves if you or the client has nonintact skin.

settings than dry heat applications to prevent injury to the client.

In *dry heat applications,* water does not come in contact with the skin. The advantages of dry heat are as follows:

- The application stays at the desired temperature longer.
- Dry heat does not penetrate as deeply as moist heat. Because water is not used, dry heat needs higher (hotter) temperatures to achieve the desired effect.

With both these applications, the client is at risk for burns. It is very important, therefore, to continually check on the client and inspect the skin under the application every 5 minutes. The applications should never be left on the skin longer than 15 minutes (see the *Focus on Home Care: Dry Heat Applications* box on page 824).

Warm Compresses

Warm compresses are moist heat applications. A **compress** is a soft pad that is moistened and applied over a body area. (Compresses can be hot or cold.)

Table 43–2 Heat and Cold Temperature Ranges

Temperature	Centigrade Range	Fahrenheit Range
Very hot	41.1°C to 46.1°C	106°F to 115°F
Hot	36.6°C to 41.1°C	98°F to 106°F
Warm	33.8°C to 36.6°C	93°F to 98°F
Tepid	26.6°C to 33.8°C	80°F to 93°F
Cool	18.3°C to 26.6°C	65°F to 80°F
Cold	10.0°C to 18.3°C	50°F to 65°F

Boxes and tables present principles, guidelines, signs and symptoms, care measures, and other information, often in a list format, and are useful study guides for reviewing.

Bulleted lists present information in a way that is easy to study and remember.

Preventing Infection Chapter 20 331

Box 20–2 Signs and Symptoms of Infection

- Fever and chills
- Increased pulse and respiratory rates
- Aches, pain, or tenderness
- Fatigue and loss of energy
- Loss of appetite
- Nausea
- Vomiting
- Diarrhea
- Rash
- Sores on mucous membranes
- Redness and swelling of a body part
- Discharge or drainage from the infected area that may have a foul odour
- New or increased cough, sore throat, or runny or stuffy nose
- Burning pain when urinating, or the need to urinate more often or with increased urgency

focus on ››OLDER ADULTS

Signs and Symptoms of Infection

Older adults are especially at risk for infections because of the normal age-related changes occurring in their bodies. If they had a serious health concern before they were infected, they are also more likely than younger adults to become seriously ill or to die from an infection. This is why, for example, pneumonia and influenza are often life-threatening illnesses in older adults.

Older adults often do not show the usual signs of infection. Fever, pain, and swelling, for instance, are usually absent in older adults because they tend to have lower body temperatures, decreased pain sensation, and less immune response to infection.

Sometimes the only sign of infection in older adults is a change in behaviour. If an older client displays any of the following, report it to your supervisor:

- New or increased confusion or delirium
- New or increased incontinence
- Loss of appetite
- Decreased ability to perform activities of daily

Focus on Older Adults boxes provide information about the needs, considerations, and special circumstances of older adults.

A **pandemic** occurs when a communicable illness or infection spreads throughout the population of a country or even throughout the world. The Canadian government, for example, is preparing for an influenza (the "flu") pandemic. Normally, people are exposed to different strains of the influenza virus many times during their lives, so even though the virus may change (or mutate), previous exposures to influenza may offer them some protection against infection. However, for unknown reasons, three to four times in a century, a radical change takes place in the influenza A virus, causing a new strain to emerge.[2] In the past, this has resulted in widespread illness and many deaths, especially among the young, ill, or the elderly. The Canadian government is involved in attempts to prevent such a disaster from happening through widespread public health teaching and influenza vaccinations.

The Chain of Infection

Many factors work together for an infection to develop. The spread of infection involves a process known as the chain of infection (Figure 20–1). The links in the chain are as follows:

Preventing Infection Chapter 20 353

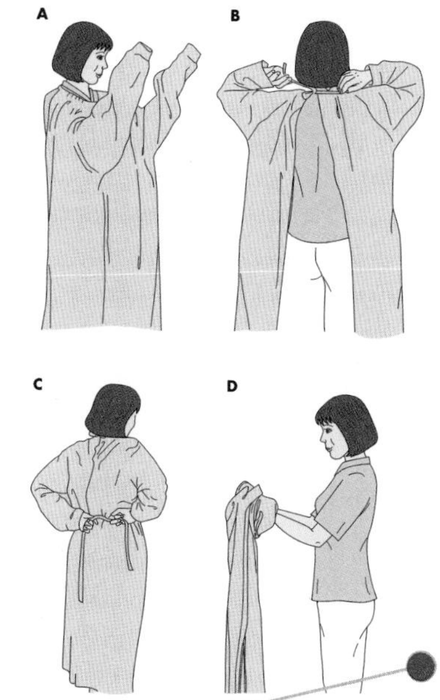

Figure 20–13 Gowning technique. **A,** Put your arms and hands through the sleeves. **B,** Tie the strings at the back of your neck. **C,** Overlap the gown in the back to cover your entire uniform. **D,** Turn the gown inside out as you remove it.

Colour illustrations and photographs visually present key ideas, concepts, and procedure steps and help you apply and remember the written material.

- The worker outside the room holds open another bag. This bag is clean. A wide cuff is made on the clean bag to protect the hands from contamination (Figure 20–15).
- The contaminated bag is placed in the clean bag at the doorway.

Bag and transport linens according to employer policy. All linen bags must have a *BIOHAZARD* symbol. Bag soiled linen in the room where it was used. Handle soiled linen as little as possible. It should not be sorted or rinsed in client care areas. Do not overfill the bag with linen. Tie the bag securely.

Linen that is very wet or soiled should be double-bagged to prevent leakage. Place the linen bag in a laundry hamper lined with a biohazard plastic bag.

Transporting Clients on Transmission-Based Precautions. When on Transmission-Based Precautions, clients usually do not leave their rooms. However, they may have to go to another area of the facility for special treatments or tests.

Transporting procedures vary among facilities. Some require transport by bed, which prevents contaminating wheelchairs and stretchers. Other facilities use wheelchairs and stretchers.

A safe transport means that other residents or patients, staff, and visitors are protected from

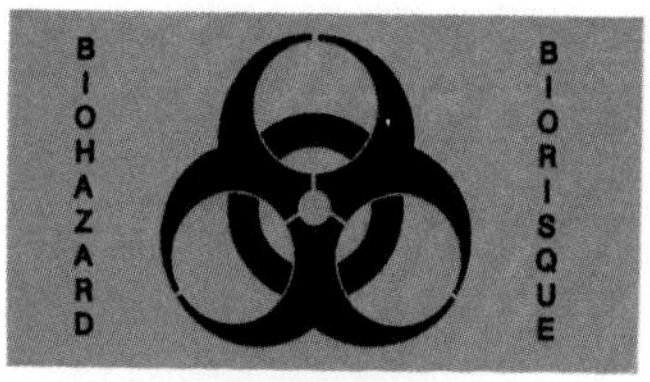

Figure 20–14 *BIOHAZARD* symbol.

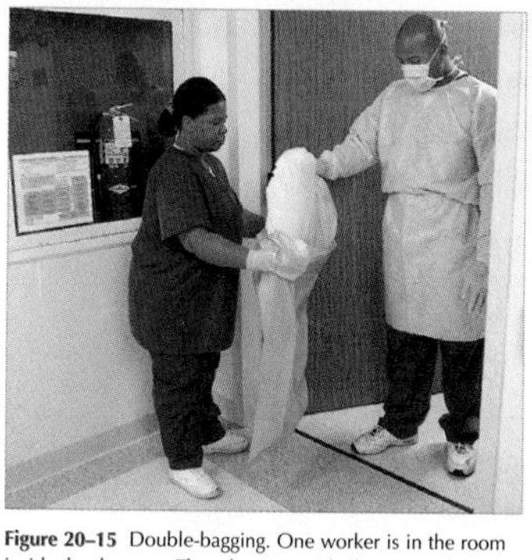

Figure 20–15 Double-bagging. One worker is in the room inside the doorway. The other is outside the room. The contaminated bag is placed inside the clean bag.

380 Chapter 22 Promoting Client Well-Being

PROVIDING COMPASSIONATE CARE

Welcoming a New Client to a Long-Term Care Facility

- **Dignity.** Treat the new client and his or her belongings with respect. Greet the client by name. Ask the client what name he or she would like the staff to use. Introduce yourself by name and title to the client and family (Figure 22–1). Do not rush into admission procedures. Treat the client and family as if they are guests in your home. Offer them refreshments, and tell them about the many good things about the facility. Listen to their concerns or questions, and do not overload them with information. Explain details about routines, recreation facilities, and other matters only if the new client seems eager to hear them. Reassure clients that they do not need to remember everything. Remind them that they can ask questions and talk to the staff at any time.
- **Independence.** A homelike setting is important to a client's independence and control. Help new clients feel at home. Show them their room, and explain how to use the various equipment in the room. Offer to help unpack and arrange their belongings (unless this has been done by the family). Make sure the client can reach the phone, TV, and light controls.
- **Preferences.** Some new clients want to arrange their own rooms, and they should always have the choice in arranging personal items. The health care team makes sure that the client's choices are safe, will not cause falls or other accidents, and do not interfere with the rights of others.
- **Privacy.** Show the new client how to draw the privacy curtains. Explain that the health care team respects all clients' right to privacy. Explain how you maintain privacy during personal care and other procedures.
- **Safety.** Explain how to use the call bell (see Chapter 19), and ensure that it is within easy reach. Show the client around the bathroom, and point out safety features, such as grab bars. Review safety and emergency procedures according to facility policy.

Providing Compassionate Care boxes highlight how to provide care discussed in the chapter in a compassionate manner. The first letters of the words in the list are bolded and coloured to help you remember DIPPS, the acronym that summarizes the five priorities of support work—providing for the client's dignity, independence, preferences, privacy, and safety.

tion, and some request a room change when room
mates do not get along. A client may or may nc
welcome a transfer, and the client's physician, nurs
or social worker usually explains the reason for th
transfer. You may assist with the transfer or carr
out the entire procedure. Clients are usually trans
ported by wheelchair or stretcher or on their bed

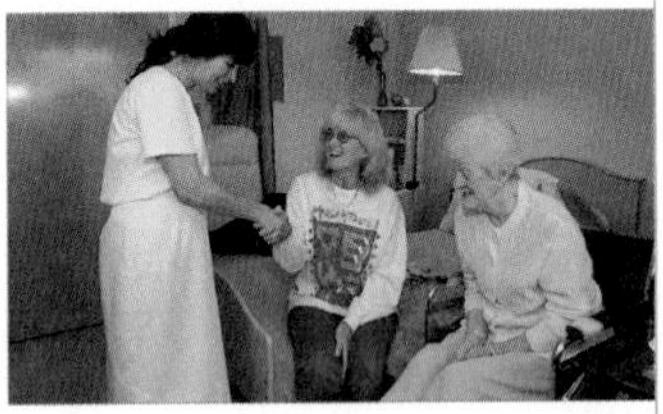

Figure 22–1 A support worker introduces herself to a new client and family member. **Source**: Sorrentino, S.A. (2000). *Mosby's textbook for nursing assistants* (5th ed., p. 552). St. Louis: Mosby.

400 Chapter 23 Body Mechanics: Moving, Positioning, Transferring, and Lifting the Client

knees. You and your helper should roll the turning sheet closely to the client's body and grasp the sheet firmly, with palms up. Check with your supervisor and the care plan to see if a turning sheet is required. Using a turning sheet will reduce possible injuries to the client.

1 2 3 MOVING THE CLIENT UP IN BED

Remember to promote:

• Dignity • Independence • Preferences • Privacy • Safety

Pre-Procedure

1 Identify the client according to employer policy.
2 Ask someone to help you.
3 Perform hand hygiene.
4 Explain the procedure to the client.
5 Provide for privacy.
6 Raise bed to a comfortable working height. Make sure bed wheels are locked. Follow the care plan for bed rail use. Lower the head of the bed to a level appropriate for the client. It should be as flat as possible.*

Procedure

7 You and your helper should stand on either side of the bed. Lower one of the bed rails.
8 Log-roll the client to one side (see the box *Log-Rolling the Client*) so that the client is facing the bed rail that is up.
9 The worker on the side facing the client should hold and support the client. Ensure that the client is in proper body alignment and safely positioned. Some clients feel better if they can hold onto the bed rail, and if this is the case, keep the bed rail up.
10 The other support worker should **fanfold** a turning sheet and place it behind the client from the back of the head to the thighs. The fanfolded sheet should be tucked as close to the client's body as possible.
11 Instruct the client that he or she will be rolling over a "bump" in the bed. Assist the client to log-roll over to the opposite side. Place the bed rail facing the client in the "up" position to allow the client to grasp it.
12 Lower the bed rail on the opposite side, grasp the turning sheet and straighten it out.
13 Assist the client to log-roll onto his or her back. Lower the raised bedrail.
14 Roll the sides of the turning sheet up close to the client.
15 Grasp the rolled up turning sheet firmly near the person (see Figure 23–7). Ensure that the client's head is supported.
16 Place the client's pillow against the headboard, if the client can do without the pillow.
17 Move the client up in bed on the count of three. Each worker should shift their weight from the rear leg to the front leg.
18 If it is more comfortable for both of you, place your knees closest to the client's head on the bed when performing steps 15 and 16 above.
19 Unroll the turning sheet.
20 Provide for safety and comfort. Position the client in good body alignment according to the care plan. Straighten linens.
21 If the client is *lying in a hospital bed,* the easiest and safest method to raise the client's head and shoulders is to raise the head of the bed. Use the electronic control to raise the head of the bed.

Post-Procedure

22 Put the pillow under the client's head and shoulders. Tidy up the bed linens. Place the call bell within reach.*
23 Provide for safety and comfort. Position the client in good body alignment. Raise the head of the bed to an appropriate level for the client.
24 Return bed to lowest position, if necessary. Follow the care plan for bed rail use.*
25 Remove privacy measures.
26 Perform hand hygiene.
27 Report and record your actions and observations according to employer policy.

*Steps marked with an asterisk may not apply in community settings.

In the **Procedures boxes,** procedures are presented in a step-by-step format and are divided into Pre-Procedure, Procedure, and Post-Procedure sections for easy studying. Those steps that do not apply in community settings are identified with an asterisk. The Compassionate Care sections in the Procedure boxes remind you of DIPPS.

520 Chapter 29 Personal Hygiene

focus on ››LONG-TERM CARE

Daily Care

Facilities provide routine hygiene care at set times of the day. The amount of care given at each time and the terminology used vary from facility to facility.

- **AM care (early morning care** and **morning care)**—routine care provided before lunch. Most clients are toileted, given a partial bath that includes perineal care, dressed, groomed, and provided mouth care before they go to the dining room for breakfast. If there is enough time, clients requiring a tub bath or shower would have this completed before breakfast. If this is not possible, these clients might go to the dining room in their pyjamas or robe. GentleCare technique involves allowing clients to continue sleeping, if they so desire, and providing them with a late breakfast.

In some facilities, tub baths or showers are done after breakfast. The client is also assisted with grooming—hair care, shaving, and dressing, mouth care, and perineal care.

- **Afternoon care**—routine care given after lunch and before the evening meal. Many clients like to have the afternoon care completed before naps, visiting time, or activity programs. Afternoon care usually includes assisting with oral hygiene, face and hand washing, and hair care.
- **HS care (evening care** or **PM care)**—care provided at bedtime. (*HS* means hour of sleep.) HS care, aimed at relaxing the client and increasing comfort, includes face and hand washing, oral hygiene, perineal care, and back massages. Bed linens and units are made neat and comfortable, and the client is helped into sleepwear.

Focus on Long Term Care boxes highlight information unique to the long-term care setting.

ORAL HYGIENE

Oral hygiene (mouth care) keeps the mouth an[d] teeth clean; prevents mouth odours, infections, an[d] *cavities* (*dental caries*); increases comfort; an[d] makes food taste better. It also prevents *periodonta[l] disease* (*gum disease, pyorrhea*), which is an inflam[m]ation of the tissues around the teeth.

Poor oral hygiene allows the buildup of biofil[m] and tartar. **Biofilm**—which contains saliv[a], microbes, and other substances—is a thin film th[at] sticks to teeth and leads to tooth decay, or cavitie[s]. When biofilm hardens, it is called **tartar.** Tart[ar] builds up at the gum line near the neck of th[e] tooth, which leads to periodontal disease. Th[e] gums become red and swollen and bleed easily. A[s] the disease progresses, bone is destroyed and teet[h] become loosened, eventually resulting in tooth los[s].

Illness and disease often cause a bad taste in th[e] mouth. Some medications and diseases cause [a] whitish coating on the mouth and tongue, an[d] some others cause redness and swelling of th[e] mouth and tongue. Dry mouth is common fro[m] oxygen administration, smoking, decreased flui[d] intake, mouth breathing, and anxiety. Some me[d]ications cause dry mouth.

Your supervisor and the care plan will tell you the type of mouth care and assistance needed. Oral

REVIEW

Answers to these questions are at the bottom of the page.

Circle the BEST answer.

1. **Which of the following is a developmental task of late adulthood?**
   A. Adjusting to increased physical strength
   B. Adjusting to physical changes
   C. Seeking employment
   D. Selecting a partner
2. **Retirement usually results in:**
   A. A lower income
   B. Physical changes due to aging
   C. Less free time
   D. Financial security
3. **Changes to the skin occur with aging. Care should include the following:**
   A. Daily baths
   B. Not applying lotion
   C. Using soap daily
   D. Providing good skin care
4. **An older adult has cold feet. You should:**
   A. Provide socks
   B. Apply a hot-water bottle
   C. Soak the feet in hot water
   D. Apply a heating pad
5. **Changes occur in the musculo-skeletal system with aging. Which is true?**
   A. Bones do not become brittle.
   B. Older adults should avoid exercise.
   C. Joints become less stiff.
   D. Range-of-motion exercises help slow the rate of musculo-skeletal changes.
6. **In older adults, arteries lose their elasticity and become narrow. These changes result in:**
   A. A slower heart rate
   B. Lower blood pressure
   C. Poor circulation to many body parts
   D. Less blood in the body
7. **Mr. Steinberg, 88, has severe circulatory problems. You should do the following:**
   A. Ignore his complaints of discomfort
   B. Follow the care plan
   C. Plan physically demanding activities
   D. Allow him to carry heavy bags
8. **Respiratory changes occur with aging. Which is *true?***
   A. Heavy bed linens prevent normal chest expansion.
   B. The person is not turned and repositioned frequently.
   C. The side-lying position is best for breathing.
   D. The person should not be physically active.
9. **Older adults should avoid fried and fatty foods because of:**
   A. Decreases in saliva
   B. Ill-fitting dentures or loss of teeth
   C. Decreased amount of digestive juices
   D. A decreased sense of taste
10. **A physician orders increased fluid intake for an older client. You should:**
    A. Give most of the fluid before 1700 (5:00 p.m.)
    B. Provide mostly water
    C. Start a bladder training program
    D. Insert an indwelling urinary catheter
11. **The health care team in a long-term care facility should:**
    A. Discourage older residents from sexual expression and activity
    B. Allow and promote sexual expression and activity in older adults
    C. Expect every resident to have the same attitudes toward sex
    D. Not allow residents to masturbate, even in private

Answers: 1.B, 2.A, 3.D, 4.A, 5.D, 6.C, 7.B, 8.C, 9.C, 10.A, 11.B

247

Review questions are a useful study guide, as they provide a means to review the main ideas presented in the chapter. Use them to study for a test or examination. Answers are placed upside down below questions.

CHAPTER 1

The Role of the Support Worker

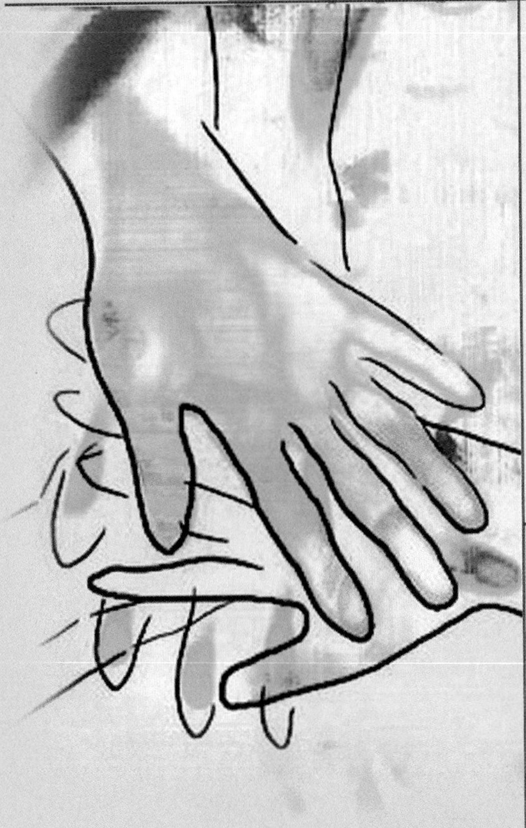

OBJECTIVES

- Define the key terms listed in this chapter.
- Describe the goal of support work.
- Describe the five main responsibilities of the support worker.
- Identify the goal of the health care team.
- Identify the common members of a health care team.
- Distinguish between regulated and unregulated health care providers.
- Describe the importance of scope of practice in support work.
- Describe the significance of having a professional approach to support work.
- List the five priorities in compassionate care.
- Identify four things to consider when solving problems.

key terms

activities of daily living (ADL) Self-care activities people perform daily to remain independent and to function in society.

caring Concern for clients', as well as their families', dignity, independence, preferences, privacy, and safety at all times. True *caring* means honesty, sensitivity, comforting, discretion, and respect while showing this concern.

chronic care Treatment and care given for a pre-existing or long-term illness or health problem. Also known as **long-term** or **continuing care**.

client A person receiving care or support services in a community setting; a general term for all people receiving health care or support services: hospital patients, facility residents, and clients in the community.

compassion Compassion is the awareness of the misfortune and suffering of another person and the desire and actions taken to reduce or alleviate the problem.

complex care This term is used in some provinces as a guide to describe the 24-hour professional care required by clients within a residential care facility. Also known as **long-term care** or **complex continuing care.**

confidentiality Respecting and guarding personal and private information about another person.

continuing care Medical, nursing, and support services provided over the course of months or years to people who cannot care for themselves. Also known as **long-term care** or **chronic care**.

dignity The state of feeling worthy, valued, and respected.

discretion Ability to use responsible judgement in order to avoid causing distress or embarrassment to a person.

empathy The ability to recognize, perceive, and have an understanding of another person's emotions by being able to "put oneself into his or her shoes."

licensed practical nurse (LPN) See **registered practical nurse.**

long-term care Medical, nursing, and support services provided over the course of months or years to people who cannot care for themselves. Also known as **complex care, chronic care,** or **continuing care.**

long-term care facility A facility that provides accommodations, 24-hour nursing care, and support services to people who cannot care for themselves at home but who do not need hospital care.

patient A person receiving care in a hospital setting.

primary care nurse A primary care nurse is responsible for the ongoing management of the health of a client, which includes liaising with other health care team members, the client/resident and her or his family. In a long-term care (complex care) environment, the primary care nurse may or may not be directly involved in providing care on a daily basis.

professionalism An approach to work that demonstrates respect for others, commitment, competence, and appropriate behaviour.

registered nurse (RN) A health care professional who is licensed and regulated by the province or territory to maintain overall responsibility for the planning and provision of client care. RNs study for a longer period of time than do RPNs/LPNs, allowing for greater depth and breadth of foundational knowledge in the areas of clinical practice, decision making, critical thinking, leadership, research utilization, and resource management.

registered practical nurse (RPN) A health care professional licensed and regulated by the province or territory to carry out nursing techniques and client care. Both categories of nurse (RNs and LPN/RPNs) study from the same body of nursing knowledge, although RPNs study for a shorter period of time than RNs, resulting in a more focused body of foundational knowledge. They can work both independently and as part of the health team along with an RN. Also known as a **licensed practical nurse (LPN)** in many provinces.

registered psychiatric nurse (RPN) A nurse who is educated and registered in his or her own province to provide care specifically to individuals whose primary needs relate to mental, emotional, and developmental health.

rehabilitation The process of restoring a person to the highest level of functioning possible through the use of therapy, exercise, or other methods.

resident A person living in a long-term care (also known as a **residential**) facility.

residential facility A facility that provides living accommodations and services; includes assisted-living facilities and retirement residences.

scope of practice The legal limits and extent of a health care worker's role. This will vary from province to province and employer to employer.

social reintegration See **social support.**

social support Equipping a person with the skills and knowledge necessary to successfully live independently outside an institution. Also known as **social integration.**

support worker Support workers provide services to people who need help with their daily needs, both in facilities and in the community.

unregulated care providers (UCPs) A broad term applied to staff who assist nurses and other health care professionals in giving care.

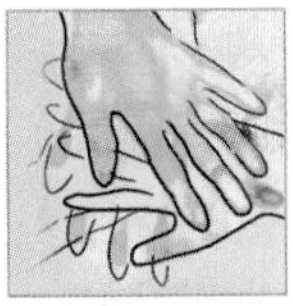

As a support worker, you provide services to people who require help with their daily needs, in facilities as well as in the community. You may work as part of a health care team, or you may work individually with a client. Legislation, employer policies, and the person's condition all influence how you function and how much supervision you need. You may collaborate with health care professionals or with professionals outside of the health care sector, depending on clients and their situations. You adapt your work according to the setting and the needs and wishes of the person receiving care.

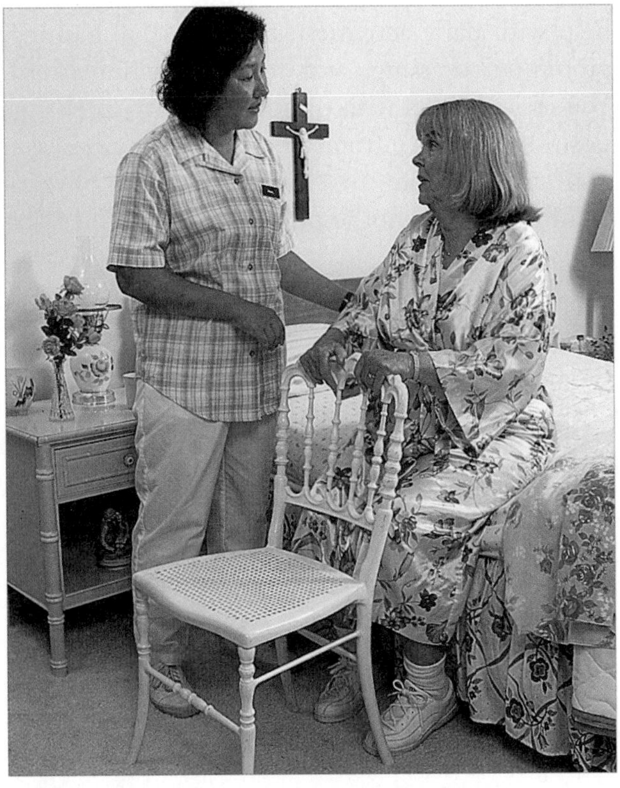

Figure 1–1 A support worker comforts a client.
Source: Birchenall, J., & Streight, E. (1997). *Mosby's textbook for the home care aide* (2nd ed., p. 221). St. Louis: Mosby.

The ultimate goal of support work is to improve the person's quality of life. **Caring** is provided in a kind, sensitive, and understanding manner. While tending to the person's physical needs, you also relieve loneliness, provide comfort, encourage independence, and promote the person's self-respect (Figure 1–1). While discussing the client with co-workers, you must use **discretion** at all times and honour the client's right to **confidentiality**. Your services to people in their homes help them remain independent and with their families. You may assist clients with **social reintegration** as they prepare to move into a home or group setting. Your services show people in facilities that you have **empathy** and that you care for and about them. You make a difference in people's lives.

SUPPORT WORK ACROSS CANADA

The nature of support work differs across the country. There are differences in educational programs, work settings, job responsibilities, and terms used to describe support workers. Some sections of this text may not apply to support work in your particular province or territory. If you are unsure about which parts apply to your area, ask your instructor.

The term **support worker** refers to the worker who provides personal care and support services. However, *assisted living worker, personal support worker, personal attendant, patient care assistant, resident care aide, resident care attendant, health care aide, home care attendant, home support worker, nursing aide, nursing attendant, community health worker,* or *continuing care assistant*—among other titles—may be used in your province or territory. The Appendix at the end of the book outlines what the support worker is called in different provinces/territories. You should be aware that the educational programs and the **scope of practice** for support workers may vary from province to province.

In some parts of Canada, *personal attendant* refers to those workers who are supervised directly by the person for whom they provide support services. Generally, if an educational program is available to become a personal attendant, it is shorter in duration than the one for a support worker. Personal attendants support people who have physical disabilities.

Settings for Support Work

You can work in facility-based as well as in community-based settings (see Chapter 3).

- *Facility-based settings*—workplaces in which accommodations, health care, and support services are provided. Several types of facilities employ support workers. These include hospitals and complex care or long-term care facilities (Figure 1–2). A **complex**, **chronic,** or **long-term care** facility is home to people who are not able to live independently or in their own homes and who require 24-hour nursing services to be available to meet their personal care needs but do not need hospital care. In some provinces, complex care or long-term care facilities are also called *nursing homes.*
- *Community-based settings*—workplaces within the community, where health care and support services are provided. Support workers sometimes assist their clients with social integration, and they may teach their clients important skills, such as doing laundry, shopping for groceries, managing their money, and doing their own banking. Other clients may need assistance with learning how to take a bus or how to apply for a job.

The most common community setting is the person's home (Figure 1–3). Clients can live in a variety of settings, such as retirement-living homes, group homes, or by themselves in their houses or apartments.

Support Worker Responsibilities

The tasks performed by support workers vary across Canada. Generally, most of your responsibilities can be grouped into five categories: (1) personal care, (2) support for nurses and other health care professionals, (3) family support, (4) **social support,** and (5) housekeeping/home management.

Personal Care. Personal care activities include assisting with **activities of daily living (ADLs)**. These are the self-care activities that people perform daily to remain independent and to function effectively in society. As a support worker, you help with daily activities such as eating, bathing, grooming, dressing, and toileting (elimination). You assist clients with limited mobility to change positions or move from one place to another. You also help promote the client's safety and physical comfort. You are not responsible for deciding what

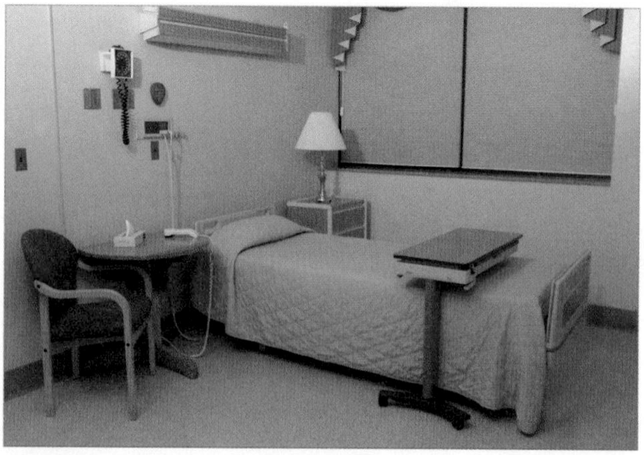

Figure 1–2 A room in a long-term care facility. Note how the table lamp can make it seem homier to the client residing there.

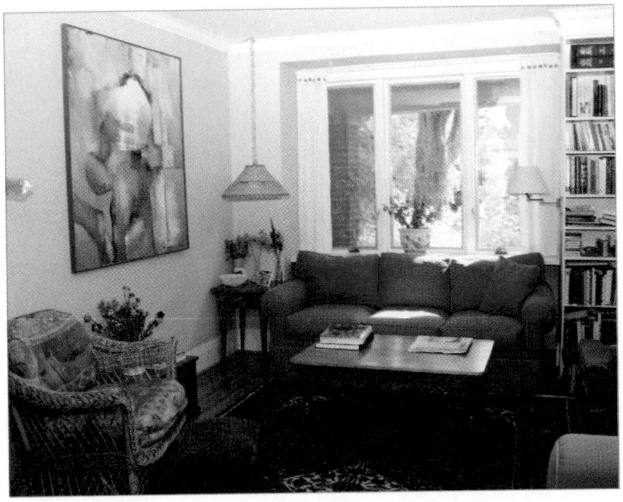

Figure 1–3 A room in a community-based setting; the person's home.

should or should not be done for the client. However, while providing personal care, you observe for and report any changes in the client's behaviour or health. This is important information for the health care team.

Support for Nurses and Other Health Care Professionals. You assist nurses or other health care team members by following the established care plan for each client. For instance, you might clean equipment, measure and report vital signs, or assist with simple wound care. You might also assist with oxygen therapy, heat or cold applications, and range-of-motion exercises. You are often the nurse's "eyes and ears." This means that because you are the person who is *most often* with the client or resident, you will very likely observe or hear things that need to be reported to the nurse. This is a very important part of your role, as it could have a great impact on your clients' care.

As a support worker, you may have to consult with other health care professionals, such as social workers or physiotherapists. You may also have to consult with other professionals, such as your client's employers, clergy, or teachers, depending on your client's individual care plan.

Family Support. In facilities, you may assist with admissions and discharges. You may introduce the person and family to the facility. You may also show them around and help the client unpack and settle in. In private homes, you help families care for loved ones with health problems or those who need assistance with ADLs. Family situations vary. Some families need help preparing meals and doing household chores. Other families need help with child care. Your services often give family caregivers a break from their duties.

Social Support. You may help clients participate in social activities. These activities provide the client with enjoyment, recreation, and a chance to meet with friends. You may organize games and outings. You may be hired privately to be a client's companion. You may also be responsible for teaching your clients to learn to live independently and to cook, clean, or shop by themselves.

Housekeeping/Home Management. You may do a variety of housekeeping tasks in a facility setting. These include making beds, delivering meals, tidying living areas, and maintaining supplies. In a private home, housekeeping is called *home management.* Services depend on the needs of the person and the resources available to provide these services. They may include doing light housekeeping, doing laundry, and preparing and serving nutritious meals.

The boxes on the following pages describe a support worker's typical work day in the community, in a long-term care facility, and in a hospital setting. In each box, the word "nurse" may mean the **RN** or the **RPN/LPN**, depending on the staffing policies of that particular agency.

A DAY IN THE LIFE OF A SUPPORT WORKER

HOME CARE

Each evening, Stephen receives his assignment for the next day from his supervisor. He uses the details in the assignment to plan his day. He consults a city map and plans his route. The people he is assigned to visit have a range of physical, emotional, and social problems and disabilities. Their major problems are briefly described below.

Ms. Lau, 32, has cerebral palsy. She uses a wheelchair. She lives alone. Two days per week she works outside the home. She receives home care to help her prepare for work.

Mr. O'Connor, 59, is recovering at home from a stroke. He is paralyzed on one side of his body and has a speech/language disorder. His wife is his primary caregiver. Mr. O'Connor receives home care three mornings a week. Mrs. O'Connor, 51, is at work during Stephen's visit.

Mr. Horowitz, 71, has dementia. His wife, 67, is caring for him at home. The couple gets emotional and social support from family and friends. Mrs. Horowitz looks after her husband's personal care needs. They receive two hours of home care per week to enable Mrs. Horowitz to have a break.

Ms. Adams, 25, is a single mother on social assistance. She is recovering from a Cesarean section. She gets very little social and emotional support. She has newborn twins and three young children aged 1, 3, and 4 years.

Below are the tasks and activities that Stephen performs on a typical day at work.

0715–0830h (7:15 A.M.–8:30 A.M.)

- Travels to first appointment. Arrives at 0730h.
- Assists Ms. Lau with showering, grooming, and dressing.
- Helps Ms. Lau to prepare breakfast, clean up kitchen, and make bed.
- Records care provided, including any relevant observations.

0830–1000 (8:30 A.M.–10:00 A.M.)

- Travels to next appointment. Arrives at 0845h.
- Assists Mr. O'Connor with elimination, bathing, shaving, hair care, and mouth care.
- Prepares breakfast for Mr. O'Connor and assists him with eating.
- Cleans up kitchen and makes bed.
- Takes Mr. O'Connor for a brief walk. He is learning to walk with a cane.
- Assists Mr. O'Connor with elimination.
- Records care provided, including any relevant observations.

1000–1215h (10:00 A.M.–12:15 P.M.)

- Travels to next appointment. Arrives at 1015h.
- The client's wife, Mrs. Horowitz, is crying and says that she is "worn out."
- Listens to Mrs. Horowitz and suggests she talk to Stephen's supervisor. Telephones supervisor, who, in turn, calls the Horowitzs' case manager. Case manager schedules a visit.
- Assists Mr. Horowitz with elimination, bathing, shaving, hair care, and mouth care.
- Cleans kitchen and does light housework in main living areas.
- Prepares lunch for Mr. Horowitz and assists him with eating.
- Records care provided, including any relevant observations.

1215–1530h (12:15 P.M.–3:30 P.M.)

- Takes break for lunch.
- Travels to next appointment. Arrives at 1300h, the same time as the public health nurse.
- Helps children wash face and hands before preparing lunch.
- Prepares lunch for the mother and the three older children while the nurse assists the mother with breastfeeding. Feeds 1-year-old.
- Helps children with oral hygiene after lunch.
- Prepares three dinners. Leaves one in the refrigerator and the others in the freezer.
- Records care provided, including any relevant observations.
- Reports unusual observations to nurse supervisor.
- Drives home.

A DAY IN THE LIFE OF A SUPPORT WORKER

LONG-TERM CARE

Claire works on a unit in which the residents, mostly older adults, require help with ADLs. The eight residents assigned to her have a range of physical, emotional, and social problems and disabilities.

Miss McDonald, 94, is partially disabled due to rheumatoid arthritis.

Mr. Schmidt, 82, is recovering from surgery. He is incontinent of urine, which causes him anxiety.

Mrs. Lawson, 88, has a heart condition and osteoarthritis.

Mr. Delgado, 63, is paralyzed on one side due to a stroke. He is unable to speak but is able to understand both written and spoken language.

Mr. Taylor, 71, is in the early stages of Parkinson's disease. He has diabetes and poor vision as well.

Mrs. Sanchez, 81, is partially disabled due to multiple leg and hip fractures. She has osteoporosis. She is also depressed.

Mr. Bouchard, 89, is recovering from pneumonia. He has age-related hearing loss.

Mrs. Khan, 44, is severely disabled due to multiple sclerosis. She is incontinent of urine and feces.

Below are the tasks and activities that Claire performs on a typical day at work.

0700–0715h (7:00 A.M.–7:15 A.M.)

- Receives report from nurse on the conditions of all residents on the unit.
- Receives assignment of care requirements, appointments, and activities scheduled for residents.
- Plans morning's tasks and activities.

0715–0845h (7:15 A.M.–8:45 A.M.)

- Helps seven of the residents get out of bed.
- Provides partial hygiene care to six residents, a shower for one resident, and a tub bath for another.
- Assists with elimination and changes their incontinence briefs.
- Assists residents with dressing and accompanies them to the dining room.
- Returns to unit. Provides partial hygiene to Mrs. Khan.
- Observes that the cut on Mrs. Khan's arm looks red and swollen and feels warm to the touch. Makes a written record of it. Makes a verbal report to the nurse.
- With help from another support worker, moves Mrs. Khan from her bed to a wheelchair.
- Transports Mrs. Khan to the dining room for breakfast.
- Records care provided, including any relevant observations.

0845–0930h (8:45 A.M.–9:30 A.M.)

- Assists residents with breakfast. Ensures that all residents have a nutritious breakfast and that special diets are followed.
- Encourages Mr. Taylor, Mrs. Lawson, and Miss McDonald to eat.
- Feeds Mrs. Khan.
- Transports Mrs. Khan back to unit.
- Returns to dining room and accompanies other residents back to unit.
- Records each resident's dietary intake in dietary intake record.

0930–1130h (9:30 A.M.–11:30 A.M.)

- Reports to nurse that Mr. Taylor (who has diabetes) did not eat.
- With assistance, lifts Mrs. Khan and settles her in bed.
- Assists residents with elimination and mouth care.
- Changes their incontinence briefs.
- Reports on condition of residents to replacement support worker. Takes 15-minute break.
- Completes hygiene and grooming care for residents who received only partial care before breakfast.
- Accompanies residents at 1030h to games room.
- Makes beds and changes linens.
- Repositions Mrs. Khan to prevent pressure ulcers.
- Tidies rooms and living areas.
- Accompanies residents back to unit from games room at 1130h.
- Records care provided, including any relevant observations.

continued

A DAY IN THE LIFE OF A SUPPORT WORKER

LONG-TERM CARE *continued*

1130–1300h (11:30 A.M.–1:00 P.M.)

- Reports on condition of residents to replacement support worker. Takes 30-minute break for lunch.
- Checks care requirements for each resident and plans the afternoon's tasks and activities.
- Accompanies residents to dining room.
- Supervises, assists, and feeds residents, as required.
- Accompanies residents back to the unit.
- Assists residents with elimination and changes their incontinence briefs.
- Assists with mouth care.
- Makes sure that residents rest after lunch, as directed.
- Records care provided, including any relevant observations.
- Records each resident's dietary intake in dietary intake record.

1300–1500h (1:00 P.M.–3:00 P.M.)

- Assists residents with elimination and changes their incontinence briefs.
- Greets new resident, Mrs. Griffiths, and her family. Introduces them to the facility. Assists Mrs. Griffiths with unpacking.
- Introduces Mrs. Griffiths to other residents.
- Repositions Mrs. Khan.
- Comforts Mrs. Griffiths, who is feeling upset and lonely.
- Takes Mrs. Sanchez and Mrs. Griffiths for a walk.
- Assists residents with elimination and changes their incontinence briefs.
- Records care provided, including any relevant observations.
- Provides a verbal report to the nurse concerning each client's care.

A DAY IN THE LIFE OF A SUPPORT WORKER

HOSPITAL CARE

Gina works on a surgical unit, which is one type of acute care. Most clients on this unit have had surgery for fractures (broken bones). Others have had hip or knee replacement surgery. A few are waiting for their surgery. Many of these clients have additional health problems. Gina assists with the care of 10 clients.

Miss Kwan, 66, thigh bone fracture

Mr. McDuff, 76, spine fracture; osteoporosis

Mrs. Sadiq, 46, shoulder and rib fractures; osteoporosis; quadriplegia

Mrs. Clark, 85, hip fracture; osteoporosis; Alzheimer's disease

Mr. Keene, 44, thigh bone and knee fractures

Mr. Cross, 55, knee replacement; arthritis

Mrs. Pocza, 82, hip fracture; osteoporosis

Ms. Hill, 35, multiple fractures: spine, thigh bone, and ankle

Mrs. Leblanc, 74, hip replacement; diabetes

Mr. Paes, 82, hip fracture; hearing loss

Below are the tasks and activities that Gina performs on a typical day at work.

0700–0710h (7:00 A.M.–7:10 A.M.)

- Receives assignment on care requirements.
- Plans morning's tasks and activities.

0710–0800h (7:10 A.M.–8:00 A.M.)

- Provides hygiene care to four clients, including assisting with oral hygiene, hair care, and providing partial bed baths.
- Assists with elimination.
- Records care provided as completed, including any relevant observations.

continued

A DAY IN THE LIFE OF A SUPPORT WORKER

HOSPITAL CARE *continued*

0800–0845h (8:00 A.M.–8:45 A.M.)

- Accompanies dietary staff as they deliver breakfast trays.
- Positions and arranges trays for clients.
- Assists clients with eating.
- Listens to Mrs. Pocza's concerns about her surgery; calls for the nurse who answers Mrs. Pocza's questions.
- Records clients' food and fluid intake.
- Assists clients with elimination.
- Records care provided, including any relevant observations.

0845–1130h (8:45 A.M.–11:30 A.M.)

- Assists clients with hygiene, elimination, showers, and baths, as required.
- Reports on condition of clients and care requirement to replacement support worker. Takes 15-minute break.
- Makes and changes beds.
- Assists with two discharges. Helps clients pack.
- Helps nurse to reposition clients, as required.
- Assists clients with leg exercises, coughing, and deep-breathing exercises.
- Records care provided, including any relevant observations.

1130–1300h (11:30 A.M.–1:00 P.M.)

- Reports on condition of clients and care requirement to replacement support worker. Takes 30-minute break for lunch.
- Checks condition and care requirements of each client and plans afternoon tasks.
- Accompanies dietary staff as they deliver lunch trays.
- Positions and arranges trays for clients.
- Assists clients with eating.
- Observes that Mr. McDuff's IV fluid is running low. Notifies nurse immediately.
- Records food and fluid intake.
- Assists clients with elimination and mouth care.
- Records care provided, including any relevant observations.

1300–1500h (1:00 P.M.–3:00 P.M.)

- Removes Mr. Paes's dentures before his medications are given.
- Assists clients with elimination.
- Observes drainage under Miss Kwan's cast. Notifies nurse immediately.
- Answers call from nurse. Provides comfort to Mrs. Clark (who is upset).
- Assists clients with leg exercises, coughing, and deep-breathing exercises.
- Assists with admitting two clients.
- Helps nurse reposition clients, as required.
- Records care provided, including any relevant observations.
- Provides a verbal report to the nurse who is responsible for each of these clients. (Note: in many hospitals, each client is assigned to a **primary care nurse**. You might be assigned to help care for the clients of several nurses, so you would have to report to *each* primary care nurse about his or her specific client).

The People You Support

People receiving health care and support services are known by different terms, depending on the workplace setting. A person receiving care in a hospital is called a **patient**. A person living in a **residential facility** is called a **resident**. A person receiving care or support services in the community is called a **client**. "Client" is also a general term for all people receiving health care or support services: hospital patients, facility residents, and clients in the community.

Whether the individual receiving care is known as a client, patient, or resident, always remember that he or she is first and foremost a *person*. Every person is unique. The people to whom you provide services have a variety of needs and abilities. They all have unique life experiences and situations. They also have unique wants and opinions. You will work with people from a variety of cultures or backgrounds (see Chapter 12). Part of your job is to accept this diversity among people. The *Respecting Diversity* boxes that appear throughout this text will help you appreciate the importance of diversity and how people's backgrounds influence who they are and what they do.

The people you support can be grouped according to their problems, needs, and ages:

- ***Older adults.*** Aging is a normal process and is not an illness or disease. Many older adults enjoy good health. However, body changes normally occur with the aging process. Social and emotional changes may also occur (see Chapter 17). The risks for contracting serious illnesses and becoming disabled increase with age. Most older adults remain at home as long as possible. Others are unable to manage even with assistance and move into a residential facility. Throughout the text, issues relevant to older adults are discussed.
- ***People with disabilities.*** Some people are disabled due to illness, injury, or conditions present at birth. Disabilities may affect physical functioning, mental functioning, or both. Many adults with disabilities live in their own homes. Many work outside the home. You might help disabled clients with their ADLs or may be responsible for teaching them how to perform the ADLs independently.
- ***People with medical problems.*** Medical problems include illnesses, diseases, and injuries. Medical problems may be short-term (such as a broken bone), long-term (such as diabetes or multiple sclerosis), or progressive and life-threatening (such as some types of cancer).
- ***People having surgery.*** Surgical clients are those being prepared for or who have recently had surgery. Preoperative care involves preparing the client for what to expect after surgery. The client's fears and anxieties are also addressed. Needs after surgery relate to relieving pain and discomfort, preventing complications, and helping the client adjust to body changes. People recover from surgeries in hospitals and in their homes.
- ***People with mental health problems.*** Mental health problems range from mild to severe. Some people function normally but need help making decisions or coping with life stresses. Others are severely affected and need assistance with ADLs.
- ***People needing rehabilitation.*** **Rehabilitation** is the process of restoring a person to the highest level of functioning possible through the use of therapy, exercise, or other methods. The person may need to regain functions lost due to surgery, illness, or accident. Some hospitals have special rehabilitation units. Many people receiving support at home and in long-term care settings require rehabilitation.
- ***Children.*** When hospital care is needed, children are admitted to the pediatric unit. Some areas of Canada hire support workers to work in pediatric units (Figure 1–4). However, most support work for children occurs in community settings and long-term care facilities. Some children who receive care have physical or intellectual disabilities. Others need care because a parent is ill or disabled or has just had a new baby. *Focus on Children* boxes discuss issues related to caring for children.
- ***Mothers and newborns.*** Complications and difficulties can occur at any time during pregnancy and even up to 6 to 8 weeks following childbirth. Some new mothers need assistance with their own care or with their newborn's care. Most support work with mothers and newborns takes place in the home.
- ***People requiring special care.*** Some people who have serious and complex medical conditions need special care and equipment. Hospitals have special care units, including intensive care units, coronary care units, kidney dialysis units, burn units, and emergency rooms. Some areas of Canada hire support workers to work in these units. You might transport people from one unit to another, take specimens to the lab, and assist with special procedures. In some parts of Canada, support workers do not provide personal care to patients in unstable or critical condition.

THE HEALTH CARE TEAM

A *team* is a group of people working together toward a common goal. Health care teams include professionals with a variety of skills and knowledge

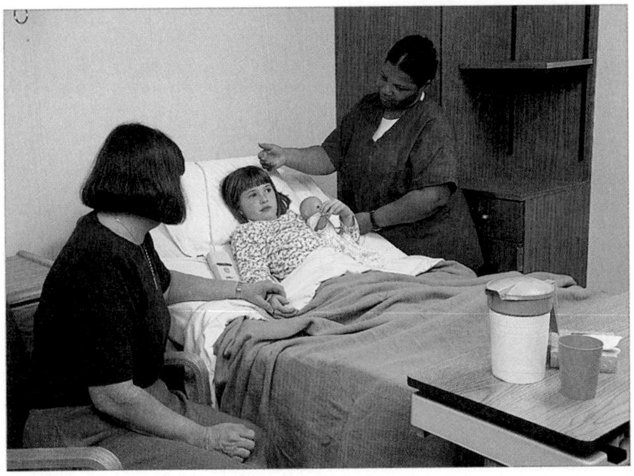

Figure 1–4 A support worker provides care to a sick child.

who work together to meet the client's needs. Their goal is to provide quality care. Many professionals are involved in the care of one client. Which professionals are involved depends on the needs of the client.

You, as the support worker, are an important member of the health care team. The client and family members are also important members of the team. The client is always the focus of the health care team's efforts (Figure 1–5).

Regulated and Unregulated Workers

Health care professions are either regulated or unregulated. A regulated profession is self-governing. It has a professional organization called a *college*, which sets education and licence requirements. It also establishes the scope of practice, codes of ethics, and standards of conduct for its members. The college investigates complaints about a member's conduct. If necessary, the college disciplines members guilty of misconduct. Each regulated health care profession has legislation that details the roles and responsibilities of its members. Nursing is one of many regulated health care professions.

An unregulated profession does not have a professional college, and it does not have legislation written specifically for it. There are no official requirements for educational programs, and there are no codes of ethics. At this point, support workers are still considered **unregulated care providers (UCPs)**. As a support worker, you do not have an organization or college that governs your role, so you are accountable to your supervisor, your employer, and your clients.

Table 1–1 describes the titles and positions of the common health care team members. It also specifies whether they are regulated or unregulated workers.

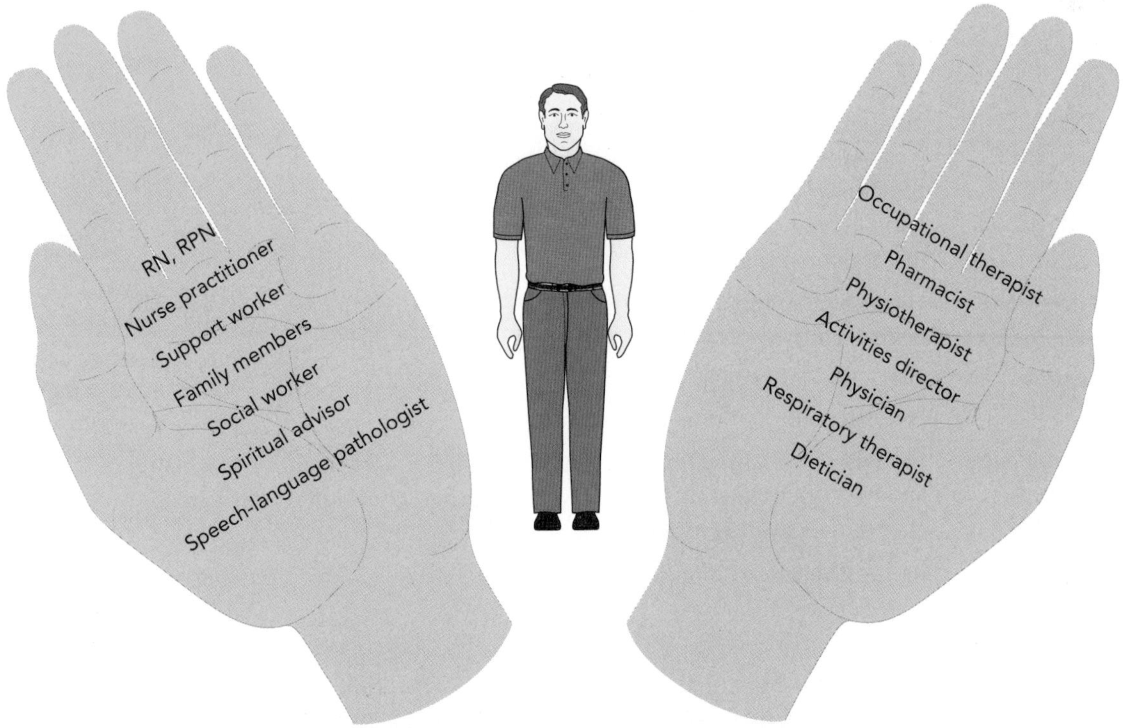

Figure 1–5 Members of the health care team, with the client as the focus of care.

Table 1–1 Support and Health Care Team Members

Title	Description	Regulated/Unregulated
Activities director	Assesses, plans, and implements recreational activities based on clients' needs	Unregulated; provincial/territorial educational requirements vary
Dietician	Assesses and plans for nutritional needs; teaches clients about nutrition, food selection, and preparation	Regulated
Nurse practitioner	Registered nurse with advanced education and additional responsibilities for management of client care	Regulated
Occupational therapist	Focuses on rehabilitation; teaches clients skills needed to perform ADLs; designs adaptive equipment for ADLs	Regulated
Pharmacist	Fills medication orders written by physicians; monitors and evaluates drug interactions; consults with physicians and nurses about drug actions and interactions	Regulated
Physiotherapist (Physical therapist)	Focuses on rehabilitation; assists clients with musculo-skeletal problems; focuses on restoring function and preventing disability from illness or injury	Regulated
Physician	Diagnoses and treats clients with illnesses and injuries	Regulated
Registered nurse (RN)	Assesses; makes nursing diagnoses; plans, implements, and evaluates nursing care; tends to clients who have unstable health conditions; provides direct client care, administers medications, supervises support workers	Regulated
Registered practical nurse/Licensed practical nurse (RPN/LPN)	Assesses; makes nursing diagnoses; plans, implements, and evaluates nursing care; tends to clients who have stable health conditions; provides direct client care, administers medications, supervises support workers	Regulated
Registered psychiatric nurse (RPN)	Provides care to individuals whose primary needs relate to mental, emotional, and developmental health. Works independently or in cooperation with other health care professionals (for example, psychiatrists, physicians, psychologists, social workers, recreational therapists, and occupational therapists) to develop or implement therapeutic programs	Regulated
Respiratory therapist	Focuses on rehabilitation; assists in treatment of lung and heart disorders; gives respiratory treatments and therapies	Regulated
Social worker	Helps clients and families deal with social and emotional issues related to illness and recovery	Varies according to province/territory
Speech–language pathologist (therapist)	Focuses on rehabilitation; evaluates speech and language; and treats people with speech, voice, hearing, communication, and swallowing disorders	Regulated
Spiritual advisor	Assists clients and families with spiritual needs	Determined by religious order
Support worker	Assists clients with personal care, family responsibilities, social and recreational activities, housekeeping/home management; provides personal care and assistance with ADLs	Unregulated

Scope of Practice

To protect clients from harm, you must understand what you can do, what you cannot do, and the legal limits of your role as a support worker. This is called **scope of practice**.

Never act beyond the legal limits of your role. Also never perform a function or task that you have not been trained to do. If you perform a task that is outside these limits, you could harm a client and create serious legal problems for yourself and your employer.

Three sources of information about scope of practice are as follows:

1. ***Your educational program.*** Your educational program includes information on scope of practice for support work in your province or territory. If you are unsure about the laws in your part of the country, ask your instructor.
2. ***Your employer's policies.*** Your employer has written policies that establish what you can and cannot do. Read these carefully before you start work.
3. ***Your supervisor.*** On the job, your supervisor is the best source of information. If you have any questions, do not hesitate to ask your supervisor. If you are unsure about how to carry out a procedure, inform your supervisor. It is far better to ask for direction than risk harming a client.

The Supervision of Support Workers

In many settings, nurses or other professionals supervise support workers. A **registered nurse (RN)** is licensed and regulated by the province or territory to maintain overall responsibility for the planning and provision of client care. Some RNs have university degrees and even postgraduate education. Others have community college diplomas. RNs assess, make nursing diagnoses, develop care plans, and implement and evaluate nursing care. They also carry out physicians' orders. An RN is usually a team leader of the health care team consisting of RPNs/LPNs (see below), support workers, and other assistive personnel.

Assistive personnel is a broad term applied to staff who assist nurses and other health care professionals in giving care or support to clients in facilities, in the community, or in private homes.

A **registered practical nurse (RPN)**, also known as a **licensed practical nurse (LPN)**, is licensed and regulated by the province or territory to carry out basic nursing procedures and client care. RPNs/LPNs have a community college diploma, and like RNs, they must hold a current nursing registration in the province that they practise in. RPNs/LPNs function in a decision-making position when caring for stable clients with uncomplicated health problems, but in providing care to clients with serious and unstable health issues, they assist RNs and help with complex procedures. They can also supervise support workers in most situations. Sometimes the client is assigned to a nurse who acts as a **primary care nurse**. A primary care nurse is responsible for the ongoing management of the health of a client, which includes liaising with other heath care team members, the client/resident, and her or his family. In a long-term care (complex care) environment, the primary care nurse may or may not be directly involved in providing care on a daily basis.

Depending on the situation, you may be supervised by a professional other than an RN or RPN/LPN. For example, if you work in the recreation department of a long-term care facility, you may report to a recreational therapist. In the community, your supervisor may be a social worker, a physiotherapist, or another health care professional. Refer to the Appendix at the end of the book for a description of some of the people who may supervise you.

Some support workers are hired and supervised directly by clients. You must be aware of provincial or territorial legislation that limits the tasks and procedures you can perform as a support worker.

BEING A PROFESSIONAL

Professionalism is an approach to work that demonstrates respect for others, commitment, competence, and appropriate behaviour. Being cheerful and friendly, keeping work schedules, performing tasks competently, and being helpful are all part of a professional approach. To be a true professional, you must demonstrate the following:

- ***A positive attitude.*** You need to show a good attitude about your job. The work you do is very important. People rely on you to give good care and support. You need to believe that you and your work are valuable. Show that you enjoy your work. This involves being enthusiastic, considerate, courteous, honest, and cooperative. Always think before you speak, do not gossip, and do not complain. Your words reveal your attitude. Box 1–1 lists some statements that show a negative attitude. These should be avoided.

- ***A sense of responsibility.*** Never blame others for your problems or mistakes at work. Admit your mistakes, accept constructive criticism, and learn from others. Always report to work when scheduled and on time. Everyone in the team including the client is affected when even one person is late. Have a plan ready for times when you are urgently needed at home or your transportation is unavailable. Inform your supervisor immediately if you will be late or unable to work. Also, be sure to finish assigned tasks before you leave for the day. The client's care cannot be neglected for any reason. Promptly explain to your supervisor if you cannot finish your assignment.
- ***A professional appearance.*** A professional, appropriate appearance shows respect for the people in your care, your co-workers, and yourself. It indicates that you take your job seriously. Your appearance includes your clothes, grooming, and hygiene (see Box 1–2 on this page and Figure 1–6 on page 15).
- ***Discretion about client information.*** **Discretion** means good judgement—being very careful about what you say, how you say it, when you say it, and where you say it. You need to judge when information should be kept private and when it should be shared. Information about a client is confidential. **Confidentiality** means respecting and guarding personal and private information about another person. Information should be shared only among the health care team members involved in the client's care. Information about your employer, your co-workers, and other clients is also private. Never talk with a client about another client, even if you avoid using names. Avoid talking about clients, co-workers, and your employer where you can be overheard. If you need to discuss a client's care with team members, make sure that other clients, families, and visitors cannot hear you. People overhearing may think you are talking about them or their family members. This can lead to misinformation and confusion, which can be very distressing.
- ***Discretion about personal matters.*** Discretion in support work includes keeping personal mat-

Box 1–1 Statements That Show a Negative Attitude

- "I can't. I'm too busy. Can't somebody else help?"
- "I didn't do it."
- "It's not my fault."
- "Don't blame me."
- "It's not my turn. I did it yesterday."
- "Nobody told me."
- "I work harder than anyone else."
- "No one appreciates what I do."

Box 1–2 Practices for a Professional Appearance

- Follow your employer's dress code policies.
- Wear a clean, well-fitting, modest uniform.
- Wear a name badge or photo ID, per your employer's policy.
- Wear clean stockings and socks that are in good repair.
- Wear comfortable, well-polished shoes that give you good support.
- Ensure that your underclothing cannot be seen through your uniform.
- Keep your hair away from your face and up off your collar.
- Use makeup sparingly to avoid a painted, severe look.
- Do not wear perfume, cologne, or aftershave. They may cause nausea or breathing problems in some clients.
- Keep fingernails clean, short, and neatly shaped. Long nails can scratch the client.
- Do not wear jewellery (even if parts of your body are pierced). Jewellery may scratch or cause injury to your client and yourself. It may offend some clients as well.
- Cover tattoos because they may be offensive to some clients.

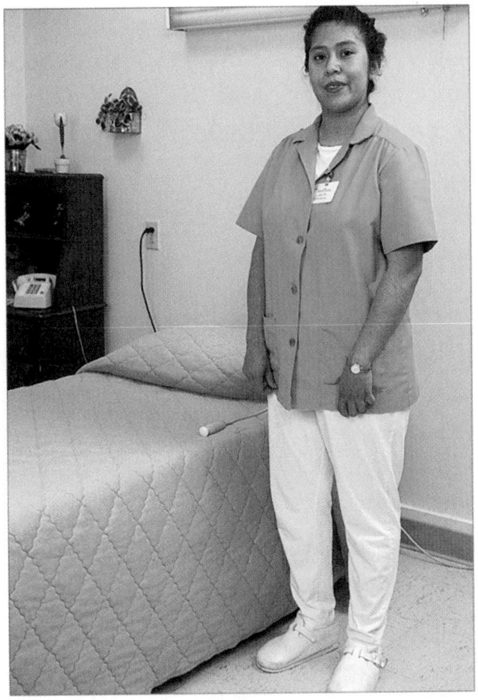

Figure 1–6 This support worker is well-groomed. Her uniform and shoes are clean. Her hair is worn in a simple style and is kept out of her face and off her collar. She is not wearing any jewellery, except a watch. Her nametag is easily visible and approved by her employer. **Source:** Sorrentino, S.A. (2000). *Mosby's textbook for nursing assistants* (5th ed., p. 37). St. Louis: Mosby.

ters out of the workplace. Your role is to focus on your clients and the task at hand. Do not discuss with clients your family matters and personal problems or the problems of others (Box 1–3). ***No matter how well you think you know a client, remember that your relationship must remain professional. It would be inappropriate to discuss your personal problems with your client.***

- ***Acceptable speech and language.*** The way you speak at home and in casual social settings may not be appropriate for a work setting. Even if you are speaking with a co-worker, others could hear you and be offended by what you say or how you say it. Your speech and language must be professional. In order not to offend clients or co-workers, never use foul, vulgar, or abusive language. Also, avoid using slang. Speak gently and clearly; never yell or shout. Never fight or argue with clients, their family members, or your co-workers.

Box 1–3 Keeping Personal Matters Out of the Workplace

- Make personal calls only during scheduled breaks. Use a client's phone only for urgent matters. Always ask for permission before using his or her phone.
- Do not discuss your personal problems at work.
- Do not let your family and friends visit you at work.
- Arrange your personal appointments outside of your scheduled work hours.
- Do not use your employer's supplies or equipment for personal matters.
- Do not try to raise funds at work, even if the funds are for a good cause.

THE PRIORITIES OF SUPPORT WORK: COMPASSIONATE CARE AND SUPPORT

Compassion means caring about another person's misfortune and suffering. **Caring** means having concern for the dignity, independence, preferences, privacy, and safety of clients and their families at all times. True *compassionate care* includes honesty, sensitivity, comforting, discretion, and respect while providing this service. Many people who require *support* are coping with serious illness, disability, personal problems, or challenges. Providing compassionate care involves treating people with respect, kindness, and understanding. No matter what kind of care or support you provide, most clients have the following needs:

- ***To preserve their dignity.*** **Dignity** is the state of feeling worthy, valued, and respected. People need to feel dignified.
- ***To live independently.*** Clients need to do what they can for themselves.
- ***To express their preferences.*** Clients need to make choices and explain how they want to have things done.
- ***To preserve their privacy.*** Clients need to know that their bodies and their affairs are treated respectfully and protected from public view (Figure 1–7).

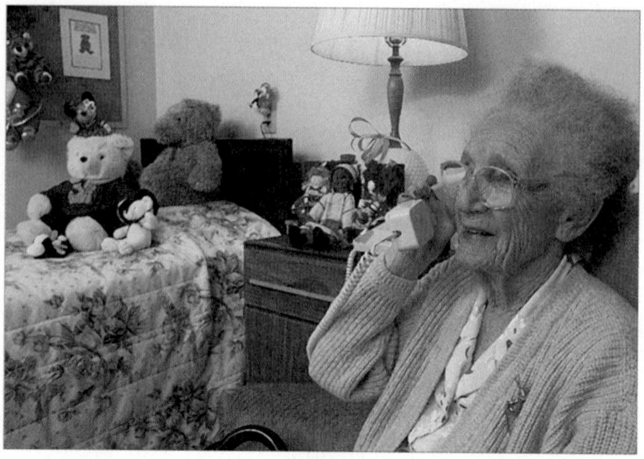

Figure 1–7 A client talks privately on a telephone.

- ***To be safe from harm.*** Clients need to live in an environment that is as hazard-free as possible. They also need to feel secure about the care provided.

When well and able-bodied, most people take the fulfillment of the five needs listed above for granted. When they become disabled or suffer a serious illness, however, these needs may be more difficult to fulfill. Those who rely on others for personal care may worry about losing their dignity. They may not feel free to express their wishes. For example, clients living in long-term care facilities may have to eat what is provided and socialize only at prearranged times. When they live in a facility and share a room with another client, they may find that private moments are rare. Safety concerns are serious issues in the lives of clients who are ill and disabled. For example, they may worry about reaching the bathroom without falling.

Not all clients who are ill and disabled have the same needs. However, most have at least some of the needs just discussed. To help you recognize these needs, *Providing Compassionate Care* boxes throughout the text discuss the priorities of support work. Most of these boxes discuss how to promote the person's **D**ignity, **I**ndependence, **P**references, **P**rivacy, and **S**afety. The acronym DIPPS reminds you of these five priorities.

DECISION MAKING AND PROBLEM SOLVING

You make many decisions in the course of your work day. For example, you estimate the time each task will take and plan the best way to complete your work on time. Many decisions involve solving problems.

When solving problems, consider the following:

- ***The priorities of support work.*** Solutions to problems should not compromise the five priorities of support work: dignity, independence, preferences, privacy, and safety.
- ***The client's viewpoint.*** Involve clients in solving problems that concern them. Examine the problem from the client's perspective.
- ***Your scope of practice.*** Learn and observe the rules of your workplace. Know the limits of your role.
- ***Your supervisor's viewpoint.*** Decide if the problem is one that you can handle on your own or one that your supervisor should handle. Your supervisor should provide guidance about which problems you can deal with on your own.

Decision making and problem solving are crucial to your role but are often difficult when you are new to the job. To help you with the problem-solving process, this text includes boxes called *Support Workers Solving Problems.* These boxes present examples of problems faced by support workers and how the problems were solved.

REVIEW

Answers to these questions are at the bottom of the page.

Circle the BEST answer.

1. **Activities of daily living (ADLs) are:**
   A. Social and recreational activities
   B. Activities that support workers perform to prevent injuries
   C. Physical exercises that people perform daily to keep themselves fit
   D. Self-care activities that people perform daily to remain independent and to function in society

2. **Which of the following is a way in which support workers assist nurses or other health care team members?**
   A. Assess the client's needs
   B. Order range-of-motion exercises
   C. Witness legal signatures on permission forms
   D. Report changes in the client's behaviour or health

3. **"Resident" is a term used to describe a person who is receiving care at:**
   A. Home
   B. A long-term care facility
   C. An outpatient clinic
   D. A hospital

4. **The main focus of the health care team is to:**
   A. See as many clients as possible
   B. Provide quality care for the client
   C. Complete assigned tasks as quickly as possible
   D. Find a cure for the client's illness or condition

5. **Support workers are:**
   A. Unregulated care providers
   B. Licensed health care workers
   C. Members of a professional college
   D. Members of a regulatory body

6. ***Scope of practice* means:**
   A. The tasks that are assigned by your supervisor
   B. The tasks that a client asks you to perform
   C. The effort you put into performing a task or procedure
   D. The legal limits of your role

7. **Professionalism is:**
   A. An approach to work used only by members of regulated professions
   B. An approach to work that demonstrates respect for others, commitment, competence, and appropriate behaviour
   C. A commitment made by regulated professionals
   D. Another term for confidentiality

8. **Which of the following is true?**
   A. You can use a client's phone to make personal calls.
   B. Friends can visit you at work.
   C. You must follow your employer's dress code policies.
   D. Sharing your personal problems with a client shows compassion.

9. **In a long-term care facility, the client's information should be shared among:**
   A. Health care team members involved in the client's care
   B. Health care team members and friends who visit the client
   C. Family and friends of the client
   D. All staff members at the facility

10. ***Compassion* means:**
    A. Keeping one's feelings to oneself
    B. Approaching your work with enthusiasm
    C. Taking pity on those who are less fortunate
    D. Caring about another's misfortune and suffering

11. **The acronym DIPPS stands for:**
    A. Danger, independence, preferences, policies, sympathy
    B. Dignity, independence, preferences, privacy, safety
    C. Difference, individuality, pity, privacy, scope of practice
    D. Disability, individuality, pity, privacy, scope of practice

12. **Which is false? When solving problems, you should:**
    A. Consider your scope of practice
    B. Consider the priorities of support work
    C. Discuss the problem with the client
    D. Not involve the client to prevent causing more problems

Answers: 1.D, 2.D, 3.B, 4.B, 5.A, 6.D, 7.B, 8.C, 9.A, 10.D, 11.B, 12.D

CHAPTER 2

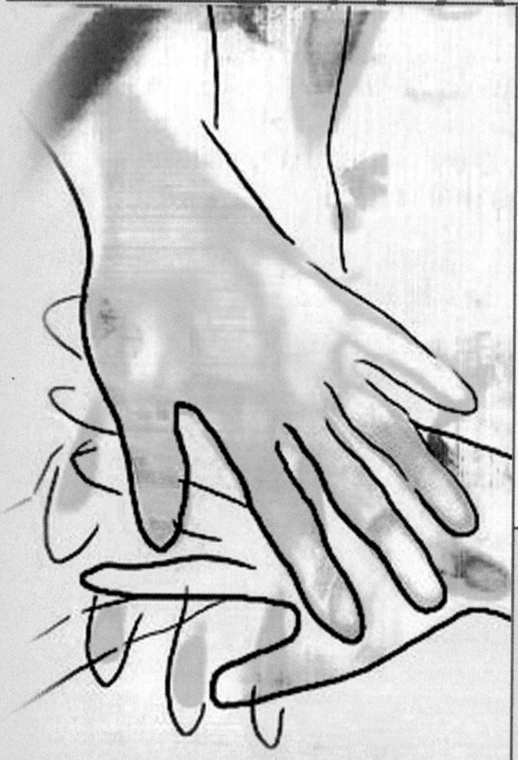

The Canadian Health Care System

OBJECTIVES

- Define the key terms listed in this chapter.
- Describe medicare and how it has evolved.
- Identify the federal, provincial, and territorial roles in the health care system.
- Summarize the five principles of medicare described in the *Canada Health Act.*
- Identify how the focus of the Canadian health care system is shifting to home care.
- Explain why health promotion and disease prevention are important functions of the Canadian health care system.
- Recognize the emerging importance of home care and the support worker's role in providing some of these services.

key terms

accessibility A principle of the *Canada Health Act* that states that people must have reasonable access to insured health care services.

benefits Types of assistance that are provided through available insurance premiums. An example of one benefit would be a medical physical examination without any additional cost to the consumer.

***Canada Health Act* (1984)** Federal legislation that clarifies the types of health care services that are insured; it also outlines five principles **(comprehensiveness, universality, portability, accessibility,** and **public administration)** that must be met by provinces and territories to qualify for federal health money.

comprehensiveness A principle of the *Canada Health Act* that states that all necessary health services, including hospitalization and access to physicians and surgical dentists, must be insured.

disease prevention Strategies that prevent the occurrence of disease or injury.

health promotion A strategy for improving the population's health by providing the necessary information and tools so that individuals, groups, and communities can make informed decisions that promote health and wellness.

home care Health care and support services provided to people in their places of residence.

medicare Canada's national health care insurance system; publicly funds all the cost of medically necessary health services.

portability A principle of the *Canada Health Act* that states that residents continue to be entitled to coverage from their home province even when they live in a different province or territory or out of the country.

public administration A principle of the *Canada Health Act* that states that provincial health insurance must be administered by a public authority on a nonprofit basis.

Telehealth Medical telephone call centres where nurses give advice to callers on health issues.

universality A principle of the *Canada Health Act* that states that all residents are entitled to the same basic level of health care services across the country.

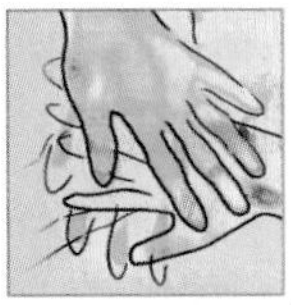

Few issues are as important to Canadians as health care. Most Canadians believe that quality health care should be available to all citizens, regardless of their ability to pay. Canada's national health insurance system, known as **medicare,** was developed to achieve this goal. Medicare uses provincial/territorial and federal taxes to pay for all medically necessary health services for all permanent residents. Faced with the ever-increasing costs of providing care, Canadians are re-examining their health care spending and priorities. Support workers have an increasingly important role within Canada's changing health care system.[1]

THE EVOLUTION OF CANADA'S HEALTH CARE SYSTEM

Canada's publicly funded health care system is best described as an interlocking set of 10 provincial and 3 territorial health insurance plans. Medicare provides access to universal, comprehensive coverage for medically necessary hospital and physician services. These services are administered and delivered by the provincial and territorial governments and are provided free of charge. The provincial and territorial governments fund health care services with assistance from the federal government.

Canadian Health Care in the Past. In the first part of the twentieth century, individuals in Canada were expected to pay the entire amount of their doctors' bills and hospital fees. Often, there were no "set fees," that is, for the same treatment, a physician could charge one patient a certain amount and another an entirely different fee, depending on what the physician thought the patient could afford to pay. As a result, people often paid different fees for similar services. Those who could not afford to pay had to find charity services through community agencies such as the Victorian Order of Nurses, the Red Cross, and local churches (Figure 2–1), and some even went without health care.

The Great Depression across Canada in the 1930s had a dramatic effect on the health care system. Families struggled to feed, clothe, and house their members and could not possibly pay their medical bills. A serious illness or stay in a hospital caused financial disaster for many. The cost of care prevented many from seeking medical treatment. Many ill and disabled people depended on family members and neighbours to provide care. Box 2–1 presents one woman's memoir of the Depression years. As a child, she witnessed the hardships people endured because of the health care system of the time.

These hardships inspired Canadians to create a prepaid medical and hospitalization insurance plan. In 1947, under then-Premier Tommy Douglas, Saskatchewan was the first province to introduce a public insurance plan that covered the costs of hospital services (Box 2–2). By 1961, all 10 provinces and 2 territories agreed to provide coverage for inpatient hospital care. The federal government paid about half the cost of hospital and diagnostic services for each province/territory. The provincial and territorial governments paid for the other half. By 1972, all provinces and territories extended their insurance plans to also cover medical services provided outside hospitals. Again, the provincial/territorial and federal governments shared the health care expenses roughly equally. Modern medicare began that year, and all permanent residents now had free access to the same quality of hospital and medical care, regardless of their personal wealth.

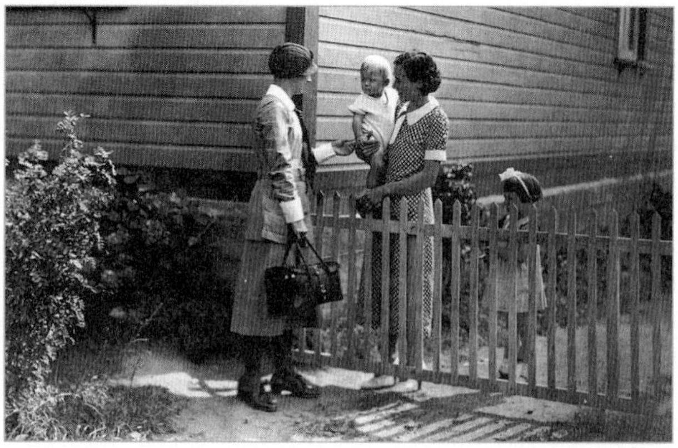

Figure 2–1 In the first part of the twentieth century, charitable services were provided by community agencies such as the Victorian Order of Nurses for Canada. **Source:** Victorian Order of Nurses (VON), Canada.

Box 2–1 Health Care During the Depression

The Depression years were the years of my growing up on an apple farm near a small village in eastern Ontario. Living in the country meant you knew the joys, pains, and sorrows of your neighbours and community. In those years, many were in very difficult circumstances.... The cost of medical care was one of the most painful situations many people faced. Proud and needy people visited the one doctor available only in times of extremity. Recently, I heard that during these years, one-half of Canadians never in all their lives received any medical attention....

The doctor in our community was caring and very hardworking. Many patients paid him in chickens, eggs, potatoes, or apples. Some were unable to make any payment. It was a situation which was devastating for both patient and doctor. The patient had to beg for medical attention for himself and loved ones. The doctor must have been overstocked with food articles beyond the needs of his family, but without the ready cash for taxes, car upkeep, or clothing for his family.

Source: Heeney, Helen (Ed.). (1995). *Life before Medicare: Canadian experiences.* Toronto: The Stories Project, p. ix.

THE MODERN HEALTH CARE SYSTEM

The federal government and the 10 provincial and 3 territorial governments share responsibilities within Canada's health care system. In order to receive their full share of federal funding for health care, the provincial and territorial health insurance plans must meet five criteria—**comprehensiveness, universality, portability, accessibility,** and **public administration** (see Box 2–3 on page 22)—that are provided in the federal government's ***Canada Health Act***. Many other organizations and groups, including health professional associations and accreditation, education, research, and voluntary organizations, contribute to health care in Canada.

Box 2–2 Tommy Douglas, the "Greatest Canadian"

In the spring of 2004, the CBC invited Canadians to submit their nominations for the "Greatest Canadian" of all time. Canadians responded with thousands of worthy suggestions, including Terry Fox, a courageous young man who ran across Canada to champion cancer research; scientists; athletes; as well as Prime Ministers who have contributed to Canada's history. After 6 weeks of voting, on November 29, 2004, Tommy Douglas won. You might be wondering who Tommy Douglas was, and why Canadians are grateful for his contributions to this country.

Thomas Clement Douglas (1904–1986) was elected to office in June, 1944, and with his party, the Cooperative Commonwealth Federation (CCF), was given the difficult task of reorganizing Saskatchewan's post-war employment, social, and health public policies. Through "humanitarian idealism and courage," over the next 40 years, his party transformed that relatively poor, remote agricultural province into the country's leader in social and health care reforms. Douglas' reforms have become his legacy, as they now form the basis for Canada's social and health care policies, which continue to exist today.

A few of the many contributions he made to the Province of Saskatchewan—and to the whole country by example—include:

- As Health Minister (1944–1948), he took the first steps towards what we now call *medicare* by establishing the following:
  - free health care for pensioners
  - free cancer treatment to those in need
  - the first comprehensive health services region
  - new health care facilities
- Creating Canada's first universal and compulsory hospital insurance program for Saskatchewan. This was the beginning of what Canadians now know as "health insurance programs."
- Under his leadership, many of the rights that workers now take for granted—such as establishing a minimum wage, ensuring a maximum 44-hour work week, and paid 2-week vacation leave—were made into policy.
- He oversaw old age pension and mother's allowance increases and legislated that free medical and hospital benefits be given to welfare recipients.

These are just a few of the many contributions that Tommy Douglas made. There is no doubt that without him, Canada would be a very different country today. We can all be grateful for the role he played in making Canada the country that it is.

Source: Tommy Douglas Research Institute. (2007). *The greatest Canadian.* Retrieved January 25, 2008, from http://www.tommydouglas.ca/tommy/greatest_canadian.

The responsibility for Aboriginal (First Nations people and Inuit) health services is shared by the federal, provincial, and territorial governments and the Aboriginal organizations. The responsibility for public health is also shared. The federal Public Health Agency of Canada acts as a focal point for disease prevention and control and for emergency response to infectious diseases; however, public health services are generally delivered at the provincial/territorial and local levels.

The Federal Role

The federal government is responsible for:

- Administering the *Canada Health Act* and providing provincial funding.
- Providing direct delivery of health care services to specific groups, such as First Nations people living on reserves; Inuit; serving members of the Canadian Forces and the Royal Canadian Mounted Police (RCMP); eligible veterans; and inmates of federal penitentiaries.[2]
- Developing and carrying out government policy and programs that promote health and prevent disease. For example, the federal government approves drugs, assesses health risks posed by environmental hazards, and provides grant money to support public health programs, such as prenatal health education.
- Transferring tax money to the provinces and territories to share the cost of medically necessary health care services.

Box 2–3 The Principles of Medicare, as Listed in the *Canada Health Act* (1984)

1. **Public administration.** The insurance plan must be run by a public organization on a nonprofit basis. The public organization must be accountable to the citizens and the government of the province or territory.
2. **Comprehensiveness.** The insurance plan must pay for all medically necessary services. In a hospital, all necessary drugs, supplies, and diagnostic tests are covered. A range of necessary services provided outside a hospital are also covered.
3. **Universality.** Every permanent resident of a province or territory is entitled to receive the insured health care services provided by the plan on similar terms and conditions.
4. **Portability.** People can keep their health care coverage even if they are unemployed, change jobs, relocate between provinces and territories, or travel within Canada or abroad.
5. **Accessibility.** People can receive medically necessary services regardless of their income, age, health status, gender, or geographical location. Additional charges for insured services are not permitted.

- Ensuring that the provinces and territories provide the same quality and type of care. The act does not allow service providers (such as physicians) to bill clients for extra charges and user fees.

The Provincial/Territorial Role

Each province and territory is responsible for developing and administering its own health care insurance plan. The provincial or territorial government finances and plans its health care services, following the five basic principles outlined in the *Canada Health Act*. For example, the provincial or territorial governments decide where hospitals or long-term care facilities will be located and organized; how many physicians, nurses, and other service providers will be needed; and how much money to spend on health care services. The provincial and territorial health insurance plans (Table 2–1) pay for hospital and physician costs.

Table 2–1 List of Provincial and Territorial Health Insurance Programs

Province	Name of Plan
Alberta	Alberta Health Care Insurance Plan
British Columbia	Medical Services Plan
Manitoba	Manitoba Health
New Brunswick	Medicare
Newfoundland and Labrador	Newfoundland and Labrador Medical Care Plan
Northwest Territories	NWT Health Care Insurance Plan
Nova Scotia	Medical Service Insurance
Nunavut	Nunavut Health Care Plan
Ontario	Ontario Health Insurance Plan
Prince Edward Island	Medicare
Quebec	Assurance maladie (Medicare)
Saskatchewan	Saskatchewan Medical Care Insurance Plan
Yukon	Yukon Health Care Insurance Plan

Source: Health Canada. Provincial/territorial role in health. Retrieved January 24, 2008, from http://www.hc-sc.gc.ca/hcs-sss/delivery-prestation/ptrole/ptmin/index_e.html.

HEALTH CARE CHALLENGES AND TRENDS

Challenges. Many factors challenge the country's ability to provide universal, quality health care, and the Canadian health care system has come under stress in recent years. These factors are expected to continue in the future.[2]

The factors that have stressed Canada's health care system include:

- Many rural or remote areas facing severe shortages of physicians, nurses, and other health care workers
- Financial issues
- Aging of the "baby boomer" generation

- Long waiting lists that are common for surgeries, diagnostics, or medical procedures
- High cost of new technology

Of these factors, the greatest challenge facing the health care system is the steadily rising cost of care. Drugs and technology now exist that treat diseases and disabilities better than ever before. However, these advances come at a high price due to the cost of developing them.

Additional (Supplementary) Services. The provinces and territories provide coverage to certain people (e.g., seniors, children, and social assistance recipients) for health services that are not generally covered under the publicly funded health care system. These supplementary health benefits often include prescription drugs, dental care, vision care, medical equipment and appliances (prostheses, wheelchairs, etc.), independent living and the services of other health professionals, such as podiatrists and chiropractors. The level of coverage varies across the country.[2]

Private Insurance. Those who do not qualify for supplementary benefits under government plans pay for these services with individual, out-of pocket payments or through private health insurance plans. Many Canadians, either through their employers or on their own, are covered by private health insurance, and the level of service provided varies according to the plan purchased. Each provincial and territorial plan of private insurance is unique. Exactly what is covered and by how much varies across the country; for example, coverage for ambulance services, drugs, and home care varies from province to province.

To help pay for services not covered by provincial or territorial insurance, people can buy extra health insurance policies. Private health insurance covers the costs that are not government funded, such as some of the costs of rehabilitation and extended care services. These costs are sometimes referred to as **benefits**. Some people have private insurance coverage that has a very comprehensive benefit plan; other people have very few benefits paid for by their private insurance company; and some people do not have any private insurance, so they receive no other funding other than what is provided by their province.

Trends. In order to reduce some of the pressures placed on our health care system, new ways of providing care have been introduced to Canadians, with the intent of providing quality care while avoiding needless spending. As a result, health care services and the way they are delivered have changed from a reliance on hospitals and doctors to the following:

- Alternative care in clinics
- Primary health care centres
- Community health centres
- Home care

As a result of changing the way health care is delivered, the number of acute care hospitals and acute care hospital beds decreased from 1995 to 2000. Medical advances have led to more procedures being done on an outpatient basis, and to a rise in the number of day surgeries. During this time, the number of nights Canadians spent in acute care hospitals fell by 10%. Postacute or hospital alternative services provided in the home and community have grown, and there have been many reforms evident, such as trends to spend less time in hospitals and more growth in day surgeries.[2]

Other reforms have focused on primary health care delivery, including setting up more community primary health care centres that provide services around-the-clock; creating primary health care teams; placing greater emphasis on promoting health, preventing illness and injury, and managing chronic diseases; increasing coordination and integration of comprehensive health services; and improving the work environments of primary health care providers.

Coordinated primary health care teams include family doctors, nurses, nurse practitioners, and other health professionals, and provide a broad range of primary health care services. These team members can vary according to the needs of the community they serve and the provincial and territorial priorities. This team approach, along with the introduction of medical telephone call centres (**Telehealth**) that provide advice and after-hours access to primary health care services, reduces the use of emergency units.

Most provinces and territories have tried to control costs and improve delivery by decentralizing decision making on health care delivery to the regional or local board level. Such regional authorities are managed by elected and appointed members who oversee hospitals, nursing homes, home care, and public health services in their area. As part of these reforms, provincial and territorial governments are now focused on two areas:

- Health promotion and disease prevention
- Home care

Health Promotion and Disease Prevention

Traditionally, the purpose of a health care system has been to diagnose, treat, and cure illnesses. A more recent approach to health care, however, involves developing ways to promote health and prevent disease. Preventing illness and injury, while keeping people healthy, is more effective and cheaper than treating them in hospitals. **Health promotion** refers to strategies that improve or maintain health and independence. **Disease prevention** refers to strategies that prevent the occurrence of disease or injury. Health promotion and disease prevention are now important functions of Canada's health care system.

Research has been done to determine the factors that most affect the health of the population. The following are key determinants that determine a person's health:[2]

- Income and social status
- Social support networks (see Chapter 4)
- Education and literacy
- Employment and working conditions
- Social environment
- Physical environment
- Personal health practices and coping skills
- Healthy child development
- Biological and genetic endowment

Government policy promotes health and prevents illness by improving these areas of people's lives. These policies occur in many sectors of government and industry. Examples of policies that promote health and prevent illness include:

- Immunization programs
- Prenatal and parenting classes
- Information campaigns to reduce drinking during pregnancy, unsafe sex, and tobacco use and to encourage healthy eating and physical activity
- Efforts to improve housing, decrease poverty, monitor safe drinking water, and protect the environment

Support workers contribute to health promotion and disease prevention. You provide nonmedical care and services that can help prevent major health problems. For example, Mr. Lukovic has been in bed rest for a long time. He is at risk for pressure ulcers, pneumonia, and blood clots. To prevent these complications, you, as his support worker, help him keep his skin clean and dry, change his position in bed frequently, and help him perform range-of-motion exercises. By doing these important things for Mr. Lukovic, you can help improve his quality of life now and prevent him from developing illness or disability in the future.

Home Care

The Canadian health care system has seen a shift in focus from hospital care to home care. Traditionally, people entered the health care system through hospitals. However, over the last two decades, the role and structure of hospitals have changed dramatically. Hospitals require a tremendous amount of money to operate. Over a third of all health care spending goes into operating the hospitals. Therefore, most provincial and territorial governments have reduced the number of hospitals to cut costs. In the last few years, hundreds of hospitals have closed, merged, or been converted to other types of care facilities.

Partly to save money and partly as a result of technological advances, clients are sent home sooner after hospital procedures. Each year, fewer clients stay in hospital overnight, and if they do stay overnight, they stay for shorter periods than they would have in the past.

To support patients who leave hospitals early, governments have gradually increased spending on home care. **Home care** is health care and support services provided to people in their places of residence, including private homes, licensed residential care facilities and homes (called retirement residences in some provinces), and assisted-living facilities (see Chapter 3). Home care is the most common of the community-based services.

Home care was first created to provide care for people who needed at-home assistance after hospital discharge. Today, home care provides community care and support to a range of people. Clients include older adults; families with children; people who have mental, physical, or developmental disabilities; people with short-term and long-term medical conditions; and people in the recovery, rehabilitative, or final, life-ending stages of a disease. Home care services provide assistance to families who need help with a new baby. They enable people with disabilities to get up in the morning and get ready for school or work. They help people adjust to a disability or recover from an illness (Figure 2–2). They enable people who are dying to remain at home rather than being admitted to hospital.

One major focus of home care is to enable people to remain in their homes, as healthy and as independent for as long as possible. For some people, home care replaces hospital or other facility care. For others, home care enables them to maintain their health and independence, thus delaying or preventing admission to a facility.

Services and Funding. Support workers provide most support services for home care. In most provinces and territories, support services are provided by both public and private agencies and are either for-profit or not-for-profit. Every province and territory has a publicly funded home care program.

The funding for the specific type of care that each client will receive will depend on his or her province's funding policies. Because the *Canada Health Act* does not say what services must be provided, each province and territory has defined and funded its own home care system. The services offered and how they are provided vary across the country (see Box 2–4).

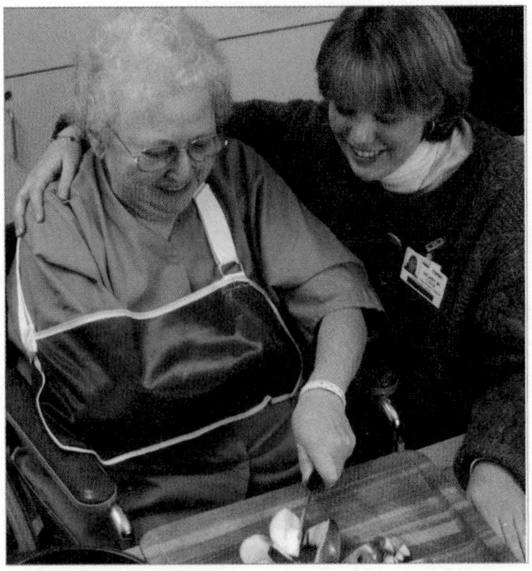

Figure 2–2 This woman receives assistance from home care services so she can continue to live by herself at home. **Source:** Tom Stewart/Corbis/Magma.

All provinces and territories, however, offer the following:

- Client assessment—determining if the person is eligible for services
- Case coordination and management (see Chapter 5)
- Nursing services
- Support services for eligible clients

Eligibility and hours of services provided will also vary, depending on the province or territory. Some people may want home care services that are not funded by their province or for which they do not qualify. They can hire a private agency and pay for these services themselves or with insurance plans (see discussion on "Private Insurance" earlier in this chapter).

Home Care services are classified into the following:

Personal care services: These are nonmedical services offered through home care, often by support workers. They include:

- Assistance with activities of daily living (ADLs, e.g., bathing, feeding, mobility, and dressing)
- Providing comfort care to clients who are dying

Home support services: These services are often provided by support workers, and they provide clients who live at home with the following:

- Assistance with home management
- Assistance with ADLs (bathing, feeding, mobility, and dressing)
- Assistance with taking medications

Nursing and professional services: Therapies and treatments provided by health care professionals include:

- Nursing care
- Physiotherapy
- Occupational therapy
- Speech therapy

- Nutrition counselling
- Social work
- Respiratory therapy

Ancillary support: These services are often provided by support workers, and include:

- Shopping with a client
- Assisting a client with banking
- Teaching a client how to shop for groceries
- Volunteer services, such as Meals on Wheels (Figure 2–3) and friendly visiting, can be provided by anyone who meets the volunteer criteria.

Box 2–4 How Home Care Is Governed and Delivered

How home care is governed and delivered varies from province to province or territory. In all provinces and territories, the ministries or departments of health and social/community services are responsible for home care services. These departments monitor the services and decide on budgets, policies, and standards of care. In Nova Scotia and the Yukon, they also administer and deliver the services. In the rest of the country, other organizations administer and deliver home care. In British Columbia, public home support services provide direct care to clients. In Alberta, Saskatchewan, Manitoba, Prince Edward Island, Newfoundland, and the Northwest Territories, local or regional health authorities administer and deliver home care services. Ontario has Community Care Access Centres (CCACs), which are overseen by Local Health Integration Networks (LHINs). Quebec has Local Community Services Centres (CLSCs), and New Brunswick has the Extra-Mural Program (EMP) to administer and deliver their services.

Service delivery involves:

- Assessing clients' needs
- Determining clients' eligibility for professional and support services
- Co-ordinating and monitoring home care services. These services are provided by private or not-for-profit agencies. Eligible clients do not have to pay for these services.
- Providing information and referrals to other long-term care services. These include volunteer-based community services, such as Meals on Wheels. Some community services charge user fees to the client.
- Providing placement services to assisted-living facilities and extended care (also known in some provinces as long-term care) facilities (some provinces only)

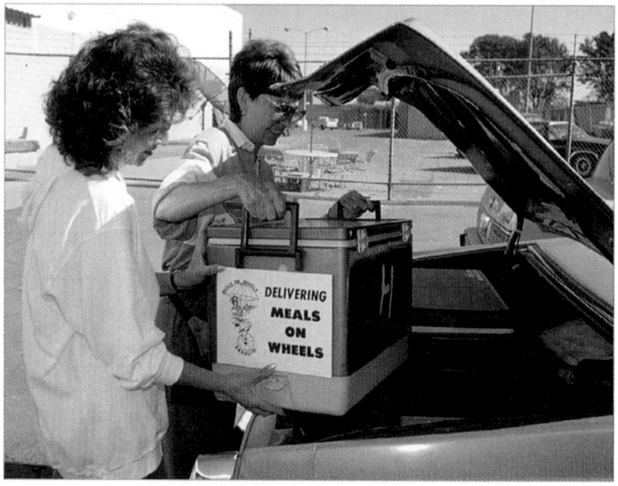

Figure 2–3 Delivery of hot meals to clients in their homes.
Source: Tony Freeman/PhotoEdit.

supporting MR. WOLOSHYN

Ivan Woloshyn is a 65-year-old widower who was seriously injured in an explosion in his factory about 6 months ago, just a few weeks before he was to retire. In the months since his accident, he has been cared for at home by nurses, physiotherapists, and occupational therapists for the severe burns he received to his face and right arm. Since he was also blinded in the accident, he requires support workers to assist him with taking a bus to his various appointments, as well as with his banking and grocery shopping.

Mr. Woloshyn, who lives in Manitoba, has decided that he would like to move in with his married daughter, who lives in Ontario. He has been told that his private insurance, through his employer, would still cover his ongoing treatments and support after he moves. He is not sure, however, about what to do about his provincial insurance coverage. What can you tell him? How can he find out about switching coverage?

REVIEW

Answers to these questions are at the bottom of the page.

Circle the **BEST** answer.

1. **Canada's health care system is:**
   - A. Strictly a federal responsibility
   - B. Delivered by government employees
   - C. Funded by private insurance companies
   - D. Publicly funded through provincial/territorial and federal taxes

2. **The provincial and territorial governments are responsible for:**
   - A. Paying the full amount of all medical procedures
   - B. Planning, financing, and delivering their own health care insurance plans
   - C. Delivering health care services to Aboriginal people and military personnel
   - D. Delivering health care services to inmates of federal penitentiaries and to the Royal Canadian Mounted Police (RCMP)

3. **Which law ensures that every citizen has access to health care?**
   - A. *The Medical Care Act*
   - B. *The Canada Health Act*
   - C. *The Long-Term Care Facilities Act*
   - D. *The Hospital Insurance and Diagnostic Services Act*

4. **Canadians who travel to other parts of the country still maintain their provincial/territorial health care coverage. This is an example of which principle of medicare?**
   - A. Portability
   - B. Universality
   - C. Comprehensiveness
   - D. Public administration

5. **The most pressing cause of health care reform has been:**
   - A. The Depression
   - B. Lack of accessibility
   - C. Lack of available technology
   - D. Rising costs of providing technology, drugs, and services

6. **A recent trend in health care is to focus on:**
   - A. Cutting back on home care services
   - B. Opening more hospitals in rural areas
   - C. Cutting back on public health policies
   - D. Public policy that promotes health and prevents disease

7. **Immunization programs are an example of a:**
   - A. Medicare system
   - B. Disease prevention program
   - C. Home care service
   - D. Facility-based treatment

8. **One major focus of home care is to:**
   - A. Diagnose and treat disease
   - B. Enable clients to remain in their own homes
   - C. Provide accommodation for people with disabilities
   - D. Provide accommodation for acutely ill people who do not want to go to hospital

9. **Home care services provided by support workers might include:**
   - A. Vacuuming and dusting
   - B. Respiratory therapy
   - C. Assisting the client with physiotherapy
   - D. Assisting the client with banking

10. **Which statement about Canadian home care programs is correct?**
    - A. All home care is free to Canadians.
    - B. Provincial government funding is shifting to home care.
    - C. Hospital care is a cheaper and better alternative for most people.
    - D. All provinces and territories govern their programs in a similar manner

11. **In most provinces and territories, types of support services are governed by:**
    - A. Regional health boards
    - B. The federal government
    - C. Private or not-for-profit agencies
    - D. The provincial or territorial government

Answers: 1.D, 2.B, 3.B, 4.A, 5.D, 6.D, 7.B, 8.B, 9.A, 10.B, 11.D

CHAPTER 3

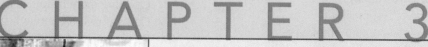

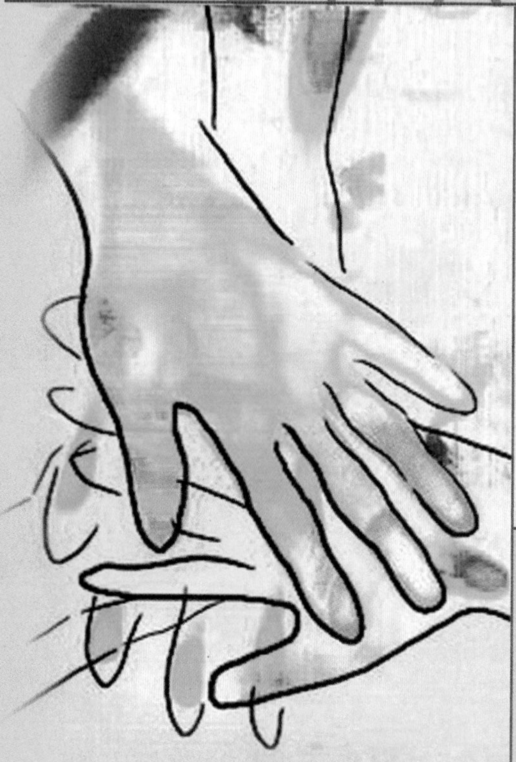

Workplace Settings

OBJECTIVES

- Define the key terms listed in this chapter.
- Differentiate between community-based care and facility-based care.
- List work settings where support workers are employed.
- Differentiate between residential facilities and other medical facilities.
- Describe the various types of residential facilities.
- Identify the issues and challenges support workers encounter in the workplace.

key terms

acute care Health care that is provided for a relatively short time (usually days to weeks) and is intended to diagnose and treat an immediate health issue.

acute illness An illness that appears suddenly and lasts a short time, usually less than 3 months; symptoms can be severe.

adult day care See **community day program**.

adult day centre See **community day program**.

assisted-living facility See **supportive housing facility**.

chronic illness An ongoing illness, slow or gradual in onset, that may or may not grow worse over time. Because chronic illness cannot be cured, the focus of care is on preventing complications of the illness.

community day program A daytime community-based program for people with physical or mental health problems or older adults who need assistance. Also known as **adult day care** and **adult day centre**.

community-based services The health care and support services provided outside of a facility setting and in a community setting.

complex care See **long-term care**.

complex care facility See **long-term care facility**.

continuing care See **long-term care**.

continuing care facility See **long-term care facility**.

convalescent care Comprehensive, inpatient care provided to people who are recovering from surgery, injury, an acute illness, or an exacerbation of a disease process. Convalescent care provides less intensive care than acute care in a hospital but more intensive care than that provided in long-term care facilities. The duration of care in a subacute care setting is time-limited. The goal is to help the client recover to be strong enough to go back into the community. If that is not possible, the client will be transferred to a long-term care facility. Also known as **subacute care** and **transitional care.**

end-of-life care See **palliative care**.

group home A residential facility in which a small number of people with physical and/or mental disabilities live together and are provided with supervision, care, and support services.

hospice A portion of palliative care that provides home, residential or in-patient care to a patient who has a terminal diagnosis and is no longer seeking life-prolonging care. The philosophy of hospice is to provide support for the patient's emotional, social, and spiritual needs as well as medical symptoms as part of treating the whole person. Hospice workers try to make the client's last days as painless, comfortable, and dignified as possible.

inpatient A patient who is assigned a bed and is admitted to stay in a facility overnight or longer.

long-term care Medical, nursing, and/or support services provided over the course of months or years to people who cannot care for themselves. Also known as **complex care** in some provinces.

mental health care services Services provided to individuals and families confronting mental illness or disorders. Also known as **psychiatric services.**

outpatient A patient who does not stay overnight in a facility.

palliative care Services for people with progressive, life-threatening illnesses or conditions; these services aim to relieve or reduce uncomfortable symptoms but not produce a cure. End-of-life care is provided in an interdisciplinary approach to care and service provision. Also known as **end-of-life care.**

psychiatric services See **mental health care services**.

rehabilitation services Therapies and educational programs designed to restore or improve the client's independence and functional abilities.

residential facility A facility that provides living accommodations and services; includes assisted-living facilities, long-term care facilities, group homes and retirement residences.

respite care Temporary care of a person who requires a high level of support, care, and supervision that gives the client's caregivers a break from their duties.

retirement residence A facility that provides accommodation and supervision for older adults.

scope of practice The legal limits of your role.

subacute care See **convalescent care**.

supportive housing facility A residential facility where residents live in their own apartments and are provided support services. Assisted living facilities are increasingly providing services to young and middle-age adults, and are not limited to a majority of older adults. Also known as an **assisted-living facility**.

transitional care See **convalescent care**.

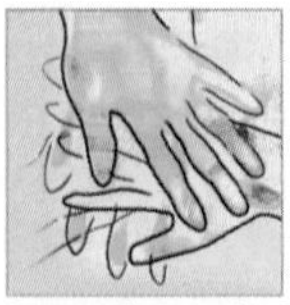

Support workers are employed in many settings. Each setting has different goals and services. This chapter describes common community-based and facility-based workplace settings. It also explores issues and challenges you may encounter in these settings. Wherever you work, you provide people with vital services that enable them to be as safe, comfortable, dignified, and independent as possible.

WORKING IN COMMUNITY-BASED SETTINGS

As discussed in Chapter 2, the current trend within the Canadian health care system is to decrease hospital costs and increase resources in **community-based services**. These include the health care and support services provided outside of a facility and in a community setting. For example, community-based services are provided in schools, community health centres, and doctors' offices. Home care agencies, day programs, and school boards are all community-based services that will likely hire support workers.

Regardless of where you work, you should be familiar with the scope of practice for support workers in your province, and you should always stay within this scope. Agreeing to perform tasks that are beyond your scope of practice can possibly risk legal actions.

Home Care

Home care is a vital part of Canada's health care system (see Chapter 2). Support workers have a central role within home care. As a support worker, you are responsible for providing a range of home care services, including assisting with personal care (Figure 3–1), activities of daily living (ADLs), child care, transportation, and home management.

Support workers providing home care services are hired on a full-time, part-time, or casual basis. You must follow your agency policies and procedures. Some agencies offer further education and many offer inservicing, to keep staff up to date with new procedures. Box 3–1 describes some of the issues and challenges associated with working in home care.

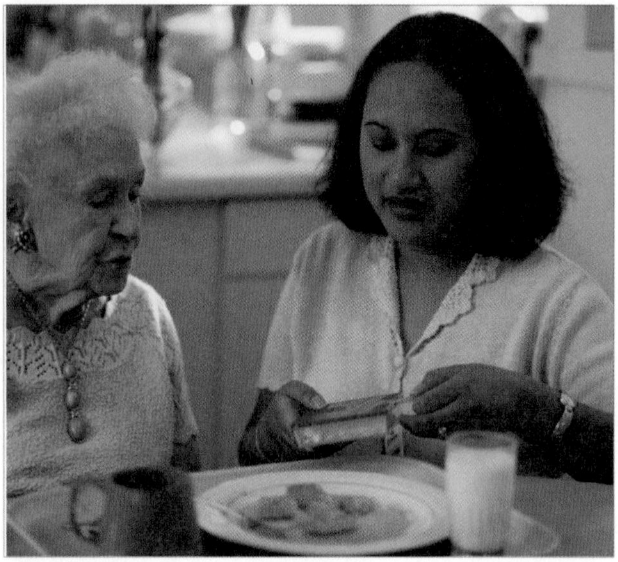

Figure 3–1 With the assistance of support workers, many clients are able to remain in their own homes. **Source:** Keith Brofsky/Photodisc/Getty Images.

Community Day Programs

In some provinces, support workers are hired by school boards to assist with a client who may be attending school instead of a day program. A **community day program** (also called **adult day care** or **adult day program**) is a daytime program for people with physical or mental health problems or for older adults who need assistance. Day programs aim to meet the client's needs and provide a break for family caregivers. These programs may be held in hospitals, nursing homes, community and recreational centres, **adult day centres**, church basements, or other settings.

Each day program is unique. Some programs offer rehabilitation to people with disabilities. Others offer counselling to people with mental illness. Many day programs offer recreational activities (Figure 3–2). Arts and crafts, social events, films, and board or card games are examples.

In addition, some provinces hire support workers to work in community day programs, while other provinces do not. If your province does hire support workers, you provide personal care and assistance to people attending the program. You may assist with recreational and social activities. Make sure that you follow all the employer policies and procedures. Box 3–2 lists common issues and challenges associated with working in a community day program.

Box 3–1 Issues and Challenges Associated With Working in Home Care

- ***Working on your own.*** Many support workers prefer the hustle and bustle of a facility setting, while others like working one-on-one with a client by providing home care services. Some support workers find home care work lonely and isolating while others enjoy the independence it offers. However, not having a supervisor around may sometimes present a challenge. Although your supervisor can be reached by phone, you sometimes need to use your own judgement to solve problems.
- ***Taking direction from different health care professionals.*** You may be expected to take directions from your supervisor and a number of different health care professionals. For example, the client's physiotherapist visits during your shift. He or she asks you to perform tasks that your supervisor has not asked you to do. These tasks are unfamiliar to you or not allowed by agency policy. In such situations, before taking on new tasks, always check with your supervisor.
- ***Maintaining professional boundaries.*** You often work closely with clients and their family members. However, it is never appropriate to become personally involved in the client's life decisions and family relationships. You should always be caring and compassionate but respect that a boundary does exist in your relationship with clients and their families. Do not confuse professionalism and empathy with friendship. Clients and their families need your skills, services, and your undivided attention. Do not discuss your personal problems or ask your clients or their family members for advice. Keep these matters private and to yourself.
- ***Providing for client safety.*** Clients' homes may present many safety hazards. Frayed electric cords and unsafe smoking practices are examples. Discuss any safety concerns you may have with the client and your supervisor.
- ***Providing for your personal safety.*** In home care, you do not have control over the environment that you will enter. You will travel to unfamiliar areas. You may have to drive in hazardous weather conditions. You may face abuse or violence in unfamiliar homes. At such times, you must look out for your own safety (see Chapter 19).

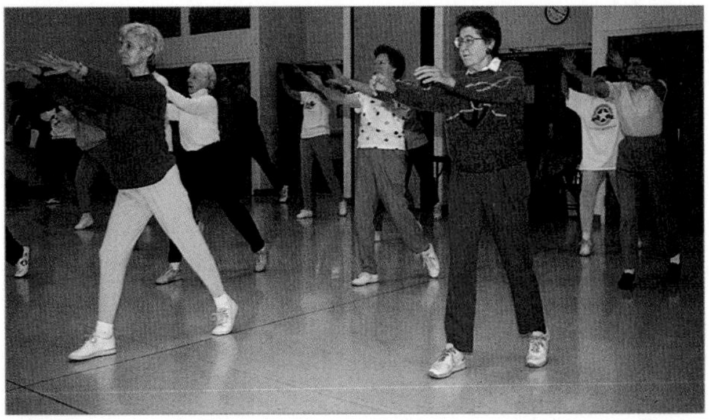

Figure 3–2 Community day programs provide recreational or other activities to clients during the day.

Working Directly for Clients

You may work directly for a client or the client's family. Such clients select and supervise their own support workers. Clients may hire their own support workers if they need a service that is not provided by the local agencies. Or their province may provide funding assistance directly to them and not through an agency. Box 3–3 describes issues and challenges associated with working directly for clients.

Box 3–2 Issues and Challenges Associated With Working in a Community Day Program

- ***Working closely with a team and a supervisor.*** In most community day programs, you work closely with a supervisor and other team members. This could be either a challenge or a benefit. Teamwork can be a success if team members have a common goal and work well together. It can be difficult if conflicts occur within the team. Effective communication skills are necessary (see Chapters 5 and 6).
- ***Working in a structured environment.*** Many day programs have a highly structured environment, particularly those that provide rehabilitation. People with such conditions as Alzheimer's disease usually benefit from having a predictable routine. To work well in a structured environment, you must be very organized and sensitive to clients' needs.
- ***Meeting multiple needs.*** You may have to attend to the needs of many people. You must be able to focus on each person and quickly decide whose needs to address first. Good judgement and time management are essential.

Box 3–3 Issues and Challenges Associated With Working Directly for Clients

- ***Clarifying the terms of employment.*** Some clients who employ you may want to have a contract signed. Read the contract carefully before signing it. Hours and pay may change from week to week. Make sure you understand how many hours you are expected to work and what pay you can expect. If you are hired directly, your employer may be required to pay benefits, such as unemployment insurance.
- ***Establishing work limits.*** Before you begin working for the client, find out what exactly is expected of you and how your performance will be evaluated. Ask for this in writing. Find out as much as you can about the client's preferences and standards.
- ***Knowing scope of practice limits.*** A private employer may ask you to do something that is beyond your scope of practice (see Chapter 1). In this event, you may feel uneasy about what to do but may not know who to contact to confirm what you are allowed to do. It is therefore important that you inform your private employer of the scope of your role and it is also important that you know someone (a former teacher or employer, for example) who can answer your questions if such a situation ever arises.

WORKING IN A FACILITY

A health care facility is a building designed or established for the delivery of specific care, treatment, and support services. Such facilities provide a range of services.

Hospitals and Other Medical Facilities

Clients in hospitals usually have serious illnesses or injuries. They require skilled professional care and complex equipment. Some hospitals hire support workers, while others do not. Support workers work in a variety of hospital departments depending on the role they fulfill. In most circumstances, you, as a support worker, report to and are supervised by a nurse.

Depending on the region where you live and the hospital's hiring policies, you may be employed in any unit in a hospital, including the intensive care unit (ICU) and the emergency room (ER). Your role may be to help people with basic care, such as feeding, and you may also be assigned to transport people, take specimens to the lab, and measure vital signs. In some hospitals, you may assist nurses before, during, or after surgical or medical procedures. You may perform other tasks, if requested and supervised by the nurse. You usually do not provide care to clients in unstable conditions but may assist the nurse in moving, turning, or bathing a client in such areas as the ICU or the ER.

Health care services are offered to **inpatients** (patients who are assigned a bed and admitted to stay in the facility overnight or longer) and to **outpatients** (patients who do not stay overnight in the facility).

Hospitals and other medical facilities provide a variety of services, including acute care, subacute care, long-term care, respite care, rehabilitation services, palliative care, and mental health services. Not all hospitals provide all these services. In some cities and towns in Canada, these services are provided in separate, specialized facilities. You may work in these or other medical facilities. Some of these facilities may require, and also provide, further education.

- ***Acute care***—health care that is provided for a relatively short time (usually days to weeks) and is intended to diagnose and treat an immediate health issue. It is provided mainly in hospitals. An **acute illness** appears suddenly and lasts a short time, usually less than 3 months. Symptoms can be severe. Examples of acute illnesses are pneumonia and influenza.
- ***Subacute care (convalescent care)***—health care or rehabilitation for people recovering from surgery, injury, or serious illness. The client's condition is stable, but he or she still needs care requiring complex equipment and

procedures. Many hospitals and **complex care** or **continuing care facilities** provide subacute care. Eventually, the client is discharged home or to another level of care. Clients who require physiotherapy and dressing changes after a hip replacement, for example, may not be ready to go home but may require subacute care during their stay in hospital. Some hospitals have wards that are dedicated to providing subacute care.

- ***Long-term care***—health and support services provided over the course of months or years to people who cannot care for themselves. Many people who require long-term care have chronic illnesses. A **chronic illness** is an ongoing illness, slow or gradual in onset, that usually grows worse over time. Examples of chronic illnesses are diabetes, multiple sclerosis, and Alzheimer's disease. Because chronic illnesses cannot be cured, the focus of care is on preventing complications of the illness. These illnesses can sometimes be controlled and complications prevented. In some cases, long-term care is provided for the remainder of the client's life. The goal of long-term care is to help the client cope with the challenges of living with a long-term illness or disability. Some hospitals provide long-term care, but more often long-term care is provided in **long-term care facilities** or through home care services.
- ***Respite care***—temporary care of a person who requires a high level of support, care, and supervision. Respite care gives the client's caregivers a break from their duties. Respite care is often provided by support workers in the client's home. However, many hospitals and other facilities also offer respite care.
- ***Rehabilitation services***—therapies and educational programs designed to restore or improve the client's independence and functional abilities. These services are for people who are or have been ill, injured, or disabled. Hospitals, long-term care facilities, and clinics offer rehabilitation services. Services may include life skills training, occupational and rehabilitation services, behavioural management, speech therapy, physiotherapy, job coaching, and family counselling. You may assist the client with personal care or activities of daily living (ADLs). You may also assist with program delivery.
- ***Palliative care***—both **palliative care** and **hospice** provide **end-of-life care**—an approach to care that emphasizes patient goals, relief of pain and suffering, and quality of life. Palliative care and hospice often work together to help the client and the family during the client's journey near the end of his or her life. **Palliative care** (also known as **end-of-life care**) are services for clients with progressive, life-threatening illnesses or conditions; these services aim to relieve or reduce uncomfortable symptoms and not to produce a cure. End-of-life care is provided with an interdisciplinary approach.

Hospice is a portion of palliative care that provides home, residential, or inpatient care to a client who has a terminal diagnosis and is no longer seeking life-prolonging care. The philosophy of **hospice** is to provide support for the client's emotional, social, and spiritual needs as well as addressing medical symptoms as part of treating the whole person. Hospice workers try to make the client's last days as painless, comfortable, and dignified as possible. You, as the support worker, assist with personal care and ADLs. You also provide emotional support and encouragement to the client and family (see Chapter 47).

- ***Mental health services*** (also known as **psychiatric services**)—services for people with mental disorders (such as schizophrenia, bipolar disorder, and addictions). Entire facilities, health care centres, and hospital units are devoted to caring for people with mental disorders. Assessment and treatment programs enable them to function as independently as possible within the community. Inpatient and outpatient services are provided in these facilities. Clients are encouraged to return to the community, rather than stay in a hospital. In the community, they have access to community-based care and support services.

Residential Facilities

A **residential facility** is a facility that provides living accommodations, care, and support services. These facilities vary in size and levels of care and support.

People using residential facilities are called *residents* because they reside, or live, in the facility. The facility is their temporary or permanent home. Therefore, these facilities provide care in a comfortable, homelike atmosphere (Figure 3–3) and ensure that they meet the social and emotional needs of the residents.

Clients need residential care when they cannot care for themselves at home but do not need acute medical care or high-level nursing care. Such clients include:

- Frail, older adults
- Individuals of all ages who have physical disabilities, mental disabilities, or both
- Individuals with mental illness
- Individuals with alcohol or drug addiction

The type of facility appropriate for a client depends on the individual's needs and level of independence. The types of residential facilities include assisted-living facilities, retirement homes, and long-term care facilities. Names of these types of facilities vary across Canada.

Supportive Housing Facilities. Also called **assisted-living facilities**, supportive housing facilities are residential facilities where people live in their own apartments and are provided support services.

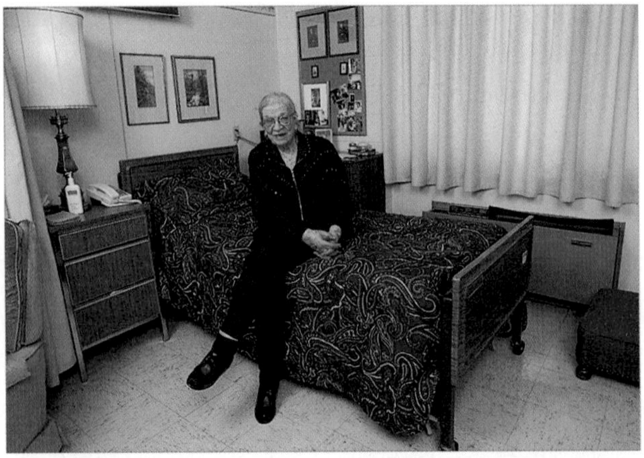

Figure 3–3 The atmosphere of a residential facility is made as homelike as possible.

Because they are located in the community, assisted-living facilities are also considered to be community-based services. Residents are usually older adults who require minimal care. Usually the setting is a multistoried apartment building or condominium complex. These apartments usually have kitchens, so residents may be able to cook their own meals. Many assisted-living facilities provide a common living area, an activity room, and a games room. Residents usually receive the following support services:

- 24-hour monitoring and emergency response services
- Social/recreational programs
- One or two daily meals
- Housekeeping and laundry

Some residents purchase extra support services, if needed. Not all residents need or want the same services. Some residents in assisted-living facilities may also qualify for home care.

Group Homes. Group homes are another type of assisted-living facility. A **group home** is a residential facility in which a small number of people with physical or mental disabilities live together and receive supervision, care, and support services. Some group homes provide services to children and adolescents with behavioural and conduct disorders. Rather than having their own apartments, residents share a house in a residential neighbourhood (Figure 3–4). Usually residents have their own bedrooms but share bathrooms and living and dining areas. They receive 24-hour supervision, meals, housekeeping and laundry services, and assistance with personal care and ADLs.

Residents of group homes are often adolescents or young adults who have disabilities or mental illness; older adults; women leaving abusive situations; and people with substance abuse problems. The number and type of staff employed by a group home depend on the residents' needs.

All assisted-living facilities must be approved and licensed by the provincial or territorial government, which provides partial funding for these services. Public or private agencies manage the facility and hire and supervise support workers. Your supervisor may be responsible for one or several assisted-living

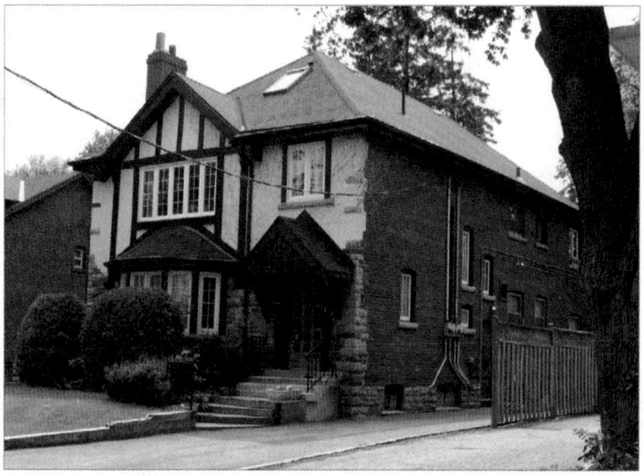

Figure 3–4 Group homes, another type of assisted-living facility, are usually situated in residential neighbourhoods. **Source:** Dick Hemingway.

facilities. Some supervisors work onsite; others visit the facility periodically. Because the level of assistance needed differs among residents, you are often required to perform a variety of tasks.

Retirement Residences. A **retirement residence** (or retirement home) is a facility that provides accommodation and supervision for older adults. Residents have their own bedrooms and bathrooms but share common living and dining areas (Figure 3–5). They may need help with housekeeping but limited supervision and little to no assistance with personal care. The goal of a retirement residence is to allow older people to live as independently as possible while providing security, support services, and varying degrees of care, as needed.

Regulations governing retirement residences vary. In some provinces and territories, they are privately operated and not regulated or financed by the government. Therefore, residents are required to pay the full cost. Standards, prices, and services vary from one facility to another. These facilities could be small, converted houses or high-rise apartment buildings.

Support workers are almost always hired directly by the facility or the resident. If hired by a resident, you provide care only for that person. You perform many functions. You may run errands; provide transportation; assist with activities or social and recreational events; or help with various tasks, such as unpacking suitcases or arranging bedrooms. In some provinces, support workers may even be required to assist the residents with taking their medications, including insulin injections.

Residents in retirement homes are not ill or disabled. Most can meet their own personal care needs. Usually personal care services are limited to a few simple tasks. For example, you may help the client get in and out of a bathtub. When residents need more than minimal daily care, they have to move to long-term care. Some retirement facilities have a retirement residence as well as a long-term care facility. When residents need more assistance than the retirement residence can provide, they move into the long-term care facility, where nursing and personal care services are available 24 hours a day.

Long-Term Care Facilities. These facilities (also called nursing homes, homes for the aged, long-term care homes, and special care homes) provide higher levels of care than do retirement residences and assisted-living facilities. **Long-term care facilities** provide accommodations, 24-hour professional nursing care, and support services to clients who cannot care for themselves at home but do not need hospital care. Most residents are frail, older adults with many health problems. Some residents are young and middle-aged adults who have severe, chronic health conditions or disabilities. The goals of these facilities are to maintain the residents' health and independence to the greatest extent possible and to meet their physical, emotional, social, intellectual, and spiritual needs.

Residents stay on a ward or in private or semi-private bedrooms. Usually each room has a

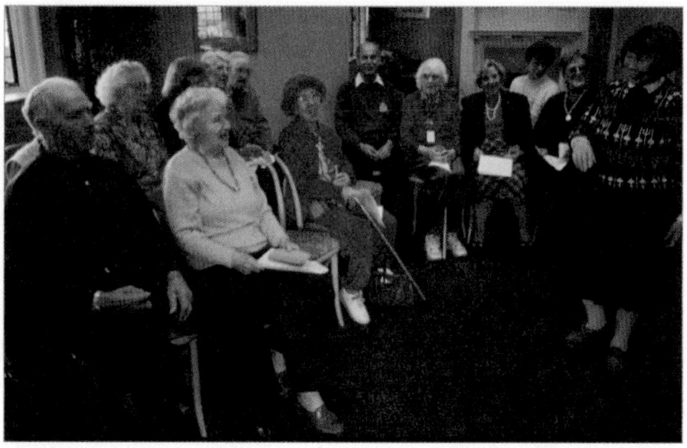

Figure 3–5 Residents living in retirement homes share common living and dining areas in a homelike environment. **Source:** Al Harvey.

bathroom with a toilet and a sink. Tubs and showers are in the common bathrooms. Besides nursing care, these facilities also provide access to medical and rehabilitative care. They also provide assistance with personal care and ADLs, meals, laundry service, and recreational and social activities.

Long-term care facilities are licensed, regulated, and funded by the province or territory in which they are located. Medicare pays for some costs. Residents are required to pay a monthly fee. They also must pay for personal clothing, toiletries, hair dressings, and other incidentals. Government or charitable organizations operate some facilities on a not-for-profit basis. Private facilities operate on a for-profit basis. Each facility hires its own staff.

Most long-term care facilities serve many residents with various physical or other disabilities. Therefore, to function efficiently, these facilities maintain highly structured work environments. Nurses plan and coordinate resident care. You, as the support worker, are a member of the health care team and report to a nurse. You provide personal care and assist clients with various ADLs (Figure 3–6). Support workers make important contributions to the clients' care plans, and during discussions in family conferences, they provide valuable feedback based on their observations of the client.

Many long-term care facilities have subacute care units. Some facilities also have special care units for residents with specific disabilities. For example, a facility may have a dementia care unit for people with Alzheimer's disease or other dementias. Respite care and palliative care units are also part of some long-term care facilities. You may work in any of these units. You may, however, need extra training to work in these units.

You may also work in the facility's recreation department. You may help organize and carry out recreational outings and activities. Here, you report to the recreation supervisor.

Issues and Challenges Associated with Facility-Based Care

As with working in the community, working in a facility also presents issues and challenges to the support worker (Box 3–4).

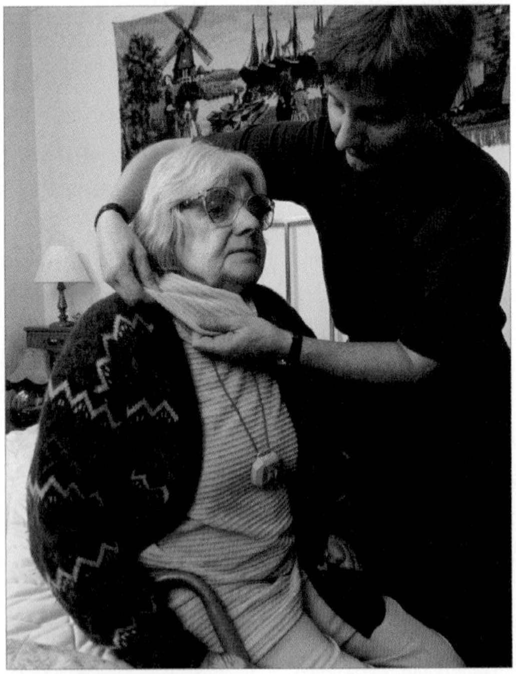

Figure 3–6 Residents in long-term care facilities may need support workers to assist them with activities of daily living. **Source:** Penny Tweedie/Stone/Getty Images.

Box 3–4 Issues and Challenges Associated With Working in a Facility

- ***Working in a structured team environment.*** You work on a team with highly skilled professionals. Some of you may feel intimidated in such an environment. Remember that you are a valuable member of the team and have much to contribute at team meetings. In residential facilities, you usually spend more time with clients than do the nurses and physicians. You have valuable insights and observations about the client's daily needs and possible changes in health.
- ***Meeting multiple needs and demands.*** You are required to respond to the many needs and demands of clients. It may not be possible to respond immediately to all demands. You should be able to prioritize clients' needs and manage your time. You must be flexible, diplomatic, and consistent. Effective organizational and communication skills are essential.
- ***Doing many tasks in a short period of time.*** You must provide thorough, competent, and respectful care within a short time. This requires self-discipline, dedication, and efficiency.
- ***Respecting your scope of practice.*** You work closely with nurses and may become familiar with many nursing procedures. You might sometimes be asked to perform a procedure that may be beyond your scope of practice. Never attempt any procedure that you are not legally allowed to perform. Only perform procedures allowed by law and facility policy. Never perform a procedure unless your supervisor is allowed to train you on that procedure and has given you sufficient training and you are comfortable doing it. The facility has written policies to guide you.
- ***Working in shifts.*** Most facilities are staffed round the clock. You may have to work evening and night shifts, and your shifts may be 8 to 12 hours long, depending on the agency. Many support workers love the variety of working different shifts, while others have difficulty adjusting to the change in sleep and lifestyle habits that shift work demands. Those who have families may also find that it is a challenge to participate in their children's activities. In time, these workers usually learn to get used to their sleep cycle and other routines in their lives.

Especially in Hospitals or Other Medical Facilities

- ***Dealing with people in distress.*** Clients admitted to hospital or other medical facilities may show signs of intense emotional or physical distress. They may be in pain, afraid, upset, or angry, and not cooperate with their care providers. Remain calm and professional, no matter how they express themselves. Also, be sensitive to their feelings. Try to imagine how they are feeling. Sometimes you can provide emotional support just by holding the client's hand or listening. In the case of palliative care, you need to be strong and supportive in the presence of intense suffering and emotions. If the client is facing a life-threatening illness, you need to be comfortable with your own feelings and attitude toward death. Otherwise you may find it very difficult to care for the client.

Especially in Residential Facilities

- ***Making the facility feel like a home.*** A residential facility is, first and foremost, the resident's home. Treat the setting with as much respect as you would your own home. Be careful with the client's personal possessions. Make all areas of the facility cheerful, comfortable places. Every staff member must contribute to creating a positive, homelike environment.
- ***Respecting the client's privacy and dignity.*** In any work setting, you must respect your client's privacy and dignity. Lack of privacy can result in loss of self-esteem, particularly during personal care. Carefully screen the area and cover the client. This may seem an obvious step, but it could be easily omitted. Sometimes it is easy to focus more on getting the job done than on respecting the need for privacy. As in other care situations, respecting privacy also includes keeping discussions about the client with co-workers confidential and professional, respecting the client's property, and recognizing the client's right to express his or her preferences.

(continued on page 38)

Box 3–4 Issues and Challenges Associated With Working in a Facility (cont'd)

- ***Maintaining professional boundaries.*** You may be providing care to residents who have no close personal relationships. When you work closely with clients, you tend to form strong attachments to them. This aspect of the job may be one of the main attractions of support work. However, do not become too personally involved with clients and their families. Always be caring and supportive, but remember that your main responsibility is providing care and maintaining a professional attitude.

Support Workers Solving Problems

Choosing a Place to Work

Theresa LeCroix is a new support worker who has just graduated from a reputable support worker program. She was a very motivated and interested student who enjoyed all of the placements that she was given during her support worker program. She is now looking for a permanent position but does not know where to begin. She has seen ads listed in her local newspaper, as well as online, for many jobs available in her town for support workers.

Theresa has decided to ask her classmates where they are going to apply for jobs. She is amazed that many of them are fairly certain of what type of support work they prefer. Some love providing home care, and some others are interested in working in long-term care facilities. Other classmates have decided to apply for positions at their local hospital, where support workers are hired. Finally, many of Theresa's classmates say that they would love working in the community for various agencies that offer day programs for special groups of clients.

Theresa finally begins to understand why it is so difficult for her to decide: it is because there are so many opportunities for support workers, in so many settings. She then decides that she should keep an open mind and apply to different agencies and settings. Theresa realizes that she is lucky to be in a line of work where there are so many different opportunities and where the workers are so much in demand!

REVIEW

Answers to these questions are at the bottom of the page.

Circle the BEST answer.

1. **A current trend in the Canadian health care system is to:**
   A. Increase public spending on hospitals
   B. Decrease spending on community-based services
   C. Focus on providing more community-based services
   D. Promote facility-based services over home care

2. **Home care is an example of:**
   A. A community-based service
   B. A facility-based service
   C. A community day program
   D. Palliative care

3. **Which work setting provides acute care?**
   A. Home care
   B. Long-term care facilities
   C. Assisted-living facilities
   D. Hospitals

4. **Which work setting may provide subacute care?**
   A. Retirement homes
   B. Long-term care facilities
   C. Group homes
   D. Hospices

5. **What type of service aims to provide a temporary break to family caregivers?**
   A. Acute care services
   B. Palliative care
   C. Respite services
   D. Outpatient services

6. **Which of the following is an example of a residential facility?**
   A. Hospital
   B. Methadone clinic
   C. Private residence
   D. Assisted-living facility

7. **Residents in retirement facilities generally include:**
   A. People with mental illness
   B. Young adults with physical or other disabilities
   C. Frail, older adults with multiple health problems
   D. Older adults with limited care needs

8. **Residents in long-term care facilities generally require:**
   A. 24-hour nursing care and support services
   B. Supervision and limited support services
   C. Acute care
   D. Housekeeping services, but not meal services

9. **In which setting is maintaining a homelike atmosphere *especially* important?**
   A. Hospital
   B. Doctor's office
   C. Community day program
   D. Long-term care facility

Answers: 1.C, 2.A, 3.D, 4.B, 5.C, 6.D, 7.D, 8.A, 9.D

CHAPTER 4

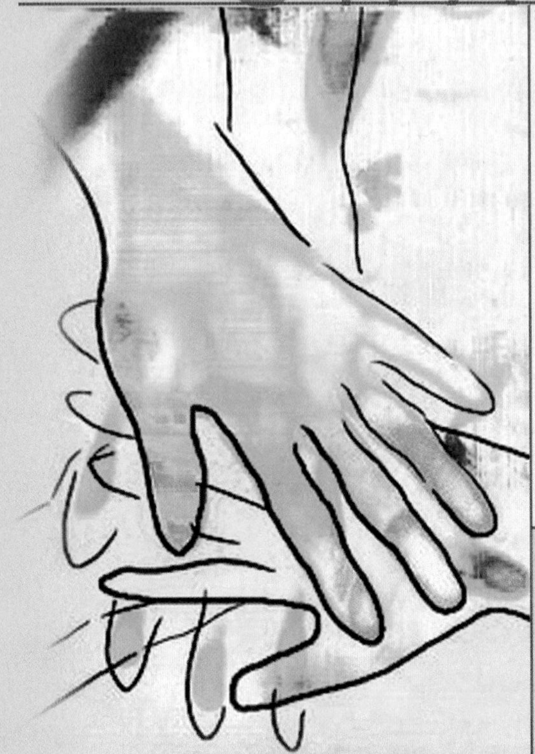

Health, Wellness, Illness, and Disability

OBJECTIVES

- Define the key terms listed in this chapter.
- Differentiate between the current definition of health and the one used in the past.
- Describe the concept of holism and explain how it affects your role as a support worker.
- Explain the current concepts of health and wellness.
- Describe how health can be achieved in all dimensions of life.
- Explain common reactions to illness and disability.
- Describe change and loss associated with illness and disability.
- Explain the effects of stigma and discrimination on clients who are ill and disabled.

key terms

acute illness Illnesses (such as influenza) and disabilities (such as a broken arm) which have a sudden onset and last for a relatively short period of time.

chronic illness Illnesses (such as AIDS) or disabilities (such as paraplegia) that are permanent and last throughout the person's life. Also called *long-term illnesses* in some provinces.

Determinants of Health The most important factors, such as lifestyle, environment, human biology, and health services, that determine health status in an individual or a population of people.

disability The loss of physical or mental function.

discrimination Behaviour that treats people unfairly based on their group membership.

emotional health Well-being in the emotional dimension, achieved when people feel good about themselves.

equitable Fair, reasonable, and just.

gender The condition of being male or female, such as the *sex* of a person.

genetic endowment The genetic makeup that predisposes individuals to a wide range of responses that affect health status.

health The state of well-being in all dimensions of one's life.

holism A concept that considers the whole person; the whole person has physical, social, emotional, intellectual, and spiritual dimensions.

illness The loss of physical or mental health.

informal giving practices Ways of giving which are not part of a formal celebration, for example, random acts of kindness.

intellectual health Well-being in the intellectual dimension achieved through an active, creative mind.

marginalize The act of excluding people who are not part of the majority culture.

physical health Well-being in the physical dimension achieved when the body is strong, fit, and free of disease.

prognosis The expected course of recovery, which may range from recovery to death, based on the usual outcome of the illness.

secondary prevention Prevention strategies designed to intervene when risk factors or early indicators of a health-related problem are present.

social health Well-being in the social dimension achieved when people have stable and satisfying relationships.

social support system An informal group of people who help each other or others.

spiritual health Well-being in the spiritual dimension achieved through the belief in a purpose greater than the self.

stigma A characteristic that marks a person as different or flawed.

wellness The achievement of the best health possible in all dimensions of one's life.

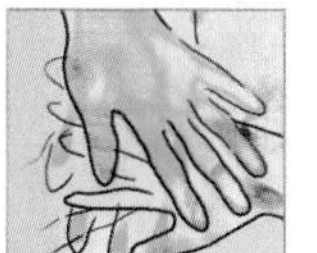

Your job as a support worker is to help clients achieve or maintain optimal **health**. But what exactly is "optimal" health? This chapter examines the concepts and experiences of health and wellness as well as illness and disability and tries to explain what optimal health is. When you are providing supporting care to a client who lives with an illness or disability, you might be tempted to focus on the medical condition rather than on the *holistic* person. However, by trying to understand what the person may be experiencing, you can provide better, more compassionate care and support.

As a support worker, you must focus your care and support on improving (or maximizing) a person's health potential, whatever that potential may be. All caregivers need to understand how health practices, lifestyle, and social status can influence a person's health, and to understand these important concepts.

> ***"I realized back then that my biggest disability was my attitude."***
> – Rick Hanson, activist and spinal cord athlete, on the days immediately following his spinal cord injury.

HEALTH AND WELLNESS

Definitions of Health in the Past. Definitions of the term "health" have changed over the years. At the end of the 1800s, "health" was defined by what it was not: health was the state of *not* being sick. At that time, the leading causes of death were diseases that spread from one person to another. Pneumonia, tuberculosis, and influenza, for example, were frequent killers. Anyone lucky enough to avoid being infected during an outbreak was considered healthy. During the first half of the twentieth century, vaccinations, antibiotics, health education, and cleaner living conditions reduced the spread of diseases. People were living longer and getting sick less often. But were they healthy? People began to realize that health is more than the absence of disease.

Modern Definitions of Health. During the latter part of the twentieth century, people recognized that health is affected by factors other than disease, such as lifestyle and environment. Discussions of health focused on the person rather than on the disease. Also, people began to place a new emphasis on holistic health. **Holism** means *whole*.

A whole person has physical, emotional, social, intellectual, and spiritual dimensions. Each dimension relates to and depends on the others. Current views on health give importance to holistic health—a state of well-being in all dimensions of one's life (Figure 4–1). When providing holistic health care, you care for all dimensions of the person, not just the physical.

A widely accepted definition of health is that of the *World Health Organization* (WHO), which states that "health is a state of complete physical, mental, and social well-being and not merely the absence of disease or infirmity." In more recent years, this statement has been modified to include the ability to lead a "socially and economically productive life."[1]

Dimensions of Health

Holism involves considering all dimensions of health. These include:

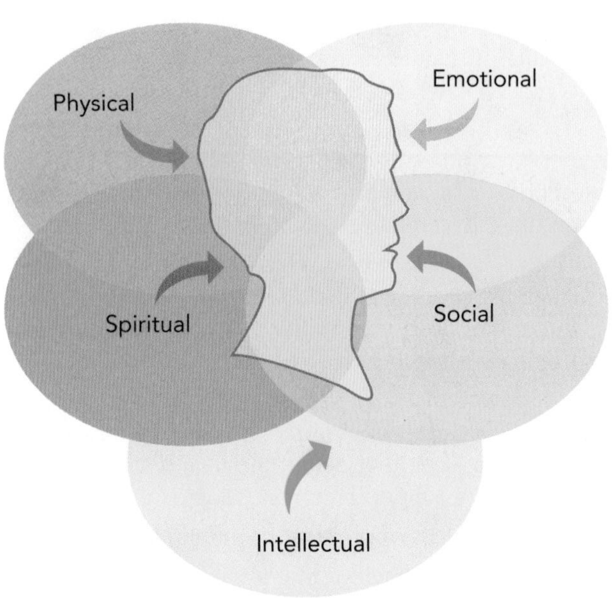

Figure 4–1 A whole person has physical, emotional, social, intellectual, and spiritual dimensions. Health is a state of well-being in all dimensions.

Physical Health. Physical health is achieved when the body is strong, fit, and free of disease. Physical health is influenced by genetics and lifestyle. The following factors contribute to the physical health of all people, including caregivers:

- Following a nutritious diet according to *Canada's Food Guide* (see Chapter 27)
- Exercising regularly
- Living in a smoke-free environment
- Drinking alcohol moderately or not at all
- Having a good night's sleep
- Following safety practices, such as using seat belts and bike helmets
- Seeking medical attention when needed

As a support worker, you have an important role in maintaining your clients' physical health. For instance, you help maintain a clean, safe, and comfortable environment. You may also prepare nutritious meals and assist clients with physical activity.

You should have healthy habits yourself with regard to drinking alcohol. For most people, more than 2 drinks a day is harmful. Women who have more than 9 drinks a week have higher rates of cancer and other problems compared with women who drink less. Men who have more than 14 drinks a week also have higher rates of alcohol-related problems.[2]

Emotional Health. Emotional health is not merely the absence of negative emotions but the ability to function well in and adapt appropriately to circumstances, whatever they may be. When people feel good about themselves, they are emotionally healthy. They have strong self-esteem, self-control, and self-awareness. They are able to give and receive from others, without worrying about being hurt or rejected. In contrast, emotionally unhealthy people are often insecure. When upset, they may feel overwhelmed and become aggressive.

Emotional health varies throughout one's life. For example, Mr. Szabo was a confident and happy person and enjoyed many social relationships. However, at the age of 60, a series of tragedies destroyed his emotional health: his daughter died in a car accident, his grandson died from a drug overdose, and Mr. Szabo himself suffered a heart attack. While recovering from the heart attack, he experienced major depression. This example shows that even emotionally strong individuals cannot always withstand misfortune and suffering.

As a support worker, you will work with emotionally healthy as well as emotionally unhealthy individuals. The behaviours of some of these clients may surprise you. For instance, a client who is usually cheerful may sometimes be irritable. Avoid judging them. Instead, learn to read their emotions so that you can respond in a caring manner.

Social Health. Social health is achieved through stable and satisfying relationships. Socially healthy people treat others with respect, warmth, and openness. They like and trust others. People with poor social health may show little regard for others and may use others for their own gain.

Few people enjoy strong social health all through life. Feelings of isolation and loneliness are common among older people and others who have lost their partners, friends, or other social relationships. New immigrants are also at risk for poor social health. Being in an unfamiliar place and not speaking the local language can be very lonely and socially isolating.

Most people have friends and acquaintances who help each other meet their needs. These needs may be practical ones, such as a ride to work. They may also be deeper, such as the need for:

- Companionship and a feeling of belonging
- Comfort, emotional support, and encouragement
- Reassurance of one's self-worth
- Help, guidance, and advice

A **social support system** is an informal group of people who help each other or others. Research has shown that social support systems help improve overall health. Indeed, social support may be as important to wellness as a nutritious diet, a smoke-free environment, and regular exercise. Social support systems can provide food, housing, financial aid, and emotional support during crises. They can make it possible for ill and frail people to continue to stay in their homes rather than move to a facility (Figure 4–2). As a support worker, you may be a key member of your client's social support system. You provide practical support, such as help with ADLs and home management. You provide emotional support by practising compassionate care.

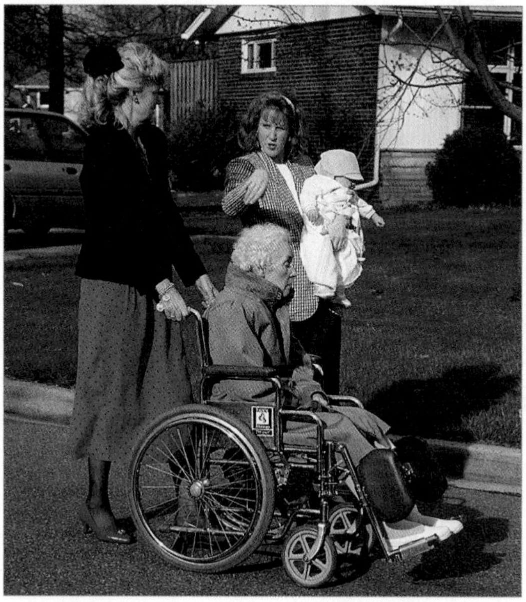

Figure 4–2 This older woman is able to stay in her own home because of her strong social support system. She has help from her daughter, her granddaughter, and support workers. **Source:** Sorrentino, S.A. (2000). *Mosby's textbook for nursing assistants* (5th ed., p. 148). St. Louis: Mosby.

Spiritual Health. Spiritual health is achieved through the belief in a purpose greater than the self. It may or may not involve being a member of a formal religion or even believing in a higher being. People who are spiritually healthy have a clear understanding of what they believe to be right and wrong, and their behaviours reflect their beliefs. They feel their life has meaning. They are more concerned about personal fulfillment than about material things. Compassion, honesty, humility, forgiveness, and charity are elements of spiritual health.

For some people, spiritual health is closely linked to religion. Being able to attend regular religious worship may be very important for their spiritual health. As a support worker, you must respect your clients' expressions of their spirituality. In a facility, you may be responsible for transporting clients to religious services conducted within the building. Make sure you are not late for this task. In a private home, you may see symbols of the person's faith, such as religious icons, displayed in many areas of the house. Always handle these items with respect. People of different cultures may express their spirituality in unique ways (see the *Respecting Diversity: Diversity, Health, and Spirituality* box on page 46.)

Intellectual Health. This type of health is achieved by keeping the mind active and creative throughout life. Recall the last time you talked with a child. You may have marvelled at the curiosity the child showed as he or she asked you endless questions. Intellectually healthy people maintain this curiosity throughout life. They are interested in what is going on around them. They analyze, reason, and solve problems. They are open-minded and eager to learn.

People who have poor intellectual health often take a passive approach to life. They do not try to participate in community and world events and avoid being involved in the lives of others. They often suffer from poor emotional, social, and physical health as well.

Many residential facilities have recreational programs and activities that promote intellectual and social health. Residents are encouraged to take part in games and outings that are organized for them. They are encouraged to continue to be intellectually active even when they are in their rooms. Activities such as reading, doing crossword puzzles, keeping indoor plants, doing crafts, and knitting all challenge the mind and keep it active. You can promote your clients' intellectual health by encouraging them to perform all these activities and by talking with them about community and world events (see Figure 4–3.

Health is sometimes referred to as wellness. **Wellness** is achieving the best health possible in all five dimensions of one's life, as mentioned earlier. It is the perfect balance of body, mind, and spirit. Although many people try to achieve wellness, few actually have it. It is difficult to be healthy in all areas of life all the time. At some point, everyone experiences ill health in one or more dimensions.

Seeking wellness is an ongoing process throughout life. It involves making choices that improve the quality of life. It also involves becoming the best a person can be in all areas of life, despite limitations. Even people with diseases or disabilities can aim to have a high level of wellness.

Interestingly, even some individuals with excellent physical health may not achieve wellness. For example, Soo Hee is an athlete in excellent shape. She eats well and trains daily. However, she does not make time for friends or family and suffers from loneliness and a lack of meaningful relation-

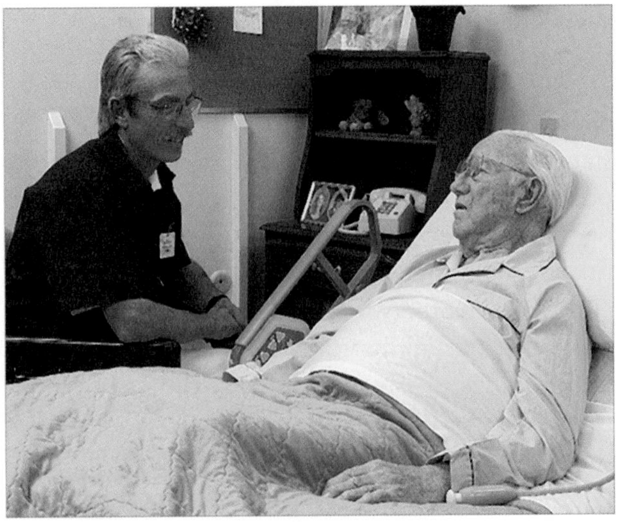

Figure 4–3 A support worker providing care to a client.

ships. So, she is not content with her life. She needs to improve the emotional and social dimensions of her life in order to achieve wellness. Compare her with Michael, who has diabetes but manages his disease well, feels good about himself, and has strong relationships and an active mind. He feels he has a meaningful, productive life. Despite his illness, he has achieved a high level of wellness.

Health is a continuum (Figure 4–4). On one end is optimal (complete) health or wellness and on the other end is extreme ill health. A person's place on the continuum shifts depending on life's circumstances. Remember that health is not constant throughout life. Everyone experiences physical illness and emotional stress during their lives, and therefore most people can be said to have only average health.

Culture and Health, Wellness, Illness, and Disability

Culture can influence whether or not a person will seek out medical treatment, take prescribed medications, take herbal or nonmedicinal supplements, or even accept care from someone who is not a family member. Culture can also influence when and how a person will accept care. For example, clients from a certain culture may view North American medicines as poisons and may therefore distrust any advice from doctors, nurses, or support workers. See "Culture," one of the Determinants of Health, on page 48.

First Nations people include such values as balance, interconnectedness, nature, and spirituality into their view of the delicate balance of health, healing, and spirituality. Mainstream psychology often focuses on only one part of the person, such as the person's thinking, feeling, or behaviour. However, First Nations people believe that interconnectedness is an important part of healing. Mainstream therapy focuses on the individual alone, while the First Nations healing practices consider the individual in the context of the family, community, culture, and all of creation. Nature and spirituality, which play a prominent role in First Nations healing practices, are almost nonexistent in mainstream therapies. Balance is important because illness occurs when a person lives life

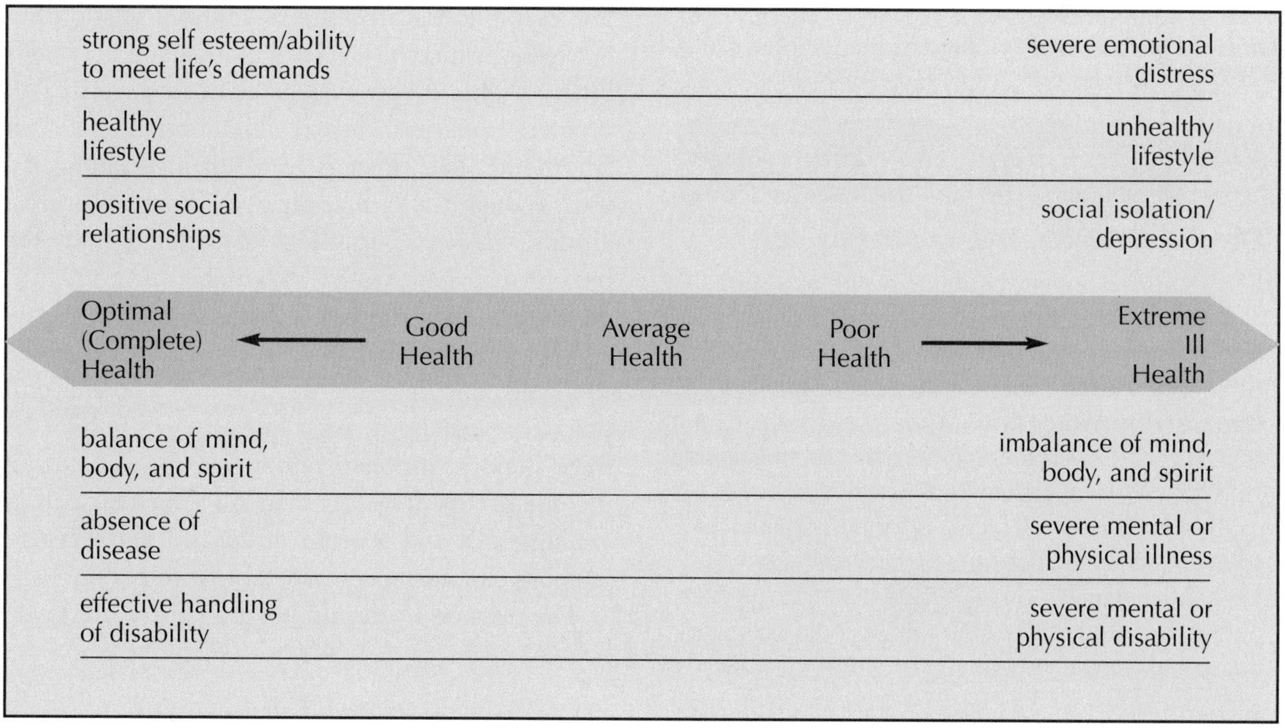

Figure 4–4 The continuum of health.

in an unbalanced way. Healing should therefore incorporate the physical, emotional, mental, and spiritual aspects of the self.[3]

Throughout history, many cultures have treated their old and sick members as important persons in need of the utmost care and respect, while some other cultures have believed that people who are unable to contribute to society should be segregated from those who can. For example, during World War II, Adolf Hitler and his followers sought to exterminate all people who were chronically ill, mentally challenged, or otherwise "unacceptable." This sort of belief goes against the fundamental principles of Canada, where people are accepted, regardless of their differences, including differences in health status (see the *Respecting Diversity: Diversity, Health and Spirituality* box). Refer to Chapter 12, which deals with diversity among clients to whom you may provide support care.

Determinants of Health

In Chapter 2, as well as earlier in this chapter, you read about the dimensions of health, which include the holistic aspects of an individual's health. **Determinants of Health** are different from dimensions of health, which identify *what makes a population of people healthy*. Determinants of Health look at the "bigger picture" of where we live. For example, a person might follow good holistic health practices for everyone in the family, but if these family members are likely to get a genetic (inherited) condition, they may still become very ill. Similarly, in spite of holistic health practices, people in a neighbourhood could become very ill if they live close to a toxic waste dump or are several hundred kilometres from the closest hospital.

In Canada, the Lalonde Report (1974) first identified key factors that determine health status—lifestyle, environment, human biology, and health services. The findings of this report are just as true today as they were then. In particular, evidence has shown that spending more on health care will not result in significant improvements in population health. On the other hand, we do know that other important factors such as good living and working conditions are vital for a healthy population. Lalonde called these 12 identified factors key Determinants of Health.[4]

RESPECTING DIVERSITY

Diversity, Health, and Spirituality

In traditional Aboriginal culture, health and spirituality are closely connected. Illness can be prevented if the mind, body, and spirit are in harmony. Aboriginal healers include herbalists, diagnosticians, and shamans. In the Cree culture, shamans have special powers to bring the Earth and the spirit world into harmony to aid in the healing process.

Aboriginal peoples recognized the mind–body–spirit connection long before people in Western cultures realized that health was more than the absence of disease. Today, many Aboriginal people combine traditional knowledge with modern health practices.

Source: Potter, P.A., Griffin Perry, A., Ross-Kerr, J.C., and Wood, M.J. (2001). *Canadian fundamentals of nursing* (2nd ed., p. 127). Toronto: Harcourt Canada.

The Interrelationship of Each Factor Is Significant. While each factor identified in the Lalonde Report is important in its own right, it is the *interrelationship* of these factors that is of particular importance. For example, research shows a strong relationship between the income level of a mother and her baby's birth weight. A low weight at birth is related to problems not just during childhood but also in adulthood. The effect is seen not just among the most economically disadvantaged groups but in all groups. However, mothers at each step *up* the income scale have babies with higher birth weights, on average, than those at a step *below*.

This indicates that these problems are not *just* a result of poor maternal nutrition and poor health practices associated with poverty, although the most serious problems do occur in the lowest income group. It seems that other factors such as coping skills and a sense of control and mastery over life circumstances also come into play.

The 12 key Determinants of Health are given below:[5]

1. ***Income and social status:*** Health status improves as you go up the ladder of income and social standing. High income determines

living conditions, such as safe housing and ability to buy sufficient nutritious food. The healthiest populations are those in societies that are prosperous and have an **equitable** distribution of wealth.

2. ***Social support networks:*** Support from families, friends, and communities is associated with better health. Such social support networks could be very important in helping people solve and deal with problems, as well as in maintaining a sense of mastery and control over life circumstances. The caring and respect that occur in social relationships and the resulting sense of satisfaction and well-being seem to act as a buffer against health problems.
3. ***Education and literacy:*** Health status improves with level of education. Education is closely connected to socioeconomic status; effective education for children and lifelong learning for adults are key contributors to health and prosperity not only of individuals but also of the country as a whole. Education contributes to health and prosperity by equipping people with knowledge and skills for problem solving. It gives people a sense of control and mastery over their life circumstances. It increases job opportunities, income security, and job satisfaction. Education improves people's ability to access and understand information that will help them keep themselves healthy.
4. ***Employment and working conditions:*** Unemployment, underemployment, stressful or unsafe work are all associated with poor health. People who have more control over their work circumstances and fewer stress-related demands in their jobs are healthier and often live longer than those in more stressful or riskier jobs and activities.
5. ***Social supports:*** The importance of social support extends to the broader community. The strength of social networks within a community, region, province, or country is reflected in the institutions, organizations, and informal giving practices that people create to share resources and build attachments with others.
6. ***Physical environments:*** The physical environment is an important determinant of health. At certain levels of exposure, contaminants in the air, water, food, and soil can cause a variety of adverse health effects, including cancer, birth defects, and respiratory and gastrointestinal ailments.
7. ***Personal health practices and coping skills:*** Personal health practices and coping skills refer to actions by individuals that can help them prevent diseases and promote self-care, cope with challenges, develop self-reliance, solve problems, and make choices that enhance health. Personal health practices are not only the outcome of individual choices but also the influence of social, economic, and environmental factors on the decisions people make about their health.

   There is a growing recognition that personal life "choices" are greatly influenced by the socioeconomic environments in which people live, learn, work, and play. These influences impact lifestyle choice through at least five areas: (1) personal life skills, (2) stress, (3) culture, (4) social relationships and belonging, and (5) a sense of control. Environments should support and encourage a person to make healthy lifestyle choices in a world where many choices are possible.
8. ***Healthy child development:*** A young person's development is greatly affected by his or her housing and neighbourhood, family income, the level of parents' education, access to nutritious foods and physical recreation, genetic makeup, and access to dental and medical care.
9. ***Biology and genetic endowment:*** Genetic makeup is a person's tendency to a wide range of individual responses that affect health status. **Genetic endowment** provides a person with the potential for easy emotional adaptation to their situations. Although socioeconomic and environmental factors are important determinants of overall health, in some circumstances, genetic endowment appears to predispose certain individuals to particular diseases or health problems.
10. ***Health services:*** Health services, particularly those designed to maintain and promote health, prevent disease, and restore health and function, contribute to population health. The health services continuum of care includes treatment and secondary prevention.

11. ***Gender:*** Gender refers to the array of society-determined roles, personality traits, attitudes, behaviours, values, and relative power and influence ascribed to the two sexes on a differential basis. "Gendered" norms influence the health system's practices and priorities. Many health issues are a function of gender-based social status or roles.
12. ***Culture:*** Certain people or groups may face additional health risks because of their socioeconomic environment that is largely determined by dominant cultural values. These values tend to **marginalize** and stigmatize these people or groups. This results in a loss or devaluation of their language and culture and a lack of access to culturally appropriate health care and services.

Secondary Prevention. Secondary prevention strategies are designed for dealing with risk factors or early indicators of a health-related problem that are present. For example, we may come to know that many children living in a particular community are developing various types of cancer, but until we make the effort to *prevent* the root cause of the problem (and not just *treat* the cancers), that community will continue have serious health problems.

supporting MRS. DAVIDSON

Emma is a support worker at a long-term care facility. She works on a floor for residents with physical problems, such as arthritis and osteoporosis. Mrs. Davidson, 92 years old, is a resident on Emma's floor. Mrs. Davidson loves to read. She reads the newspaper every morning, and listens to an audio book in the afternoon. One day, Mrs. Davidson tells Emma that she misses talking about books with other people. Emma knows some other residents who also like to read and listen to stories. She wonders if there is a way to bring these clients together as a group.

Emma suggests to her supervisor that the facility start a book club. Emma explains that discussing books will help the residents maintain their cognitive function. Belonging to a book club will also help them develop friendships. Emma's supervisor likes her idea and speaks to the recreation director about it. By the end of the month, a weekly book club meeting is up and running, with Mrs. Davidson as leader. The book club becomes so popular that within a year the members form two separate clubs—one for fiction and another for nonfiction.

ILLNESS AND DISABILITY

Illness is the loss of physical or mental health, whereas **disability** is the loss of physical or mental function. Illness and disability may limit a person's ability to communicate, move, or perform ADLs without assistance. Some illnesses (such as influenza) and disabilities (such as a broken arm) last for a relatively short period of time. These are **acute illnesses** and disabilities. Other illnesses or disabilities (such as paraplegia) are **chronic (permanent)** and last for the person's life. Some chronic illnesses and disabilities are progressive, that is, they become worse with time. Others can be managed to prevent further medical problems. Both acute and chronic illnesses are discussed in Chapter 18.

It is important to remember that clients with illnesses and disabilities are whole persons with many dimensions. They are more than their medical conditions. As a support worker, while you help them achieve their best physical health possible, you must also consider their emotional, social, intellectual, and spiritual health.

SUPPORTING CLIENTS WITH ILLNESS AND DISABILITY

Illness and disability usually affect all aspects of a client's life. For example, Mr. Spinelli recently suffered severe vision loss. As a result, his intellectual health suffers because he can no longer read or pursue his other hobbies; his social health is affected because he can no longer travel to meet friends; his emotional health suffers because he is frustrated and depressed; and his spiritual life is affected because he is angry at God and no longer wants to attend his church services.

No two clients will experience illness and disability in the same way. Some severely ill clients remain cheerful and calm throughout their illness; some who are not seriously ill complain constantly or grow easily sad or frustrated. Many clients who are disabled are not ill, and they do not consider themselves to be ill. Clients who are born with disabilities have never known life any other way, and many clients disabled later in life learn to adjust to their situation and need no further medical care. Although clients' experiences vary, health care professionals have identified some common reactions to newly diagnosed illness or a recently acquired disability (see Box 4–1).

Box 4–1 Common Reactions to Illness and Disability

- ***Fear and anxiety.*** When even minor illness can cause anxiety, it is understandable that clients with serious illnesses will have many fears and anxieties—the effects of their illness on their family; how they will manage their daily responsibilities; financial problems; their families' future; and death. Some clients worry about what their role will be within the family unit. Clients with disabilities, disfigurements, or speech or memory problems may worry about embarrassing themselves in front of others. Clients with mental illnesses often experience severe anxiety. Some clients' fears may make sense to you as a support worker; others may not. To the person experiencing the fear, however, it is real. Some clients will communicate their fear and anxiety to you, but many will not and prefer to keep their concerns to themselves.
- ***Sadness and grief.*** Clients facing loss are usually sad. Those with serious illness and disabilities often deal with many kinds of losses—loss of position, loss of independence, loss of confidence. For some, there is loss of their dreams for the future. These losses can cause intense grief. These clients who are grieving need to mourn. Observe and listen to your clients so you can understand their needs. Some clients may not want to talk about their feelings, while others may find it helpful to talk to an understanding, caring person.
- ***Depression.*** Fear, anxiety, sadness, and grief can cause anyone to feel depressed. This is called *reactive depression* (see Chapter 34). However, clients coping with serious illness, progressive disability, or, in the case of some elderly clients, the losses of life-long friends and family members are at risk for more serious depression called *clinical depression*. Clients who are depressed are often tired, anxious, and uninterested in life. They may avoid contact with other people. Clients who are severely depressed may be suicidal. Observe closely for any changes in a client's mood, energy levels, and behaviour. Report these changes to your supervisor immediately (see Chapter 34).
- ***Denial.*** Denial is a refusal to recognize and admit the truth. Clients who are afraid that they might be seriously ill may downplay or deny symptoms. Even clients who know that they are seriously ill may deny their situation. For example, a diabetic teenager may refuse to take her insulin or may demand foods that she should avoid. A middle-aged man with heart disease may continue to shovel his driveway in spite of strict doctor's orders not to do such heavy work. Their way of coping may be to deny they have serious health problems. If you think a client is denying his or her condition, be understanding and show a positive attitude. If the person's denial may cause harm, let your supervisor know.
- ***Anger.*** Some clients may be angry because they resent their limitations, their illnesses, and their inability to have control over their life. They may direct their anger toward their physician, family, friends, or caregivers. Some clients may direct their anger toward their support worker. If this happens, you should remain calm, patient, and gentle with the client. Avoid becoming angry yourself. That will only make the situation worse. Try to understand the client's needs and problems. Imagine what life must be like for him or her. However, you do not have to accept abuse. Learn what to do when faced with an angry client (see Chapters 21 and 35).

Factors affecting a client's experience of illness and disability include:

- The nature of the illness or condition
- The client's age
- The client's level of physical fitness
- The amount and degree of pain and discomfort the client experiences
- The **prognosis** (the expected course of recovery based on the usual outcome of the illness)
- The client's emotional, social, intellectual, and spiritual health
- The client's personality and ability to cope with difficulties
- The client's cultural background, which may influence how he or she perceives the illness, seeks treatment, and interacts with caregivers and health care workers (see Chapter 12)
- The presence of emotional, social, and financial support

Change and Loss Associated With Illness and Disability

Clients with serious illness or recent disability must cope with change and loss. The following are just a few of the many changes these clients must face:

Change in Routine. Daily routines almost always change. Time previously spent at work or with friends and family is often now filled with doctors' appointments, tests, and treatments. For many clients, what used to be simple ADLs suddenly become challenges. Such routine matters as getting to the bathroom, making meals, eating, and controlling pain now become serious issues.

Change in Work Life. Many clients with serious illnesses or disabilities quit or limit work. Clients who used to feel rewarded and fulfilled by their work may suddenly feel worthless when they can no longer work (see Box 4–1 on page 49). The loss of work may also result in financial problems and loss of social interactions.

Change in Family Life. Serious illness or disability almost always disrupts family life. When one family member is ill, often the lives of everyone at home change greatly. Every family member must make adjustments to the new situation and take on new roles. For example, Mrs. Kim has survived a severe stroke. She can no longer be the sole provider and caregiver for her teenage children. Her role changes to that of a patient. While she recovers, her children must now take care of her, with help from professional caregivers. The children may have to give up after-school activities or time with their friends. Changes and new roles often create stress. Sometimes the stress on family members is so severe that their own health suffers as a result (see Chapter 6).

Change in Sexual Function. Disability and illness often affect sexual function. The client may feel unfit for closeness and love and may become uninterested in sex. He or she may be physically unable to have sex because of the side effects of the medications or the illness. Reproductive surgery, heart disease, stroke, spinal cord injuries, and nervous disorders are some of the conditions that can affect sexual function in men and women. Changes in sexual function can significantly affect clients and their partners. Fear, anger, worry, and depression are common but normal and expected reactions. Time, understanding, and a caring partner will be helpful to the client. Professional counselling may help the client and the partner adjust to the situation.

Loss of Independence. Independence is the state of being able to do things for oneself. Losing one's independence can be very hard. It is particularly distressing when the onset of the illness or disability is sudden and there is little or no hope for recovery. As the support worker, you must try at all times to enable your clients to be as independent as they can be.

Loss of Dignity. Independence and dignity are closely related. For some clients, loss of independence can lead to loss of dignity. This is particularly true when they need help with personal care. It can be extremely difficult for some clients to have to depend on others to perform private functions, including bodily functions. Always be sensitive to your clients' need for dignity.

Change in Self-Image. Self-image is the individual's perception of himself or herself. Changes to a person's body caused by illness may affect self-image. Clients who have lost body parts or have scars due to surgery or accidents may feel unattractive or even repulsive. Others who have conditions that negatively affect the way they look, move, walk, or speak may feel very self-conscious.

You can help clients who are ill and disabled by understanding how their condition affects every aspect of their lives. Do not make assumptions. Do not judge the person's behaviour or compare one client's reaction to illness with another's. Do everything you can to communicate warmth, acceptance, and respect to clients. Always keep the priorities of support work (DIPPS) in mind. (See *Providing Compassionate Care: Caring for Clients Who Are Ill or Disabled* box.)

Attitudes of Others Toward Illness and Disability

Some people are uncomfortable or fearful when they are with ill or disabled people. They may stare or avoid eye contact. They may treat ill and disabled people differently from the way they treat the well and able-bodied.

Ms. Leblanc used a wheelchair after an injury to her spinal cord. She said that it was very hard getting used to the way some people treated her. "The first time my husband and I went out to dinner after the accident, the waiter asked my husband

PROVIDING COMPASSIONATE CARE

Caring for Clients Who Are Ill or Disabled

- **Dignity.** Being helped with bathing, toileting, and other ADLs can be extremely embarrassing and can affect a client's dignity. Never expose a client's body unnecessarily. Be aware of your facial expressions and gestures while you are providing care, as they may reveal that you are disturbed by the client's disfigurement or body odours. This will cause feelings of shame in the client.
- **Independence.** Encourage clients to participate in their care. Tell them what you are about to do, and ask if they can help. Clients may be able to carry out some of the steps in a procedure themselves. Let clients make decisions for themselves, if they are able. For example, clients who are paralyzed may not be able to dress themselves, but they can decide what to wear.
- **Preferences.** Ask clients how they want tasks done. You may have to ask for specific information. For example, ask them what is important to them, what they enjoy doing, what they are able to do, what they find easy, and what they find difficult.
- **Privacy.** Clients may, in some situations, feel that their privacy has been violated. They may need to adjust to all the people around who are providing care. Never snoop around and look at your client's belongings when you are in a client's room or house. The following actions promote privacy: knocking before entering, drawing curtains and blinds, closing doors and windows, covering the client during personal care activities, and keeping client information confidential. Clients who are ill and disabled still have sexual needs, including the need for touching, caressing, and embracing. Allow privacy for the client to fulfill his or her sexual needs.
- **Safety.** All clients need to feel safe from harm. Clients who are ill or disabled have special safety needs. Check with your supervisor and the care plan for specific safety measures for each client. Follow the safety measures described in Chapter 19. When you recognize signs and symptoms that your client may be tired or has overexerted himself or herself, allow some time for rest. View the room from their perspective. Ask yourself if there is a safe passage to the bathroom, or if any items could be in the way and cause falls or injuries. If you are not sure the client's safety needs are being met, talk to the client and to your supervisor.

what I wanted for dinner. To the waiter, I was invisible. Since then I have met many people who ignore me or treat me like a child. I've learned to live with it, but it still hurts."

Some ill and disabled clients experience stigma and discrimination. A **stigma** is a characteristic that marks a person as different or flawed, and is often associated with shame or disgrace. **Discrimination** is behaviour that treats people unfairly based on their group membership. Some clients with AIDS, mental illness, and substance abuse disorders are vulnerable to discrimination. Sometimes they are blamed for their misfortunes, and they and their families are deprived of much-needed social support. Such rejection can lead to isolation, loneliness, and depression, as well as feelings of self-blame and guilt in these clients.

supporting
MR. VITALE

The Effect of Serious Illness on Self-Esteem

On Wednesday, Tony Vitale felt on top of the world. He got up at 6:00 A.M., as usual, and ran for half an hour. Over breakfast, he reviewed the speech he was to give at his company's annual meeting. He was looking forward to announcing that profits were up. At the age of 46, he had achieved his life's goal of becoming the chief executive officer (CEO) of a major corporation.

Mr. Vitale never gave his speech. As he stepped up to the podium, he let out a short gasp and collapsed to the floor. When he awoke 10 hours later, he did not recognize his wife or his two children. He could not speak or understand anything that was said. He had suffered a severe stroke.

Within 4 months, it became clear that Mr. Vitale would never recover sufficiently to be able to return to his job. Although his memory eventually returned, his speech remained difficult for others to understand. He also had difficulty understanding others. The news that his position had been filled by a new CEO overwhelmed him with sadness and anger. Throughout his adult life, Mr. Vitale's job had given him the recognition, prestige, and status that he craved. Without it, he felt useless and depressed. He slowly began to be consumed by anger. He was angry at his body for "betraying" him and at his caregivers for not being able to "make him better." He shouted at his family each time they came to visit him. He was angry that they were able to survive without him.

During 8 months of therapy and rehabilitation, Mr. Vitale made impressive progress. Although he found long sentences difficult to understand, other people could now understand much of what he said. With the support of his family and a caring health care team, his depression was gradually reduced. He began to realize that he still had something to offer to the world. This realization also helped lift the anger that pressed him down. He understood that his family loved him, and he began to feel pride that they were independent enough to survive without his financial support. He discovered that he enjoyed painting. He spent time volunteering with people suffering from brain injury. His newfound self-esteem came from the knowledge that he was making a useful contribution.

REVIEW

Answers to these questions are at the bottom of the page.

Circle the BEST answer.

1. **In the 1800s, good health was considered to be:**
   A. Well-being in all dimensions of life
   B. Optimal wellness
   C. The absence of disease
   D. Physical, emotional, and social well-being

2. **A holistic approach to health is one that:**
   A. Takes a realistic view of a person's health problems
   B. Takes into account the whole person
   C. Focuses on the person's illness or disability
   D. Focuses on the person's physical health

3. **Which of the following is one of the five dimensions of health?**
   A. Recreational health
   B. Income and social status
   C. Emotional health
   D. Education and literacy

4. **Which of the following is one of the key Determinants of Health?**
   A. Intellectual health
   B. Biology and genetic endowment
   C. Fear and anxiety
   D. Change in sexual functioning

5. **What is the difference between *dimensions* of health and *Determinants* of Health?**
   A. One is a Canadian term and the other is an American term.
   B. One involves men and the other involves women.
   C. One is an older, outdated term and the other is a new, current term.
   D. One is about an individual's health and the other is about population health.

6. **Which factor *best* contributes to good physical health?**
   A. A high-fat diet
   B. Smoking outside
   C. The regular use of seat belts
   D. Avoiding all animal protein

7. **People with strong emotional health:**
   A. Exhibit self-control
   B. Read the paper and are curious about life
   C. Can become angry easily when provoked
   D. Practise good eating habits

8. **A social support system is:**
   A. A group of people who volunteer in the community
   B. A system of social welfare
   C. An informal network of people who help each other or others
   D. Another term for a health care team

9. **An acute illness:**
   A. Appears suddenly and lasts a short time
   B. Is a slow, progressive illness
   C. Results in disability
   D. Is another term for influenza

10. **Which of the following is true of chronic illness?**
    A. People usually recover.
    B. The symptoms often appear quickly.
    C. Most of us have a chronic illness.
    D. It is a slow, progressive illness.

11. **Which of the following is a true statement?**
    A. People respond to illness and disability in much the same way.
    B. People's responses to illness and disability vary.
    C. Almost all ill and disabled people are depressed.
    D. Most ill and disabled people are in denial.

12. **The term *stigma* means:**
    A. Denial
    B. An artificial opening between the colon and the abdominal wall
    C. A characteristic that marks a person as different or flawed
    D. A refusal to admit the truth

Answers: 1.C, 2.B, 3.C, 4.B, 5.C, 6.C, 7.A, 8.C, 9.A, 10.D, 11.B, 12.C

CHAPTER 5

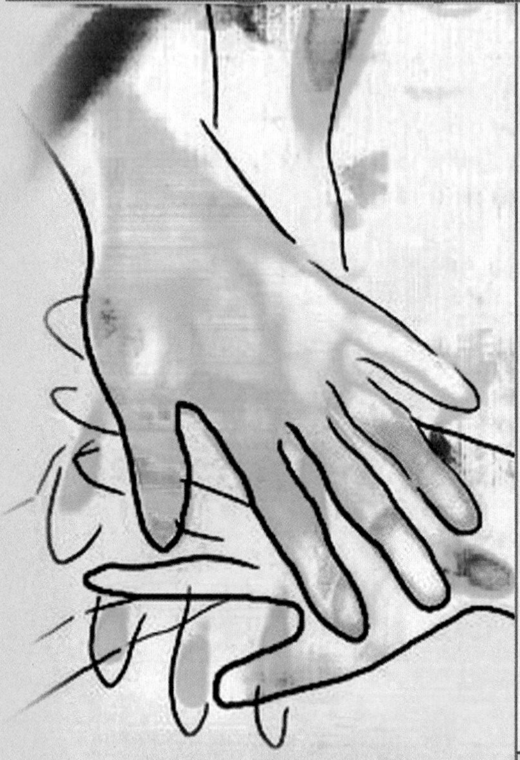

Working With Others: Teamwork, Supervision, and Delegation

OBJECTIVES

- Define the key terms listed in this chapter.
- List the benefits and challenges in working on a health care team.
- Explain your role on the health care team.
- Describe how teams function in different health care settings.
- Explain how delegation applies to you.
- Describe the delegation process and your role in it.

key terms

accountable Being willing to accept responsibility and to explain your actions, inactions, or omissions, intentions, and decisions. Accountability cannot be shared; it rests solely on an individual.

assigning Giving responsibility for providing care.

authority The legal right to do something.

care conference A meeting that occurs on admission and on an ongoing basis, usually once or twice a year. The purpose of the meeting is to discuss a client's care. It is attended by the client (if able), family/significant others/advocate, and members of the health care team. Also known as **family conference**.

case manager See **team leader**.

delegation A process by which an RN authorizes another health care provider to perform certain tasks.

family conference See **care conference**.

interdisciplinary team See **multidisciplinary team**.

intradisciplinary team A team of providers from the same specialty.

multidisciplinary team A team of health care providers from a variety of backgrounds and specialties who work together to meet the client's needs. Also known as **interdisciplinary team**.

task A function, procedure, or activity that you assist with or perform for the client.

team leader A health care professional who assesses, monitors, and evaluates a client's needs in a community care setting; also coordinates team services. In a care facility setting, a team leader, usually a nurse, is responsible for managing the care of the clients. The team leader also provides direction to support workers. Support workers report to the team leader. Also known as **case manager**.

transfer of function A process by which an RN authorizes another health care provider to perform certain tasks

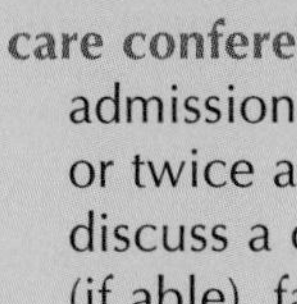

This chapter discusses the health care team and your role as the support worker. It also discusses the relationship between you and your supervisor. All health care workers must protect their clients from harm. Understanding the delegation process will help you protect clients and prevent potential legal problems.

THE HEALTH CARE TEAM

In most health care settings, you work on a team. A team is a group of people who work together toward a common goal (see Chapter 1). The goal of a health care team is to provide the client with the best possible care and support. When providing care, team members must consider the whole client. You must promote health in all five dimensions of the client's life: physical, emotional, social, intellectual, and spiritual (see Chapter 4). Health care team members depend on each other to perform their roles to the best of their abilities. Members of effective teams support one another, understand each other's scope of practice, and communicate with each other effectively.

Members of health care teams vary from setting to setting and from team to team. The client's needs determine who will be on the team. For example, Tom Brown, 15, has mental health problems. Tom, his parents, an RN, a psychiatrist, a social worker, and a support worker work together as a team. Tom's team is different from Mrs. Darby's team. Mrs. Darby, 86, is recovering from hip surgery. She and her daughter are on a team that also has an RN, a social worker, a physiotherapist, and support workers. The client is an active member of the team unless he or she is not mentally capable of being involved in the team work or chooses not to participate.

In some situations, you and a nurse may be the only health care providers on the team. In others, you may be part of a multidisciplinary team. A **multidisciplinary team** includes health care providers from a variety of backgrounds and specialties who work together to meet the client's needs.

Benefits of Working on a Team

There are many benefits to the team approach to health care. A group of people is more effective at making decisions and solving problems than one person. The many benefits of a team approach to care include:

- ***Opportunities for collaboration.*** All team members are encouraged to *collaborate* (to work together toward a common goal). Successful collaboration creates a positive atmosphere that even the client can sense. Staff and clients both benefit when team members share information. For example, you may find a way to ease a client's discomfort during a bed bath. You share this information with the nurse. The nurse asks other support workers to use your method.
- ***Opportunities for communication.*** Team meetings provide the opportunity for all team members to share experiences, opinions, and ideas. Without the meetings, valuable ideas might be missed. Box 5–1 contains part of a dialogue from a team meeting. Note how each team member contributes to the complete picture of the client's health.
- ***A wide range of abilities, skills, and perspectives.*** Team members include individuals with a range of abilities, skills, training, and experience. Each team member, based on scope of practice, has ideas and viewpoints that he or she brings to the team. In Box 5–1, note the support worker's contributions. Because she is the only person who has daily contact with Mrs. Darby, she is able to provide important information. The other team members know more about the health and medical conditions that are discussed. However, only the support worker is in a position to share daily observations about Mrs. Darby.
- ***Better decision making and problem solving.*** When team members discuss issues, they are more likely to make sound decisions and find appropriate solutions to problems. When information is shared, workable solutions are found.
- ***A positive, trusting atmosphere.*** Trust develops when team members can be relied upon to do their jobs well, to respect each other, and to share responsibility. The team leader is responsible for fostering a high level of trust. The leader should encourage team members to openly discuss problems. Team members also play a role in creating trust. They must not blame others for their own mistakes. They should take responsibility for their own actions. An effective team provides support to each other during difficult emotional situations, such as the death of a client.

Just as there are many benefits to working on a team, there are also challenges:

- ***Recognizing role boundaries.*** In successful teams, team members understand each other's role. You may become familiar with tasks that support workers are not permitted to perform. However, never attempt any task that you are not allowed to perform. You must be aware of your scope of practice and your employer's policies and procedures.
- ***Being flexible.*** Teams function best when members are willing to meet each other's needs. This requires flexibility. For example, you can help co-workers by exchanging shifts. You might also assist them with certain tasks. Remember, you might need your supervisor's permission first.
- ***Handling conflict.*** Any group of people is bound to have disagreements. The way conflict is handled affects the whole team. The team leader plays a critical role in the resolution of conflict. Team members should feel comfortable discussing problems with their leader. They should address conflict rather than hope it will go away. This may mean talking to a co-worker with whom you are having problems. If you have hurt someone's feelings, you need to apologize. You also need to be accountable for your actions and admit your mistakes.
- ***Expressing your needs and views.*** Support workers may sometimes feel intimidated on a

Box 5–1 Contributions to a Team Meeting

A health care team in a long-term care facility is meeting to discuss a client's rehabilitation following her hip surgery. Mrs. Darby is 86 years old. The team consists of Mrs. Darby, her daughter, an RN, two support workers, a social worker, and a physical therapist. At the previous meeting, the physical therapist had suggested exercises to help Mrs. Darby regain mobility. Since then, the physical therapist has shown Mrs. Darby how to do the exercises. A support worker has helped her practise the exercises. Mrs. Darby has chosen not to attend the team meeting. The following team members are attending the meeting:

- The RN, who is also the team leader
- The support worker (Meredith)
- The physiotherapist
- The social worker
- Mrs. Darby's daughter (Sandra)

RN: I understand that Mrs. Darby is having difficulty with some of her exercises. Meredith, could you please tell the team what you have observed?

Support worker: Well, Mrs. Darby has been having trouble with all the exercises. They give her great pain. She has such a grimace on her face when she attempts them. Let me tell you what she said on Tuesday morning. (Checks notes.) *"I can't do these exercises. It feels like someone is boring holes in my hip."*

Physical therapist: Can you tell me how high she is able to lift her leg?

Support worker: About 5 cm off the bed.

Physical therapist: Is she taking her pain medication?

RN: Yes, I help her with her medication. She takes it regularly. To me, Mrs. Darby seems much less cheerful than usual. Has anyone else noticed this?

Support worker: Yes, I've noticed that she is much less outgoing than usual. She used to read the newspaper in the mornings. Now, she just sits in her chair. When I ask her how she is feeling, she says she is tired. She told me that she is not attending this meeting because she is very tired.

RN: Perhaps Mrs. Darby is depressed. Sandra, what do you think?

Daughter: I'd say that Mom is definitely feeling down. I just thought it was because of the broken hip and the surgery. Who wouldn't be after what she has been through? She used to be so cheerful and outgoing. Perhaps Mom is depressed. I haven't heard her mention any of her friends lately. Are they keeping in touch?

Social worker: Didn't your mother tell you that she is worried about her roommate, Mrs. Martino, who has been in hospital for 2 weeks? Your mom is worried that she might not be coming back here.

Daughter: No, she didn't mention it. That's odd. Gosh, she is so close to Mrs. Martino.

RN: I think someone needs to talk to Mrs. Darby to find out how she is feeling. Maybe she'll have some ideas about how we can help her. She might benefit from some outings and other social activities.

Social worker: I'll talk with Mrs. Darby. We may also need to discuss this with her family physician.

The discussion continues.

team that includes physicians and other health care professionals. You *are* a valuable team member. You spend more time with the client than do other team members. You have a great deal to contribute to team meetings (see *Supporting Mr. Rodriguez*). Your day-to-day reporting of concerns are heard by registered staff and reported.

Teamwork in Facilities

Teams in facilities vary as much as the settings themselves. For example, a team at a retirement home functions differently from a team at a hospital. A hospital team functions differently from a team in a long-term care facility. However, most teams in facilities have one thing in common: team members work in the same location. This makes communication easy. Team members have many opportunities to meet and collaborate.

Long-Term Care Facilities. Most long-term care facilities use a multidisciplinary team approach to care. Teams include physicians, nurses, social workers, support workers, therapists, the client, and the

supporting MR. RODRIGUEZ

Mario Rodriguez is a 52-year-old client with your home care agency. You are giving him support care for several weeks, ever since he was discharged from the hospital following his cerebro-vascular accident (CVA, or stroke). You have been able to develop a good relationship with him because you speak his native language. In addition to the support services that you provide in his home, he goes for physiotherapy at the local hospital three times a week. In order to get there, he has to take a taxi.

On the day of your last visit, Mr. Rodriguez seemed a little depressed. He tearfully confided in you that he used to work as a cement mason before his stroke and was self-employed, and being out of work now, it was financially hard on him and his family to pay for his taxi. Because of that, he has only gone for his physiotherapy once that week. He told you that he wants to get better but cannot afford to spend any more money in this way.

As a support worker, you knew that you have to report this information to your supervisor and the rest of the team at your weekly conference. After reporting this information, arrangements are being made through a church volunteer group to drive Mr. Rodriguez to and from the hospital.

client's family. In a large facility, the team may also include the pharmacist, activity director, and other staff members. Usually, the team leader is an RN. Often, one RN is team leader for all the clients. The same team provides care to all clients. Support workers have many opportunities to work with other team members (Figure 5–1).

Hospitals. Team functions and members vary from hospital to hospital and department to department. Many departments use a multidisciplinary team approach. Specialists and other health care providers are brought together, as needed.

Hospices and Palliative Care Units. Most hospices and palliative care units use a multidisciplinary approach. A team usually consists of nurses, support workers, physicians, social workers, volunteers, the client, and family members. Depending on the client's wishes, other individuals, such as a spiritual adviser, may be on the team.

Although hospices and palliative care units are facilities, they are also considered community-based services. They have outreach programs that provide palliative care to people at home. Team members of such programs meet in the facility or in the client's home.

You may be asked to attend a family conference. A **family conference** is a meeting attended by the health care team and family members to discuss the client's care. Family conferences are usually held when difficult situations arise. Family members can ask questions, express feelings, and make difficult decisions. Family conferences are common in hospice and community care settings. They are also held in hospitals and other facilities.

Assisted-Living Facilities. These community-based facilities are usually located in a single building. Being in one building makes communication easier. The number of staff in assisted-living facilities (including group homes) is small. They are often multidisciplinary. The makeup of the team depends on the needs of the clients. Teams usually have a supervisor (who may be an RN, an RPN/LPN, a social worker, or a qualified youth care worker), and one or two support workers. There may also be other assistive personnel.

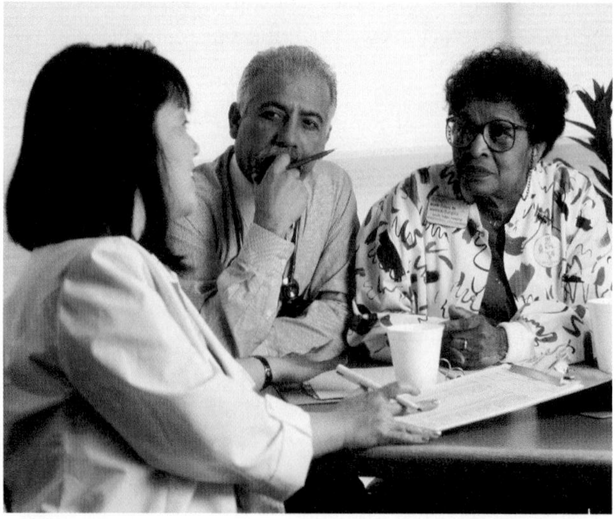

Figure 5–1 A team in a long-term care facility meets to discuss a client's care. **Source:** Patricia Barry Levy/Maxx Images.

Teamwork in Community Settings

Teams in community settings also vary in membership and function.

Home Care. The home care team usually includes the client, family members, the case manager, the family physician, nurses, and support workers and their supervisors. Social workers and therapists may also be on the team.

The **case manager/team leader** assesses, monitors, and evaluates a client's needs in a community care setting. He or she also coordinates the services of the team. A case manager could be a nurse but may be a social worker or another professional. Occasionally, the client chooses to be the case manager (see Chapter 8).

Home care teams do not always meet regularly. Team members may communicate with each other by telephone or written reports. The case manager schedules a team meeting when the need arises.

Community Day Programs. Teams in community day programs function differently from home care teams. A rehabilitative program team may include a supervisor (who is often a nurse or another health care professional), other professionals, and support workers. A recreational program team may include a supervisor (who is usually a recreational or occupational therapist) and support workers. In a day program, you will probably work with the same team every day. There are regular opportunities to discuss your client's progress. You may meet before the program starts, after it is over, or once a week.

WORKING UNDER SUPERVISION

You are responsible to the client and to your co-workers. You are accountable to your supervisor. The supervisor is usually an RN. Some provinces allow RPNs to supervise support workers in long-term care facilities. In some community care settings, you may occasionally be supervised by an RPN, a social worker, or another health care professional.

- ***Supervision in a facility.*** In many facilities, the team leader is also your supervisor. The team leader (usually an RN) has overall responsibility and accountability for the client's care, the work of other RNs, RPN/LPNs, support workers, and assistive personnel. The team leader may not be on duty when you are working. You then report to the *charge nurse* (the nurse on duty for that shift).
- ***Supervision in a community setting.*** In these settings, you report to a supervisor, who is responsible and accountable for your work performance. You and your supervisor work for the same agency. Your agency may be hired by a health district or community services organization. When this happens, a case manager will arrange with the agency to provide care or support for the client. The case manager is usually, but not always, an RN. The case manager communicates with your supervisor. Your supervisor then gives you information and instructions about specific clients.

In some cases, your agency's services may be purchased privately by a client or a client's family. In this case, your supervisor will be given the overall instructions from the client and the family. Your supervisor then gives you information and instructions about the client.

In some situations, clients directly hire their own support worker. In these circumstances, there is no agency supervisor. The client is your supervisor. It is advisable to have a written contract outlining each person's responsibilities, compensation, hours of work, and so on. The contract must be acceptable to both the support worker and the client. This contract would prevent unethical clients and their families from taking advantage of you. Do not hesitate to have the contract reviewed by a lawyer.

Respecting Your Supervisor and Employer

You must respect your supervisor and your employer. Avoid talking with others about your clients or co-workers. Your negative, disrespectful attitude toward your employer could decrease your clients' trust, resulting in less cooperation in their plan of care. Try not to be negative, even if co-workers complain about a policy or a situation. If you are unhappy with a situation, talk to your supervisor. If you have difficulties communicating with your supervisor, try some of the strategies discussed in Chapters 9 and 13. If you remain unhappy, it might be best for you to find a position with a different agency.

Do not discuss your work problems with your clients. You represent your employer. The client trusts the facility or agency to provide quality care. A negative, disrespectful attitude could destroy this trust and harm your client's health.

DELEGATION

A **task** is a function, procedure, or activity that you assist the client with or perform for the client. Your supervisor *assigns* most of your daily tasks. **Assigning** means giving responsibility for providing care or support. The assigned tasks are listed on your assignment sheet. Assigned tasks do not require a nurse's education and professional judgement, as the tasks will be within the support worker's scope of practice. For example, you are assigned to assist with or perform the following tasks:

- Activities of daily living (ADLs)—dressing, personal hygiene, mobility, feeding, toileting
- Social and recreational activities
- Household management—housecleaning, meal preparation
- Basic nursing care tasks—measuring height, weight, and vital signs

Some care tasks could harm a client if done by unqualified workers. Only nurses have the **authority** (the legal right) to do these tasks. Inserting catheters and giving insulin are examples. However, in certain situations, these tasks may be *delegated* to you. **Delegation (transfer of function)** is a process by which an RN authorizes another health care provider to perform certain tasks. The RN transfers to you the authority to perform a task. This frees the nurse to perform other tasks. It is important to remember that the nurse maintains the authority to delegate to others. The support worker does not. The Regulated Health Professional legislation states that if the controlled act is determined to be a routine ADL for a particular client, delegation can occur.

During the delegation process, you are taught how to perform the task. You are then supervised and monitored to make sure you are performing the task correctly. You are delegated tasks that are routine, require little supervision, and are done for stable clients. Some tasks that you may be delegated to perform include suctioning of permanent tracheotomy, in-and-out catheterization, and administering glucometers, dressings, tube feedings, and medication.

Only some nursing tasks can be delegated. ***Your employer's policies and guidelines, your job description, and provincial or territorial legislation determine what tasks can be delegated to you.*** They also determine when and how tasks can be delegated. Although there are many similarities across the country, each province and territory has its own rules for delegation (see the examples described in Box 5–2).

Who Can Delegate?

In most parts of the country, only RNs can delegate to support workers. When making delegating decisions, RNs must protect the client's health and safety. The delegating RN remains **accountable** for the delegated task. The RN is accountable for the outcome of the delegated task. If necessary, the RN must answer questions about and explain the actions and decisions involved in the delegated task. However, you are also accountable for your own actions.

Health care professionals other than RNs may *assign* tasks to you. However, only an RN can *delegate* tasks to you. For example, a physician can ask you to help a client with elimination but cannot ask you to give an enema. Only an RN can delegate this task to you.

Delegation in a Facility

When an RN delegates a task in a facility, he or she is required to:

- ***Teach you the task.*** The delegating RN is responsible for providing all necessary teaching. The RN may teach you the delegated task, or the RN may have a qualified RPN teach you.

Box 5–2 Delegation in British Columbia, Alberta, and Ontario

All provinces and territories have legislation that guides nursing practice, usually called a *nursing act.* British Columbia, Alberta, and Ontario also have legislation that applies to all regulated health professions. This legislation prevents unqualified people from performing professional functions.

Regulated health professions legislation and nursing acts list tasks that only nurses are legally able (authorized) to perform. In British Columbia, these authorized tasks are called *reserved acts;* in Alberta, they are known as *restricted activities;* and in Ontario, they are called *controlled acts.* Only nurses—and not support workers—are authorized to do the following:

- Perform a procedure below the skin or mucous membrane (e.g., cleaning and dressing an open wound)
- Administer a substance by injection or inhalation (e.g., giving an insulin injection)
- Insert an instrument, hand, or finger into a client's body openings, including the client's bladder, esophagus, trachea, nose, ears, bloodstream, or surgically created body openings (e.g., inserting urinary catheters and rectal tubes)

Unregulated health care workers (including support workers) are not normally allowed to perform authorized acts. However, unregulated workers may perform an authorized act if an RN properly delegates it. In the delegation process, the RN transfers authority to the unregulated health care worker. However, you are delegated an authorized act only if it is allowed within your job description and employer policy. It remains the responsibility of the RN to determine how and when an unregulated care provider can perform these acts.

Regulated health professions legislation also states that in certain situations, delegation is not necessary. Unregulated workers can be assigned the last two of the above-listed authorized acts if the task is a routine activity of living. A routine activity of living is an activity that:

- The client needs done on a regular basis
- Has already been done for the client by a nurse, with consistent and safe results

For example, administering an enema is an authorized act. For example, (a) Mr. Patel is paralyzed. He requires regular enemas to aid elimination. Because the procedure is a predictable and safe part of his routine, his support worker is assigned to perform the procedure; (b) Ms. Wolfe requires an enema before her surgery. She has never had an enema before. In her situation, the enema is not routine. Therefore, a support worker is not legally allowed to administer it. In this case, only a nurse is authorized to give the enema. Support workers are not responsible for deciding when to do a task. You will be assigned or delegated the task, as appropriate.

- ***Assess your performance.*** The RN must determine if you are able to perform the task correctly. If an RPN is teaching you, the delegating RN is still responsible for determining if you are competent.
- ***Monitor you over time to ensure you remain able to perform the task correctly and safely.*** The monitoring may be done in a number of ways, at the discretion of the RN.

Support workers cannot assign or delegate. You cannot authorize someone to perform a task that has been assigned or delegated to you. A co-worker can help you with tasks that have been *assigned* to you. However, only an RN or RPN can help you with tasks that have been *delegated* to you.

Delegation in the Community

In the community, your supervisor may or may not be an RN. If your supervisor is an RN, he or she follows the same delegation process used in facilities. This involves teaching you the delegated task, assessing your performance, and monitoring your performance over time. The RN should also provide you with written instructions on how to carry out the task, the predicted outcome, and what you need to record.

You may have a client who requires in-and-out catheterization. The RN determines that this is a routine activity of living by answering the questions in Box 5–3. The RN will then teach you the task, assess your performance, provide you with written instructions on how the task is to be done, when to ask for assistance, and what you need to record (the results of the in-and-out catheterization). The RN will then monitor your performance on a regular basis.

If your supervisor is not an RN and you need to learn a delegated task, the agency may send out an instructor (an RN) to teach you. The instructor teaches you the task. He or she assesses and monitors your performance over time or asks your supervisor to do so. The instructor or your supervisor may consult with the client or the client's family to determine if you are performing the task correctly.

Some agencies provide educational programs or workshops for support workers. These programs educate workers about specific activities or daily living tasks. For example, you might attend a program given by an RN on how to do catheterizations for clients with paraplegia. You graduate from the program only after the RN is satisfied that you can perform the task safely and competently. The agency is responsible for monitoring your performance over time.

You may be asked to perform tasks by a professional who is not an RN and not your supervisor. Before taking on a task requested by another professional, use your judgement. Usually, you can do a simple, noninvasive task that you have done for the client before. Tell the person who made the request that you cannot fulfill the request if:

- You have concerns about your ability to do the task
- It is beyond your scope of practice

Be aware of your employer's policies. If you need clarification, contact your supervisor.

The client and caregivers may ask you to do certain tasks. This is common in home settings when no health care professionals are present. You must never perform a task that is beyond your scope of practice. Explain that you are not allowed to perform the task without the authorization of your supervisor. Call your supervisor to discuss the situation.

The Delegation Process

The RN considers factors that are unique to the client's situation when delegating tasks to you. A task that has been delegated is rarely transferable to another client. It must be retaught and redelegated before you can carry it out on another client. For example, you have been taught how to give an enema to Mr. Lau. Mr. Davis is also your client and requires an enema. You cannot give an enema to Mr. Davis without being taught again.

Delegated tasks must be within the legal limits of what you can do. Before delegating tasks to you, the RN must know:

- What tasks your province or territory allows support workers to perform
- The tasks included in your job description
- What you were taught in your training program
- What skills you learned and how they were evaluated
- Your work experience

Even if a task is in your job description and you have done it before, the RN may or may not decide to assign or delegate it to you. The RN must consider the circumstances when delegating. The RN makes delegation decisions after considering the questions in Box 5–3. The circumstances, the client's needs, the task, and the support worker performing the task must all be right. If the client's needs and the task require the knowledge, judgement, and skill of an RN or RPN, a nurse must perform the task. You may, however, be asked to assist.

Do not get offended or angry if you are not allowed to perform a task that is part of your job description and that you usually do. The RN makes a decision that is best for the client at that time. This decision is also best for you at that time. You do not want to perform a task that requires a nurse's judgement and critical thinking skills. For example, you often care for Mrs. Mills. You provide personal care to her and assist her with walking.

Box 5–3 Factors Affecting Delegation Decisions

- What is the client's condition? Is it stable or likely to change?
- What level of knowledge, skill, and judgement is required by the support worker to safely perform the task? Does the support worker have the ability to learn the task?
- What are the risks involved in performing the task? Can the support worker recognize these risks and respond to them appropriately?
- Will the support worker be required to perform the task frequently enough to maintain competency?
- Can the support worker be adequately supervised in the setting?
- Is a nurse available to help or take over if the client's condition changes or problems arise?
- Does the support worker have the time to perform the task safely?
- Does legislation restrict the kinds of acts and procedures support workers are able to perform?
- What tasks are included in the support worker's job description?

Source: College of Nurses of Ontario. (1999). *Guidelines for working with unregulated care providers: For registered nurses and registered practical nurses in Ontario.* Toronto, ON: College of Nurses of Ontario.

She visits with her son during the weekend. When she returns to the long-term care facility, she has bruises on her face and arms. She reports that she fell down the stairs. The RN suspects abuse. Instead of assigning you the task of bathing Mrs. Mills, the RN does it herself. The RN wants to assess Mrs. Mills for other signs of abuse and to talk with her. Although you are able to give Mrs. Mills a bath, at this time she needs the RN's knowledge and judgement.

The client's circumstances are central factors in making assignment and delegation decisions. These decisions should always result in the best care for the client. Poor decisions could place a client's health and safety at risk and result in serious legal problems.

The Five Rights of Delegation. In the United States, the National Council of State Boards of Nursing identifies five rights of delegation. These rights are relevant in Canada as well.

1. ***The right task***—Can the task be delegated? Does the provincial nursing act or regulated health professions act allow the RN to delegate the act? Is the task in your job description? Have you been trained to do the task? A written job description and job routine for a particular shift should be available to support workers when they are hired and in the procedure manual for review.
2. ***The right circumstances***—What are the client's physical, emotional, social, intellectual, and spiritual needs at this time? Do you understand the purpose of the task for the client? Do you have the equipment and supplies to perform the task? Do you know how to use the equipment and supplies?
3. ***The right person***—Do you have the training and experience to safely perform the task for this client? Do you have concerns about performing the task?
4. ***The right directions and communication***—Does the nurse provide clear directions and instructions? Does the nurse tell you what to do, when to do it, what observations to make, and when to report back? Are the directions legal, ethical, and consistent with employer policies? Can you review the task with the nurse? Do you understand what the nurse expects?
5. ***The right supervision***—Is a nurse available to answer questions? Is a nurse available if the client's condition changes or if problems occur? After the task is completed, does the nurse assess how the task affected the client? Does the nurse discuss your performance with you, telling you what you did well and how you can improve your work?

Your Role in Delegation

Although the RN is responsible for teaching, supervising, and monitoring your performance, you are responsible for your own actions. You must perform the task safely to protect the client from harm. You are *responsible and accountable* for performing the task correctly and safely.

You have two choices when delegated a task. You either *agree* or *refuse* to do the task. Before accepting a delegated task, ask yourself the questions listed in "The Five Rights of Delegation."

Accepting a Task. When you agree to perform a task, you are accountable for your own actions. Remember, what you do or fail to do can harm the client. *You must complete the task safely.* Do not hesitate to ask for help if you are unsure or if you have questions about a task. Always report what you did and your observations.

Refusing a Task. You have the right to say "no." If you have good reasons for not doing a task, refusing to follow the nurse's directions is your right and duty. Use "The Five Rights of Delegation" as a guide, and protect clients and yourself by using common sense. Ask yourself if what you are doing is safe for the client.

You must never ignore an order or request to do something. You must communicate your concerns to the delegating RN. With good communication, you and the nurse should be able to solve the problem. If problems continue, talk to your supervisor, instructor, or another professional to help you sort them out (see Chapters 9 and 13).

You must not refuse a delegated task simply because you do not like or want to do the task. You must have sound reasons for your refusal. Otherwise, you could place the client at risk for harm. You also risk losing your job.

REVIEW

Answers to these questions are at the bottom of the page.

Circle the BEST answer.

1. **The membership of a health care team is determined by:**
   - A. The client's needs
   - B. The RN's needs
   - C. The physician's needs
   - D. The needs of the client's family
2. **Which of the following is a benefit to the team approach to health care?**
   - A. Opportunities for confidentiality
   - B. Opportunities for delegation
   - C. Opportunities for collaboration
   - D. Opportunities for assignment of tasks
3. **The following statements are about health care teams and facilities. Which is true?**
   - A. Teams are often multidisciplinary.
   - B. Family conferences do not include the client.
   - C. Team members usually work in different locations.
   - D. Team members have few opportunities to meet.
4. **In a community setting, who usually assesses, monitors, and evaluates a client's needs and co-ordinates the services of the health care team?**
   - A. The family physician
   - B. The case manager
   - C. The occupational therapist
   - D. The social worker
5. **Delegation means:**
   - A. Giving responsibility for providing care
   - B. Authorizing another worker to perform a task
   - C. Transferring responsibility to another worker
   - D. Giving another worker the power or right to enforce an act, function, or role
6. **Which factor affects delegation decisions made by an RN?**
   - A. What is the client's condition? Is it stable or likely to change?
   - B. Has the support worker done the task before?
   - C. Is the support worker at risk doing the task?
   - D. Would the support worker's feelings be hurt if the RN does not delegate the task to him or her?
7. **If an RN delegates a task to you, which of the following is *true*?**
   - A. The RN is completely responsible for your actions; you are not responsible.
   - B. The RN has overall responsibility for your actions; you are also responsible.
   - C. You are completely responsible for your actions; the RN is not responsible.
   - D. Neither you nor the RN is responsible.
8. **A procedure can be delegated to you:**
   - A. By any regulated health care professional
   - B. By a physician
   - C. By the client
   - D. By an RN
9. **An RN delegates a task to you that you are not comfortable doing. Which of the following is a true statement?**
   - A. You must perform the task.
   - B. You can refuse to perform the task.
   - C. You cannot ask for further training on how to perform the task.
   - D. You cannot ask the nurse to stay while you perform the task.
10. **You are assisting Mr. Chiang with personal care in his home. Mrs. Chiang asks you to change her husband's dressing. RNs have delegated dressing changes to you for other clients. What should you do?**
    - A. Tell Mrs. Chiang that you are not allowed to perform the procedure without the authorization of your supervisor. Call your supervisor.
    - B. Tell Mrs. Chiang that you can change the dressing if her husband (your client) asks you to do it.
    - C. Tell Mrs. Chiang that you can change the dressing if she stays in the room during the procedure.
    - D. Tell Mrs. Chiang she has to obtain permission from your supervisor.

Answers: 1.A, 2.C, 3.A, 4.B, 5.B, 6.D, 7.B, 8.D, 9.B, 10.A

CHAPTER 6

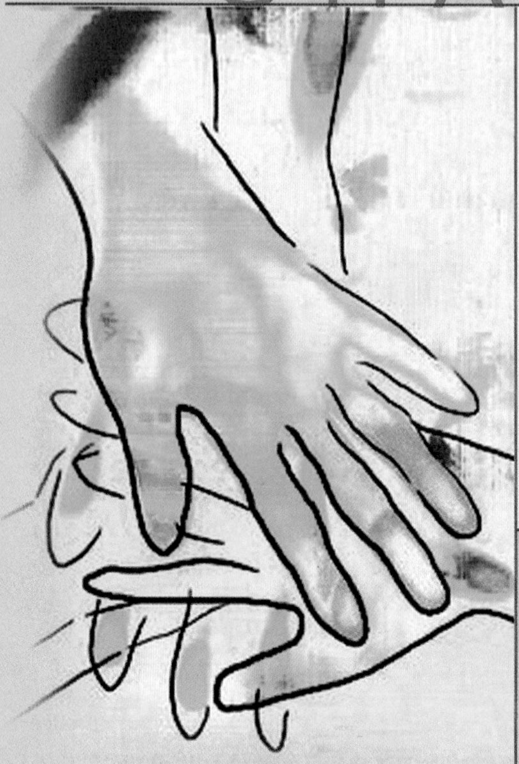

Working With Clients and Their Families

OBJECTIVES

- Define the key terms listed in this chapter.
- Recognize that each client is an individual and a whole person.
- Describe Erikson's developmental stages.
- Explain how Maslow's hierarchy of needs applies to support work.
- Explain the difference between a professional helping relationship and a friendship.
- Explain independence, dependence, and interdependence.
- Describe common family patterns.
- Explain how the health care team assists the family.

key terms

compassion Is characterized by a person's awareness of the misfortune and suffering of another and the desire and actions taken to reduce or alleviate the problem.

competence Performing one's job safely and within one's scope of practice or legal limits.

dependence The state of relying on others for support; being unable to manage without help.

empathy The ability to recognize, perceive, and have an understanding of another's emotions by being able to "put oneself into another person's shoes."

family A biological, legal, or social network of people who provide support for one another.

independence The state of not depending on others for control or authority.

interdependence The state of depending on one another.

need (basic human) That which is necessary or desirable for maintaining life and psychosocial well-being.

primary caregiver A person—usually a family member or close friend—who assumes the responsibilities of caring for an ill or disabled client in the home.

psychosocial health Well-being in the social, emotional, intellectual, and spiritual dimensions of one's life.

relationship The connection between two or more people, shaped by the roles, feelings, and interactions of those involved.

respect Showing acceptance and regard for another person.

self-actualization Experiencing one's potential.

self-awareness Understanding one's own feelings, moods, attitudes, preferences, biases, qualities, and limitations.

self-esteem Thinking well of oneself and being well thought of by others.

sympathy Feeling compassion for, or commiseration with, another person.

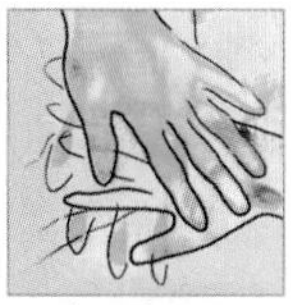

Every person is an individual shaped by a unique blend of genetics and experiences. Health care workers sometimes overlook a client's individuality, and too often, they tend to focus on the disease or problem rather than on the client. For example, to the health care worker, Mrs. Porter might be just "the client with colon cancer" rather than "Mrs. Porter." Most clients of support workers have physical problems, but to provide good care, it is necessary to have a holistic approach to care. Considering only the physical part ignores the client's ability to think, make decisions, and interact with others. It also ignores the client's experiences, joys, sorrows, and needs.

The client is usually part of a family, and your job as a support worker often involves helping the client's family as well. What you do affects not only the client but also the client's family. It is, therefore, important to understand your role when working with a client and his or her family.

PSYCHOSOCIAL HEALTH

A holistic approach to health care takes into account the whole client (see Chapter 4). It considers a client's physical as well as psychosocial health. **Psychosocial health** is well-being in the social, emotional, intellectual, and spiritual dimensions of one's life. Few people enjoy perfect psychosocial health throughout life. Factors that influence psychosocial health include:

- ***Personality.*** Personality is the blend of thought patterns, feelings, characteristics, and behaviour that makes a person unique.
- ***Family background.*** People who grew up in caring, loving families are more likely to have good psychosocial health than those who did not. When there are serious family problems, children growing up in that family may be harmed psychosocially. Problems that such children face include abuse, neglect, distrust, anger, and substance abuse. As they grow

older, these children may have problems with trust and intimacy. They may repeat the patterns learned in childhood. Abused children, when they become adults, may abuse their own children. Children of substance abusers may develop their own substance abuse problems in adulthood.

- ***Environment.*** Experiences outside the family setting also strongly influence psychosocial health. For children and adolescents, such experiences include school, the influence of the media, and interactions with friends and acquaintances. For adults, they include experiences at work and in the community. Access to social support systems, such as health care and social welfare, can also influence psychosocial health.
- ***Life circumstances.*** Some people experience devastating loss or tragedy in their lives, for example, the death of a parent during childhood, or the death of a child. People who experience such losses may never enjoy strong psychosocial health after the experience.

Erikson's Developmental Stages

Erik Erikson was a psychologist who strongly influenced ideas about the development of psychosocial health. In the 1960s, he developed a theory that people move through a series of stages throughout their lives (Table 6–1). Each stage is necessary for a person's identity and psychosocial health. Every stage consists of a task that must be completed successfully before the person can move on to the next stage. For example, a child who never learns to trust others will likely have difficulties forming trusting, intimate relationships later in life.

Table 6–1 Erikson's Theory of Psychosocial Development, from Birth Through Old Age

Stage	Age (years)	Psychosocial Task	Description of Task
1	0–1	Trust versus mistrust	Babies learn to trust that their needs will be met. This shows the infant that the world is a safe place.
2	1–3	Autonomy versus doubt	The toddler learns to become independent and develops self-confidence. Not learning independence creates feelings of shame and doubt.
3	3–6	Initiative versus guilt	The young child learns to initiate his or her activities. Accomplishing this task teaches the child to seek challenges later in life.
4	6–12	Competence versus inferiority	The child develops skill in physical, cognitive, and social areas. This task teaches independence and responsibility.
5	12–19	Identity versus role confusion	The adolescent tries out several roles and forms a single, unique identity.
6	20–40	Intimacy versus isolation	The young adult forms close, permanent relationships and makes career commitments.
7	40–65	Generativity versus stagnation	The person in middle adulthood helps younger people develop their lives.
8	65 on	Integrity versus despair	The older adult thinks back on life, experiencing satisfaction or disappointment.

Source: Matlin, M.W. (1999). *Psychology* (3rd ed.), p. 370. Fort Worth, Texas: Harcourt Brace.

Maslow's Hierarchy of Needs

Abraham Maslow is another psychologist who has influenced ideas about psychosocial health. Maslow is best known for his theory of needs. A **need** is that which is necessary or desirable for maintaining life and psychosocial well-being. According to Maslow, certain basic needs must be met for a person to survive and function. These needs are arranged in a *hierarchy*, or order of importance (Figure 6–1). Lower-level needs must be met before higher-level needs are met. These basic needs are, from the lowest level to the highest level:

- Physical needs—must be met first
- The need for safety
- The need for love and belonging
- The need for self-esteem
- The need for self-actualization—last need to be met

Some people will deliberately ignore a particular need for a period of time in order to meet another need. An example would be a person who spends his or her money on street drugs instead of food.

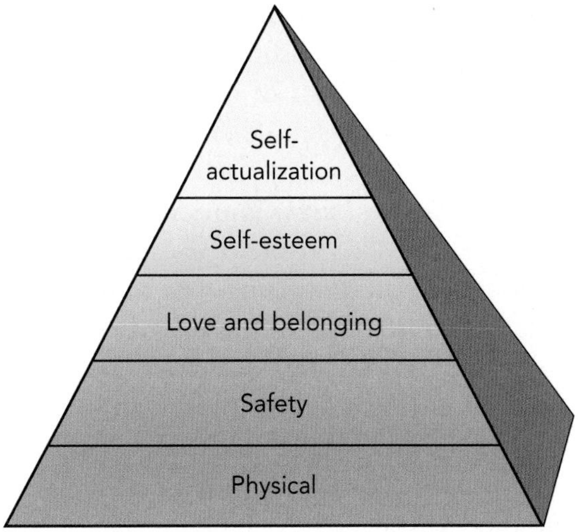

Figure 6–1 Maslow's hierarchy of needs. These needs, from the lowest to the highest level, are physical needs, the need for safety, the need for love and belonging, the need for self-esteem, and the need for self-actualization (the fulfillment of one's potential). **Source:** Maslow, Abraham H., Frager, Robert D (Editor), & Fadiman, James (Editor). (1987). *Motivation and personality* (3rd ed.). Reproduced by permission of Pearson Education, Inc., Upper Saddle River, New Jersey.

Physical Needs. The most basic needs in Maslow's hierarchy are physical needs. Oxygen, food, water, elimination, rest, and shelter are necessary for life, and since they are the most important for survival, they must be met before other needs. For example, people who are starving need food before they become concerned about their need for safety, self-esteem, and love.

Most adults are able to satisfy their own physical needs. However, children and seriously ill or disabled adults may depend on others to fulfill these needs. You, as the support worker, are often involved in meeting your clients' physical needs. For example, you feed clients who cannot feed themselves.

Safety Needs. Safety needs relate to protection from harm, danger, fear, and pain. Even minor illness and surgery can make people feel afraid. Most seriously ill clients feel extremely fearful. Many clients may be afraid of even health care procedures, as many of them involve frightening equipment, require invasive techniques, and cause pain and discomfort. Clients feel safer and more secure when they are able to understand these procedures. Even in the case of a simple bed bath, clients should be informed about:

- Why the procedure is to be done
- Who will do it
- How it will be performed
- What sensations or feelings to expect

Love and Belonging Needs. Love is a powerful human emotion that includes deep affection, tenderness, and devotion. Romantic love also involves physical desire. The need for belonging includes the need for a rightful place in society, in a peer group, and in a family. A peer group is a group of friends or acquaintances. Human beings are social creatures who need to be around others. When love and belonging needs are unfulfilled, people often feel lonely and rejected. Many cases have been reported where clients were slow to recover or died because of lack of love and belonging. This is particularly true of children and older adults (see *Supporting Mr. Cohen*).

Maslow believed that unfamiliar surroundings create a greater need for love and belonging. Clients in long-term care facilities have left their homes, friends, neighbours, pets, belongings, and familiar surroundings, so, as their support worker, you must be sensitive to the needs of those clients who are struggling with settling into their new environment.

Self-Esteem Needs. Esteem is the worth, value, or opinion one has of a person. **Self-esteem** is thinking well of oneself and being well thought of by others. When self-esteem needs are fulfilled, a person feels confident, adequate, and useful. Unmet self-esteem needs can result in feelings of inferiority, worthlessness, helplessness, and possibly depression. Clients often lose their self-esteem when they become ill or injured. Think about the following:

- How do ill parents feel when they cannot support or care for their children?
- Does a woman feel whole and attractive after a breast has been removed?
- Does a person who had a leg amputation feel complete, useful, and attractive?

You can help meet clients' self-esteem needs by being sensitive to their feelings and encouraging them to be as independent as possible.

Self-Actualization Needs. **Self-actualization** means realizing one's full potential. It involves learning, understanding, and creating to the best of one's ability. It is the highest need in the hierarchy and is rarely, if ever, met. Most people constantly try to learn more and understand more. However, the need for self-actualization can be postponed, and life will continue.

YOUR RELATIONSHIP WITH THE CLIENT

A **relationship** is the connection between two or more people and is shaped by the roles, feelings, and interactions of those involved. Relationships can be either personal or professional. It is unethical to mix a professional relationship with a personal relationship. As a support worker, you may get to know some of your clients very well. However, your relationship with your clients must remain professional at all times.

A Professional Helping Relationship

Your relationship with your clients is a professional helping relationship that is established to benefit the client. It is different from a friendship, which is a personal social relationship that benefits both persons involved. You relate to a client as a professional helper, not as a friend. Box 6–1 compares professional helping relationships with friendships.

supporting MR. COHEN

Isaac Cohen, a 92-year-old man, was brought to the hospital by the police, after neighbours reported that they had not seen him for several months. The police found him in his home alive but very thin and poorly nourished. He had not been able to go to the grocery store for over 2 months because he had fallen and broken his ankle while going to the bathroom. He managed to survive by eating the food he had in his house, and when he ran out of food, he ate dry cat food.

According to his neighbours, Mr. Cohen always lived alone and never had any visitors. He never spoke to his neighbours, but he always took care of his house and garden. His next door neighbour said that occasionally Mr. Cohen would give him bags of potatoes, beets, or other produce from his garden. Mr. Cohen would just ring the doorbell and silently hand the bag of produce to the person that answered the door. He never had a pet but would feed stray cats that wandered into his yard.

The hospital staff found out that before immigrating to Canada, he used to be a very religious man but stopped going to the synagogue after he lost his wife, his two children, his brother, and his nephew at Auschwitz, a concentration camp, during World War II. In Canada, he worked in a bakery. He never talked to anyone at work or elsewhere about what he had to endure at Auschwitz. Mr. Cohen would be going home once his ankle had healed but would require a support worker to assist him with shopping and light housework.

Box 6–1 Professional Helping Relationships Versus Friendships

Professional Helping Relationships	Friendships
One person takes the responsibility for helping the other.	The people involved are not responsible for helping each other. However, it is a choice they can make.
There is a specific goal to the relationship.	The relationship is not necessarily goal directed.
Behaviours are based on professional roles, such as support worker and client.	Behaviours are based on personal roles.
The people involved may not choose the relationship.	The people involved choose to have the relationship.
The helper seeks to fulfill the needs of the person being helped.	Both people in the relationship seek to have their needs fulfilled.
The helper is nonjudgemental.	Both people may be judgemental.

Adapted from: Arnold, E., & Underman Boggs, E. (1999). *Interpersonal relationships: Professional communication skills* (3rd ed., p. 82). Philadelphia: Saunders.

Although your professional relationship with a client is not a friendship, you should still show that you care about him or her. Treat the client with compassion and consideration, and recognize that each client is a unique individual. When working with clients, demonstrate the following:

- ***Respect***—showing acceptance and regard for another person. Accept your client's values, feelings, lifestyle, and decisions. When clients are treated with respect, they feel valued and important and when treated with disrespect, they feel ashamed, rejected, or hurt. Being respectful to clients means always being courteous and polite. For example, remember to say "please" and "thank you," as appropriate. Being overly familiar with clients can be seen as lack of respect. Calling clients by their first names without permission is an example of behaviour showing a lack of respect. Failing to recognize a client's need for privacy and independence can also be seen as lack of respect. Respect your client's preferences for how tasks should be done. As you perform the tasks, make sure that the client is comfortable, safe, and satisfied. Encourage clients to express preferences, make personal choices, and do as much as they can for themselves.
- ***Compassion***—is characterized by a person's awareness of the misfortune and suffering of another and the desire and actions taken to reduce or alleviate the problem. Compassion requires an understanding that bad things can happen to people through no fault of their own. Compassion is not the same as pity. To pity someone may imply that you feel superior to that person. (See the *Support Workers Solving Problems: Demonstrating Compassion* box on page 72.)
- ***Empathy***—is the ability to recognize, perceive, and have an understanding of another's emotions by being able to put oneself in another person's shoes. Empathy involves being receptive to others and not being judgemental. Compassion and empathy are similar. Compassion is felt in response to suffering, whereas empathy may be felt in response to a full range of emotions. For example, a client is told that her son has successfully come through a potentially dangerous heart operation. You, as her support worker, feel great joy and relief at the news. Your feelings show that you are sensitive to your client's situation and share her reactions. It is not enough to *feel* empathy for a person. You must also *show* the client that you empathize. Eye contact and physical closeness can show empathy. So can a smile or a kind word. An empathetic response can

SUPPORT WORKERS SOLVING PROBLEMS

Demonstrating Compassion

<< Scenario >>

Mark Vickers, 16, has Down syndrome. His mother recently died of cancer, and since Mark's father abandoned the family long ago and Mark has no siblings or other family nearby, he has been moved into a group home.

Cynthia is a support worker in the group home. She notices that Mark sits all day in his room, staring at the wall. He refuses to join the other clients in the common room.

<< Discussion >>

Cynthia has great compassion for Mark. She tries to imagine what it must be like to lose the only person you had in the world and to be moved to a strange, new place. Cynthia recognizes that Mark needs time to deal with his grief and loneliness. She spends as much time as she can with Mark, sometimes simply sitting with him and holding his hand. Her quiet acceptance of his sadness comforts Mark. After a few days, he begins to open up to Cynthia.

decrease loneliness and create feelings of well-being and belonging in a client.

- ***Sympathy***—sympathy differs from empathy. Empathy involves listening and understanding, whereas sympathy involves reacting. When you sympathize with your clients, you identify with their feelings to the point where you take on their pain. Instead of merely listening, a sympathetic person often offers advice and solutions. You must remember that the role of a professional caregiver is to provide the information the client needs in order to make informed decisions. Taking on the problems of your clients on yourself can leave you tense, tired, and anxious.
- ***Competence***—performing your job well. You must perform your tasks as a support worker safely and skillfully. You must be well-organized, punctual, and reliable. You must know your scope of practice and personal limits. At the same time, you should be flexible and responsive to the client's needs. By being competent, you will earn the client's trust.
- ***Self-Awareness***—understanding one's own feelings, moods, attitudes, preferences, biases, qualities, and limitations. You must know yourself well in order to be genuine and nonjudgemental with others, and this requires examining your own feelings and behaviours in an honest manner. (See the *Support Workers Solving Problems: Demonstrating Self-Awareness* box.)

Independence, Dependence, and Interdependence

Independence, dependence, and interdependence are fundamental concepts in professional helping relationships.

SUPPORT WORKERS SOLVING PROBLEMS

Demonstrating Self-Awareness

<< Scenario >>

Mr. Raftis requires assistance with self-care. Maia is the support worker who has been providing care for 8 days. One morning, Mr. Raftis complains to Maia that she is too rough when shaving him. Maia feels that Mr. Raftis is questioning her competence and is hurt by his comment. She becomes quiet and withdrawn.

<< Discussion >>

Later, Maia thinks about her reaction to Mr. Raftis's comment and feels upset with herself for having let the comment affect how she treated Mr. Raftis. Mr. Raftis and Maia usually carry on a lively conversation while she is providing care, but after his comment, she barely said a word. She realizes that this may have had something to do with the fact that when she was a child, her father used to criticize her constantly, making her feel incompetent. Once she understands the reason for her hurt feelings, Maia understands that Mr. Raftis's comment was constructive rather than critical. The next day, she asks Mr. Raftis to explain how he would like to be shaved, and together they decide how she can make it more comfortable for him.

- **Independence** is the state of not depending on others for control or authority. People who are independent control and direct their own lives, and can do things for themselves.
- **Dependence** is the state of relying on others for support and being unable to manage without help.
- **Interdependence** is the state of depending on each other. In most interdependent relationships, each person relies upon the other for some things.

The above terms must be considered in relation to one another. No one is completely independent, and only infants, very young children, and unconscious people are completely dependent. Most people's relationships have elements of all three.

For example, Julie considers herself independent. She feels she is in control of her busy and rewarding life as a support worker, wife, and mother of two young boys. She works full-time and drives her children to day care. Julie is independent because she is in control of her career and her home life. However, she also depends on others. Without reliable child care, she cannot work full time. Julie and her husband have an interdependent relationship—they rely on each other for emotional support and companionship and also for help with childrearing, housework, grocery shopping, and cooking.

An important goal of most clients' care is to achieve or maintain as much independence as possible (Figure 6–2). Everyone makes choices about when to do things for themselves and when to rely on others. These choices involve setting goals and priorities. As a support worker, you must respect your client's choices to do some things independently and to accept help with other things, even though you may not fully understand the reason for these choices.

For example, Elena is hired to help Ms. Godin, 31, who has cerebral palsy. Elena's role is to help Ms. Godin get ready for work in the morning. Elena knows that Ms. Godin is capable of dressing, showering, and preparing breakfast without help. However, each task takes a long time for Ms. Godin. She chooses to put her energies into her work, not into getting ready for work. Elena respectfully accepts Ms. Godin's choices. Clients, like everyone else, make choices according to their wishes and capabilities and must never feel that you are judging their decisions.

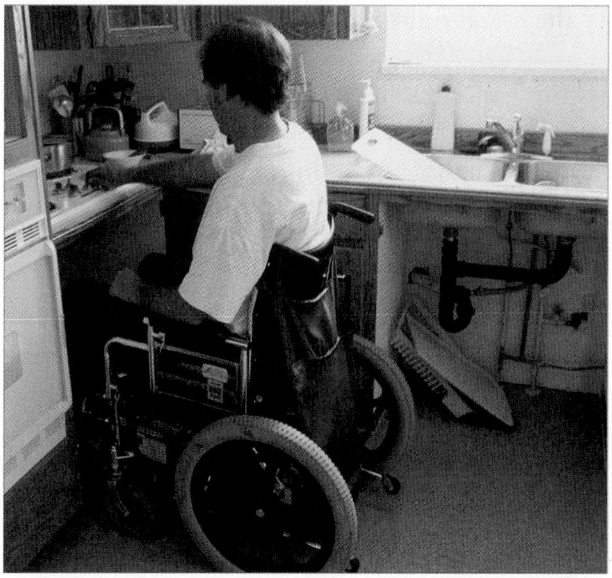

Figure 6–2 This client is able to function independently at home. **Source:** Al Harvey.

Independence and Self-Esteem

What makes you feel good about yourself? Working hard at your job or school? Playing a sport? Caring for your family? How would you feel if you could no longer do these things? Self-esteem often develops when people feel that their lives have meaning for themselves and others. Self-esteem is also closely associated with independence.

For children, attaining power and control over their bodies and their environments helps develop self-esteem. Self-esteem can suffer when independence is limited or lost. People's roles and identities can change when they are no longer in control of their lives (see Chapter 4). You must be sensitive to how clients feel when they lose their independence because of illness or disability.

Clients who have lost their independence need to find ways to rebuild their self-esteem. While some clients who cannot do this become frustrated or depressed, others are able to find a new purpose in life. For example, Ricardo became quadriplegic at the age of 17. He and two friends had been drinking at a party. On the way home, the driver lost control of the car and hit a telephone pole. Ricardo's two friends died at the scene, and Ricardo was in hospital for 7 months. He became so depressed that he wished he had died with his friends in the accident. Then his high school principal asked him to speak to the students about the dangers of drinking and driving. Ricardo agreed, and since then, he has spoken to students at every school in his community, which has given him a purpose in life.

You can reinforce a client's self-esteem by offering encouragement and praising the client's successes. If the client is not successful yet, you should recognize the efforts made. You might say, "I can see how hard you are trying." Give the client honest, constructive feedback, in a gentle, supportive fashion.

Independence and Balance of Power

In any relationship in which one person is dependent on the other, the balance of power may not be equal. The strong, independent person may control the vulnerable, dependent person. In some situations, this may lead to the stronger person abusing the dependent person (see Chapter 21).

Be aware of the balance of power in your relationships with your clients. It is important to avoid any controlling behaviour, since it is easy to be controlling without being aware of it. For example, Lynn's client, Mrs. Kerr, insists on wearing a blouse with 10 tiny buttons and doing them up herself. Mrs. Kerr takes 3 minutes to do up the first button. Lynn does not have 30 minutes to help Mrs. Kerr dress. She suggests to Mrs. Kerr that she wear something else but Mrs. Kerr refuses. She is expecting visitors and wants to look good. Lynn undoes the button, removes the blouse, and hands Mrs. Kerr another garment, while saying, "You will look just as nice in this sweater."

Instead of imposing your will on your clients, involve them in solving problems that may arise. For example, Lynn could have explained to Mrs. Kerr that her time was limited, and together they could have thought of some solutions. Lynn might have suggested that they take turns to do up the buttons. Or she might have suggested that she carry on with doing other tasks (like tidying the room) while Mrs. Kerr dressed herself. Or Lynn could set some guidelines at the very beginning of the day's schedule. "Mrs. Kerr, I have 20 minutes today, and this is what we have to accomplish in that time frame."

THE CLIENT'S FAMILY

Close personal and family relationships are central to the lives of most people and involve some forms of dependency. Spouses depend on one another for emotional support, companionship, and financial support. Children depend on their parents to meet their physical, emotional, and financial needs. Older parents may depend on their adult children to help them with physical and emotional needs.

The **family** is a biological, legal, or social network of people who provide support for one another. Families can take many forms and may include people related by blood or marriage or unrelated people who have formed a close personal relationship. Examples of families include:

- A married couple with or without children or stepchildren
- An unmarried couple living together, with or without children
- A widowed grandmother raising two grandchildren
- A divorced parent living with a partner, who has children living elsewhere
- Two women or two men living together in a same-sex relationship
- Older parents, adult children, and grandchildren living together

You may have different ideas about what a family is. However, as a support worker, you must always respect your client's definition of family. Your client will determine who he or she regards as family. Do not impose your values on the person.

Your Role in Assisting the Family

There are many situations in which you help families in your role as a support worker. You may care for new mothers and their babies. You may care for toddlers or older children when their parent is ill or unavailable. You may assist or provide needed respite for a **primary caregiver**. A primary caregiver is the person (usually a family member or close friend) who assumes the responsibilities of caring for an ill or disabled person in the home (see the *Focus on Home Care: Assisting the Primary Caregiver* box). Whatever the situation, when working with a family, you indirectly support their relationships. By providing a family with basic care and support services, you enable family members to invest more time and energy in their relationships.

Chapter 4 discussed how roles change when illness or disability strikes a family. Very often, one family member becomes the primary caregiver of another family member. They form a different relationship, with new patterns of dependency, and this is rarely easy. The ill client may feel angry at having to depend on the caregiver. The caregiver may feel burdened by the new responsibility in addition to other family and work demands.

Professionals on the health care team prepare family members to take on care responsibilities. When helping families cope, they consider the physical, emotional, social, spiritual, and intellectual health of all family members. They also consider relationships within the family, including any conflict and potential for conflict. They may help the family deal with stress by working on improving communication skills and problem-solving abilities of family members. This sometimes involves bringing them together in a family conference to discuss the ill person's care and its impact on the entire family. As a support worker, you may sometimes be asked to attend such family conferences.

focus on
›› HOME CARE

Assisting the Primary Caregiver

Sometimes you work closely with the client's primary caregiver. For example, you assist Mrs. Kalopsis with housekeeping and meal preparation so that she can spend more time caring for her ill husband.

Primary caregivers are often relieved to have assistance from the health care team. However, some may have mixed feelings about your presence in their home. Some people may resent the interruption to their routine, and others may feel that you are invading their privacy. Some caregivers may also feel that they are failures for needing help or may regret that someone else is accomplishing tasks that they wish they had accomplished themselves.

Try to put the family caregivers at ease by showing that you are there to help, not to take over or judge their housekeeping or caregiving skills. Do not take on tasks that have not been assigned to you.

Adapt your support work to suit the family's standards and preferences, not your own. Respect the family's routines, schedules, and way of doing things. Consult with your supervisor if you think the family's wishes may affect safety.

Families in Conflict

When illness or disability occurs, the stress on all family members may be great and they have to cope with conflict. Conflicts may take the form of expressions of irritation, anger, bickering, and arguments. Conflict may sometimes be hidden. Adult children may care for aging parents with whom they have unresolved conflicts. Siblings who have not spoken in years may be forced to see one another during a parent's illness. Sometimes the health care team can help families resolve their difficulties in such situations. Members of palliative care teams are specially trained to help people resolve emotional problems that are causing them distress.

When working with a family, be aware of family relationships and any conflicts, communication difficulties, and stressful situations (Figure 6–3). It is not part of your role to help families deal with their interpersonal problems, but there are some things you can do in a stressful situation. You could encourage communication without taking sides, or you can defuse (calm) a tense situation—for example, when angry words have been exchanged between the client and a family member, you may suggest to the family member to go out for a coffee (see Chapter 9). Agencies and facilities have policies to guide you in dealing with conflicts you might encounter. You must observe and report on family interactions (see the

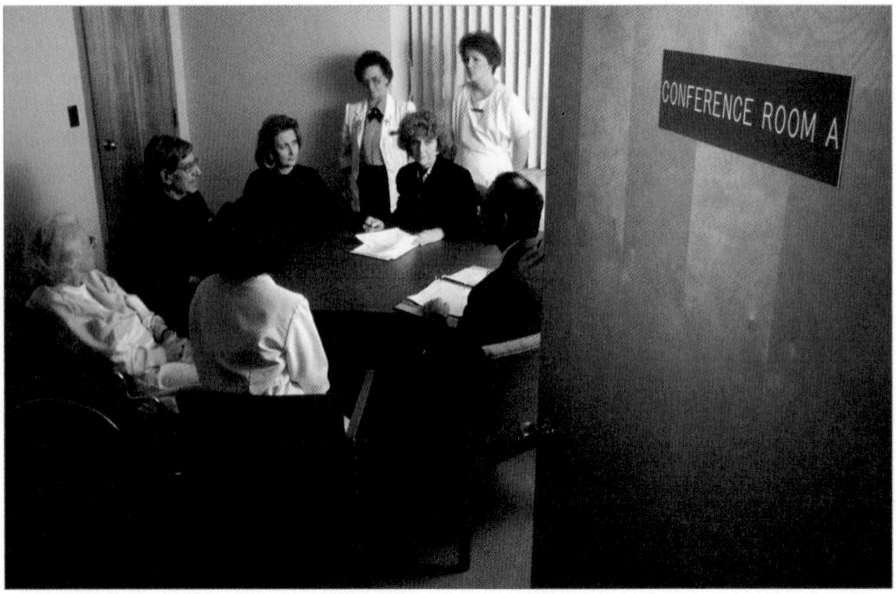

Figure 6–3 A family conference discusses a loved one's needs and care requirements and their effect on the family. The client, client's family, case manager, support workers, and any other health professionals involved in the client's care may attend.
Source: Frank Siteman/Rainbow.

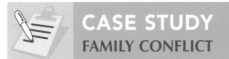

CASE STUDY
FAMILY CONFLICT

Mei is a support worker. She tells the following story about her experience working with a family in conflict.

"When I look back on the families I've worked with, one in particular stands out. Mr. Skala was an older man with cancer. His wife was his primary caregiver. They had a daughter living nearby who had a family of her own. Just before Mr. Skala became ill, there was a major argument over the family business. The result was that their daughter refused to speak to her parents. The Skalas' son-in-law brought their two young grandchildren to visit, but their daughter never came. She refused all attempts to resolve the conflict.

Mrs. Skala found this situation extremely hard to bear. She asked me to talk to her daughter to try to mend the rift. I felt for Mrs. Skala and wanted to help, but I had to tell Mrs. Skala that it wasn't my role to get involved in the family's problems. The case manager arranged for a social worker to talk with them. Eventually, the daughter resolved her differences with her parents. In the last 3 weeks of Mr. Skala's life, the family spent meaningful time together."

REVIEW

Answers to these questions are at the bottom of the page.

Circle the BEST answer.

1. **Which of the following is *true?***
   A. Every client is a unique individual
   B. Clients of the same age with the same condition are much the same
   C. Support workers should only focus on the client's physical problems
   D. People are not influenced by their genetics and their environments

2. **Psychosocial health is the achievement of:**
   A. Well-being in the social, emotional, intellectual, and spiritual dimensions of one's life
   B. Secure, intimate love relationships
   C. Good physical health
   D. Strong social bonds in the community

3. **Which is part of Erikson's theory of psychosocial development?**
   A. People must successfully complete a task in each stage before moving on to the next
   B. Babies do not learn to trust that their needs will be met
   C. People do not need to move through a series of stages throughout their lives
   D. Moving to unfamiliar surroundings creates love and belonging needs

4. **Maslow's hierarchy of needs can best be described as:**
   A. Another term for psychosocial health
   B. A system that arranges human needs into categories
   C. Physiological and safety needs
   D. Love and belonging needs

5. **Which of the following is part of Maslow's hierarchy of needs?**
   A. Financial needs
   B. Trust needs
   C. Intimacy needs
   D. Physical needs

6. **A professional helping relationship is established for the benefit of the:**
   A. Client and support worker
   B. Client, support worker, and health care team
   C. Client
   D. Client's family

7. **Empathy is:**
   A. Feelings of pity for another person
   B. Being open to and trying to understand the experiences and feelings of others
   C. Showing acceptance and regard for another person
   D. The process of enabling others to set and achieve goals

8. **Common courtesy is a sign of:**
   A. Empathy
   B. Interdependence
   C. Respect
   D. Need

9. **Independence is:**
   A. Not depending on others for control or authority
   B. Being unable to manage without help
   C. Relying on others for support
   D. Showing acceptance for another person

10. **When supporting clients from families in conflict, your supervisor expects you to:**
   A. Help family members resolve conflict
   B. Observe and report on family interactions
   C. Ignore any conflict you witness
   D. Take sides in family arguments

Circle T if the answer is true or circle F if the answer is false.

11. T F **Conflict in families may be hidden.**

12. T F **Part of your role is to help families deal with their interpersonal problems.**

13. T F **You should always take your client's side in a disagreement.**

Answers: 1.A, 2.A, 3.A, 4.B, 5.D, 6.C, 7.B, 8.C, 9.A, 10.B, 11.T, 12.F, 13.F

CHAPTER 7

Medical Terminology

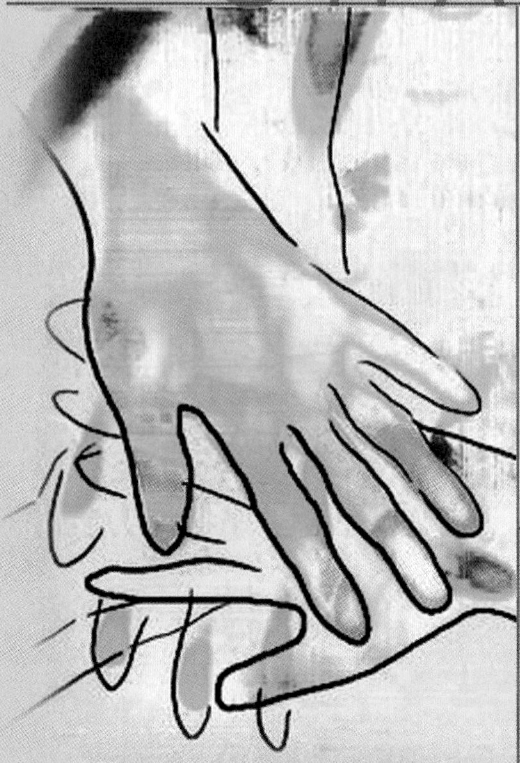

OBJECTIVES

- Define the key terms listed in this chapter.
- Identify three word elements used in medical terms.
- Learn the meanings of common Greek and Latin prefixes, roots, and suffixes.
- Combine word elements into medical terms.
- Learn the meanings of common medical terms.
- Identify the four abdominal regions.
- Define the directional terms that describe the positions of the body in relation to other body parts.
- Identify and define some of the abbreviations used in health care.

key terms

abbreviation A shortened form of a word or phrase.

anterior Located at or toward the front of the body or body part; ventral.

combining vowel A vowel added between two roots or between a root and a suffix to make pronunciation easier.

distal The part farthest from the centre or from the point of attachment.

dorsal Located at or toward the back of the body or body part; posterior.

lateral Relating to or located at the side of the body or body part.

medial Relating to or located at or near the middle or midline of the body or body part.

posterior See **dorsal**.

prefix A word element placed at the beginning of a word to change the meaning of the word.

proximal The part nearest to the centre or to the point of origin.

root A word element containing the basic meaning of the word.

suffix A word element placed at the end of a root to change the meaning of the word.

ventral See **anterior**.

word element A part of a word.

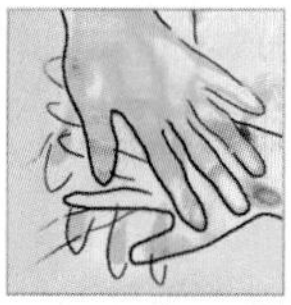

Many people find medical language mysterious and secretive—the private code of physicians and nurses—and yet people use medical terms every day. Examples are *flu*, *diarrhea*, *cancer*, *appendectomy*, *cardiac*, and *pneumonia.* Health and medicine get a lot of attention in the media, and because of so much coverage, many medical terms are understood by most people.

Knowing medical terminology is important in your work as a support worker. As you gain more knowledge and experience, you will understand and use medical terms often and with ease. Learning medical terms for illnesses, diseases, and common things like bruises, baldness, and a "runny nose" can be fun and educational. This chapter introduces medical terminology and the common abbreviations used in health care. It is very important that you use correct terms and abbreviations for creating clear charts. There could be legal consequences if incorrect terms are used, as charts are legal documents.

WORD ELEMENTS

Like all words, medical terms are made up of parts, or **word elements,** that are combined in various ways to form medical terms. A term is translated by separating the word into its elements. Important word elements are prefixes, roots, and suffixes, which are all based in the Greek and Latin languages.

Prefixes

A **prefix** is a word element placed at the beginning of a word and changes the meaning of the word. The prefix *olig* (scant, small amount) is placed before the word *uria* (urine) to make *oliguria*—meaning a scant amount of urine. Prefixes are always combined with other word elements. They are never used alone. You need to learn the following prefixes to begin understanding medical terminology:

Prefix	**Meaning**
a-, an-	without, not, lack of
ab-	away from
ad-	to, toward, near
ante-	before, forward, in front of
anti-	against
auto-	self
bi-	double, two, twice
brady-	slow
circum-	around
contra-	against, opposite

Prefix	Meaning
de-	down, from
dia-	across, through, apart
dis-	apart, free from
dys-	difficult, abnormal
ecto-	outer, outside
en-	in, into, within
endo-	inner, inside
epi-	over, on, upon
eryth-	red
eu-	normal, good, well, healthy
ex-	out, out of, from, away from
hemi-	half
hyper-	excessive, too much, high
hypo-	under, decreased, less than normal
in-	in, into, within, not
infra-	within
inter-	between
intra-	into, within
leuk-	white
macro-	large
mal-	illness, disease
meg-	large
micro-	small
mono-	one, single
neo-	new
non-	not
olig-	small, scant
para-	beside, beyond, after
per-	by, through
peri-	around
poly-	many, much
post-	after, behind
pre-	before, in front of, prior to
pro-	before, in front of
re-	again, backward
retro-	backward, behind
semi-	half
sub-	under, beneath
super-	above, over, excess
supra-	above, over
tachy-	fast, rapid
trans-	across, over
uni-	one

Roots

The **root** contains the basic meaning of the word. It is combined with another root, with prefixes, and with suffixes in various combinations to form a medical term.

A vowel is added when two roots are combined or when a suffix is added to a root. The vowel is called a **combining vowel** and is usually an *o*. An *i* is sometimes used when there is no vowel between the two combined roots or between the root and the suffix. A combining vowel makes pronunciation easier.

The most common roots and their combining vowels are listed here:

Root (combining vowel)	Meaning
abdomin(o)	abdomen
aden(o)	gland
adren(o)	adrenal gland
angi(o)	vessel
arteri(o)	artery
arthr(o)	joint
bronch(o)	bronchus, bronchi
card, cardi(o)	heart
cephal(o)	head
chole, chol(o)	bile
chondr(o)	cartilage
colo	colon, large intestine
cost(o)	rib
crani(o)	skull
cyan(o)	blue
cyst(o)	bladder, cyst
cyt(o)	cell
dent(o)	tooth
derma	skin
duoden(o)	duodenum
encephal(o)	brain
enter(o)	intestines
fibr(o)	fibre, fibrous
gastr(o)	stomach
gloss(o)	tongue
gluc(o)	sweetness, glucose
glyc(o)	sugar
gyn, gyne, gyneco	woman
hem, hema, hemo, hemat(o)	blood
hepat(o)	liver
hydr(o)	water
hyster(o)	uterus
ile(o), ili(o)	ileum
laparo	abdomen, loin, or flank

Root (combining vowel)	Meaning
laryng(o)	larynx
lith(o)	stone
mamm(o)	breast, mammary gland
mast(o)	mammary gland, breast
meno	menstruation
my(o)	muscle
myel(o)	spinal cord, bone marrow
necro	death
nephr(o)	kidney
neur(o)	nerve
ocul(o)	eye
oophor(o)	ovary
ophthalm(o)	eye
orth(o)	straight, normal, correct
oste(o)	bone
ot(o)	ear
ped(o)	child, foot
pharyng(o)	pharynx
phleb(o)	vein
pnea	breathing, respiration
pneum(o)	lung, air, gas
proct(o)	rectum
psych(o)	mind
pulmo	lung
py(o)	pus
rect(o)	rectum
rhin(o)	nose
salping(o)	eustachian tube, uterine tube
splen(o)	spleen
sten(o)	narrow, constriction
stern(o)	sternum
stomat(o)	mouth
therm(o)	heat
thoraco	chest
thromb(o)	clot, thrombus
thyr(o)	thyroid
toxic(o)	poison, poisonous
toxo	poison
trache(o)	trachea
urethr(o)	urethra
urin(o)	urine
uro	urine, urinary tract, urination
uter(o)	uterus
vas(o)	blood vessel, vas deferens
ven(o)	vein
vertebr(o)	spine, vertebrae

Suffixes

A **suffix** is placed at the end of a root to change the meaning of the word, but it is not used alone. For example, *nephritis* means inflammation of the kidney. It is formed by combining *nephro* (kidney) and *itis* (inflammation).

You need to learn the suffixes listed below:

Suffix	Meaning
-algia	pain
-asis	condition, usually abnormal
-cele	hernia, herniation, pouching
-centesis	puncture and aspiration of
-cyte	cell
-ectasis	dilation, stretching
-ectomy	excision, removal of
-emia	blood condition
-genesis	development, production, creation
-genic	producing, causing
-gram	record
-graph	a diagram, a recording instrument
-graphy	making a recording
-iasis	condition of
-ism	a condition
-itis	inflammation
-logy	the study of
-lysis	destruction of, decomposition
-megaly	enlargement
-meter	measuring instrument
-metry	measurement
-oma	tumour
-osis	condition
-pathy	disease
-penia	lack, deficiency
-phasia	speaking
-phobia	an exaggerated fear
-plasty	surgical repair or reshaping
-plegia	paralysis
-ptosis	falling, sagging, dropping, down
-rrhage, -rrhagia	excessive flow
-rrhaphy	stitching, suturing
-rrhea	profuse flow, discharge
-scope	examination instrument
-scopy	examination using a scope
-stasis	maintenance, maintaining a constant level

Suffix	Meaning
-stomy, -ostomy	creation of an opening
-tomy, -otomy	incision, cutting into
-uria	condition of the urine

COMBINING WORD ELEMENTS

Medical terms are formed by combining word elements. A root can be combined with prefixes, roots, or suffixes. The prefix *dys* (difficult) can be combined with the root *pnea* (breathing) to form the term *dyspnea,* meaning "difficulty in breathing."

Roots can be combined with suffixes. The root *mast* (breast) combined with the suffix *ectomy* (excision or removal) forms the term *mastectomy,* which means "removal of a breast."

Combining a prefix, root, and suffix is another way to form medical terms. *Endocarditis* (meaning "inflammation of the inner part of the heart") consists of the prefix *endo* (inner), the root *card* (heart), and the suffix *itis* (inflammation).

More complex combinations of prefixes, roots, and suffixes can be created:

- Two prefixes, a root, and a suffix
- A prefix, two roots, and a suffix
- Two roots and a suffix

The important things to remember are that (a) prefixes always come before roots, and (b) suffixes always come after roots. You can practise forming medical terms by combining the word elements listed in this chapter.

ABDOMINAL REGIONS

The abdomen is divided into regions (Figure 7–1) in order to help describe the location of body structures, pain, or discomfort. The regions are:

- Right upper quadrant (RUQ)
- Left upper quadrant (LUQ)
- Right lower quadrant (RLQ)
- Left lower quadrant (LLQ)

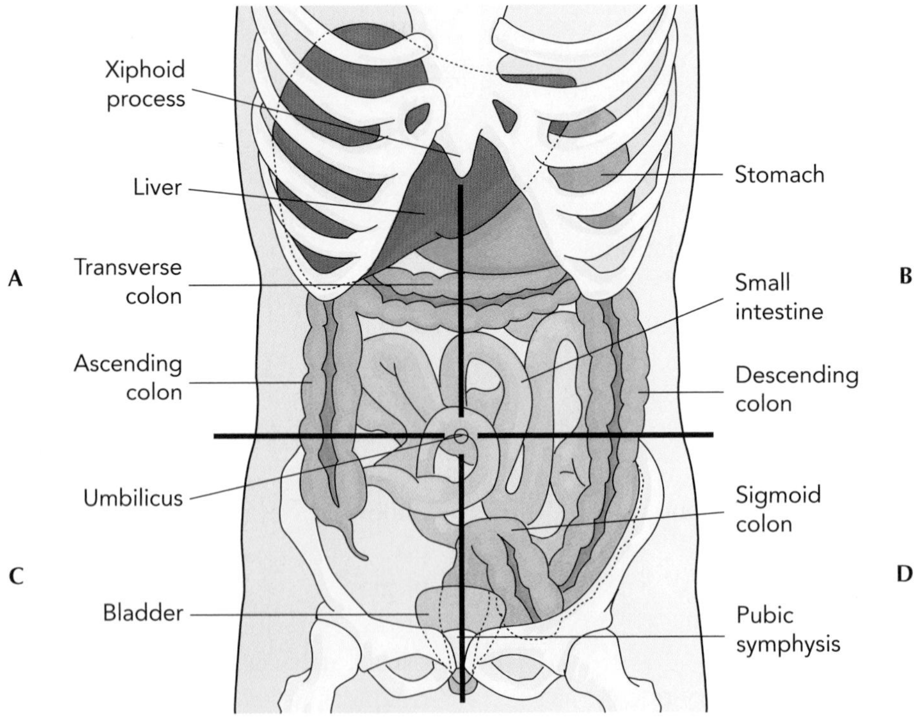

Figure 7–1 The four regions of the abdomen. **A,** Right upper quadrant. **B,** Left upper quadrant. **C,** Right lower quadrant. **D,** Left lower quadrant.

DIRECTIONAL TERMS

Certain terms describe the position of one body part in relation to another. These terms indicate the direction of the body part when a person is standing and facing forward. The following directional terms come from some of the prefixes listed earlier in this chapter:

- ***Anterior (ventral)***—located at or toward the front of the body or body part
- ***Distal***—the part farthest from the centre or from the point of attachment; for example, the foot is distal to the knee.
- ***Lateral***—relating to or located at the side of the body or body part
- ***Medial***—relating to or located at or near the middle or midline of the body or body part.
- ***Posterior (dorsal)***—located at or toward the back of the body or body part
- ***Proximal***—the part nearest to the centre or to the point of origin

ABBREVIATIONS

Abbreviations are shortened forms of words or phrases and save time and space in written communication (see table on the following page). Each employer has a list of accepted abbreviations. Obtain the list when you are hired as a support worker, and use only the abbreviations accepted by your employer. If you are unsure whether an abbreviation is acceptable, write the term out in full to communicate accurately.

COMMON ABBREVIATIONS

ABBREV.	MEANING
abd	abdomen
ac	before meals
ADL	activities of daily living
ad lib	as desired
AM (am)	morning
amb	ambulatory
amt	amount
ap	apical
bid	twice a day
BM (bm)	bowel movement
BP	blood pressure
BRP	bathroom privileges
$\bar{c}$	with
C	centigrade
CA	cancer
cath	catheter
CBC	complete blood count
CBR	complete bed rest
cc	cubic centimetre
c/o	complains of
CO_2	carbon dioxide
CPR	cardiopulmonary resuscitation
dc (d/c)	discontinue
DOA	dead on arrival
DON	director of nursing
drsg	dressing
dx	diagnosis
ECG (EKG)	electrocardiogram
EEG	electroencephalogram
ER	emergency room
F	Fahrenheit
FBS	fasting blood sugar
fl (fld)	fluid
gal	gallon
GB	gallbladder
GI	gastrointestinal
h (hr)	hour
H_2O	water
HS (hs)	hour of sleep
ht	height
in	inch
I&O	intake and output
IV	intravenous
L	left, litre
lab	laboratory
liq	liquid
LLQ	left lower quadrant
lt	left
LPN	licensed practical nurse
LVN	licensed vocational nurse
LUQ	left upper quadrant
meds	medications
mid noc	midnight

ABBREV.	MEANING
min	minute
mL	millilitre
neg	negative
noc	night
NPO (npo)	nothing by mouth
O_2	oxygen
OB	obstetrics
OOB	out of bed
OR	operating room
OT	occupational therapy
oz (Oz)	ounce
pc	after meals
peds	pediatrics
per	by, through
PM (pm)	after noon
po (per os)	by mouth
postop (post op)	postoperative
preop (pre op)	preoperative
prep	preparation
prn	when necessary
Pt (pt)	patient
PT	physiotherapy
$\bar{q}$	every
qd	every day
qh	every hour
q2h, q3h, etc.	every 2 hours, every 3 hours, and so on
qhs	every night at bedtime
qid	four times a day
qod	every other day
R	rectal temperature; respiration; right
RBC	red blood cell; red blood count
RLQ	right lower quadrant
RN	registered nurse
ROM	range of motion
RPN	registered practical nurse; registered psychiatric nurse
RUQ	right upper quadrant
$\bar{s}$	without
SOB	shortness of breath
Spec (spec)	specimen
SSE	soap suds enema
stat	at once, immediately
tbsp	tablespoon
tid	three times a day
TLC	tender loving care
TPR	temperature, pulse, and respirations
tsp	teaspoon
U/a (U/A, u/a)	urinalysis
VS (vs)	vital signs
WBC	white blood cell; white blood count
w/c	wheel chair
wt	weight

REVIEW

Answers to these questions are on page 87.

Fill in the blanks.

1. **Word elements used in medical terminology are:**
   A. PREFIX
   B. ROOT
   C. SUFFIX
2. **A** PREFIX **is placed at the beginning of a word to change the meaning of the word.**
3. **A** SUFFIX **is placed at the end of a word to change the meaning of the word.**
4. **The four regions of the abdomen are:**
   A. RUQ
   B. LUQ
   C. RLQ
   D. LUQ

Match the item in column A with its meaning in column B.

Column A	Column B
5. Distal	6 A. The part nearest to the centre or point of origin
6. Proximal	10 B. Relating to or located at the side of the body or body part
7. Anterior (ventral)	7 C. Located at or toward the front part of the body or body part
8. Medial	5 D. The part farthest from the centre or point of attachment
9. Posterior (dorsal)	9 E. Located at or toward the back of the body or body part
10. Lateral	8 F. Relating to or located at or near the middle or the midline of the body or body part

Write the definition of the following prefixes.

11. **a-** WITHOUT
12. **dys-** DIFFICULT
13. **bi-** DOUBLE, TWO, TWICE
14. **ab-** AWAY FROM
15. **trans-** ACROSS, OVER
16. **post-** AFTER, BEHIND
17. **olig-** SCANT, SMALL
18. **hyper-** EXCESSIVE, TOO MUCH
19. **per-** BY, THROUGH
20. **hemi-** HALF
21. **hypo-** UNDER, DECREASED
22. **ad-** TO, TOWARD, NEAR

Write the definition of the following suffixes.

23. **-algia** PAIN
24. **-itis** INFLAMMATION
25. **-ostomy** CREATION OF AN OPENING
26. **-ectomy** REMOVAL OF
27. **-emia** BLOOD CONDITION
28. **-osis** CONDITION
29. **-rrhage** EXCESSIVE FLOW
30. **-penia** LACK, DEFICIENCY
31. **-pathy** DISEASE
32. **-otomy** INCISION, CUTTING INTO
33. **-rrhea** DISCHARGE
34. **-plasty** SURGICAL REPAIR

REVIEW

Answers to these questions are on page 87.

Write the definition of the following roots.

35. cranio SKULL
36. cardio HEART
37. mammo BREAST
38. veno VEIN
39. urino URINE
40. pnea BREATHING, RESPIRATION
41. cyano BLUE
42. arterio ARTERY
43. colo COLON; LARGE INTESTINE
44. arthro JOINT
45. litho STONE
46. gastro STOMACH
47. encephalo BRAIN
48. gluco GLUCOSE, SWEETNESS
49. hemo BLOOD
50. hystero UTERUS
51. hepato LIVER
52. myo MUSCLE
53. nephro KIDNEY
54. phlebo VEIN
55. oculo EYE
56. osteo BONE
57. neuro NERVE
58. pneumo LUNG
59. toxico POISON
60. psycho MIND
61. thoraco CHEST

Match the item in column A with the item in column B.

Column A	Column B
62. Intravenous	66 A. Inflammation of a joint
63. Apnea	69 B. Blood in the urine
64. Hemiplegia	71 C. Excessive flow of blood
65. Thoracotomy	64 D. Paralysis on one side
66. Arthritis	70 E. Surgical removal of the uterus
67. Bronchitis	63 F. No breathing
68. Anuria	67 G. Inflammation of the bronchi
69. Hematuria	65 H. Incision into the chest
70. Hysterectomy	68 I. No urine
71. Hemorrhage	62 J. Within a vein

Write the abbreviation for the following terms.

72. Bathroom privileges BPR
73. As desired Ad lib
74. Complains of C/O
75. Twice a day bid
76. Hour of sleep HS
77. Intake and output I&O
78. Nothing by mouth NPO
79. When necessary PRN
80. Postoperative POSTOP
81. Every q̄
82. Wheelchair W/W
83. At once, immediately STAT.

Answers:

1. A. Prefix, B. Root, C. Suffix
2. Prefix
3. Suffix
4. A. Right upper quadrant, B. Left upper quadrant, C. Right lower quadrant, D. Left lower quadrant
5. D
6. A
7. C
8. F
9. E
10. B
11. Without, not, lack of
12. Difficult, abnormal
13. Double, two, twice
14. Away from
15. Across, over
16. After, behind
17. Scant, small
18. Excessive, too much
19. By, through
20. Half
21. Under, decreased, less than normal
22. To, toward, near
23. Pain
24. Inflammation
25. Creation of an opening
26. Removal of, excision
27. Blood condition
28. Condition
29. Excessive flow
30. Lack, deficiency
31. Disease
32. Incision, cutting into
33. Profuse flow, discharge
34. Surgical repair or reshaping
35. Skull
36. Heart
37. Breast
38. Vein
39. Urine
40. Breathing, respiration
41. Blue
42. Artery
43. Colon, large intestine
44. Joint
45. Stone
46. Stomach
47. Brain
48. Glucose, sweetness
49. Blood
50. Uterus
51. Liver
52. Muscle
53. Kidney
54. Vein
55. Eye
56. Bone
57. Nerve
58. Lung
59. Poison
60. Mind
61. Chest
62. J
63. F
64. D
65. H
66. A
67. G
68. I
69. B
70. E
71. C
72. BRP
73. Ad lib
74. c/o
75. bid
76. HS (hs)
77. I&O
78. NPO (npo)
79. prn
80. postop (post op)
81. $\overline{q}$
82. w/c
83. stat

CHAPTER 8

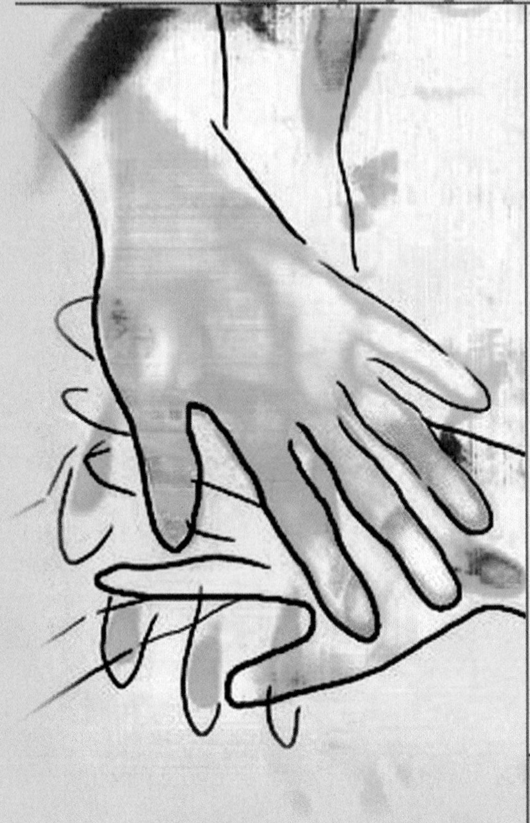

Client Care: Planning, Processes, Reporting, and Recording

OBJECTIVES

- Define the key terms listed in this chapter.
- Explain the steps in the care planning process in facilities.
- Explain the steps in the care planning process in the community.
- Explain the function of the care plan.
- Describe your role in the care planning process.
- Explain why observation is an important part of the support worker's role.
- Describe the difference between objective data and subjective data.
- Explain what makes an observation effective.
- Describe how reporting differs in a facility and in a community setting.
- List the four functions of a client's chart.
- Identify the types of documents found in a client's chart.
- List the basic rules for recording.
- Use the 24-hour clock.
- Explain why confidentiality is important in all aspects of the client's care.
- Describe how computers have affected the care planning process.

key terms

assessment Collecting information about the client; a step in the care planning process.

care plan A document that details the care and services the client should receive.

care planning process The method used by nurses and case managers to plan the client's care with the team. Also known as the **nursing process**.

chart A legal document that details a client's condition or illness and responses to care; **record.**

charting See **documentation.**

documentation Recording the care you have given the client and the observations you have made during care. Documentation is a legal requirement for health care providers. Support workers working in the community or the home care setting are required to document the care provided. In facilities, support workers may or may not document care, depending on the agency's policy.

evaluation Assessing and measuring; a step in the care planning process.

implementation Carrying out or performing; a step in the care planning process.

intervention An action or measure taken by the health care team to help the client meet a goal in the care plan.

medical diagnosis The identification of a disease or condition by a physician.

nursing diagnosis A statement describing a health problem that is treated by nursing measures.

objective data See **signs**.

observation The active process of sensing and assimilating information within the context that has been constructed from past experiences.

planning Establishing priorities and goals and developing measures or actions to help the client meet the goals; a step in the care planning process.

record See **chart**.

recording The process of documenting care provided and observations made. Also known as **charting** and **documentation**.

signs Objective data gained through observation and the use of other senses about a client's health. Also known as **objective data**.

subjective data See **symptoms**.

symptoms Information reported by a client that cannot be directly observed by others. Also known as **subjective data**.

verbal report A spoken account of care provided and observations made.

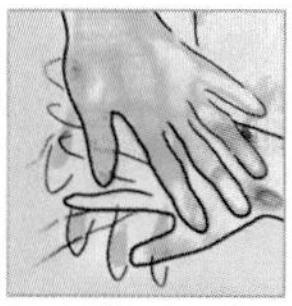

Safe and effective care requires careful planning and coordination. It does not just happen. Facilities and agencies put systems and processes in place to protect clients from harm and to ensure high-quality care. This chapter discusses systems and processes you need to know as a support worker, including care planning, reporting, and recording.

THE CARE PLANNING PROCESS IN FACILITIES

Nurses in facilities use a method called the **care planning process** (also known as the **nursing process**) to plan and deliver care to clients. Its purpose is to meet the client's need for care and support. The care planning process in facilities has the following steps:

1. Assessment
2. Nursing diagnosis
3. Planning
4. Implementation
5. Evaluation

Assessment

Assessment involves collecting information about the client. The nurse meets with the client and takes a health history, which records details of the client's past and present health problems. The nurse conducts a physical assessment by taking the client's vital signs and making observations about the client's physical health. The nurse also assesses the client's emotional, social, intellectual, and spiritual health. The nurse gathers as much information as possible from various sources, which includes information collected by the physician, the social worker, and other health care providers. The report also includes information recorded in past medical documents and test results. The nurse usually meets with members of the client's family. The nurse considers the client's needs and the family's needs when preparing the care plan.

Nursing Diagnosis

The nurse uses information from the assessment to make a nursing diagnosis. A **nursing diagnosis** is a statement describing a health problem that is treated by nursing measures. Nursing diagnoses take into account the whole client. Psychosocial health is as important as physical health. For example, a nursing diagnosis may be *low self-esteem, social isolation,* or *spiritual distress.* Most Canadian nurses use nursing diagnoses from the North American Nursing Diagnosis Association or similar lists of diagnoses (see Box 8–1, which contains a partial list).

The client may have a specific health problem or may be at risk for developing a health problem. Some clients have many health problems and nursing diagnoses. A nursing diagnosis and a medical diagnosis are different. A **medical diagnosis** is the identification of a disease or condition by a physician, for example, cancer, pneumonia, bipolar disorder, stroke, heart attack, acquired immune deficiency syndrome (AIDS), or diabetes. Medications, therapies, and surgery are ordered only by physicians to treat diseases or conditions.

Planning

Planning involves establishing priorities and goals and developing measures or actions to help the client meet these goals.

Establishing Priorities. The client and the nurse discuss the client's needs and then decide on the client's priorities. Often family members and the health care team take part in this stage of the planning process. Nurses use Maslow's theory of basic needs to help set priorities (see Chapter 6). The needs necessary for life and survival have priority and must be met before the other needs can be considered.

Setting Goals. After the nurse and the client agree on priorities, they discuss the goals for the client's care. Goals are practical, achievable, measurable outcomes (results) of the care (Figure 8–1) and contain

Box 8–1 Nursing Examples of Diagnoses Approved by the North American Nursing Diagnosis Association (NANDA)

- Anxiety
- Breastfeeding, Ineffective
- Cardiac Output, Decreased
- Caregiver Role Strain
- Communication, Impaired Verbal
- Community Coping, Ineffective
- Constipation
- Diarrhea
- Family Coping, Compromised
- Fatigue
- Grieving, Dysfunctional
- Home Maintenance, Impaired
- Hopelessness
- Incontinence, Urinary, Stress
- Infant Feeding Pattern, Ineffective
- Infection, Risk for
- Injury, Risk for
- Loneliness, Risk for
- Pain, Chronic
- Physical Mobility, Impaired
- Powerlessness
- Social Interaction, Impaired
- Swallowing, Impaired
- Urinary Elimination, Impaired

Adapted from: NANDA International. (2002). *NANDA Nursing diagnosis: Definitions and classification 2003–2004.* Philadelphia: NANDA.

Nursing diagnosis	Goal	Intervention
Constipation related to lack of privacy.	Resident will have regular bowel movement by 6/30.	Ask resident to use call bell when urge to have bowel movement is felt.
		Answer call promptly.
		Assist resident to bathroom.
		Close bathroom door for privacy.
		Leave room if resident can be alone; tell resident you are leaving and that you will return if the call bell is turned on.
Sleep pattern disturbance related to noisy environment.	Resident will report a restful sleep by 6/29.	Perform necessary care measures before bedtime.
		Close door to resident's room.
		Turn off television or keep volume low if the resident prefers.
		Ask staff to avoid talking outside the resident's room.
		Ask staff to speak in low voices.
		Turn off unneeded equipment.

Figure 8–1 Partial client care plan in a long-term care facility. Each nursing diagnosis has a goal, with nursing measures for each goal.

specific actions and dates. If the client does not achieve the goal by the date, the nurse and client will re-evaluate the goal. Sometimes the family is involved in setting goals. Goals focus on promoting health, preventing health problems, rehabilitation, and promoting independence and are aimed at maintaining or improving the client's physical, emotional, social, spiritual, and intellectual health.

Determining Interventions. After the nurse and client have set goals, they discuss interventions. An **intervention** is an action or measure taken by the health care team to help the client meet the goal. An intervention does not need a physician's order but some can come from a physician's order. For example, if a physician orders that Mrs. Jacob walk 100 metres twice a day, the nurse will include this order in the care plan.

Establishing the Care Plan. The **care plan** is a two part system consisting of a Kardex (a card file that summarizes information in the chart) as well as a care plan. The care plan is a document that details the care and services the client should receive. The plan contains the client's diagnosis, goals, and interventions required to achieve each goal. The care plan has several important functions:

- It lists the care and services the client receives.
- It ensures that the client's care is consistent, no matter who provides the care. For example, Mr. Sayeed's care plan details methods for helping him overcome swallowing difficulties. Each care provider uses the same methods.
- It enables the health care team to communicate details about the client's care. For example, as a support worker, when you start your shift in a long-term care facility, you see on the care plan that Mrs. Desormo has achieved the goal of dressing herself.

The care plan is not a finished document. It is continually reviewed and revised, depending on the client's needs, condition, and progress. For example, Mrs. Atkins' care plan is modified when she does not achieve the goal of bathing herself by May 20.

Usually only the nurse who has the overall responsibility for the client's care makes changes to the care plan. Your input, as the client's support worker, regarding any changes in your client will assist the nurse in changing the plan.

Implementation

Implementation means carrying out or performing, and at this stage of the process, the actions listed in the care plan take place. The nurse in charge of the client's care assigns or delegates tasks to members of the health care team. As the support worker, you are only assigned or delegated tasks that are within the legal limits of your role and job description. To communicate tasks assigned or delegated to you, the nurse uses an assignment sheet. This tells you what tasks you need to perform for each client.

There are four main functions of the implementation process:

- Providing the care
- Observing the client during the care
- Reporting and recording that the care has been completed
- Reporting and recording observations made during the care

Observing the client is an important part of the implementation process. Support workers must report and record their actions and observations after care is completed, according to employer policy.

Evaluation

Evaluation means assessing and measuring. This step involves determining whether the goals in the care plan have been met; that is, the nurse measures the progress made. Goals may be met totally, partly, or not at all. The nurse assesses the reasons why a client may have made no progress or only partial progress toward reaching a goal. Evaluation is an ongoing process, and as the client's condition or needs change, revisions are made to the diagnoses, goals, and interventions. Changes to the care plan are made in consultation with the client and other members of the health care team.

Team meetings are often part of the evaluation process. The nurse conducts a meeting to share information and ideas about the client's care. The purpose is to develop, evaluate, or revise the client's care plan. You and other members of the health care team are usually included in the meeting. You are encouraged to share your suggestions and observations. You are an important part of the team as you are often with the client more than any other member of the health care team (see Chapter 5).

THE CARE PLANNING PROCESS IN COMMUNITY SETTINGS

Case managers coordinate and manage client care. The care planning process used by case managers usually involves four steps: assessment, planning, implementation, and evaluation.

Assessment

The case manager meets with the client and family members to identify the client's problems and needs. Usually the meeting takes place in the client's home. If the client is coming home from the hospital, the case manager uses information from the hospital record or information obtained through a referral sent to the case manager's agency. The referral information may, in some cases, have been completed by a hospital case manager or discharge planner.

The family is very important to the assessment process in community care settings. Serious illness and disability greatly affect family life (see Chapter 4). Family members take on new roles, including the role of caregiver to the ill client. The case manager considers the needs, health, and well-being of the entire family. He or she also considers whether family members need help adjusting to the situation or training to help them care for the ill client. Together, the case manager, client, and family members decide what care and services are needed. For example, they consider nursing and personal care needs and services, such as Meals on Wheels, housekeeping, and transportation, as well as the need for special equipment, such as for oxygen therapy.

The case manager also considers whether the client's home is a safe environment. For example, the home must be reasonably clean, free of pest infestations, and have hand-washing facilities and adequate heating and cooling systems. The case manager assesses whether the home needs modifications to accommodate the client's safety needs. For example, the home may need grab bars installed in the bathroom or a mechanical lifting device in the bedroom. Often, further safety assessments by other specialists are needed. For example, an occupational therapist may assess a home for wheelchair accessibility (see Chapter 33).

Planning

In community care settings, the planning stage can be lengthy and complicated. First, the case manager, client, and family establish priorities, set goals, and determine available resources. Then the case manager develops a master care plan based on the goals and puts together a health care team (Figure 8–2).

The case manager and family members consider resources available for the care. The case manager determines how much publicly funded home care the client and family are eligible for. The family may choose to pay for additional care and services from a private agency.

The care plan includes the care and services provided by family members, outside professionals, and agencies. These professionals and agencies often develop their own care plans, but the case manager is in charge of the master plan. For example, the nursing care plan may be one part of the master care plan.

The case manager schedules all outside services and arranges financing for them. If the client needs help from a support worker, the case manager contacts an agency. A supervisor assigns the support worker to provide care or support for the client. The assignment may be communicated to the support worker by phone or on an assignment sheet.

When clients have multiple needs, several agencies may be involved. For example, Mr. Tremblay is recovering from a stroke. His wife is his primary caregiver. He needs four hours of nursing care a week and visits from respiratory, occupational, speech, and physical therapists. A support worker is also needed to help Mr. Tremblay prepare for bed when his wife is at work. Arrangements are made for Meals on Wheels so that Mrs. Tremblay does not have to prepare every meal.

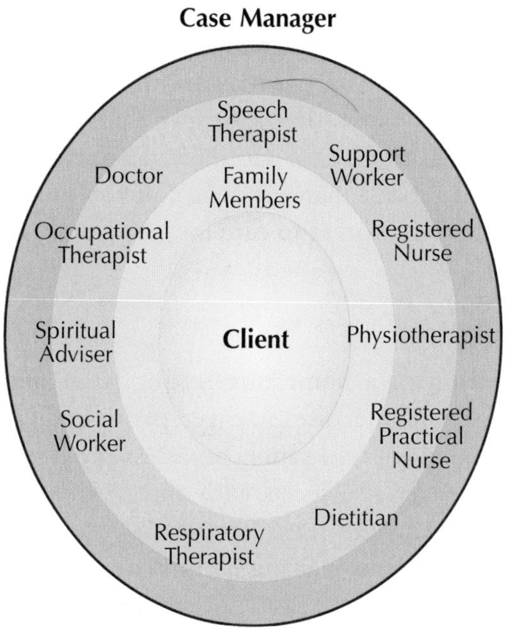

Figure 8–2 The circle of community care. This circle indicates the central role of the case manager, client, and family members on a health care team. **Source:** Birchenall, J., & Streight, E. (2003). *Mosby's textbook for the home care aide,* (2nd ed., p.17). St. Louis: Mosby.

Some clients choose to coordinate and manage their own care. They may develop their own written care plan, or they may not write anything down. If there are no written directions for the support worker, you need detailed instructions from the client. You must ensure that you know exactly what you are allowed to do according to your employer's policies and what to do if the client's expectations are beyond your scope of practice. If you are hired privately, then you must decide whether you can or cannot provide the care requested based on your education, since you are liable for legal actions if hired privately.

Implementation

Agency staff provide care and services on the dates and times arranged by the case manager. If any unforeseen needs arise, the client or a family member calls the case manager. After assessing the situation, the case manager may ask the agency for an unscheduled visit. For example, Mrs. Tremblay feels too ill to care for her husband one morning. She calls her case manager, who contacts the agency for a support worker to care for Mr. Tremblay.

Evaulation

Evaluation in a home care setting is an ongoing process, and the case manager periodically meets with the client and family to assess progress. The case manager also meets with and receives reports from the care and service providers, who continually monitor and evaluate their own care plans.

YOUR ROLE IN THE CARE PLANNING PROCESS

In any health care setting, you have an important role in the care planning process. You make observations and provide feedback, and others on the team use this information when reassessing the client's progress, revising goals, and changing the care plan.

Developing Observation Skills

You are often with clients more than are other care providers. Sometimes you are the first to notice a change in a client's condition, and you observe the client's preferences and reactions to interventions. You are expected to make careful and accurate reports of these observations for use in the care planning process.

Observation is an active process of sensing and assimilating information within the context that has been constructed from past experience. Observation requires you to use your sight, hearing, touch, and smell. You see the way the client lies, sits, or walks. You see flushed or pale skin and reddened or swollen body areas. You listen to the client breathe, talk, and cough. You feel changes in the client's skin temperature. With smell, you detect body, wound, and breath odours and unusual odours from urine and bowel movements.

Information observed about a client is called **objective data** (or **signs**). You can feel a pulse and see urine. However, you cannot feel or see the client's pain, fear, or nausea. **Subjective data** (or **symptoms**) are information reported by a client that is not directly observed by others. The following comments are examples of subjective data:

- "I hardly slept last night. I lay awake from 1:00 a.m. until the sun came up."
- "With George gone, I just don't feel like living any more. I feel so hopeless."
- "The pain is worse when I move. It is a sharp pain that goes up from my ankle to my hip. Thankfully, it comes and goes. I couldn't stand it if I felt it all the time."

When you report or record subjective data, do not interpret the client's comments. Use the client's exact words.

Box 8–2 is a guide for making observations. It contains some basic observations, but you may observe other conditions and situations. Be alert to changes in your client's condition or behaviour. Focus your observations on the client's physical, mental, emotional, and social condition. Look for:

- Changes in physical condition—the client's skin is red and blistering
- Changes in mental condition—the client forgets how to use a toothbrush
- Changes in emotional states—the client is crying
- Changes in social condition—the client's friend does not visit at the usual time
- New conditions that you observe—the client develops diarrhea

Describing Your Observations

Your observations are critical to the care planning process, since nurses and case managers use them for the assessment and evaluation steps. Remember these points when describing your observations:

- ***Be precise and accurate.*** Provide details of what you actually see, hear, touch, and smell. Measurements, calculations, and times must be accurate. When describing subjective data, report or record the client's exact words.

Box 8–2 Basic Observations

Ability to Respond

- Is the client easy or difficult to rouse?
- Can the client give his or her name, the time, and location when asked?
- Does the client identify others accurately?
- Does the client answer questions correctly?
- Does the client speak clearly?
- Does the client follow instructions correctly?
- Is the client calm, restless, or excited?
- Is the client conversing, quiet, or talking a lot?

Movement

- Can the client squeeze your fingers with each hand?
- Can the client walk?
- Can the client move arms and legs?
- Are the client's movements shaky or jerky?
- Does the client complain of stiff or painful joints?

Pain or Discomfort

- Where is the pain located? (Ask the client to point to the pain.)
- Does the pain go anywhere else?
- When did the pain begin?
- What was the client doing when the pain began?
- How long does the pain last?
- How does the client describe the pain?
  - Sharp
  - Severe
  - Knifelike
  - Dull
  - Burning
  - Aching
  - Comes and goes
  - Depends on position
- Has the client felt this pain before?
- If the client has felt this pain before, what helped relieve the pain?
- Was medication given?
- Did the medication help relieve the pain? Is pain still present?
- Is the client able to sleep and rest?
- What is the position of comfort?

Skin

- Is the skin pale or flushed?
- Is the skin cool, warm, or hot?
- Is the skin moist or dry?
- What colour are the lips and nails?
- Is the skin intact? Are there broken areas? If so, where?
- Are sores or reddened areas present?
- Are bruises present? Where are they located?
- Does the person complain of itching?

Eyes, Ears, Nose, and Mouth

- Is there drainage from the eyes? What colour is the drainage?
- Are the eyelids closed?
- Are the eyes reddened?
- Does the client complain of spots, flashes, or blurring?
- Is the client sensitive to bright lights?
- Is there drainage from the ears? What colour is the drainage?
- Can the client hear? Is repeating questions necessary? Are questions answered appropriately?
- Is there drainage from the nose? What colour is the drainage?
- Can the client breathe through the nose?
- Is there breath odour?
- Does the client complain of a bad taste in the mouth?
- Does the client complain of painful gums or teeth?

Respirations

- Do both sides of the client's chest rise and fall with respirations?
- Is breathing noisy?
- Does the client complain of difficulty breathing?
- What is the amount and colour of the sputum?
- What is the frequency of the client's cough? Is it dry or productive?

Bowels and Bladder

- Is the abdomen firm or soft?
- Does the client complain of gas?
- What are the amount, colour, and consistency of bowel movements?
- What is the frequency of bowel movements?
- Can the client control bowel movements?
- Does the client have pain or difficulty urinating?
- What is the amount and colour of the urine?

(continued on page 96)

Box 8–2 **Basic Observations** (cont'd)

- Is the urine clear or cloudy?
- Does the urine have a foul smell?
- Can the client control the passage of urine?
- What is the frequency of urination?

Appetite

- Does the client like the diet?
- How much of the meal is eaten?
- What are the client's food preferences?
- Can the person chew food?
- How much liquid was taken?
- What are the client's liquid preferences?
- How often does the client drink liquids?
- Can the person swallow food and fluids?
- Does the client complain of nausea?
- What is the amount and colour of material vomited?
- Does the client have hiccups?
- Is the client belching?

Activities of Daily Living

- Can the client perform personal care without help?
  - Bathing?
  - Brushing teeth?
  - Combing and brushing hair?
  - Shaving?
- Does the client use the toilet, commode, bedpan, or urinal?
- Does the client feed himself or herself?
- Can the client walk?
- What amount and kind of assistance are needed?

Box 8–3 **Ineffective and Effective Observations Made by Support Workers**

Ineffective Observation	Reasons the Observation Is Ineffective	Effective Observation	Reasons the Observation Is Effective
Mrs. Demarco is having trouble going to the bathroom this morning.	Correct terminology is not used. The statement is vague. No details are provided.	Mrs. Demarco urinated 3 times between 0900 and 0920. She said, "I feel a burning pain when I try to go to the bathroom, and only a trickle of urine is coming out."	Correct terminology is used. The statement is a direct, precise observation. Both objective and subjective data are used.
Mr. Quennell is having trouble remembering things.	The statement is an assumption. There is no supporting evidence.	Mr. Quennell did not remember eating his breakfast. He asked me to make breakfast 30 minutes after he had eaten. I told him he had already had breakfast. He said, "I don't remember."	The statement is an observation supported by detailed examples. Both objective and subjective data are used.
Mrs. Witowski seems under the weather today.	Correct terminology is not used. There is no supporting evidence.	Mrs. Witowski did not play bridge today. She took only two bites of her lunch (a turkey sandwich). She said, "I'm not hungry. I feel tired, and I don't feel like doing anything."	The statement about Mrs. Witowski's behaviour and condition are observations supported by evidence. Mrs. Witowski's words are quoted exactly.

- ***Do not interpret or make assumptions.*** In most cases, your observations are sufficient, and you do not need to interpret them. Do not make assumptions. An *assumption* is a guess, usually based on insufficient evidence. When you make assumptions, you may be jumping to conclusions.

Box 8–3 contains some examples of ineffective and effective reporting of observations. After you have read the contents of the box, read the dialogue from the team meeting. Note that the support worker's contributions to the meeting are her observations of the client. She provides precise, accurate details but does not make any assumptions. The social worker and the nurse use the support worker's observations to make a judgement about the client's mental health.

VERBAL REPORTING

As a support worker, you need to report and record your actions and observations. A **verbal report** is the spoken account of care provided and observations made. Employers use different methods for verbal reporting, and all have policies about how often to report and what to report. So, you need to know your employer's policies. There are certain circumstances in which you always need to contact your supervisor. These are listed in Box 8–4.

Remember that information about a client is confidential. Be careful when communicating client information to members of the health care team. Choose a quiet area where you cannot be overheard by others. Do not discuss a client in his/her room or a common area. Keep all your conversations about clients on a professional level. When making reports by phone to your supervisor from your own home, make sure your family cannot hear you.

Box 8–4 When to Contact Your Supervisor

Contact your supervisor whenever:

- There is an emergency, such as finding your client unconscious on the floor.
- You observe a change in the client's condition or normal functioning.
- The client becomes ill. For example, the client vomits, has diarrhea, or develops a fever.
- The client is in distress, either physical or emotional.
- You believe the client's safety is at risk.
- A problem arises involving medications.
- The client complains about his or her condition or care.
- The client asks you a question about his or her diagnosis, condition, or treatment plans.
- The client or family member asks you to do something that contradicts the care plan.
- You have a conflict with a client or a family member.
- A question or problem arises with which you need help.

Verbal Reporting in a Facility

In a facility, you report your actions and observations to the charge nurse. Reports must be prompt, thorough, and accurate. Always give the client's name, the room and bed number, and the time you made the observation or gave the care. Report only what you observed or did yourself. Prioritize items by starting your report with the most important points. Give reports as often as the client's condition requires or as often as requested by the nurse. Immediately report any changes from normal or changes in the person's condition.

The charge nurse gives a report at the end of shift to the incoming charge nurse (called the *end-of-shift report*). The report includes information about each client's condition, the care given, and the care that must be given on the next shift. Some facilities expect all team members to hear the end-of-shift report as they come on duty.

Verbal Reporting in a Community Setting

Employers have their own policies for verbal reports. Most employers do not require support workers to make daily verbal reports. Usually, you call your employer if something out of the ordinary occurs. However, call your supervisor immediately if something unexpected happens. Follow employer policy and the guidelines in Box 8–4 and Box 8–5.

CHARTS

A **chart** (also known as a **record)** is a written account of a client's condition or illness and responses to care. The chart is a permanent, legal record of care provided from admission to discharge or death. The chart is filed and kept for future reference. It is used as a reference for future admissions, or it could be subpoenaed for a court case involving malpractice. It provides for the following:

- ***Communication.*** Health care teams rely on charts to relay information about their clients (Figure 8–3). All team members must be informed about the client's condition and care. The chart is a method to ensure that all members of the team are aware of the care the client has received. Recording is an accurate way to communicate information about the client. The care plan is one part of the chart. Other parts are discussed in the next section, Documents Used in Charts.
- ***Currency.*** Care plans change as the client's needs, preferences, and condition change. Charts enable staff to keep the client's information up-to-date. Other areas of the chart are also kept up to date, for example, the latest reports of laboratory tests and doctors' orders.
- ***Accountability.*** Charts are signed and dated by members of the health care team. This allows information to be tracked. All team members are accountable for their words and actions. ***In a legal case, you may need to testify regarding what you wrote on the chart.***
- ***Continuity of care.*** Written documentation contains information on the client's past health problems and treatments. This information enables health care providers to detect patterns and changes in the client's health. Team members change over time. Without a written record, care might become fragmented and unreliable.
- ***Funding.*** In some provinces, the amount of funding dollars long-term care facilities receive is based on reviews of each client's chart. It is very important that charting is accurate. In Ontario, many employers have faced funding cuts because of inadequate reporting and documentation of actual client care needs. Your role is very important in recording and describing the care you provide to your client.

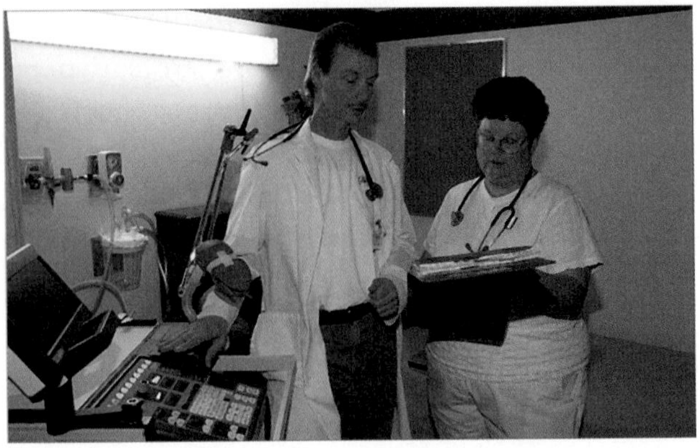

Figure 8–3 The nurse and respiratory therapist review a client's chart. **Source:** Sorrentino, S.A. (2000). *Mosby's textbook for nursing assistants* (5th ed., p. 56). St. Louis: Mosby.

Box 8–5 Guidelines for Making Telephone Reports to Your Supervisor

- Keep agency phone numbers and extensions handy.
- Make sure you have a pen and paper handy.
- Identify yourself, the date, and the time of your call.
- Give a concise, accurate, and descriptive report. For example, say what you observed, (client has bruises on buttocks), when you made the observation (when bathing the client), and what the client said ("I fell down the stairs last night").
- Use the client's exact words.
- Speak clearly and slowly. Pause between sentences.
- Write down the instructions from your supervisor.
- Repeat the instructions back to your supervisor.
- Write the instructions on the appropriate document in the client's chart.
- Remember that the client's information is confidential. It is shared only with the health care team members involved in the client's care.

Documents Used in Charts

Charts vary, depending on the employer, as most employers design their own documents. This section describes some common documents contained in a client's chart.

- ***Data forms***—include details about the client's physical, emotional, social, and intellectual health. Long-term care facilities use these forms to record information about residents' health. Activities, interests, medications, treatments, and therapies are examples of information that is recorded.
- ***Assessment forms***—used by nurses and case managers to record a client's health problems and needs. Assessments are based on information from the data form and other sources, including observations made by the health care team (Figure 8–4).
- ***Home assessment forms***—document changes that need to be made to the client's home during rehabilitation (see Box 34–3 on page 659).
- ***Care plans***—contain goals and interventions (action plan) based on the assessment. Sometimes the assessment and the care plan are on the same form.
- ***Progress notes***—record information about the care given, the client's response to care, observations, the client's activities, special treatments, and medications. Progress notes also contain areas for the date, time, and initials (Figure 8–5). Health care team members from various disciplines may or may not record care and treatment on one set of notes. In some circumstances, progress notes may be separated into disciplines (for example, a section for nursing, a section for physiotherapy, and so on). This enables the disciplines to easily access information for their own disciplines or to learn about the client's progress in a certain area of their health goals. Whether or not you record information on progress notes depends on your employer's policy.
- ***Activities-of-daily-living (ADLs) checklists and flow sheets***—record actions relating to hygiene, food and fluids, elimination, rest and sleep, mobility, activity, and social interactions. ADL checklists require you to place a check mark in a box. ADL flow sheets use codes for actions, such as "I" for independent and "A" for assist. ADL checklists and flow sheets provide little or no space for writing details. ADL checklists are sometimes called "tick sheets." Some of the items in an ADL flow sheet are shown in Figure 8–6.
- ***Task sheets (Log Notes)***—used by employers in community settings to record care and services provided. The form has boxes for each day and for care and support activities. You check the box for the day the care or service was given (Figure 8–7).
- ***Graphic sheets***—record measurements and observations made every shift, or three to four times per day. Information may include the client's blood pressure, temperature, pulse, respirations, height, and weight. Some graphic sheets have places to chart the intake and output, routine care, bowel movements, and physician's visits. An example is shown in Figure 8–8.
- ***Other flow sheets***—record frequent measurements and observations. Some record blood pressure, pulse, and respirations every 15 minutes or more often. Others record intake and output. Flow sheets are used to monitor the condition of seriously ill people.
- ***Summary reports***—summarize care and service provided over a period of time. These are used in community settings and by some long-term care facilities to provide summaries of the client's condition monthly or every second or third month.
- ***Incident reports***—written accounts made after an accident, error, or unexpected event. In the community, these reports are commonly called occurrence reports (see Chapter 19).
- ***Kardex***—a card file that summarizes information in the chart. It usually includes the person's current diagnosis, medications and treatments, any special equipment needs, and routine care measures. The Kardex system provides a quick source of current information and can be frequently updated to reflect changes. The Kardex is used in some facilities, but is rarely used in community settings.

7 Day Observation Record – St Joseph's at Fleming

Resident Name: ____________________

Dates of 7 Day Assessment **From:** ____________ **To:** ____________

PLEASE USE TICK MARKS UNLESS OTHERWISE INDICATED

*INDICATE THE **MOST** ASSISTANCE THE RESIDENT REQUIRED FOR EACH SHIFT*

	0			1			2			3			4			5			6			7		
Date:																								
Code Section: Shift:	**N**	**D**	**E**	**N**	**D**	**E**	**N**	**D**	**E**	**N**	**D**	**E**	**N**	**D**	**E**	**N**	**D**	**E**	**N**	**D**	**E**	**N**	**D**	**E**
B5 – Cognitive patterns																								
Distracted Easily *(becomes sidetracked)*																								
Periods of altered awareness*(talks to someone not there, believes He/she is somewhere else, confuses night and day)*																								
Disorganized speech *(rambling, incoherent, loses train of Thought)*																								
Restlessness *(fidgeting, frequent position changes, calling out)*																								
Lethargy *(sluggish, tired, moving slower than normal)*																								
Mental Function varies during the day																								
Initials:																								
E1 – Indicators of Depression, Anxiety, Sad Mood																								
Negative statements ("What's the use?")																								
Repetitive questions (Where do I go?)																								
Repetitive statements (calling for help etc.)																								
Persistent anger (with self or others)																								
Self-deprecation ("I'm no good")																								
Unrealistic Fears (being alone or in a crowd)																								
Comments something bad will happen ("I'll die")																								
Complains repetitively re: health																								
Non-health complaints *(attention seeking, repetitive reassurance Re: schedules, meals, clothing, relationship issues)*																								
Unpleasant mood in the morning																								
Insomnia																								
Facial expression sad, pained, worried																								
Crying/tearful																								
Repetitive movements *(pacing, exit-seeking, elopement, tapping)*																								
New onset or worsening of behaviours? (Y – Yes)																								
Withdrawal from activities of interest																								
Reduced social interaction																								
Initials:																								

Form #

7 Day Observation Record – St Joseph's at Fleming

Resident Name: ____________________

Dates of 7 Day Assessment **From:** ____________ **To:** ____________

PLEASE USE TICK MARKS UNLESS OTHERWISE INDICATED

*INDICATE THE **MOST** ASSISTANCE THE RESIDENT REQUIRED FOR EACH SHIFT*

	0			1			2			3			4			5			6			7		
Date:																								
Code Section: Shift:	N	D	E	N	D	E	N	D	E	N	D	E	N	D	E	N	D	E	N	D	E	N	D	E
E4 – Behavioral Symptoms																								
Wandering *(no rational purpose)*																								
Verbally abusive *(others were threatened, screamed at, cursed at)*																								
Physically Abusive *(others were hit, shoved, scratched, sexually Abused)*																								
Socially inappropriate or disruptive																								
Resists care *(resisted taking meds, ADL assistance, or eating)*																								
Behaviours easily altered? *(Y – Yes; N – No)*																								
Initials:																								
G1 (a) – Mobility While in Bed																								
Self; Needs no help to move in bed																								
Staff cue resident																								
Guided maneuvering of limbs – no weight-bearing help																								
Some Weight-bearing assistance *(e.g. staff lift legs into bed)*																								
Staff totally reposition while in bed																								
# of staff required? *(1 or 2)*																								
Initials:																								
G1 (b) – Transfer																								
Self; Needs no help to transfer																								
Staff locks equipment or sets up equipment or Cues resident; resident transfers self																								
Guided maneuvering of limbs – no weight-bearing help																								
Some weight-bearing assistance (record # of staff)																								
Mechanical transfer/ Totally dependent on staff																								
Initials:																								

Form #

Figure 8–4 Assessment forms that may be used in long-term care facilities by support workers.
Courtesy: St. Joseph's at Fleming, Peterborough, Ontario.

7 Day Observation Record – St Joseph's at Fleming

Resident Name ______________________________

Dates of 7 Day Assessment **From:** ______________ **To:** ______________

PLEASE USE TICK MARKS UNLESS OTHERWISE INDICATED

*INDICATE THE **MOST** ASSISTANCE THE RESIDENT REQUIRED FOR EACH SHIFT*

	0			1			2			3			4			5			6			7		
Date:																								
Code Section: Shift:	N	D	E	N	D	E	N	D	E	N	D	E	N	D	E	N	D	E	N	D	E	N	D	E
G1 (c) - Walking in Room																								
Independent; requires no help																								
Staff cue resident only; requires no physical assistance																								
Guided maneuvering *(e.g. staff holds resident's hand)*																								
Weight-bearing assistance required *(# of staff?)*																								
Resident does not walk in room																								
Initials:																								
G1 (d) – Walking in Corridor																								
Independent; requires no help																								
Staff cue resident only: requires no physical assistance																								
Guided maneuvering *(e.g. staff holds resident's hand)*																								
Weight-bearing assistance required *(# of staff?)*																								
Resident does not walk in corridor																								
Initials:																								
G1 (e) – Locomotion on Unit by Wheelchair																								
Independent; requires no help																								
Staff cue resident only; requires no physical assistance																								
Guided maneuvering																								
Weight-bearing assistance required *(# of staff?)*																								
Not applicable																								
Initials:																								
G1(g) – Dressing																								
Self; no staff help required																								
Staff cue resident only; requires no physical assistance																								
Guided maneuvering																								
Staff do up buttons, zippers, tie laces etc.																								
Weight-bearing assistance required *(e.g. lift arm or lift leg to Apply KED stockings or prosthesis)*																								
Total assist																								
Number of staff required																								
Initials:																								

Form #

7 Day Observation Record – St Joseph's at Fleming

Resident Name: ______________________________

Dates of 7 Day Assessment **From:** ______________ **To:** ______________

PLEASE USE TICK MARKS UNLESS OTHERWISE INDICATED

*INDICATE THE **MOST** ASSISTANCE THE RESIDENT REQUIRED FOR EACH SHIFT*

	0			1			2			3			4			5			6			7		
Date:																								
Code Section: Shift:	N	D	E	N	D	E	N	D	E	N	D	E	N	D	E	N	D	E	N	D	E	N	D	E
G1(h) – Eating ***(How resident eats or drinks, regardless of skill)***																								
Supervision only																								
Guided maneuvering of food or utensil to mouth																								
Weight-bearing assistance *(e.g. staff lifts resident's arm or hand To mouth)*																								
Total assist																								
Initials:																								
G1 (i) – Toileting ***(includes transfers on/off toilet)***																								
Independent; requires no help																								
Staff supervise/cue resident only; no physical assistance																								
Guided maneuvering of limbs, non weight-bearing help																								
Some weight-bearing assistance required *(# of staff?)*																								
Mechanical Lift/ Total assist (# of staff?)																								
Activity did not occur																								
Initials:																								
G1 (j) – Personal Hygiene ***(excludes baths or showers)***																								
Independent																								
Supervision or cueing or set-up required																								
Guided maneuvering of limbs, non weight-bearing help,																								
Weight-bearing assistance *(e.g. staff lift arm so resident can Brush hair or teeth)*																								
Total dependence																								
Resident refused hygiene care																								
Initials:																								

Form #

Figure 8–4 continued

7 Day Observation Record – St Joseph's at Fleming

Resident Name: ____________________

Dates of 7 Day Assessment **From:** ____________ **To:** ________________

PLEASE USE TICK MARKS UNLESS OTHERWISE INDICATED

*INDICATE THE **MOST** ASSISTANCE THE RESIDENT REQUIRED FOR EACH SHIFT*

	0			1			2			3			4			5			6			7		
Date:																								
Code Section: Shift:	N	D	E	N	D	E	N	D	E	N	D	E	N	D	E	N	D	E	N	D	E	N	D	E
G2 – Bathing																								
Independent																								
Bath/shower with supervision only																								
Physical assistance for transfer *(# of staff?)*																								
Physical assistance for part of bathing activity *(excluding back and hair)*																								
Total dependence *(# of staff?)*																								
Refused bath																								
Initials:																								
G8 – ADL Self-Performance																								
Resident states could/ wants to do more for self																								
Staff feel resident could do more for self																								
Resident would be able to do more for self but is very slow																								
Initials:																								
H1 (b) – Urinary Continence *(control of urine with appliances or continence program)*																								
Uses pads/incontinent products																								
Continent – Skin remains dry/catheter did not leak																								
Incontinent occasional or frequent *(put check-mark for each episode)*																								
Totally incontinent																								
Is incontinence new for resident? *(Y – Yes; N – No)*																								
Initials:																								

Form #

7 Day Observation Record – St Joseph's at Fleming

Resident Name: ____________________

Dates of 7 Day Assessment **From:** ____________ **To:** ________________

PLEASE USE TICK MARKS UNLESS OTHERWISE INDICATED

*INDICATE THE **MOST** ASSISTANCE THE RESIDENT REQUIRED FOR EACH SHIFT*

	0			1			2			3			4			5			6			7		
Date:																								
Code Section: Shift:	N	D	E	N	D	E	N	D	E	N	D	E	N	D	E	N	D	E	N	D	E	N	D	E
H1 (a) – Bowel Continence ***(control of bowels with appliance or bowel continence program)***																								
Continent - Skin remained dry; BM on toilet/commode *(# of BM's/shift; small (S), medium (M), large (L))*																								
Incontinent of stool in product, lining; or colostomy leak																								
Initials:																								
K – Oral/Nutritional Problems																								
Record food consumed: 100%=1, 75%=2, 50%=3, 25%=4, R=Refused (***Use N column for breakfast)***																								
Record fluid consumed: 1G=1 glass=125ml, 2G=2, 3G=3 4G=4***(Use N column for breakfast)***																								
Record snack fluid consumed: 1G=1 glass, 2G=2, 3G=3 4G=4 (***Use N column for breakfast)***																								
Record snack taken ***(Use N column for breakfast)***																								
Complains about the taste of food																								
Complains of hunger																								
Initials:																								
N1 – Personal Activities																								
Naps more than 1 hour in morning, afternoon, evening																								
Initials:																								
P4 – Devices and Restraints																								
Full bed rails on all open sides of bed																								
Half-rail or 1 side-rail up																								
Trunk Restraint *(e.g. lap belt that cannot be removed by resident)*																								
Limb Restraint																								
Geri-chair																								
DID THE RESIDENT FALL?																								
Initials:																								

Form #

PLEASE FILE IN RESIDENT'S CHART UPON COMPLETION OF ASSESSMENT PERIOD

Figure 8–4 continued

NNR – NARRATIVE NOTES – Client: ______________________

TIME	DATE (D/M/Y):

Supplied by Nightingale Nursing

Figure 8–5 Narrative notes from a community agency. **Courtesy:** Nightingale Nursing Registry, Peterborough, Ontario.

Activities of Daily Living Flow Sheet

JAN FEB (MAR) APR MAY JUN JUL AUG SEP OCT NOV DEC

ORDER/INSTRUCTION	TIME	1	2	3	4	5	6	7	8	9	10	11	12	13	14	15	16	17	18	19	20	21	22	23	24	25	26	27	28	29	30	31
Bowel Movements L = Large M = Medium S = Small IC = Incontinent	11-7	M																														
	7-3			L																												
	3-11																															
Bladder Elimination I = Independent IC = Incontinent FC = Foley Catheter	11-7	I	I	I	I																											
	7-3	I	I	I	I																											
	3-11	I	IC	I	I																											
Weight Bearing Status TT = Toe Touch AT = As tol. P = Partial F = Full NWB = No wt. Bearing	11-7	AT	AT	AT	AT																											
	7-3	AT	AT	AT	AT																											
	3-11	AT	AT	AT	AT																											
Transfer Status ML = Medilift SBA = Stand By Assist; Assist of 1 or 2	11-7	SBA	SBA	SBA	SBA																											
	7-3	SBA	SBA	SBA	SBA																											
	3-11	SBA	SBA	SBA	A-1																											
Activity A = Ambulate GC = Gerichair T = Turn every 2 hrs. W/C = Wheelchair	11-7	T	T	T	T																											
	7-3	A	A	A	A																											
	3-11	A	A	A	A																											
Safety LT = Lap Tray SR = Siderails BA = Bed Alarm SB = Seat Belt	11-7																															
	7-3																															
	3-11																															
Feeding Status I = Independent S = Set up F = Staff feed SP = Swallow precautions TL = Thickened Liquids	Breakfast	S	S	S	S																											
	Lunch	S	S	S	S																											
	Supper	S	S	S	S																											
Amount of food taken in %	Breakfast	75	100	100	75																											
	Lunch	75	75	100	75																											
	Supper	50	50	50	75																											
Bath and Shampoo every Monday & Thursday on 7-3 shift T = Tub S = Shower B = Bedbath	11-7																															
	7-3		T																													
	3-11																															
Oral Care Own/(Dentures)/None I = Independent S = Set up A = Assist	11-7	S	S	S	S																											
	7-3	S	S	S	S																											
	3-11	S	S	S	S																											
Dressing I = Independent S = Set up A = Assist T = Total Care	11-7	A	A	S	S																											
	7-3																															
	3-11	A	A	A	A																											
Grooming: Washing Face and Hands Combing Hair I = Independent S = Set up A = Assist T = Total Care	11-7	A	A	A	A																											
	7-3	A	A	A	A																											
	3-11	A	A	A	A																											
Trim Nails Weekly	11-7																															
	7-3		✓																													
	3-11																															
Lotion Arms and Legs twice daily	11-7																															
	7-3	✓	✓	✓	✓																											
	3-11	✓	✓	✓	✓																											
Shave Men Daily Shave Women every 3 days	11-7																															
	7-3	✓			✓																											
	3-11																															
Amount snacks taken in %	AM	100	75	100	50																											
	PM	100	100	75	75																											
	HS	50	75	75	75																											
Intake and Output	11-7																															
	7-3																															
	3-11																															
Vital Signs Every Week	11-7																															
	7-3		✓																													
	3-11																															
Weight Every Week	11-7		✓																													
	7-3																															

Figure 8–6 Some of the items in an activities-of-daily-living flow sheet. **Courtesy:** Nightingale Nursing Registry, Peterborough, Ontario.

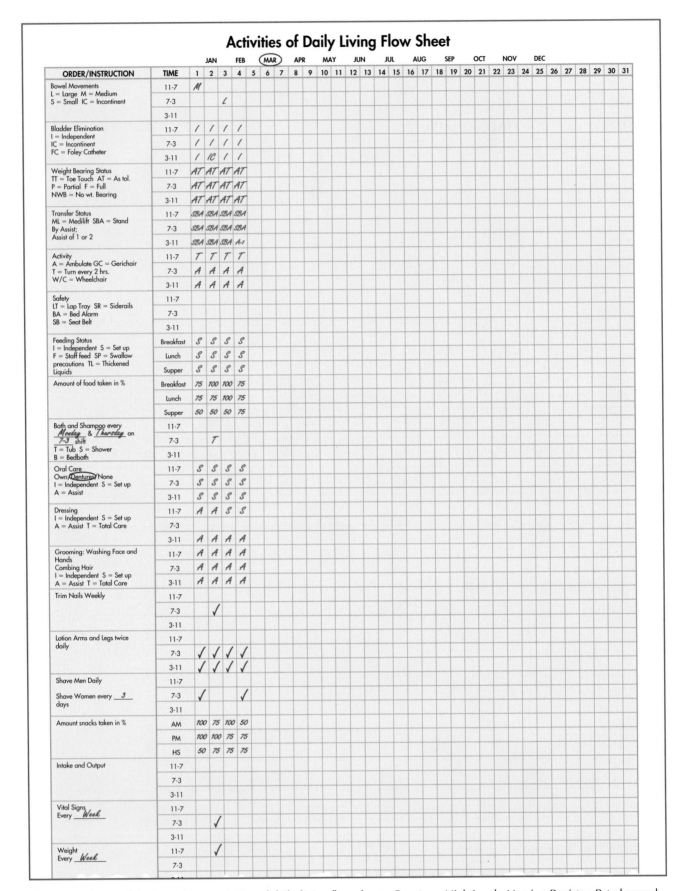

LOG NOTES

Client: ____________________

Date: ____________________

PSW: ____________________

Activity/Task	**3pm–11pm**	**7am–3pm**	**11pm–7am**	**Comments**
Personal Care				
Awake				
Asleep				
Napping/In Bed				
Bed/Sponge Bath				
Shower				
Spa Tub				
Transfer to Wheelchair (specify times)				
Transfer to Bed (specify times)				
White Board on Tray				
Personal Hygiene				
teeth				
hair				
nose				
ears				
deodorant				
cut nails				
other				
Pericare				
Dressing				

Meals & Snacks				
Meals/Snacks/Flush, etc.:				
11:00am Meal & Flush				
4:00pm Juice				
10:00pm Meal & Flush				
1:15am Meal & Flush				

Medical/Health/Safety				
Report from Previous Shift (5 min)				
Read Log Notes (5–10 min)				
Location & Condition (arrival)				
Location & Condition (departure)				
Check on client (every 15 minutes if				
not around client specify times)				
Meds:				
9:30am				
3:00pm–5:00pm				
9:00pm–11:00pm				

Figure 8–7 Log Notes/Agency client care task sheet. **Courtesy:** Nightingale Nursing Registry, Peterborough, Ontario.

The Credit Valley Hospital

SALUS ET SPES

VITAL SIGNS FLOWSHEET

Signature/Status	Initials	Signature/Status	Initials

	Date :												
	Time :												
Temperature (C°)	: 40												
	39												
	38												
	37												
	36												
	35												
Pulse :													
Respirations :													
B.P. :	Lying :												
	Sitting :												
	Standing :												
Weight :													
	Initials												

Figure 8–8 Graphic sheet. **Courtesy:** Credit Valley Hospital, Mississauga, Ontario. Reprinted with permission.

Recording

Recording (charting, documentation) is documenting care and observations. Employers have their own policies for recording, including when to record, how often to record, what should be recorded, and who should record. Policies address such issues as how to abbreviate, what colour of ink to use, and how to make corrections. When recording, focus on:

- What you observed, including symptoms the client reports to you
- What you did
- When you did it
- The client's response

When recording on a document or form, communicate clearly and thoroughly. Make sure that measurements and numbers recorded are absolutely accurate. If there is a space for observations, you should record them in a precise, accurate, and relevant manner. You should use the third person and focus specifically on the client—for example, "Abrasion, 5 cm by 3 cm, noted on left knee" rather than "I saw an abrasion on Mrs. Smith's left knee." Appropriate charting that follows standardized documentation guidelines is becoming very important as Canadians are suing care facilities and their staff more frequently for malpractice, neglect, and so on. Use the guidelines in Box 8–6, and follow your employer's policies.[1]

Box 8–6 Guidelines: Recording

- Always use ink. Follow employer policy for the colour of ink to use.
- Include the date and the time whenever a recording is made. Use conventional time (a.m. or p.m.) or 24-hour clock time according to employer policy.
- Make sure that your writing is legible and neat.
- Use only employer-approved abbreviations.
- Use correct spelling, grammar, and punctuation.
- Never erase or use correction fluid if you make an error. Make a single line through the error. Write "error" or "mistaken entry" over it, and sign your initials. Then rewrite the part. Follow your employer's policies for correcting errors.
- Sign all entries with your name and title, as required by your employer's policy.
- Do not skip lines. Draw a line through the blank space of a partially completed line or to the end of a page. This prevents others from recording in a space that has your signature.
- Make sure each form is stamped with the client's name and other identifying information.
- Record only what you observed and did yourself.
- Never chart a procedure or treatment until after its completion.
- Be accurate, concise, and factual. Do not record assumptions or opinions.
- Record in a logical manner and in the order in which tasks and procedures occurred.
- Be descriptive. Avoid terms with more than one meaning.
- Use the client's exact words. Use quotation marks to show that the statement is a direct quote.
- Chart any changes from normal or changes in the client's condition. Also, chart that you informed your supervisor and the time you made the report.
- Do not omit information.
- Record all safety measures used, such as assisting a client when he or she is up or reminding a client not to get out of bed. This will help protect you from legal action if the client has a fall.

Recording Time. The 24-hour clock is used to document care. The 24-hour clock involves using a four-digit number for time (Figure 8–9). The first two digits are for the hour: 0100 = 1:00 a.m.; 1300 = 1:00 p.m. The last two digits are for minutes: 0110 = 1:10 a.m. The abbreviations a.m. and p.m. are not used.

As Box 8–7 shows, morning hours are the same in the 24-hour clock as they are in the conventional clock, except that a.m. is not used. For p.m. times, add 12 to the first two digits (the hours) of clock time. If it is 2:00 p.m., add 12 to 2 to make 1400. For 8:35 p.m., add 12 to 8 to make 2035.

The 24-hour clock helps make communication more accurate. Since health care team members do not have to write a.m. or p.m., there is less chance for confusion.

Terminology and Abbreviations. In health care, medical terminology and abbreviations are used to communicate effectively and clearly (see Chapter 7). If a member of your health care team uses a word that you do not understand, be sure to ask the person what the word means. It is a good idea to buy a medical dictionary to constantly look up meanings

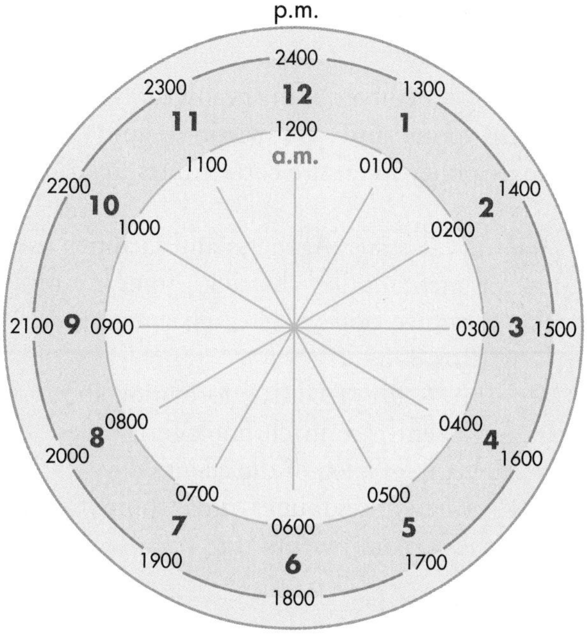

Figure 8–9 The 24-hour clock.

Box 8–7 24-Hour Clock

Conventional Time	24-hour Clock
1:00 a.m.	0100
2:00 a.m.	0200
3:00 a.m.	0300
4:00 a.m.	0400
5:00 a.m.	0500
6:00 a.m.	0600
7:00 a.m.	0700
8:00 a.m.	0800
9:00 a.m.	0900
10:00 a.m.	1000
11:00 a.m.	1100
12:00 noon	1200
1:00 p.m.	1300
2:00 p.m.	1400
3:00 p.m.	1500
4:00 p.m.	1600
5:00 p.m.	1700
6:00 p.m.	1800
7:00 p.m.	1900
8:00 p.m.	2000
9:00 p.m.	2100
10:00 p.m.	2200
11:00 p.m.	2300
12:00 midnight	2400 or 0000

of words. All members of the health care team must use only terms and abbreviations approved by employer policy to ensure correct interpretations.

Methods of Charting. Agencies and facilities use a variety of methods for charting. Some examples include narrative notes, SOAP charting, and PIE charting (Box 8–8).

Narrative charting records information about the client and client care in chronological order. The content resembles a log of the client's day.

SOAP charting uses four essential components in recording. The components are:

S—subjective data
O—objective data
A—assessment or analysis of the data
P—plan of care

PIE charting uses three essential components in recording. The components are:

P—problem
I—intervention
E—evaluation

See the examples in Box 8–8.

Recording in a Facility

In an acute care setting, you most likely will document care on graphic sheets, flow sheets, and progress notes. You may be expected to document, for example, temperature, blood pressure, intake and output, bowel movements, and routine care.

In a long-term care setting, you will likely document care on ADL checklists or flow sheets. If a resident's health status needs frequent monitoring, you may also document on graphic sheets and flow sheets. You may be expected to give summary reports on care provided to residents. Or your supervisor will ask for your input for the preparation of a summary report from the health care team. These written reports are usually required monthly or every 3 months.

Recording in the Community

Every agency and case manager keep separate client charts in their organizations. Some parts of the client's chart are usually, but not always, kept in the client's home, often in a binder. The forms in the binder vary according to agency policy and the client's condition and needs. Among other documents, the binder usually contains the care plan, progress notes, ADL checklists, flow sheets, or task sheets. Agency policies differ—some do not allow support workers to enter anything on the documents in the binder, while others expect support workers to record tasks and observations on the forms in the binder.

Most agencies have forms called *client care task sheets* that you carry with you to every assignment (see Figure 8–7 on page 105). You start a new task sheet for each client, and as you complete tasks, you check off relevant areas of the form.

Most task sheets contain space for you to record special circumstances or observations. You may be

Box 8–8 Examples of Progress Notes Written in Different Formats

SOAP (Subjective – Objective – Assessment – Plan)

1/19/05 Knowledge deficit related to inexperience regarding surgery 1630

S "I'm so worried about what it will be like after surgery."

O Client asking frequent questions about surgery. Has had no previous experience with surgery. Wife present, acts as a support person.

A Knowledge deficit regarding surgery related to inexperience. Client also expressing anxiety.

P Explain routine preoperative preparation. Demonstrate and explain rationale for turning, coughing, and deep breathing (TCDB) exercises. Provide explanation and teaching booklet on postoperative nursing care. S. Lazarus, RPN

PIE (Problem – Intervention – Evaluation)

P Knowledge deficit regarding surgery related to inexperience.

I Explained to client normal preoperative preparations for surgery. Demonstrated TCDB exercises. Provided booklet to client on postoperative nursing care.

E Client demonstrates TCDB exercises correctly. Needs review of postoperative nursing care. S. Lazarus, RPN

Focus Charting (Data – Action – Response)

D Client states, "I'm so worried about what it will be like after surgery." Client asking frequent questions about surgery. Has no previous experience with surgery. Wife present; acts as a support person.

A Explained to client normal preoperative preparations for surgery. Demonstrated TCDB exercises. Provided booklet to client on postoperative nursing care.

R Client demonstrates TCDB exercises correctly. Needs review of postoperative nursing care.

Note: Some agencies also add P (Plan).

Source: Potter, P.A, Perry, A., Ross-Kerr, J.C., & Wood, M.J. (2001). *Canadian fundamentals of nursing* (2nd ed., p. 240). Toronto: Harcourt Canada.

expected to identify whether the client was independent, dependent, or needed some assistance with activities. As mentioned, any changes you observe in a client's normal functioning or condition should be reported by phone to your supervisor. Record on the task sheet any verbal reports that you make as well as phone instructions received from your supervisor.

You hand in your task sheets monthly or weekly, depending on agency policy, along with forms that track mileage and other work expenses. Your supervisor may use your task sheets to prepare a report on each client. You may be asked for additional information on some of your clients.

Confidentiality

The client chart is a confidential document. You are ethically and legally bound to keep client information confidential. This includes information about the client that you record. All employers have strict guidelines about the confidentiality of charts and client information. You must be particularly careful to observe guidelines on accessing, reporting, and transporting information.

Only health care team members involved in the client's care have access to confidential information. Those not directly involved usually are not allowed access to the client's chart. Housekeeping staff, kitchen staff, and office clerks do not need to see charts or to hear any confidential details about a client. In a home care setting, only certain family members have access to these details. Your supervisor will tell you who can look at the chart.

You may transport a document from a central file area to a client's room or other location in a facility, and you may carry with you confidential information about a client in a community setting. Be very careful when transporting confidential documents. Concentrate on what you are doing and remind yourself of the importance of your task. If you become distracted, you could easily leave the documents in an inappropriate place.

Computerized Charts

Charts are maintained on computers in many agencies and facilities. Using a computer is easier, faster, and more efficient than writing on the chart (Figure 8–10), and the recordings are more accurate, legible, and reliable. Information can be accessed at the nurse's station, at the agency, and even at the bedside. These computer links reduce clerical work and telephone calls.

In a community setting, you might be expected to send in reports by e-mail. In the future, support workers may be required to have computer literacy and to own a computer for working in these settings.

Computer information is easy to access, so the client's right to privacy must be protected. Only certain staff members are allowed to access the computer. They have their own codes (passwords) to access computer files. If you are allowed access, you will be trained on how to use the computer system in your work setting. Follow the ethical and legal considerations relating to privacy and confidentiality (see Chapters 10 and 11).

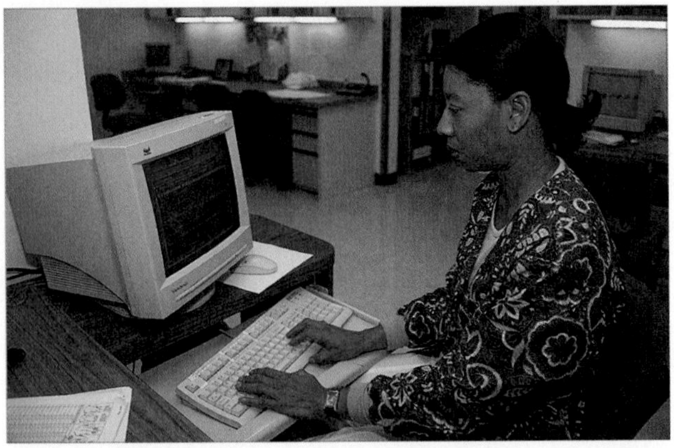

Figure 8–10 A nurse enters information into the computer. **Source:** Sorrentino, S.A. (2000). *Mosby's textbook for nursing assistants* (5th ed. p. 85). St. Louis: Mosby.

We have discussed three methods of reporting—verbal reports, written reports, and computerized reports. Each method has advantages as well as disadvantages. Verbal reports allow for quick, up-to-date information sharing; however, there is no permanent record of what you have reported. Written reports provide a permanent record of what you report, but they are time consuming and sometimes can be difficult to read if the handwriting is not clear. Computerized reports are fast and efficient but confidentiality is more difficult to maintain because data could be accessed by unauthorized people.

REVIEW

Answers to these questions are at the bottom of the page.

Circle the BEST answer.

1. **Assessment involves:**
   A. Collecting information about the client
   B. Carrying out or performing the elements of the care plan
   C. Implementing the care plan
   D. Evaluating and measuring the effectiveness of the care plan

2. **The statement, "Urinary Elimination, Impaired" is on a care plan. This statement is a(n):**
   A. Nursing diagnosis
   B. Assessment
   C. Evaluation
   D. Medical diagnosis

3. **Mrs. Muryama says, "I didn't sleep at all last night because of the pain in my back." This is:**
   A. A nursing diagnosis
   B. Subjective data
   C. An intervention
   D. Objective data

4. **You record the following: "Mr. Munro was better today." What is wrong with this observation?**
   A. It does not say better than what.
   B. It is an assumption.
   C. It is an assessment.
   D. Nothing is wrong with this observation.

5. **Which statement is *false*?**
   A. A chart is discarded after the client is discharged from hospital.
   B. A chart is a permanent, legal document.
   C. A chart is updated as a client's needs and condition change.
   D. A chart provides a record of accountability for health care providers.

6. **A graphic sheet:**
   A. Records a client's activities of daily living (ADLs)
   B. Is used to record measurements and observations made three to four times per day
   C. Contains information about the care given, the client's responses to care, and observations about the client's condition
   D. Summarizes a client's care and services over a period of time

7. **A data form:**
   A. Is used in long-term care settings to detail a person's physical, emotional, social, and intellectual health
   B. Is used in home care settings to assess changes that may be needed to the home
   C. Includes boxes that are checked for the day on which care or services were given
   D. Is another name for Kardex

8. **In 24-hour time, 1330 is:**
   A. 3:30 p.m.
   B. 3:30 a.m.
   C. 1:30 p.m.
   D. 1:30 a.m.

9. **If you make an error when recording, you should:**
   A. Put an X though the error, and write "error" over it.
   B. Erase the error.
   C. Draw a single line through the error, and write "error" over it.
   D. Use correction fluid.

10. **In a long-term care facility, who has access to residents' charts?**
    A. All staff members
    B. Only the office staff and nursing staff
    C. Nurses, support workers, physiotherapists, occupational therapists, and dieticians
    D. It depends on facility policy and procedures.

Answers: 1.A, 2.A, 3.B, 4.B, 5.A, 6.B, 7.A, 8.C, 9.C, 10.D

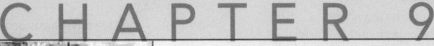

CHAPTER 9

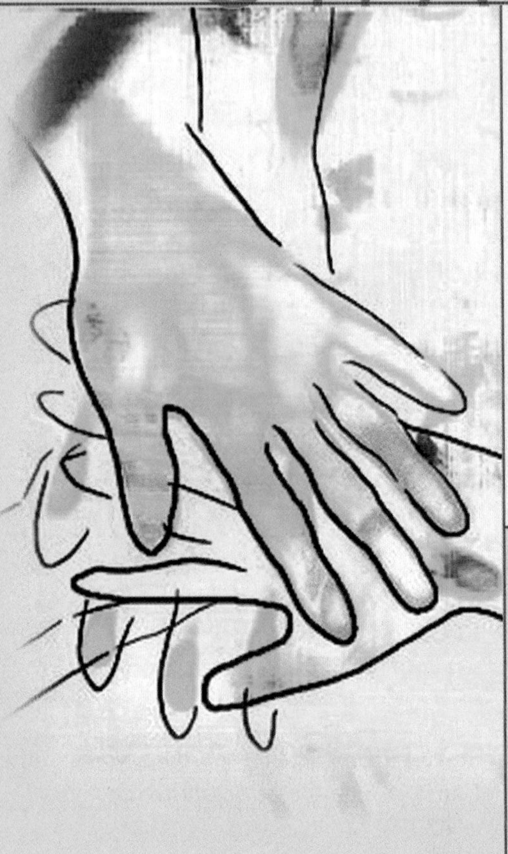

Managing Stress, Time, and Problems

OBJECTIVES

- Define the key terms listed in this chapter.
- Describe how stress can affect all dimensions of life.
- List the signs of stress.
- Discuss defence mechanisms.
- Describe the common stressors.
- Describe ways to manage stress.
- Define SMART goals.
- Describe methods that will improve your decision-making and problem-solving abilities.
- Identify ways to deal with conflict.

key terms

anxiety A vague, uneasy feeling, including a sense of impending danger or harm.

burnout A state of physical, emotional, and mental exhaustion.

conflict A clash between opposing interests and ideas.

defence mechanism An unconscious reaction that blocks unpleasant or threatening feelings.

empathy The ability to recognize, perceive, and have an understanding of another's emotions by being able to put oneself into another person's shoes.

stress The emotional, behavioural, or physical response to an event or situation.

stressor An event or situation that causes stress.

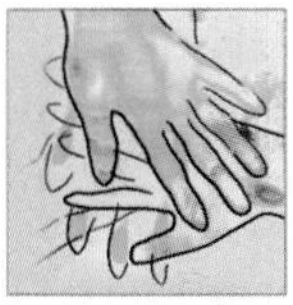

Marissa became a support worker because she likes helping people. She feels great compassion for her clients. Most of the time, she likes her job, but she sometimes worries that she is not doing her best. She feels stressed and rushed and has trouble making decisions. She discusses her feelings with her supervisor, who encourages her to take a time-management course. Her supervisor also offers to help Marissa become a better decision maker and problem solver.

This chapter deals with four key challenges faced by support workers: (1) handling stress, (2) managing time, (3) making decisions, and (4) solving problems. As a support worker, if you can manage time, make wise decisions, and solve problems, you will have less stress.

STRESS

Stress is a normal part of life, and everyone experiences stress at one time or another. **Stress** is the emotional, behavioural, or physical response to an event or situation. The event or situation that causes stress is a **stressor**. Events or situations that are perceived to be threatening, new, or exciting, and physical conditions such as illness, fever, or pregnancy are all stressors.

Although most people do not like stress, sometimes it can be helpful because it can encourage people to function effectively. For example, the stress caused by a busy schedule can motivate a person to work efficiently. However, stress that lasts for a long time or is very intense can cause illness. Headaches, upset stomach, depression, heart disease, and some cancers are examples of illness caused by stress.

Stress affects the whole person. It can have positive or negative effects in all dimensions—the physical, emotional, social, intellectual, and spiritual (Table 9–1). Severe and prolonged stress can lead to **burnout**—a state of physical, emotional, and mental exhaustion. A person experiencing burnout feels discouraged, negative, and powerless. We discuss the topic of burnout in more detail on page 117.

Responses to Stress

Different people respond differently to the same stressor. A person's responses to stressors are influenced by several factors, including:

- Health
- Temperament or personality
- Past experiences with the same or similar stressors
- The number of other stressors the person is experiencing
- The nature, severity, and duration of the stressor

People respond to stress in different ways. There are physical responses to stress (Box 9–1 on page 115) and emotional and behavioural responses (Box 9–2 on page 115). Physical responses are the same for most people, but emotional and behavioural responses vary among individuals. Often a person's

Table 9–1 Stress Can Affect All Dimensions

Dimension	Example of Stressor	Example of a Negative Effect	Example of a Positive Effect
Physical	Pneumonia	Death	Infection resolved
	Breast cancer	Death	Successful treatment
Emotional	Sexual assault by a man	Fear of men; depression	Finding fulfillment as a mentor for others at sexual assault crisis centre
	Divorce	Anger, resentment, crying, unable to work	Seeking help through employment. assistance program
Intellectual	Diagnosis of cancer	Denying presence of cancer and refusing to consider treatment	Learning about the disease to make decisions about care
	Final exam	Deciding not to continue to study	Planning a study schedule
Social	Alcoholism	Withdrawal from family and other social contacts	Participation in Alcoholics Anonymous support group
	Move to new city; knowing no one	Remaining isolated, becoming depressed	Joining a group that shares similar interests, e.g., ski club, or taking a course
Spiritual	Injury	Feeling abandoned by God	Seeking counselling from spiritual adviser; finding comfort in faith
	Death of a family member	Abandoning faith	Seeking comfort from faith or from other people

Source: Adapted from Potter, P.A., Perry, A.G., Ross-Kerr, J.C., & Wood, M.J. (2001). *Canadian fundamentals of nursing,* (2nd ed., p. 647). Toronto: Harcourt Canada.

behaviour is his or her way of coping with stress. Some behaviours relieve stress, for example, crying and talking. Some other behaviours, for example, smoking and drinking, are unhealthy, and these may eventually increase rather than decrease stress.

As a support worker, it is important to recognize the common responses to stress both in yourself and in your clients. Tell your supervisor if you notice a client is showing signs of stress. Remember, your role is to observe and report, not to assess or diagnose. So, report only your observations, and do not make assumptions based on your observations. For example, when a client complains of headaches and nausea, do not assume that the client is suffering from stress, as it could be just a physical condition. However, it is necessary to note and report these symptoms, since professionals such as nurses and social workers can help clients cope with stress.

Defence Mechanisms

A **defence mechanism** is an unconscious reaction that blocks unpleasant or threatening feelings. Most people use defence mechanisms, at one time or another, especially when they are under stress, as defence mechanisms help relieve stress by helping the person avoid facing a troubling reality. For example, a client in a facility is upset that his daughter cannot visit him frequently. He blames the city bus system, since he believes that if the buses were more reliable, his

Box 9–1 Physical Signs of Stress

- Rapid pulse
- Rapid respirations
- Increased blood pressure
- Rapid speech, higher-pitched voice
- A "lump" in the throat
- "Butterflies" in the stomach
- Dry mouth
- Sweaty palms
- Sore muscles in neck, arms, and back
- Perspiration
- Nausea
- Diarrhea
- Urinary frequency
- Urinary urgency
- Difficulty sleeping
- Change in appetite
- Change in weight

daughter would visit more often. Even though he focuses his anger on the bus system, he really is disappointed with his daughter.

When working with clients under stress, it is useful to be able to recognize their defence mechanisms. Understanding defence mechanisms gives you insight into what they may really be feeling. You can help clients by being empathetic to their feelings and providing compassionate care. Report your observations. The following are examples of defence mechanisms:

- ***Conversion***—changing an emotion into a physical symptom. *Example:* The mother of a seriously ill boy notices she is losing large amounts of hair. Although she appears to be handling the situation very well, her hair loss is a response to the intense stress she is experiencing.
- ***Denial***—refusing to accept an unpleasant or threatening reality. *Example:* A man in a retirement facility has been told that his roommate John has died. The man insists that his new roommate *is* John.
- ***Displacement***—directing emotions toward a person or thing that seems safe instead of toward the person or thing that is the source of the emotions. *Example:* A client is angry with her husband. Instead of expressing anger at him, she shouts at her support worker.
- ***Projection***—assigning one's feelings to someone or something else. *Example:* A child says that she needs a night-light because her doll is afraid of the dark.
- ***Rationalization***—making excuses for one's behaviour or a situation while ignoring the real reason. *Example:* An older man experiences hearing loss. He says he cannot understand what his granddaughter is saying because she is mumbling.
- ***Reaction formation***—acting in a way that is opposite to what one feels. *Example:* A woman ignores a man to whom she is attracted.
- ***Regression***—reverting or moving back to earlier behaviours. *Example:* A 3-year-old wants a bottle when a new baby comes into the family.
- ***Repression***—keeping unpleasant or painful thoughts or experiences from the conscious mind. *Example:* A woman who was sexually abused as a child has no memory of the abuse.

Box 9–2 Emotional and Behavioural Signs of Stress

- **Anxiety**—a vague, uneasy feeling, including a sense of impending danger or harm
- Depression
- Anger
- Worry
- Fear
- Burnout
- Irritability
- Loss of self-esteem
- Fatigue
- Dissatisfaction
- Forgetfulness
- Poor concentration
- Difficulty focusing or following directions
- Emotional outbursts, including yelling or crying
- Smoking
- Drinking
- Talking about the stressor

Sources of Stress

Many factors cause stress. Common stressors include the following:

Change. Whether it is positive or negative, change is always a source of stress. For example, getting a promotion, having a baby, and becoming ill all cause life changes and may cause stress.

Pressure. Pressure is feeling pushed beyond one's limits or abilities. People feel pressured for many reasons. Being rushed, having too many demands, and feeling unable to fulfill expectations are examples (Figure 9–1). People sometimes put pressure on themselves by setting goals that are very difficult or impossible to achieve. For example, Penelope is frustrated with herself because she fails to lose 15 pounds in one month, and this causes stress. Clearly, her goal was too difficult to achieve.

Lack of Control. People feel stress when they feel they cannot control what happens to them and to their environment around them and they have to depend on someone else. For example, loss of work, economic hardships, violence, illness, discrimination, and death of a loved one all cause stress. Not being able to control one's own behaviour is also a stressor. For example, Ms. Kumar wants to quit smoking. She tries and fails, and she is angry at her apparent lack of self-control. This causes stress, to which she responds by smoking.

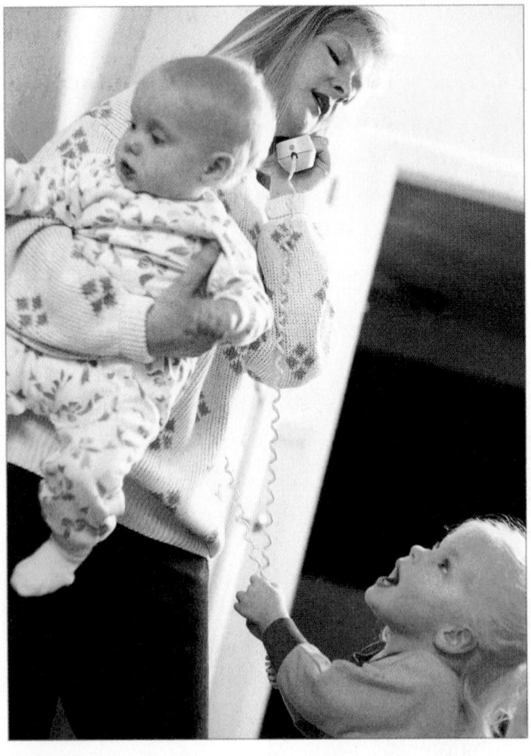

Figure 9–1 This woman feels pressured because she is unable to fulfill the demands made on her by both her children and her job. **Source:** Chris Lowe/Index Stock Imagery/Maxx Images.

Conflict. **Conflict** is a clash between opposing interests and ideas. Conflicts with a partner, friend, child, co-worker, or client are serious sources of stress. People also experience conflict within themselves when sorting out their problems or making decisions.

School. When you are studying to become a support worker, you may become stressed by numerous assignments, tests, exams, and clinical placements that you have to complete.

Daily Irritations. The seemingly minor incidents that occur every day sometimes cause stress—for example, not finding the car keys, being stuck in traffic, or oversleeping. As a support worker, you may encounter minor irritants, such as having to manage with insufficient staff to complete all the required care or being sent to another floor to cover for someone else when you do not know the residents. Depending on how you usually react to a frustrating situation, any incident can cause stress.

The more frequently the stressor occurs and the longer it lasts, the more likely it is that the person's health will suffer. Stressors that last for a few minutes to a few hours usually create only mild stress, for example, daily irritations. Stressors that last for months or years, such as chronic illness, disability, and family relationship problems, cause severe stress (see the *Focus on Older Adults: Stress* and the *Focus on Children: Stress* boxes).

Managing Stress in Your Life

Burnout is common among health care workers, particularly in support work, which can be very demanding. You may feel stress from all the lifting, moving, and carrying that you are required to do

focus on
>>OLDER ADULTS

Stress

Older adults may face many stressors, including:

- Health problems
- Economic worries, since most older adults are on a limited, fixed income
- Increased dependency if the person becomes frail
- Loneliness and isolation
- Decline in abilities due to the normal aging process

Although they may be faced with many stressors, most older adults can cope with stress equally well as other adults do. Many older adults are likely to rely on their spirituality to cope with illness or severe stress.

Source: Potter, P.A., Perry, A.G., Ross-Kerr, J.C., & Wood, M.J. (2001). *Canadian fundamentals of nursing* (2nd ed., p. 655). Toronto: Harcourt Canada.

every day. You may feel stress while trying to do many things at once. For example, a client asks for the bedpan every time you walk by the room, and another needs to be turned and repositioned every 15 minutes. You may feel emotional stress from working with clients who are sick, lonely, frail, or dying. You may also work with clients or family members who are angry or distressed. For example, a wife who is the primary caregiver for her ill husband is angry with her boss for insisting that she always stay late at work. She may direct her anger toward you or you might feel upset for her. Depending on how you react, situations like this could cause severe stress.

Managing stress is essential, so do not ignore the signs of stress. Letting stress build can result in burnout or illness. Not dealing properly and immediately with stress can cause some support workers to take out their frustrations on their clients or someone in their personal lives. This may lead to abuse or neglect, which cannot be allowed to happen.

focus on
>>CHILDREN

Stress

Infants and children also react to stressors and may show the same signs of stress as do adults. For example, a child under stress might have stomachaches, irritability, changes in appetite, or changes in sleep patterns.

Children might not be able to communicate their feelings in words very well. They are more likely to indicate how they feel with their actions. Whenever a child behaves out of the ordinary, the behaviour may be a sign of stress—for example, a normally content baby cries for an hour after she was overstimulated; a fully toilet-trained 4-year-old suddenly begins to wet the bed after his mother becomes seriously ill; or a usually calm adolescent begins to engage in physical fights with peers after his parents divorce.

Job Burnout

Burnout is common among health care workers, since these helping professions can be very demanding physically, emotionally, and mentally. As we discussed earlier, severe or prolonged stress can lead to burnout, which is a state of physical, emotional, and mental exhaustion caused by long-term exposure to demanding work situations. Like stress, burnout can have negative consequences for your health, such as insomnia, weight gain or loss, depression, anxiety, and other emotional difficulties.

The following are some of the signs of burnout:

- You find yourself more critical or sarcastic at work.
- Your sleep habits have changed.
- Your appetite has changed.
- You drag yourself to work and have trouble getting started once you arrive.
- You have less patience with your clients and co-workers.
- You are self-medicating—using food, drugs, or alcohol to make yourself feel better.

If you are showing signs of burnout, do not ignore them. Talk to your supervisor, doctor, or employee assistance program counselor. Recovery can take time, but keep an open mind and consider all of your options.

supporting KATHY

Kathy is a support worker, who has been working at the same continuing care facility for over 20 years. If asked if she likes her job, she would say, "It pays the bills." You have noticed that she arrives at work a few minutes late every day and takes longer breaks than the other employees do. When everyone else is getting up to go back to work after their break time ends, Kathy announces, "Well, I'm going to the bathroom." She then returns to the unit 5 to 10 minutes after everyone else. You suspect that she goes outside to have another cigarette because she usually smells strongly of tobacco upon her return.

You do not enjoy working with Kathy because she is opinionated and occasionally rude to you when you ask her questions. You have seen her being "short" with some of the more challenging or demanding residents. Kathy rarely smiles and hardly ever speaks to you. She usually only talks to the other senior staff.

Today, at change-of-shift report, the nurse reports that Mrs. Price—a client who you liked very much—has died. Kathy says loudly, "Good, one less person I've got to toilet." Lately, you have been thinking about doing something to address Kathy's altitude but do not know where to begin. You do not want to quit because the agency is located conveniently just down the street from where you live. What should you do?

The following strategies will help in managing stress:

- ***Develop self-awareness.*** Know what causes your stress. Think about when you felt under stress. What was the source? Does it occur often? After determining your stressors, you need to decide how to eliminate them, avoid them, or cope with them.
- ***Take care of your needs.*** A healthy mind and body enable people to cope better with stress. Getting enough sleep is important. Mild irritations may seem like serious problems if you are sleep deprived. Exercising regularly and following a nutritious diet are also important. Do not ignore your social, intellectual, and spiritual needs. For many people, the key to managing stress is finding ways to balance family, work, relaxation, and recreation. Keep track of how you spend your time. Which parts of your life get too much time? Which parts are neglected? How might you achieve a better balance?
- ***Think positively.*** A positive attitude can help you manage stress. Focus on what you do well and what you can control. Remember that every person perceives stress differently. Try to change your perspective to see how a stressor can create a positive outcome. Put the stressor into perspective. Try not to let a minor stressor become a major one. Keeping a sense of humour also helps reduce tension.
- ***Assert yourself.*** Nonassertive people say yes to things when they really want to say no. They take on tasks when they have no time for them. They also give in to the demands of others, without considering their own needs. Never agree to do more than you are able (see Chapter 13).
- ***Ask others for help and support.*** To avoid stress, you have to accept that you cannot do everything yourself. Assert yourself at work and in your home life. If you need help with an assignment, tell your supervisor. At home, let your family know that you need their help and support. Discuss sharing household duties with your spouse and children. Let them know what you need and expect, and take the time to explain to them how things are done. Be encouraging, and avoid being critical if things are not done to your standard.
- ***Practise calming exercises.*** As soon as you feel the first sign of stress, find a way to calm yourself (see Box 9–3). Some people do daily meditation to help cope with stress (see Box 9–4).

TIME MANAGEMENT

Time management, which is essential to reducing stress, is also important in support work. You can use time-management strategies in all aspects of

Box 9–3 Calming Yourself When Feeling Stress

- Shut your eyes (if safe to do so) and take deep, slow breaths. Relax your stomach muscles. Breathe in through your nose and out through your mouth. Your stomach should rise about 3 cm (1 inch) as you breathe in. As you inhale, count slowly up to 4. As you exhale, count slowly back down to 1. Pause between breaths. Continue breathing slowly and rhythmically until you can feel yourself relaxing.
- If you feel your muscles tensing, relax them. People tend to clench their jaws and tighten their necks and backs when they are under stress. Relax your muscles, from your face down to your feet.
- If possible, take a few minutes to yourself. Remove yourself from the stressful situation. ***However, never leave a client unless it is safe to do so.***

your life. If you reduce your overall stress levels, stress at work will also decline.

To manage your time, you must identify your priorities. They help you stay focused on what is important to you. While at work, providing competent, compassionate care is a priority. To determine your priorities outside of work, ask yourself these questions:

- What do I value most in life?
- What gives me satisfaction?
- What principles do I want to live my life by?

You may identify a large number of priorities. Take some time to decide which ones are the most important. Assign a number to each, with 1 being the most important and 10 being the least important. Now you are ready to turn your priorities into goals.[1]

Setting Smart Goals

Setting goals for yourself will help you manage time and stress. Your goals should motivate you to take action and give you direction. Start with your priority number 1 and work down the list to number 10. Do not set more than 10 goals, or you may lose your focus. Your goals should be SMART: **S**pecific, **M**easurable, **A**chievable, **R**ealistic, and **T**imely.[1]

- ***Specific.*** Goals must be clear. For example, "losing weight" is not a specific goal. The goal of "losing 5 kilograms by the end of March" is specific and gives direction and focus.
- ***Measurable.*** Measurable goals tell you if you are making progress. The goal stated above is measurable in two ways: "5 kilograms" and "by the end of March."
- ***Achievable.*** Goals should be challenging, yet achievable. When setting goals, consider how much time and effort you can put into them. A goal may need two or more parts to be achievable. For example, to lose the weight you are going to need to investigate a diet plan or an exercise plan and how much time will be needed to put your plan into action.
- ***Realistic.*** A realistic goal accounts for time, resources, and skills. For example, losing 5 kilograms in 3 months is realistic. It would not be realistic if you are planning on a vacation during this time.

Box 9–4 Meditation

- At home, sit in a comfortable position in a quiet place. Turn the ringer off the phone.
- Pick a word that can be repeated during meditation. Single-syllable words, such as "one," are very effective.
- Relax all muscle groups, beginning with the head and working progressively down to your feet.
- Breathe in slowly through the nose, and exhale slowly through your mouth.
- Silently repeat the chosen word while inhaling and exhaling.
- Focus thoughts on this rhythmic chanting and breathing for 10 minutes.
- Allow images and thoughts to flow freely.

Source: Adapted from Potter, P.A., Perry, A., Ross-Kerr, J.C., & Wood, M.J. (2001). *Canadian fundamentals of nursing,* (2nd ed., p. 655). Toronto: Harcourt Canada.

- ***Timely.*** A target date for meeting goals increases commitment. Break goals into parts, and set time schedules. As each part is achieved, you will gain confidence and be motivated to reach higher goals. For example, your goal can be broken down into losing 1.5 kilograms a month.

Planning Your Life and Your Work

Well-organized people have weekly and daily plans and include their personal and professional goals in their planning. Goals are easier to achieve if you spend some time planning at the start of each week. For example, every Sunday, Raj, a busy support worker who has a wife and two children, plans his week. He is working the evening shift this week, which means his wife must pick up the children, make dinner, and take them to after-school activities. Since Raj's wife is going to be out of town on Thursday, Raj makes a note to arrange for his sister to look after the children that day. One of Raj's goals is to build a backyard hockey rink, as he promised his children. He decides to do this during the day every day before leaving for work. Raj reviews his work schedule for the week. His supervisor has asked him to coach a new support worker this week, which means he will be taking the new support worker on client visits. Since this may cause concern for one of his clients, his supervisor has asked him to call the client ahead to prepare him for the new worker. Raj makes a note to telephone this client on Monday.

Daily planning and scheduling are important to meeting goals. Review your assignment sheet and the care plan for each client, and decide how you will approach each task. If you do this ahead of time (the night before or just before your shift), you will not have to waste the valuable time you have with clients scheduling tasks. This does not mean that you should never change a schedule once it has been set. You must stay flexible and responsive to the needs of the client (see the *Support Workers Solving Problems: Daily Planning* box).

Use your planning and scheduling time to think about problems that might arise. Review the tasks on your list. Plan how much time each task will take. To improve scheduling, ask yourself these questions:

SUPPORT WORKERS SOLVING PROBLEMS

Daily Planning

<< Scenario >>

Chona is a support worker in a long-term care facility. Before her morning shift begins, she reviews her assignment sheet and the care plans for each of the clients she supports. The care plan notes that Mrs. Paget, a new client, requires assistance in making decisions for herself. The care plan identifies that all care providers should help Mrs. Paget make decisions by providing choices.

<< Discussion >>

Chona considers the choices that she could provide for Mrs. Paget during the day. She decides that she can offer Mrs. Paget two sets of clothes to wear for the day, two different items for breakfast, two different items for lunch. As she provides A.M. care, Chona can familiarize Mrs. Paget to the activities that are available during the morning and offer Mrs. Paget her choices. After lunch she can talk to her about activities available for the afternoon and again offer her choices. Planning for these choices in advance will help Chona plan her day. There may be many other opportunities during the day when Mrs. Paget can be given choices as situations occur. Chona will need to plan on time for completing flow charts and reporting to the charge nurse.

- What are the client's needs and priorities?
- How much time will each task or activity require?
- When will I do each task or activity?
- Can I organize my time so that some of the tasks overlap?
- Have I allowed time for the unexpected?
- Is there anyone with whom I should co-ordinate these activities?

Give each task a time limit. This helps you stay focused and complete a task in good time. See Box 9–5 for ways to manage your time and stay organized. At the end of your work day, compare what you planned to do with what you actually did. Did you accomplish what you planned? If not, try to

Box 9–5 Tips to Save Time and Stay Organized

- Follow the assignment sheet and the care plan.
- Remember the client's needs and priorities.
- Know what your supervisor expects you to do and when.
- Know what tasks need to be done at a certain time.
- Set yourself time limits; work within those limits, unless a client's needs are more pressing.
- Develop routines that work for you and the client.
- Allow for more time than you need, when possible.
- Remain flexible at all times.
- Start with the tasks that must get done.
- Remind yourself not to get sidetracked by nonessential things.
- Learn to say no—firmly, positively, and tactfully.
- Use a calendar to note down important dates and reminders.
- Make sure that you have equipment and supplies before you start a task.
- Put equipment and supplies back in their proper place.

identify the reasons. Did problems arise? Were there interruptions? Was it a poor schedule?

DECISION MAKING

As a support worker, you make many decisions in the course of your work day—when you organize your time, make a schedule, and provide care to a client. For example, you decide:

- The order in which you are going to carry out tasks
- The equipment and supplies you need for each task
- The amount of time to spend with a client
- When a problem or an observation needs to be reported immediately
- If you need help to complete a task
- If you need to consult with your supervisor
- If you will accept or refuse a delegated task

Skills You Need to Make Decisions

Do you know people who always seem to make the right decisions? They are usually decisive and calm. The following skills will help improve your decision making:

- ***Focus.*** Focus requires concentration, involvement, and commitment. Focus on the client and the task at hand to make the right decisions. This involves asking questions and active listening (Figure 9–2).
- ***Flexibility.*** You need to be flexible and responsive. Involve clients in decisions that affect them. Be ready to adapt in response to a client's needs. Remember, each client is an individual with unique needs. Age, culture, and health status affect the client's needs. For example, (a) Mr. Johnston, 91, lives in a facility and has no family or friends living nearby. He tells you he feels lonely. You decide to chat with him while helping him bathe; (b) Ms. Chow, 35, is recovering at home after surgery. She tells you she feels exhausted. Since listening and talking can

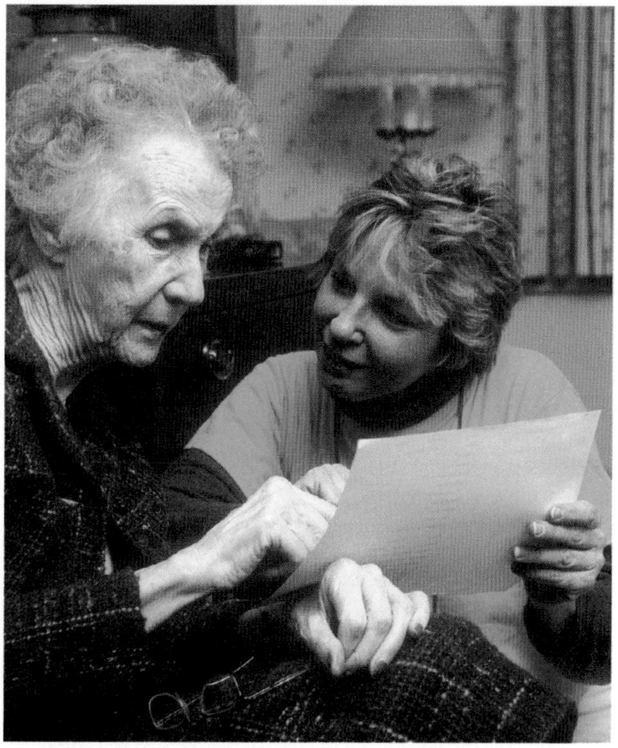

Figure 9–2 This support worker listens carefully to a client in order to make the right decision. **Source:** Frank Siteman/Rainbow.

be tiring, you remain quiet while helping Ms. Chow with her bath. You ask her if she would like to rest afterward and she agrees. The same task is done differently because you responded to each client's unique needs.

- ***Decisiveness.*** Stick to your decisions unless they are not working, since indecisiveness on your part can upset clients. Clients expect you to be confident and competent.

Decision Making in Different Health Care Settings

You will face similar kinds of decisions in most settings, even though some differences exist between facilities and private homes. In a facility, you care for several clients and also assist nurses, as needed. Sometimes you have to decide which person's needs are to be met first. For example, you see a client shouting angrily at her roommate. Another client needs to be shaved. You need to decide who should be helped first.

In a home care setting, you must plan your time so that you can be on time for the next client. Since your supervisor is not on site, you have to make many decisions on your own.

PROBLEM SOLVING

Problem solving is a process—you identify and analyze a problem, find a solution, and devise a plan to apply that solution.

Identify the Problem

You must first determine *if* you have a problem and *what* it is. Ask yourself the following questions:

- Is the situation or issue affecting you, a co-worker, your supervisor, or one of your clients?
- Should you be concerned about the situation?
- Can you influence or contribute to a positive outcome?
- Does the issue require immediate attention?

Consider the following examples. (a) Miles helps Mr. Rossi, 85, get dressed in the mornings. Most days, Mr. Rossi chooses to wear the same tattered sweater. Miles is tired of seeing it on him. He knows that Mr. Rossi has many other sweaters. However, when Miles considers the above questions, he answers "no" to each question. He knows that the sweater is clean, that Mr. Rossi enjoys wearing it, and that he has the right to choose what he wears. Miles decides that this situation is not a problem. (b) Cheryl assists Mr. McDonald, 88, with lunch in the dining room of a long-term care facility. He chooses tomato soup for lunch. After one spoonful, he refuses to eat. Cheryl is concerned about the situation. She knows that if Mr. McDonald does not eat, he tends to get dizzy and may fall. She knows this is a problem that requires her immediate attention.

Analyze the Problem

Once you know you have a problem, think about what kind of problem it is. Decide if it is one that you can solve on your own. Consult the assignment sheet and care plan to make sure you know what is expected of you. Remember, consult your supervisor when:

- There is an emergency.
- You observe a change in the client's condition or normal functioning.
- The client becomes ill. For example, the client vomits, has diarrhea, or develops a fever.
- The client is in distress.
- You believe the client's safety is at risk.
- A problem arises involving medications.
- The client complains about his or her condition or care.
- The client asks you a question about his or her diagnosis, condition, or treatment plans.
- The client or family member asks you to do something that goes against the care plan.
- You have a conflict with a client or family member.
- A question or problem arises with which you need help.

Your supervisor is always available to provide guidance and solve problems. Even in a community setting, your supervisor is just a phone call away.

Analyzing a problem involves communication. Ask the client questions about the problem, and listen attentively to the answers. Remember to pay attention to verbal as well as nonverbal messages (see *Support Workers Solving Problems: Asking, Listening, and Observing* box.) Do not make assumptions about the cause of a problem.

For example, when Cheryl asks Mr. McDonald why he does not want to eat, he says that he has a sore on the inside of his cheek where he bit himself the other day. She can tell by his expression that his mouth is sore. Cheryl knows that Mr. McDonald's care plan does not specify a special diet. He is able to eat anything from the available menu. She therefore decides that she can try to solve the problem herself. She does not need to involve her supervisor right now.

SUPPORT WORKERS SOLVING PROBLEMS

Asking, Listening, and Observing

<< Scenario >>

Salman, a support worker on a surgical ward in a hospital, is assigned to help Mrs. Kao do range-of-motion (ROM) exercises following surgery. When Mrs. Kao refuses, Salman asks her why she does not want to do the exercises. Mrs. Kao says her legs ache and she does not feel like moving them. Salman tries to encourage Mrs. Kao and asks her if the nurse explained why the exercises are important. Mrs. Kao says she knows why the exercises are important. Salman suggests that Mrs. Kao start by moving her toes, and when Mrs. Kao moves her toes, she grimaces. Salman asks Mrs. Kao if she is in pain, and Mrs. Kao says, "No, I'm not in pain."

<< Discussion >>

Salman realizes that there is nothing more that he can do or say. He has asked Mrs. Kao the right questions, listened to her responses, and observed her behaviour. It is not his job to assess or diagnose Mrs. Kao's problem. So he informs his supervisor of his conversation with Mrs. Kao and reports to his supervisor that Mrs. Kao grimaced when she moved her toes. He is careful to report Mrs. Kao's exact words.

Devise a Plan

Think of as many solutions as you can. Decide which is the most practical and helpful, but always be sure that it is safe. Try the solution and see if it works. For example, Cheryl thinks that the tomato soup is too hot and acidic for Mr. McDonald's sore mouth. She suggests he try a cooler, blander meal. He chooses the macaroni and cheese. He is able to eat this without discomfort. Cheryl later reports to her supervisor that Mr. McDonald has a sore in his mouth.

The planning part of the problem-solving process may involve creativity. Do not be afraid to try a plan, as long as it is safe. Consider Ruth's creative solution to a problem. Ruth's client, Mrs. Klassen, is in the early stages of Alzheimer's disease. Mrs. Klassen is upset because she cannot remember her grandson's name. He will be visiting the next day, and she wants to be able to call him by his name. Ruth has the grandson's name listed on the care plan. She then gently suggests a way to help Mrs. Klassen remember it. They find a picture of her grandson and write his name on it. Ruth then tapes the picture to the wall by the phone. Mrs. Klassen will have the picture handy when her grandson visits. Ruth records this on the task sheet. At her next visit with Mrs. Klassen, she asks her if their solution worked (see the *Support Workers Solving Problems: Creative Solutions* box for another example of a support worker devising a plan to solve a problem).

DEALING WITH CONFLICT

Some problems can be resolved at once, but others take longer. Interpersonal problems, which are a common cause of stress, may take weeks to solve. People bring their own values, attitudes, opinions, experiences, and expectations to the work setting. Differences often lead to conflict, and disagreements, misunderstandings, arguments, and unrest can occur. Conflicts may arise over issues or events, for example, work schedules, absences, and the amount and quality of work performed. The problems must be worked out to avoid unkind words or actions. When the work environment becomes unpleasant, providing effective care to clients is affected.

Support Workers Solving Problems

Creative Solutions

<< Scenario >>

Josephine's client Mrs. Samuels, 34, is a single mother who is receiving chemotherapy for ovarian cancer. Mrs. Samuels has three boys, ages 9 years, 5 years, and 20 months. Mrs. Samuels tells Josephine that ever since she became ill she does not feel that she is doing enough for her children.

<< Discussion >>

Josephine asks Mrs. Samuels what sorts of things she misses doing for her children. Mrs. Samuels says that she wishes she could dress her two little boys in the morning. She also regrets not being able to drive her older boy to after-school activities. Josephine decides to look for opportunities to consult and involve Mrs. Samuels in the care of her children. As the 5-year-old gets ready for school that morning, Josephine suggests to him that he ask his mother to zip up his jacket and help him put on his mittens and hat. Later she asks Mrs. Samuels what she would like the baby to wear that day.

Sometimes you may experience conflict with clients, their families, or co-workers. In dealing with any conflict, it is imperative to remember that caring for the client's needs is always your first priority.

Conflict between you and a client could occur if a client is too tired, overstimulated, confused, or having difficulty communicating. For example, Mrs. Jones had been out to a doctor's appointment in the morning and is refusing to eat her lunch. You know it is important that she eat something. If you do not recognize that Mrs. Jones is too tired and you persist in trying to get her to eat, the conflict could escalate. Perhaps you should allow Mrs. Jones to rest first and eat later, and you should report this to your supervisor. Report all conflicts with clients to your supervisor, including the ones where you have resolved the problem. You can prevent conflict from escalating by remaining calm and respectful, understanding the client's needs and feelings, and recognizing the reason for the client's behaviour.

Conflict can also occur between you and the client's family. It is important to remember that in most cases, they are only trying to ensure the best care for their ill family member. The conflict usually occurs because of failure to understand the nursing care plan, the reasons for a change in the client's condition or treatment, or the policies of the facility or agency. You should listen to their concerns in a calm, nonjudgemental way. If your explanation does not satisfy them, contact your supervisor to ensure that the situation does not worsen. Even if you have defused the situation, you must still report the family member's concern to your supervisor.

Conflict between co-workers can have a negative effect on the care of clients. Unresolved conflict causes stress and hinders communication and team work. To some extent, this is unavoidable, since you are not always going to agree with your supervisors or team members. Applying some of the principles outlined in Box 9–6 can help you resolve conflict in many situations. You do not need to report conflicts with co-workers if the problem has been resolved. However, if you cannot resolve a conflict, discuss it with your supervisor.

Communication and a good work ethic are essential in preventing and resolving conflicts. Identify and solve problems before they become major issues.

Box 9–6 Managing Conflict

- Approach the co-worker with whom you have a conflict, and ask to talk with him or her privately. Be polite and professional in your approach.
- Agree on a time and place to talk.
- Talk in a private setting. Others should not see or hear you and your co-worker having what might seem like an argument.
- Explain the problem and what is bothering you. Give facts, and describe specific behaviours. Focus on the problem, not on the person. For example, say, "I need to know when you cannot help me so I can make other plans." Avoid criticizing the person—for example, saying, "You are always late and never call to let me know."
- Listen to the co-worker's response. Do not interrupt.
- Identify ways to resolve the problem. Offer your own thoughts, and ask for the person's ideas.
- Schedule a date and a time to review the situation.
- Thank the person for meeting with you.
- Implement the solutions.
- Review the situation, as needed.
- If you are unable to resolve the conflict, ask your supervisor for some time to talk privately. Explain the situation, and ask for advice in solving the problem. Give facts and specific examples.

Scenario: Your teacher has just handed back a major assignment, and you do not understand why you have received such a low mark. You face the choice of becoming very upset, complaining to other students about the teacher, becoming discouraged and dropping out of the program, or managing this conflict. To manage this conflicting you should do the following:

- Ask to talk privately with the teacher.
- Set a time and private place to talk.
- Explain the problem, and ask the teacher to review the assignment with you so that you can understand where you made errors or did not meet the required standards.
- Listen carefully to the teacher's explanation.
- Calmly explain why you feel your mark should be higher.
- Offer your ideas on how to resolve the problem, and ask for the teacher's ideas.
- Set a time to review the situation.
- Thank the teacher for meeting with you.
- Implement the solution you have arrived at.

REVIEW

Answers to these questions are at the bottom of the page.

Circle the **BEST** answer.

1. **Stress is:**
   - A. The way you cope with and adjust to everyday living
   - B. The emotional, behavioural, or physical response to an event or situation
   - C. A mental or emotional disorder
   - D. A thought or idea

2. **A stressor is:**
   - A. An event or situation that causes stress
   - B. A coping strategy
   - C. A defence mechanism
   - D. A reaction to stress

3. **Which influences a person's reaction to a stressor?**
   - A. Past experiences with the same stressor
   - B. The person's sex
   - C. A and D
   - D. The person's temperament or personality

4. **Which of the following is a physical sign of stress?**
   - A. Fatigue
   - B. Depression
   - C. Diarrhea
   - D. Irritability

5. **A defence mechanism is used to:**
   - A. Blame others
   - B. Block unpleasant or threatening feelings
   - C. Solve problems
   - D. Make excuses for behaviour

6. **You are angry with a co-worker. Instead of responding appropriately to the situation, you yell at a friend. Which defence mechanism is this?**
   - A. Denial
   - B. Conversion
   - C. Displacement
   - D. Compensation

7. **Goals should be SMART. What does SMART stand for?**
   - A. Simple, monthly, allowable, reasonable, timely
   - B. Specific, measurable, achievable, realistic, timely
   - C. Simple, measurable, achievable, reasonable, topical
   - D. Specific, monthly, allowable, realistic, topical

8. **When trying to stay organized and save time, it is best to:**
   - A. Save the important tasks until last
   - B. Not set yourself a time limit for each task
   - C. Develop a routine that works for you
   - D. Remain inflexible

9. **The first step in the problem-solving process is to:**
   - A. Call for help
   - B. Learn to say no assertively
   - C. Identify the problem
   - D. Think of as many solutions as you can

10. **What is an important part of resolving conflict?**
    - A. Communication and good work ethics
    - B. Focusing on the person, not the problem
    - C. Avoiding the person with whom you have a conflict
    - D. Confronting the person with your supervisor for support

Answers: 1.B, 2.A, 3.C, 4.C, 5.B, 6.C, 7.B, 8.C, 9.C, 10.A

CHAPTER 10

Ethics

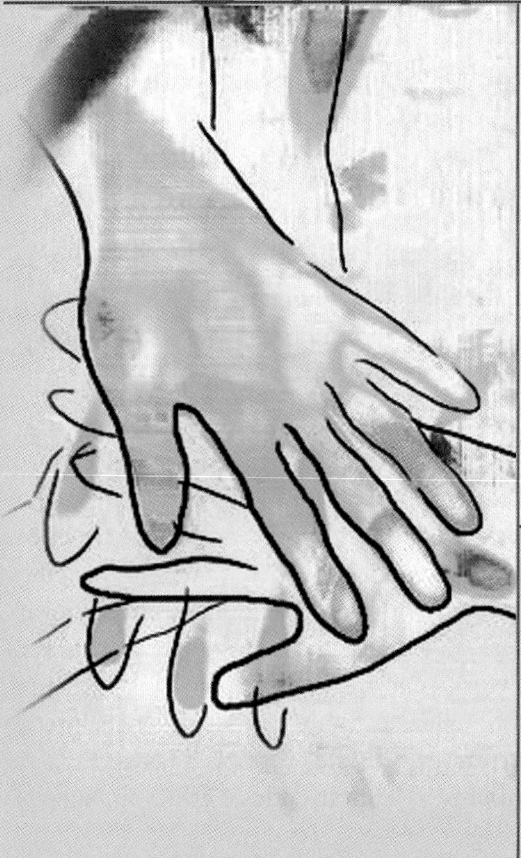

OBJECTIVES

- Define the key terms listed in this chapter.
- Explain the purpose of a code of ethics.
- Differentiate between ethics and morals.
- Identify the four basic principles of health care ethics.
- Describe how each of the four principles applies to support work.
- Define the term "ethical dilemma."
- Apply the principles to solve ethical dilemmas.

key terms

autonomy Having free choice to make decisions that affect one's life. Also known as **self-determination**.

beneficence Doing or promoting good.

conduct Personal behaviour that is based on moral principles.

ethics The principles or values that guide us when deciding what is right and what is wrong, and what is good and what is bad.

ethical dilemma A situation that will often involve an apparent conflict between opposing moral choices, and choosing one would result in going against another moral choice.

health care ethics The philosophical study of what is morally right and wrong when providing health care services.

immoral Actions conflicting with traditionally held moral principles and are often regarded as indecent or deviant.

justice Treating people in a fair and equal manner.

morals Actions that are founded on the fundamental principles of right and virtuous conduct, rather than legalities or customs. The opposite of moral is **immoral**.

nonmaleficence The ethical principle of doing no harm.

self-determination See **autonomy**.

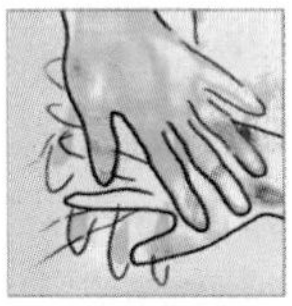

The term **ethics** refers to the principles or values that guide us when deciding what is right and what is wrong (**immoral**), and what is good and what is bad. Ethics and **morals** are often used to mean the same thing, although some people also think of morals as including values related to sexual behaviour. Ethics play a part in your everyday life, and we apply them when making both big and small decisions. Whether we realize it or not, ethics have a great impact on our personal and professional relationships. As a support worker, when you have to make difficult choices or decisions, you will rely on your ethics to guide your conduct.

CODES OF ETHICS

Members of the health care team have special responsibilities as they form professional helping relationships with clients who require care and services. To guide health care workers' interactions with clients, ethical standards have been established.

Regulated professionals (such as physicians and nurses) have codes of ethics provided by their governing colleges. These codes describe the ideals of the profession as well as standards of conduct that group members must follow.

Support workers do not have a formal code of ethics. However, many employers have their own code of ethics for their employees that describes the values and personal qualities that should guide your work and your **conduct**. Codes of ethics vary among employers, but most verify the priorities of support work that are identified in this text: promoting the client's dignity, independence, preferences, privacy, and safety, as well as a right to confidentiality. A sample code of ethics for support workers is given in Box 10–1.

supporting MR. CREISHILO

Sam Creishilo is a 32-year-old client to whom you have provided support care in his home for several months after a motor vehicle accident. Mr. Creishilo is a bachelor and lives alone. He has always been very pleasant to you, and you have developed a professional relationship with him. On your last visit, he asked if he could have your home phone number so that he could invite you "...out for a coffee sometime." You do not know what your response to him should be. You are also wondering whether the fact that you are single and have no family responsibilities has any bearing in this situation.

Box 10–1 A Sample Code of Ethics for Support Workers

- ***Support workers provide high-quality personal care and support services.*** They work within their scope of practice. They promptly report to their supervisors any concerns and observations about clients' health and well-being. They perform only those tasks for which they have received the necessary education. They know and follow employer policies as well as federal, provincial, or territorial laws. They work within the parameters of national and provincial or territorial laws at all times.
- ***The support worker needs to be aware of the policies and procedures for each area.*** If the support worker is employed for more than one client or agency, the required skills may vary. It should never be assumed that the skills allowed at one agency can be automatically transferred to another agency.
- ***Support workers provide compassionate care to all clients.*** They promote the client's physical, emotional, intellectual, social, and spiritual well-being. They encourage clients to maintain as much independence as possible, during times of normal health and in situations of illness, injury, disability, or while dying. They respect and promote the family's roles and relationships.
- ***Support workers value the dignity and worth of all clients.*** They strive to treat all clients in an honest, fair, and just manner. They do not discriminate against a client on the basis of age, race/ethnicity, colour, religion, sexual orientation, or culture.
- ***Support workers respect their clients' choices about how they receive or participate in their care.*** They respect and promote the client's wishes.
- *Support workers respect their clients' right to privacy and confidentiality.* Information about the client learned while providing care is not shared with anyone outside the health care team.
- ***Support workers do not misuse their position of trust.*** They do not accept gifts or tips from their clients. They do not buy property from their clients, nor do they sell products to them. They do not try to impose their own religious or other beliefs on their clients. Their behaviour toward clients and co-workers is professional at all times (see the box *Supporting Mr. Creishilo*).
- ***Support workers are reliable.*** They arrive at work on time and complete all assignments. They are patient and courteous with clients. They notify their supervisor if they are going to be late or are unable to work, or inform their client if they are working in the community or home care setting. Their conduct is professional and based on ethical principals.
- ***Support workers promote and maintain their clients' safety.*** They report mistakes and unsafe situations immediately to their supervisors. They consider their clients' safety when performing all tasks and activities.

THE PRINCIPLES OF HEALTH CARE ETHICS

Most codes of ethics are based on the principles of health care ethics. **Health care ethics** is the philosophical study of what is morally right and wrong when providing *health care services.* Sometimes you will find that ethical decisions are easy to make, such as assisting an unsteady but ambulatory client who requests your help with toileting. However, at other times you will find that certain other ethical decisions are more difficult. An **ethical dilemma** is a situation that will often involve an apparent conflict between opposing moral choices, in which choosing one would result in going against another moral choice (see the *Support Workers Solving Problems: Ethical Dilemmas* box on page 132).

The four basic principles of health care ethics are:

- Autonomy—respecting the client's right to make choices for himself or herself
- Justice—being fair
- Beneficence—doing good
- Nonmaleficence—doing no harm

Understanding the principles of health care ethics will help you think and behave ethically toward your clients and co-workers.

Autonomy

Autonomy (also called **self-determination**) means having free choice to make decisions that affect one's life and refers to a person's independence. As long as a person is mentally competent, he or she has the right to make decisions about lifestyle and medical care and services. This concept is critical to health care ethics. There are laws that protect the client's right to autonomy (see Chapter 11). For example, physicians, facilities, and agencies must, by law, ensure that clients give informed consent before any procedure is done to them. Clients decide what kind of treatment they want or do not want.

As a support worker, you must always respect your clients' choices and preferences. The client has autonomy even with routine tasks; for example, if a client asks you to use her own blue sheets to make her bed, it is important that you do so. Using other sheets shows a lack of respect for the client's choice. Even if a client wants a certain hair style that you think is unattractive, you must respect her choice. It would be unethical to ignore her preference and style her hair according to your own taste.

Respecting your clients' autonomy is more complicated if you think their decisions are unsafe. The client has the right to make choices and to take risks. For example, an older client may refuse to use his cane in spite of knowing that he is at risk for falling. After explaining why he should use the cane, you should accept his decision, whatever it may be. Always consult with your supervisor if you have concerns about the client's safety.

Respecting your clients' autonomy also means that you do not judge their choices or lifestyles. You base your judgements and opinions on your own values and standards. Your clients may have values and standards different from yours. For example:

- A daughter decides that her elderly mother needs nursing home care. In your culture, children usually take care of their aging parents at home. You do not understand why the daughter will not care for her mother at home.
- A client has multiple tattoos and body piercings. You do not approve of tattooing or body piercing.
- A client mentions to you that he has decided not to seek treatment for his cancer. You believe he should try everything possible to save his life.

You should avoid judging your clients and their decisions by your values or standards and set aside your biases. Do not give clients advice, and never express your disapproval or opinions about their choices, preferences, politics, religion, or lifestyle.

Justice

The principle of **justice** means that all people should be treated in a fair and equal manner. Justice is an ideal that is central to Canada's universal health care system—all Canadians, regardless of ability to pay, receive equal access to the same medical services. Unfortunately, this is not always true for all people across Canada. Some clients who can afford it can buy services that are not readily available to everyone. Examples of these services include private clinics, medical tests and procedures (such as MRI and hip replacement), as well as elective procedures (such as plastic surgery).

You can uphold the principle of justice by being concerned for all clients, regardless of their conditions or temperaments. Some people are easier to work with than are others. You may be tempted to spend less time with a client who is demanding and ungrateful. You may wish to avoid a client whose lifestyle is very different from your own. However, doing so would be unjust and unethical. Every client deserves your attention and care equally.

Treating people justly also means that you do not betray their trust. Clients trust that you will handle their possessions with care, respect their privacy, perform your services competently and skillfully, and keep all conversations and health information confidential. Do not snoop in the clients' homes, pry into their personal lives, or gossip with your friends or coworkers about them. Share information about the client only with your supervisor and the health care team. Never speak about a client where others may overhear you. This includes public areas such as dining rooms, lounges, locker rooms, and elevators. Confidentiality is a basic right. It is so important that laws have been passed to protect it (see Chapter 11).

Beneficence

Beneficence means doing or promoting good. The principle of beneficence is central to your work.

Support work is about promoting wellness, helping people in their daily lives, and supporting them during difficult times.

To apply the principle of beneficence in your work life, always consider meeting the client's needs to be your most important function. The client's needs come before those of his or her family. Consider the following: Mr. Mijovick lives with his son and daughter-in-law in their home and receives home care services. Marcia is assigned to give Mr. Mijovick a bed bath. His son, however, insists that Marcia does not bathe Mr. Mijovick and finish early that day because he is expecting a visitor. When deciding what to do, Marcia focuses on Mr. Mijovick's needs, not on his son's. She calls her supervisor to report the situation and seek guidance.

The concept of beneficence and professionalism are closely related. To meet your clients' needs, stay within the boundaries of a professional helping relationship (see Chapter 6). Do not ask clients to do something that is in your interests rather than in theirs. For example, if your child is selling chocolate bars to raise money for a school trip, do not ask your client to buy a chocolate bar. Avoid asking clients to do something for you, even if it aims to benefit others more than yourself or your family. For example, even if you are canvassing for United Way, do not ask your client to contribute to the campaign.

When caring for a client, avoid focusing on yourself or burdening the client with your problems and worries. Never take advantage of a client's compassion and generosity. If you tell a client your problems, he or she may try to help you. For example, if you tell a client you are in financial difficulties, the client may offer you money. ***Never ask for or accept money or loans from clients regardless of how long you have been working with them. To do so is unethical.***

Never forget that your relationship with your clients is professional. Clients can become very attached to their support workers. If family relationships are strained, the client may see the relationship with you as replacing the relationship with a family member. Never take advantage of strained family relationships. Do not take sides with a client against a family member. Never flirt, date, or accept invitations made by a client or the client's partner. When support workers become entangled in their clients' affairs, serious consequences can result. For example, you could be named as a beneficiary in a client's will. This could lead to legal problems for you and your employer.

To do the most good for your clients, always give your best effort at work. Unless the person has unexpected problems or needs that require your attention, finish all your assigned tasks. Be careful, alert, and exact when following instructions. Also, be compassionate and empathetic. Self-discipline is essential, especially when working in home care. Avoid any temptation to use your work time for your own interests. This includes watching television, talking on the telephone, and stopping for an extra cup of coffee.

Nonmaleficence

Nonmaleficence is seeking to do no harm. Harm can be intentional (abuse) or unintentional (accidental injury or negligence). To avoid harming a client, only perform tasks that you have been trained to do. By recognizing the limits of your role and knowledge, you are protecting your clients from the risk of harm. Clients or family members may ask you to perform functions that could be dangerous if not performed correctly. Often such requests are made innocently. The client may forget that you are not qualified to do certain tasks. While this confidence in you as a support worker is to be appreciated, it is not safe or wise to take on tasks that you are not trained to do, even if you have the best of intentions.

Clients and their family members may also ask you for information about diagnosis or medical, surgical, or treatment plans. You must never reveal these details, whether or not you are asked. You could give the wrong information and cause harm or distress. Giving or discussing medical information is not only outside your scope of practice, it is also unethical. Refer all such questions to your supervisor.

To provide safe and effective care, you must keep your skills and knowledge current. Participate in educational programs offered by your employer. Consider enrolling in courses or workshops relevant to your work. Support work is continually changing, so you must keep your skills and abilities up to date. What you are trained to do this year may become outdated in a few years. The more knowledge and practice you get, the better and safer your skills will be.

You must keep clients as safe as possible. You can protect them from harm by practising infection control techniques (see Chapter 20) and by recognizing common safety hazards and knowing how to prevent them (see Chapter 19).

DEALING WITH ETHICAL DILEMMAS

Codes of ethics only provide guidelines for ethical behaviour. They do not have the answers or rules for every situation. Occasionally, you may come across a situation that will involve a conflict between two opposing moral choices, and choosing one would result in going against the other. When confronted with such an ethical dilemma, you need to know how to decide on the right thing to do.

When making an ethical decision, carefully consider the four principles of health care ethics. Collect as much information about the situation as possible. Consider all possible options to resolve the dilemma. Ask yourself these questions about each option:

- Does the option respect the client's wishes and preferences?
- Does the option treat the client justly and fairly?
- Does the option provide the client with a short-term benefit or a long-term benefit?
- Could the option cause harm or increase the client's risk of harm?

Answers to these questions may contradict each other. For example, one option may benefit the client but go against his or her wishes. Another option may reflect the client's preferences but increase the risk of harm. If any one option could harm the client, you *must* involve your supervisor in the solution. You must protect the client from harm and also avoid serious legal problems for yourself and your employer.

See the *Support Workers Solving Problems: Ethical Dilemmas* box for a discussion on how support workers deal with ethical dilemmas, and then read *Supporting Mr. Adamson* on page 134. What would *you* do in these situations? Remember to consider the four principles of health care ethics when making your decision.

SUPPORT WORKERS SOLVING PROBLEMS

Ethical Dilemmas

<< Scenario 1 >>

You are assigned to work for a family with a 2-year-old boy and newborn twins. You are responsible for helping with care of the 2-year-old. The mother mentions that since the birth of the twins, the toddler has been throwing temper tantrums around lunch time. She wants to stop this problem behaviour and tells you that if the toddler throws a tantrum or misbehaves, he is to be sent to his room alone for 15 minutes, or longer if he has not settled down by the end of that time.

Discussion: Consider how applying the main principles of health care can seem to cause conflict. What should you do?

Autonomy: The mother has the right to make parenting decisions.

Justice: Would it be fair to the child to leave him in his room for so long?

Beneficence: Will the disciplining help the child improve his behaviour? Can other actions improve his behaviour?

Nonmaleficence: Could leaving the child in his room cause harm?

<< Scenario 2 >>

Miki works in a long-term care facility. Mr. Petrova is a resident on her Resident Care Unit. Miki smells alcohol on Mr. Petrova's breath after his son has visited him. She comments on this to Mr. Petrova, and he tells her that his son had brought him a bottle of liquor. Residents keeping alcohol in their rooms is against facility rules. Mr. Petrova says that alcohol eases his pain and asks Miki to promise not to tell anyone about the liquor.

Discussion: Telling her supervisor about the liquor would disregard Mr. Petrova's wishes and autonomy.

(cont'd)

Support Workers Solving Problems (cont'd)

However, not telling her supervisor could harm Mr. Petrova. For example, alcohol may interfere with his medications or cause adverse reactions. Not telling could also harm Miki. She could be fired for not following facility rules.

Miki explains to Mr. Petrova that she is ethically and legally obligated to tell her supervisor about the bottle of liquor in his room. She explains her reasons but Mr. Petrova still gets upset. Miki, however, knows that she has followed the ethical principle of nonmaleficence. Also, she has avoided betraying Mr. Petrova's trust by refusing to make a promise she cannot keep.

<< Scenario 3 >>

John's home care client is Mrs. Jessop, whose care plan states that she is not allowed sugary foods. Today is Mrs. Jessop's birthday, and her neighbour brings her a cake. Mrs. Jessop tells John that every year on her birthday she chooses to go off her diet. She asks him to cut her a piece of cake. Serving Mrs. Jessop a piece of cake would respect her autonomy. However, the cake could harm Mrs. Jessop's physical health.

Discussion: John decides not to serve the cake to Mrs. Jessop. He knows that she can serve herself or her neighbour can serve it to her. John says that he should perhaps call Mrs. Jessop's case manager about the situation, but Mrs. Jessop does not want John to make the call. She goes ahead and eats the cake. John observes her carefully for any ill effects but notices no change in her condition. Later, he telephones his supervisor to report the incident. His written notes also include exactly what happened.

John upholds the principle of autonomy by allowing Mrs. Jessop to decide to eat the cake. He also upholds the principle of nonmaleficence by not serving her the cake and by encouraging her to consult her case manager before she has a piece. Because he has reported what happened, he has also followed the principle of beneficence.

<< Scenario 4 >>

Tomas is a support worker in a long-term care facility. One afternoon, he observes that Mrs. O'Brian seems upset. He asks Mrs. O'Brian if anything is wrong, and she starts to cry. She tells Tomas that her 17-year-old grandson has been arrested for drunk driving. She asks Tomas not to tell anyone because the family wants to keep the matter private. She also asks Tomas not to tell the nursing staff that she is upset.

Keeping the information confidential and telling no one about her emotional state would respect Mrs. O'Brian's privacy. However, Tomas is expected to report his observations about residents' emotional health. Not doing so could cause Mrs. O'Brian harm. She may suffer from the effects of stress.

Discussion: Tomas decides to tell the charge nurse that Mrs. O'Brian is upset about a private family matter. First, Tomas explains to Mrs. O'Brian that he is required to report his observations of his clients' emotional health. He also assures her that anything he reports will be kept confidential by the health care team.

Tomas's solution respects the ethical principles of autonomy and justice. It also upholds the principle of nonmaleficence. By reporting that Mrs. O'Brian is upset, Tomas ensures that someone with authority will take responsibility for Mrs. O'Brian's emotional health.

<< Scenario 5 >>

P.J. is a support worker caring for Mrs. Osillo, an elderly woman who has a "G-tube" for feeding. As P.J.'s supervisor explained to him, this tube goes directly into Mrs. Osillo's stomach through an opening made in her abdomen, and all of her foods and nutrients are given through it. She cannot have anything to drink, as she has severe swallowing problems and any food or fluids would go into her lungs, resulting in respiratory problems and pneumonia. Mrs. Osillo has already been admitted to the hospital for pneumonia twice this year.

Mrs. Osillo complains that she feels thirsty all the time and begs P.J. to give her something to drink.

Discussion: P.J. cannot give Mrs. Osillo anything to drink, as this would violate the principle of nonmaleficence. Anything that is orally taken can cause severe problems for Mrs. Osillo. P.J. decides that he should discuss this dilemma with the supervisor so that they both can come up with a solution that respects Mrs. Osillo's right to autonomy and is in keeping with the principle of beneficence.

After a discussion with the supervisor and Mrs. Osillo's doctor, P.J. is told to give Mrs. Osillo ice chips to suck on several times a day. In between the ice chips, Mrs. Osillo is given mouthwashes to gargle and spit out. Mrs. Osillo says that this helps get rid of the dry mouth feeling that she had been experiencing all of the time.

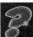

supporting MR. ADAMSON

Mick Adamson is a 62-year-old man who has amyotrophic lateral sclerosis (ALS, also known as Lou Gehrig's disease). ALS is a devastating neurodegenerative disease which causes clients living with the disease become progressively paralyzed as the upper and lower motor neurons in their brain and spinal cord begin to degenerate.[1] Mr. Adamson's family was told that 80% of people with ALS die within 2 to 5 years of diagnosis gradually becoming unable to breathe or swallow.

Mr. Adamson's illness has progressed to a point when he is unable to stand, turn himself in bed, or toilet himself. He is being cared for at home, and you are one of the support workers working for the agency that his family has contracted with to provide care and support for him.

Today, Mr. Adamson has told your supervisor that he just "wants to die." During your work with him, he refuses both his food and his fluids whenever you try to feed him. While you empathize with Mr. Adamson, you do not want to watch him and do nothing as he tries to starve himself to death. You feel frustrated by the situation and by your inability to change Mr. Adamson's situation. You are also frightened by the thought that you might be assisting Mr. Adamson to commit suicide, something that you never imagined that you could ever do and you know is illegal in Canada. How can you handle this ethical dilemma? Who do you turn to for support?

REVIEW

Answers to these questions are at the bottom of the page.

Circle T if the answer is true or circle F if the answer is false.

1. T F **Ethics apply only to life-and-death situations.**
2. T F **Codes of ethics provide rules and answers to ethical dilemmas.**
3. T F **Ethics are a guide when deciding between right and wrong, and good and bad.**
4. T F **Keeping a resident's information confidential is ethical behaviour.**
5. T F **Any decision regarding a client's care is ethical if it does not harm the person.**

Circle the BEST answer.

6. **Providing a safe environment is an example of:**
   - A. Autonomy
   - B. Justice
   - C. Beneficence
   - D. Nonmaleficence
7. **Showing respect and protecting a client's dignity is an example of:**
   - A. Autonomy
   - B. Justice
   - C. Beneficence
   - D. Nonmaleficence
8. **Treating all clients with equal care and attention, regardless of their condition or temperament, is an example of:**
   - A. Autonomy
   - B. Justice
   - C. Beneficence
   - D. Nonmaleficence
9. **Respecting personal preferences is an example of:**
   - A. Autonomy
   - B. Justice
   - C. Beneficence
   - D. Nonmaleficence
10. **Which question is *not* helpful when deciding on an ethical solution to a problem?**
    - A. Does the solution respect the client's wishes and stated preferences?
    - B. Does the solution treat the client justly and fairly?
    - C. Does the solution provide a short-term or long-term benefit to the client?
    - D. Does the solution benefit you?

Answers: 1.F, 2.F, 3.T, 4.T, 5.F, 6.D, 7.C, 8.B, 9.A, 10.D

CHAPTER 11

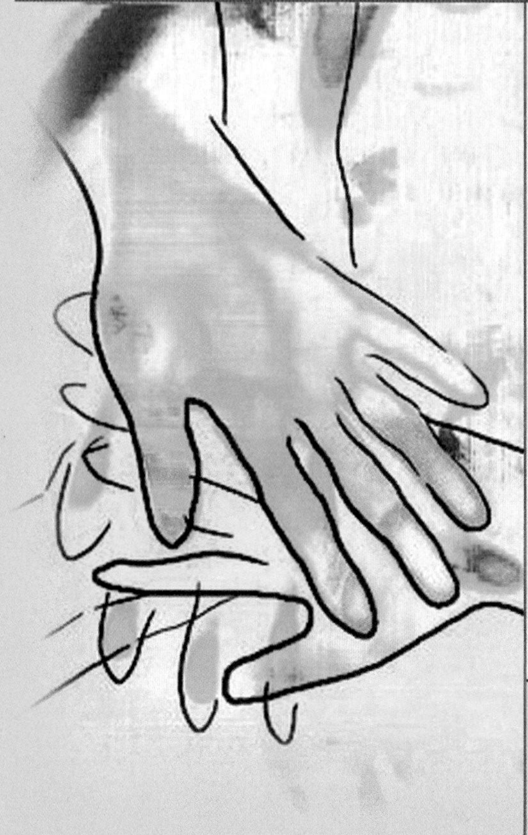

Legislation: The Client's Rights and Your Rights

OBJECTIVES

- Define the key terms listed in this chapter.
- Explain the basic rights protected by the *Canadian Charter of Rights and Freedoms* and the provincial and territorial human rights codes.
- Describe client rights.
- Identify ways you can respect your client's rights.
- Describe the difference between criminal law and civil law.
- Describe how negligence, defamation, assault, battery, false imprisonment, and invasion of privacy apply to your job.
- Define electronic privacy and describe how to maintain confidentiality electronically.
- List the types of legislation that address support workers' rights and duties.
- Apply the information in this chapter to your clinical practice properly.

key terms

act A specific law that has passed through the required legislative steps.

administrator The name given to the person appointed by that province's Provincial Courts to administer the estate of a client who has died without leaving a will.

advance care directive See **advance directive.**

advance directive Legal documents that allow people to convey their decisions about their own end-of-life care. These documents are signed ahead of time, usually when the client is admitted to a long-term care facility. They are usually done in consultation with the client, his or her next of kin (usually one with power of attorney), the client's physician, and the agency's Director of Care (usually the nurse or supervisor in charge). Also known as an **advance care directive.**

assault Intentionally attempting or threatening to touch a client's body to cause harm without the client's consent.

autonomy Having free choice to make decisions that affect one's life. Also known as **self-determination**.

battery The touching of a client's body without the client's consent.

Canadian Charter of Rights and Freedoms The *Charter* is part of the Canadian Constitution and is a constitutional document. It applies at the federal level, and all other laws must be consistent with its rules. The *Charter* lists the basic rights and freedoms to which all Canadians are entitled.

civil laws Laws that deal with relationships between people.

confidentiality Respecting, guarding, and using discretion with personal and private information about a client.

consent Agreeing or giving approval, such as to medical treatment, health care, or personal care services.

crime A violation of a criminal law.

criminal law Laws concerned with offences against the public and against society in general.

defamation Injuring the name and reputation of a client by making false statements to a third person.

electronic privacy Not disseminating a client's image, words, character description, or comments about his or her reputation by electronic means, including posting or forwarding these on any Web site, chat room, or e-mail address on the Internet, by way of cell phones, electronic listening devices, spy cameras, computers, or personal messaging devices of any sort.

executor, executrix See **guardian of property.**

false imprisonment Unlawful restraint or restrictions of a client's freedom of movement.

guardian of property The person chosen by the deceased client to deal with his or her possessions, as it states in the will. Also known as **executer** and **executrix.**

harassment Troubling, tormenting, offending, or worrying a client by one's behaviour or comments.

informed consent Legal condition whereby a client has been given the relevant information so that she or he can appreciate and understand the situation and the potential implications and still consent to an action or procedure.

invasion of privacy Violating a client's right not to have his or her name, photograph, private affairs, health information, or any personal information exposed or made public without consent.

legislation A body of laws that govern the behaviour of a country's residents.

liable Being legally responsible.

libel Making false statements that hurt the reputation of another client. Statements are in the form of a permanent record and are usually in print, writing, or through pictures or drawings.

living will A document that lets the reader (for example, health care professionals or family members) know one's preferences about care intended to sustain life. In most long-term care facilities, it is part of an **advanced directive**. Anyone can have a living will. However, it is not legally enforceable.

negligence Failing to act in a careful or competent manner and thereby harming a client or damaging property.

oath of confidentiality A pledge that all health care workers must sign, which promises that the signer will respect and guard personal and private information about a client, family, or agency. Signing the document obligates you to not reveal information obtained in the course of your work.

key terms

proxy See **substitute decision maker**.

regulations Detailed rules that implement the requirements of a legislative act.

right Something to which a client is justly entitled.

self-determination See **autonomy**.

slander Making false statements that hurt the reputation of another client. Statements are usually verbalized and have no permanent record.

substitute decision maker for health care A person authorized to make health decisions, such as to give or withhold consent on behalf if the client is unable to do so. Also known as **proxy**.

substitute decision maker for property The person who would represent the incapable client's interests regarding his or her property.

tort A wrongful act committed by an individual against another person or the person's property.

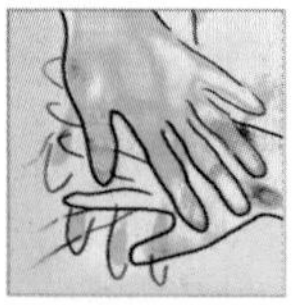

The foundation of a good client–worker relationship is a basic understanding of the client's rights and the worker's rights and legal responsibilities. As a support worker, how you conduct yourself at work and how you relate to your clients are determined by:

- Your code of ethics
- Your employer's policies
- Federal and provincial or territorial laws

Remember, ethics is concerned with what you *should* or *should not do*. Legislation tells you what you *can* and *cannot do*. **Legislation** is a body of laws that govern the behaviour of a country's residents. In Canada, legislation helps to make sure that all clients receive safe and skillful care and to help them enjoy the privacy that all people deserve. Enforced by the courts, legislation also protects clients' rights and your rights.

UNDERSTANDING RIGHTS

A **right** is something to which a person is justly entitled. Some rights are based on a sense of fairness or ethics and are sometimes called *moral rights*. For example, when you and a classmate arrange to study together, you have the right to expect that the classmate will show up and be prepared to work. In another example, if you discussed a personal matter with a friend, you have the right to expect that your friend will not repeat this information to others. These rights are not based on written laws. They are based on moral principles: commitments should be honoured and secrets should be kept.

Rights that are formally recognized in law are *legal rights* based on rules and principles outlined in the law and enforced by society. For example, various laws give you the right to vote, to receive medical care, to own property, and to receive fair treatment if accused of a crime. Laws reflect the values of the society that created them. Canadians enjoy many rights and freedoms that enable a life of equality and dignity.

BASIC HUMAN RIGHTS IN CANADA

The ***Canadian Charter of Rights and Freedoms*** is federal legislation that applies to all Canadians regardless of where they live. The *Charter* is part of the Canadian Constitution and is a constitutional document. It applies at the federal level, and all provincial and territorial laws must be consistent with its rules. The *Charter* lists the basic rights and freedoms to which all Canadians are entitled. They include:

- Freedom of conscience and religion
- Freedom of thought, belief, opinion, and expression

- Freedom of peaceful assembly and association (usually these freedoms are associated with the right to form a union or engage in a strike)
- The right to vote
- The right to enter, stay in, or leave Canada
- The right to life, liberty, and security
- The right to equality before and under the law, without discrimination based on race, ethnic origin, colour, religion, sex, age, or mental or physical disability

The *Canadian Charter of Rights and Freedoms* is also discussed in Chapter 12: Caring about Culture and Diversity and Chapter 21: Abuse, as this legislation also pertains to those areas.

All Canadian provinces and territories also have human rights codes. These codes affirm the principle that all people are entitled to equal rights and opportunities without discrimination. Your provincial human rights code protects you and your clients from being treated unfairly because of race, ethnicity, religion, sex, age, or disability. The human rights code affirms that all clients have a right to receive the same type and quality of support services and to be free from discrimination.

BASIC RIGHTS OF PEOPLE RECEIVING HEALTH SERVICES

The Human Rights Code is provincial legislation based on the *Canadian Human Rights Act* and applies to its specific provincial or territorial jurisdiction. The Human Rights Code of each province and territory is intended to: (a) prevent discrimination, and (b) promote and advance human rights for that province and territory. Some of the issues addressed by the Human Rights Code of each province or territory include:

- Aboriginal rights
- Age discrimination
- Disability
- Employment
- Gender identity
- Hiring practices
- Housing
- Pregnancy and breastfeeding
- Racism
- Religious rights
- Sexual harassment
- Sexual orientation

All provinces and territories have legislation that addresses the rights and freedoms of people using health care services. Your clients may be unable to exercise their rights due to:

- Illness or injury
- Physical, cognitive, or mental disabilities
- Old age, if the client is frail, confused, or isolated

The laws governing health care have different titles across the country and may differ in detail. Examples of this legislation are given in Box 11–1. Provincial and territorial governments constantly revise health care legislation and introduce new laws in order to protect the rights of people receiving care in facilities and in the community.

Health care legislation consists of acts and regulations. An **act** is another term for a specific law. **Regulations** consist of detailed rules that implement the requirements of the act. Most health care acts consist of general requirements for maintaining health, safety, and well-being. For example, British Columbia's *Community Care and Assisted Living Act* sets out general requirements for the licensing, administration, operation, and inspection of long-term care facilities and also sets out broad standards of care. *Adult Care Regulations* that accompany the *Community Care and Assisted Living Act* set out detailed rules for meeting those broad standards of care. Box 11–2 on page 141 outlines some of the detailed rules covered in British Columbia's *Adult Care Regulations.*

Some provincial and territorial governments do not have regulations that lay out detailed rules. Instead, they issue standards that expand on their legislation. For example, Alberta's long-term care legislation is accompanied by standards called *Basic Service Standards for Continuing Care Centres.* Regardless of whether detailed rules are contained in regulations or standards, all residential facilities in a province or territory must abide by these rules. Not to do so could result in removal of their licences.

Box 11–1 Examples of Extended, Continuing Care, and Community Care Legislation

Refer to each provincial or territorial government Web site for further information regarding each act.

British Columbia
Community Care and Assisted Living Act (2004)

Alberta
Nursing Homes Act (2000)
Social Care Facilities Licensing Act (2007)

Saskatchewan
Housing and Special-Care Homes Act (2002)
Personal Care Homes Act (2006)
Residential Services Act (2006)

Manitoba
Public Health Act (2006)
Health Services Insurance Act (2005)
The Vulnerable Clients Living with a Mental Disability Act (1996)
Protection for Persons in Care Act (2001)

Ontario
Long-Term Care Act (2006)
Long-Term Care Homes Act (2007)

Quebec
An Act Respecting Health Services and Social Services (2007)
An Act Respecting Health Services and Social Services for Cree Native Clients (2002)

New Brunswick
Family Services Act (2007)
Nursing Homes Act (1985)

Nova Scotia
Homes for Special Care Act (1995)

Newfoundland/Labrador
Homes for Special Care Act (2006)
Private Homes for Special Care Allowances Act (2006)
Self-Managed Home Support Services Act (2007)
Personal Care Homes Regulations under the Health and Community Services Act (2005)

Prince Edward Island
Community Care Facilities and Nursing Homes Act (2007)

Yukon
Health Act (2006)

Northwest Territories/Nunavut
Hospital Insurance and Health and Social Services Administration Act (2005)

BILLS OF RIGHTS

There is no single list of rights afforded to all Canadians receiving care in facilities and in the community. However, some provinces, such as Manitoba and Ontario, have created a bill of rights for clients. These bills of rights take the lengthy rules contained in regulations and standards and condense them into a list of basic rights for people receiving care. For example, consider Ontario's *Resident's Bill of Rights* for long-term care (see Box 11–3 on page 142) and *Bill of Rights* for community care clients (see Box 11–4 on page 143).

Some facilities and agencies write their own bills of rights based on provincial or territorial laws. Clients must receive a written list of their rights. You must know your provincial or territorial laws and employer policy regarding client rights. Generally, all clients have the following rights, which are a combination of moral and legal rights:

- The right to be treated with dignity and respect
- The right to privacy and confidentiality
- The right to give or withhold informed consent
- The right to autonomy

Recently, the Aphasia Society of Ontario introduced the first-ever pictographic version of the *Ontario Residents' Bill of Rights*. It was designed by the Aphasia Institute and funded by the Ontario Ministry of Health and Long-Term Care through the Seniors' Health Research Transfer Network (SHRTN) initiative (Figure 11–1). It is required to be posted near the text version of the *Residents' Bill of Rights*. This guide outlines effective ways to communicate with clients who retain thinking and social skills but have difficulty with expressing

Box 11–2 Some Complex Care Facility Issues Controlled by Legislation (British Columbia)

- Bedroom requirements—space, furnishings, privacy, windows, and lighting
- Room and water temperature
- Bathrooms and bathing facilities
- Safety requirements, including fire safety and call systems
- Mobility and access
- Dining area, lounges, recreation, and outside activity area
- Social activities and recreation programs
- Care and supervision; care plans
- Confidentiality and privacy
- Neglect and abuse
- Restrictions on the use of restraints
- Preparation and service of food
- Medication safety; administration of medication; medication records
- Access to health services; oral health

Source: Province of British Columbia. (2002). *BILL 73: Community care and assisted living act,* Adult care regulations. Copyright © Queen's Printer Victoria BC. See http://www.qp.gov.bc.ca/statreg/reg/C/CommuCareAssisted/536-80.htm

themselves when speaking, with understanding the speech of others, and with reading and writing.

THE RIGHT TO BE TREATED WITH DIGNITY AND RESPECT

All people have the right to be treated with dignity and respect, and generally all health care laws aim to protect and promote the client's dignity. It is an ethical principle and a legal obligation throughout Canada. This right is a guiding principle of caregiving and is emphasized throughout this textbook under the acronym DIPPS (dignity, independence, preferences, privacy, and safety).

Most health care legislation refers to the client's right to be treated with dignity. For example, British Columbia's *Community Care and Assisted Living Act* states that facilities must be operated "in a manner that will maintain the spirit, dignity, and individuality of the client being cared for."[1] Ontario's *Long-Term Care Act* states that the client has the right to be dealt with "in a courteous and respectful manner . . . that respects the client's dignity." The *Act* also states that workers must deal with the client in a manner that "recognizes the client's individuality and that is sensitive to and

Figure 11–1 Pictographic version of the *Resident's Bill of Rights.* **Source:** Aphasia Institute, Toronto, ON. Retrieved November 2, 2007, from http://www.oanhss.org/staticcontent/staticpages/members/fullmembers/Full_Member_pdf/Residents_Rights_Pictograph_March2007.pdf

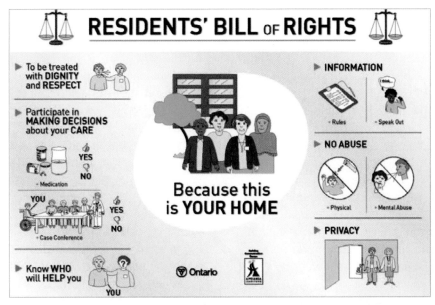

Box 11–3 Ontario's *Resident's Bill of Rights*

1. Every resident has the right to be treated with courtesy and respect and in a way that fully recognizes the resident's dignity and individuality and to be free from mental and physical abuse.
2. Every resident has the right to be properly sheltered, fed, clothed, groomed, and cared for in a manner consistent with his or her needs.
3. Every resident has the right to be told who is responsible for and who is providing the resident's direct care.
4. Every resident has the right to be afforded privacy in treatment and in caring for his or her personal needs.
5. Every resident has the right to keep in his or her room and display personal possessions, pictures, and furnishings in keeping with safety requirements and rights of other residents of the home.
6. Every resident has the right:
   - to be informed of his or her medical condition, treatment, and proposed course of treatment;
   - to give or refuse consent to treatment, including medication, in accordance with the law and to be informed of the consequences of giving or refusing consent;
   - to have the opportunity to participate fully in making any decision and obtaining an independent medical opinion concerning any aspect of his or her care, including any decision concerning his or her admission, discharge or transfer to or from a home; and
   - to have his or her medical records kept confidential in accordance with the law.
7. Every resident has the right to receive reactivation and assistance toward independence consistent with his or her requirements.
8. Every resident who is being considered for restraints has the right to be fully informed about the procedures and the consequences of receiving or refusing them.
9. Every resident has the right to communicate in confidence, to receive visitors of his or her choice, and to consult in private with any client without interference.
10. Every resident whose death is likely to be imminent has the right to have members of the resident's family present 24 hours per day.
11. Every resident has the right to designate a person to receive information concerning any transfer or emergency hospitalization of the resident and, if a person is so designated, to have that person so informed forthwith.
12. Every resident has the right to exercise the rights of a citizen and to raise concerns or recommend changes in policies and services on behalf of himself or herself or others to the resident's council, staff of the home, government officials or any other client inside or outside the home, without fear of restraint, interference, coercion, discrimination, or reprisal.
13. Every resident has the right to form friendships, to enjoy relationships, and to participate in the resident's council.
14. Every resident has the right to meet privately with his or her spouse or same-sex partner in a room that assures privacy, and, if both spouses or same-sex partners are residents in the same home, they have a right to share a room according to their wishes, if an appropriate room is available.
15. Every resident has the right to pursue social, cultural, religious, and other interests, to develop his or her potential, and to be given reasonable provisions by the home to accommodate these pursuits.
16. Every resident has the right to be informed in writing of any law, rule, or policy affecting the operation of the institution and of the procedures for initiating complaints.
17. Every resident has the right to manage his or her own financial affairs if the resident is able to do so and, if the resident's financial affairs are managed by the institution, to receive a quarterly accounting of any transactions undertaken on his or her behalf and to be assured that the resident's property is managed solely on the resident's behalf.
18. Every resident has the right to live in a safe and clean environment.
19. Every resident has the right to be given access to protected areas outside the home in order to enjoy outdoor activity, unless the physical setting makes this impossible.

Source: (2005). *Every resident: Bill of rights for people who live in Ontario long-term care homes.* © Advocacy Centre for the Elderly (ACE) and Community Legal Education Ontario (CLEO). ISBN 0-88903-244-0 http://www.cleo.on.ca/english/pub/onpub/PDF/seniors/everyres.pdf

Box 11–4 Ontario's *Bill of Rights* for Community Care Clients

Note: The term "service provider" refers to either an agency or a client paid to provide the community service; in other words, a support worker is a service provider.

1. A client receiving a community service has the right to be dealt with by the service provider in a courteous and respectful manner and to be free from mental, physical, and financial abuse by the service provider.
2. A client receiving a community service has the right to be dealt with by the service provider in a manner that respects the client's dignity and privacy and that promotes the client's autonomy.
3. A client receiving a community service has the right to be dealt with by the service provider in a manner that recognizes the client's individuality and that is sensitive to and responds to the client's needs and preferences, including preferences based on ethnic, spiritual, linguistic, familial, and cultural factors.
4. A client receiving a community service has the right to information about the community services provided to him or her and to be told who will be providing the community services.
5. A client applying for a community service has the right to participate in the service provider's assessment of his or her requirements and a client who is determined under this *Act* to be eligible for a community service has the right to participate in the service provider's development of the client's plan of service, the service provider's review of the client's requirements, and the service provider's evaluation and revision of the client's plan of service.
6. A client receiving a community service has the right to give or refuse consent to the provision of any community service.
7. A client receiving a community service has the right to raise concerns or recommend changes in connection with the community service provided to him or her and in connection with policies and decisions that affect his or her interests, to the service provider, government officials or any other client, without fear of interference, coercion, discrimination, or reprisal.
8. A client receiving a community service has the right to be informed of the laws, rules and policies affecting the operation of the service provider and to be informed in writing of the procedures for initiating complaints about the service provider.
9. A client receiving a community service has the right to have his or her records kept confidential in accordance with the law.

Source: Government of Ontario. (Consolidated as of: January 1, 2005). *Long-term care act*, 1994, S.O. 1994, c. 26, s. 3(1). Retrieved January 25, 2008, from http://www.e-laws.gov.on.ca/html/statutes/english/elaws_statutes_94l26_e.htm.

responds to the client's needs and preferences, including preferences based on ethnic, spiritual, linguistic, familial, and cultural factors."[2]

Many long-term care facilities have policies that promote the dignity of the residents. Because the facility is the residents' home, residents are guaranteed the same freedoms they would have in their own homes. Many long-term care acts, regulations, standards, and facility policies recognize that residents have the following rights:

- To live in a safe and clean environment
- To be properly sheltered, fed, clothed, groomed, and cared for according to their needs
- To keep and display personal possessions, pictures, and furnishings in their rooms
- To have their families present 24 hours a day if they are dying
- To be free from emotional, physical, sexual, and financial abuse
- To discuss problems with or suggest changes to any aspect of the services provided to them

Respecting the client's dignity is a basic and important part of support work. For most people, dignity and independence go together. To respect a client's dignity, encourage the client to be independent. Allow clients to do as much for themselves as possible (Figure 11–2). For example, if a frail older man can put on his shoes, let him do so. It may be faster for you to put his shoes on for him. However, letting him do so helps him maintain some independence.

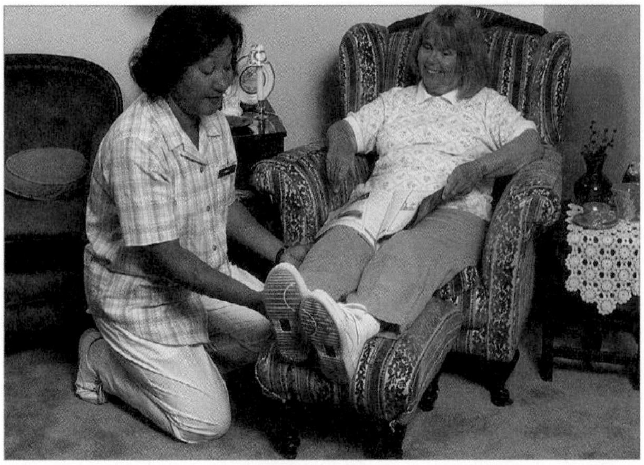

Figure 11–2 Support workers should treat their clients with dignity and respect. **Source:** Birchenall, J., & Streight, E. (2003). *Mosby's textbook for the home care aide* (2nd ed., p. 14). St. Louis: Mosby.

Be careful not to make assumptions about client's abilities, interests and limitations. By making assumptions, you may discourage them from doing tasks and activities that they *can* do. Observe what your client is capable of doing, and check the care plan. A client who is dependent in one area is not necessarily dependent in all areas. For example, Mrs. Mukherjee needs help getting up out of a chair. However, she can feed herself. Mr. Simpson needs help shaving, but he can comb his hair and brush his teeth. Mrs. MacDonald can easily walk by herself, but because of Alzheimer's disease, she may wander off and therefore needs to be supported in a secure environment.

Respecting people's dignity means relating to them the way you would want to be related to if you were in their position. Speak respectfully to them, keeping in mind their hearing or sight limitations, if they have any (Figure 11–3). In support work, how you relate to a client is just as important as the care you provide. Treating clients with dignity provides them with emotional support and greatly contributes to quality of life. Box 11–5 *Respecting the Client's Right to Dignity* lists ways of respecting the client's dignity.

THE RIGHT TO PRIVACY AND CONFIDENTIALITY

People using health care services have the right to personal privacy. They have the right to receive care in private and in a way that does not expose their bodies unnecessarily. Only staff members involved in the client's care should see, handle, or examine the client's body.

Information about the client's care, treatment, and condition is confidential. **Confidentiality** is respecting, guarding, and using discretion with personal and private information about a client.

Health information must be kept confidential. All provinces and territories have legislation that protects the privacy and confidentiality of clients' health information. This legislation is usually called a Privacy Act. Privacy acts provide guidelines to facilities and agencies on how to collect, use, and disclose personal health information. All agencies require that all staff (and usually volunteers and students) sign an **oath of confidentiality**. This is a pledge that all health care workers must sign, and it promises that the signer will respect and guard personal and private information about a client, family, or agency. When in doubt about whether or not to discuss something that you saw with regard to the client, you should always follow your employer's policies.

Providing for privacy and confidentiality shows respect for the client and protects the client's dignity. Box 11–6 lists measures that show respect for privacy and confidentiality.

Electronic Privacy

These days more and more people communicate electronically—they use their home computers or cell phones to talk to others and send pictures

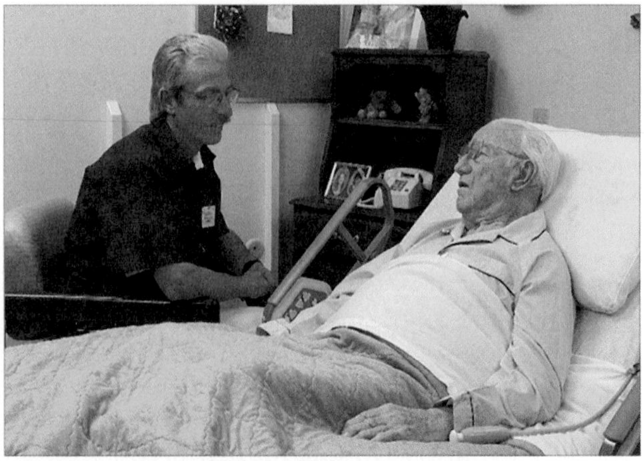

Figure 11–3 Listen to the client by facing the client, having good eye contact, and leaning toward the client.

Box 11–5 Respecting the Client's Right to Dignity

- Make eye contact with the client, if culturally appropriate, and listen attentively (see Figure 11–3).
- Stand or sit close enough to the client, as appropriate. Use touch if you are sure the client would approve. Respect cultural differences regarding touching and personal space preferences (see Chapter 12).
- Be patient. Provide kind and thoughtful care.
- Say "please" and "thank you," and practise other common acts of courtesy.
- Never yell, scold, embarrass, laugh at, or be sarcastic toward the client.
- Respect the client's belongings and property. Do not touch personal possessions unless you have a reason to and have the client's permission. Be sure to put items back where you found them.
- Address an adult client by title and last name, unless the client tells you otherwise. Never call a client honey, sweetie, dear, grandma, grandpa, or by any other such terms.
- Tell your supervisor about the client's complaints or concerns about the agency, facility, or services.
- Reinforce clients' independence by allowing them to do things for themselves. Avoid creating dependency.
- Assist the client with personal care and grooming, whenever necessary. Make sure the client has:
  - A neat and clean appearance
  - A clean-shaven face or groomed beard
  - Trimmed and clean nails
  - Dentures, hearing aids, glasses, and other prostheses available, as appropriate
  - Clean and properly fitted and fastened clothing
  - Shoes and socks or hose properly applied and fastened
  - Extra clothing for warmth, as needed, such as a sweater or lap blanket

electronically to each other. There are dedicated Web sites that allow the browser to look at pictures or clips of other people doing things. When a movie star was photographed with a woman other than his wife, this image was quickly disseminated through various Internet sites throughout the world and this led to the movie star's devastated wife filing for divorce immediately.

Box 11–6 Respecting the Client's Right to Privacy

- Knock on the client's door and wait for permission to enter.
- Ask others in the room to leave before giving care to the client. In order to stay, they must have the client's permission.
- Close the door, and use curtains or screens when providing care or whenever the client requests it. Also, close drapes and window shades.
- Drape the client properly during personal care and procedures. Expose only the body part involved in the treatment or procedure.
- Keep the client covered when moving him or her through a facility's corridors and elevators.
- Close the bathroom door when the client is using the bathroom. If the client needs help, stay in the bathroom with the client and keep the door closed.
- Do not open or read the client's mail or personal documents (Figure 11–4).
- Do not touch or examine the client's belongings without permission.
- Allow the client to visit with others in the facility and to use the telephone in private.
- Do not pry into the client's private life or ask for personal information that is not necessary for your work.
- Keep all personal and health care information about the client confidential.
- Do not discuss a client with your family, friends, or the client's family. Only talk about the client with your supervisor and members of the health care team who need to know.

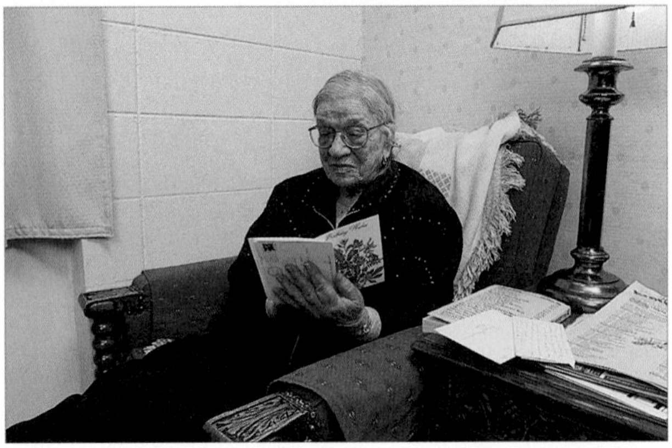

Figure 11–4 A client is reading her mail. Clients have a right to privacy, so never open or read their mail. **Source:** Sorrentino, S.A. (2004). *Mosby's textbook for nursing assistants* (2nd ed., p. 339). St. Louis: Mosby.

In today's age of electronic distribution of images and words, many people forget that people have the right to privacy. In health care, **electronic privacy** could be defined as not disseminating a client's image, words, character description or comments about his or her reputation by electronic means, including forwarding these through any Web site, chat room, or e-mail, by way of cell phones, electronic listening devices, spy cameras, computers, or personal messaging devices of any sort. It is wrong, both ethically and now legally in many provinces, to post pictures, names, or discussions about your clients, no matter how "nice" you think you are being to that client (see the *Supporting Mrs. Jones* box for an example of how one client's privacy rights were violated).

supporting MRS. JONES

Jane (not her real name) was a student support worker who was really very fond of one particular client, Mrs. Jones, to whom she provided support care in the home. On the client's birthday, Jane took a picture of her on her cell phone and posted the picture on a Web site that displays other pictures. The picture showed Mrs. Jones smiling and wearing a hat with a cellophane bow that had been taken from the wrapping of a birthday present.

Mrs. Jones' teenage grandchildren, who live in another city, happened to come across this site, where they saw the picture of their grandmother. The grandchildren showed it to their parents, who were shocked and horrified that their mother (usually a very proper woman) was displayed in such an undignified manner. When they questioned their mother, she recalled that it was the student who took her picture. The client's children called the student's school and filed a formal complaint.

The school's lawyer agreed that the student violated the client's right to privacy by posting her picture on the Internet without her permission. The lawyer also reminded the school that they have an obligation to inform the students that ***they must destroy any client information (printed or electronic) in such a way that it cannot be retrieved or reassembled.*** The student was eventually asked to leave her support worker program because her actions went against the oath of confidentiality that she had signed in the first week of her program.

THE RIGHT TO GIVE OR WITHHOLD INFORMED CONSENT

All people have the right to decide for themselves whether or not they agree to medical treatment, health care, or personal care services. This is called **consent**. ***All provinces and territories have legislation that describes when and how consent is to be obtained.***

For consent to be valid, it must be **informed consent,** which is based on accurate and complete information.[3] This information is provided to the client by the facility, agency, or physician.[3] Consent is informed when the client clearly understands the following:[3]

- The reason for the treatment or service
- What will be done
- How it will be done
- Who will be doing it
- The expected outcomes
- Potential risks and side effects of the treatment
- Other treatment options
- The likely consequences of not having the treatment

Consent is given when the client enters a facility or hires an agency. A form is signed giving general consent to treatment (see "Advanced Care Directive," below). Special consent forms are required for surgery and other complex and invasive procedures. The physician is responsible for informing the client about all aspects of the surgery or procedure.

The support worker is never responsible for obtaining written consent or giving medical information. As a support worker, you may or may not be allowed to witness clients' signatures on consent forms. Know your employer's policy.

Advanced Care Directive

Advanced care directives (also known as **advanced directives)** are legal documents that allow clients to convey their decisions about their own end-of-life care. These documents are signed ahead of time, usually when the client is admitted to an extended care facility, and are usually done in consultation with the client, their next of kin (usually their **substitute decision maker**) and the agency's director of care.[3]

Advanced care directives provide a way for the client to communicate his or her wishes to family, friends, and health care professionals and are intended to avoid confusion later on, perhaps when the client is less cognitively aware of his or her surroundings.[3]

Living Will. Sometimes people who are still living at home will want their family and friends to know their thoughts on whether or not they want care that is intended to sustain their life and will sometimes write these thoughts down. This is called a **living will**. In a living will, a person can state whether or not he or she wishes to accept or refuse medical care when the time comes. There are many issues that a living will can address, such as:

- The use of dialysis and breathing machines
- Resuscitation if breathing or heartbeat stops
- Tube feeding
- Organ or tissue donation

A living will is ***not*** legally enforceable (see *Supporting Mme. LeBrun*) but is merely used to encourage family members to make decisions that respect the client's wishes.

supporting MME. LEBRUN

Mme. Violette LeBrun had signed her organ donor card, and had indicated that her organs should be donated upon her death. She always kept this card in her purse, next to her driver's licence. She also instructed her friends and family that when the time came, she did not want to be kept alive on life support. Mme. LeBrun even purchased over the Internet a "living will kit," filled it out, and gave it to her lawyer for safekeeping until the time came for her family to make this decision.

Later, Mme. LeBrun was involved in a head-on motor vehicle accident and was declared "brain dead" by the emergency room doctor. She was placed on life support until her family could be notified. Her family immediately rushed to the emergency room and then were shown Mme. LeBrun's organ donor card that indicated that Mme. LeBrun wished to donate her organs. Her family was then asked if they would give permission for Mme. LeBrun's organs to be taken from her body.

Mme. LeBrun's husband and daughter, both in a state of shock, refused to allow the doctors to retrieve any of Mme. LeBrun's organs. They decided that "Mom had been through enough pain" and asked for her to be taken off the life support system. Her body was then sent to the funeral home that her family specified.

Substitute Decision Maker

Consent is often needed for clients under the legal age (usually 18 years of age) and for clients who are unable to make informed decisions for themselves or their property. The generally accepted generic term for this in Canada is substitute decision maker. In some provinces, the legal term for a substitute decision maker is *power of attorney.*

Substitute Decision Maker for Personal Care. People with certain mental illnesses, confusion, dementia, or intellectual disabilities may not be able to give informed consent. In some situations, for example, an unconscious client cannot give consent for a procedure. Such situations require a **substitute decision maker for health care.** In some provinces, the word **proxy** is used instead. The substitute decision maker for health care makes health care decisions if the client is unable to do so, such as giving or withholding consent for treatments. Usually the substitute decision maker is a husband, wife, daughter, son, or legal representative. As with consent given by the client, consent given by a substitute decision maker must be an **informed consent**.

If your client has a substitute decision maker, this person will consult with the health care team to make decisions on the client's behalf. All provinces and territories have legislation that addresses substitute decision making.

Substitute Decision Maker for Property. As in situations that require a substitute decision maker for health care, there are situations when the client is unable to make decisions regarding his or her property. In this case, the client's interests would be represented by a **substitute decision maker for property**. This person may or may not have been chosen by the client when he or she was able to make these decisions.

Sometimes, if the client does not have a substitute decision maker, the Provincial Court of that province might appoint someone to act as one. The appointed person would be legally bound to act in the client's best interests. Although terms may vary from province to province, a generally accepted term in Canada for the person who acts on behalf of a client with regard to property is an *estate trustee*.

Many people have a *will*—a legal document that states one's wishes about where (or to whom) his or her property should go. It should be drawn (or written) while the client is cognitively intact, witnessed by a lawyer, and kept in the lawyer's office. Most people also keep a copy of their will in a safe, fireproof place, such as in a safe or a safety deposit box.

It becomes the duty of the **guardian of property** (depending on the province, this person is sometimes called an **executor** if the person is a man and an **executrix** if the person is a woman) to deal with the deceased client's possessions according to his or her wishes, as stated in the will. If the client dies without leaving a will, the Provincial Courts will appoint an **administrator** to divide up the client's property.

THE RIGHT TO AUTONOMY

Autonomy (also called **self-determination**) means having free choice to make decisions that affect one's life. People using health care services also have their right to autonomy and have the right to make decisions and choices concerning their care and lifestyle. Clients have the right to be involved with issues concerning their admission, discharge, or transfer to or from a facility (see the *Focus on Long-Term Care: Autonomy* box). All clients have the right to participate fully in assessing and planning their own care and treatment, whether receiving care in a facility or at home.

To have autonomy, people need (and have the right to) complete and accurate information about their health condition, care, and treatment. Make sure your clients know your name and title. Remember to explain procedures before doing them. Clients may ask you about their condition, care, or your employer's policies. Inform your supervisor, and he or she will provide this information. Remember, you must not discuss diagnoses or health conditions with clients.

Personal choice is important for quality of life, dignity, and self-respect, so respect for an individual's personal preference is emphasized throughout this book. As a support worker, you must allow your clients to make choices whenever it is safely possible.

focus on ›› LONG-TERM CARE

Autonomy

Long-term care residents have the right to choose activities, schedules, and care based on personal preferences. They have the right to choose when to get up and go to bed, what to wear, how to spend their time, and what to eat (Figure 11–5). They are also free to form friendships and receive visitors inside and outside the facility. They have the right to share a room with their spouse or partner if they wish to and if a room is available. They also have the right to manage their own financial affairs or receive an accounting of transactions done on their behalf.

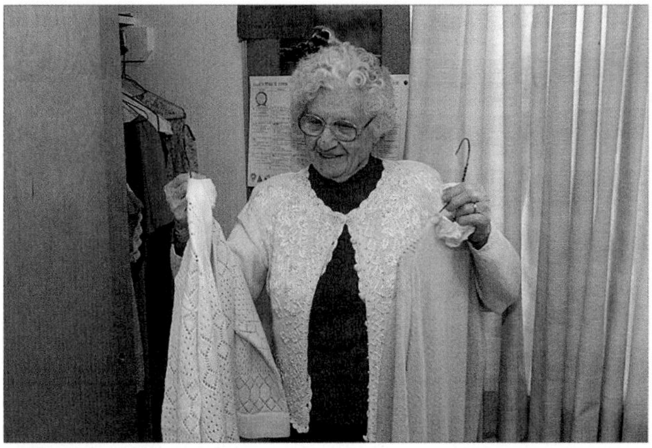

Figure 11–5 The client chooses what clothing to wear.

UNDERSTANDING LEGAL ISSUES

Many client rights are based on laws. Like all health care team members, you, as the support worker, must act in a legally appropriate manner. If you break the law or violate someone's rights, you are legally responsible (**liable**) for your actions and you could be fined, sued, or even imprisoned.

You must obey both criminal and civil laws. **Criminal laws** are concerned with offences against the public and against society in general. A violation of criminal law is called a **crime**—for example, theft, murder, rape, and abuse—and a person found guilty of a crime is fined or sent to prison.

Civil laws deal with relationships between people. For example, laws relating to business disputes, divorce, or adoption are civil laws. A **tort** is a wrongful act committed by an individual against another person or the person's property. A person who commits such an act can be sued by the injured person. Torts may be intentional or unintentional. An example of an unintentional tort is negligence. Examples of intentional torts are assault, battery, false imprisonment, invasion of privacy, and defamation of character.

Negligence

Your clients expect that you will do your job competently and carefully. **Negligence** occurs when you fail to act in a careful or competent manner and thereby harm the client or damage property. Negligence is an unintentional wrong because the person at fault did not mean or intend to cause harm. He or she failed to do what a reasonable and careful person would have done, or did what a reasonable and careful person would *not* have done. The negligent individual may have to pay damages (a sum of money) to the person that they injured. The causes of negligence are given below.

Not performing a task or procedure correctly: As a support worker, always perform your tasks and procedures exactly as you have been taught. Not following procedures can harm the client. For example, you are taught to keep a urinary drainage bag below the client's bladder level. If you keep it above the bladder, urine will not drain and the client could develop a urinary tract infection. Such negligence could harm the client and charges could result.

Performing a task or procedure that you are not qualified to do: You are legally allowed to do only those tasks and procedures that you are qualified to do. Do not do more than is allowed within your job description, your employer's policies, and legislation within your province or territory. You may be asked to do something beyond your scope of practice, for example, giving medications. Even if you are assured that you are not liable, you should remember that *you are responsible for your own actions.* You may, in fact, be liable. In such situations, remember that refusing to follow such requests is your right and duty.

Making a mistake due to carelessness that causes harm to a client: Everyone makes mistakes sometime or another, but a mistake that results from carelessness and causes harm is a negligent act. For example, if you do not mop up a spill, you could cause a client to slip and fall, and your carelessness could be considered negligent.

Box 11–7 contains examples of negligent acts committed by support workers.

A client could be harmed even though you do your job competently and carefully. It is important to accurately record every procedure, following your employer's policy. What you record may later on protect you from charges of negligence. For example, a client confined to bed develops serious bed sores. The family thinks she was left lying in the same position for too long. Your charting shows that you repositioned her every hour, as stated in

Box 11–7 Examples of Negligent Acts Committed by Support Workers

- A support worker leaves the bed in the raised position. The client falls out of bed and breaks a hip.
- A support worker raises the bed rails when the care plan states that they should be left down. The client falls while trying to climb over the bed rails.
- A support worker does not raise the bed rails when the care plan states they should be raised. The client falls out of bed.
- A support worker does not check the temperature of the bath water. The client is burned.
- A support worker drops a client's dentures. The dentures break.
- A client complains to the support worker of chest pain and difficulty breathing. The support worker does not report the complaints to the supervisor. The client has a heart attack and dies.
- A client calls for help using the call bell. The support worker ignores the call. The client goes into shock because of sudden, severe bleeding.
- A support worker does not secure a client's garden gate. The client (who has Alzheimer's disease) wanders out on the street and is hit by a car.

her care plan. This proves that you gave the required care and did not cause the bed sores. If you did not record that you repositioned her every hour, it could have been presumed that you did not do it (see Chapter 8 for further discussion of recording).

Assault and Battery

Assault and battery may result in both civil and criminal charges. **Assault** is intentionally attempting or threatening to touch a client's body without the client's consent, causing the client to fear bodily harm. Threatening to "tie down" an uncooperative client is an example of assault. **Battery** is the actual touching of a client's body without the client's consent. You do not have to have intent to injure a client in order to commit a battery; you are committing a battery if you touch the client without his or her permission. Force-feeding a client is an example of battery. Another example of battery is giving a treatment (such as a blood transfusion) to a person who has refused the treatment, even if you think it will "help" the person.

You are not required to obtain written consent before you perform a task or procedure. However, you must always be aware of the client's wishes. Also, a client who has signed a consent form has the right to withdraw his or her consent at any time. Always explain the procedure and what you are going to do, and make sure the client agrees to it. Consent may be verbal ("yes" or "okay") or a gesture (a nod, turning over for a back rub, or holding out an arm for a blood pressure measurement). If the client objects to or declines your services, respect his or her wishes and stop the procedure or task, and immediately inform your supervisor, since the client's decision may affect his or her well-being.

In some provinces, registered staff may sometimes delegate support workers to perform duties that are beyond the scope of their practice (see Chapter 5: Working with Others: Teamwork, Supervision and Delegation; Chapter 40: Assisting with Medications; and Chapter 43: Heat and Cold Applications). ***If a support worker performs duties that are beyond the scope of his or her practice, and these duties were never delegated and taught by the registered staff, the support worker is actually assaulting the client. It is the responsibility of the support worker to understand the responsibilities within his or her role and to safely act within these boundaries!***

False Imprisonment

False imprisonment is the unlawful restraint or restrictions on a client's freedom of movement. Preventing a client from leaving a facility is false imprisonment. So is the unnecessary use of restraints (they are discussed in Chapter 19: Safety).

Invasion of Privacy

Every client has the right not to have his or her name, photograph, private affairs, health information, or any personal information exposed or made public without having given consent. Violating this right is an **invasion of privacy** and is punishable by law. Your employer may require you to sign a document binding you to confidentiality in all dealings with clients and your employer. This is called an oath of confidentiality. This document may refer to the provincial or territorial privacy act that protects the privacy of individuals. Signing the document obligates you to not reveal information about clients obtained in the course of your work.

Freedom of Information. Canada is on the rapidly growing list of countries that have freedom of information and data protection legislation.[4] There are many federal laws that govern access to information and privacy, with the two main laws being the *Access to Information Act* and *Privacy Act.* In Canada, the *Access to Information Act* allows citizens to demand records from federal bodies. This is enforced by the Information Commissioner of Canada.

There is also a complementary *Privacy Act*, which was introduced in 1983. The *Privacy Act*'s purpose is to (a) extend the present laws of Canada that protect the privacy of individuals with respect to personal information about themselves held by a federal government institution, and (b) to provide individuals with a right of access to that information. Complaints for possible violations of the *Act* may be reported to the Privacy Commissioner of Canada.

The various provinces and territories of Canada also have legislation governing access to government information; in many cases, this is also the provincial privacy legislation. For example, the *Freedom of Information and Protection of Privacy Act* applies to the province of Ontario's provincial ministries and agencies, boards and most commissions, as well as community colleges and district health councils. In Quebec, the *Act* respecting access to documents held by public bodies and the protection of personal information governs access to government information.

Defamation of Character

Defamation is injuring the name and reputation of a client by making false statements to a third person. **Libel** is making false statements in print, writing, or through pictures or drawings. **Slander** is making false statements orally. As a support worker, protect yourself from defamation by never making false statements about a client, co-worker, or any other person. Examples of defamation include:

- Implying or suggesting that a client has a sexually transmitted disease
- Saying that a client is insane or mentally ill
- Implying or suggesting that a client is corrupt or dishonest

YOUR LEGAL RIGHTS

Federal, provincial, and territorial legislation ensures that Canadian workers receive fair wages and work in a fair and safe environment. There are laws that protect workers' rights and clarify their requirements and duties. These laws have different names across the country and vary in their details. In general, however, all provinces and territories have legislation that addresses human rights, occupational health and safety, employment, labour relations, workers' compensation, long-term care services, and community services legislation.

Human Rights Legislation. Human rights codes protect workers' basic human rights. This legislation states that employers must treat all workers equally and not discriminate on the basis of the worker's race, colour, sex, sexual orientation, religion, age, or disability. Employers and employment agencies also cannot discriminate at the request of a client. Human rights legislation also declares that workers have the right to be free from harassment in the workplace by the employer, client, or fellow worker. **Harassment** means troubling, tormenting, offending, or worrying a client by one's behaviour or comments.

Occupational Health and Safety Legislation. All provinces and territories have occupational health and safety (OH&S) legislation. This legislation outlines the rights and responsibilities of workers, employers, and supervisors in creating and maintaining a safe work environment. OH&S legislation, however, is not enforceable in a home care environment and does not protect the support worker in home care.

Employers must "take every precaution reasonable in the circumstances for the protection of a worker."[2] Workers have a right to receive (and employers must provide) proper education, instruction, and supervision to ensure their safety. Employers who do not fulfill these duties may be fined. Workers have the right to refuse to work if the work poses a danger to themselves or others.

In some provinces, however, health care workers cannot refuse to work if in so doing they endanger a client's health or safety.[3] OH&S legislation also details how hazardous materials used in the workplace are to be identified and managed. WHMIS (Workplace Hazardous Materials Information System) is a national plan developed to provide information on the safe use and potential health risks of hazardous materials (see Chapter 19).

Employment Standards and Legislation. Employment standards legislation states the minimum employment standards acceptable within the workplace. This legislation covers basic rules about issues such as minimum wage, how wages are paid, how many hours of work per day and per week are acceptable, what is fair overtime pay, how many holidays and vacation days are required, and what situations qualify a worker for a leave of absence.

Labour Relations Legislation. Provinces and territories have legislation that addresses how employers and employees can resolve workplace issues. According to these laws, all employees have a basic right to form or join a trade union of their choice and to participate in lawful union activities. These unions can negotiate wages and other issues with the employer on all union members' behalf. Labour relations legislation sets out the rules for these negotiations (also called collective bargaining), identifies what obligations must be fulfilled before a legal strike can take place, and identifies unfair labour and employee conduct.

Workers' Compensation Legislation. The provinces and territories have workers' compensation legislation about how workers are financially compensated for accidental injuries on the job. Generally, an employee is considered on the job from the time of reporting to work until the end of the shift. If travel is work-related, accidents that happen while travelling may also be covered by workers' compensation. This legislation also discusses worker and employer rights when an injury occurs.

Long-term Care Facilities Legislation. All long-term care facilities are regulated by provincial and territorial legislation. These laws address the basic rights of residents and describe requirements for the operation of the facility. Licensing and placement requirements, funding structures, accountability systems, guidelines about creating and maintaining health care records, and the level of training required of the staff are all listed as well.

Community Services Legislation. This legislation sets out the rules and procedures for accessing and providing community services, including support work. It defines the different types of community services and details how the services are to be provided.

REVIEW

Answers to these questions are at the bottom of the page.

Circle the BEST answer.

1. **Which statement about the *Canadian Charter of Rights and Freedoms* is *true*?**
   A. The *Charter* is still awaiting final passage in the courts.
   B. It lists the basic rights and freedoms to which all Canadians are entitled.
   C. It protects Canadians' right to equality as long as they are citizens.
   D. It was made to protect all adults over the age of 18.
2. **Provincial and territorial human rights codes promote:**
   A. Freedom from poverty by reducing taxes
   B. Unequal treatment with respect to services and facilities
   C. The right to vote
   D. Equal treatment with respect to age, sex, and ethnicity
3. **Which is an example of treating a client with respect and dignity?**
   A. Assuming that the client needs your help before he or she asks
   B. Forgetting to insert the hearing aids for the client
   C. Ordering the client's food at mealtime
   D. Being careful with the client's personal possessions
4. **Which of the following is required to help a client give informed consent?**
   A. Asking the client politely to hurry up and make a decision
   B. Ignoring details about the potential risks and side effects of the treatment
   C. Reassurance that the proposed treatment is the only option
   D. Information about the likely consequences of not having the treatment
5. **Who decides on the kind of recreation activities for a long-term care resident?**
   A. The client's family
   B. The client's physician or nurse
   C. The facility
   D. The client
6. **If a client complains to you about the home care agency's policy, you should:**
   A. Inform your supervisor about the complaint
   B. Advise the client to speak to your supervisor
   C. Ignore the client's complaint
   D. Try to distract the client
7. **Which of the following statements about negligence is true?**
   A. It is an intentional tort.
   B. The client acted in a reasonable manner.
   C. Harm was caused to a client or a client's property.
   D. A prison term may result.
8. **The intentional attempt or threat to touch a client's body without the client's consent is:**
   A. Assault
   B. Battery
   C. Defamation
   D. False imprisonment
9. **The illegal restraint of another client's movement is:**
   A. Assault
   B. Battery
   C. Defamation
   D. False imprisonment
10. **Mr. Mohammed's photograph is made public on the Internet without his consent. This is:**
    A. Battery
    B. Unintentional tort
    C. Invasion of privacy
    D. Libel
11. **Informed consent is obtained by the:**
    A. Client's family
    B. Registered staff
    C. Client's substitute decision maker
    D. Support worker
12. **The basic rules about wages, work hours, and vacation days are covered in:**
    A. Labour relations legislation
    B. Workers' compensation legislation
    C. Employment standards legislation
    D. Regulated health professions legislation

Answers: 1.B, 2.D, 3.D, 4.D, 5.D, 6.A, 7.C, 8.A, 9.D, 10.C, 11.B, 12.C

CHAPTER 12

Caring About Culture and Diversity

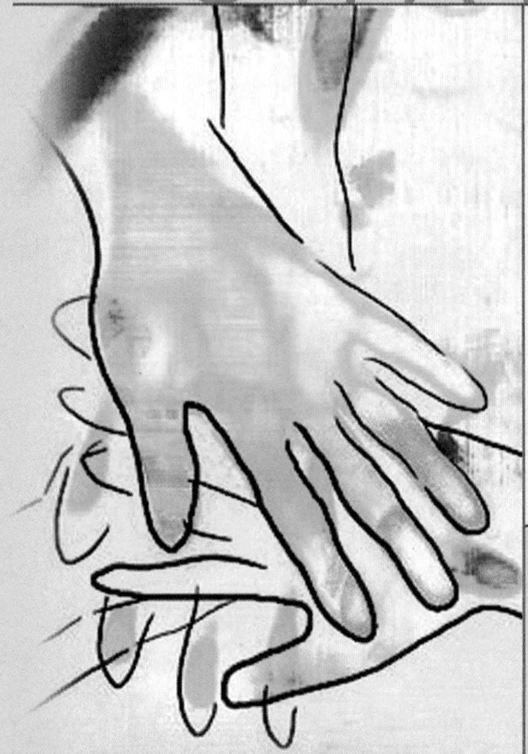

OBJECTIVES

- Define the key terms listed in this chapter.
- Distinguish among race, ethnicity, and culture.
- Describe the factors that influence a person's culture.
- Summarize how culture influences a person's attitudes and behaviours in many areas.
- Describe how culture may affect communication, family organization, religious convictions, and perceptions about illness and health care.
- Analyze how your own cultural biases may affect your relationships with your clients.
- Apply the information in this chapter in your work by providing culturally sensitive care.

key terms

ageism Feelings of intolerance or prejudice toward a person or group of people because of their age.

bias When one person's point of view prevents him or her from impartially judging the issues relating to the subject being considered.

blended family A couple with two or more children, and at least one of the children is the natural child of both members of the couple, and at least one child is the stepchild of either member of the couple.

Canadian Charter of Rights and Freedoms The *Charter* is part of the Canadian Constitution and is therefore a constitutional document. It applies at the federal and provincial/territorial levels. All other laws must be consistent with its rules. The *Charter* lists the basic rights and freedoms to which all Canadians are entitled.

culture The characteristics of a group of people—the language, values, beliefs, customs, habits, ways of life, rules of behaviour, and traditions—that are passed from one person to the next and from one generation to the next. Culture is not limited to ethnic background but can extend to any group of interacting individuals that share similar learned characteristics.

cultural conflict This term refers to negative feelings and conduct that can result when people from one culture try to assert their own set of values and behaviours onto another culture. In individuals, feelings of cultural conflict can also be caused by living within different cultures at the same time.

DIPPS This acronym stands for **dignity, independence, preferences, privacy,** and **safety**. All clients have the right to compassionate care, which includes dignity, respect for their independence, respect for their own preferences, respect for their need for privacy, and need for safety.

discrimination Behaviour that prejudges or treats people unfairly, based on their group membership.

diversity The state of different individuals and cultures coexisting together.

ethnicity Groups of people who share a common history, language, geography, national origin, religion, or identity.

ethnic identity The ethnic background a person considers himself or herself to be part of, based usually on similar language and customs. Ethnic identity is not the same as citizenship, as people can be a citizens of one country but consider themselves to be part of another ethnic group.

homophobia The irrational fear of, aversion to, discrimination and contempt against homosexuality and homosexuals.

nuclear family A family consisting of a father, a mother, and children.

personal space The area immediately around one's body.

prejudice An attitude that forms an opinion on a person based on his or her membership in a group. It is formed from the word "prejudge," which implies that value assumptions regarding a person are formed before meeting or knowing that person.

racism Feelings of superiority over, and intolerance or prejudice toward, a person or group of people who may have different physical appearances or cultural practices.

same-sex families A family in which both adults who live together in a loving, intimate relationship are of the same gender.

sexism Feelings of intolerance or prejudice toward a person or group of people because of their gender.

single-parent families Families in which the adult head of the household does not have a partner who shares the home.

stereotype Assumptions made of a certain ethnic or cultural group by assuming that they are "all alike" or by believing that everyone in that group acts or behaves in a certain way.

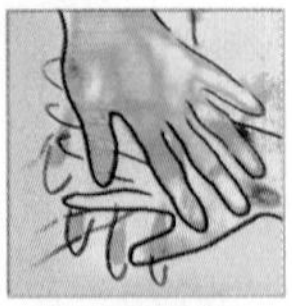

This chapter addresses one of the most important values that all support workers—and all caregivers, for that matter—must possess. That is respect for **diversity**. During your career as a support worker, you will care for and work with people whose lifestyles, beliefs, customs, and rituals are different from your own. It is necessary that you are always respectful of a person's age, race, gender, occupation, sexual orientation, or lifestyle. ***This is a theme that will be repeated throughout this textbook and will be reinforced throughout your career as a support worker.***

Canada has a very diverse population. Your client (or a co-worker) may be a third-generation Canadian, an Aboriginal Canadian, or a new immigrant and you will see that each has a unique culture and perspective. When giving support care, you should never try to change the client to fit in with your care but rather adapt your care and support to fit him or her. To provide the best care possible, you should be aware of and respectful toward that client's cultural background. Your supportive care should never be less respectful for one client than it is for any other client for any reason.

DIVERSITY: ETHNICITY AND CULTURE

Two terms are often confused when discussing *diversity*—"ethnicity" and "culture." Because of the number of people who find the term "race" insulting or misleading, this chapter will avoid this term and use the word *ethnicity* instead. While the authors agree that it is not a seamless replacement, it is the one that is usually used.

According to the ***Canadian Charter of Rights and Freedoms* (*"The Charter"*)**, all Canadians have the right to equality before and under the law, without discrimination based on race, ethnic origin, colour, religion, sex, age, or mental or physical disability. *The Charter* is part of the Canadian Constitution and is therefore a constitutional document. It applies at the federal and provincial/territorial levels, and all other laws must be consistent with its rules.

If you look around you, you will notice many people with different skin and facial features that show that they come from a variety of ethnicities and backgrounds. This is another example of the ever-increasing diversity of our country. **Racism** results when people have feelings of intolerance or prejudice toward a person or group of people because of their racial or ethnic backgrounds.

Ethnicity. **Ethnicity** refers to groups of people who share a common history, language, geography, national origin, religion, or identity. Examples of ethnic groups include the Irish, the Inuit, and the Chinese. An ethnic group is not necessarily a nationality. For example, you may have been born in Canada, so your nationality is Canadian, but you may consider your **ethnic identity** to be Ukrainian. This might be because your family came from the Ukraine and you still speak that language or practise some or many Ukrainian ethnic customs. Canada can be proud that it has many interesting ethnic groups within it.

Culture. Culture makes a society distinctive. **Culture** refers to the characteristics of a group of people—the language, values, beliefs, habits, ways of life, implied rules of behaviour, and traditions—that are shared among groups of people or perhaps even passed from one generation to the next. Culture is influenced by your age, race, gender, occupation, sexual orientation, or lifestyle.

Cultural characteristics are learned from living within the group and influence a person's attitudes and behaviours. Some examples of cultural groups include high school students (there are many subgroups within this main group!), farmers, or snowboarders. Everyone is part of a culture. Some people belong to many cultures at once. For example, you might be a college student, belong to a religious organization, have parents with whom you speak another language, and go jogging with a set of friends regularly. Each of these groups of people that you associate with can have its own "culture."

Ethnicity is an important influence on a person's culture, but it is not the only influence. You might have come from China as a young child, have always spoken Chinese at home, and love Chinese food and customs. Having grown up in Canada, however, you might be very different from your parents, who came to this country as adults. Your ethnicity has influenced you, but so has being schooled in Canada, having outside interests, and making friends from different social, cultural, and religious backgrounds. Because your experiences are different from your parents', you have been subject to different cultural influences than they have been.

Figure 12–1 shows some of the main factors that shape an individual's culture. As the figure depicts, every person reacts to the various cultural factors in his or her own way, and because of this, each person is culturally unique. A person's culture can change over time when the person leaves one group and joins another or encounters new life experiences.

Prejudice and Discrimination. Making assumptions about a person based on his or her cultural or ethnic group is always wrong and often hurtful. Unfortunately, prejudice and discrimination exist throughout the world. **Prejudice** is an attitude toward or opinion of a person based on his or her membership in a group. It is formed from the word "prejudge," which implies that value assumptions regarding a person are formed before even meeting or knowing that person. Prejudice frequently leads to discrimination, as some people cannot be fair and impartial because of their prejudices. A **bias** occurs when one person's point of view prevents him or her from impartially judging the issues relating to whatever is being considered.

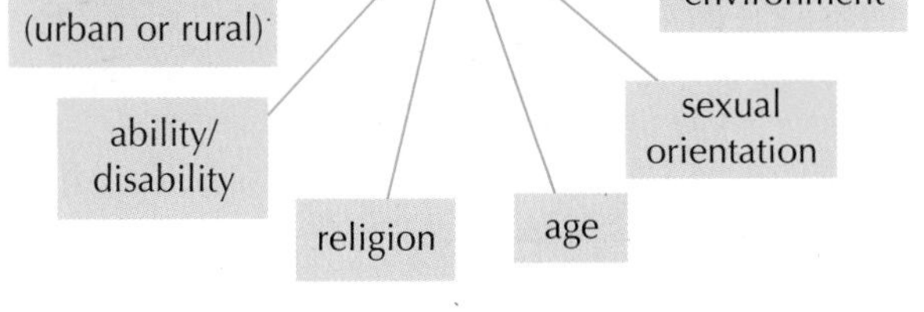

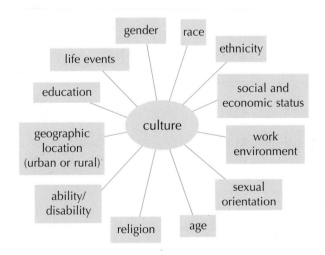

Figure 12–1 Culture is influenced by a number of factors.

Stereotyping People. Some people **stereotype** racial or cultural groups by assuming they are "all alike" or by believing that everyone in that group acts or behaves in a certain way. People can be prejudiced against other people just because they belong to a different race, religion, culture, gender, or age. When people act on their prejudices, it is known as discrimination. An example of this is not hiring someone because they are a certain race. **Discrimination** is behaviour that treats people unfairly on the basis of their group membership.

Other Types of Prejudice. There are many types of prejudice and discrimination other than racism. **Sexism** is a term that describes feelings of intolerance or prejudice toward a person or group of people because of their gender. Some people are **homophobic**, meaning they fear or feel contempt for gay men or lesbian women.

Ageism refers to feelings of intolerance or prejudice toward others because of their age. In an ethnically and culturally diverse society such as Canada's, prejudices and discrimination should not be tolerated. As a support worker, you will be caring for and supporting all types of people and must be prepared to give all your clients the same high quality of care, regardless of their differences.

Cultural Conflict. **Cultural conflict** occurs when a person tries to dictate to another person what his or her culture should be. Unfortunately, we often see examples of cultural conflict existing even in our multicultural society. For example, a person may be forced by another not to wear certain religious symbols or articles of clothing that indicate religious affiliation. In another instance, a caregiver might serve foods that a client would not normally eat because of beliefs existing in his or her ethnic background.

Feelings of cultural conflict can also be caused within an individual by living within different cultures at the same time. A child raised in a very modest, religious family may experience cultural conflict when he or she grows up and moves out of the house to go to school. This person may struggle with trying to live by the family's rules as expected by his or her parents, while trying to enjoy some of the newly-found freedoms. Refer to the *Case Study* box below for an example of cultural conflict experienced by an individual.

THE EFFECT OF CULTURE

A person's culture affects how he or she deals with daily situations and problems. It is not possible to understand the beliefs and practices of all cultures. However, it is important to realize that culture affects a person's beliefs and behaviours toward such issues as:

- Family and social organization
- Religion and worship
- Health care practices and reactions to illness
- Communication

The Effect of Culture on Family

In your career as a support worker, you will meet many different kinds of families. Culture affects family structure as well as the roles and responsibilities of various family members during times of illness. For example, in some cultures, adult children (especially daughters) are expected to be responsible for caring for their older parents.

The Many Types of Families. In Western culture, the most common family structure is the traditional **nuclear family**, which consists of a mother, father, and children (Figure 12–2). The nuclear family arrangement of the last generation is very different from what it is in today's Canada. Now there is an increasing number of **single-parent families**, in which the adult head of the household does not have a partner who shares the home. Many other families are **blended families**, meaning the family consists of a couple with two or more children, at least one of which is the natural child of both members of the couple, and at least one is the stepchild of one of the partners. Another common family structure, the **same-sex family**, is one in which both partners living together in a loving, intimate relationship are of the same gender.

CASE STUDY
CULTURAL CONFLICT

Salvanna Di Silva is a 75-year-old widow receiving home care. She and her husband moved from Portugal to Canada in the 1960s with their three young children. For the next 30 years, Mr. Di Silva worked on the assembly line of an automobile factory, while Mrs. Di Silva worked as a dressmaker. They worked long hours to pay for their children's education. All three children now have successful careers and their own families.

Mrs. Di Silva's health began to decline after her husband died. Severe arthritis in her leg and hip progressed to a point where she could no longer walk. A family conference was held and the children agreed that their mother no longer could care for herself, even with the aid of a support worker. They thought it was unsafe for her to live alone. None of the children felt that they could manage their mother's care and the demands of their own families and careers, so they told their mother that she should consider moving into a long-term care facility.

This came as a great shock to Mrs. Di Silva. She and her husband had taken care of her mother years ago, until her mother's death. Mrs. Di Silva had assumed that one of her children would do the same for her. In Portugal, it was common for children to take care of their older parents. Mrs. Di Silva felt as if she was being cast aside. The idea of leaving her home and moving into a facility with strangers depressed her greatly.

This is an example of conflict between two cultures. Mr. and Mrs. Di Silva had given their children opportunities to enter and succeed in a new culture. Because the children believe they are now a part of the new culture, they feel that they would have to give up too much in order to care for their mother in their own homes. They see many of their friends' parents enjoying living in a retirement facility with other people of their own age. They believe their mother will also eventually settle in and feel at home there.

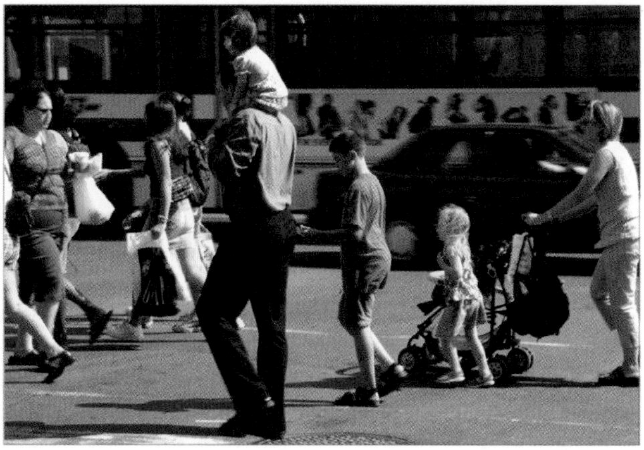

Figure 12–2 A traditional nuclear family. **Source:** Dick Hemingway.

Western culture emphasizes self-reliance and independence. Children are usually encouraged to be self-sufficient, and most young adults leave the family home and live independently of their parents and siblings. Care of family members outside the nuclear family—such as that of grandparents, aunts, or uncles—is often entrusted to others outside the family.

In other cultures, such as in the Asian, South Asian, and Aboriginal cultures, extended families are common. A family in one household may include parents and their children, grandparents, aunts, uncles, and cousins (Figure 12–3). In extended families, the needs of the entire family are more important than individual needs. Elders and the sick are often taken care of by family members. For example, in Vietnam and China, all family members are involved in the ill person's care.[1]

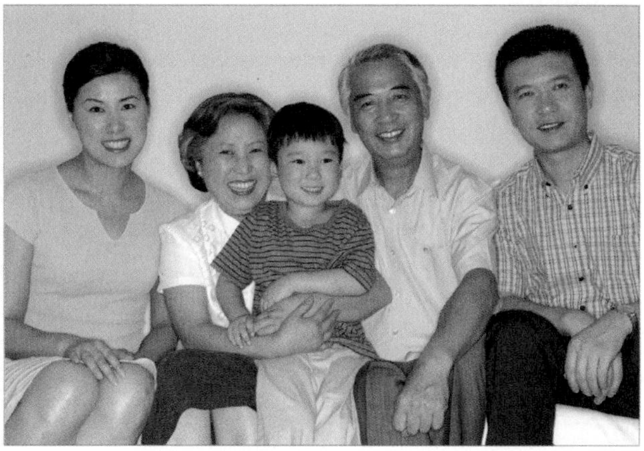

Figure 12–3 An extended family. **Source:** Leland Bobbé/Magma/Corbis.

Family members bathe, feed, and comfort the ill person. People from these and other such cultures continue this custom even in Canada and are often surrounded by family during illness.

Sometimes children rebel against the culture of their parents. Children of first-generation immigrants often reject the roles and behaviours expected of them in favour of those of the new culture. This can cause great stress for the parents and family. The *Case Study* box on page 158 describes how cultural conflict affected one older person.

The Effect of Culture on Religion

In most cultures, religion is an extremely important influence. Religion relates to spiritual beliefs, needs, and practices and may promote beliefs and practices related to daily living habits, behaviours, relationships with others, diet, healing, days of worship, birth and birth control, medicine, and death.

Many people rely on religion for support and comfort during illness. They may want to pray and observe certain religious practices and may find it helpful to have a visit from their spiritual leader or adviser. If a client asks to see a religious leader, promptly report the request to your supervisor. Make sure the client's room is neat and orderly for the visit. Ensure privacy during the visit.

Many religions, including Christianity (Catholic and Protestant faiths), Judaism, Buddhism, Islam, Hinduism, Sikhism, and the Baha'i faith, among others, are practised by various groups within Canada. You will care for clients who have religious beliefs that are different from yours, and some who may not follow any religion. Never try to convert your clients to your own belief system. You must always respect the client's beliefs, practices, and religious symbols and items (such as a rosary, yarmulke, prayer rug, or religious medal). Religious items should be treated with the greatest of respect and never moved or touched unless you are given permission to do so by the client.

The Effect of Culture on Perceptions of Health Care and Illness

Culture greatly affects how people view health care and illness and how they cope with their symptoms and the stresses of being ill. Some cultures have beliefs about the causes of illnesses. In Western culture, the general belief is that disease and illness are caused by biological or environmental factors. Illness and disease can often be prevented, and people can be cared for or cured with scientifically proven methods. Other cultures believe that illness is caused by supernatural forces, an imbalance with nature, or disharmony among mind, body, and spirit. People from these cultures may use charms, rituals, alternative medicines, or traditional or folk medicine that may include ancient remedies and rituals, passed down through many generations. Many folk remedies involve herbs or a traditional healer or shaman.

Folk remedies may help the person or may not have any effect on the person's health. If the practice does not harm the client and promotes his or her emotional well-being, the nurse or case manager may include it in the care plan. Some folk remedies, however, may interfere with the client's medical treatment. For example, some herbal medicines may interact with prescription drugs and produce harmful results. Often clients try alternative therapies or cultural health care practices without telling their physician, nurse, or case manager.[2] The health care team must be aware of all health care practices to make sure they are not harmful to the client. Tell your supervisor if:

- Your client tells you that he or she is using alternative or folk remedies
- You observe a client using alternative or folk remedies

The Effect of Culture on Communication

Many of your clients may speak languages or dialects different from yours. With some clients, you will work with an interpreter, but in many situations, you may not have an interpreter handy when you need to communicate with clients who do not speak your language (see box below).

Speaking the same language is only part of communicating with someone from an ethnic group different from yours. Information and messages are also sent using many nonverbal cues, such as the use of touch, space, eye contact, facial expressions, and even silence. It must be remembered that the meanings of these cues vary among cultures.

Touch. Touch is a very important form of nonverbal communication. It can convey comfort, caring, love, affection, interest, trust, concern, and reassurance. Clients are often comforted by being stroked or having their hands held. However, many cultural groups have rules or expectations regarding who can touch, when touch can occur, and which parts of the body can be touched (Figure 12–4). Some cultures, for example, the Spanish, Italian, French, and South American cultures, freely use touch.[3] People in some other cultures, for example, the English, German, and Chinese cultures, are embarrassed or uncomfortable with any casual touch by strangers and tend to avoid it.[4]

Sometimes the cultural rules of touch depend on the person's gender. For example, in the Indian and

Communicating With Clients Who Speak a Language Different From Yours

- Convey comfort to the client by your tone of voice and body language.
- Do not speak loudly or shout. It will not help the client understand English.
- Speak slowly and distinctly.
- Keep messages short and simple.
- Be alert to identify words the client seems to understand.
- Use gestures and pictures to convey the message.
- Repeat the message in different ways.
- Avoid using technical terms, abbreviations, and slang.
- Be certain that the client understands what is going to be done to him or her and consents to it before you begin a procedure. Be alert for signs that the client is only pretending to understand. Nodding and answering "yes" to all questions are signs that the client may not be really understanding what you are saying.
- Learn a few useful phrases in the client's language.

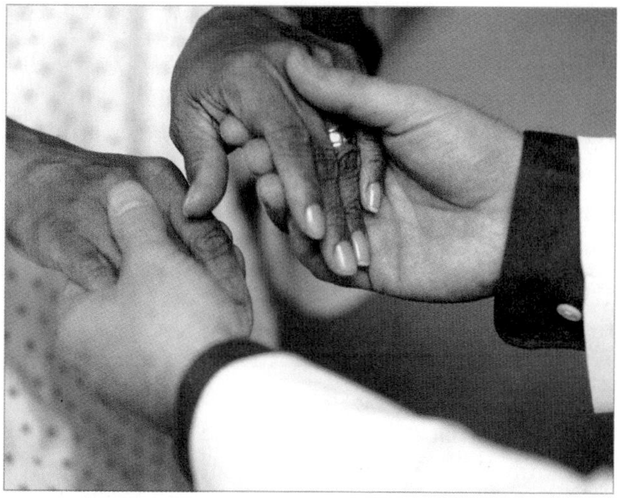

Figure 12–4 Culture may influence how a client responds to touch. **Source:** Tom and Dee Ann McCarthy/Corbis/Magma.

Vietnamese cultures, men shake hands with other men but not with women.[4] You must be aware of what kind of touch and how much touch the client is comfortable with. Ask your supervisor for guidance, and watch the client interact with family or other people. ***Regardless of the situation, a support worker's touch should be gentle, not hurried or rough, and never sexual in nature.***

Personal Space. If someone stands too close to you, you would probably feel uncomfortable or anxious because your personal space has been invaded. The same is true for your clients. **Personal space** is the area immediately around one's body. Everyone has personal space preferences, and it is not always dictated by their culture. Some people prefer more personal space than do others because of their own life experiences (see *Supporting Emmy Lou*).

The exact distance requirements vary among individuals and situations. However, people in the same cultural group tend to have similar personal space requirements.[5] In Western cultures, most people prefer to stand and speak at a distance of about 90 cm (3 feet). People in other cultures may prefer to stand closer or farther away when interacting with others. When providing care, it is important to not invade your client's personal space. If the client steps back from you, does not face you directly, or pulls his or her chair away from you, the client may be sending a message that you are too close.[6]

supporting EMMY LOU

Emmy Lou is an attractive 32-year-old woman who grew up in a family that always hugged, kissed, and displayed affection. When Emmy Lou was in high school, one night she was babysitting her neighbour's two children, as she often did. She was upstairs putting the children to bed and did not hear the children's father come into the house and up the stairs. She greeted him when she walked out of the children's bedroom and asked him where his wife was. He explained that she was going to be late coming home from their meeting. At that point Emmy Lou said that she should go home, as it was a school night and she had to get up early the next day for school.

The neighbour prevented her from going down the stairs, and he forced her to the floor in the hallway and sexually assaulted her. Later, Emmy Lou ran home and showered. She always blamed herself for what had happened and has never told anyone what happened that night. Since that incident, Emmy Lou has always hated being touched or to have anybody stand close to her.

Last month, Emmy Lou was injured in a head-on collision caused by a drunk driver and became permanently paralyzed from her neck down (quadriplegia). As a support worker, you are assigned to provide basic care to her now that she is out of the hospital and at home with her parents. One day, when you are providing personal care to her, Emmy Lou begins to tear up. She shakes her head, and her lips are quivering. How would you proceed?

Eye Contact. Eye contact has different meanings within different cultures. In Western culture, eye contact is a sign of good self-concept, openness, interest in others, attention, and honesty, and it also communicates warmth. Lack of eye contact can communicate rudeness, guilt, dishonesty, shyness, or embarrassment. Some other cultures, however, are not comfortable with direct eye contact. In some Asian and Aboriginal cultures, eye contact is considered disrespectful and an invasion of privacy.[6] In certain Indian cultures, eye contact with people of a higher or lower social and economic class is avoided.[6]

Facial Expressions. Many facial expressions are universal. Expressions of pain, surprise, embarrassment, and happiness are similar around the world, but some cultures are more expressive than others. It therefore may be hard to judge what others are feeling based only on their facial expressions. For example, Italian and Spanish people tend to use many facial expressions and gestures to communicate happiness, pain, or displeasure. In contrast, Irish, English, and northern European people usually use fewer facial expressions, especially with strangers.[5] In some cultures, certain facial expressions may mean the opposite of what the person is feeling. For example, in some Asian cultures, people may smile to hide negative emotions.[6]

Silence. Even the use of silence varies among cultural groups. In some cultures, such as the English and Arabic cultures, silence is used for privacy.[7] Among Russian, French, and Spanish cultures, silence means agreement between parties.[7] In some Asian cultures, silence is used as a sign of respect, particularly in interactions with an older person.[7] In some Aboriginal cultures, silence is considered a virtue. Speaking is reserved only for matters of extreme importance.[8] Among Aboriginal, Chinese, and Japanese people, silence is used as a way to understand a person's needs. For example, if the person is speaking and suddenly stops, his or her silence may be intended to allow the listener to think about what has just been said before the speaker continues.[9]

PROVIDING CULTURALLY SENSITIVE CARE AND SUPPORT

Providing culturally sensitive care is important in support work. Remember that each client is an individual and that each client responds to cultural influences in his or her own unique way. Do not stereotype a person based on his or her ethnicity, religion, or any other factor. ***You cannot apply the cultural behaviours of a given culture to all members of the group. Individuals may not follow every belief and practice of their culture and religion. Each person is unique.***

How to Care for Clients in a Nonjudgemental Way. Sometimes people do not realize that they are prejudiced or that they discriminate against people. Remember that everyone has a culture and that attitudes and behaviours are shaped by culture. Some clients may react negatively or fearfully to cultural differences. You, as a support worker, however, must resist displaying such reactions and accept a client's differences. You do not have to agree with the client's beliefs and practices. However, you must be tolerant and not make judgements. To be tolerant and understanding of others, you need to understand how your own culture influences you.

Consider the following questions:

- Do you judge people by your own cultural standards?
- Do you have any prejudices or biases?
- Do you assume that if something works for you, it must work for others as well?
- Do you think there are "right" and "wrong" ways of doing things?
- Are you ever critical of another person's lifestyle because it is different from your own?
- Do you sometimes consider that other people's lifestyles, religious beliefs, superstitions, and beliefs are silly or odd?
- Do you try to convert others to your religion or way of thinking and doing things?
- Do you believe that people from one race, ethnic group, or religion should not marry people from another?
- Do you avoid trying new things?
- Do you draw conclusions too quickly?
- Do you respect people as individuals, or do stereotypes sometimes get in the way?

To accept people of different cultures, you need to learn from them about them. Communicate with them, and listen to them attentively. Learn as much as possible about their thoughts, beliefs, and values. Respect and show interest in their traditions, foods, dress, and customs. Your clients will feel valued and respected.

DIPPS. The acronym **DIPPS** stands for dignity, independence, preferences, privacy, and safety. ***It is an important concept and will be addressed throughout this textbook.*** It is necessary for support workers to provide care and support that is free from all prejudice and discrimination. All clients have the right to compassionate care, which includes dignity, respect for their independence, respect for their own preferences, respect for their need for privacy, and need for safety. Support workers who respect their clients' cultural and ethnic backgrounds practise the fundamental principles of DIPPS.

supporting MRS. COUTURE

Yvonne Couture is a client with a severe burn on the bottom of her foot. She mentions to her support worker Nancy that she has placed a medal of Saint John the Apostle under the top layer of bandage around her foot. Mrs. Couture also explains that Saint John the Apostle is known for healing burns, and she believes that placing the medal in the dressing will help her wound heal quickly and safely.

Nancy knows that Mrs. Couture has the right to make her own choices about her care. She also knows that Mrs. Couture's strong spiritual beliefs may help her during her healing process. Nancy is concerned, however, that having the religious medal so close to the wound may be harmful. She calls her supervisor to report the conversation. The supervisor relates the message to the case manager, who is not aware of the situation. The case manager asks Mrs. Couture's nurse to discuss the situation with her.

Based on: College of Nurses of Ontario. (2005). *Practice guideline: Culturally sensitive care* (p. 11). Toronto, ON: College of Nurses Ontario.

REVIEW

Answers to these questions are at the bottom of the page.

Circle T if the answer is true or circle F if the answer is false.

1. T F **Culture influences people's attitudes and beliefs but not their behaviours.**
2. T F **Believing that all members of a group share the same characteristics is an example of stereotyping.**
3. T F **Everyone has a culture.**
4. T F **Everyone within an ethnic group shares the same culture.**
5. T F **Each individual responds differently to cultural influences.**
6. T F **Everyone responds positively to a hug or pat on the back.**
7. T F **Although a person's experiences and situation may change over time, his or her culture never changes.**

Circle the BEST answer.

8. **Which of the following statements is true?**
   - A. Ethnicity refers to a group of people who share similar interests.
   - B. A country usually has one ethnic group.
   - C. A person's culture influences health and illness practices.
   - D. People within an ethnic community always dress and think alike.

9. **Which of the following statements is true?**
   - A. Culture rarely influences communication.
   - B. Culture may affect roles and responsibilities within families.
   - C. All people respond to cultural influences in the same way.
   - D. Canadians view health care and illness in usually the same way.

10. **Mr. Greene asks to see his spiritual adviser. You should:**
    - A. Report his request to your supervisor
    - B. Question why he wants the meeting
    - C. Offer to introduce him to your spiritual adviser
    - D. Tell him to phone his spiritual advisor himself

11. **Which statement is correct?**
    - A. We should all judge people based on their group membership.
    - B. In some situations, prejudice is acceptable.
    - C. Prejudice frequently leads to respect.
    - D. Stereotypes are often associated with prejudice.

12. **Mr. Jones rides a motorcycle and refers to himself as a "biker." He likes to wear clothing that signifies membership in his motorcycle club, and he prefers to spend time with his other "biker" friends. This is a description of a(n) _____________ group.**
    - A. ethnic
    - B. cultural
    - C. religious
    - D. racial

Answers: 1.F, 2.T, 3.T, 4.F, 5.T, 6.F, 7.F, 8.C, 9.B, 10.A, 11.D, 12.B

CHAPTER 13

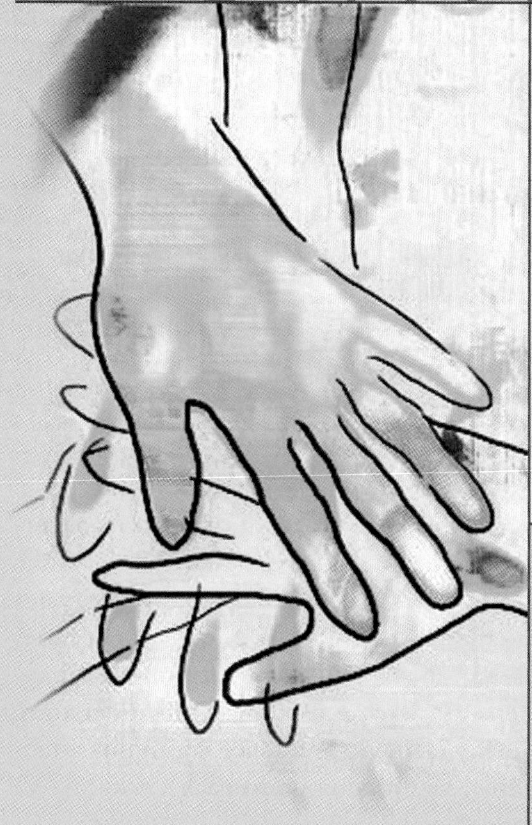

Interpersonal Communication

OBJECTIVES

- Define the key terms listed in this chapter.
- Describe the communication process.
- Describe verbal and nonverbal communication.
- Explain the methods of and barriers to effective communication.
- Explain how to communicate with an angry client.
- Explain why assertive communication is important.
- Learn to explain procedures and tasks to clients.

key terms

active listening A nonjudgemental communication technique that focuses not only on understanding the content of what is being said but also on the underlying emotions and feelings conveyed by the sender. This technique helps develop rapport and fosters a trusting relationship.

assertiveness A style of communication in which thoughts and feelings are expressed positively and directly without offending others.

body language Posture, appearance, facial expressions, body movements, eye contact, and gestures that send messages to others.

closed questions Questions that are structured so that the response can be restricted to one word, such as "yes" or "no," or a few words.

empathetic listening A nonjudgemental technique that requires the listener to be attentive to the sender's feelings.

focusing Limiting the conversation to a certain topic.

interpersonal communication The exchange of information between two people, usually face to face.

nonverbal communication Messages sent without words.

open-ended questions Questions that invite a person to share thoughts, feelings, or ideas.

paraphrasing Restating someone's message in one's own words.

verbal communication Messages sent through the spoken word.

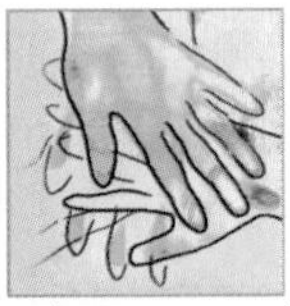

Good interpersonal communication is needed to provide safe and effective health care. Health care team members share information about what was done, what needs to be done for the client, and the client's response to care and treatment. Good communication means better relationships with clients, families, and co-workers. As a support worker, when you communicate with clients, you find out about their needs, feelings, likes, and dislikes. You also express your thoughts and ideas. *What* you say and *how* you say it are equally important.

THE COMMUNICATION PROCESS

Interpersonal communication is the exchange of information between two people, usually face to face. A message is sent by one person (the *sender*) and is received and interpreted by another person (the *receiver*). Often the receiver provides information in response to the message (*feedback*). During the exchange of information, each person usually acts as both a sender and a receiver.

Successful interpersonal communication occurs when the receiver understands the meaning of the message. However, sometimes the receiver does not interpret the message in the way the sender intended, and mistakes and hurt feelings can happen. Messages are sometimes misunderstood because many elements influence communication. For example, factors unique to each person affect communication. These include the following:

- Perceptions (how a person views events and understands messages)
- Experiences
- Physical and mental health
- Emotions
- Values
- Beliefs
- Culture
- Gender
- Age

The relationship between the sender and the receiver also affects their communication. Communication is easier when the people involved understand and respect each other (Figure 13–1).

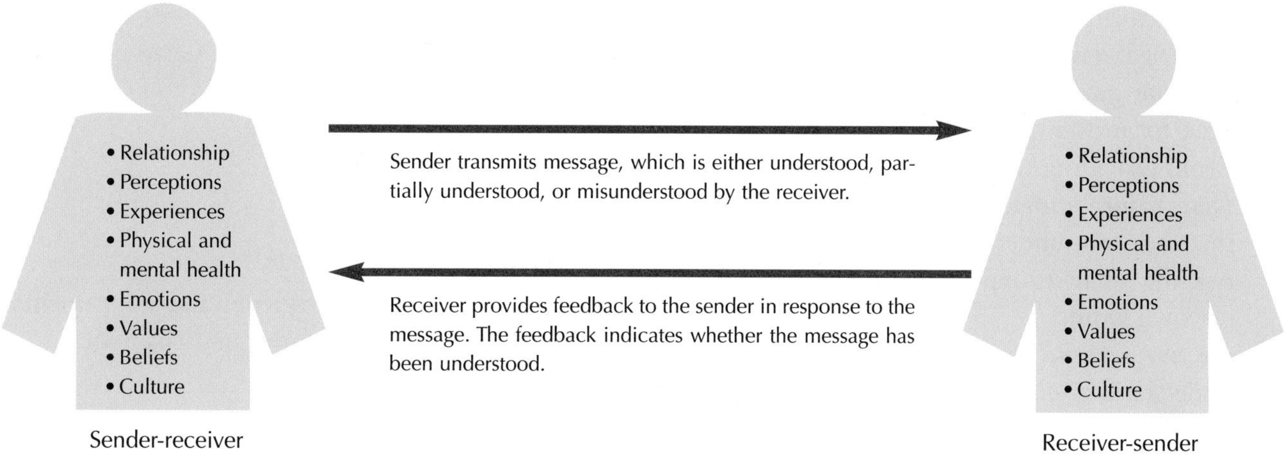

Figure 13–1 Communication is affected by the sender and receiver's relationship, as well as by many other factors.

To effectively communicate with your clients, you need to understand and respect them and be sensitive to each client's unique situation and needs. You must accept and respect the client's culture and religion. You also must understand that stresses, problems, and frustrations affect how a message is sent and received. For example, if a client is worried, he or she may not be able to pay close attention to what you are saying.

Remember that clients are whole persons. They are physical, emotional, intellectual, social, and spiritual human beings. With this in mind, you must try to understand the real meaning behind their words.

VERBAL COMMUNICATION

In **verbal communication**, messages are sent through the spoken word. Sometimes symbols substitute for spoken words; for example, sign language is used to speak with a person who cannot hear.

To effectively communicate with words, you need to:

- ***Choose your words carefully.*** Words must have the same meaning for both you and the other person. Try to avoid words with more than one meaning. For example, the words "small," "moderate," and "large" mean different things to different people. Is "small" the size of a pea or the size of a walnut? Use words that are specific and descriptive. For example, telling your supervisor that a client's temperature is 37.9°C is clearer than saying, "the temperature is up."
- ***Use simple, everyday language.*** You will become familiar with medical terminology as you study and gain experience in health care. However, do not use these medical terms when communicating with clients and their families because these terms may be unfamiliar to them. Use correct grammar, and avoid vulgar words and slang.
- ***Speak clearly, slowly, and distinctly.*** Do not mumble or speak quickly. Move your lips as you speak, slow down your speech, and pause between sentences.
- ***Control the volume and tone of your voice.*** How your voice sounds sends a message. Do not shout because shouting can mean irritation or anger. Do not talk in a harsh or abrupt manner. Avoid speaking to adults in high-pitched tones, as this may seem like you are treating them like children.
- ***Be brief and concise.*** Do not add unrelated or unneeded information. Focus on what you are saying, stay on the subject, and do not get wordy. Being brief reduces the possibility of omitting important details. Speak in short sentences to emphasize your words, as short sentences are more clearly understood.
- ***Present information in a logical manner.*** Organize your thoughts before you speak, and

present them in sequence. Think about what has happened or what is going to happen step by step.

- ***Ask one question at a time.*** Give the client time to answer, and do not rush him or her. Avoid providing the answer for the client.
- ***Determine understanding.*** Do not assume that the client understands what you are saying. Ask the client to repeat the message in his or her own words.
- ***Do not pretend to understand.*** If you do not understand a term or what the client has said, ask him or her to restate or rephrase the message. Repeat the message, if needed.

Professional Communication

When communicating with clients, their families, and the health care team, it is important to be professional. Being courteous is one part of communicating in a professional manner. It is very important that you are professional when communicating at team conferences and reporting at the start and end of shifts (see Chapter 5).

Some other ways you can show courtesy are knocking on closed doors before entering, calling people by their names, and saying "please" and "thank you." You should introduce yourself to the client first and explain what you are going to be doing. Initially, it is respectful to address clients by their last name until they ask you to call them by their first name.

Ensuring confidentiality is an important part of professional communication. In the course of your work, you will learn private and sensitive information about your clients, and this information should be protected. Only pertinent information should be shared with other team members. Gossiping about clients or other team members is unprofessional and unethical.

NONVERBAL COMMUNICATION

In **nonverbal communication**, messages are sent without words through body language, touch, and the use of silence. The meaning of messages sent through nonverbal communication varies depending on the sender's age, gender, and life experiences, as well as the person's culture (see Chapter 12).

Body Language

Body language includes:

- Posture
- Appearance (dress, hygiene, and adornments, such as jewellery, perfume, and cosmetics)
- Facial expressions
- Body movements
- Eye contact
- Gestures

Body language greatly affects communication and can change the meaning of a verbal message. For example, someone can say, "Yes, I can do that" smiling in a friendly manner or rolling the eyes and sighing. In both cases, the body language sends a message. When a person says one thing with words but another with body language, he or she sends *mixed messages,* which are confusing and unhelpful.

Be sensitive to your clients' body language, as it can help you understand them better. For example, slumped posture and a slow, shuffling walk may indicate that the client is not happy or is not feeling well. Sometimes clients may say they feel fine, but their facial expressions may show that they are in pain.

Nonverbal clues often reflect a person's true feelings, and because they are usually involuntary and unconscious, they may send messages more accurately than words can.

You need to be aware of the messages you send with your body language as well. You send messages by the way you act and move. Your facial expressions and how you stand, sit, walk, and look at a person all send messages. Your body language should show interest and enthusiasm for your work and caring and respect for your clients. For example, show respect to the client by physically positioning yourself at his or her level when talking. If the client is in a bed or wheelchair, sit or squat so that you are at eye level.

In many instances, you may need to control your body language when providing care to clients. Do not react visibly, for example, to bodily odours, as often such odours are beyond the control of

supporting MR. REYES

You have been giving support care to Jim Reyes in his home for several months. His physical condition has deteriorated, and he now requires 24-hour care. You are making your last home visit today and ask him how he is doing. Mr. Reyes says, "I am looking forward to moving to the nursing home. I am sure I will make some new friends." However, you see tears in his eyes and he looks away from you. His verbal communication suggests that he is happy, but his nonverbal communication shows sadness. How can you give him support and comfort?

clients. Your reaction is likely to increase the client's embarrassment and humiliation.

Touch

Touch is a very important form of nonverbal communication. It conveys warmth, comfort, concern, affection, trust, and reassurance. Most people respond well to touch because it helps them feel less lonely. Holding a person's hand can provide comfort. Gently stroking a person's shoulder or back can promote rest and relaxation. Your touch should be gentle, not hurried or rushed.

Touch can mean different things to different people. Some people may not want to be touched. Pulling away or tensing the body may indicate that the client does not want to be touched because he or she is in pain and it hurts to be touched. Be sure to find out whether your client wants to be touched or not.

Silence

The use of silence can convey messages of acceptance, rejection, fear, or the need for quiet and time to think. Sometimes, especially during sad times, you do not need to say anything. Just being there shows that you care. Silence can give you and others time to organize thoughts or choose words. Silence is useful when the client is making difficult decisions or is upset and is trying to regain control. In these situations, silence on your part shows respect and empathy for the client (see the *Case Study* box on page 170).

COMMUNICATION METHODS

Certain methods help you communicate well with others, which results in better relationships with people.

Active Listening

Active listening means paying close attention to a client's verbal as well as nonverbal communication. You listen to the content, the intent, and the feelings behind a client's words. You must concentrate on what a client is saying and observe nonverbal clues. Remember, nonverbal clues may show you the client's true feelings. For example, Mrs. Gorecki tells you that her knees do not hurt today. However, you observe that she is rubbing her knees and grimacing. Her nonverbal behaviour indicates that she is in pain.

Active listening requires you to be interested in your client and to show that you care. The following are guidelines for active listening:

- Face the client.
- Make eye contact. (Consider cultural preferences for eye contact.) (Figure 13–2)
- Lean toward the client. Do not sit back with your arms crossed.

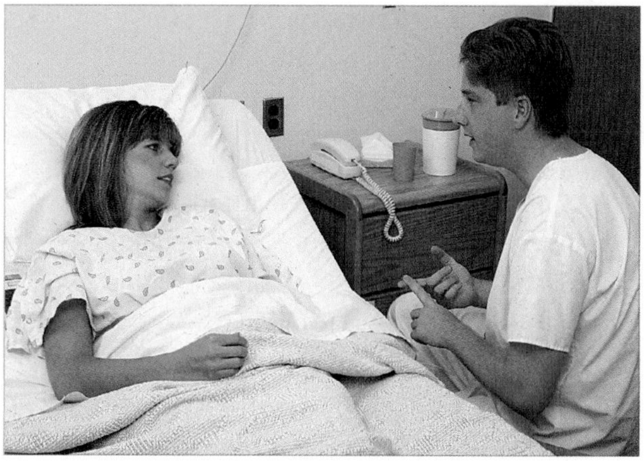

Figure 13–2 Face the client, make eye contact when conversing, and position yourself at eye level.

CASE STUDY
SILENCE AND TOUCH DURING SAD TIMES

How do you show a client that you care? Words may not be enough. You may have to be completely silent and comfort the client just with your touch. Often holding a client's hand can provide more comfort than words can. Jessica, a support worker in a long-term care facility, relates this experience:

"Mrs. Robinson has lived in our facility for 3 years. She is severely disabled by osteoarthritis. She is a friendly, cheerful woman, who rarely complains. One morning, she didn't reply when I knocked on her door. After knocking three times, I opened the door. I was afraid that she was ill. She was sitting in her wheelchair. She looked very sad. I sensed that something was wrong.

I sat down in a chair beside her and asked if I could help. When there was no reply, I placed my hand on hers. I didn't say anything. After a few minutes, she told me that her son had just called. Her grandson had been killed in a car accident. He was 19, and he had just finished his first year at university. I told Mrs. Robinson that I felt very sad for her. We sat there quietly, my hand on hers, for 5 minutes. I asked her if anyone else at the facility knew, and if there was anything that I could do. She asked me to tell the nurse. Then she said, 'You are very kind to sit with me. I know how busy you are.' "

- Respond to the client. Nod your head and say, "uh huh," "mmm," and "I see." Repeat what the client says, and ask questions.
- Avoid communication barriers (see pages 172–174).

Paraphrasing

Paraphrasing is restating a person's message in your own words. When paraphrasing, use fewer words than the person used to send the message. Paraphrasing serves three purposes:

1. It shows that you are listening.
2. It lets both you and the person know if you understood the message.
3. It promotes further communication.

People usually respond well to a paraphrased statement. For example:

Mrs. Cummings: I was a keen reader when I could see. I miss books so much. Those talking books are hard to follow.

You: You love stories, but talking books are not as good as real books.

Mrs. Cummings: Exactly. I wish you had time to read to me.

When paraphrasing, try not to interpret the client's words. Guide the conversation in such a way that the client feels comfortable expressing thoughts or feelings. If you misinterpret a client's meaning, you could put an end to the conversation or cause offence (see the *Support Workers Solving Problems: Using Paraphrasing and Questioning Skills* box for an example of effective paraphrasing).

Empathetic Listening

Empathetic listening means being attentive to a person's feelings. Empathy means being open to and trying to understand the experiences and feelings of others. It involves acknowledging the other person's point of view without judging the person. Clients need to know that they are understood. Empathy can help reduce feelings of loneliness and can create bonds of trust between you and the clients you support.

When paraphrasing, you acknowledge other people's words. When empathizing, you acknowledge their feelings. To show empathy, follow the person's lead. While the person speaks, listen quietly. Do not rush the person or change the subject. Stay focused on the person and not on your own opinions. For example, if a client mentions a difficult situation, you could say, "I can see you are upset. Do you want to talk about it?" This comment shows that you recognize and care about how the person feels.

Support Workers Solving Problems

Using Paraphrasing and Questioning Skills

<< Scenario >>

Sophia provides personal care to 48-year-old Mr. Dupuis. He is severely disabled by multiple sclerosis. On her first visit, she had helped Mr. Dupuis shave and dress. On this second visit, she is to assist him with bathing and preparing breakfast.

Mr. Dupuis: Oh, it's you. I was still asleep. It's awfully early.
Sophia: A 7:30 start is a little early for you. You're not ready for me. *(paraphrasing)*
Mr. Dupuis: Yes, I've asked the case manager to start the morning care at 8:00 instead.
Sophia: Perhaps she is working on the schedule change. I will check with the agency.
Mr. Dupuis: Thanks.
Sophia: The care plan calls for a bath today. Would you like to have your bath now or after breakfast? *(closed question)*
Mr. Dupuis: It doesn't matter much. I wish I didn't need to take a bath. Being bathed by someone else is not much fun.
Sophia: Can you tell me what you dislike about it? *(open-ended question)*
Mr. Dupuis: The lack of privacy really gets to me.
Sophia: We can work together on giving you privacy.
Mr. Dupuis: That would be a good idea. I don't think my last support worker cared much about my privacy.

<< Discussion >>

Paraphrasing and questioning skills can help you improve the care you provide to your clients. In this case, Sophia listens to Mr. Dupuis and uses paraphrasing, closed questions, and open-ended questions in her responses. Sophia uses paraphrasing *(A 7:30 start is a little early for you. You're not ready for me.)* to show Mr. Dupuis she has understood his concern and to prompt him to provide more information. She asks a closed question *(Would you like to have your bath now or after breakfast?)* because she needs specific information about Mr. Dupuis's preferences. She asks an open-ended question *(Can you tell me what you dislike about it?)* to encourage Mr. Dupuis to share his feelings about being given baths. Once Sophia understands Mr. Dupuis's worries about privacy, she can take steps to solve this problem.

Avoid these pat responses:

- "I know how you feel." *(Nobody can ever know how another person feels.)*
- "I feel sorry for you." *(This implies pity.)*
- "I wouldn't want to be in your shoes." *(This suggests superiority and implies pity.)*

Consider these two responses to a complaint:

Mr. Witowski: I can't believe they have made me move to this new room. I felt settled in the other room, and I liked the view of the lawn and the pond. Now, all I see when I look out the window is an asphalt parking lot.
Jane: The move can't be helped, unfortunately. The old wing was falling apart.
Carlos: Being moved can be upsetting. Your old room had a lovely view. I can see why you miss it.

Jane's response is not empathetic—she focuses on facts, not on Mr. Witowski's feelings. Carlos' response is empathetic—he paraphrases Mr. Witowski's statement, which lets Mr. Witowski know Carlos has understood his message and has acknowledged Mr. Witowski's feelings about moving.

Asking Closed Questions

Closed questions focus on specific information, so use them when you need to learn something precise. Some closed questions have "yes" or "no" answers. Others require a brief response. For example:

You: Would you like butter on your toast this morning, Mrs. Cummings?
Mrs. Cummings: Yes, please.
You: Would you like strawberry jam or marmalade?
Mrs. Cummings: Marmalade, please.

Asking Open-Ended Questions

Open-ended questions invite a person to share thoughts, feelings, or ideas. Answers require more than a "yes" or "no." However, the person being questioned chooses and controls what is talked about and the information given. Consider these questions: "What was it like growing up in Scotland, Mrs. Cummings?" (open-ended question) and "Did you like living in Scotland?" (closed question). The first question encourages Mrs. Cummings to talk about herself. It may start a conversation by showing Mrs. Cummings that you are interested in hearing about her life. The second question requires a "yes" or a "no" answer. It does not encourage Mrs. Cummings to talk about herself. Nor does it communicate as much interest in Mrs. Cummings' life.

Use open-ended questions in combination with closed questions to find out about a client's needs and preferences and to find out if a client is satisfied with your care. For example, a closed question ("Are you comfortable?") can give you the necessary information. An open-ended question ("Is there anything I can do to make you more comfortable?") can encourage a client to express thoughts or feelings. The *Support Workers Solving Problems: Using Paraphrasing and Questioning Skills* box on page 171 shows an example of a support worker using both types of questions to improve a client's care.

Clarifying

Clarifying helps you make sure that you have understood a person's message. You can ask the person to repeat the message, say that you do not understand, or restate the message as a question. For example:

- "Could you say that again?"
- "I'm sorry, Mr. Hart. I don't understand what you mean."
- "Are you saying that you want to go home?"

Focusing

Focusing is limiting the conversation to a certain topic. It is useful when a client rambles or wanders in thought. Consider these examples: (1) Mr. Reyes talks at length about his favourite foods and places to eat. You need to know why he did not feel like eating dinner. You focus the conversation on the subject of dinner by saying, "Let's talk about today's dinner. You said you didn't feel like eating." (2) The care plan for Mrs. Hooda directs you to provide two choices when helping her dress. She becomes distracted by the pattern on one of the dresses. You guide the conversation back to the task of dressing by saying, "Would you like to wear the dress with the pretty pattern?" (3) Mrs. Cummings has just told you that she does not want to go for a walk. She then reminisces about her early life. Your response encourages her to focus on her reason for not wanting to walk:

Mrs. Cummings: We used to walk for miles in the Lake District. It was usually raining. It rained constantly in Edinburgh, too.

You: There is no rain today, and the sun is shining. Is there a reason why you don't feel like walking?

COMMUNICATION BARRIERS

Communication barriers prevent sending and receiving messages, causing communication to be limited or to fail completely. Some barriers cannot be avoided, so you must work around these. For example, some clients have hearing and vision problems that interfere with communication, and some clients have nervous system disorders that limit communication. As a support worker, you must learn special techniques to communicate effectively in these situations (Figure 13–3; see Chapters 36 and 37). Cultural differences can also interfere with communication, since clients may attach different meanings to verbal and nonverbal communication (see Chapter 12).

Factors in the environment, such as loud noises, lack of privacy, and distractions, can limit communication. Try to ensure a calm, quiet setting when talking with a client.

Certain behaviours can also create communication barriers. Improve communication with clients by avoiding the following: interrupting, answering your own questions, giving advice, minimizing problems, using patronizing language, and failing to listen.

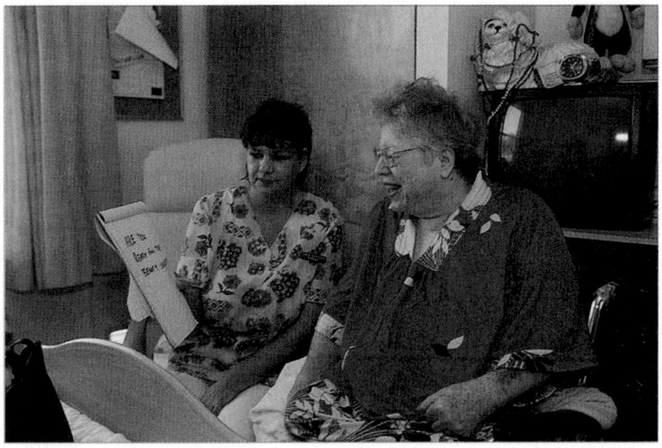

Figure 13–3 The support worker writes a note to a client who is hearing impaired.

Interrupting

Interrupting a person stops communication. People usually interrupt when they:

- Jump to conclusions about what the speaker is trying to say
- Become impatient with the speaker or the way the story is being told
- Become bored and wish to change the subject to something more interesting
- Wish to change the subject because the topic is upsetting
- Feel hurried or stressed
- Focus on a task, not on the person

Answering Your Own Questions

Avoid answering your own questions. Some people do this routinely in conversation, while others do it only with people who take a long time to respond. Answering questions or completing thoughts for people discourages openness. Note the following different responses to the same question, phrased slightly differently:

You: How did you sleep last night? Okay? *(answer provided)*

Mrs. Cummings: Yes.

You: How did you sleep last night? *(answer not provided)*

Mrs. Cummings: I was pretty restless. It took me a long time to fall asleep. The last time I looked at the clock, it was 3:00 a.m.

Giving Advice

Avoid giving advice to clients and their family members. Let people express their feelings and concerns without offering your opinion. You could create confusion, anxiety, and resentment. Your advice could go against the family's wishes, the physician's orders, or the care plan. Even if a client asks for your advice, do not give it. You could instead suggest that the client speak to your supervisor or the case manager. In the following example, the support worker tactfully avoids giving advice to Mrs. Van Doorne:

Mrs. Van Doorne: I don't feel ready to leave my home, but I'm too much of a burden on my daughter. I just don't know what do to. Sometimes I feel that we'd all be better off if I moved into a nursing home. At other times I hate the thought of it. What do you think I should do?

Support worker: I can see what a difficult decision it is, Mrs. Van Doorne. I wish I could help, but it's not my role to give you advice. Is there anyone else you can talk to about it?

Mrs. Van Doorne: I've tried to talk to Anne *(her daughter)*, but she would never admit that I'm a burden.

Support worker: What about talking to Mrs. Stainer *(the case manager)*? I'm sure she could help.

Mrs. Van Doorne: That's a good idea. I'll do that.

Minimizing Problems

Do not minimize a client's problems. Avoid making comments like these: "Everything will be fine," "Don't worry," "It's not really that bad," "Look on the bright side," and "It could be worse." These comments block communication and imply that the client is complaining or exaggerating the problem. They also show that you are judging the client or the situation when you have no right to do so. Minimizing problems makes people feel that you are ridiculing their concerns, feelings, and fears. Clients could believe that you do not care about what they think or feel. Consider these two responses to a hospital patient's concerns:

Mr. Lam: I'm so nervous about this operation. I've never even been in a hospital before.

Eduardo: Believe me, you have nothing to worry about. These surgeons could do this operation with their eyes closed. You will be just fine. (*Walks away.*)

Helga: Having surgery is frightening, especially when it's your first operation. The doctors and nurses will explain everything to you so that you know what to expect. *(Reports Mr. Lam's concerns immediately to the nurse, who reassures him about the surgery.)*

Eduardo's response minimizes Mr. Lam's worries about his surgery, whereas Helga's response is empathetic. She uses paraphrasing to let Mr. Lam know that she understands his concerns and also reassures him by expressing confidence in the health care team.

Using Patronizing Language

Sometimes the words you use can make a person feel unimportant and inferior. These words are *patronizing*. They imply that you are better than the other person. To avoid using patronizing language:

- Do not address clients as "love," "dear," "honey," or by other endearments.
- Do not use a client's first name without his or her permission.
- Do not use terms such as "good girl" or "good boy" or "you guys" with adults.
- Do not use the term "we" when you really mean "you."
- Do not use "baby talk" or expressions such as "there, there."
- Do not talk to co-workers or family members as if the client were not present.
- Do not correct a client's speech or language.

Some health care workers mistake patronizing language for warmth and friendliness (Box 13–1).

Failing to Listen

Communication is blocked if you fail to listen with interest and sincerity (Figure 13–4). Do not pretend to listen, as this conveys a lack of interest and caring. You can miss important complaints of pain, discomfort, or other abnormal sensations that must be reported to your supervisor.

Box 13–1 Avoiding Patronizing Language

Poor Communication Skills

Support worker: Hello, Doris. How are we feeling today, dear?

Mrs. Crossley: I'm feeling much better, thank you.

Support worker: Have you been doing your exercises?

Mrs. Crossley: Yes.

Support worker: Good girl!

Improved Communication Skills

Support worker: Hello, Mrs. Crossley. How are you feeling today?

Mrs. Crossley: I'm feeling much better, thank you.

Support worker: How have your exercises been going?

Mrs. Crossley: Very well, thank you. I'm up to half an hour a day now.

Support worker: That's excellent progress!

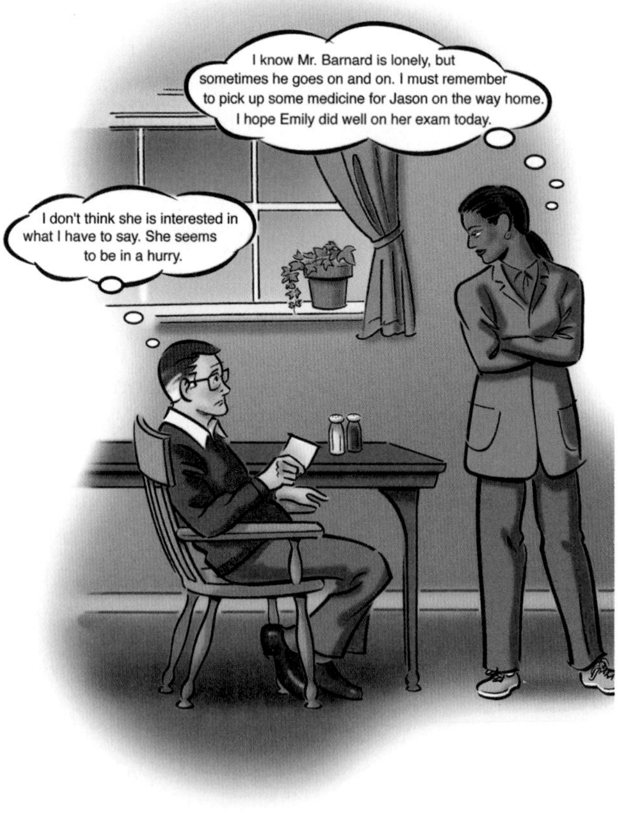

Figure 13–4 This client senses that his support worker is not listening to him.

COMMUNICATING WITH ANGRY PEOPLE

Anger is a common response to illness and disability (see Chapter 4). It is an emotion often expressed by clients and family members. The many causes of anger include frustration, anxiety, fear, and pain. Another common cause of anger is hurt feelings. People may react in anger if they feel their self-esteem is attacked. Loss of body function and losing one's independence can also cause anger. People who are angry are often feeling helpless about a situation.

Anger also is a symptom of diseases that affect thinking and behaviour. People who abuse alcohol and drugs are likely to show anger. Some people are often angry or unhappy. Few things please them or make them happy. There could be many reasons for their behaviour. Do not judge an angry client. Provide the same high-quality, compassionate care that you provide for all your clients. Report a client's angry behaviour to your supervisor.

Anger can be communicated verbally or nonverbally. Verbal expression of anger includes outbursts, shouting, raised voices, and rapid speech. An angry client may tell you what to do or may threaten you. Some clients may remain silent when angry, while some others become uncooperative and refuse to answer questions. Nonverbal signs of anger include rapid movements, pacing, clenched fists, and a reddened face or neck. The angry client may glare at you or get too close to you when speaking (see Chapter 6), and violent behaviours can occur.

Good communication is important to prevent and deal with anger. Follow the guidelines in Box 13–2 when communicating with an angry client.

Box 13–2 Communicating With an Angry Client

- Recognize that the client is feeling frustrated or frightened. Put yourself in the client's situation. How would you feel? How would you want to be treated?
- Treat the client with respect and dignity.
- Answer the client's questions clearly and thoroughly. Tell the client that your supervisor will answer questions that you cannot answer.
- Keep the client informed. Tell the client what you are going to do and when.
- Do not keep the client waiting for long periods. If you tell the client that you will do something for him or her, do it promptly.
- Stay calm and professional. Speak in a normal tone. Do not respond to a client's anger with your own anger. Try not to take the client's anger personally. Often the anger has more to do with the client's own feelings than with you or the care you give.
- Do not argue with the client.
- Listen, and use silence. The client may feel better after expressing angry feelings.
- Protect yourself from violent behaviours. Leave the client, and call your supervisor if you think you are in danger (see Chapter 19).
- Report the client's behaviour to your supervisor. Discuss how you should deal with the client.

COMMUNICATING ASSERTIVELY

Assertiveness is a style of communication in which thoughts and feelings are expressed positively and directly without offending others. You stand up for your rights while respecting the rights of others.

When you communicate assertively, you appear confident, calm, and composed. You speak gently, firmly, and positively. You do not hesitate or appear anxious. You are respectful.

Being assertive is different from being aggressive and from being passive. When you communicate aggressively, you appear upset, cold, or angry, and you may sound threatening. Aggressive communication is usually not respectful.

When you communicate passively, you appear hesitant, apologetic, and timid. A passive person does not want to hurt or offend others. But passive behaviour can make others feel uncomfortable. Assertiveness rarely has this effect because people usually like direct, honest, and sincere communication.

Some people have trouble communicating assertively with people in authority. They feel intimidated. You will have regular contact with physicians, nurses, and other members of the health care team. You need to be confident and assertive when you communicate with them.

The *Case Study* box below describes three responses to a situation that requires assertiveness.

EXPLAINING PROCEDURES AND TASKS

One of your responsibilities as a support worker is to explain procedures and tasks to clients, as some procedures may be unfamiliar or frightening to them. Some personal care activities may require staff who are strangers touching the client's private body parts. Clients feel safer and more secure if they understand what is going to be done before the procedure is performed. They should know why the procedure is done, who will do it, how it will be done, and what sensations or feelings they can expect. They should also know which parts of the procedure (if any) they will participate in and which parts you, as the support worker, will perform. For many procedures, you also need to find out your client's preferences *before* you begin.

You may help clients practise tasks they have been taught by health care professionals. For example, Mr. Krueger, 88, has osteoporosis. His physiotherapist has shown him how to do muscle-strengthening exercises. The physiotherapist has also shown you how to help him with the exercises. As part of Mr. Krueger's care plan, you work with him daily on these exercises.

You may be expected to teach simple tasks to your clients. For example, Mrs. Ali has hemiplegia (paralysis on one side of her body) and needs to learn a new method for dressing herself. You have been taught a method for dressing clients with hemiplegia. The care plan calls for you to teach this method to Mrs. Ali and to practise it with her until she is able to dress herself.

Whatever the situation, you must give clear, precise explanations and instructions that the client can understand. Organize your thoughts before you speak. Use simple, everyday language. Give your client the chance to discuss the task and to ask questions.

Most clients learn tasks best when they are shown how to do them. The following four-step teaching method works for many clients:

CASE STUDY
COMMUNICATING ASSERTIVELY

Kara just graduated as a support worker. Her first job is at a long-term care facility, where she was hired to replace Debbie. Mr. Beruti is a 28-year-old client, who had both his arms amputated. While Kara is shaving him, he shouts, "Be careful! You almost nicked me. You obviously don't know what you're doing. The nurse told me this is your first job. You're not nearly as good as Debbie. If you don't get better at this, I'll report you."

Consider the following responses:

- "Report me if you like, Mr. Beruti. I wouldn't have been assigned to you if I were useless. You're just missing Debbie. I can assure you that I am just as qualified as she is. I won't tolerate your abuse." (This is an aggressive and hostile response. It makes a judgement by assuming that Mr. Beruti misses Debbie. It shows no empathy or respect, and it disregards his safety needs.)
- "I'm so sorry, Mr. Beruti. I am so clumsy and rough. I'll try to do better." (This is a passive response. It suggests that Kara lacks confidence and also implies that Kara has doubts about her ability to provide safe and competent care.)
- "I'm sorry, Mr. Beruti. It's hard when caregivers do things in different ways. I can assure you that your safety and comfort are important to me. Can you tell me how you like to be shaved?" (This is a compassionate yet assertive response. It should reassure Mr. Beruti. It shows that Kara is confident in her ability to adapt her shaving method and also that she is open to Mr. Beruti's preferences for care.)

- Tell the client the steps in the task.
- Show the client how to do each step.
- Have the client try each step.
- Review the client's success with each step.

Follow the guidelines in Box 13–3. Break tasks into steps. Teach one step at a time. Observe your client and listen carefully to make sure he or she understands you. Recognize that people learn in different ways. Recognize as well that illness, disability, and fatigue can affect a person's ability to learn. You may have to explain a task several times and in different ways before the client understands. Even if the client understands, he or she may not be able to do it. You may have to demonstrate a task many times.

Box 13–3 Guidelines for Teaching Tasks to Clients

- ***Put the client at ease.*** Relax and smile. Do not give the impression that you are in a hurry. If the client senses you are tense or rushed, learning will be difficult.
- ***Start with small steps.*** Break the task into small steps. Focus the client's attention on one step at a time.
- ***Start with easy steps.*** Confidence increases with success. If possible, start with the steps the client is most likely to achieve.
- ***Observe and listen.*** Clients do not always tell you when they do not understand something. Or they may say they understand it when they actually do not. Watch body language, and listen actively. Be alert for signs of fatigue.
- ***Use positive statements.*** Positive statements are easier to follow than are negative statements. For example, saying "Bend your arm" is more effective than saying "Don't use a straight arm."
- ***Let the client set the pace.*** Be patient, and do not rush the client. Allow time for rest.
- ***Provide support and offer encouragement.*** Positive comments help the client feel successful and also encourage the client to continue trying. It is important to recognize what the client has achieved. Even small achievements deserve recognition and a positive comment.
- ***Give time for practice.*** Allow time for practising a task. Practice helps a client remember.

REVIEW

Answers to these questions are at the bottom of the page.

Circle the BEST answer.

1. **During an exchange of information, a message is sent:**
   - A. From a speaker to a receiver
   - B. From a receiver to a speaker
   - C. From a speaker to a speaker
   - D. Without feedback

2. **Which is *true?***
   - A. Verbal communication does not involve the spoken word.
   - B. Verbal communication is the truest reflection of a person's feelings.
   - C. Messages can be sent by facial expressions, gestures, posture, body movements, appearance, and eye contact.
   - D. All people like to be touched.

3. **To communicate with your client, Mr. Lam, you should:**
   - A. Use medical words and phrases
   - B. Listen to his concerns and report to charge nurse who can answer his questions
   - C. Give your opinion when he is sharing fears and concerns
   - D. Ask closed questions when you need specific information

4. **When talking with Mr. Long, which of the following might indicate that you are listening?**
   - A. You continue making the bed with your back to him.
   - B. You have good eye contact with him.
   - C. You cross your arms and look away.
   - D. You roll your eyes at what he has said.

5. **You and Ms. Jones are talking about her surgery. Which of the following is a closed question?**
   - A. "Do you feel better now?"
   - B. "Tell me what your plans are for home."
   - C. "What will you do when you fully recover?"
   - D. "You said that you will be off work for a while."

6. **Your client tells you she is not happy that she has to use a walker. Which of the following responses shows empathy?**
   - A. You tell her about the time you had to use crutches.
   - B. You suggest methods that might help her use her walker more efficiently.
   - C. You quickly try to change the subject to something happier.
   - D. You listen to her and acknowledge her feelings.

7. **Focusing is a useful communication tool when:**
   - A. A person is rambling
   - B. You want to make sure you understand the message
   - C. You want the person to share thoughts and feelings
   - D. You need information

8. **Which statement will promote communication?**
   - A. "Don't worry."
   - B. "Everything will be just fine."
   - C. "This is a good facility."
   - D. "I see you are upset. Do you want to talk about this?"

9. **Which is a barrier to communication?**
   - A. Interrupting
   - B. Repeating what the person says
   - C. Giving advice
   - D. A and C

10. **A client is angry. Which of the following statements is *true*?**
    - A. The person probably has a disease that affects thinking and behaviour.
    - B. Drug or alcohol abuse is likely.
    - C. You should tell the person to calm down and that everything will be fine.
    - D. Listening and the use of silence are important.

11. **With assertive communication, which is *true*?**
    - A. You appear upset, cold, or angry.
    - B. You appear confident, calm, and composed.
    - C. You are usually not respectful.
    - D. You appear hesitant, apologetic, and timid.

Answers: 1.A, 2.C, 3.B, 4.B, 5.A, 6.D, 7.A, 8.D, 9.D, 10.D, 11.B

CHAPTER 14

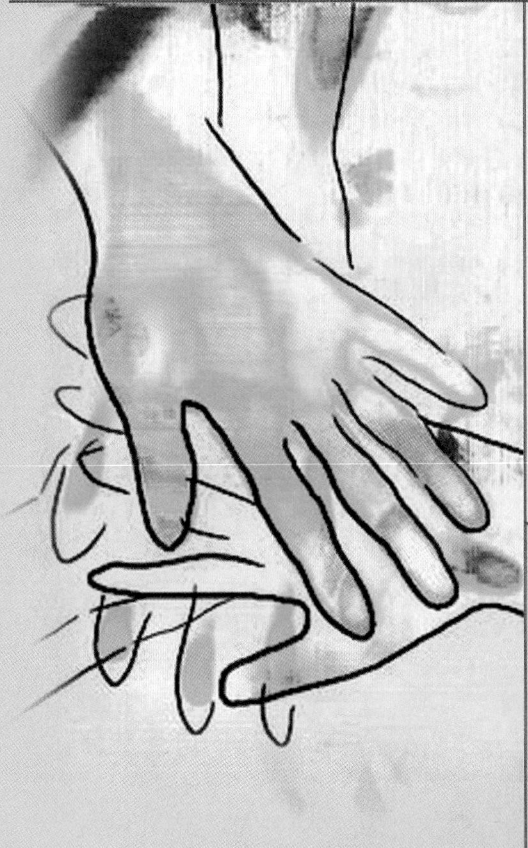

Body Structure and Function

OBJECTIVES

- Define the key terms listed in this chapter.
- Identify the basic structures of the cell, and explain how cells divide.
- Describe four types of tissue.
- Identify the structures of each body system.
- Describe the functions of each body system.

key terms

anatomical position The body is standing erect, with face forward, arms at the sides and palms of the hands facing outward.

anterior The front surface of the body—often used to indicate the position of one structure to another.

arteries Blood vessels that carry blood away from the heart.

ball-and-socket joint A joint that allows movement in all directions. It is made up of the rounded end of one bone and the hollow end of another bone. The rounded end of one fits into the hollow end of the other.

capillaries Tiny blood vessels; food, oxygen, and other substances pass from the capillaries to the cells.

cartilage Connective tissue, which cushions the joint.

cell The basic functional unit of body structure.

deep Distant from the surface of the body.

digestion The process of physically and chemically breaking down food so that it can be absorbed for use by the cells.

distal The farthest away from the trunk of the body or the point of origin.

hemoglobin The substance in red blood cells that carries oxygen and gives blood its colour.

hinge joint A joint that allows movement in one direction.

homeostasis A stable internal environment in our bodies.

hormone A chemical substance secreted by specialized glands into the bloodstream.

immunity Protection against a certain disease or infection; the person with immunity will not get or be affected by the disease.

inferior The lower parts of the body or indicating below a superior surface.

lateral The farthest away from the midline of the body.

medial The closest to the midline of the body.

menstruation The process in which the lining of the uterus breaks up and is discharged from the body through the vagina.

metabolism The burning of food for heat and energy by the cells.

organs Groups of tissues that work together to perform special functions.

peripheral Away from the centre of the body.

peristalsis Involuntary muscle contractions in the digestive system that move food through the alimentary canal.

pivot joint A joint that allows turning from side to side.

posterior The back surface of the body—often used to indicate the position of one structure to another.

proximal Nearest to the trunk of the body or the point of origin

respiration The process of supplying the cells with oxygen and removing carbon dioxide from them.

superficial Near the surface of the body.

superior Situated above.

systems Organs that work together to perform special functions.

tissue A group of cells with similar functions.

veins Blood vessels that carry blood back to the heart.

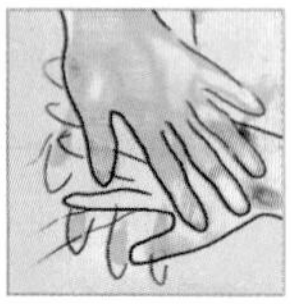

In your role as support worker, you will help clients meet their basic needs because their bodies are not working at peak efficiency due to disability, illness, disease, or injury. In order to provide care to promote comfort, healing, and recovery to clients, you need a basic understanding of the body's normal structure and function— that is, anatomy and physiology. *Anatomy* is the study of body structures, and *physiology* is the study of how the body structures work. Understanding the normal functioning of the body will help you understand and identify changes in the body. See Chapter 17 for changes in body structure and function that occur with aging.

ANATOMICAL TERMS

The terms used in the study of anatomy relate to the body in its **anatomical position.** In this position the body is standing erect, with the face forward, the arms at the sides and the toes and palms of the hands facing outward (Figure 14–1). The medical community uses specific terms to describe the position of body parts, areas of pain, and regions of the body (Box 14–1).

Box 14–1 Anatomical Terms

Superior—upper parts of the body or an organ or tissue can have a superior surface
Inferior—lower parts of the body or indicating below a superior surface
Anterior—the front surface of the body, often used to indicate the position of one structure to another
Posterior—the back surface of the body, often used to indicate the position of one structure to another
Medial—closest to the midline of the body
Lateral—farthest away from the midline of the body
Proximal—nearest the trunk of the body or the point of origin
Distal—farthest away from the trunk of the body or the point of origin
Superficial—near the surface of the body
Deep—distant from the surface of the body
Peripheral—away from the centre of the body

CELLS, TISSUES, AND ORGANS

The basic functional unit of body structure is the **cell.** Each cell has the same basic structure, but the function, size, and shape of cells may be different. Cells are so small that you need a microscope to see them. Cells need food, water, and oxygen to live and perform their functions.

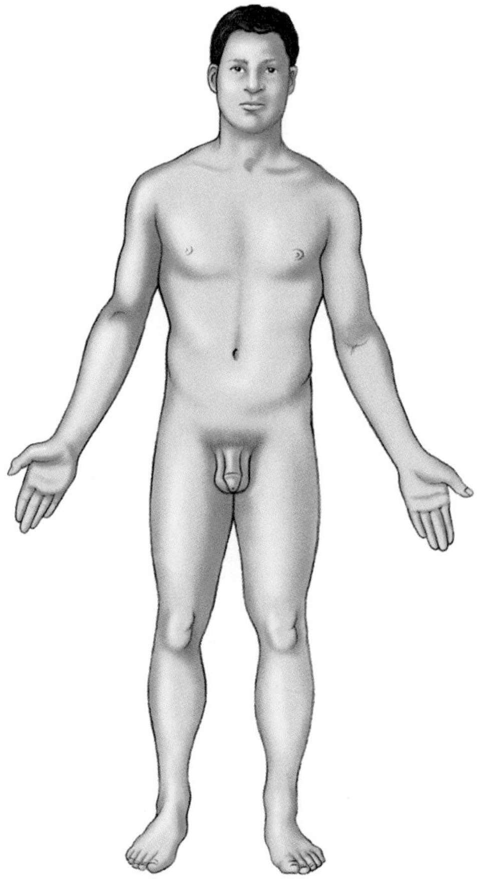

Figure 14–1 Anatomical position. **Source:** Herlihy, B. (2007). *The human body in health and illness* (3rd ed., p. 7). Philadelphia: Elsevier/Saunders.

The cell and its basic structures are shown in Figure 14–2 on page 182. The *cell membrane* is the outer covering that encloses the cell and helps it hold its shape. The *nucleus*—the control centre of the cell—directs the cell's activities and is located in the centre of the cell. The *cytoplasm* surrounds the nucleus. Cytoplasm contains many smaller structures that perform cell functions. The *protoplasm,* which means "living substance," refers to all of the structures, substances, and water within the cell. Protoplasm is a semi-liquid substance much like an egg white.

Chromosomes are threadlike structures within the nucleus. Each cell has 46 chromosomes that contain *genes.* Genes control the physical and chemical traits inherited by children from their parents. Inherited traits include height, eye colour, and skin colour.

Besides controlling the cell's activities, the nucleus is also responsible for cell reproduction. Cells reproduce by dividing in half, and each half becomes a new cell. The process of cell division, called *mitosis,* is needed for growth and repair of body tissues. During mitosis, the 46 chromosomes arrange themselves in 23 pairs. As the cell divides, the 23 pairs of chromosomes are pulled in half. The

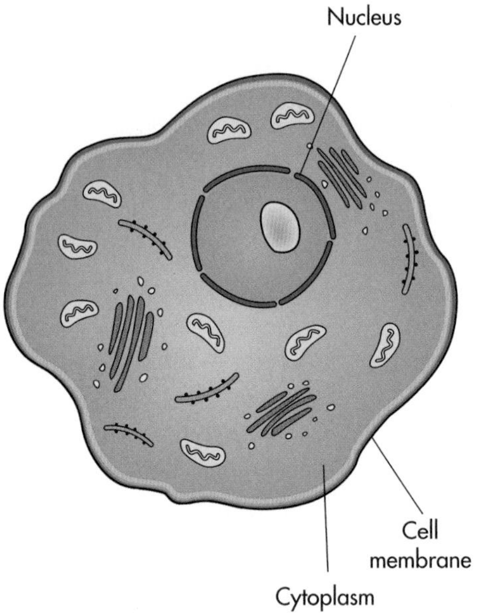

Figure 14–2 Parts of a cell.

two new cells are identical, each containing 46 chromosomes (Figure 14–3).

The cells are the body's building blocks. Groups of cells with similar functions combine to form **tissues.** The body has four basic types of tissue:

- *Epithelial cells* cover internal and external body surfaces. Tissue that lines the nose, mouth, respiratory tract, stomach, and intestines is epithelial tissue. The skin, hair, nails, and glands are also epithelial tissue.
- *Connective tissue* anchors, connects, and supports other body tissues. Connective tissue is found in every part of the body. *Tendons* (tissue that attaches muscles to bones), *ligaments* (tissue that connects bones and supports joints), and *cartilage* (tissue that cushions joints) are examples of connective tissue.
- *Muscle tissue* allows the body to move by stretching and contracting. There are three types of muscle tissue (see page 186).
- *Nerve tissue* relays information to and from the brain and throughout the body.

Organs are groups of tissue that work together to perform special functions. An organ performs one or more functions. Examples of organs are the heart, brain, liver, lungs, and kidneys. Organs are located within body cavities. The two major cavities are the dorsal cavity and the ventral cavity. The *dorsal cavity* has two cavities—the *cranial cavity* and *spinal cavity*.

The *ventral cavity* comprises the *thoracic cavity*, the *abdominal cavity*, and the *pelvic cavity* (Figure 14–4).

Systems are formed by organs that work together to perform special functions (Figure 14–5).

All of the systems in the human body work together to maintain a stable internal environment. This is called **homeostasis**. If the external temperature drops, our bodies start to shiver to keep our internal temperature at the normal level.

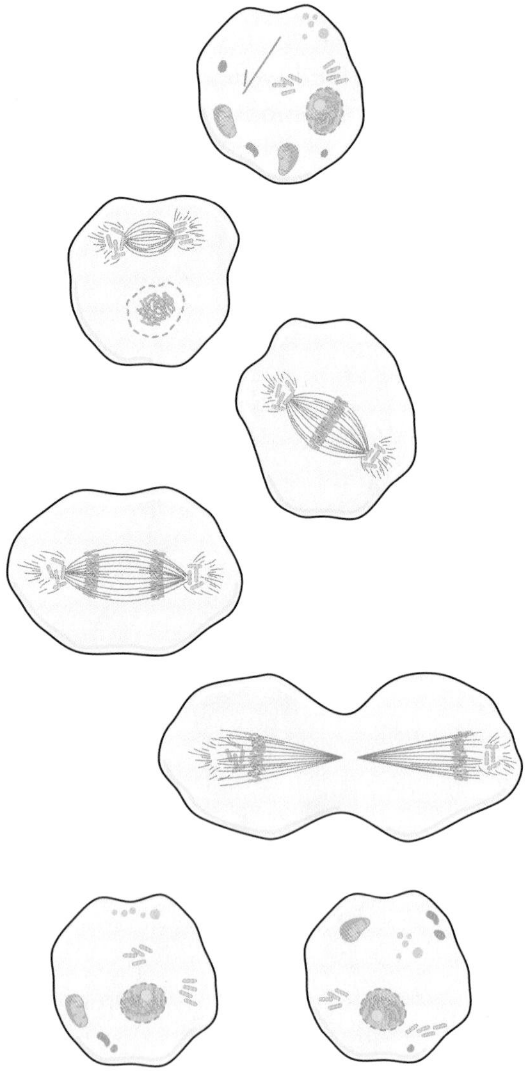

Figure 14–3 Cell division.

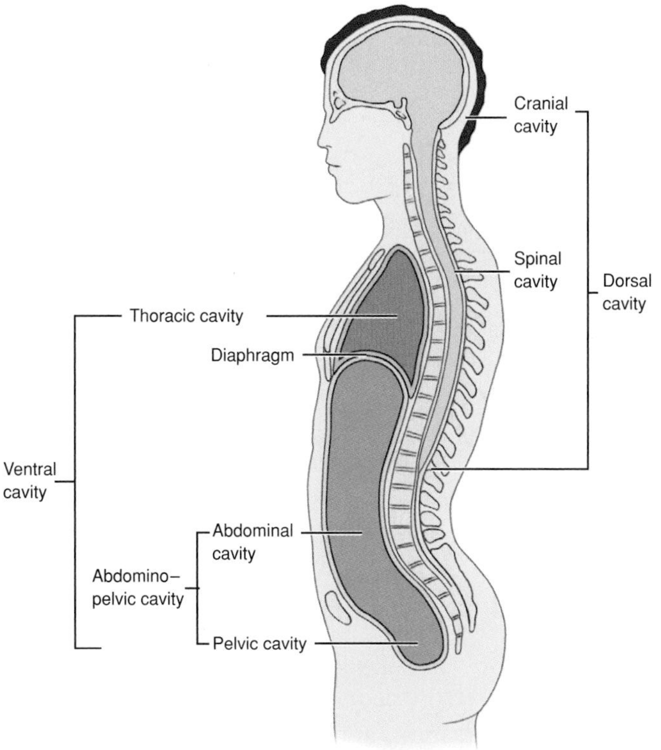

Figure 14–4 Major body cavities.

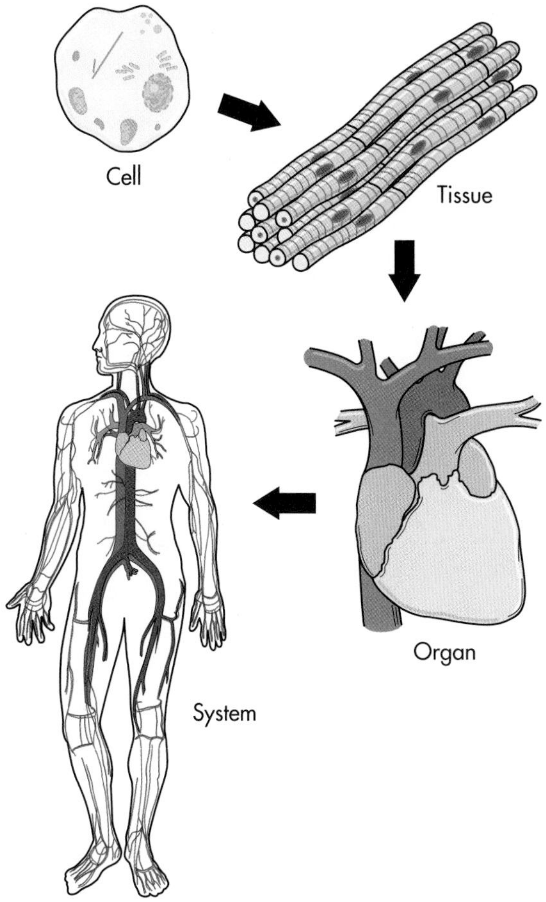

Figure 14–5 Organization of the body. **Source:** Herlihy, B. (2007). *The human body in health and illness* (3rd ed., p. 10). Philadelphia: Elsevier/Saunders.

THE INTEGUMENTARY SYSTEM

The *integumentary system* contains the skin and its appendages—hair, nails, and sweat and oil glands. (A *gland* is a group of cells that produces and secretes a substance. Glands in the skin produce and secrete sweat and oil.)

The integumentary system is the largest system of the body. *Integument* means covering. The skin is the body's natural covering. Skin is made up of epithelial, connective, and nerve tissue. There are two skin layers—the epidermis and the dermis (Figure 14–6). The *epidermis* is the outer layer and contains living and dead cells. The dead cells were once deeper in the epidermis and were pushed upward as other cells divided. Dead cells constantly flake off and are replaced by living cells. Living cells also eventually die and flake off. Living cells of the epidermis contain *pigment,* which gives skin its colour. The epidermis has no blood vessels and few nerve endings. The *dermis* is the inner layer of the skin and is made up of connective tissue. Blood vessels, nerves, sweat and oil glands, and hair roots are found in the dermis.

The skin has many important functions: (a) It is the protective covering of the body. It prevents bacteria and other substances from entering the body, prevents excessive amounts of water from leaving the body, and protects organs from injury. (b) Vitamin D and other products, such as some medications delivered in patches, are absorbed through the skin. (c) Nerve endings in the skin sense both pleasant and unpleasant stimulations. There are nerve endings over the entire body. The body is protected because heat, cold, pain, touch, and pressure are sensed. (d) The skin helps regulate body temperature. Blood vessels dilate (widen) when the temperature outside the body is high. More blood is brought to the body surface for cooling during evaporation. During exercise the blood vessels

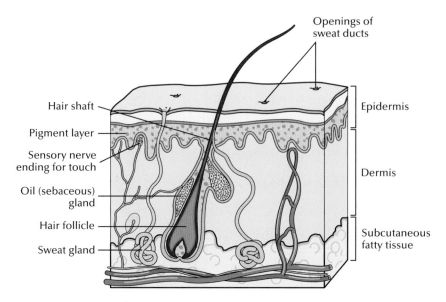

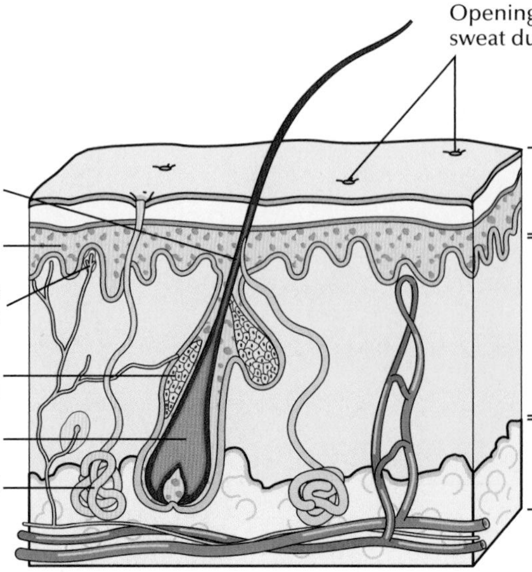

Figure 14–6 Layers of the skin.

dilate in order to cool the body. When blood vessels constrict (narrow), the body retains heat because less blood reaches the skin, for example, shivering and goose bumps.

Therefore, observing the condition of the skin can tell you several things about your client. The colour of the skin can indicate a physical condition. For example, if your client's skin or nails has a bluish tone, it could indicate a circulation problem. If the client's skin is very dry, it could indicate dehydration.

The entire body, except the palms of the hands and the soles of the feet, is covered with hair. Hair in the nose, eyes, and ears protects these organs from dust, insects, and other foreign objects getting in. Hair on the head helps retain heat.

Nails protect the tips of fingers and toes and help fingers pick up and handle small objects. A client's general state of health and nutritional status can be reflected by the condition of the nails. Nail beds are generally pink, so a bluish tinge to the nail beds can indicate poor oxygenation. Clubbing of the fingernails—when the fingertips enlarge and the nails curve down—can be caused by chronic lung and heart disease.

Sweat glands help the body regulate temperature. Sweat consists of water, salt, and a small amount of wastes. Sweat is secreted through pores in the skin, and the body is cooled as sweat evaporates. Oil glands lie near hair shafts, and they secrete an oily substance into the space near the hair shaft. Oil travels to the skin's surface, helping to keep the hair and skin soft and shiny, and also inhibits the growth of bacteria on the surface of the skin.

THE MUSCULO-SKELETAL SYSTEM

The musculo-skeletal system provides the framework for the body and allows the body to move. This system also protects and gives the body shape. Besides bones and muscles, the system has ligaments, tendons, and cartilage.

Bones

The human body has 206 bones (Figure 14–7). There are four types of bones:

- *Long bones* bear the weight of the body. The femur is a long bone.
- *Short bones* allow skill and ease in movement. Bones in the wrists, fingers, ankles, and toes are short bones.
- *Flat bones* protect the organs. Such bones include the ribs, skull, pelvic bones, and shoulder blades.
- *Irregular bones* are the vertebrae in the spinal column. They allow various degrees of movement and flexibility.

Bones are hard, rigid structures that are made up of living cells. They are covered by a membrane

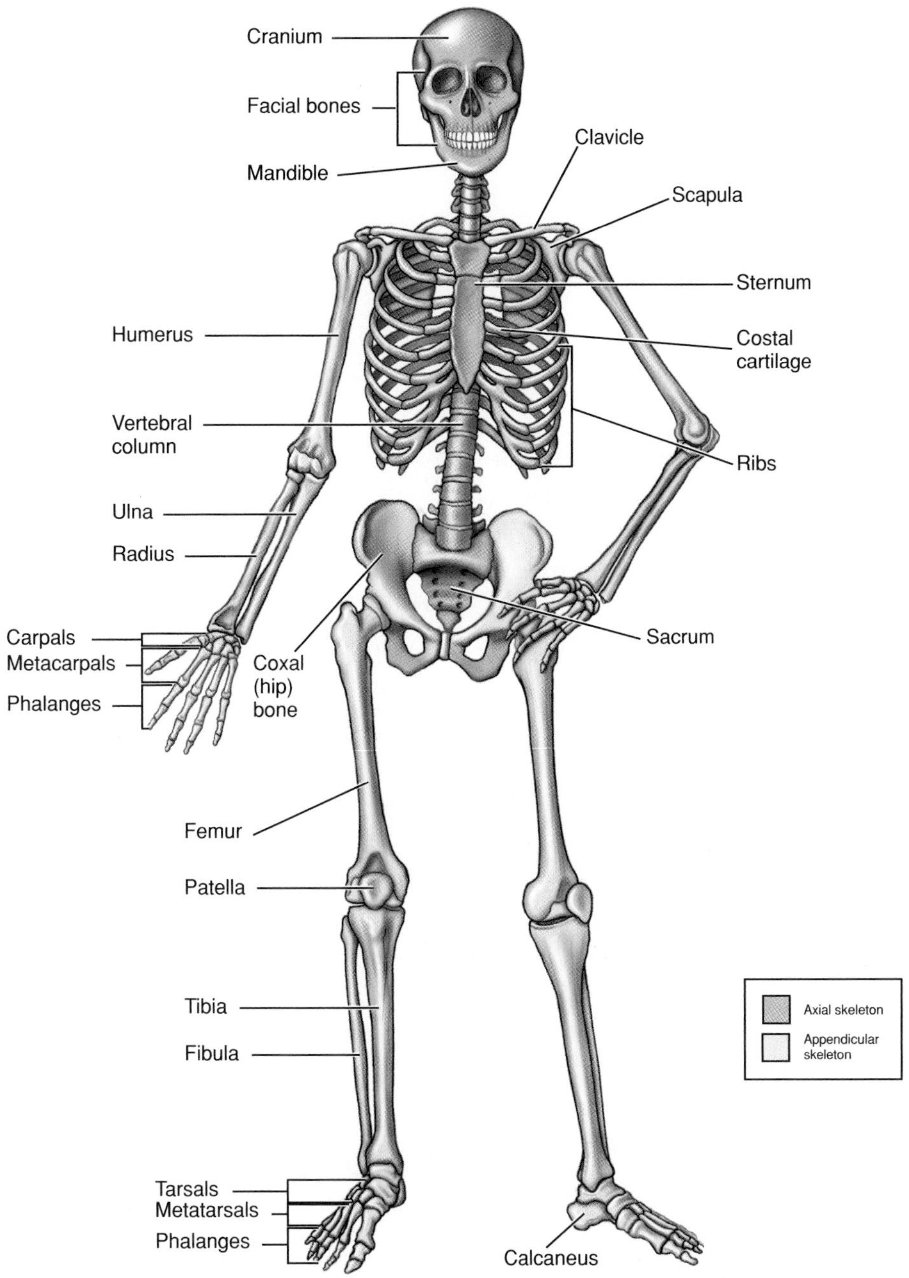

Figure 14–7 Bones of the body. **Source:** Herlihy, B. (2007). *The human body in health and illness* (3rd ed., p. 108). Philadelphia: Elsevier/Saunders.

called *periosteum*. Periosteum contains blood vessels that supply bone cells with oxygen and food. Inside the hollow centres of the bones is a substance called *bone marrow*. Blood cells are manufactured in the bone marrow.

Joints

A *joint* is the point at which two or more bones meet. Joints allow movement (see Chapter 24). **Cartilage** is connective tissue that cushions the joint so that bone ends do not rub together. The *synovial membrane* lines the joints and secretes *synovial fluid*, which acts as a lubricant so that the joint can move smoothly. Bones are held together at the joint by strong bands of connective tissue called *ligaments*.

There are three main types of joints (Figure 14–8):

- ***Ball-and-socket joint***—allows movement in all directions. It is made up of the rounded end of one bone and the hollow end of another bone. The rounded end of one fits into the hollow end of the other. The joints of the hips and shoulders are ball-and-socket joints.

- ***Hinge joint***—allows movement in one direction. The elbow is a hinge joint.
- ***Pivot joint***—allows turning from side to side. The skull is connected to the spine by a pivot joint.

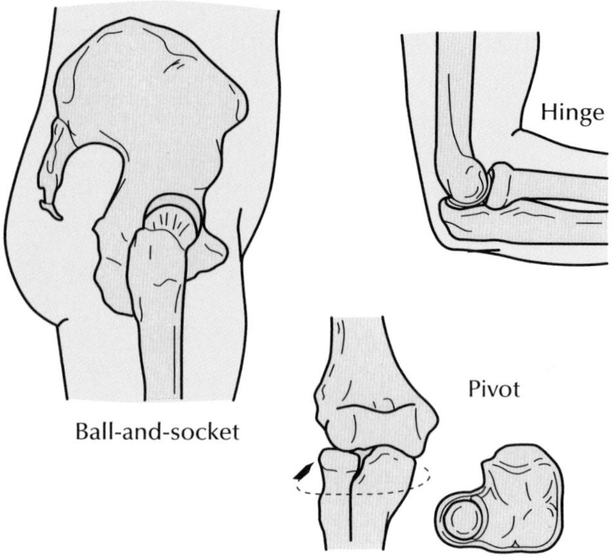

Figure 14–8 Types of joints.

Muscles

There are more than 500 muscles in the human body (Figures 14–9 through 14–11). Some are voluntary, while others are involuntary.

Voluntary muscles can be consciously controlled. Muscles attached to bones *(skeletal muscles)* are

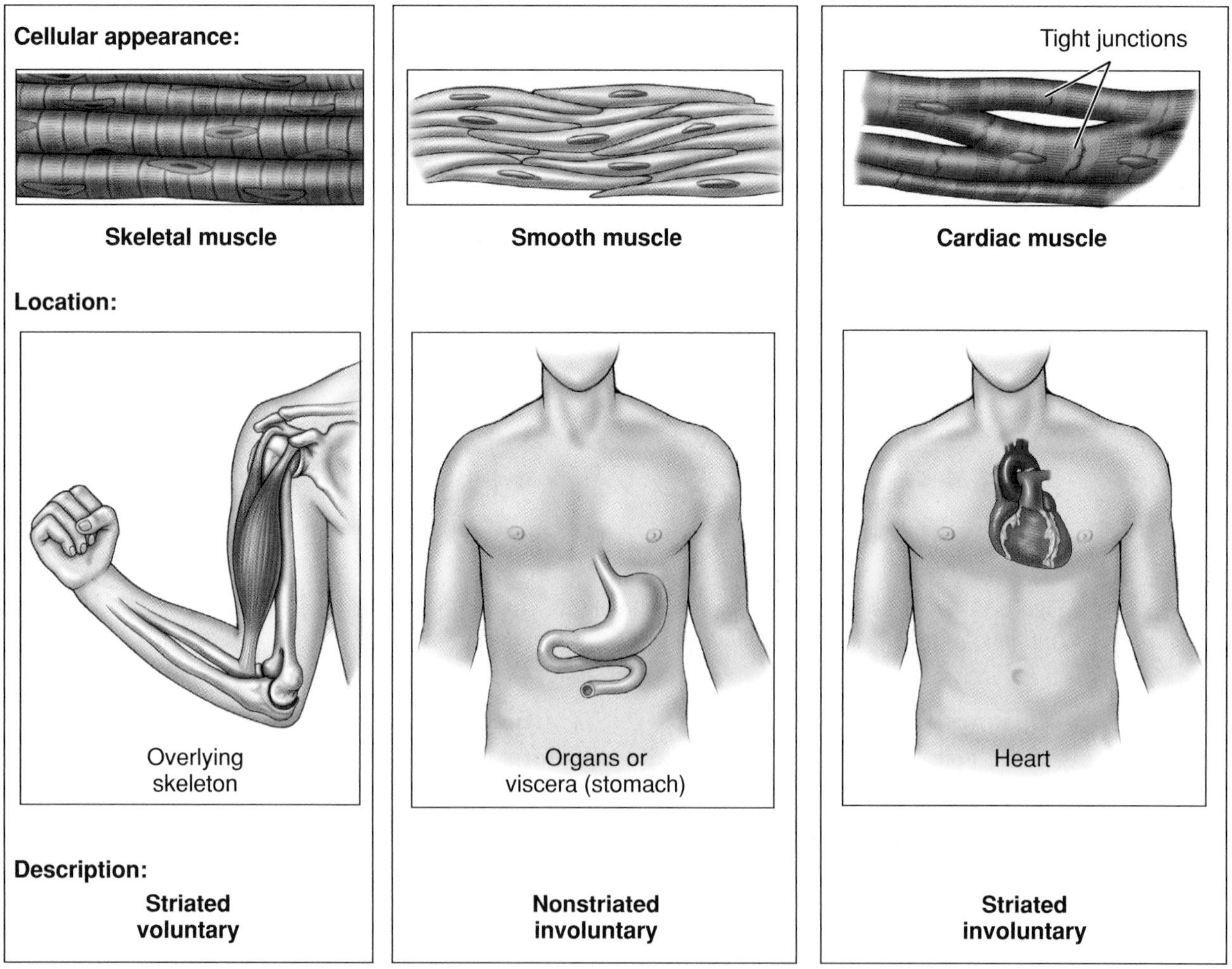

Figure 14–9 Three types of muscles. **Source:** Herlihy, B. (2007). *The human body in health and illness* (3rd ed., p. 138). Philadelphia: Elsevier/Saunders.

voluntary. Arm muscles or leg muscles do not work unless you move your arm or your leg. Skeletal muscles are *striated*; that is, they look striped or streaked.

Involuntary muscles work automatically and cannot be consciously controlled. Involuntary muscles control the action of the stomach, intestines, blood vessels, and other body organs. Involuntary muscles are also called *smooth muscles.* They look smooth, not streaked or striped. *Cardiac muscle* is found only in the heart. Although it is an involuntary muscle, it appears striated like skeletal muscle.

Muscles can do only two things: contract and relax. Most muscles contract and relax quickly. Muscles perform three important body functions:

1. Movement of body parts
2. Maintenance of posture
3. Production of body heat

Strong, tough connective tissues called *tendons* connect muscles to bones. When muscles contract (shorten), tendons at each end of the muscle cause the bone to move. The body has many tendons; the Achilles tendon is shown in Figure 14–11. Some muscles constantly contract to maintain the body's posture. When muscles contract, they burn food for energy, resulting in the production of heat. The greater the muscular activity, the greater the amount of heat produced in the body. Shivering is a way the body produces heat when exposed to cold. The shivering sensation is from rapid, general muscle contractions.

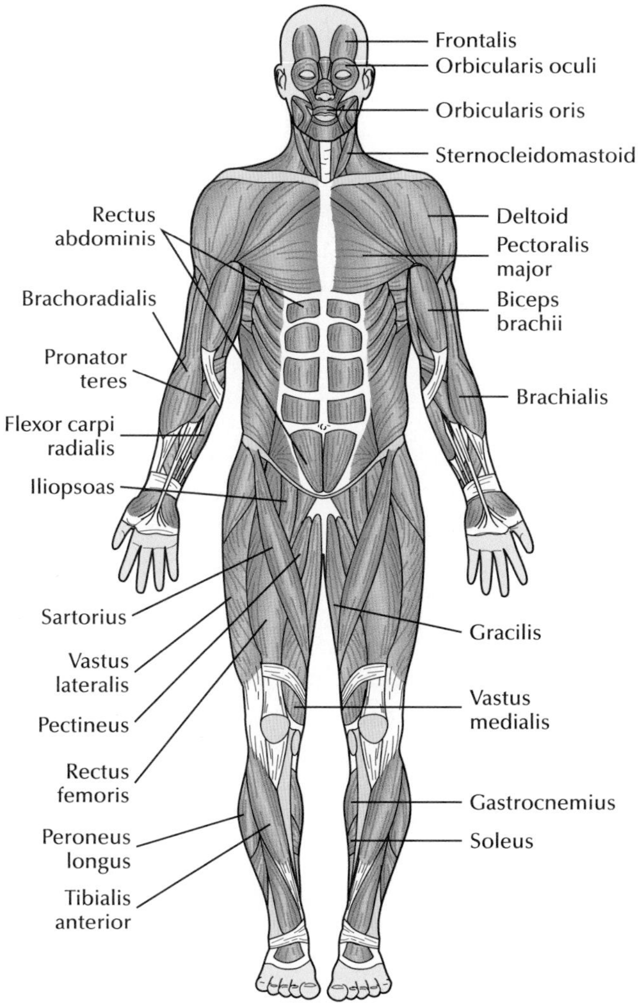

Figure 14–10 Anterior (front) view of the muscles of the body.

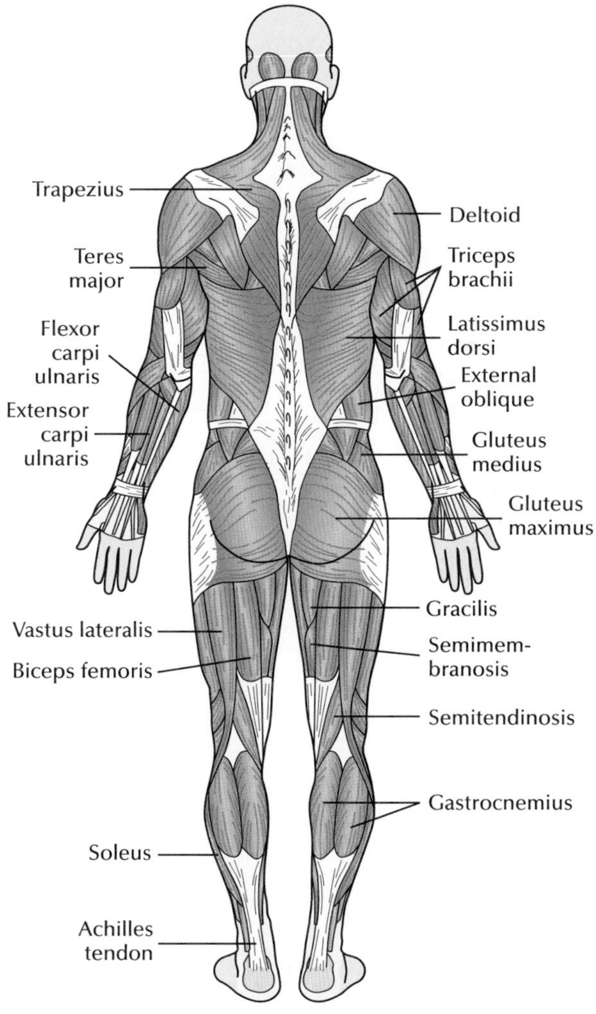

Figure 14–11 Posterior (back) view of the muscles of the body.

THE NERVOUS SYSTEM

The nervous system controls, directs, and coordinates body functions. The two main divisions of the nervous system are the *central nervous system* (CNS) and the *peripheral nervous system* (PNS). The central nervous system consists of the *brain* and *spinal cord* (Figure 14–12) and involves the *nerves* throughout the body (Figure 14–13), which carry messages or impulses to and from the brain. Nerves are connected to the spinal cord. Nerve tissue is composed of two types of cells—(1) *neuroglia* cells that nourish, protect and insulate the neurons; and (2) *neurons* that transmit information. The three parts of a neuron (Figure 14-14) are: (1) dendrites, which have branches that receive information from other neurons and send on the information to the cell body; (2) the nucleus in the cell body, which keeps the cell alive; and (3) the axon, which is a longer extension and carries information away from the cell down to the axon terminals. Chemical neurotransmitters are stored in the axon terminals. There is a space between neurons called a *synapse.* In summary, information is received in a dendrite, passes through the cell body, travels down the axon, out the axon terminals, over the synapse, and on to the next dendrite.

Nerves are easily damaged but take a long time to heal. Some nerve fibres have a protective covering called a *myelin sheath,* which also insulates the nerve fibre. Nerve fibres covered with myelin can conduct impulses faster than those fibres without the protective covering.

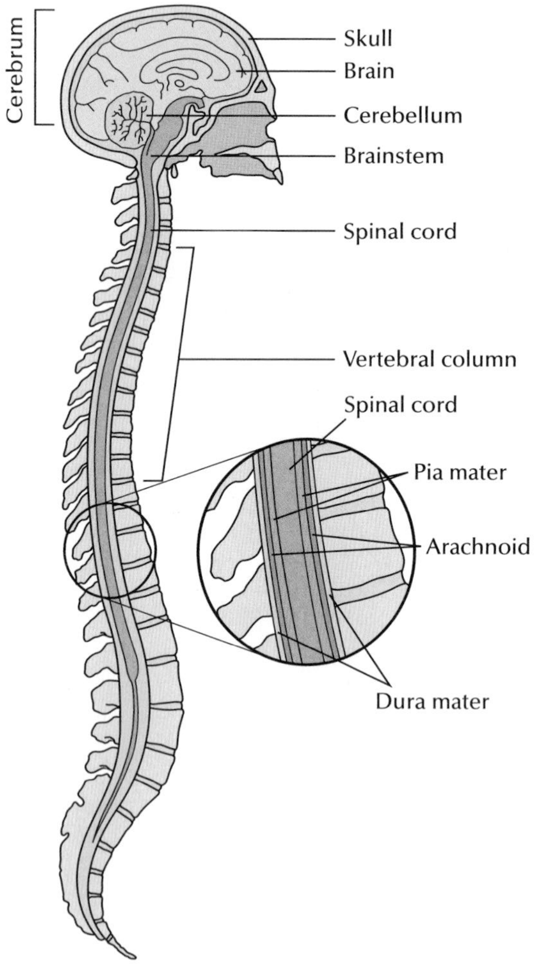

Figure 14–12 The central nervous system. **Source:** Herlihy, B. (2007). *The human body in health and illness* (3rd ed., p. 165). Philadelphia: Elsevier/Saunders.

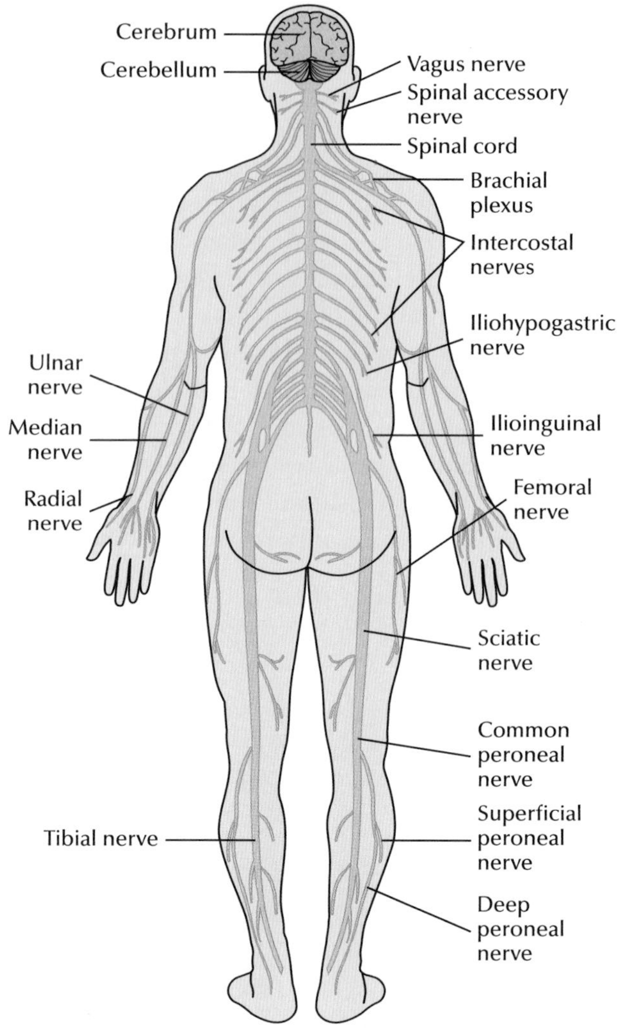

Figure 14–13 The peripheral nervous system.

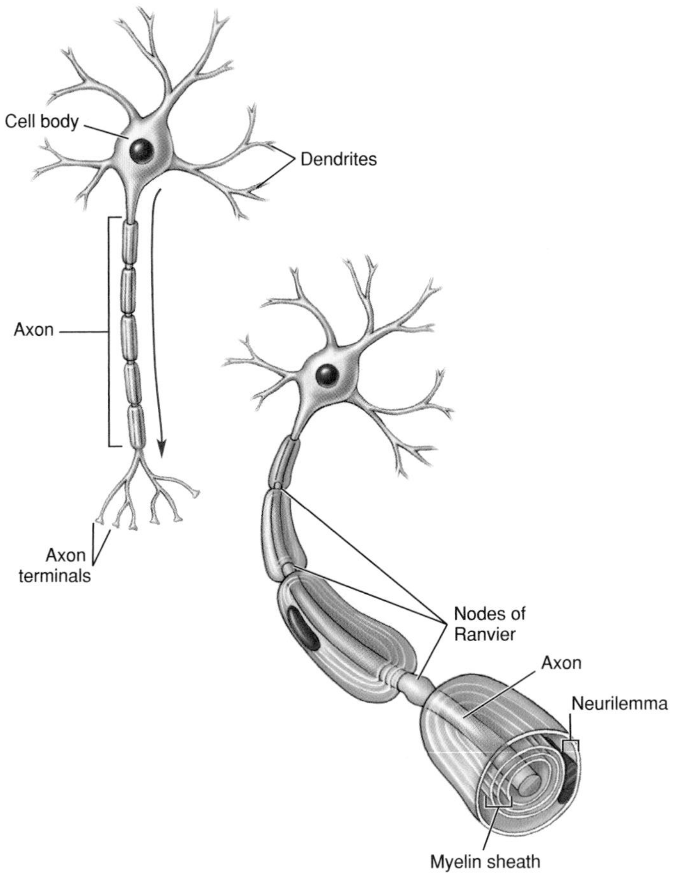

Figure 14–14 The structure of a neuron.

The Central Nervous System

The central nervous system consists of the brain and spinal cord. The brain is contained in and protected by the skull. The three main parts of the brain are the *cerebrum,* the *cerebellum,* and the *brainstem* (see Figure 14–12).

The cerebrum is the largest part of the brain and is the centre of thought and intelligence. The cerebrum is divided into two halves called the right and left *hemispheres.* The right hemisphere controls movement and activities on the body's left side. The left hemisphere controls the body's right side. The outside of the cerebrum is called the *cerebral cortex* (Figure 14–15). The cerebral cortex controls the highest functions of the brain. These include reasoning, memory, consciousness, speech, voluntary muscle movement, vision, hearing, sensation, and other activities.

The cerebellum regulates and coordinates body movements. The smooth movements of voluntary muscles and balance are possible because of control by the cerebellum. Injury to the cerebellum results in jerky movements, loss of coordination, and muscle weakness.

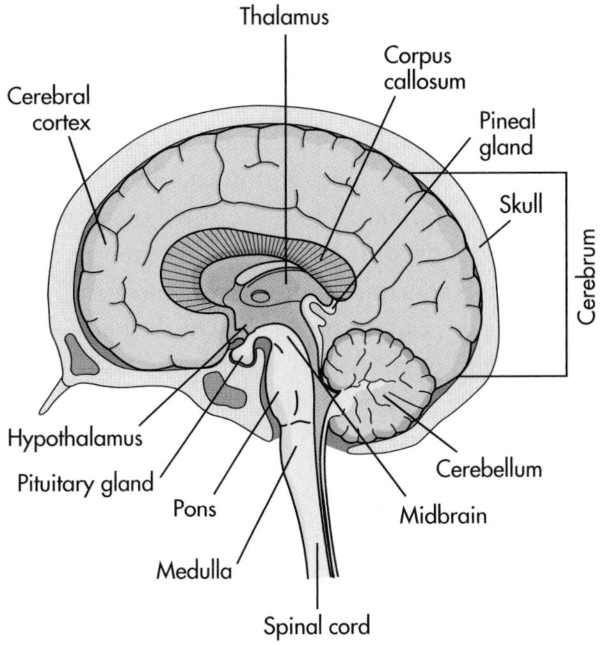

Figure 14–15 The brain.

The brainstem connects the cerebrum to the spinal cord. Important structures within the brainstem are the *midbrain, pons,* and *medulla.* The midbrain and pons relay messages between the medulla and the cerebrum. The medulla is directly below the pons. The medulla controls heart rate, breathing, blood vessel size, swallowing, coughing, and vomiting. The brain connects to the spinal cord at the lower end of the medulla.

The spinal cord lies within and is protected by the spinal column. The cord is about 45 cm (18 inches) long. It contains pathways that conduct messages to and from the brain. The brain and spinal cord are covered and protected by three layers of connective tissue called *meninges.* The outer layer, a tough covering called the *dura mater,* lies next to the skull. The middle layer is called the *arachnoid,* and the inner layer is the *pia mater.* The space between the middle and inner layers is the *arachnoid space,* and this space is filled with a fluid called *cerebrospinal fluid* that circulates around the brain and spinal cord. Cerebrospinal fluid protects the central nervous system and cushions shocks that could easily injure structures of the brain and spinal cord.

The Peripheral Nervous System

The peripheral nervous system has 12 pairs of *cranial nerves* and 31 pairs of *spinal nerves.* Cranial nerves conduct impulses between the brain and the head, neck, chest, and abdomen, and thus the impulses for smell, vision, hearing, pain, touch, temperature, pressure, and voluntary and involuntary muscle control. Spinal nerves carry impulses from the skin, extremities (a limb of the body, especially a hand or foot), and the internal body structures not supplied by cranial nerves.

Peripheral nerves with special functions form the *autonomic nervous system.* This system controls involuntary muscles and certain body functions that occur automatically, including the heartbeat, blood pressure, intestinal contractions, and glandular secretions.

The autonomic nervous system is divided into the *sympathetic nervous system* and the *parasympathetic nervous system.* These divisions balance each other. The sympathetic nervous system tends to speed up functions, and the parasympathetic nervous system slows them down. When you are angry, frightened, excited, or when you are exercising, the sympathetic nervous system is stimulated. The parasympathetic system is activated when you relax or when the sympathetic system is under stimulation for too long.

THE SENSORY SYSTEM

The five senses are sight, hearing, taste, smell, and touch. Receptors for taste are in the tongue and are called *taste buds.* Receptors for smell are in the nose. Touch receptors are found in the dermis, especially in the toes and fingertips.

The Eye. Receptors for vision are in the eyes. The eye is easily injured. Bones of the skull, eyelids and eyelashes, and tears protect the eyes from injury. Eye structures are shown in Figure 14–16. The eye has three layers:

- The *sclera,* the white of the eye, is the outer layer except for its anterior one sixth, which is the cornea. The sclera is made of tough connective tissue.
- The *choroid* is the second layer. Blood vessels, the *ciliary muscle,* and the *iris* make up the choroid. The iris gives the eye its colour. The opening in the middle of the iris is the *pupil.* Pupil size varies with the amount of light entering the eye. The pupil constricts (narrows) in bright light and dilates (widens) in dim or dark places.
- The *retina* is the inner layer of the eye. It contains receptors for vision and the nerve fibres of the optic nerve.

Light enters the eye through the *cornea.* The cornea is the transparent part of the outer layer that lies over the eye. Light rays pass to the *lens,* which lies behind the pupil. The light is then reflected to the retina and carried to the brain by the *optic nerve* for its interpretation of what is being seen.

The *aqueous chamber* separates the cornea from the lens. The chamber is filled with a fluid called *aqueous humor.* The fluid helps the cornea keep its shape and position. The *vitreous humor* is behind the lens. The vitreous body is a gelatin-like substance that supports the retina and maintains the eye's shape.

The Ear. The ear is a sense organ that functions in hearing and balance. It is divided into the *external ear, middle ear,* and *inner ear.* Ear structures are shown in Figure 14–17.

The external ear (outer part) is called the *pinna* or *auricle.* Sound waves are guided through the external ear into the *auditory canal.* Glands in the auditory canal secrete a waxy substance called

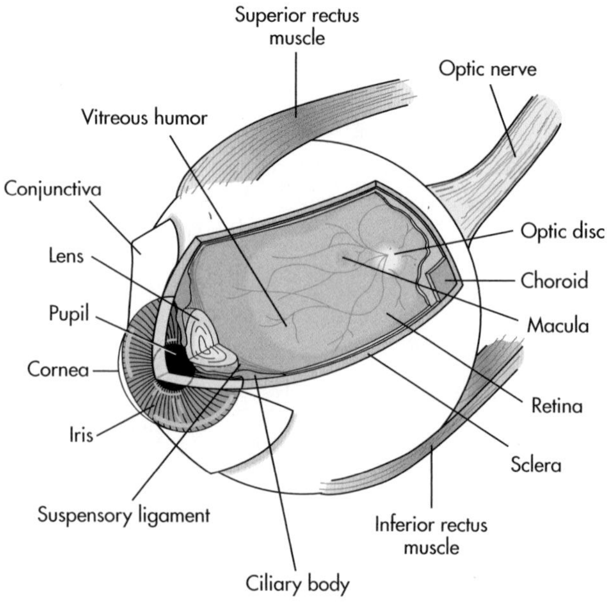

Figure 14–16 The eye.

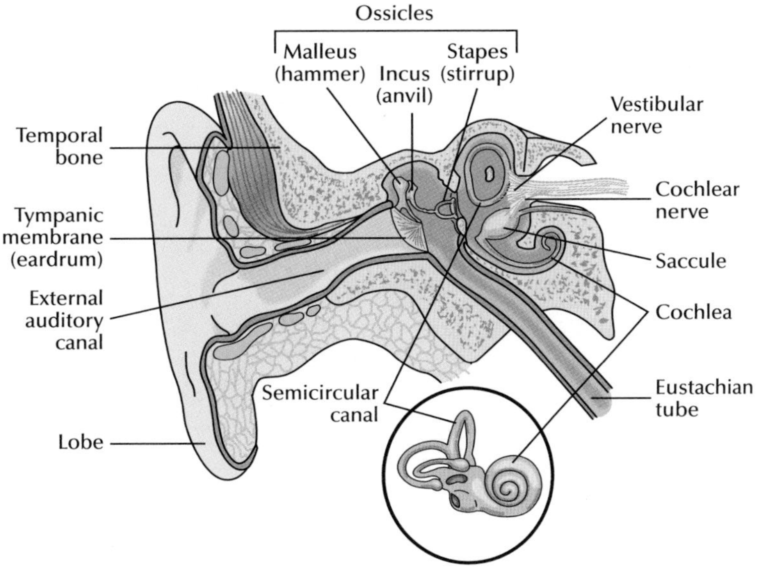

Figure 14–17 The ear.

cerumen, which catches particles that enter the ear. The auditory canal extends about 2.5 cm (1 inch) to the *eardrum.* The eardrum *(tympanic membrane)* separates the external ear and middle ear.

The middle ear is a small space that contains the *eustachian tube* and three small bones called *ossicles.* The eustachian tube connects the middle ear and the throat. Air enters the eustachian tube so that there is equal pressure on both sides of the eardrum. The ossicles amplify sound received from the eardrum and transmit the sound to the inner ear. The three ossicles are:

1. The *malleus,* which looks like a hammer
2. The *incus,* which resembles an anvil
3. The *stapes,* which is shaped like a stirrup

The inner ear consists of the *semicircular canals* and the *cochlea.* The cochlea, which looks like a snail shell, contains fluid. The fluid carries sound waves received from the middle ear to the *auditory nerve.* The auditory nerve then carries the message to the brain for interpretation of what is being heard.

The three semicircular canals are involved in maintaining balance. They sense the head's position and changes in position and send messages to the brain.

The Sense of Taste. Receptors for taste are located across the back of the tongue and are called *taste buds.* The taste buds relay sensations of different tastes to the brain for interpretation. The four basic taste sensations are salty, sweet, sour, and bitter. The receptors for each sensation are located on a particular area of the tongue. Sweet sensation receptors are on the tip of the tongue. Salty receptors are on the sides near the front. Sour receptors are located on the sides near the back, and bitter sensation receptors are across the back of the tongue.

The Sense of Smell. Receptors for smell are located on the roof of the nasal cavity. These are called *olfactory receptors.* These receptors are stimulated by the fluid in the mucous membrane in the nose. The impulses are sent to the brain, where they are interpreted as smell. Smell and taste are very connected. When we have a cold and are nasally congested, food often does not taste the same.

THE CIRCULATORY SYSTEM

The circulatory system is made up of the blood, heart, and blood vessels. The heart works as a pump to push blood through the blood vessels. The circulatory system has many important functions:

- Blood carries food, oxygen, and other substances to the cells throughout the body so they can live and function.
- Blood removes waste products from the cells.

- Blood and blood vessels help regulate body temperature. Heat from muscle activity is carried by the blood to other body parts. Blood vessels in the skin dilate if the body needs to be cooled. They constrict if heat needs to be kept in the body.
- The circulatory system also produces and carries cells that defend the body from disease-causing micro-organisms.

The Blood

The blood consists of blood cells and a liquid called *plasma.* Plasma is mostly water. It carries blood cells to other body cells. Plasma also carries other substances needed by cells for proper functioning. Food (proteins, fats, and carbohydrates), hormones, chemicals, and waste products are among the many substances carried in the plasma.

Red blood cells are called *erythrocytes.* They give the blood its red colour because of a substance in the cell called **hemoglobin**. As red blood cells circulate through the lungs, hemoglobin picks up oxygen and carries it to the cells. When the blood is bright red, hemoglobin in the red blood cells is saturated (filled) with oxygen. As blood circulates through the body, oxygen is given to the cells. The cells release carbon dioxide (a waste product), which is picked up by the hemoglobin. Red blood cells saturated with carbon dioxide make the blood look dark red.

There are about 25 trillion (25,000,000,000,000) red blood cells in the body. In a cubic millimetre of blood (the size of a tiny drop), there are about 4.5 to 5 million cells. These cells live for 3 or 4 months and are then destroyed by the liver and spleen as they wear out. Bone marrow produces new red blood cells, about one million every second.

White blood cells, called *leukocytes,* are colourless. They protect the body against infection. There are 5000 to 10,000 white blood cells in a cubic millimetre of blood. At the first sign of infection, white blood cells rush to the site of the infection and begin to multiply rapidly to kill the invading micro-organisms to fight the infection. The number of white blood cells increases when there is an infection in the body. White blood cells are also produced by the bone marrow and live about 9 days.

Platelets (thrombocytes) are necessary for the clotting of blood. They are also produced by the bone marrow. There are about 200,000 to 400,000 platelets in a cubic millimetre of blood. A platelet lives about 4 days.

The Heart

The heart is a muscle that works as a two-sided pump to push blood through the blood vessels to the tissues and cells. The heart lies in the middle to lower part of the chest cavity toward the left side (Figure 14–18). The heart is hollow and has three layers (Figure 14–19):

1. The *pericardium* is the outer layer. It is a thin sac covering the heart.
2. The *myocardium* is the second layer. This layer is the thick, muscular portion of the heart.
3. The *endocardium* is the inner layer. The endocardium is the membrane lining the inner surface of the heart.

The heart has four chambers (see Figure 14–19). Upper chambers receive blood and are called the *atria.* The *right atrium* receives blood from body tissues and the *left atrium* from the lungs. Lower chambers are called *ventricles,* which pump blood. The *right ventricle* pumps blood to the lungs for oxygen, and the *left ventricle* pumps blood to all parts of the body.

Valves, located between the atria and ventricles, allow blood to flow in only one direction, preventing blood from flowing back into the atria from

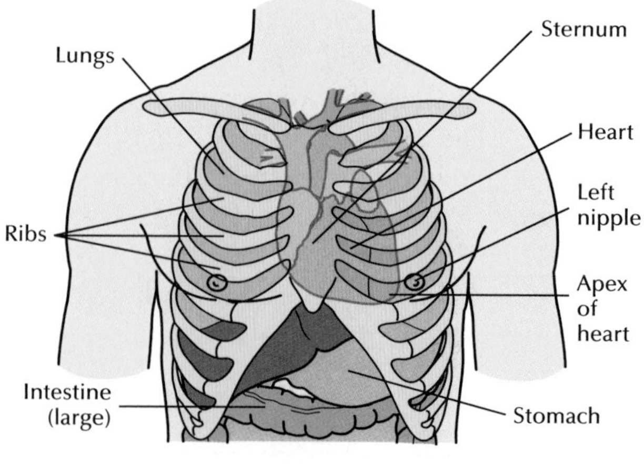

Figure 14–18 Location of the heart in the chest cavity.

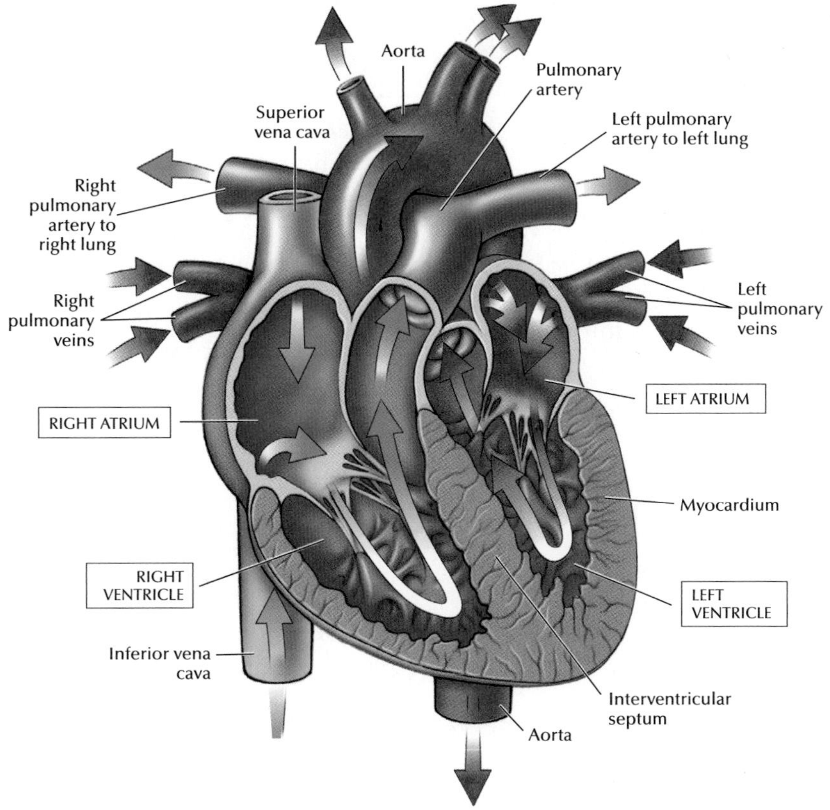

Figure 14–19 Structures of the heart. **Source:** Herlihy, B. (2007). *The human body in health and illness* (3rd ed., p. 287). Philadelphia: Elsevier/Saunders.

the ventricles. The *tricuspid valve* is between the right atrium and right ventricle, and the *mitral valve (bicuspid valve)* is between the left atrium and left ventricle.

There are two phases of heart action. During *diastole,* the resting phase, heart chambers fill with blood, and during *systole,* the working phase, the heart contracts. Blood is pumped through the blood vessels when the heart contracts.

The rate the heart beats can differ for many reasons. Generally, the larger the body size, the slower is the rate. Men have slower heart rates than do women, and the heart rate generally slows with age. Disease, fever, exercise, and some medications can also influence the heart rate. The *pulse* measures the heart rate (refer to Chapter 41 for more information on pulse rate).

The Blood Vessels

Blood flows to body tissues and cells through the blood vessels. There are four groups of blood vessels: arteries, capillaries, veins, and venules. **Arteries** carry blood away from the heart. Arterial blood is rich in oxygen. The *aorta* is the largest artery and receives blood directly from the left ventricle. The aorta branches into other arteries that carry blood to all parts of the body (Figure 14–20), and these arteries, in turn, branch into smaller parts within the tissues. The smallest branch of an artery is an *arteriole.*

Arterioles connect with blood vessels called **capillaries,** which are tiny vessels. Food, oxygen, and other substances pass from capillaries into the cells, and waste products, including carbon dioxide, are picked up from cells by the capillaries and are carried back to the heart by the veins.

Veins return blood to the heart. They are connected to the capillaries by *venules,* which are small veins. Venules begin branching together to form veins. The many branches of veins also branch together as they near the heart to form two main veins (see Figure 14–20). The two main veins are the *inferior vena cava* and the *superior vena cava.* Both empty into the right atrium. The inferior vena cava carries blood from the legs and trunk, and the superior vena cava carries blood from the head and arms. Venous blood is dark red because it contains little oxygen and a lot of carbon dioxide.

Blood flow through the circulatory system (see Figure 14–19) can be summarized as follows:

- Venous blood, poor in oxygen, empties into the right atrium.
- Blood flows through the tricuspid valve into the right ventricle.
- The right ventricle pumps blood into the lungs to pick up oxygen.
- Oxygen-rich blood from the lungs enters the left atrium.
- Blood from the left atrium passes through the mitral valve into the left ventricle.
- The left ventricle pumps the blood to the aorta, which branches off to form other arteries.
- The arterial blood is carried to the tissues by arterioles and to the cells by capillaries.
- The cells and capillaries exchange oxygen and nutrients for carbon dioxide and waste products.
- Capillaries connect with venules.
- Venules carry blood that contains carbon dioxide and waste products.
- The venules form veins.
- Veins return blood to the heart, into the right atrium.

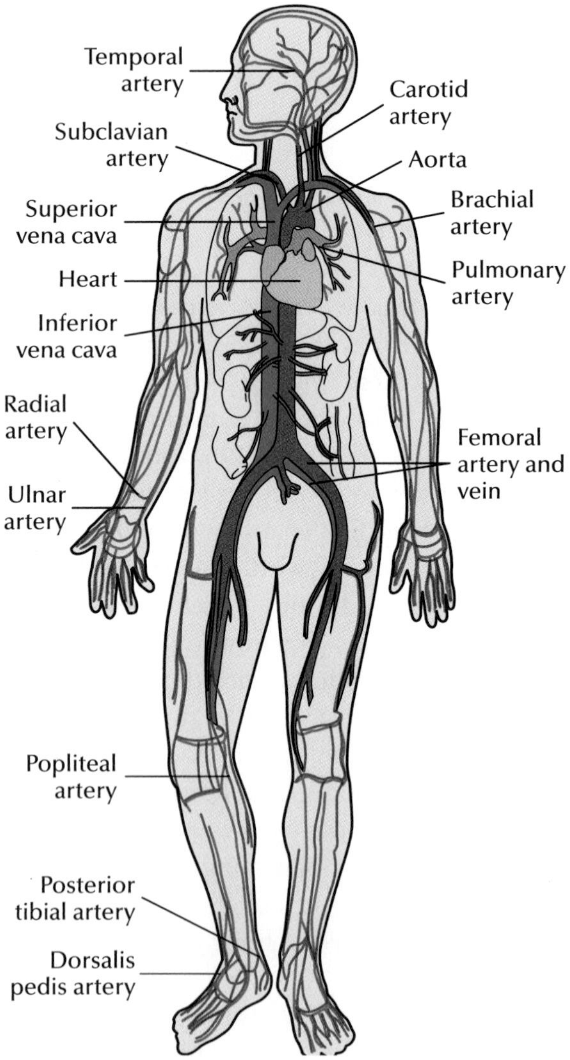

Figure 14–20 Some of the major arteries and veins in the body.

THE LYMPHATIC SYSTEM

The lymphatic system comprises lymphoid organs, lymph nodes, lymph ducts, lymphatic tissue, lymph capillaries, and lymph vessels. As blood circulates through the capillaries, blood plasma leaks out into the spaces between the cells. About 85% of the fluid is absorbed back into the blood capillaries. The other 15% drains into the lymphatic capillaries that surround the blood capillaries. This fluid is called *lymph* and is composed primarily of water, electrolytes, waste from metabolizing cells and some protein. The lymphatic capillaries empty into larger lymph vessels.

The lymphatic vessels are distributed around the entire body running beside the veins. The lymph flows through larger and larger vessels until it reaches one of the lymph ducts. Both of these ducts drain into the subclavian veins.

Blood moves because it is pumped by the heart, but lymph depends on other means for movement. Lymph moves in response to contraction of the skeletal muscles, the movement of the chest during respiration, and contraction of smooth muscles.

The lymphoid organs include the lymph nodes, tonsils, thymus gland and spleen.

Lymph nodes are small pea-shaped patches of lymphatic tissue. The cervical lymph nodes drain and filter lymph from the head and neck area. The axillary lymph nodes drain and cleanse the lymph from the upper extremities, shoulders, and breasts. The inguinal lymph nodes are located in the groin and drain and cleanse the lymph from the lower extremities and external genitalia (Figure 14–21).

The tonsils, which are located in the throat, filter tissue fluid contaminated by pathogens that enter the body through the nose or mouth or both.

The thymus is located in the thoracic cavity. It plays a crucial role in the development of the immune system before birth and in the first few months after birth. After puberty, the gland shrinks but remains active. It secretes a hormone which aids the immune system.

The spleen filters blood rather than lymph. It cleanses the blood and destroys micro-organisms. The spleen also produces disease-preventing cells, such as lymphocytes and macrophages.

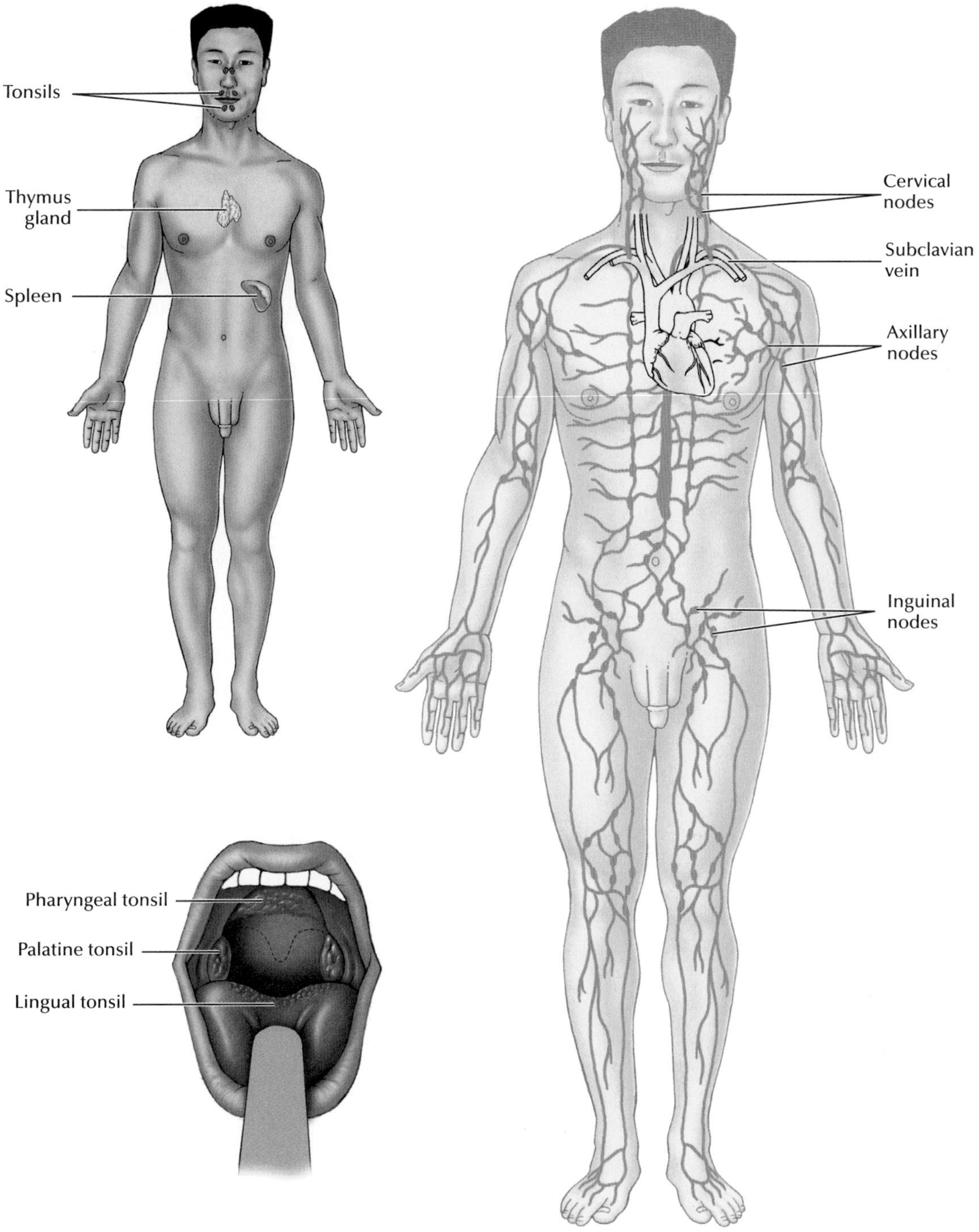

Figure 14–21 The distribution of lymph nodes. **Source:** Herlihy, B. (2007). *The human body in health and illness* (3rd ed., p. 349). Philadelphia: Elsevier/Saunders.

THE RESPIRATORY SYSTEM

Oxygen is needed for survival, and every cell needs oxygen. Air contains about 21% oxygen—enough to meet the needs of the body under normal conditions. The respiratory system (Figure 14–22) brings oxygen into the lungs and eliminates carbon dioxide. The process of supplying the cells with oxygen and removing carbon dioxide from them is called **respiration.** Respiration involves *inhalation* (breathing in) and *exhalation* (breathing out). The terms *inspiration* (breathing in) and *expiration* (breathing out) are also used. The respiratory system is divided into the *upper respiratory tract* and the *lower respiratory tract.* The upper respiratory tract includes the nose and nasal cavities, pharynx, and upper trachea. The lower respiratory tract includes the lower trachea, bronchi, bronchioles, alveoli, and the lungs.

Air enters the body through the *nose* and passes into the *pharynx* (throat), a tube-shaped passageway for both air and food. It then passes from the pharynx into the *larynx* (the voice box). A piece of cartilage called the *epiglottis* acts like a lid over the larynx. The epiglottis prevents food from entering the airway during swallowing. During inhalation, the epiglottis lifts up so that air passes over the larynx and into the *trachea* (the windpipe).

The trachea divides at its lower end into the *right bronchus* and *left bronchus.* Each bronchus enters a lung and further divides several times into smaller branches called *bronchioles.* Eventually, the bronchioles subdivide and end in tiny one-celled air sacs called *alveoli.*

Alveoli look like small clusters of grapes. They are supplied by capillaries. Oxygen and carbon dioxide are exchanged between the alveoli and capillaries. Blood in the capillaries picks up oxygen from the alveoli and is returned to the left side of the heart and pumped to the rest of the body. Alveoli pick up carbon dioxide from the capillaries for exhalation.

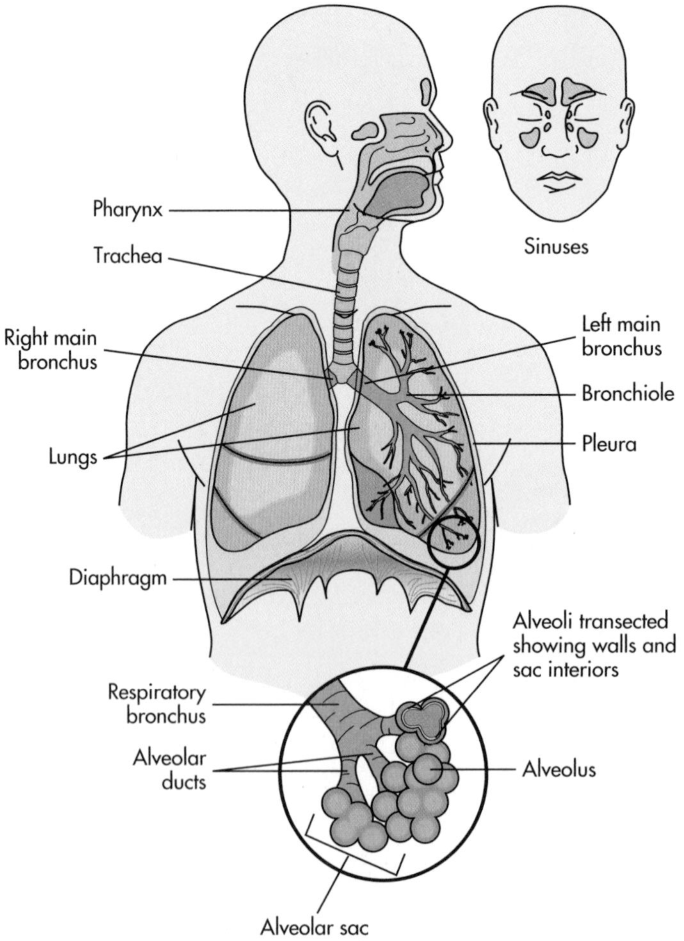

Figure 14–22 The respiratory system.

The lungs are spongy tissues filled with alveoli, blood vessels, and nerves. Each lung is divided into lobes. The right lung has three lobes; the left lung has two. The lungs are separated from the abdominal cavity by a muscle called the *diaphragm.*

Each lung is covered by a two-layered sac called the *pleura.* One layer is attached to the lung and the other to the chest wall. The pleura secretes a very thin fluid that fills the space between the layers. The fluid prevents the layers from rubbing together during inhalation and exhalation. A bony framework consisting of the ribs, sternum, and vertebrae protects the lungs.

THE DIGESTIVE SYSTEM

The digestive system, also called the *gastrointestinal system (GI system),* breaks down food physically and chemically so it can be absorbed for use by the cells—a process called **digestion**—and also eliminates solid wastes from the body.

The digestive system consists of the *alimentary canal (GI tract)* and the accessory organs of digestion (Figure 14–23). The alimentary canal is a long tube extending from the mouth to the anus. Its major parts are the mouth, pharynx, esophagus, stomach, small intestine, and large intestine. The accessory organs of digestion are the teeth, tongue, salivary glands, liver, gallbladder, and pancreas.

Digestion begins in the *mouth*—also called the *oral cavity*—which receives food and prepares it for digestion. Using chewing motions, the *teeth* cut, chop, and grind food into smaller particles for digestion and swallowing. The *tongue* aids in chewing and swallowing. *Taste buds* on the tongue's surface contain nerve endings and allow sweet, sour, bitter, and salty tastes to be sensed. *Salivary glands* in the mouth secrete *saliva,* which moistens food particles for easier swallowing and begins the

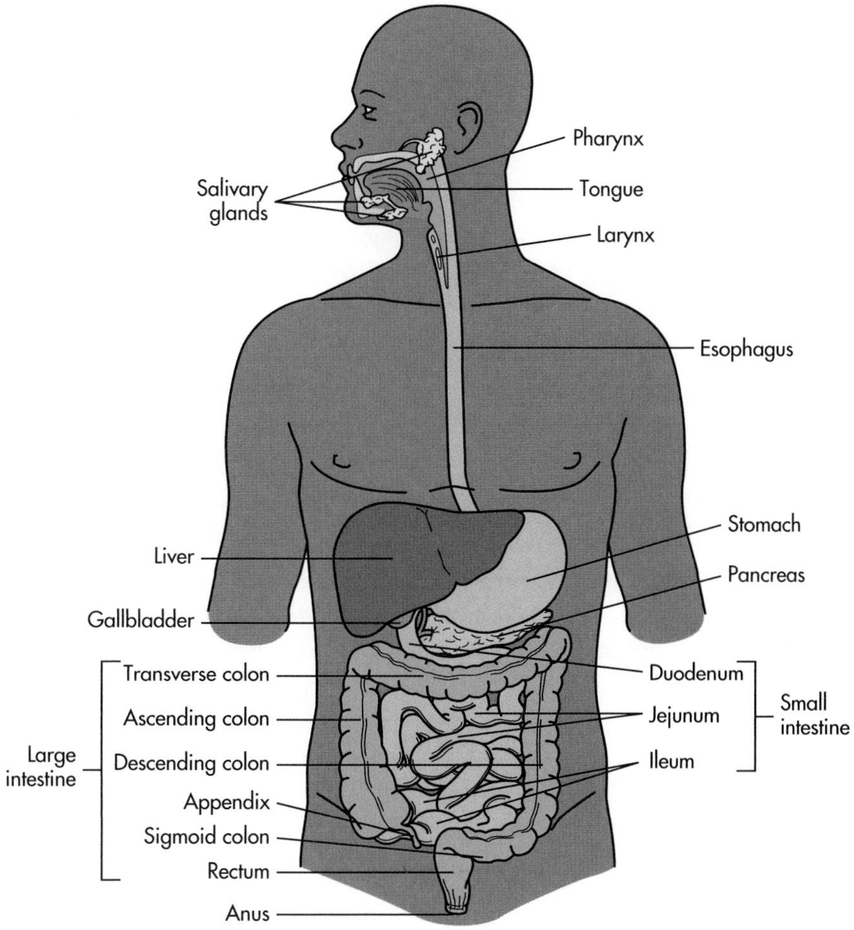

Figure 14–23 The digestive system.

digestion of food. During swallowing, the tongue pushes food into the pharynx.

The *pharynx* (throat) is a muscular tube. The act of swallowing is continued as the pharynx contracts, which pushes food into the *esophagus.* The esophagus is a muscular tube about 25 cm (10 inches) long. It extends from the pharynx to the stomach. Involuntary muscle contractions—called **peristalsis**—move food down the esophagus into the stomach.

The *stomach* is a muscular, pouchlike sac in the upper left portion of the abdominal cavity. Strong stomach muscles stir and churn food to break it up into even smaller particles. The stomach is lined with a mucous membrane containing glands that secrete *gastric juices.* Gastric juices contain strong acids that kill most micro-organisms in the food that has been eaten. Food is mixed and churned with the gastric juices to form a semi-liquid substance called *chyme.* Through peristalsis, the chyme is pushed from the stomach into the small intestine.

The *small intestine* is about 6 metres (20 feet) long and has three parts. The first part is the *duodenum,* where more digestive juices are added to the chyme.

One of the digestive juices is *bile,* which is a greenish liquid produced by the *liver* and stored in the *gallbladder.* Bile aids not only in the digestion of fat but also in the absorption of fat-soluble vitamins. It gives stool its brownish colour. The liver has many important functions: (1) it metabolizes fats, proteins, and carbohydrates; (2) detoxifies substances from the blood; (3) stores fat-soluble vitamins; and (4) excretes bile, cholesterol, and bilirubin.

The *pancreas* secretes enzymes that are the most important of all the digestive enzymes. Juices from the pancreas and small intestine are also added to the chyme.

The digestive juices chemically break down food so that it can be absorbed. Peristalsis moves the chyme through the two remaining portions of the small intestine: the *jejunum* and the *ileum.* Tiny projections called *villi* line the small intestine. Villi absorb the digested food into the capillaries. Most of the absorption of food takes place in the jejunum and ileum.

Some chyme remains undigested and passes from the small intestine into the *large intestine (large bowel* or *colon).* The colon absorbs most of the water from the chyme. The remaining semi-solid material is called *feces,* consisting of a small amount of water, solid wastes, and some mucus and micro-organisms—the waste products of digestion. Feces pass through the colon into the *rectum* by peristalsis. *Defecation* (bowel movement) is the process of excreting feces from the rectum through the anus. The term *stool* refers to excreted feces.

THE URINARY SYSTEM

Waste products are removed from the body through the respiratory system, the digestive system, the skin, and the urinary system: the digestive system rids the body of solid wastes; the lungs rid the body of carbon dioxide; water and other substances are excreted in sweat. There are other waste products in the blood as a result of body cells burning food for energy. The functions of the urinary system are to remove waste products from the blood and to maintain water balance within the body. The structures of the urinary system are shown in Figure 14–24.

The *kidneys* are two bean-shaped organs in the upper abdomen. They lie against the muscles of the back on each side of the spine and are protected by the lower edge of the rib cage. The kidneys act as a filtration system for the blood and cleanse the waste products and toxins (poisons) from the blood.

Each kidney has about a million tiny *nephrons,* which is the basic working unit of the kidney (Figure 14–25). Nephrons separate nutrients and minerals in the blood (water, sodium, amino acids, glucose) from the toxins and waste products. Every nephron has a *convoluted tubule* that ends in a *Bowman's capsule.* A cluster of capillaries called *glomerulus* is contained in this capsule. As blood passes through the glomerulus, it is filtered by the capillaries. The fluid part of the blood returns to the Bowman's capsule and then into the tubule. Most of the water and other necessary substances are reabsorbed by the blood and recirculated in the body. The toxins and waste products stay in the kidney and form *urine.* The urine flows through the tubule to a collecting tubule which drains into the renal pelvis in the kidney.

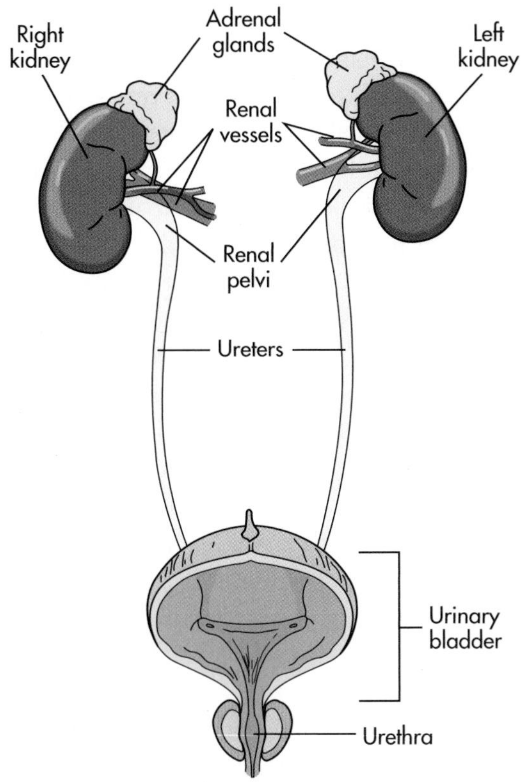

Figure 14–24 The urinary system.

The urine is transported from the kidneys to the *bladder* through the *ureters*. The two ureters are narrow tubes, each about 25 to 30 cm (10 to 12 inches) long. They run from the renal pelvis of the kidneys to the bladder. The bladder is a hollow, muscular sac situated toward the front in the lower part of the abdominal cavity.

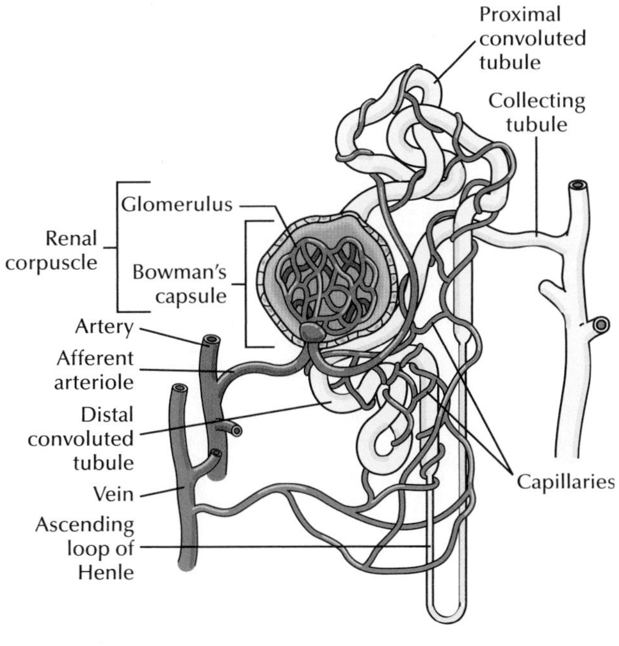

Figure 14–25 A nephron.

Urine is stored in the bladder until the urge to urinate is felt, usually when there is about 250 mL (an 8 oz. cupful or half a pint) of urine in the bladder. Urine passes from the bladder through the *urethra.* The opening at the end of the urethra is the *meatus.* Urine passes from the body through the meatus. Urine is a clear, yellowish fluid. The amount of urine eliminated over a 24-hour period should be close to the amount of fluid consumed. The average output of urine is 1500 mL/24 hr.

THE REPRODUCTIVE SYSTEM

Human reproduction results from the union of a female sex cell and a male sex cell. Structures of the male reproductive system and female reproductive system are different, which allows for the process of reproduction.

The Male Reproductive System

The structures of the male reproductive system are shown in Figure 14–26. The *testes (testicles)* are the male sex glands, also called *gonads.* The two testes are oval- or almond-shaped glands, where the male sex cells, called *sperm*, are produced. *Testosterone,* the male hormone, is also produced in the testes. This hormone is needed for the functioning of the reproductive organs and for the development of the male secondary sex characteristics (see Chapter 15). The testes are suspended between the thighs in a sac called the *scrotum,* which is made of skin and muscle.

Sperm travel from each testis to the *epididymis,* a coiled tube (6 m/20 ft in length) on the top and to the side of the testis. From the epididymis, sperm travel through a tube called the *vas deferens.* Eventually, each vas deferens joins a *seminal vesicle.* The two seminal vesicles store sperm and produce *semen,* a fluid that carries sperm from the male reproductive tract. The ducts of the seminal vesicles unite to form the *ejaculatory duct,* which passes through the prostate gland.

The *prostate gland,* shaped like a doughnut, lies just below the bladder and secretes fluid into the semen. This fluid plays a role in increasing the mobility of sperm. As the ejaculatory ducts leave the prostate, they join the *urethra,* which also runs through the prostate. The urethra, contained within the penis, is the outlet for both urine and semen.

The *penis* is outside of the body and has *erectile* tissue. When a man becomes sexually aroused, blood fills the erectile tissue causing the penis to become enlarged, hard, and erect. The erect penis can enter the vagina of the female reproductive tract. The semen, which contains sperm, is then released into the female vagina.

The Female Reproductive System

The structures of the female reproductive system are shown in Figure 14–27. The female gonads are two almond-shaped glands called *ovaries.* Ovaries are situated on each side of the uterus in the abdominal cavity and contain *ova,* or eggs, which are the female sex cells. During the woman's reproductive years, one ovum (egg) is released monthly, which is called *ovulation.* The ovaries also secrete the female hormones *estrogen* and *progesterone.* These hormones are needed for the functioning of the reproductive system and the development of secondary sex characteristics in the female (see Chapter 15).

When an ovum is released from an ovary, it travels through the *fallopian tube,* situated on either side of the uterus and attached at one end to the uterus. The ovum travels through the fallopian tube to the *uterus.* The uterus is a hollow, muscular organ shaped like a pear and located in the centre of the pelvic cavity behind the bladder and in front of the rectum. The main part of the uterus is the *fundus.* The neck or narrow section of the uterus is the *cervix.* Tissue lining the uterus is called the *endometrium.* There are many blood vessels in the endometrium. If the sex cells from the male and the female (semen and ovum) unite into one cell, that cell implants itself into the endometrium, where it develops into a baby. The uterus serves as a place for the unborn baby (the fetus) to grow and receive nourishment.

The cervix of the uterus projects into a muscular canal called the *vagina.* The vagina opens to the outside of the body and is located just behind the urethra. The vagina receives the penis during sexual intercourse and also serves as part of the birth canal. Glands in the vaginal wall keep it moistened with secretions. In young girls, the external vaginal opening is partially closed by a membrane called the *hymen.* The hymen ruptures when the female has intercourse for the first time.

The external genitalia of the female are referred to as the *vulva* (Figure 14–28). The *mons pubis* is a rounded, fatty pad over a bone called the *symphysis pubis* and is covered with hair in the adult female. The *labia majora* and *labia minora* are two folds of tissue on either side of the vaginal opening. The *clitoris* is a small organ composed of erectile tissue and becomes hard when sexually stimulated.

The *mammary glands* (*breasts*) secrete milk after childbirth. They are made up of glandular tissue and fat (Figure 14–29). The milk drains into ducts that open onto the nipple.

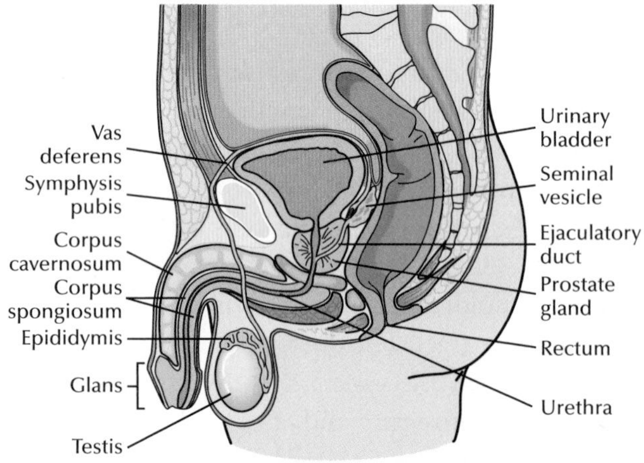

Figure 14–26 The male reproductive system.

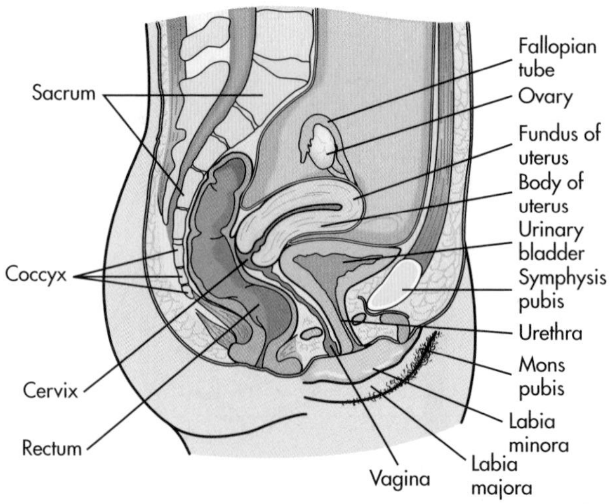

Figure 14–27 The female reproductive system.

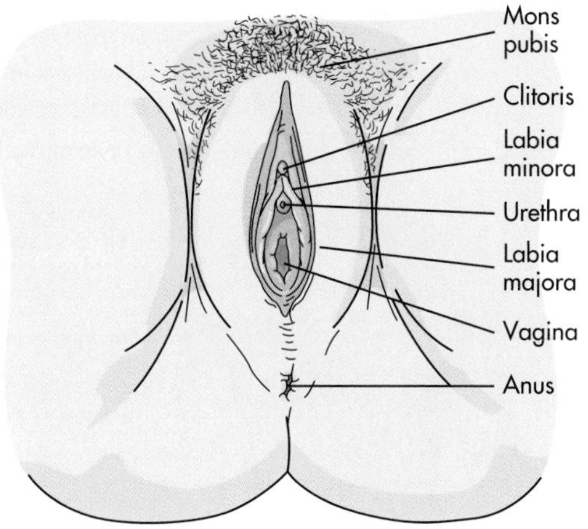

Figure 14–28 External female genitalia.

Menstruation. The endometrium is rich in blood to nourish the cell that grows into the fetus. If pregnancy does not occur, the endometrium breaks down and is discharged through the vagina to the outside of the body. This process, called **menstruation**, occurs about every 28 days and is therefore called the *menstrual cycle.*

The first day of the cycle begins with menstruation. Blood flows from the uterus through the vaginal opening, usually lasting 3 to 7 days. During the next phase—ovulation—which occurs usually on or about day 14 of the cycle, an ovum matures in an ovary and is released.

Meanwhile, estrogen and progesterone (the female hormones) are secreted by the ovaries. These hormones cause the endometrium to thicken for possible pregnancy. If pregnancy does not occur, the hormones decrease in amount, and blood supply to the endometrium decreases because of that. The endometrium then breaks down and is discharged through the vagina, and another menstrual cycle begins.

Fertilization

For reproduction to occur, a male sex cell (sperm) must unite with a female sex cell (ovum). The uniting of the sperm and ovum into one cell is called *fertilization.* A sperm and an ovum have only 23 chromosomes each, which is exactly half the number that all other cells have. When the two sex cells unite, the fertilized cell has 46 chromosomes.

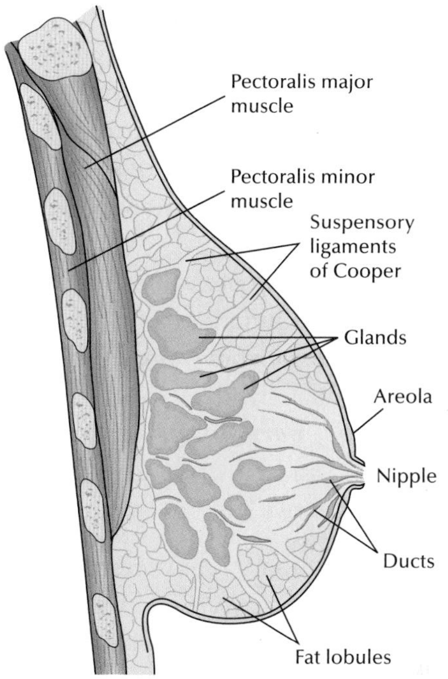

Figure 14–29 The female breast.

During intercourse, millions of sperm are deposited in the vagina. Sperm travel up the cervix, through the uterus, and into the fallopian tubes. If a sperm and an ovum unite in the fallopian tube, fertilization occurs and results in pregnancy. The fertilized cell then travels down the fallopian tube to the uterus. After a short time, the fertilized cell implants itself in the thick endometrium and grows during pregnancy.

THE ENDOCRINE SYSTEM

The endocrine system is made up of glands called the *endocrine glands* (Figure 14–30). The endocrine glands secrete chemical substances called **hormones** into the bloodstream. Hormones regulate the activities of other organs and glands in the body, the metabolic processes involving fats, proteins, and carbohydrates, and the water and electrolyte balance. Hormones play an important role in growth and reproduction.

The *pituitary gland* is called the *master gland.* About the size of a cherry, it is at the base of the brain behind the eyes. The pituitary gland is divided into the *anterior pituitary lobe* and the *posterior pituitary lobe.* The anterior pituitary lobe secretes:

- ***Growth hormone***—needed for the growth of muscles, bones, and other organs. It is needed throughout life to maintain normal-size bones and muscles. Growth is stunted if a baby is born with deficient amounts of the growth hormone. Too much of the hormone causes excessive growth.
- ***Thyroid-stimulating hormone*** (TSH)—needed for thyroid gland function.
- ***Adrenocorticotropic hormone*** (ACTH)—stimulates the adrenal gland.
- ***Reproductive hormones***—regulate growth, development, and function of the male and female reproductive systems.

The posterior pituitary lobe secretes *antidiuretic hormone* (ADH) and *oxytocin.* ADH prevents the kidneys from excreting excessive amounts of water. Oxytocin causes the uterine muscles to contract during childbirth. These two hormones are produced in the *hypothalamus.* The hypothalamus is part of the brain, but it secretes several hormones and so is considered part of the endocrine system. The hormones produced in the hypothalamus control or inhibit the release of other hormones.

The *thyroid gland,* shaped like a butterfly, is situated in the neck in front of the larynx and secretes the *thyroid hormone* (TH), also called *thyroxine.* The thyroid hormone regulates **metabolism**, which is the burning of food for heat and energy by the cells. This hormone is necessary for the proper functioning of all other hormones, the maturation of the nervous system, and normal growth and development.

Too little of the thyroid hormone results in slowed body processes, slowed movements, and weight gain. Too much of it causes increased metabolism, excess energy, and weight loss. If a baby is born with deficient amounts of thyroid hormone, physical and mental growth will be stunted.

The *parathyroid glands* secrete *parathormone.* There are four parathyroid glands, two each on either side of the thyroid gland. Parathormone regulates the body's use of calcium. Calcium is needed for the proper functioning of nerves and muscles. Insufficient amounts of calcium cause *tetany*—a state of severe muscle contraction and spasm—which, if untreated, can result in death.

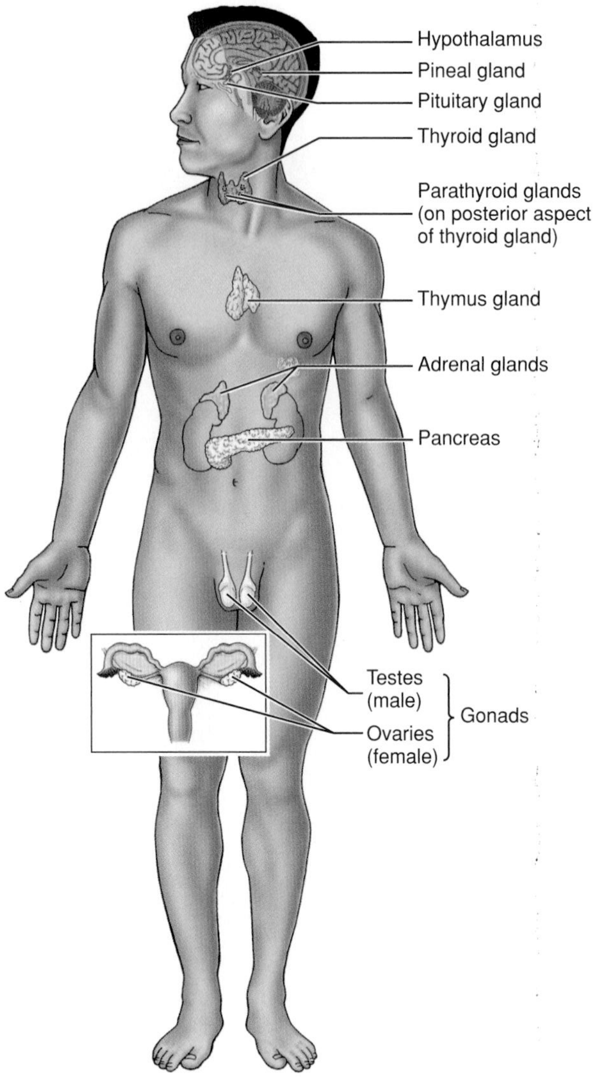

Figure 14–30 The endocrine system. **Source:** Herlihy, B. (2007). *The human body in health and illness* (3rd ed., p. 240). Philadelphia: Elsevier/Saunders.

There are two *adrenal glands,* one on the top of each kidney. The adrenal gland has two parts: the *adrenal medulla* and the *adrenal cortex.* The adrenal medulla secretes *epinephrine* and *norepinephrine.* These hormones stimulate the body to quickly produce energy during emergencies, so heart rate, blood pressure, muscle power, and energy all increase. The adrenal cortex secretes three groups of hormones that are essential for life: (1) the *glucocorticoids* regulate metabolism of carbohydrates. They also control the body's response to stress and inflammation; (2) the *mineralocorticoids* regulate the amount of salt and water that is absorbed and lost by the kidneys; and (3) the adrenal cortex also secretes small amounts of male and female sex hormones.

The *pancreas* secretes *insulin*, which regulates the amount of sugar in the blood available for use by the cells. Insulin is needed for sugar to enter the cells. If there is too little insulin, sugar cannot enter the cells, and excess amounts of sugar build up in the blood. This condition is called *diabetes*.

The *gonads* are the glands of human reproduction. Male sex glands (testes) secrete *testosterone*. Female sex glands (ovaries) secrete *estrogen* and *progesterone*.

THE IMMUNE SYSTEM

The immune system defends the body against threats from inside and outside. Some of these threats include pollens, toxins, and our own cells gone astray (cancer). We have two types of defence mechanisms classified as nonspecific **immunity** and specific immunity.

Nonspecific immunity is the body's reaction to anything it does not recognize as a normal body substance. There are two lines of defence in fighting threats.

The first line of defence includes:

- ***Mechanical barriers***—for example, intact skin and mucous membranes
- ***Chemical barriers***—for example, tears, stomach acids, saliva, perspiration
- ***Reflexes***—for example, cough, sneeze, vomiting, and diarrhea

The second line of defence includes:

- ***Phagocytes***—white blood cells that digest and destroy micro-organisms and other unwanted substances
- ***Inflammation***—when tissues are injured or irritated, *histamine* is released, causing the blood vessels to dilate and bring more blood to the area; this causes redness and heat. Histamine also causes the blood vessels to leak fluid, which causes swelling. With increased blood flow, more phagocytes arrive at the site and destroy the micro-organisms
- ***Fever***—stimulates the phagocytosis and decreases the ability of certain pathogens to multiply.

Specific immunity is the body's reaction to a specific foreign agent. Special cells and substances provide immunity.

- ***Antibodies***—normal body substances that recognize abnormal or unwanted substances. Antibodies attack and destroy such substances.
- ***Antigens***—abnormal or unwanted substances. An antigen causes the body to produce antibodies, which attack and destroy the antigens.
- ***Lymphocytes***—white blood cells that produce antibodies. Lymphocyte production increases as the body responds to an infection.
- ***B lymphocytes (B cells)***—cells that cause the production of antibodies that circulate in the plasma. The antibodies react to specific antigens.
- ***T lymphocytes (T cells)***—cells that destroy invading cells. *Killer T cells* produce poisonous substances near the invading cells. Some T cells attract other cells that destroy the invaders.

When the body senses an antigen (an unwanted substance), the immune system is activated, and phagocyte and lymphocyte production increases. Phagocytes destroy the invaders through digestion, and the lymphocytes produce antibodies that attack and destroy the unwanted substances.

Immunity to diseases can be classified as *genetic immunity* and *acquired immunity*. Genetic immunity protects a person from many diseases that afflict other species, for example, your cat will not catch chickenpox from you.

A person can get *acquired immunity* either naturally or artificially. Natural immunity can be acquired in two ways: (1) the first way is by having the disease such as chickenpox. Once you have chickenpox, your body develops the antibodies to protect you from contracting it again. This type of immunity is called active immunity; and (2) the second way is by passive immunity. This is a short-lived immunity passed from mother to fetus through the placenta and to the baby through breast milk. This protection lasts for about the first 6 months after birth.

Artificially acquired immunity is by way of *vaccine* or *immune globulin*. A vaccine is an antigen-bearing substance (pathogen) that is injected into a person to stimulate the production of antibodies. Immune globulin is obtained from a donor who already has the antibodies and is injected into a person to provide passive immunity.

REVIEW

Answers to these questions are at the bottom of the page.

Circle the **BEST** answer.

1. **The basic unit of body structure is the:**
   - A. Cell
   - B. Neuron
   - C. Nephron
   - D. Ovum
2. **The outer layer of the skin is called the:**
   - A. Dermis
   - B. Epidermis
   - C. Integument
   - D. Myelin
3. **Which parts allow movement?**
   - A. Bone marrow and periosteum
   - B. Synovial membrane and tendons
   - C. Joints
   - D. Ligaments
4. **Skeletal muscles:**
   - A. Are under involuntary control
   - B. Appear smooth
   - C. Are under voluntary control
   - D. Appear striped and smooth
5. **The highest functions of the brain take place in the:**
   - A. Cerebral cortex
   - B. Medulla
   - C. Brain stem
   - D. Spinal nerves
6. **Besides hearing, the ear is involved with:**
   - A. Regulating body movements
   - B. Balance
   - C. Smoothness of body movements
   - D. Controlling involuntary muscles
7. **The liquid part of the blood is the:**
   - A. Hemoglobin
   - B. Red blood cells
   - C. Plasma
   - D. Alveolus
8. **Which part of the heart pumps blood to the body?**
   - A. Right atrium
   - B. Right ventricle
   - C. Left atrium
   - D. Left ventricle
9. **Which carry blood away from the heart?**
   - A. Capillaries
   - B. Veins
   - C. Venules
   - D. Arteries
10. **Oxygen and carbon dioxide are exchanged:**
    - A. In the bronchi
    - B. Between the alveoli and capillaries
    - C. Between the lungs and the pleura
    - D. In the trachea
11. **The process of digestion begins in the:**
    - A. Mouth
    - B. Stomach
    - C. Small intestine
    - D. Colon
12. **Most food absorption takes place in the:**
    - A. Stomach
    - B. Small intestine
    - C. Colon
    - D. Large intestine
13. **Urine is formed by the:**
    - A. Jejunum
    - B. Kidneys
    - C. Bladder
    - D. Liver
14. **The male sex gland is called the:**
    - A. Penis
    - B. Semen
    - C. Testis
    - D. Scrotum
15. **The endocrine glands secrete substances called:**
    - A. Hormones
    - B. Mucus
    - C. Semen
    - D. Insulin
16. **The immune system protects the body from:**
    - A. Low blood sugar
    - B. Disease and infection
    - C. Falling and loss of balance
    - D. Stunted growth and loss of fluid

Answers: 1.A, 2.B, 3.C, 4.D, 5.A, 6.B, 7.C, 8.D, 9.D, 10.B, 11.A, 12.B, 13.B, 14.C, 15.A, 16.B

CHAPTER 15

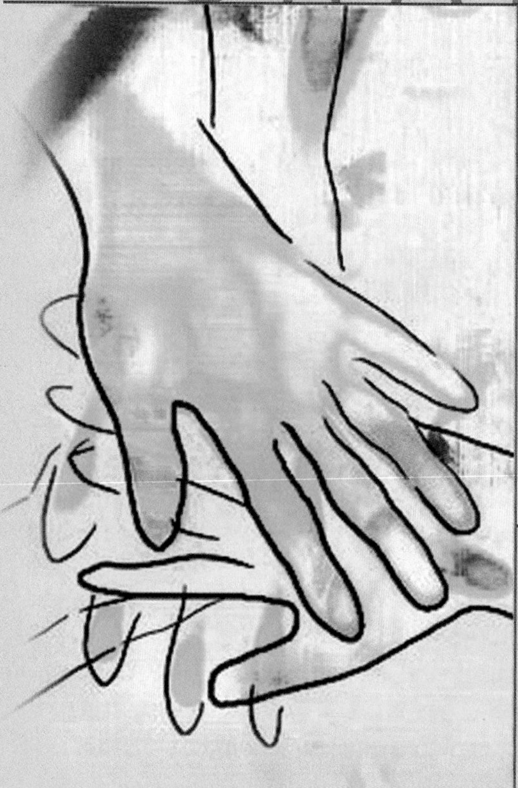

Growth and Development

OBJECTIVES

- Define the key terms listed in this chapter.
- Understand the principles of growth and development.
- Identify the stages of growth and development and the normal age ranges for each stage.
- Identify the developmental tasks for each age group.
- Describe the normal and typical growth and development for each age group.

key terms

adolescence A time of rapid growth and psychological and social maturity that occurs with puberty. Because the start of puberty varies between the genders and between individuals, the approximate age range is from 10 years old for girls and 12 years old for boys until the age of 18.

development The maturation toward adulthood that is usually characterized by physical changes and increased ability and functionality.

developmental task An activity that must be mastered during a stage of development.

growth Increase in physical size and weight. It occurs in a slow and steady manner but has marked times of acceleration that occur after birth and during puberty.

infancy The first year of life that is characterized by rapid physical, psychological, and social growth and development.

late adulthood Occurs approximately at the age of 65 years and older. This stage is characterized by adjusting to decreased physical strength and loss of health, retirement and reduced income, coping with the death of a partner, developing new friends and relationships, and preparing for one's own death.

late childhood Occurs between leaving childhood and dependency on others and entering adolescence. The approximate age range is 9 to 12 years. It is characterized by becoming independent of adults and learning to depend on oneself, developing and keeping friendships with peers, understanding the physical, psychological, and social roles of one's gender, developing moral and ethical behaviour, developing greater muscular strength, coordination and balance, and learning how to study.

menarche The time when menstruation first begins.

menopause The time when menstruation stops.

middle adulthood Occurs approximately between 40 to 65 years of age. This stage is characterized by seeing children growing up and moving away from home, adjusting to physical changes, developing leisure activities, and relating to aging parents.

middle childhood Ages 6 to 8 years, characterized by developing the social and physical skills needed for playing games, learning to get along with peers, learning behaviours and attitudes appropriate to one's own gender, learning basic reading, writing, and arithmetic skills, developing a conscience and morals, and developing a good feeling and attitude about oneself.

newborn During **infancy**, a baby is called a newborn, or **neonate**.

preschool Ages 3 to 5 years, characterized by increasing ability to communicate and understand others, the ability to perform self-care activities, learning the differences between the sexes, learning right from wrong and good from bad, learning to play with others, and developing family relationships.

primary caregiver A person who is responsible for providing care to a dependent individual, regardless of the dependant's age.

puberty The period when the reproductive organs begin to function and secondary sex characteristics appear.

reflex An involuntary movement in response to a stimulus.

toddlerhood Occurs between the age of 1 to 3 years. Characterized by tolerating separation from the primary caregiver, gaining control of bowel and bladder functions, using words to communicate, and starting to assert independence.

young adulthood Ages approximately 18 to 40 years, characterized by choosing an education and an occupation, selecting and learning to live with a partner, becoming a parent and raising children, and developing a satisfactory sex life.

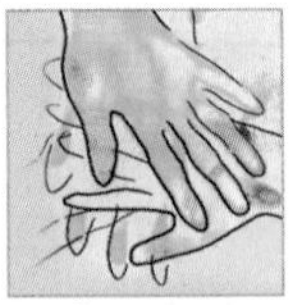

As a support worker, since you will care for clients in different stages of their development, a basic understanding of growth and development in humans will help you give better care, with easier understanding of the client's needs. This chapter presents the basic changes that occur in normal, healthy people from birth through old age.

Human growth and development are presented in nine stages, and age ranges and normal and basic descriptions of typical characteristics are given for each stage. Since the stages overlap, it is hard to see clear-cut endings and beginnings of the stages. Also, the rate of growth and development varies with each client.

Children grow and develop within the structure of the family. In Canadian society, the family can take many forms (see Chapter 6). Sometimes when parents are unable to raise their children, another person, such as a grandparent, aunt, uncle, or court-appointed guardian, takes on the parental role.

In this chapter, the term **primary caregiver** is often used when referring to the person who is mainly responsible for providing for the child's basic needs. The primary caregiver may be a parent or another person assuming the parental role.

PRINCIPLES

Growth refers to the physical changes that can be measured and that occur in a steady and orderly manner. Growth is measured in height and weight, as well as by changes in physical appearance and body functions.

Development refers to changes in psychological and social functioning. A person behaves and thinks in certain ways at different stages of development. A 2-year-old thinks in simple terms and needs a primary caregiver for meeting many basic needs. A 40-year-old thinks in complex ways and meets most of his or her own basic needs without help from others.

Growth and development affect the entire person. Although each has its own definition, growth and development:

- Overlap
- Depend on each other
- Occur at the same time

For example, an infant cannot say simple syllables (development) until the physical structures needed for speech are strong enough (growth). The basic principles of growth and development are:

- Growth and development occur from the moment of fertilization until death.
- The process goes from the simple to the complex. A baby learns to sit before standing, to stand before walking, and to walk before running. An adolescent learns to develop from dependence to independence.
- Growth and development occur in certain directions:
  - From the head to the foot—babies learn to hold up their heads before they learn to sit. After learning to sit, they learn to stand.
  - From the centre of the body outward—babies learn to control shoulder movements before they can control hand movements.
- Growth and development occur in a sequence, order, and pattern. Certain **developmental tasks** must be completed during each stage, and no stage can be skipped, as each stage lays the foundation for the next stage.
- The rate of growth and development is uneven—it does not occur at a set pace. Growth is more rapid during infancy. Also, children have growth spurts: some children develop rapidly, while others develop slowly.
- Each stage of growth and development has its own characteristics and developmental tasks.

INFANCY (BIRTH TO 1 YEAR)

Infancy is the first year of life, when rapid physical, psychological, and social growth and development occur. The developmental tasks of infancy are:

- Learning to walk
- Learning to eat solid foods
- Beginning to talk and communicate with others
- Beginning to have emotional relationships with primary caregivers, brothers, and sisters
- Developing stable sleep and feeding patterns

The *neonatal period* of infancy is the first 28 days after birth, and during this time, a baby is called a *neonate* or a **newborn**.

The average newborn is 48 to 53 cm (19 to 21 in.) long and weighs 3200 to 3600 g (7 to 8 lb) at birth. Birth weight usually doubles by the age of 5 to 6 months and triples by the first birthday. Babies are usually 51 to 76 cm (20 to 30 in.) long at the end of the first year.

The newborn's head is large compared with the rest of the body, and the skin is wrinkled. Arms and legs seem short compared with the trunk. The abdomen is large and round. Skin and eye colour vary depending on the baby's genetic background and may change during the first year. The newborn has fat, pudgy cheeks, a flat nose, and a receding chin (Figure 15–1).

The infant's central nervous system is not well developed. Movements are uncoordinated and lack purpose. Infants can see at birth, although vision is not clear. They seem attracted to patterns, and as they develop, they prefer colours. Infants hear well—they are startled by loud noises and soothed by soft sounds. They respond more often to female voices than to male voices. Infants react to touch, and the senses of smell and taste are well-developed.

Newborns have certain **reflexes** (involuntary movements in response to a stimulus). These reflexes decline and then disappear as the central nervous system develops.

- The *Moro reflex (startle reflex)* occurs when an infant is frightened by a loud noise or sudden movement. The arms are thrown apart, the legs extend, and the head is thrown back.
- The *rooting reflex* is stimulated when the infant's cheek is touched at or near the mouth. The infant's head turns toward the touch. The rooting reflex is necessary for feeding; it helps guide the infant's mouth to the nipple.
- The *sucking reflex* is produced by touching the cheeks or the sides of the lips.
- The *grasping reflex* occurs when the infant's palm is stimulated, causing the fingers to close around the object. This reflex begins to decline around the second month and disappears by the third month.

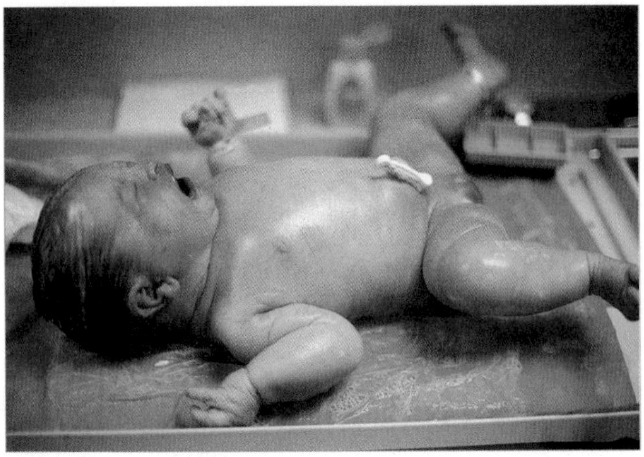

Figure 15–1 A newborn.

Infants sleep most of the time during the first few weeks of life. They awaken when hungry and fall asleep right after eating. The time between feedings lengthens as infants grow and develop. They stay awake more and sleep less as growth and development occur.

Body movements are initially uncoordinated and without purpose and are generally involuntary. As the central nervous system and muscular system develop, infants develop specific, voluntary, and coordinated movements. Newborns cannot hold their heads up. At 1 month, infants can hold their heads up when held and can lift and turn their heads when lying on their stomachs. At 2 months, they can smile and follow the movement of objects with their eyes.

Three-month-old infants can raise their heads and shoulders when lying on their stomachs. They can sit for a short while when supported and can hold a rattle. Infants 4 months of age are usually able to roll over and can sit up if supported. They may also sleep through the night by this time. The Moro and rooting reflexes disappear at this stage. Infants can hold objects with both hands, put objects into their mouths, and babble when spoken to. At 5 months, infants can grasp objects and play with their toes. Teeth start to appear.

Six-month-old infants usually have two lower front teeth and start to chew and bite finger foods. They can hold a bottle for feeding and can sit alone for a short time. At 7 months, the upper teeth start to erupt. Infants at this age respond to their names, can say "dada" and "mama," and fear strangers. At 8 months, infants may be able to stand when holding onto something. They respond to the word "no." Infants at this age often do not like to be dressed or have diapers changed. Nine-month-old infants usually crawl, and more upper teeth appear.

At 10 months, most infants can walk around while holding on to furniture (Figure 15–2). They can understand a number of words but can say only a few, and they indicate what they want by pointing or gesturing. They smile when looking into a mirror. Infants may begin to take a few steps at 11 months, and at 1 year of age, many start to walk and can hold a cup for drinking. One-year-olds know more words, can say "no," and shake their heads for "no." They try to imitate words spoken by adults around them.

During the first 6 months, the infant's diet is mainly breast or formula milk. Solid foods (strained fruits and vegetables) are usually added to their diet at 5 to 7 months. Finely chopped foods are added during the ninth and tenth months, and a 1-year-old can eat table foods.

TODDLERHOOD (1 TO 3 YEARS)

Physical growth during the second year of life is not as rapid as during infancy. The developmental tasks during **toddlerhood** are:

- Tolerating separation from the primary caregiver
- Gaining control of bowel and bladder functions
- Using words to communicate with others
- Becoming less dependent on the primary caregiver

Toddlers have the need to assert independence, and their ability to move about and walk and their curiosity increase. Toddlers get into anything and everything: they touch, smell, and taste everything within reach. As toddlers become more coordinated, they start to climb on to things and their new and increasing skills allow them to explore the environment. The child begins to venture farther away from the primary caregiver and also learns that some things can be done without the help of the primary caregiver. By 3 years, the toddler can run, jump, climb, ride a tricycle, and walk up and down stairs.

Increased hand coordination gives toddlers new skills. Their need to feel, smell, and taste things is shown in their increasing ability to feed themselves. They progress from eating with fingers to using a spoon (Figure 15–3). Toddlers can drink from cups. They can scribble, build towers with blocks, string beads, and turn book pages. Right- or left-handedness is seen during the second year.

Toilet training is a major developmental task for toddlers. Since bowel and bladder control is related to central nervous system development, children must be psychologically and physically ready for toilet training. The process starts with bowel control, which is easier because bowel movements are less frequent per day than urination. Bowel training may be completed at about $2^1/_2$ years of age. Bladder control during the day is achieved before bladder control at night. Bladder training may be completed around 3 years of age.

Speech and language skills increase: speech is clearer, and vocabulary increases. Words are learned by imitating others. Toddlers understand more words than they use. They are capable of forming two- or three-word sentences. By 3 years of age, children should be able to speak in short sentences.

Play ability increases. The 2-year-old plays alongside other children but does not usually play with them. The toddler is very possessive and does not understand the concept of sharing, and the word "mine" is often used.

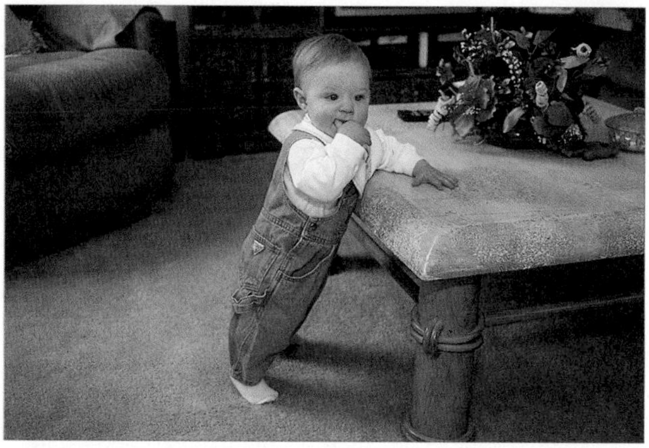

Figure 15–2 A 10-month-old infant can walk while holding on to furniture.

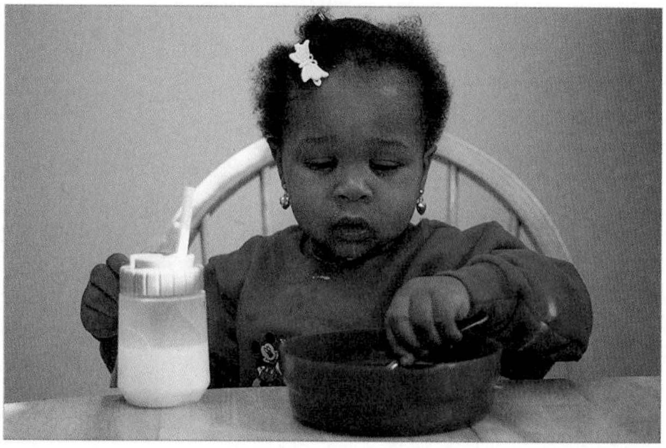

Figure 15–3 A toddler is able to use a spoon to eat food.

Temper tantrums and saying "no" are common during this stage. When disciplined, the toddler may kick and scream. The temper tantrum is the child's way of objecting to having his or her independence challenged, and this can frustrate their primary caregivers. The toddler years have many such power struggles between caregiver and child and are commonly referred to as the "terrible twos."

Another developmental task for toddlers is tolerating separation from the primary caregiver. As toddlers start to explore their environments, they tend to venture away from their primary caregivers. However, when they experience discomfort, frustration, or injury, they quickly return to primary caregivers or cry for their attention. If the primary caregiver is consistently present whenever needed, a child learns to feel secure and to tolerate brief periods of separation.

PRESCHOOL (3 TO 6 YEARS)

Ages 3 to 6 years are considered the **preschool** years (early childhood). At this stage, children grow taller but gain little weight. Preschoolers are thinner, more coordinated, and more graceful than toddlers. The developmental tasks of the preschool years include:

- Increasing the ability to communicate and understand others
- Performing self-care activities
- Learning the differences between the sexes
- Learning right from wrong and good from bad
- Learning to play with others
- Developing family relationships

The 3-Year-Old

Three-year-olds are more coordinated and can walk on tiptoe, balance on one foot for a few seconds, and run, jump, and climb with ease. Personal care skills increase—they can put on their shoes, dress themselves, manage buttons, wash their hands, and brush their teeth with help. They can feed themselves, pour from a bottle, and help set the table without breaking the dishes. Hand skills also include drawing circles and crosses.

Most 3-year-olds know roughly 1000 words, imitate new words, and talk and ask questions constantly. A favourite question repeated many times a day is "Why?" Sentences are brief—usually 3 or 4 words long. Three-year-olds can name body parts, family members, friends, and animals.

Play is important at this stage, and 3-year-olds are able to play *with* other children and not just *beside* them. They are developing an understanding that others have feelings and are more cooperative than toddlers. With an adult's encouragement, they are able to share toys and take turns. They play simple games and can follow simple rules. They enjoy using colouring books and crayons, doing crafts with child-safe scissors and paper, doing age-appropriate puzzles, and participating in role-playing games, such as "house" and "dress-up" (Figure 15–4).

Three-year-olds have vivid imaginations and often play make-believe games. Imaginary friends are common at this age. They may be so involved in their make-believe worlds that they sometimes confuse fantasy and reality. For example, a child may believe that a character in a picture book is real. Their developing imaginations may cause some children at this age to have nightmares or daytime fears and insecurities. Some may need a night-light by their beds.

At 3 years, children know that there are two sexes and begin to identify with their own sex. During role-playing games, girls will often pretend to be

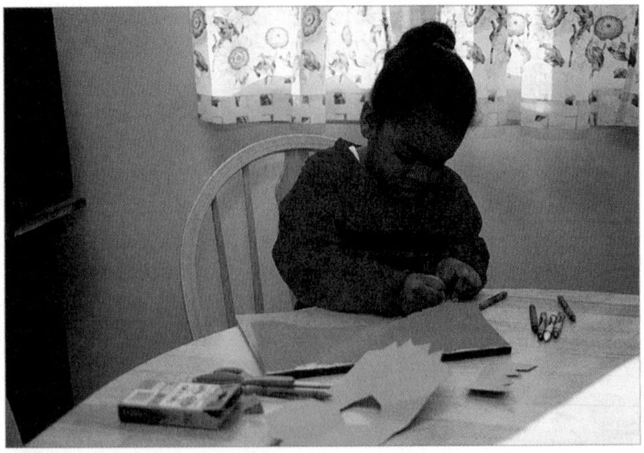

Figure 15–4 Three-year-olds have increased coordination. Many enjoy doing crafts, such as cutting paper, and using colouring books and crayons.

women (such as a mom or a princess) and boys will pretend to be men (such as a dad or a cowboy). This is their way of exploring the gender differences seen in their families and in the world around them (such as in books, television, and videos).

The concept of time develops, and 3-year-olds may speak of the past, present, and future. However, "yesterday" and "tomorrow" are still confusing to them.

Three-year-olds are less fearful of strangers and can tolerate separation from primary caregivers for short periods. They are less jealous of a new baby than are toddlers. They show that they want to please their primary caregivers.

The 4-Year-Old

Four-year-olds can hop, skip, and throw and catch a ball. They can lace shoes, draw faces, copy a square, and try to print letters. They can bathe with some help and usually tend to their toileting needs with help.

Vocabulary increases to about 1500 words, and the 4-year-old can sing simple songs, repeat four numbers, count to three, and name a few colours. The child continues to ask many questions and tends to exaggerate when telling stories. Many 4-year-olds can tell long and complex stories. Their constant chatter shows that they are learning the power of words. Sometimes they may seem bossy as they use their developing language skills to tease, tattle, or tell others (including caregivers) what to do.

A 4-year-old's hand and finger coordinations are well developed. They like to make crafts, build with blocks, and try to "write" with a pencil or pen. Children in this age group still enjoy playing "dress-up" and imitating adults (Figure 15–5). They still have vivid imaginations but are now better able to differentiate between reality and fantasy. They are more social than they were at 3 years of age and usually enjoy playing in groups of two or three. They also begin to develop close friendships and may try to be like their friends or show off to impress them.

At this age, many children express curiosity about sexuality. They may ask persistent questions about how babies are made and why boys' and girls' genitals are different. Playing "doctor and nurse" is common as curiosity about sexuality continues.

Four-year-olds may show a strong preference for the parent of the opposite sex. They show rivalries with their brothers and sisters, especially when they take the 4-year-old's possessions or when the older children have more and different privileges.

The 5-Year-Old

Coordination continues to develop, and 5-year-olds can jump rope, skate, tie shoelaces, dress, and bathe. They can use a pencil well and copy diamond and triangle shapes. They can print a few letters and numbers and their first names. Drawings of people include the body, head, arms, legs, and feet.

Communication skills also increase. Vocabulary consists of about 14,000 words, and sentences have six to eight words. Five-year-olds ask fewer questions than they used to, but now the questions have more meaning. They want definitions for unknown terms and wish to take part in conversations. They can name four or more colours, coins, days of the week, and months. They can identify the objects that they draw and give detailed descriptions of drawings.

Five-year-olds are generally responsible and truthful, and they quarrel less than before. There is greater awareness of rules and an eagerness to do things the right way, and they are proud of their accomplishments. They want to please others, especially teachers and caregivers, and display good manners. They are independent and can be trusted

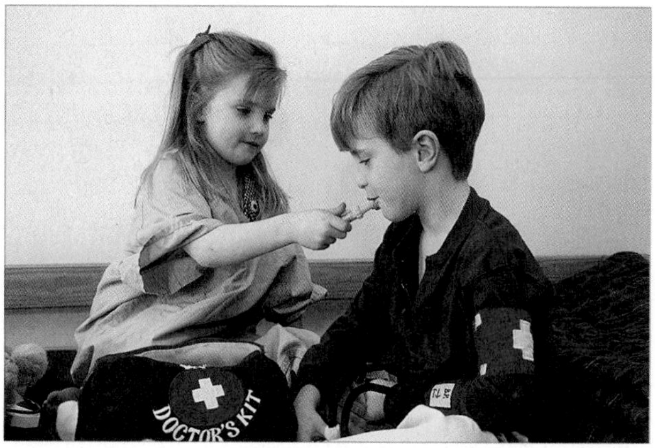

Figure 15–5 Four-year-olds play "dress-up" and imitate adults.

within limits. Five-year-olds have fewer fears but may continue to have nightmares.

Many 5-year-olds enjoy simple number and word games. Although they may cheat to win, they like having rules and try to follow them. They imitate adults during play and show a greater interest in watching television. They also enjoy activities with the primary caregiver of the same sex (Figure 15–6). Such activities include cooking, housecleaning, shopping, yard work, and sports.

Children at this age tolerate their brothers and sisters well. Although they consider younger children to be a nuisance, 5-year-olds usually are protective of them and enjoy playing with them.

MIDDLE CHILDHOOD (6 TO 8 YEARS)

Preschoolers often have nursery school and kindergarten experiences. However, **middle childhood** is the time school experiences begin in earnest. Children enter the world of peer groups, games, and learning.

The developmental tasks of middle childhood are:

- Developing the social and physical skills needed for playing games
- Learning to get along with other children of the same age and background (peers)
- Learning behaviours and attitudes appropriate to one's own sex
- Learning basic reading, writing, and arithmetic skills
- Developing a conscience and morals
- Developing a good feeling and attitude about self

The 6-Year-Old

Between the sixth and seventh birthdays, a child will grow about 5 cm (2 in.) and gain 1 to 3 kg (3 to 6 lb). Baby teeth are lost, and permanent teeth begin to erupt. Children at this stage are very active—they are skilled at running, jumping, skipping, hopping, and riding a bicycle and seem to be constantly on the go. They are content to sit only for a short time.

Six-year-olds enter Grade 1 and the world of school, activities, and interactions with other children. Children this age are often described as bossy, opinionated, charming, argumentative, and "know-it-alls." They have set ways of doing things and like to have their own way, so when they are frustrated, they may have temper tantrums. Six-year-olds play well with children of both sexes. However, they begin to prefer playing with children of the same sex (Figure 15–7). They share more with others and may have a "best friend." They may cheat to win, or may leave a game before it is over in order to avoid losing. Tattling is common at this stage.

Six-year-olds have a vocabulary of about 16,500 words. They know the alphabet and begin to read

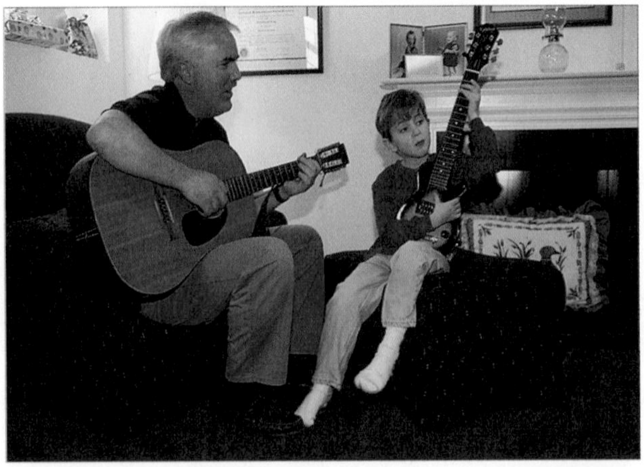

Figure 15–6 Five-year-olds enjoy doing things with the parent of the same sex.

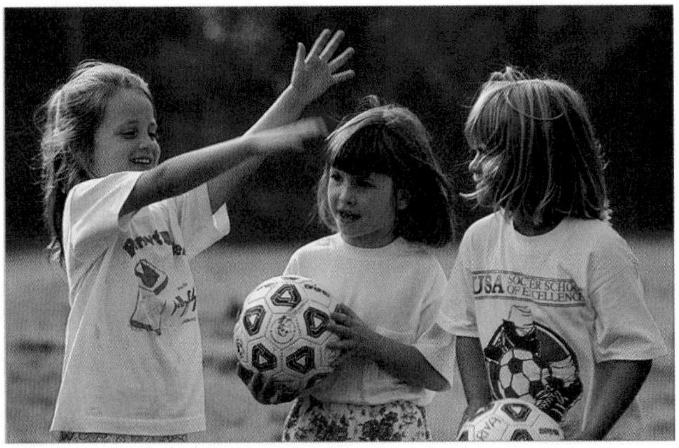

Figure 15–7 In middle childhood, belonging to a peer group is important. Children usually prefer playing with peers of the same sex.

and spell. They communicate thoughts and feelings better than before.

Play interests range from rough play to quiet activities, such as playing with cards, paints, and clay, and playing computer games. They start collections of odds and ends rather than specific things like stamps, rocks, or butterflies. More active play includes tag, hide-and-seek, playing with balls, skating, and playing in mud or sand.

The 7-Year-Old

Seven-year-olds grow about 5 cm (2 in.) in height during the year. The average 7-year-old weighs about 22 to 25 kg (49 to 56 lb) and is 119 to 124 cm (47 to 49 in.) tall. Hand coordination increases, so they are able to write and not just print. They are quieter than 6-year-olds and spend more time alone. They are more serious, less stubborn, and more concerned about being well liked by others. Seven-year-olds are more aware of themselves, their bodies, and the reactions of others. They do not like being teased or criticized and are sensitive about how others treat them. They usually like going to school, learning, and reading but may worry about grades and what the teacher thinks of them. Reading skills increase, and the child can tell time.

Play includes swimming, biking, collecting and trading objects, playing ball and games with rules, and working puzzles and video games, usually in groups. However, boys prefer to play with boys and girls prefer to play with girls.

The 8-Year-Old

The 8-year-old enters Grade 3. Increase in height and weight continues, and more permanent teeth appear. Movements are faster and more graceful.

Peer group activities and opinions are important at this stage in development. Being accepted and included in peer groups is vital for the fulfillment of the needs for love, belonging, and self-esteem. Children this age get along with adults but they give more importance to peer group fads, opinions, and activities. Boys and girls continue to play separately, and their interests relate to group games, collections, television, and movies.

Eight-year-olds are sometimes described as defensive, opinionated, practical, and outgoing. They give advice freely to others but do not accept criticism well. They are able to help with many household tasks, such as vacuuming, cooking, and yard work but also expect more privileges than those given to younger brothers and sisters.

Learning continues, and these children are curious about science, history, and other places and countries. School provides social opportunities with peers. Eight-year-olds are more daring in the classroom and may pass notes or talk with others when they think the teacher is not looking. However, they are well-mannered, relate well to adults, take part in adult conversations, and are friendly and affectionate.

LATE CHILDHOOD (9 TO 12 YEARS)

Late childhood (preadolescence) is between leaving childhood and dependency on others and entering adolescence. Developmental tasks at this stage are similar to those of middle childhood. However, a preadolescent is expected to show more refinement and maturity in achieving the following tasks:

- Becoming independent of adults and learning to depend on oneself
- Developing and keeping friendships with peers
- Understanding the physical, psychological, and social roles of one's sex
- Developing moral and ethical behaviour
- Developing greater muscular strength, coordination, and balance
- Learning how to study

Boys grow about 2.5 cm (1 in.) per year. Girls grow about 5 cm (2 in.) per year. Boys gain about 1.8 kg (4 lb) each year. Girls gain about 2.3 kg (5 lb) each year. Girls are usually taller than boys during late preadolescence. Many permanent teeth have erupted by now.

Body movements are more graceful and coordinated (Figure 15–8). Muscular strength and physical skills increase. Skill in team sports is often important to the child.

Body changes begin to occur as the onset of puberty nears. In girls, the pelvis becomes broader,

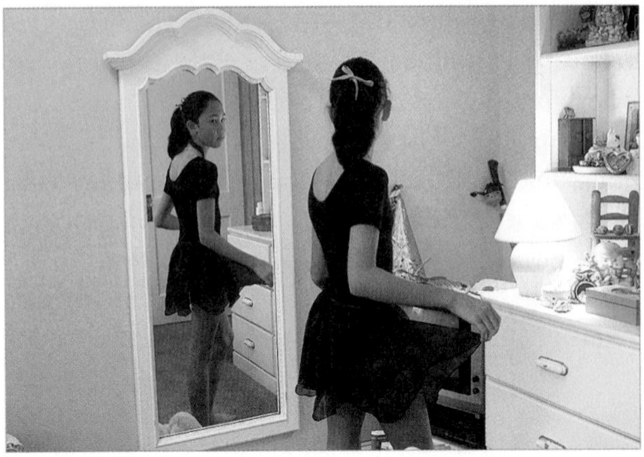

Figure 15–8 Movements are smooth and graceful in late childhood.

fat appears on the hips and chest, and the budding of breasts occurs. Boys show fewer signs of maturing sexually during this time, but genital organs begin to grow.

Children of this age must be given factual sex education. Information that is shared among friends about sex is often incomplete and inaccurate. Parents and children may be uncomfortable discussing sex with each other and may avoid the subject. When children do ask questions, honest and complete answers must be given in terms that the children can understand.

Peer groups, which are the centre of preadolescent activities, begin to affect the child's attitudes and behaviour. Preference for companions of the same sex continues. Boys need to show their strength and toughness and may give each other nicknames. Arguments between boys and girls are common, and they often tease each other.

At this stage, preadolescents are more aware of the mistakes and weaknesses of adults. They do not accept adult standards and rules without question, and rebellion against adults is common. Disagreements between parents and children increase, although the parents continue to be important for the child's development.

ADOLESCENCE (12 TO 18 YEARS)

Adolescence is a time of rapid growth and psychological and social maturity. The stage begins with puberty. **Puberty** is the period during which the reproductive organs begin to function and the secondary sex characteristics appear. Girls experience puberty between the ages of 10 and 14. Most boys reach puberty between the ages of 12 and 16. Knowing or questioning sexual orientation can occur at this stage of development.

Because the age of puberty varies, adolescence ranges from the ages of 12 to 18 years. The developmental tasks of adolescence include:

- Accepting changes in the body and appearance
- Developing appropriate relationships with males and females of the same age
- Accepting the male or female role appropriate for one's age
- Becoming independent from parents and adults
- Developing morals, attitudes, and values needed for functioning in society

Menarche, the beginning of menstruation, marks the onset of puberty in girls and the appearance of secondary sex characteristics, which include:

- Increase in breast size
- Appearance of pubic and axillary (underarm) hair
- Slight deepening of the voice
- Widening and rounding of the hips

During late childhood, male sex organs begin to increase in size. This growth continues during adolescence. *Ejaculation* (the release of semen) signals the onset of puberty in boys, and *nocturnal emissions* ("wet dreams") occur. During sleep *(nocturnal)*, the penis becomes erect and semen is released *(emission)*. Secondary sex characteristics also appear. These include:

- Appearance of facial hair
- Pubic and axillary (underarm) hair
- Hair on the arms, chest, and legs
- Deepening of the voice
- Increases in neck and shoulder size

A growth spurt occurs during adolescence. Boys grow about 10 to 41 cm (4 to 16 in.) and gain 7 to 27 kg (15 to 60 lb). They usually stop growing between the ages of 18 and 21. Some continue to grow until about 25. Girls grow about 5 to 23 cm (2 to 9 in.) and gain between 7 and 23 kg (15 and

50 lb). They usually stop growing between the ages of 17 and 18, but some girls continue to grow until about age 21.

Adolescence is described as the "awkward stage." Awkwardness and clumsiness are caused by the uneven growth of muscles and bones. Coordination and graceful body movements eventually develop as muscle and bone growth even out.

Children at this stage often find changes in physical appearance hard to accept. Some girls are embarrassed about breast development, especially about very large or small breast size, and genital size may be a concern for some boys. Height may cause concern in both boys and girls—boys do not like being much shorter than their peers, and tall girls may feel embarrassed about being taller than other girls and boys. Many adolescents, especially girls, worry about their weight, and thinking that they weigh too much, many try to diet and some develop eating disorders.

Teenagers often feel intense emotions, and their emotional reactions vary from high to low. Adolescents can be happy one moment and sad the next, so predicting their reaction to a comment or event can be difficult. Teenagers can control their emotions better later in this stage. Older adolescents (15- to 18-year-olds) can still become sad and depressed, but they can better control the time and place of their emotional reactions.

Adolescents need to become independent of adults, especially their parents. They must learn to function, make decisions, and act in a responsible manner without adult supervision. Many teenagers work toward this independence through part-time jobs, babysitting, going to dances and parties, dating, taking part in school clubs and organizations, shopping without an adult, and staying home alone (Figure 15–9).

Adolescents are increasingly able to use logic and reasoning, and they often form passionate opinions on many issues. However, their judgement and reasoning are not always sound. Guidance, discipline, and emotional and financial support are still needed from parents. Disagreements with parents are common, especially about behaviour and activity restrictions and limits. Teenagers would rather be with peers than do things with parents and other family members. Adolescents tend to confide in and seek advice from peers or from adults other than their parents.

Teenage interests and activities reflect the need to become independent, to develop relationships with the opposite sex, and to act like males or females. Both sexes are often interested in parties, dances, and other social activities. Clothing, makeup, and hairstyles are often important to teenagers because their appearance enables them to define their identity and fit in with a group. Parents and teenagers often disagree about clothing and hairstyles. Teenagers may spend a lot of time with friends or conversing with them through e-mail, in chat rooms, or on the phone. They also spend time participating in sports or in club activities, listening to music, or playing video games.

Dating begins during adolescence, and although the age when dating begins varies, there is usually a dating pattern. "Crowd" dates are common in Grades 7 and 8. They are usually related to school activities, such as a dance or basketball game. The same group of girls just happens to be with the same group of boys during these social events. In Grade 9, pairing off is common during crowd dating. Grade 10 is usually when boy–girl couples go to social events together and then join other couples. Double dating occurs in Grade 11. Dates involve one couple during Grade 12, although there is some double dating occasionally.

Many difficult decisions and conflicts result as the adolescent matures physically, psychologically, and emotionally. Parents and teenagers often disagree about dating because parents worry that dating will

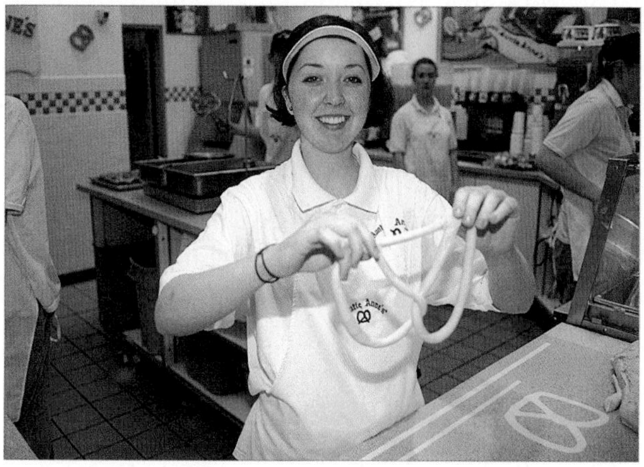

Figure 15–9 This teenager has a part-time job.

lead to sexual activities, pregnancies, and sexually transmitted infections. Teenagers usually do not understand or appreciate these concerns. "Going steady" helps the teenager meet needs for security, love and belonging, and self-esteem. Teenagers sometimes have difficulty controlling sexual urges and considering the consequences of sexual activity.

Adolescents begin to think about careers and what to do after high school graduation. Interests, skills, and talents are some of the factors that influence the choice of further education or a job. Adolescents also need to develop morals, values, and attitudes for living in society. They need to develop a sense about what is good and bad, right and wrong, and important and unimportant. Parents, peers, culture, religion, television, school, and movies are among the many factors that influence teenagers. Drug abuse, unwanted pregnancy, alcoholism, and criminal acts are common problems among troubled adolescents.

YOUNG ADULTHOOD (18 TO 40 YEARS)

Psychological and social development continue during **young adulthood**. There is little physical growth because by this time adult height has already been reached and body systems are fully developed. Developmental tasks of young adulthood include:

- Choosing further education and a career
- Selecting a partner
- Learning to live with a partner
- Becoming a parent and raising children
- Developing a satisfactory sex life

Education and occupation are so closely related that they can rarely be separated. Most jobs require specific knowledge and skills, so the amount and kind of education needed depend on the career choice. Most adults find that job choices are greater with adequate educational preparation and that employment is necessary for economic independence and for supporting a family.

At this stage of development, young adults choose to marry their partner, remain single, or live in a common-law relationship.

The many reasons for marriage or common-law relationship include love, emotional security, wanting a family, sex, wanting to leave an unhappy home life, social status, companionship, and financial security. Some marry to feel wanted, needed, and desirable. Many factors, including age, religion, interests, education, race, personality, and love, affect the selection of a spouse. Some marriages are happy and successful, while others are not. There are no guarantees that a marriage will work, so the couple must work together to build a marriage based on trust, respect, caring, and friendship.

Partners (married or unmarried) must learn to live with each other. Habits, routines, household management, meal preparation, and pastimes may need to be changed or adjusted to "fit" each other's needs. They must learn how to solve problems and make decisions together and need to work toward the same goals. Open and honest communication is essential to create a successful partnership (Figure 15–10).

Young adults also need to develop a satisfactory sex life. Frequency of sex, desires, practices, and preferences vary among couples. Understanding and accepting a partner's needs are necessary for a satisfying and intimate relationship.

Most couples decide to have children, and modern birth control methods allow them to plan the number of children they want to have and when to have them. However, some pregnancies are unplanned. Many couples have a child during the first few years of marriage; some wait several years

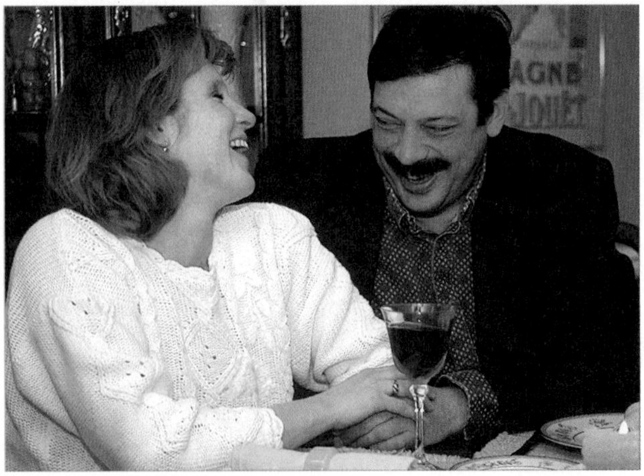

Figure 15–10 Communication is necessary for a successful partnership and a satisfactory sex life.

before starting a family. Some couples decide not to have children at all, and some experience difficulty or inability to have children because of physical problems in one or both partners. Those couples deciding to have children need to agree on methods of childrearing and discipline and need to adjust to the child and his or her need for time, energy, and parental attention.

MIDDLE ADULTHOOD (40 TO 65 YEARS)

This stage of development is often stable and comfortable, when children have grown up and moved away. Partners now have time to spend alone with each other. There are fewer worries about children and money. The developmental tasks of **middle adulthood** include:

- Adjusting to physical changes
- Having grown-up children
- Developing leisure activities
- Relating to aging parents

Of the several physical changes that occur, many are gradual and go unnoticed, while some others are seen early. People in their early forties may feel energetic and able to function as they did in their twenties. However, energy and endurance begin to decrease. Weight control becomes a problem as metabolism and physical activities slow down. Facial wrinkles and grey hair appear. The need for eyeglasses is common at this stage, and there may be hearing loss or deterioration. In women, menstruation stops between the ages of 42 and 55; this is called **menopause**. The ovaries stop producing eggs and secreting hormones, and the woman can no longer become pregnant. Many diseases and illnesses can develop, some of them chronic or life-threatening.

Children leave home for school, marry, move to homes of their own, and start their own families. Middle-aged adults have to cope with letting children go, being in-laws, and becoming grandparents. Parents must let children lead their own lives, but they need to be available to their children for emotional support in their times of need.

Middle-aged adults often discover that they have a lot more spare time when the demands of parenthood decrease. Hobbies and pastimes, such as gardening, fishing, painting, golfing, volunteer work, and membership in clubs and organizations, are sources of pleasure (Figure 15–11). Hobbies and pastimes become even more important after retirement and during late adulthood.

Some middle-aged adults have parents who are very old and developing poor health; they have the responsibility for their parents' care and often have to deal with the death of parents. See Chapter 15 for a more detailed discussion on middle-aged adults.

LATE ADULTHOOD (65 YEARS AND OLDER)

Chapter 17 describes the many physical, psychological, and social changes that occur during **late adulthood**, as well as the care that older adults may need.

The developmental tasks of this stage are:

- Adjusting to decreased physical strength and loss of health
- Adjusting to retirement and reduced income
- Coping with the death of a partner
- Developing new friends and relationships
- Preparing for one's own death

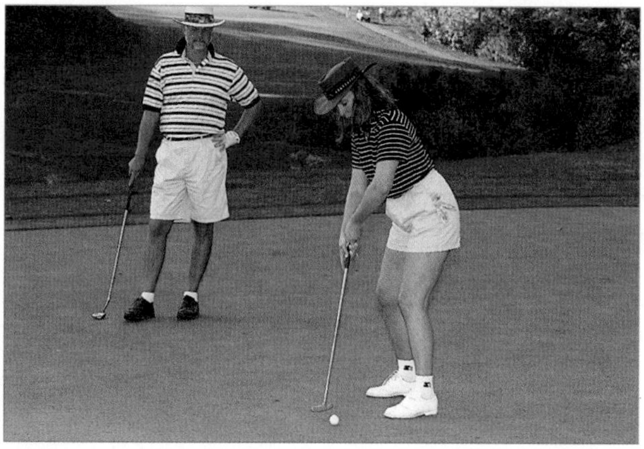

Figure 15–11 Middle-aged adults usually have more time for hobbies.

REVIEW

Answers to these questions are at the bottom of the page.

Circle the BEST answer.

1. **Changes in psychological and social functioning are called:**
   A. Growth
   B. Development
   C. A reflex
   D. A stage

2. **Which is true?**
   A. Growth and development do not occur from the simple to the complex.
   B. Growth and development do not occur in an orderly pattern.
   C. Growth and development occur at specific rates.
   D. Each stage has its own characteristics.

3. **The stage of infancy is the first:**
   A. 4 weeks of life
   B. 3 months of life
   C. 6 months of life
   D. 1 year of life

4. **Which reflexes are needed for feeding in the infant?**
   A. The Moro and startle reflexes
   B. The rooting and sucking reflexes
   C. The grasping and Moro reflexes
   D. The rooting and grasping reflexes

5. **Solid foods are usually given to an infant during the:**
   A. Fifth to seventh month
   B. Eighth month
   C. Ninth or tenth month
   D. Eleventh or twelfth month

6. **The toddler can:**
   A. Use a spoon and cup
   B. Ride a bike
   C. Help set the table
   D. Name parts of the body

7. **Playing with other children begins during:**
   A. Infancy
   B. The toddler years
   C. The preschool years
   D. Middle childhood

8. **Peer group activities become more important at the age of:**
   A. 6
   B. 7
   C. 8
   D. 9

9. **Reproductive organs begin to function and secondary sex characteristics appear during:**
   A. Late childhood
   B. Preadolescence
   C. Puberty
   D. Early adulthood

10. **Which is true?**
   A. Boys reach puberty earlier than girls do.
   B. Most girls reach puberty between the ages of 10 and 14.
   C. Menopause marks the onset of puberty in girls.
   D. A growth spurt occurs during the toddler stage.

11. **Dating usually begins:**
   A. During late childhood
   B. With "crowd" dating
   C. With "pairing off"
   D. During late adolescence

12. **Adolescence is usually a time when parents and children:**
   A. Talk openly about sex
   B. Express love and affection
   C. Disagree
   D. Do things as a family

13. **Which is a developmental task of young adulthood?**
   A. Adjusting to changes in the body and in physical appearance
   B. Becoming independent
   C. Choosing an occupation
   D. Relating to aging parents

14. **Middle adulthood is from about:**
   A. 25 to 35 years
   B. 30 to 40 years
   C. 40 to 50 years
   D. 40 to 65 years

15. **Middle adulthood is usually a time when:**
   A. Families are started
   B. Physical energy and free time are gained
   C. Children have grown up and leave home
   D. People need to prepare for death

Answers: 1.B, 2.B, 3.D, 4.B, 5.A, 6.A, 7.C, 8.C, 9.C, 10.B, 11.B, 12.C, 13.C, 14.D, 15.C

CHAPTER 16

Caring for the Young

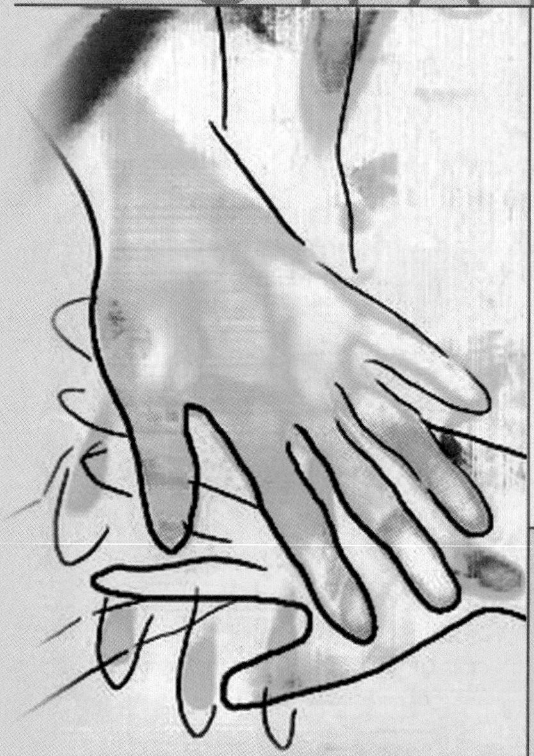

OBJECTIVES

- Define the key terms listed in this chapter.
- Identify the role of the support worker when caring for the young.
- List ways to assist an infant or child to meet nutritional needs.
- Identify the twelve principles for dealing with a challenging child.
- Identify causes of early childhood deaths from injury.
- List ways to prevent falls in children.
- List ways to prevent choking in children.
- List ways to prevent burns in infants and children.
- List ways to prevent accidental poisoning in children.
- Explain how developmental levels of children can influence their risk for injury.
- Describe ways to prevent or minimize childhood infections.
- List the five most common reasons for children missing school.
- Properly apply the information in this chapter to your clinical practice.

key terms

activities of daily living (ADLs) Self-care activities people perform daily to remain independent and to function in society.

conjunctivitis An inflammation of the clear membrane that covers the white part of the eye and lines the inner surface of the eyelids. The nonmedical term for this is **pink eye.**

ear infection See **otitis media**.

eustachian tube The name for the tiny drainage pipe in the middle ear.

gastroenteritis More commonly known as "stomach flu," this illness causes vomiting and diarrhea and can lead to dehydration, particularly in very young children and the frail older adult.

negative reinforcement Encouraging a behaviour by penalizing the person when that behaviour is not demonstrated.

otitis media Middle ear infections, caused by either a virus or a bacteria, that most often occur in children under the age of 2 but are also common between the ages of 5 and 6; they are triggered by respiratory illnesses picked up in kindergarten or first grade. Also known as **ear infection.**

physical abuse The deliberate application of force to any part of a child's body, which may result in a nonaccidental injury.

pink eye See **conjunctivitis.**

positive reinforcement Encouraging a behaviour by rewarding the desired behaviour after it is demonstrated.

Reye's syndrome A rare but potentially fatal disease causing inflammation of the brain, which can occur during the recovery stage of flu or chickenpox. It has been seen in children who take aspirin.

sexual abuse Occurs when a child is used for sexual purposes by an adult or an adolescent. It involves exposing a child to any sexual activity or behaviour.

strep throat A throat that is infected with **streptococci.**

streptococci (singular, *streptococcus*) A type of bacteria that cause **strep throat** and other problems.

upper respiratory infections (URIs) The medical term for colds and other viral illnesses that affect the throat, nose, and sinuses.

As a support worker, you will be expected to provide care and support to people of all ages, including the young. The young person that you are assigned to support may have physical or developmental challenges; may be a family member of your primary client (see *Supporting Jane Smith*); or may be your assigned client (see *Supporting Jamie*). Always consult your supervisor if you have questions or concerns when working with children (Figure 16–1).

This chapter presents discussions on the role of the support worker when dealing with the family, as well as a list of ways to deal with a challenging child. In addition, this chapter also includes a discussion on the need to provide a safe environment for the young and the common causes for children missing school.

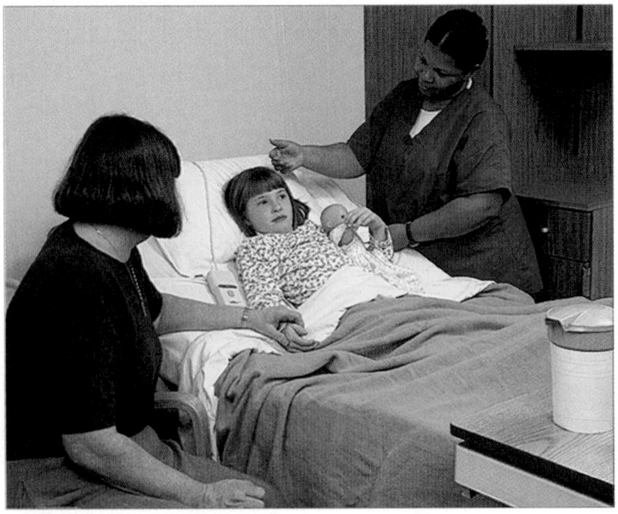

Figure 16–1 The support worker provides care to a sick child. **Source:** Sorrentino, S.A. (2004). *Mosby's textbook for nursing assistants* (7th ed., p. 86). St. Louis: Mosby.

When providing support to the young, you must always remember that they have rights, too. Promote the priorities of support work when working with children. When dealing with both the young and their family, you must remember to follow the principles of DIPPS (dignity, independence, privacy, preferences, and safety) just as you would for any other client (see the *Providing Compassionate Care: Working with Children* box).

SUPPORTING THE INFANT, CHILD, OR TEEN

Your Role

As a support worker, your goal is to provide a stable, secure, and safe atmosphere for the family. This is very important for sick children and for those who are experiencing stress when a family member is ill.

supporting JANE SMITH

Jane Smith is a 29-year-old woman who has terminal cancer. She is the mother of four young children, aged 6 months to 4 years. Her husband is a truck driver and is often away from home during the week but takes care of Jane and the children on weekends. During the week, Jane's mother (who is herself not well) takes the three older children to and from day care and assists with the family's shopping and laundry.

Jane was diagnosed with ovarian cancer during her pregnancy but waited till after her baby was born before starting any cancer treatments. Last month, Jane tripped over one of her children's toys, fell, and broke her ankle. While her ankle was being X-rayed, it was discovered that Jane's cancer had spread (metastasized) to her bones. Further tests revealed that it had also spread to her liver and brain. The doctors gave Jane only months to live.

Jane has a support worker in her home for 4 hours a day to assist with morning care for her and her baby. Jane's baby is a happy, active infant who is beginning to crawl. The support worker's responsibilities also include caring for the baby while Jane sleeps (she takes frequent naps throughout the day), light housekeeping (which includes ensuring that toys are not left on the floor), and preparing the family's dinner. Because Jane's husband's insurance only covers the cost of a support worker for up to 20 hours per week, Jane is worried about what will happen to her family when her condition declines further. Jane has often told the support worker just how grateful she is to have this assistance.

supporting JAMIE

Jamie is a happy, fun-loving guy who has just celebrated his twelfth birthday. Like many preteens his age, he likes to watch television and listen to music. Jamie is in Grade 8 and is looking forward to attending high school next year. He does well in school, but he is not sure yet about the career he wants to pursue. Jamie is just beginning his growth spurt. His family has noticed that he has grown taller and his voice is getting deeper. He has three younger brothers and his mother and stepfather who care for Jamie when he is home from school.

Jamie has cerebral palsy and is wheelchair dependent. He is often incontinent of urine, so he must wear incontinence products. Because of his ever-increasing size, his mother (who has always been his primary caregiver) has rented a mechanical lifter and is able to use it to toilet, bathe, and move Jamie from the bed to his chair. Jamie also requires assistance with eating. He communicates by way of a computer which sounds out words that he types using the keyboard.

After putting off surgery on her knee for several years, Jamie's mother is now going to have a total knee replacement and will therefore not be able to care for Jamie for several weeks. You are one of the support workers who will be caring for Jamie in his home during this time. Your duties are to assist with his **activities of daily living (ADLs)** and occasionally, arrange for his wheelchair taxi to drive him to school. You will get to know all of Jamie's family, as they will be home during the afternoon and evening hours when you are there.

PROVIDING COMPASSIONATE CARE

Working With Children

- **Dignity.** Children have the right to be treated with respect and in a manner that promotes their dignity. Never tease or laugh at a child, as their feelings are easily hurt. Remember to include children in conversations, when appropriate. Do not talk about the child in front of him or her. Also, remember to say "please" and "thank you" to children. Treat each child as an individual of worth.
- **Independence.** Even very young children should be allowed and encouraged to do what they can for themselves.
- **Preferences.** It is usually not difficult to find out a child's preferences. However, many times, the child cannot have what he or she wants. The child's wishes may be unsafe or unhealthy. Whenever possible, offer limited choices that are equally acceptable. For example, instead of saying, "What do you want for a snack?" say, "Would you like an apple or an orange for your snack?" This way, you are able to accept the child's preference.
- **Privacy.** Privacy is especially important to middle-school-aged children and adolescents. Unless the care plan directs otherwise, let them have privacy when using the bathroom, bathing, and using the phone. Do not pry into their affairs, and respect their belongings.
- **Safety.** Ensuring the child's safety is essential. Children are at high risk for accidental injuries. Young children are curious about everything around them, and most are very active, but they do not usually understand danger. Provide constant supervision for babies, toddlers, and young children. When you are responsible for them, do not let them out of your sight. Review the safety measures in Chapter 19.

Your responsibilities will vary in each family situation. However, the following are usually included:

- Developing positive relationships with all family members
- Maintaining the existing rules of behaviour
- Maintaining daily routines as much as possible
- Being alert to situations that may create stress or cause harm to the family. Report these situations to your supervisor (Box 16–1).

Follow the guidelines in Box 16–2 when interacting with children. Check with your supervisor and the care plan for instructions for each child.

Discipline

When supervising or caring for children, you need to reinforce the rules of acceptable behaviour in the home. The system of rules that governs how we act is called *discipline*. Discipline is a positive way of teaching responsible behaviour. It sets limits and provides guidelines so that children can learn how to behave in an appropriate way.

Box 16–1 Family Situations That Must Be Reported

- Violent behaviour of a family member (see Chapter 21)
- Frequent visits by "strangers," who seem to make the members of the household fearful or uneasy
- Suspected drug abuse; for example, when you notice the presence of drug paraphernalia
- Excessive drinking, as evidenced by the presence of liquor bottles hidden away throughout the house or the child's parent or caregiver being inebriated
- Electricity, heat, or water turned off
- Severe shortage of food or clothing. There is no food in the cupboards or refrigerator and the child is dressed inappropriately for the weather (such as no coat in winter)
- Illness of a child that has been unreported to you
- Sudden departure of caregiver
- Unexpected return of a family member

Box 16–2 Guidelines for Caring for Children in the Home

Communication

- Use active listening skills. Maintain eye contact, and concentrate on what is being said.
- Watch for nonverbal communication cues from the child. These include frowning, lack of eye contact, and lack of smiling.
- Provide nonverbal communication by way of comforting the child with a hug or touch on the shoulder or arm (according to acceptable custom and culture).
- Speak to the child in a manner that is appropriate for their developmental level or age. If the child (or teen) has a developmental delay, speak to the child using clear instructions, being careful about your body language and nonverbal cues. Ask the child's family for suggestions on how to best communicate with him or her.
- Answer the child's questions simply, honestly, and clearly. Difficult questions about a family member's illness or death should be handled carefully. Ask your supervisor for guidance in advance.
- Offer praise for something well done.
- Give encouragement when the child attempts to improve behaviour, even when there is only slight progress.
- Use positive suggestions rather than negative words. Avoid using "Don't" and "No."

Rest, Sleep, Play, and Exercise

- Maintain the child's bedtime and naptime routines. Routines and rituals are usually very important to the child, as they give the child comfort. Going to sleep at the right time is also very important for most children because they will become overtired, overactive, or cranky without enough sleep.
- Supervise playtime. Encourage active exercise, if allowed.
- Avoid taking sides when a disagreement occurs among children.
- Do not give more attention to one child and ignore others.
- Ignore tattling, if it is used to get attention.
- Distract the child if he or she begins to misbehave. If possible, play with the child or provide a different toy or activity.

Mealtime

- Prepare foods that the child will eat. Follow the care plan. Check if the child has food allergies or sensitivities (see Chapter 27).
- Do not force a child to eat. When the child feels full, the meal is over.
- Serve meals and snacks on time. Many children become cranky if they do not eat on time.

Discipline should be consistent. Each time a rule is broken, the consequence should be the same. For example, Noah (age 4) forgets to remove his boots and gets the floor dirty. He must get a cloth and help clean the floor, and he is not allowed to play until it is done. Noah knows the rules and what will happen if a rule is broken. The child feels safe when he or she knows the caregiver's expectations.

Recognize the child's efforts when he or she tries to follow the rules of the household. Praising these efforts encourages acceptable behaviour. Being positive with children is always more effective than being negative. For example, if Noah gets the floor dirty, it is better to say, "Let's clean up the mess" than "Shame on you for making that big mess." After he cleans up the mess, you could say, "Thank you for doing such a fine job." This would help to make Noah feel good about his accomplishment. Praise and acknowledgement also promote a child's dignity and show respect for the child.

Your role in disciplining the child is to:

- Know the rules of acceptable behaviour in each family situation
- Ask an appropriate family member to clarify the rules if you are unsure
- Reinforce existing rules
- Be consistent when using discipline
- Praise the child's efforts to follow the rules

Some parents may have very few rules of discipline, or the existing rules may seem too harsh or too loose. If this is the case, you should contact your supervisor. New rules may need to be set, and you should not set discipline rules without the guidance of your supervisor.

Punishment

Punishment is a harsh response that occurs when a discipline rule is broken. Punishing a child for failing to follow the rules of the household is *not* your responsibility. If a family member asks you to do so, explain that it is not your agency's policy to carry out punishment. Ask the family member to contact your supervisor if he or she has further questions. Record this information, and tell your supervisor about the situation.

SUPPORTING THE CHALLENGING CHILD

Many children raised in troubled environments become troubled themselves. These challenging children may be verbally aggressive, resistant to rules and regulations, or have difficulty forming bonds with others.

Why Do Some Children "Act Out"? Children of all ages sometimes express their feelings of anger, frustration, fear, guilt, or shame through their behaviour because this is the only way they know how to convey what they feel. Some children display emotional or behavioural outbursts, while others will demonstrate that they feel overwhelmed, tired, or physically unwell. Children can behave this way if there are too many changes in their lives; if they have recently experienced painful losses, or if they have problems at school, such as difficulty learning, too much peer pressure, or bullying.

Other children may have suffered or witnessed **physical abuse**, emotional or **sexual abuse**, or they may be using drugs or alcohol. In a few cases where children have been hospitalized for most of their lives, they may have difficulty accepting limits, especially if his or her parents tend to overindulge the child, which parents are tempted to do if they think the child is going to die or to reduce their own guilt feelings regarding the child's illnesses.

These are some of the more common reasons that may cause a child to "act out." As a support worker, it is your responsibility to provide care in a nonjudgemental and supportive manner. Some ways to successfully manage the challenging child are discussed in Box 16–3.

ASSISTING INFANTS AND CHILDREN TO MEET NUTRITIONAL NEEDS

Infants and children require proper, nutritional food in order to grow and develop each body system to its maximum potential. The nutritional requirements for children are discussed in Chapter 27: Basic Nutrition and Fluids. However, for many parents and caregivers, getting children to eat properly is an ongoing challenge. As a support worker, you should be aware that many children in Canada face nutritional challenges, not just the ones you may be supporting.

Understanding the Challenges.

- More than 1.2 million Canadian children live in poverty, including one in five under the age of 7. Poor children are more likely to have chronic health problems and difficulties at school and less likely to feel good about themselves.
- Almost 40% of the Aboriginal population is under the age of 15; they are more likely to face food shortages, and their social and economic conditions are significant barriers to healthy eating and positive self-esteem.[1]

One fifth of school children spend some time alone at home and tend to make many decisions about what and when to eat. Almost 30% of these "latch-key" kids are between 6 and 9 years of age.

Obesity appears to be increasingly prevalent among Canadian children, mainly because of their limited physical activity.

Many young people, especially girls, are concerned about their appearance and weight and about dieting. Many also report low self-esteem, increasing their risk for eating disorders. By Grade 9, only 26% of girls report high self-esteem compared with 40% of boys.

Box 16–3 Twelve Principles for Supporting a Challenging Child

1. Be specific about your expectations, and stick to them!
2. Put first things first. Keep your focus on important issues and choose your battles wisely. This will teach the child to make *good decisions*, not to win power struggles.
3. Praise, praise, and praise some more! **Positive reinforcement** (encouraging a behaviour by rewarding the desired behaviour after it is demonstrated) is much more effective than **negative reinforcement.**
4. Be knowledgeable about the child's specific problem(s) and difficulties. The child's parents, siblings, or caregivers may be able to assist you with finding solutions.
5. Follow the client's care plan for the amount of time and activity you should provide for the child. If you can, spend some "one-on-one" time focusing only on positives.
6. Be specific about positive and negative consequences ("rewards and punishments"), and follow through with them *consistently*. You should also consistently allow your words and actions to be straightforward and clear, so that the child cannot misinterpret you.
7. Act quickly and speak calmly. Never yell, scream, or swear, as this will only aggravate the situation.
8. Give bonuses, and focus on the positive. For example, if a child puts his clothing away, reward him by placing a gold star on his "Activities" sheet. Display the sheet where others can see it.
9. Seek out the middle ground. Know when to negotiate and when to stand firm. For example, if a child wants to watch television for some more time and her request is reasonable, negotiate with her how much extra time she can have.
10. Practise forgiveness and patience. Children need to know that they are still valued and cared for in spite of their naughty behaviour.
11. Use others for support, and seek assistance, when appropriate. Consult your supervisor if the child's behaviour worsens or if you are unsure about what you should do.
12. Remember to take care of yourself. You have needs, too! Pay attention to your own cues that you may be losing patience. It is better to silently "count to ten" than to lose your cool!

Source: The Maryland Institute for Individual & Family Therapy. *Twelve principles for dealing with a difficult child.* Retrieved June 11, 2007, from http://personal.boo.net/~dpfago/difficult_children.htm

About 13% of Canadians speak a language other than English or French at home and come from different backgrounds, and the cultural diversity is reflected in eating patterns.

Helping a Child Eat Well

Setting the Stage for Pleasant Mealtimes.

- The family should make it a point to eat as many meals together at home as possible and have regular mealtimes. A regular mealtime gives the family a chance to talk and relax together and helps them develop positive relationships with food.
- The meal table should be viewed as a positive, conflict-free zone. Problem solving and difficult discussions should be saved for a different time and place.
- Distractions, such as reading, toys, watching television, or answering the phone, should be avoided. The family should relax, eat, and talk together instead.
- Adults must teach and model good table manners and respectful behaviour.[2]

Avoiding Power Struggles and Learning to Trust the Child's Food Choices.

- Most children self-correct their undereating, overeating, and weight problems when the power struggle is taken out of their mealtimes. Parents and caregivers should avoid using comments such as "Eat at least one bite of vegetable"; "That's a lot of bread you're eating"; "Clean your plate"; "No seconds." Children have an internal hunger gauge that controls how much they eat. By overriding the child's signals, you will prevent the child from easily tuning into that internal hunger gauge.

- If the child skips over certain foods, eats lightly, or eats more than you would like him or her to:
  - As the support worker, check the family's diet, and ask: Are there any foods that the family eats that are not good for them? Is the child watching the behaviours of adults? If so, you can politely make suggestions to the family to improve the situation.
  - Let the child decide when he or she is full. You can remind him or her of the next scheduled meal or snack time: "Just make sure that you've eaten enough to hold you till snack time, which is after we get back from your swim class." This can help the child make a wise decision about what and how much to eat now.
- Although it can be tempting to give in to the child's demands, if you give consistent messages to him or her about eating and mealtimes, the child will eventually become more comfortable with the division of responsibility.
- Gradually, the child's eating habits will balance out. You will notice that as long as you provide nutritious choices, the child will eat a healthy variety and amount of food each week. Try to relax through this change in roles, and you will see that the child relaxes, too.

Adjusting Your Approach Based on the Child's Age.

- ***Feeding an infant.*** From birth, infants follow their internal hunger and fullness cues. They eat when they are hungry, and they stop eating when they are full. Experts recommend that newborns be fed on demand, and not on a schedule.
- ***Feeding a child.*** As you introduce new foods to a young child's diet, you are encouraging a love of variety, texture, and taste in foods. This is essential because the more adventurous a child feels about foods, the more balanced and nutritious his or her weekly intake will be. Remember that you may need to present a new or different food as many as 15 times or more before a child will be comfortable trying it, and this is normal. The key is to offer the new food in a relaxed manner without pressuring the child.

Getting Help for a Child's Eating Habits. As the support worker providing care to a child, if you are worried about the child's eating habits, you can call your supervisor, who may suggest that you ask his or her family doctor for help. This is especially important if the child has a major change in appetite or weight. This could include eating too much or too little, or gaining or losing weight. Other concerns might include:[1]

- Eating issues have turned the family's mealtimes into a battleground.
- The child may have an eating disorder, such as anorexia or bulimia (see Chapter 34).

Your supervisor (or the child's doctor) can advise you on actions you can take or direct you to seek out assistance from someone with specific expertise, such as:

- ***Registered dietitians***, who teach people about nutrition or develop diets to promote health. They also specialize in counselling to help treat food-related problems, including eating disorders.
- ***Pediatricians***, who may have special training and experience in caring for children with eating issues.
- ***Therapists or counsellors***, who can help the family cope with power struggles over eating.
- ***Psychiatrists***, who can provide counselling and medication.
- ***Pediatric gastroenterologists***, who can rule out or treat conditions of the digestive system that could cause an eating problem.
- ***Pediatric endocrinologists***, who can rule out or treat hormone conditions that can lead to weight problems.

PROTECTING CHILDREN FROM INJURY

As a support worker, it is your responsibility to ensure that children (regardless of age) are protected from harm. Injuries (from accidents, falls, choking, burns, abuse, poisonings, and other causes) are the leading causes of death in children over 1 year and are responsible for more deaths and disabilities in children than all causes of disease combined.[3] The developmental stage of the child (see Chapter 15) can help predict the injuries that a child may be prone to.

Despite various safety efforts, one of the leading causes of death for children over the age of one in North America is motor vehicle (MV)–related fatalities, including occupant, pedestrian, bicycle, and motorcycle deaths. Box 16–4 lists the causes of early childhood deaths from injury, and Box 16–5 lists risk factors for childhood injuries. You should also refer to Chapter 19 for further discussion of potential hazards in the home.

Preventing Falls in Children

Falls are the leading cause of injuries in children, and accidental injuries are the leading cause of death among Canadian children.[3] Infants can easily roll off a change table or bed. Falls out of highchairs and infant seats and falls down the stairs are also common accidents among babies and children. Older children often fall when running or playing. When children are tired, they may not pay close attention to the potential dangers around them and may also have a delay in their reaction time, which contributes to an injury.

Children are at an increased risk of being accidentally hurt during times of stress or changes in the family's routine. This is because the caregiver's attention is divided and supervision may not be as careful as usual. For example, when a family member is ill, the caregiver may be focused on the ill person rather than on the child. Support workers can provide care and support to clients and their families at such times of stress and at times of change.

As a support worker, when you are working with or around children, you must always be aware of possible dangers to them. It is your responsibility to always practise safety measures to prevent falls, burns, poisoning, and suffocation. Use common sense and follow the safety rules of your agency and the client's care plan at all times. Refer to Box 16–6 (on page 229) for a discussion of ways to prevent falls and injuries in children. Box 16–7 (on page 230) discusses ways to prevent choking in children.

Protecting Children From Burns

Burns are common in children and can cause significant morbidity (illness) and mortality (deaths). They constitute one of the leading causes of accidental death in children.[4] Varying degrees of burns can occur, depending on the extent of tissue damage. Children and older adults are both at great risk for burns.

Hot liquids, such as coffee or tap water, are responsible for many childhood burns. For example, a child may get in the way when an adult is carrying a hot drink, and the adult may trip over the child and spill the hot liquid on the child (see Box 16–8 on page 231).

Preventing Accidental Poisoning in Children

All children, especially when they are very young, put things in their mouths as part of learning and exploring their world. This is one reason why hundreds of children every year are victims of accidental poisonings.[3] Parents, guardians, and caregivers can prevent many of these accidents by identifying and locking away toxic materials.

Accidental poisoning is most common in children between the ages of 1 and 4, when they are crawling or walking and exploring their environment. Eating substances such as aspirin, cigarette butts, or vitamin pills is a common cause of childhood poisoning. Poisoning also occurs when certain poisonous substances, such as oven cleaner or pesticide, spill on the skin and are absorbed into the body.[3] Refer to Box 16–9 (on page 232) for ways to prevent accidental poisoning.

PREVENTING INFECTIONS IN CHILDREN

When a child starts child care or school, it may seem as if he or she is sick all the time. This pattern is normal, as all children's immune systems are developing, and their resistance to infection develops only after exposure to a multitude of germs. Young children in large groups are breeding grounds for the organisms that cause illness. Little

Box 16–4 Causes of Early Childhood Deaths (ages 2–7) From Injury in North America

Homicide	22.6%
Suffocation (see Box 16–7)	17.7%
Motor vehicle accident	15.2%
Fire and burns (see Box 16–8)	9.5%
Drowning	7.2%
Choking on food	7.1%
Choking on objects	5.9%
Other unintentional injuries	10.6%
Injuries of undetermined intent	4.2%

Source: National Institute of Child Health and Human Development. (2003). Retrieved June 11, 2007, from http://www.cnn.com/HEALTH/9905/03/infant.deaths/

Box 16–5 Risk Factors for Childhood Injuries

- **Sex:** The majority are males mainly due to behavioural characteristics, such as aggression.
- **Temperament:** This is especially true for children who have persistent or high activity temperament.
- **Stress:** Predisposes the child to increased risk-taking and self-destructive behaviour, usually combined with a general lack of self-protection.
- **Alcohol and drug use:** This is associated with higher incidence of motor vehicle injuries, drownings, homicides, and suicides.
- **History of previous injury:** This is associated with an increased likelihood of another injury, especially if initial injury required hospitalization.
- **Developmental characteristics:**
  - Mismatch between the child's developmental level and skill required for the activity (such as driving all-terrain vehicles)
  - Natural curiosity to explore environment
  - Desire to assert self and challenge rules
  - In older child, desire for peer approval and peer acceptance
- **Cognitive characteristics (age specific):**
  - ***Infancy***—this age group explores the environment through taste and touch, which may lead to accidental poisonings or burns.
  - ***Young child***—this age group:
    - tends to actively search for attractive objects
    - is unaware of "cause and effect" consequential dangers
    - may fail to learn from experiences (for example, falling from a step is not perceived as the same type of danger as climbing a tree)
    - cannot comprehend dangers to themselves or others (for example, children may accidentally poison themselves)
  - ***School-age child***—this age group is generally unable to fully comprehend "cause and effect," so they may attempt dangerous acts without thinking of the consequences (for example, too few children wear safety helmets when bicycle riding).
  - ***Adolescent***—adolescents' preoccupation with abstract thinking may cause them to feel invulnerable (for example, drowning, diving in shallow water).
- **Anatomic characteristics (especially in young children)**
  - ***Large head***—predisposes to cranial injury
  - ***Large spleen and liver***—predisposes to trauma in these areas
  - ***Small and light body***—may be thrown easily, especially out of a moving vehicle
  - ***Left-handedness***—environmental biases (things built for people who are right-handed) may predispose them to injury
- **Other factors:**
  - Poverty (and living in substandard housing), family stress (such as maternal illness or recent environmental change), substandard alternative child care, young maternal age, low maternal education, and multiple siblings may also increase a child's risk for injury.

Sources: Hockenbury, M., Wilson, D., Winkelstein, M., & Kline, N. (2003). *Wong's nursing care of infants and children* (7th ed., p. 7). St. Louis, Missouri: Mosby.

Box 16–6 Safety Measures to Prevent Falls Among Infants and Children

- Do not leave infants and young children unsupervised. Never leave them unattended in highchairs or on a table, couch, bed, or any other high surface.
- Secure the child in a highchair or infant seat. Use both the waist and crotch straps. Lock the highchair tray after securing the child in the chair. Keep highchairs away from stoves, tables, and counters. The child could push off against these and fall.
- Do not use baby walkers; they have caused many serious falls and injuries.
- Use safety gates at the top and bottom of stairs. Make sure the child cannot get caught in the slats.
- Keep one hand on a child lying on a scale, bed, change table, or other furniture (Figure 16–2).
- Keep one hand on the baby when changing diapers. Gather supplies before changing diapers or bathing an infant. Place supplies within easy reach.
- Keep crib rails up and in the locked position. Frequently check children in cribs.
- Make sure there is nothing in the crib that the baby can stand on (like large stuffed toys or firm bumper pads). Standing on something in the crib could cause the baby to fall over the top of the railing.
- Do not let children under 6 years of age sleep or play on the top bed of a bunk bed.
- Keep children away from windows. Do not let them sit on window sills or lean on windows. Window screens are not strong enough to prevent a child from falling out. Do not put furniture underneath or near windows. Children could climb on them to reach the window.
- Do not let children run with objects in their hands or mouths (like baby bottles, soothers, or sticks). The object could cause injury if the child falls.
- Prevent furniture, such as TVs, bookcases, dressers, and tables, from falling on children. Injuries and deaths can occur when children climb, pull on, sit on, lean on, or try to move furniture. Heavy furniture should be anchored to the wall.

hands rub drippy noses and then transfer infectious agents to other children or to shared toys.

Children who have physical or developmental delays may be even more prone to infectious illnesses, as they may have a fragile immune system. As a support worker, it is your responsibility to ensure that you always practise hand hygiene (see Chapter 20) to prevent spreading infections from yourself to these children. By simply following proper hygiene practices, you may reduce the likelihood that a contagious infection will keep the child home from school or child care. The guidelines for hand hygiene should also be followed in your own household, to reduce transmission of germs and infectious illnesses from your client's home, to you or your own family.

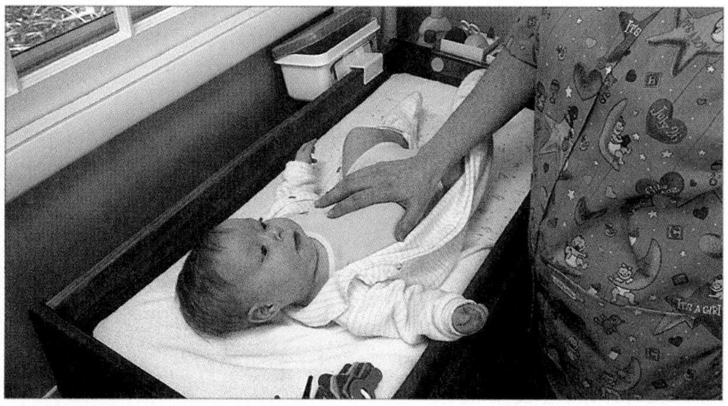

Figure 16–2 Keep one hand on a child on a change table.

Prevention of Childhood Infections

When a child or a young person sneezes and coughs, he or she sprays germs into the air, sometimes landing right on other children, who are then infected. A child's hand can become a vehicle for carrying viruses and bacteria from toys and other frequently handled objects to other children's eyes, noses, or mouths, the usual points of entry for germs that cause illness.

The single most important thing anyone can do to prevent illness is to wash his or her hands thoroughly and frequently. The Centers for Disease Control and Prevention recommends that people wash their hands with soap and warm water for 15

Box 16–7 Ways to Prevent Choking in Children

- Always supervise children while they are eating. Grate, mash, blend, or chop food into very small pieces before giving it to a baby. Do not give infants and young children hot dogs, raw carrots, peanuts, popcorn, whole grapes, raisins, hard candy, or gum.
- Do not prop bottles on a rolled towel or blanket. Hold the baby and bottle during feedings.
- Check for small objects like coins, buttons, marbles, pins, and paper clips lying on the floor and remove them. Children can choke on them.
- Do not allow children to blow up balloons or put one in their mouths. Immediately dispose of any broken balloon pieces.
- Keep all plastic bags and wrappings away from children.
- Do not let children wear necklaces, strings, cords, or other items round their necks. These can become tightly twisted or get caught on furniture. Remove bibs before placing infants in cribs.
- Remove or tie up cords or drawstrings on all articles of children's clothing. This includes drawstrings in the hood, at the neckline, and at the waist.
- Keep cords for blinds, curtains, and drapes out of children's reach. Tie cords up or use a cord shortener. Make sure cribs and playpens are placed far away from blinds, shades, or drapes. Do not hang items with strings, cords, or elastic around cribs or playpens.
- Position infants on their backs for sleep.
- Make sure crib mattresses fit snugly and are very firm. The space between crib rail slats must be no more than 6.3 cm ($2\frac{1}{2}$ in.). Never let infants sleep on a waterbed. They should sleep only on firm, flat surfaces.
- Do not use pillows to position infants or prevent them from falling off beds or furniture.
- Remove pillows, comforters, quilts, sheepskin, stuffed toys, and other soft items from the crib when the baby is sleeping.
- Always supervise children who are in or near water. This includes tubs, toilets, sinks, buckets and containers, wading pools, and swimming pools.
- Keep bathroom doors closed to prevent children from entering the bathroom without supervision and drowning in toilets or bathtubs. Keep toilet seats down, and use toilet safety locks.
- Keep sinks, tubs, basins, and buckets empty when not in use.
- Keep diaper pails locked.
- Do not leave children unattended in a vehicle. They can suffocate very quickly in high temperatures in the summer or suffer from extreme cold temperatures in the winter inside the vehicle.

seconds—about as long as it takes to sing the "Happy Birthday" song twice. Alcohol-based hand sanitizers come in disposable hand wipes or in gel form and require no water; they also can help keep hands clean (see Chapter 20).

Vaccinations to Prevent Serious Infectious Illnesses

Canadian babies and children require various vaccinations in order to fend off contagious infections and illnesses such as measles, mumps, pertussis (whooping cough), diphtheria, tetanus, certain types of meningitis, and polio by being routinely vaccinated.[5] Refer to Table 16–1 (on page 233) for the immunization schedule suggested by Health Canada. Vaccines are so effective that most of the diseases that they help prevent are now rare in Canada.

What Would Happen If We Stopped Vaccinating? In other countries, when fewer people were immunized, diseases quickly returned. For example:

- In 2000, the number of measles cases in Ireland increased from 148 to more than 1200 in just 1 year because vaccination was reduced to 76%, and several children died as a result.
- In 1999, there was a large outbreak of rubella (German measles) in Nebraska. All 83 adults who were affected had not previously been vaccinated, and most of them came from countries where rubella vaccine is not routine.

Box 16–8 Protecting Children From Burns

- Do not drink or carry hot liquids near infants and children. Make sure children are not in your way when you are carrying anything hot, including drinks, clothes irons, or dishes from the oven.
- Do not heat a baby bottle or baby food in a microwave. Always shake the bottle or stir the food and test the temperature before giving it to the baby.
- Keep hot foods and liquids away from counter and table edges where children can reach them.
- Avoid using tablecloths or placemats that can be pulled down by a child.
- Always test the temperature of the bath water before bathing a child. Position the child facing away from water faucets, and do not let children touch faucet handles.
- Never leave a "live" extension cord lying out (that is, one end is plugged in and the other end is free). A child could pick it up and put it in the mouth, resulting in severe burns to the mouth.
- Put safety plugs in all unused electrical outlets (Figure 16–3).
- Keep pot handles pointed toward the back of the stove. Use the back burners on the stove rather than the front, whenever possible, when children are around. Turn off stove and burners when they are not in use.
- Do not let very young children help you cook on the stove.
- Do not let electrical cords from irons, coffee pots, toasters, and so on, hang down where children could pull on them.
- Do not let children play near hot stoves, space heaters, fireplaces, and other heat sources.

▣ After a routine vaccination was cancelled in Russia, there were 5000 deaths in 1994 due to diphtheria. In previous years, Russia, like Canada, had only a few cases of diphtheria each year and no deaths.[5]

Do the Benefits of Vaccination Outweigh the Possible Side Effects? The short answer is yes. If there were no vaccines, there would be many more cases of disease, more serious side effects from disease, and more deaths. ***The diseases that vaccines help prevent lead to pneumonia, deafness, brain damage, heart problems, blindness, and paralysis in children who are not vaccinated.*** Canadian children are very fortunate to have vaccines that prevent diseases that still kill and disable children in many other parts of the world every day. The risks of not being vaccinated are much greater than any risk of vaccination itself.

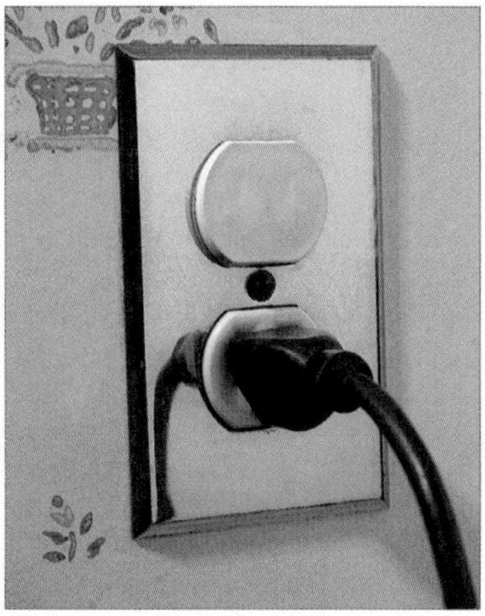
Figure 16–3 Safety plug in an outlet.

Reye's Syndrome. In cooperation with the Canadian Pediatric Association, Health and Welfare Canada has issued a warning asking that ASA (commonly referred to as "aspirin" or acetylsalicylic acid) and products containing ASA not be used for treating the symptoms of flu or chickenpox in those younger than 20 years of age.[6] In addition, manufacturers of products containing ASA are now putting warnings on their labels saying that a doctor should be consulted before giving ASA to children or teenagers who have the flu or chickenpox.

These warnings have resulted from research which has linked the use of ASA for flu or chickenpox symptoms and the development of a condition involving inflammation of the brain called **Reye's syndrome,** which is a rare but often fatal condition that can occur during the recovery stage of flu or chickenpox. There is no evidence to suggest that Reye's syndrome is associated with the use of acetaminophen (brand name Tylenol).[6] Therefore, acetaminophen may be safely used to treat the symptoms of flu or chickenpox, such as fever and headache.

Box 16–9 Ways to Prevent Accidental Poisoning

- ***Read the labels on all household products before buying them, and try to use the least-toxic ones.*** Among the household products generally considered less hazardous are nonchlorine bleaches, vinegar, borax, beeswax, mineral oil, and compressed air drain openers (rather than corrosive liquids).
- ***Lock up all medicines and harmful substances.*** Secure all cupboards that contain poisons, even those you might assume to be out of range. Poison experts have come across many cases of toddlers dragging a chair over to a kitchen counter, climbing onto the counter or even the refrigerator, and opening a cupboard that is at eye level.
- ***Do not rely on child-resistant containers.*** These are not always childproof. No bottle top can be made so fail-safe that a child cannot find a way to get it off. It is not unusual for a 2-year-old, left alone for 30 minutes, to break down even the safest devices of a manufacturer.
- ***Keep medicines, pesticides, and even detergents, in their original containers.*** Rewrite any labels that get smudged so that you know exactly what is in each bottle. Never put poisonous or toxic products in containers that were once used for food. Ambulance staff have heard far too many horror stories of toxic liquid put into an unmarked container and having been mistaken for juice.
- ***Never refer to any kind of medicine as sweets.*** Even if you are trying to get a reluctant toddler to take his cough syrup, do not present it as something good to eat. Children learn by imitation, so when you take your own medications, make sure that they are not watching.
- ***Never let children play with chipped or flaking paint.*** Old paint contains lead, which is a toxic substance known to cause neurological problems in children. Remove all chipped paint and consult your local poison control centre or reputable paint store for ways to remove the lead paint from your walls and woodwork.

Examples of Materials Found in the Home That Are Toxic to Children

- ***Household cleaning products.*** Assume that they are all dangerous. The list should include drain cleaner, oven cleaner, toilet cleaner, dishwasher detergent, and rust remover, but there are so many more that the safest thing to do is to keep them *all* out of the way of children. Even if they do not ingest them, they may spray themselves with them, burning their eyes or skin.
- ***Pills and medicines.*** Always assume that any medicine your child takes, whether prescribed for you or for him, can be dangerous. Even vitamin supplements can be fatal in large doses, so keep them locked in the cupboard. Prescription drugs, especially antidepressants and time-release drugs, have a cumulative effect. Even travel medicines can be dangerous; put them all in the locked medicine cupboard.
- ***Cosmetics.*** Lock them in the medicine cabinet. Even an everyday product, such as hair remover, can be dangerous if swallowed.
- ***Household plants.*** Many garden plants are poisonous, especially philodendron, rue, privet, and laurel berries, Yew berries, and Laburnum seeds. Make sure that you and all of the child's caregivers know the names of all the plants and trees inside and outside the home, just in case. It is a good idea for caregivers to leave the tags on all items that are brought home from a plant nursery. An expert from a plant nursery may be able to help identify the plant and also provide tags to place near the plants.
- ***Paint thinner and paint remover, gasoline, paraffin, and metal polishes.*** Keep them locked out of children's way in the garage, and do not let them into the workshop unsupervised.
- ***Pesticides.*** Lock them away.
- ***Adult substances.*** Alcohol and tobacco can be lethal to a child. One cigarette could kill a 1-year old, if swallowed, and a large mouthful of a strong alcoholic drink could kill a toddler.

The symptoms of Reye's syndrome are:[6]

- A viral illness (such as the flu or chickenpox) that seems to last longer than in others who have the same illness
- Frequent or persistent nausea and vomiting
- A change in personality, confusion, agitation, or combativeness
- Coma
- Seizures

Table 16–1 Recommended Immunization Schedule for Infants, Children, and Youth*

Age of Vaccination	D	P	T	IPV	Pneu-C	Hib	MMR	Men-C	Flu	Var	HepB
2 months	X	X	X	X	X	X					
4 months	X	X	X	X	X	X					
6 months	X	X	X	X	X	X			**		
12 months							X	X	**		
15 months					X				**	X	
18 months	X	X	X	X		X	X		**		
4–6 years	X	X	X	X						X ***	
12 years (Grade 7)								X			X
14–16 years	X	X	X								

Abbreviations:

D	Diptheria vaccine
P	Pertussis vaccine
T	Tetanus vaccine
IPV	Inactivated polio vaccine
Pneu-C	Pneumococcal conjugate vaccine
Hib	*Hemophilus influenzae* type b conjugate vaccine
MMR	Measles, mumps, rubella vaccine
Men-C	Meningococcal C conjugate vaccine
Flu	Influenza Vaccine
Var	Varicella (chickenpox) vaccine
HepB	Hepatitis B vaccine*

Notes:
* These are recommended guidelines only. You must check with your health care practitioner in your area for confirmation.
** Previously unvaccinated children in the 6–23-month age group require two doses with an interval of at least 4 weeks.
*** If your child has not had chickenpox (varicella zoster) or the vaccine, he or she can receive the chickenpox vaccine at 5 years of age.

Source: Public Health Agency of Canada. (2006). *Canadian immunization guide* (7th ed., pp. 93–94). (Catalogue no. HP40-3/2006E). Ottawa: Minister of Public Works and Government Services Canada. Retrieved February 2, 2007, from http://www.phac-aspc.gc.ca/naci-ccni/is-si/recimmsche-icy_e.html; http://www.phac-aspc.gc.ca/naci-ccni/is-si/recimmsche-icy_e.html

If these symptoms occur in a child or teenager who has been given ASA for the symptoms of flu or chickenpox, you should seek medical attention immediately.

How Long Should Sick Children Stay Home?

Each facility generally has its own rules, but most will not let children attend school or child care if they have a fever of more than 38°C, are vomiting, or have diarrhea. In addition, some facilities require that children with **strep throat** or bacterial **conjunctivitis** be on antibiotic therapy for 24 hours before returning.

Generally, however, children can return to school when they:

- Have no fever
- Can eat and drink normally
- Are rested and alert enough to pay attention in class
- Have completed any period of medically recommended isolation

Resistance Comes With Time. Despite our best efforts, most children will get sick, especially during the first few years of contact with larger groups of children. Most children's immunity does improve with time, with school-age children gradually becoming less prone to common illnesses and recovering more quickly from the diseases they do catch. If you have any questions about the child that you are supporting and his or her immunity, you should ask your supervisor.

The Top Five Reasons Why Children Miss School or Child Care

1. ***Colds:*** The most common childhood illnesses are **upper respiratory infections (URIs),** the medical term for colds and other viral ailments that affect the throat, nose, and sinuses. While adults average 2 to 4 colds a year, children typically have 6 to 10. Children also tend to have more severe and longer-lasting symptoms than do adults.

   Studies have shown that there is no benefit in treating children's colds with antihistamines, decongestants, or cough suppressants. If it is *your* child who is ill, you should discuss the appropriate medication to give in order to reduce fever. Children should never be given aspirin because it may trigger Reye's syndrome, a rare but potentially fatal disease (see page 231).
2. ***The stomach flu (gastroenteritis):*** The second most common childhood illness is **gastroenteritis**, more commonly known as the "stomach flu." This childhood illness causes vomiting and diarrhea and can lead to dehydration, particularly in very young children. Signs and symptoms of dehydration include:
   - Excessive thirst
   - Dry mouth
   - Little or no urine, or dark yellow urine
   - Decreased tears
   - Severe weakness or lethargy

   Your client may be required to drink an oral rehydration solution (e.g., special frozen treats, or Pedialyte) that can help replace lost fluids, minerals, and salts. (***These items would be on the client's care plan and should not be given unless it is specified there.***) When food *is* reintroduced, easy-to-digest items should be given first, such as broth, toast, bananas, and rice. Avoid dairy products, which can be hard to digest.

   Many parents assume that any kind of stomach upset in a child is the result of a contagious illness, when the real culprit is simple indigestion or constipation. Some children get stomachaches when they are worried about things, either at home or at school. The dread of facing a bully or taking a test, for example, can make a child's stomach hurt. It is important for a doctor to determine the cause of a child's digestive symptoms before prescribing treatment.
3. ***Ear infection (otitis media):*** Ear infections most often occur in children under the age of 2, but the problem can also be common between the ages of 5 and 6, triggered by the respiratory illnesses picked up in kindergarten or first grade. Colds or allergies cause congestion, which may squeeze shut the child's **eustachian**

tube, the tiny drainage pipe for the middle ear. Fluid trapped in the middle ear can become a breeding ground for viruses or bacteria.

It can be difficult to distinguish between ear infections caused by bacteria and those caused by viruses. The distinction is important, however, because antibiotics will cure bacterial—but not viral—infections. And using antibiotics when they are not necessary has serious consequences, most notably causing the emergence of bacteria strains with built-in resistance to many of the drugs that fight infection. For that reason, doctors today often wait to see if an ear infection will clear up on its own before prescribing antibiotics.

4. ***Pink eye (conjunctivitis):*** **Pink eye (conjunctivitis)** is an inflammation of the clear membrane that covers the white part of the eye and lines the inner surface of the eyelids. When caused by viruses or bacteria, conjunctivitis is highly contagious. It is typically treated with antibiotic eye drops or ointment. Warm or cool compresses may ease the child's discomfort.
5. ***Sore throat:*** Most sore throats are caused by viruses and are usually associated with other respiratory signs and symptoms, such as a runny nose and cough. But about 15% of children's sore throats are caused by *Streptococcus*, a bacterium that causes strep throat.

   Fevers above 38°C are common in strep throat, and swallowing can be so painful that the child may have difficulty eating. Antibiotics are required to combat strep throat. Left untreated, strep bacteria eventually can trigger an abnormal immune response, which can lead to rheumatic fever. Complications of rheumatic fever include damaged heart valves and stiff, swollen joints.[7]

REVIEW

Answers to these questions are at the bottom of the page.

Circle the **BEST** answer.

1. **Your role when providing child care includes:**
   A. Maintaining your rules of behaviour
   B. Providing punishment when necessary
   C. Maintaining the family's daily routines
   D. Ignoring situations that may add stress or cause harm to the family

2. **The leading cause of death in children over the age of one is:**
   A. Cancer
   B. Starvation
   C. Injuries
   D. Pneumonia

3. **Why is it important to understand the relationship between a child's developmental level and his or her risk factors for injuries?**
   A. You can more easily anticipate which injuries they are more likely to get.
   B. The older the child, the less likely he or she will get injured.
   C. Older children are more likely to get injured than are toddlers.
   D. There is no relationship between a child's developmental level and the risk for injuries.

4. **Why are boys more likely to become injured than are girls?**
   A. Girls have smaller heads.
   B. Girls play more computer games.
   C. Boys are usually more physically aggressive.
   D. Boys are usually poorer eaters than are girls, and this subjects them to injury.

5. **A teen who is under stress is more at risk for injury because he or she:**
   A. Is less active
   B. Engages in riskier behaviours
   C. Eats more fast food
   D. Has more friends than happy teens

6. **How can an infant most likely be injured while in his own crib or playpen?**
   A. He can burn himself on a cigarette lighter.
   B. He can get head and neck injuries by crawling around.
   C. He can get a shock from his MP3 player.
   D. He might choke on his toys.

7. **Young children are at risk for injuries because they:**
   A. Do not know that some things may be poisonous
   B. Usually engage in risk-taking behaviours
   C. Are prone to depression and suicidal behaviours
   D. Want peer acceptance and approval

8. **You are caring for an infant and some young children. Which measure is safe?**
   A. Using a safety strap when putting a child in a highchair
   B. Ironing the clothes while the children play near your feet
   C. Placing stuffed animals and toys in the crib at naptime
   D. Allowing a child to play with empty pill bottles

9. **One of the main illnesses that cause children to miss school or child care is:**
   A. Stomach flu
   B. Headaches
   C. Chickenpox
   D. Head lice

10. **Children can usually return to school after a contagious illness when:**
   A. They have a fever of just below 38°C
   B. Their parents must go to work
   C. They can eat and drink normally
   D. They miss a day of school

11. **In time, most school age children become less prone to common infectious diseases because:**
   A. Older children eat more vegetables
   B. They eventually know how to avoid getting sick.
   C. Their immune system matures, and this makes them more resistant to illnesses
   D. They are given decongestants and antihistamines by their parents

Answers: 1.C, 2.C, 3.A, 4.C, 5.B, 6.D, 7.A, 8.A, 9.A, 10.C, 11.C

CHAPTER 17

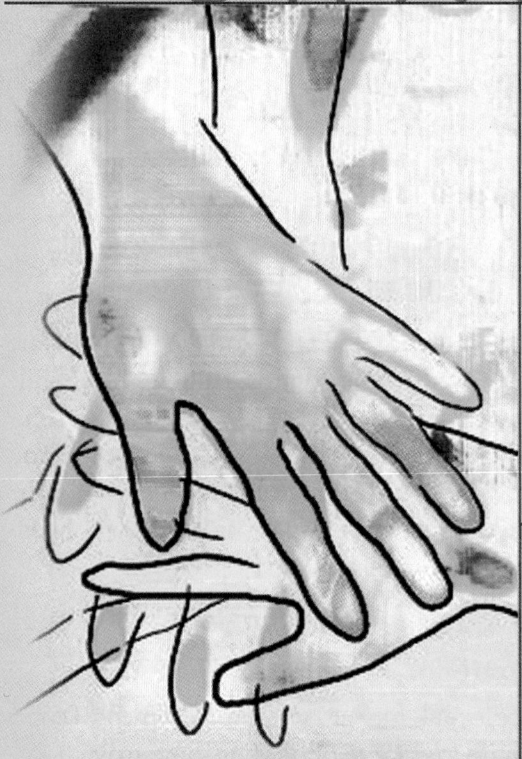

Caring for Older Adults

OBJECTIVES

- Define the key terms listed in this chapter.
- Describe the effects of retirement.
- Identify the social changes common in older adulthood.
- Describe how a partner's death affects the survivor.
- Describe the changes that occur in the body's systems during aging and the care required.
- Explain how aging affects sexuality in older adults.
- Describe how the health care team promotes the client's sexuality.
- Explain the effect of ageism on older adults.

key terms

ageism Bias and discrimination against older adults.

atrophy A decrease in size or wasting away of tissue.

discrimination Behaviour that treats people unfairly based on their group membership.

dysphagia Difficulty swallowing.

dyspnea Difficult, laboured, or painful breathing.

geriatrics The branch of medicine that provides care for older adults.

gerontology The study of the aging process.

stereotype An overly simple or exaggerated view of a group of people.

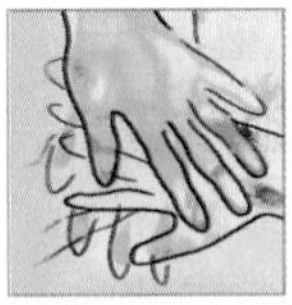

The number of older adults is increasing every day in today's society. People live longer and are healthier and more active than ever before, so most people can expect to live into their seventies, or even into their eighties and nineties. There are more 100-year-olds now than ever before.

Gerontology is the study of the aging process. **Geriatrics** is the branch of medicine that provides care for older adults. Aging, or growing old, is a normal process, when normal changes in body structure and function occur, increasing the risk for illness, injury, chronic disease, and disability. These changes, however, are usually gradual. Emotional and social changes also occur, and most older adults adjust to these changes well and live healthy and happy lives. Older adults may continue to live in their own homes by themselves or with their partners or live with their adult children or other family members. Some move into assisted-living facilities, and some others who require 24-hour care move into long-term care facilities.

As stated in Chapter 15, the developmental tasks of late adulthood are:

- Adjusting to decreased physical strength and loss of health
- Adjusting to retirement and reduced income
- Coping with the death of a partner
- Developing new friends and relationships
- Preparing for one's own death

EMOTIONAL AND SOCIAL CHANGES

Greying hair, wrinkles, and slow movements are physical reminders that one is growing old, while retirement and the deaths of partners, family members, and friends are social reminders. Physical and social changes have emotional effects on older adults and also have an impact on their basic needs of love and belonging and self-esteem.

Retirement

Most people look forward to their retirement. People usually retire at the age of 65, but some may choose to retire earlier or work until the age of 70 and beyond. Retirement is a reward for a lifetime of work. The person has earned the right not to work any more and can now relax and enjoy life. Travel, leisure, spending time with family, and doing only what one wants to do are retirement "benefits." Nowadays more and more retired people are interested in furthering their education.

Many people enjoy their retirement, but some are not so fortunate. Some are forced to retire because of chronic disease or disability, and poor health can make retirement very difficult. Retirement is often a person's first real experience with aging.

Work has social and emotional effects. It helps meet the basic needs of love and belonging and self-esteem and brings fulfillment and a feeling of usefulness. There is pride in a day's work or a job well done. Friendships form; co-workers share daily events; and leisure time, recreation, and companionship often involve co-workers. Some people thus need work for emotional and social fulfillment, and for such people, retirement can be hard. Some retired people therefore take on part-time jobs or volunteer work (Figure 17–1) because such activities promote a sense of usefulness and well-being.

Reduced Income. Retirement income is often less than half of the person's full income during their work years. For some retired people, the Canada Pension Plan (CPP) may be the only source of income, but, unfortunately, CPP has not kept pace with the rising cost of living.

Retirement and being an older adult do not mean fewer expenses. Older adults still need to make rent or mortgage payments, buy food and clothing, spend on transportation and utilities, and pay taxes. They must also pay for medications that are not covered under government drug plans.

Reduced income during retirement may force lifestyle changes, such as limiting social and leisure activities and finding cheaper housing or moving in with children or other relatives. Some older adults must rely on family for money or needed items; others live in poverty if they do not have an adequate pension income or assets. As the cost of living rises in Canada, the old age pension does not increase at the same rate, so the gap between income and need is widening each year.

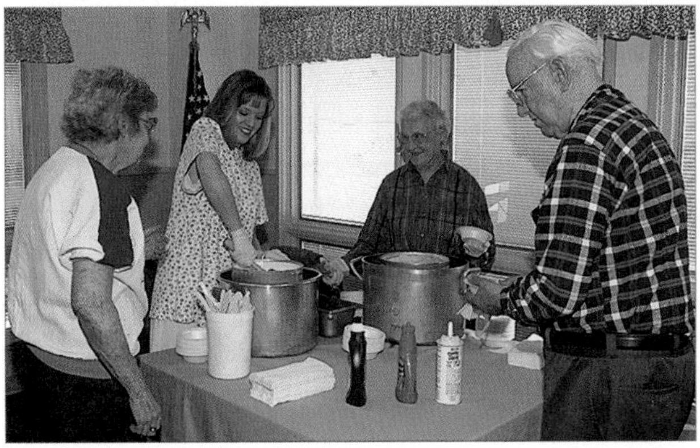

Figure 17–1 These retired people volunteer at a local food bank.

Some older adults do not face a reduction in their income because when they were working, they were able to provide for their retirement through their savings, investments, retirement plans, and insurance. For these older adults, the retirement years are financially comfortable.

Social Relationships

Social relationships change throughout life (see the *Respecting Diversity: Older Adults Born in Other Countries* box). Children grow up, leave home, and have their own families. Many live far away from parents. Older friends and family move away, die, or become disabled. While many older people have regular contact with children, grandchildren, brothers and sisters, nieces and nephews, and other relatives and friends, some are lonely due to separation from children and lack of companionship.

Many older adults adjust well to changes. Hobbies, religious and community activities, and new friends help prevent loneliness. Grandchildren can bring great love and enjoyment. Taking part in family activities not only gives companionship but also allows the older person to feel useful and wanted. Some home care plans include a "friendly visitor" program for older adults living alone. Older adults who move into retirement homes and long-term care facilities often make new friends

RESPECTING DIVERSITY

Older Adults Born in Other Countries

Some of the older adults who have moved to Canada from another country may not speak English or French. In Canada, they may have lived and worked in a community of people from their home country. When family and friends move away or die, these people may be left with no one to talk to. If the health care workers also do not speak the same language or understand their culture, these older adults feel lonely and isolated. As a support worker, you need to be sensitive to clients in this situation.

and take part in social activities that are offered in the facilities (Figure 17–2).

Children as Caregivers

Sometimes when adult children care for their older parents, parents and children exchange roles and the child cares for the parent. This role exchange and dependency on a child can make some older adults feel more secure, but some others may feel unwanted, in the way, and useless. Some may feel that they have lost their dignity and self-respect, so tensions may develop among the child, parent, and other household members. Being a caregiver to an elderly parent can be very stressful. Caregivers often have to meet the needs of the parent as well as those of their own children. If the parent has a medical condition, the caregiver has even more responsibilities; he or she may need to quit work to care for the ill parent, and the resulting loss of income may cause financial difficulties. Lack of privacy is also a common problem for both the caregiver and the parent.

Death of a Partner

As a couple grows older, the chances that one partner will die increase. Women usually live longer than men do, so many older women will become widows.

Even when a person tries to be emotionally prepared for a partner's death, when death occurs, the loss is still devastating. No amount of preparation is ever enough to cope with the emptiness that results. The surviving partner loses a friend, lover, companion, and confidant, so the grief is great, leading to serious physical and mental health problems. The grieving partner may lose the will to live or even attempt suicide. Support from family, friends, and church, social, or recreational groups is very important at this time to help the older person cope.

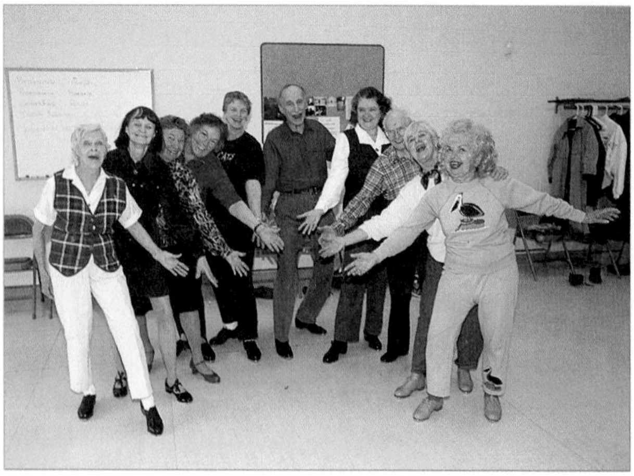

Figure 17–2 Older adults enjoy companionship with people their own age.

PHYSICAL CHANGES

Certain physical changes are a normal part of aging and occur in everyone (Table 17–1). Physical processes slow down, and energy level and body efficiency decline. The rate and degree of change vary with each person. Influencing factors include diet, general health, exercise, stress, environment, and heredity. Many of these normal changes are gradual and not noticed for a long time. Some older adults also have physical changes caused by disease, illness, or injury.

Normal aging does not mean loss of health, so quality of life does not have to change with aging. The older person can adjust to many of the normal changes, but some have at least one chronic illness.

The Integumentary System

In older adulthood, the skin loses its elasticity, strength, and fatty-tissue layer. This causes the skin to thin and sag, and folds, lines, and wrinkles appear. Dry skin develops because of decreased secretions from oil and sweat glands, so the skin becomes fragile and is easily injured. Skin breakdown, skin tears, and pressure ulcers are some of the risks older adults face (see Chapter 42). Brown spots, often called "age spots" or "liver spots," appear on the skin, usually on the wrists and hands.

The skin has fewer nerve endings, which affects the client's ability to sense heat, cold, and pain. Bruising and delayed healing can result from a decreased number of blood vessels.

Loss of fatty tissues beneath the skin increases sensitivity to cold, so the client needs to be protected from drafts and extreme cold. Sweaters, lap blankets, socks, and higher thermostat settings are often needed.

Table 17–1 Physical Changes That May Occur During the Aging Process

System	Changes
Integumentary	Skin becomes less elastic Skin loses its strength Brown spots ("age spots" or "liver spots") on the wrists and hands Fewer nerve endings Fewer blood vessels Fatty-tissue layer is lost Skin thins and sags Skin is fragile and easily injured Folds, lines, and wrinkles appear Secretion from oil and sweat glands decreases Dry skin Itching Sensitivity to extreme heat and cold environments decreases Sensitivity to pain decreases Nails become thick and tough Whitening or greying hair Loss or thinning of hair Facial hair in some women Drier hair
Musculo-skeletal	Muscles atrophy Strength decreases Bones become brittle; can break easily Joints become stiff and painful Gradual loss of height Mobility decreases
Nervous	Vision and hearing decrease Senses of taste, smell, and touch decrease Sensitivity to pain is reduced Blood flow to the brain is reduced Cells shrink Shorter memory; forgetfulness Slower ability to respond Changes in sleep patterns Dizziness
Circulatory	Heart pumps with less force Arteries narrow and are less elastic Less blood flows through narrowed arteries Weakened heart has to work harder to pump blood through narrowed vessels
Respiratory	Respiratory muscles weaken Lung tissue becomes less elastic Difficulty breathing Strength for coughing decreases
Digestive	Saliva production decreases Difficulty swallowing Appetite decreases Secretion of digestive juices decreases Difficulty digesting fried and fatty foods Indigestion Loss of teeth Peristalsis decreases, causing flatulence and constipation
Urinary	Blood supply to kidneys is reduced Kidneys atrophy Kidney function decreases Urine becomes concentrated Urinary frequency, urgency, and incontinence may occur Night-time urination may occur
Reproductive Female	Menstruation stops Estrogen production decreases Ovaries and uterus decrease in size Vaginal walls become thinner, drier, and less elastic Loss of fat and elastic tissue in external genitalia Breasts are less firm
Male	Testosterone production decreases Force of ejaculation decreases Sperm count is reduced Testes are smaller Prostate gland enlarges Erections develop more slowly

Nails become thick and tough, and the feet usually have poor circulation. A nick or cut can lead to a serious infection (see Chapter 30 for a description of nail and foot care).

Dry skin is easily damaged, and it causes itching, so older adults with dry skin should avoid daily showers or tub baths. A complete bath once a week and partial baths on the other days should be enough to maintain hygiene. Wash the client's face with water only, as soap can dry the skin too much. Use mild soaps when washing the other parts of the body. Lotions, oils, and creams are often recommended to prevent drying and itching. Deodorants usually are not needed because sweat gland secretion decreases (see Chapter 29 for a discussion on hygiene). Be sure to follow the care plan for these older clients.

Older clients may complain of cold feet. Provide socks for warmth, but do not use hot-water bottles and heating pads because of the risk of burns. Fragile skin, poor circulation, and decreased sensitivity to heat can all increase the risk of burns.

Most older adults have grey or white hair, and some of them may want to colour their hair. Hair loss and thinning occur in both men and women as they age. Thinning occurs on the head, in the pubic area, and under the arms. Facial hair grows above the lips and on the chin of some older women. Decreased scalp oils lead to dry hair in older adults. Brushing helps stimulate circulation and oil production. Even though the frequency of shampooing is a matter of personal choice, shampooing should be done as often as necessary for the client's hygiene and comfort. Follow the care plan for the client regarding this.

Signs of age are often visible on a person's skin. Older adults themselves and others can see grey hair, bald patches, brown spots, wrinkles, and sagging skin, and these reminders of old age can affect an older adult's self-esteem and body image.

The Musculo-skeletal System

Muscles **atrophy** (shrink) and decrease in strength. Bones lose strength, become brittle, and break easily, so sometimes just turning in bed can cause fractures (broken bones). Vertebrae shorten, joints become stiff and painful, and hip and knee joints flex (bend) only slightly. These changes result in a gradual loss of height, loss of strength, and decreased mobility.

Activity and diet can help slow the rate of these changes, so older adults need to be as active as possible. A regular exercise program, including range-of-motion (ROM) exercises, is helpful; bathing, dressing, grooming, and other activities of daily living (ADLs) are forms of physical activity that are also helpful (see Chapter 24). In addition, an older adult's diet should be high in protein, calcium, and vitamins.

Remember, the bones of older adults can break easily, so protect these clients from injury and prevent falls (see Chapter 19). Turn and move your client gently and carefully. Some older clients need help and support to get out of bed or for walking.

The Nervous System

Aging affects the senses—hearing and vision losses may occur (see Chapter 37); the senses of taste and smell may become dull; and touch and sensitivity to pain and pressure and the ability to feel heat and cold are reduced. These changes increase the risk for injury, as the older adult may not feel pain when ill or injured, or pain may be felt by the client as only minor. Protect older clients from injury (see Chapter 19), provide skin care, check for signs of skin breakdown, and prevent pressure ulcers (see Chapters 29 and 42).

Aging affects the cells in the brain—they shrink, and blood flow to the brain is reduced. These changes affect response time, energy levels, and memory, and reflexes become slower. The client may tire more easily. Forgetfulness may occur, but it is not a normal part of aging. The reduction in blood flow to the brain may also cause dizziness, which increases the risk for falls. As a support worker, practise measures to prevent falls (see Chapter 19). Remind your older clients to rise slowly from their beds or chairs, as this helps prevent dizziness.

Sleep patterns may change with age. Many older adults have difficulty falling asleep or wake often during the night, so they may rest or nap during the day to prevent fatigue.

The Circulatory System

The heart muscle weakens with age, so the heart pumps blood through the body with less force. This may not cause problems at rest, but when activity, exercise, excitement, and illness increase the body's need for oxygen and nutrients, a weak heart may not be able to meet these needs.

In the older adult, arteries narrow and become less elastic, and less blood flows through them, causing poor circulation in many body parts. A weak heart must worker harder to pump blood through narrow vessels. Clients with severe circulatory problems need rest periods throughout the day. Their activities should not cause overexertion, so they should not walk long distances, climb many stairs, or carry heavy things. Personal care items, television controls, and other needed items should be kept close at hand.

Moderate daily exercise, however, stimulates circulatory, respiratory, digestive, and musculo-skeletal functions and helps prevent blood clots (thrombi) in the leg veins. Many older adults are able to engage in activities such as walking, biking, golf, tennis, swimming, and other forms of exercise. Active or passive ROM exercises are necessary for clients in bed rest (see Chapter 24). Follow the care plan for exercise and activity levels.

The Respiratory System

Respiratory muscles weaken with age, and lung tissue becomes less elastic. These changes may not be noticed at rest, but difficult, laboured, or painful breathing (**dyspnea;** *dys* means difficult, and *pnea* means breathing) may occur with activity. Older clients may lack the strength to cough and clear the airway of secretions, which puts them at risk for respiratory infections (such as pneumonia) and other diseases that can be life-threatening.

Normal breathing should be promoted in older clients. Heavy bed linens should not cover the client's chest because they can prevent normal chest expansion. Turning, repositioning, and deep breathing help prevent respiratory complications that can arise from continuous bed rest. Breathing is usually easier in semi-Fowler's position (see Chapter 26). As the support worker, make sure that the client is as active as possible.

The Digestive System

Changes in the digestive system due to aging include the following: (a) salivary glands produce less saliva, causing difficulty swallowing (**dysphagia**); (b) secretion of digestive juices decreases, resulting in difficulty in digesting fried and fatty foods; and (c) peristalsis decreases, so the stomach and colon empty at a slower rate, which leads to flatulence and constipation. Other physical changes, such as dulled senses of taste and smell, affect appetite and enjoyment of food. Loss of teeth and ill-fitting dentures make chewing difficult (see Chapter 27 for a discussion on diet changes that help older adults address eating and digestive problems).

The Urinary System

Kidney function declines with age. Blood flow to the kidneys is reduced and the kidneys atrophy. As a result, the removal of body wastes is less efficient, and urine is more concentrated. This is also caused by not drinking enough fluids.

Since bladder muscles weaken and the size of the bladder decreases, it is able to hold very little urine, resulting in urinary frequency or urgency. Many older adults need to urinate several times during the night. In some, urinary incontinence (the inability to control passing urine) may occur, but it is not a normal part of aging (see Chapter 31).

In older men, the prostate gland enlarges, which causes pressure on the urethra. As a result, difficulty urinating and frequent urination are common problems.

Older adults, especially women, are at risk for urinary tract infections. To avoid this, drinking adequate fluids, including water, fruit juices, and milk, is necessary. As a support worker, you should allow clients personal choice in beverages. Most fluids should be ingested before 1700 (5:00 p.m.), as this helps reduce the need to urinate during the night. Bladder control training programs may be necessary for those with urinary incontinence. However, fluids should never be restricted just to reduce the need to urinate at night (see Chapter 31 for a discussion on urinary elimination).

The Reproductive System

In older men, the hormone testosterone decreases. Since the decrease in this hormone affects physical strength, sperm production, and reproductive tissues, it has a negative impact on sexual activity. It takes longer for erection and orgasm to occur, and orgasm is weaker than in younger years. The erection is lost quickly after orgasm and the time between erections gets longer. Older men may need to have the penis stimulated for sexual arousal. These changes result in decreased frequency of sexual activity.

Mental and physical fatigue, overeating, and excessive drinking can also affect erections. Some men fear performance problems and may avoid sexual activity.

In women, menopause occurs around 50 years of age. At menopause, a woman stops menstruating, and her reproductive years come to an end. Female hormones (estrogen and progesterone) decrease, and this affects the reproductive tissues. The uterus, vagina, and external genitalia all begin to atrophy. Intercourse may be uncomfortable or painful because of thinning vaginal walls and vaginal dryness. Older women also experience changes in sexual excitement. Arousal takes longer, and the time between arousal and orgasm is longer. Orgasm is less intense, and the pre-excitement state returns more quickly.

Frequency of sexual activity decreases for many older men and women because of weakness, mental and physical fatigue, pain, chronic illness, and reduced mobility.

THE OLDER ADULT AND SEXUALITY

Love, affection, and intimacy are needed throughout life, as sexuality is part of the whole person. These needs do not disappear in older adults (Figure 17–3); they have the right, and it is normal, to be sexual and to form sexual relationships throughout their lives.

Some people are not able to have sexual intercourse, but this does not mean that they have lost their sexual needs or desires. They can express their feelings in other ways, such as hand-holding, touching, caressing, and embracing, that bring closeness and intimacy.

Members of the health care team must respect their clients' sexuality and allow and promote the meeting of sexual needs (see Box 17–1 and the *Focus on Long-Term Care: Residents' Sexual Rights* box).

CARING FOR OLDER CLIENTS

Mainstream North American culture tends to overvalue youth, and this is reflected in media messages that stress the importance of looking and acting young. There are ads for hair dyes that cover grey hair and lotions that reduce wrinkles. Greeting cards and cartoons often show older adults as grouchy, unproductive, simple, and slow.

Media images like these stereotype older adults. A **stereotype** is an overly simple or exaggerated view of a group of people. Stereotyping encourages discrimination against older adults. **Discrimination** is behaviour that treats people unfairly based on their group membership. **Ageism** is bias and discrimination against older adults. Treating all older people as boring, useless, or childlike is ageism. Remember, older adults are not all alike. Every person—young, middle-aged, or old—is unique, and every person develops and ages in his or her own way.

Older adults can think and make decisions for themselves. Failure to recognize this can make the

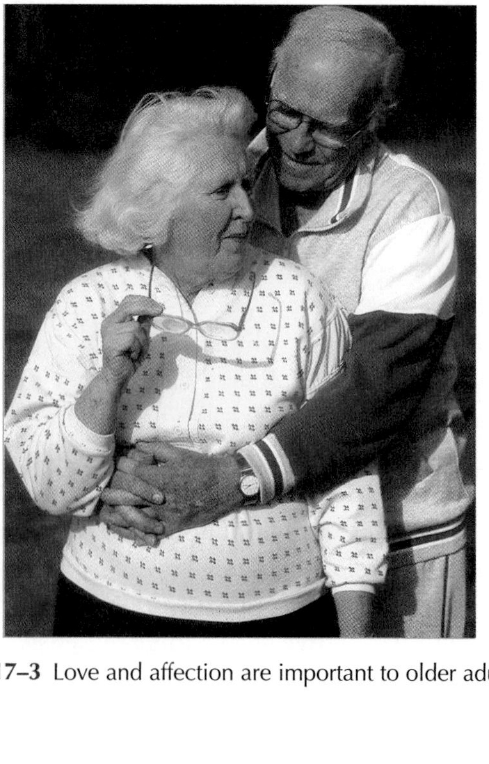

Figure 17–3 Love and affection are important to older adults.

person feel that he or she is being treated like a child. How would you feel if a younger person made decisions for you? Would you feel insulted or angry? Would you feel useless?

Box 17–1 Respecting and Promoting the Client's Sexuality

- ***Respect your client's clothing and grooming routines.*** Appearance is often an important part of sexual identity and expression. The client may want to spend extra time on grooming. Assist, as needed.
- ***Accept the client's sexual relationships.*** He or she may not share your sexual attitudes, values, practices, or standards. The older person may have a marital, premarital (before marriage), extramarital (outside marriage), or homosexual (same sex) relationship. Do not judge or gossip about relationships.
- ***Allow privacy.*** Privacy is key to sexual expression. Knock before entering the client's room, as this shows respect for privacy. It also saves you and the client possible embarrassment. Privacy is sometimes hard to find, especially in a facility. Remember the following if you work in a facility:
  - You can usually tell when two people want to be alone. If the client has a private room, close the door for privacy. It is ideal for facilities to have *Do Not Disturb* signs for doors. Let the client and partner know how much time they have alone. For example, remind them about meal times or medications. Tell other staff members to avoid disturbing the couple.
  - Consider the client's roommate. Privacy curtains provide little privacy. Arrange for privacy when the roommate is out of the room. Sometimes roommates offer to leave the room for a while. If the roommate cannot leave, the nurse should find other private areas for the client.
  - Allow privacy for masturbation. It is a normal form of sexual expression and release. Close the privacy curtain and the door. Sometimes people who are confused masturbate in public areas. Lead the person to a private area. Or distract him or her with an activity.

Treating older adults with disrespect threatens their dignity and sends the message that they are no longer useful, productive members of society. Many older people are coping with the loss of loved ones, friends, and health. Added to that, loss of dignity and self-esteem can be too much for them to bear, and they face risks of withdrawal from social contact and depression. As a support worker, by treating older clients with respect, you help them maintain emotional and social health.

To care for older clients effectively, you need to understand the emotional, social, and physical changes that occur with aging and also be aware of each client's health status and needs. Always follow the individual care plan for each older client (see the *Providing Compassionate Care: Supporting Older Clients* box).

focus on ››LONG-TERM CARE

Residents' Sexual Rights

Married couples in long-term care facilities are allowed to share the same room, if one is available. This is required in long-term care legislation (see Chapter 11). The couple has lived together for many years, and they have the right to stay together in a facility. They can share the same bed if their conditions permit.

When a sexual partner is lost through death and divorce, a resident may develop a relationship with another resident. The couple have the right to spend time together (Figure 17–4).

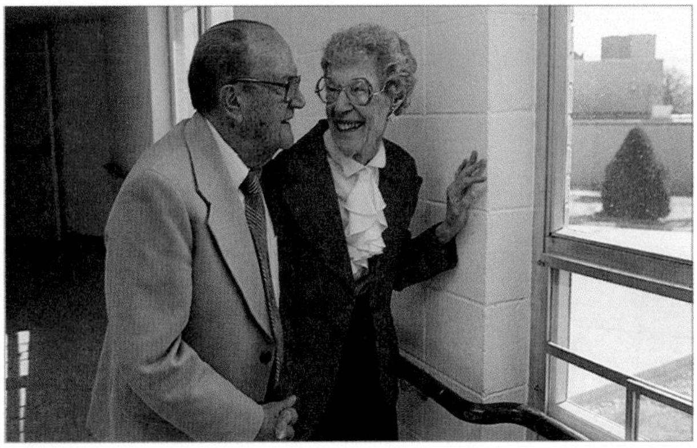

Figure 17–4 Relationships can be formed in long-term care facilities.

PROVIDING COMPASSIONATE CARE

Supporting Older Clients

- **Dignity.** Show respect for your older clients. Avoid using terms, gestures, or a tone of voice that could be considered patronizing (see Chapter 12). For example, never use the term "girl" when addressing an older female client. Some older clients find it rude to be addressed by their first names, especially by younger people. Ask your clients how they would like to be addressed. Never assume you can use a client's first name, even if you have heard your co-workers use it. Do not talk about the client with others. Do not exchange glances with co-workers when reacting to something an older client has said or done.
- **Independence.** Help the client only when necessary. Respect the client's routine. Do things in the way the client is used to doing them. Allow time for rest, and avoid rushing him or her.
- **Preferences.** Older clients have the right to make choices, so you must have their consent for all procedures. They can make decisions regarding their care and also choose when to get up and go to bed, what to wear, what activities to participate in, and what to eat. Always ask about and accommodate a client's preferences.
- **Privacy.** Provide for privacy, and keep information about the client confidential. All clients should be given privacy when they are visiting with others or using the telephone. Do not expose the client's body. Drape and screen the client during procedures. Provide for privacy during elimination.
- **Safety.** Be alert to safety hazards in the client's environment. Practise the safety measures in Chapter 17 to prevent falls, burns, poisonings, and suffocation. Apply restraints only if ordered by a physician and properly delegated.

  Older clients may not show the usual signs of infection, such as fever, pain, inflammation, and swelling (see Chapter 20). The only signs may be changes in behaviour, so observe for any changes in behaviour, including sudden confusion, urinary incontinence, a fall, or a change in mood, energy levels, or eating habits. Be aware that some older clients who are lonely and isolated are at risk for depression. Immediately report all changes in their behaviour and health to your supervisor.

REVIEW

Answers to these questions are at the bottom of the page.

Circle the BEST answer.

1. **Which of the following is a developmental task of late adulthood?**
   A. Adjusting to increased physical strength
   B. Adjusting to physical changes
   C. Seeking employment
   D. Selecting a partner

2. **Retirement usually results in:**
   A. A lower income
   B. Physical changes due to aging
   C. Less free time
   D. Financial security

3. **Changes to the skin occur with aging. Care should include the following:**
   A. Daily baths
   B. Not applying lotion
   C. Using soap daily
   D. Providing good skin care

4. **An older adult has cold feet. You should:**
   A. Provide socks
   B. Apply a hot-water bottle
   C. Soak the feet in hot water
   D. Apply a heating pad

5. **Changes occur in the musculo-skeletal system with aging. Which is true?**
   A. Bones do not become brittle.
   B. Older adults should avoid exercise.
   C. Joints become less stiff.
   D. Range-of-motion exercises help slow the rate of musculo-skeletal changes.

6. **In older adults, arteries lose their elasticity and become narrow. These changes result in:**
   A. A slower heart rate
   B. Lower blood pressure
   C. Poor circulation to many body parts
   D. Less blood in the body

7. **Mr. Steinberg, 88, has severe circulatory problems. You should do the following:**
   A. Ignore his complaints of discomfort
   B. Follow the care plan
   C. Plan physically demanding activities
   D. Allow him to carry heavy bags

8. **Respiratory changes occur with aging. Which is *true?***
   A. Heavy bed linens prevent normal chest expansion.
   B. The person is not turned and repositioned frequently.
   C. The side-lying position is best for breathing.
   D. The person should not be physically active.

9. **Older adults should avoid fried and fatty foods because of:**
   A. Decreases in saliva
   B. Ill-fitting dentures or loss of teeth
   C. Decreased amount of digestive juices
   D. A decreased sense of taste

10. **A physician orders increased fluid intake for an older client. You should:**
    A. Give most of the fluid before 1700 (5:00 p.m.)
    B. Provide mostly water
    C. Start a bladder training program
    D. Insert an indwelling urinary catheter

11. **The health care team in a long-term care facility should:**
    A. Discourage older residents from sexual expression and activity
    B. Allow and promote sexual expression and activity in older adults
    C. Expect every resident to have the same attitudes toward sex
    D. Not allow residents to masturbate, even in private

Answers: 1.B, 2.A, 3.D, 4.A, 5.D, 6.C, 7.B, 8.C, 9.C, 10.A, 11.B

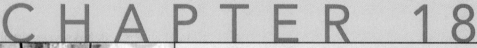

CHAPTER 18

Common Diseases and Conditions

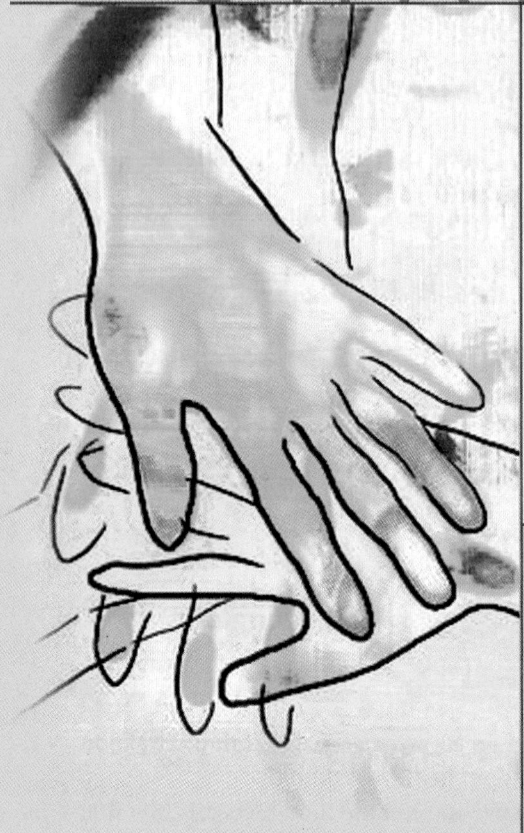

OBJECTIVES

- Define the key terms listed in this chapter.
- Describe cancer and its treatment.
- Describe common cardiovascular disorders and the care required.
- Describe common respiratory disorders and the care required.
- Describe common neurological disorders and the care required.
- Identify the causes and effects of brain and spinal cord injuries and the care required.
- Describe common musculo-skeletal disorders and the care required.
- Explain how to care for clients in casts, in traction, and with fractures.
- Describe the effects of amputation.
- Describe common endocrine disorders and the care required.
- Describe common digestive disorders and the care required.
- Describe common disorders of the integumentary system and the care required.
- Describe common urinary disorders and the care required.
- Describe common communicable diseases and the care required.

key terms

abduction Movement of a body part away from the median plane.

acquired brain injury Damage to brain tissue caused by disease, medical condition, accident, or violence.

acquired immune deficiency syndrome (AIDS) Immune system disease caused by the human immunodeficiency virus (HIV).

adduction Movement of a body part toward the median plane.

amputation The removal of all or part of an extremity.

amyotrophic lateral sclerosis (ALS) A neurological disorder that results in the loss of all muscle control but does not affect intelligence. Also known as **Lou Gehrig's disease.**

angina pectoris Chest (*pectoris*) pain (*angina*) due to ischemia, a lack of blood supply to the heart muscle that is usually caused by an obstruction or spasm of the coronary arteries because of coronary artery disease.

arrhythmia Abnormal (*a*) heart rhythm (*rhythmia*).

arthritis Joint (*arthr*) inflammation (*itis*).

arthroplasty Surgical replacement (*plasty*) of a joint (*arthro*).

asthma Respiratory disease characterized by narrowed air passages; episodes of difficulty breathing (asthma attacks) occur.

benign Noncancerous.

boil A skin disorder caused by the infection of a hair follicle. Also known as **furuncle.**

cancer A group of diseases characterized by out-of-control cell division and growth.

celiac disease A disorder of the small intestine caused by a reaction to gluten protein.

cerebral vascular accident (CVA) Stroke.

cholecystitis Inflammation of the gallbladder.

chronic obstructive pulmonary disease (COPD) A chronic lung disorder that obstructs (blocks) the airways; refers to chronic bronchitis and emphysema.

cirrhosis Chronic liver disease characterized by normal liver cells being replaced by scar tissue.

colitis Inflammation of the bowel.

communicable disease A disease caused by microbes that spread easily.

congestive heart failure (CHF) Condition occurring when the heart cannot pump blood normally; causes a buildup (congestion) of fluid in the tissues.

coronary artery disease (CAD) A condition in which the coronary arteries are narrowed or blocked.

Crohn's disease A chronic, inflammatory condition of the gastro-intestinal tract.

cyst An abnormal closed sac, which may contain air, fluids, or semi-solid material.

cystitis A bladder infection.

dermatitis Inflammation of the skin caused by direct contact with an irritating or allergy-causing substance.

diabetes A metabolic disorder characterized by hyperglycemia (high blood sugar levels) and resulting from low levels of insulin or a resistance to insulin's effect on a cellular level.

diverticulosis The condition (*osis*) of having small pouches in the colon that bulge outward (*diverticulum*).

eczema A persistent inflammatory condition of the skin that can include recurring skin rashes.

epilepsy A chronic disorder of recurring seizures.

fibromyalgia A condition associated with aching, stiffness, and fatigue in muscles, ligaments, and tendons.

fracture A broken bone.

furuncle A skin disorder caused by the infection of a hair follicle. Also called a **boil.**

gangrene A condition in which there is tissue death.

gastro-esophageal reflux disease (GERD) A disorder of the digestive system which causes heart burn.

gout A painful disease caused by the accumulation of uric acid in the cartilage of a joint.

heart attack See **myocardial infarction**.

hemiplegia Paralysis (*plegia*) of one side (*hemi*) of the body; the arm and leg, body organs, vision, the tongue, and the swallowing mechanisms on the affected side can all be compromised.

hepatitis Inflammation (*itis*) of the liver (*hepat*) caused by a viral infection.

hives (wheals) A common form of an allergic reaction that causes raised red skin welts.

key terms

Huntington's disease An inherited neurological disorder; causes uncontrolled movements, emotional disturbances, and cognitive losses.

hypertension High blood pressure.

hyperthyroidism A condition caused by an overactive thyroid gland.

hypothyroidism A condition caused by an underactive thyroid gland.

impetigo A contagious skin disorder caused by bacteria.

influenza Respiratory tract infection; the "flu."

irritable bowel syndrome (IBS) A disorder of the bowel characterized by abdominal pain and changes in bowel habits.

Lou Gehrig's disease See **amyotrophic lateral sclerosis**.

malignant Cancerous; characterized by progressive and uncontrolled growth.

metastasis The spread of cancer to other parts of the body.

multiple sclerosis (MS) Progressive neurological disease, in which nerve impulses are not sent to and from the brain in a normal manner.

myocardial infarction (MI) Death (*infarction*) of heart tissue (*myocardium*) caused by lack of oxygen to the heart. Also known as **heart attack**.

osteomyelitis Inflammation or infection of the bone.

osteoporosis A bone disorder (*osteo*) in which the bone becomes porous and brittle (*poros*).

paralysis Complete or partial loss of ability to move a limb or muscle group.

paraplegia Paralysis (*plegia*) from the waist down.

Parkinson's disease Neurological disorder in which cells in certain parts of the brain are gradually destroyed; causes tremors, muscle stiffness, slow movement, and poor balance.

phlebitis An inflammation of a vein.

pneumonia Infection of the lung tissue.

psoriasis A chronic skin disorder which affects the skin and joints. It commonly causes red scaly patches to appear on the skin.

pyelonephritis Inflammation of the pelvis or of the kidney

quadriplegia Paralysis (*plegia*) of all four (*quad*) limbs and the trunk; paralysis from the neck down.

renal calculi Kidney (*renal*) stones (*calculi*).

scabies A highly contagious skin infection caused by a mite.

scleroderma A chronic disease caused by excessive deposits of collagen in the skin or other organs.

sexually transmitted infections (STIs) Diseases that are spread by sexual contact.

stroke Sudden loss of brain function due to the disruption of blood supply to the brain. Also known as **cerebral vascular accident (CVA).**

thrombus A blood clot that forms in a blood vessel.

transient ischemic attack (TIA) A temporary interruption of blood flow in the brain.

tuberculosis (TB) A bacterial infection, usually affecting the lungs.

tumour An abnormal lump or mass caused by cells growing out of control; tumours are benign or malignant.

urinary tract infection (UTI) An infection in the urinary system.

urticaria A common form of an allergic reaction that causes raised red skin welts (**wheals**). Also known as **hives**.

wheals Raised red skin welts.

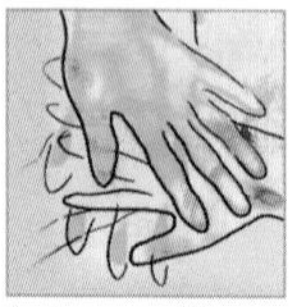

This chapter gives basic information about common diseases and conditions. While some diseases and conditions are acute, others are chronic. Many diseases are progressive—that is, they gradually get worse over time. Some clients become immobile and confined to bed, and some others have physician's orders to stay in bed. Follow the guidelines listed in Box 18–1 when caring for clients confined to bed. These measures prevent complications of bedrest.

As a support worker, understanding the disease or the health condition is important when providing care. Your supervisor gives you more information, as needed. While caring for clients, a good attitude is important. Many diseases and health conditions are very disabling or life-threatening. Be positive when with clients, and always remember the priorities of support work (see the *Providing Compassionate Care: Caring for Clients With Diseases or Conditions* box.)

A review of Chapter 14 will be helpful when you study this chapter. See Chapters 34 through 37 and Chapter 39 for descriptions of other health problems.

Box 18–1 Guidelines for Caring for Clients Confined to Bed

- Practise safety precautions. Check with your supervisor and the care plan about the use of bed rails.
- Give good skin care, as skin breakdown can occur rapidly (see Chapter 29).
- Turn and reposition the client, as directed by the care plan. The client must be repositioned at least every 2 hours.
- Keep the client in good body alignment. Use pillows, trochanter rolls, foot boards, and other devices, as needed (see Chapter 23).
- Make sure the client can call for assistance. In facilities, keep the call bell within easy reach. In private homes, stay within hearing distance or provide a tap bell, horn, or other device that helps the client call for you. Infant monitors may be used for clients to call for assistance. Answer calls for assistance promptly.
- Meet food, fluid, and elimination needs.
- Change damp, soiled, or wet linen and garments immediately.
- Straighten wrinkled linen, as needed.
- Perform range-of-motion exercises, as directed by the care plan (see Chapter 24). These and other exercises maintain muscle function and prevent contractures.
- Encourage coughing and deep breathing exercises, as directed by the care plan. These prevent respiratory complications (see Chapter 44).
- Ensure proper setup and application of specialty mattresses, such as proper inflation and positioning.

CANCER

Cells reproduce for tissue growth and repair and usually divide in an orderly and controlled way. **Cancer** is a group of diseases characterized by out-of-control cell division and growth leading to the development of a lump or mass of cells. This new growth of abnormal cells is called a **tumour**. Tumours can be **benign** (noncancerous) or **malignant** (cancerous). Benign tumours grow slowly and are contained in one area. They do not usually cause death. Malignant tumours grow rapidly and invade other tissues (Figure 18–1).

Metastasis is the spread of cancer to other body parts (Figure 18–2). Cancer cells break off from the tumour and travel to other body parts where new tumours grow. Death occurs if the cancer cannot be treated or controlled.

Cancer can occur in almost any body part. Common cancer sites are the lungs, breast, prostate, colon and rectum, uterus, urinary tract, and skin. Cancer is the second leading cause of death in Canada and occurs in all age groups.[1] *Leukemia* (a type of blood cancer) is the most common cancer in children.

The exact causes of cancer are unknown. However, certain factors contribute to its development. They include:

- A family history of cancer
- Smoking
- Alcohol abuse
- High-fat, high-calorie, low-fibre diet
- Exposure to radiation (including the sun)
- Exposure to certain chemicals (carcinogenic agents)
- Hormones
- Viruses

Treatment is most successful when the cancer is detected as early as possible. The warning signs identified by the Canadian Cancer Society are listed in Box 18–2.

Treatment depends on the type of tumour, its location and size, and whether it has spread. One or a combination of treatments is used. The treatment can be used to:

- Cure the cancer
- Keep the cancer from spreading

PROVIDING COMPASSIONATE CARE

Caring for Clients With Diseases or Conditions

- **Dignity.** The care you give impacts the client's life. While the physical support you provide is very important, clients also need emotional support, as it promotes the client's dignity. It shows that you care about the whole client, not just his or her physical needs. Remember, many clients dealing with serious health problems are coping with change, loss, and fear. Imagine what life must be like for the client. Whenever the client needs someone to talk to, being there for him or her is important. You may not have to say anything. Just be a good listener, and use touch, if appropriate. Do not avoid being near the client out of fear of getting the disease. Do not judge the client or assume that he or she "deserves" the disease. This is very important, especially in caring for clients with communicable diseases.

  Many clients with health problems rely on their spiritual faith to help them cope. Respect all expressions of spirituality. Tell your supervisor if the client asks to speak with a spiritual adviser.
- **Independence.** The more clients can do for themselves, the better off they are. Always encourage clients to do what they can for themselves. This includes even clients in advanced stages of disease.
- **Preferences.** Protect the right to personal choice. Always explain what you are going to do. The client's consent is necessary. Also, involve the client in deciding when to begin care or procedures. Always ask clients about their preferences, and respect them. If they conflict with the care plan, notify your supervisor.
- **Privacy.** Protect the client's right to privacy and confidentiality. Remember to close doors and privacy curtains before procedures. Expose only the body part involved in the procedure. Always keep your conversations private. Discuss the client's health problems only with your supervisor and the health team members involved in the client's care. Do not give information to families and visitors. Do not discuss clients with your family and friends.
- **Safety.** Clients with health problems are at high risk for falls, choking, and other accidents (see Chapter 19). Know the safety measures required for each client. Also, follow the guidelines listed in Box 18–1. Always remember to follow Standard Practices. They protect you and others.

- Slow the cancer's growth
- Relieve symptoms caused by the cancer

The three major cancer treatments are surgery, radiation therapy, and chemotherapy.

Surgery is often the first treatment if the cancer is localized (contained to one area). Malignant tissue as well as the surrounding tissue that might contain cancer cells are removed. If the tumour has not spread to other areas, surgery is more likely to be successful.

Radiation therapy destroys living cells, and, like surgery, it is used for treating localized cancers. Radiation therapy uses high-energy rays directed at the tumour to destroy cancer cells. Radiation therapy can be used alone or in combination with

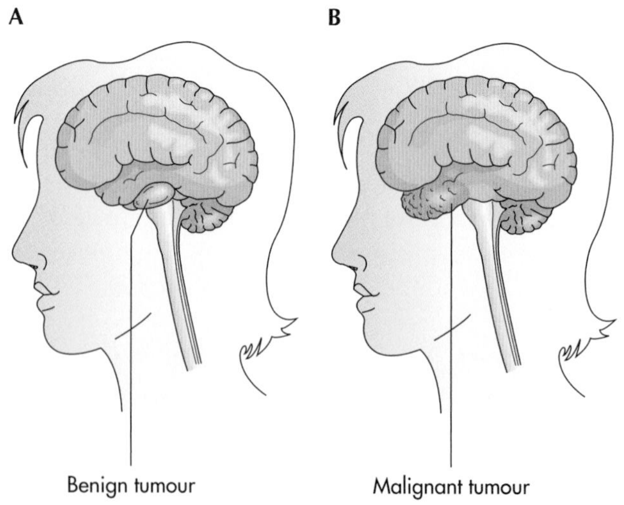

Figure 18–1 **A,** Benign tumours grow within a localized area. **B,** Malignant tumours invade other tissues.

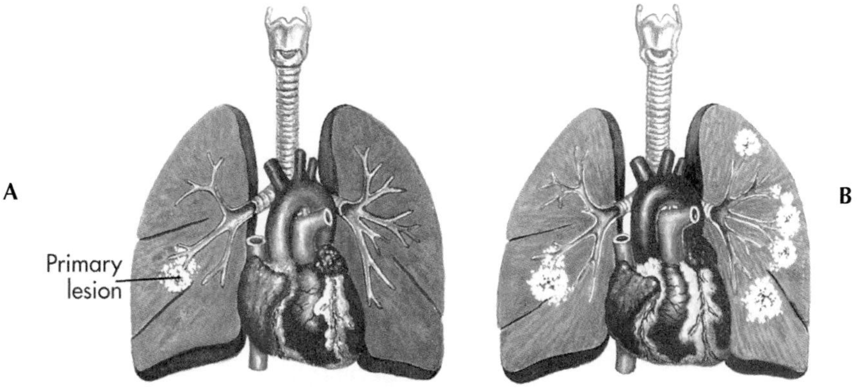

Figure 18–2 **A,** A tumour in the lung. **B,** The tumour has metastasized to the other lung.
Source: Belcher, A.E. (1992) *Cancer nursing.* St. Louis: Mosby.

surgery and chemotherapy. Treatment is usually given over a period of weeks. During treatment, normal cells are also destroyed along with cancer cells. Side effects of radiation therapy include discomfort, nausea and vomiting, fatigue (tiredness), anorexia (loss of appetite), and diarrhea. Skin breakdown can occur in the exposed area, so the physician may order special skin care procedures.

Box 18–2 Warning Signs of Cancer

- A cough that goes on for more than 2 weeks
- Blood in the stool
- Any change in bowel habits (constipation or diarrhea) that continues for more than a few days
- Indigestion that continues for more than 2 weeks
- Unexplained aches and pains that go on for more than 2 weeks
- Difficulty urinating or blood in the urine
- Unexplained bleeding of any sort
- Any lump or mass, especially in the breasts or testicles
- Any sore that does not heal
- Any new growth on the skin
- Patches of skin that bleed, itch, or become red
- Any change in the colour, shape, surface appearance, or size of moles or birthmarks

Source: Canadian Cancer Society. (2003). *When to call your doctor.* Retrieved February 15, 2007, from http://www.cancer.ca/ccs/internet/standard/0,3182,3172_13307__langId-en,00.html

Chemotherapy involves powerful drugs that kill cancer cells. These drugs can be administered orally or intravenously. Like radiation, chemotherapy affects normal cells as well as cancer cells, so side effects can be severe. The digestive tract may be irritated, and nausea, vomiting, and diarrhea may result. Some other side effects are an inflammation of the mouth (*stomatitis*) and hair loss (*alopecia*), and due to the decreased production of blood cells, the client may tire easily and is at risk for bruising, bleeding, and infection.

Clients with cancer have many needs, and their care often includes:

- Providing relief or control of the pain
- Ensuring adequate rest and exercise
- Providing fluids and good nutrition
- Preventing skin breakdown
- Preventing bowel elimination problems (constipation occurs from pain medications; diarrhea occurs from chemotherapy)
- Managing the side effects of radiation therapy and chemotherapy

The client with cancer has great emotional and social needs. Anger, fear, and depression are common in these clients. The appearance of the affected area following surgery may cause the client to feel unwhole, unattractive, or unclean. The client and family need much emotional support. Talk to the client. Do not avoid him or her because you feel uncomfortable.

INTEGUMENTARY DISORDERS

The integumentary system is the skin and its appendages, such as hair, nails, and sweat and oil glands. Many skin disorders cause discomfort to your client (also refer to Chapter 42).

Hives

Hives or **urticaria** is a relatively common form of an allergic reaction that causes raised red skin welts (**wheals**). These wheals vary in size, 5 mm (0.2 in.) or more, and cause severe itching. Hives can be caused by allergies to many things. Common allergic reactions are to foods such as shellfish or to drugs. If you observe hives on your client, report this immediately to your supervisor. Treatments may include antihistamines as well as topical application of a lotion or cream to relieve the itching. It is important to record what your client has ingested (eaten) and any substances they have been in contact with, such as powders or creams. Hives usually disappear in a matter of hours.

Dermatitis

Dermatitis is an inflammation of the skin caused by direct contact with an irritating or allergy-causing substance. Irritant dermatitis can be caused by reaction to materials such as soaps, detergents, or chemicals and usually resembles a burn. Contact dermatitis can also be caused by exposure to a material that the client has become allergic to. Some other common allergens that can cause dermatitis are poison ivy, poison oak, latex, cosmetics, perfumes, and plants. Symptoms can include itching, skin redness, skin tenderness, swelling, or warmth of the exposed area. Your role as the support worker will be to follow the care plan and ensure that further exposure to the irritant is prevented.

Eczema

Eczema is an inflammatory condition of the skin. Eczema may look different from person to person. In most cases, it is characterized by dry, red, and extremely itchy patches of skin. In other cases, it can involve papular (solid elevation of the skin) or vesicular (solid elevation of the skin containing fluid) lesions. Eczema occurs in both children and adults and often first appears in infancy. Treatment usually focuses on preventing scratching. The care plan will tell you what treatments are to be carried out. One of the most common treatments is to apply lotions or creams to keep the skin as moist as possible. Eczema is a chronic condition, and research is ongoing to find medications to control outbreaks.

Scabies

Scabies is a highly contagious skin infection caused by a mite. The mite burrows under the skin to deposit its eggs, and this causes intense, itchy skin rashes. Scabies is transmitted by skin-to-skin contact between people. Since it takes approximately 4 to 6 weeks to develop symptoms after the initial infestation, a client can be contagious for at least a month before the condition is diagnosed. This is the reason it can spread through a family or facility. The mites and burrows are difficult to see, so scabies is frequently misdiagnosed as intense itching of the skin before the papular eruptions (red, elevated area on the skin) form. Treatment usually involves a topical application to kill the mites. Some applications are repeated a week later. Ensure that you follow the manufacturer's instructions if you are carrying out the treatment. After the treatment, it is recommended to wash all material (such as bedding and clothing) that has been in contact with the infected client in the last 4 days.

Psoriasis

Psoriasis is a chronic skin disorder that causes red scaly plaques (patches) on the skin that can be found anywhere on the body. These scaly patches are areas of excessive skin production that accumulate and become inflamed. As the skin accumulates, it takes on a silvery-white appearance. The cause of psoriasis has not been identified. Stress and excessive alcohol consumption can aggravate this condition. A client suffering from psoriasis can suffer from physical discomfort, itching, and poor self-image because of the appearance of the skin. There are many types of treatments available and will be different for each client. You need to follow the care plan for the treatments of the affected areas.

Boil

A **boil** or **furuncle** is a skin disorder caused by the infection of a hair follicle, usually by *Staphylococcus* bacteria. Boils present as red, pus-filled lumps, which are painful. The most common sites for boils are the back, underarms, shoulders, thighs, and buttocks. When the boil is ready to drain or discharge the pus, a yellow or white point will appear in the middle of the boil. The care plan may include applying warm compresses to the boil, referred to as bringing it to a head. You cannot predict when the boil may break, so use Standard Precautions when providing care to the area of the boil. Your supervisor will inform you about the nursing care required when the boil drains.

Cyst

A **cyst** is an abnormal closed sac that can occur anywhere in the body. The sac may contain air, fluids, or semi-solid material and has a distinct membrane enclosing it. Once the cyst has formed, it will remain in the tissue unless it is removed by surgery or by taking medication that will dissolve the sac.

Impetigo

Impetigo is a contagious skin disorder that is caused by either *Streptococcus* or *Staphylococcus* bacteria. A cut or scratch can become infected, and the bacteria are spread by the client scratching the area and touching another part of the body. The infected area forms a crust which then drains and can spread. It is commonly found on the hands and face of children. The most common way of getting impetigo is by coming in contact with an infected person. If you are caring for a client with impetigo, use Standard Precautions when washing around the area. Encourage the client to perform frequent hand hygiene. Separate washing of the client's linens and dishes will help avoid contact with the discharge. Usual treatment of small areas is application of an antibiotic ointment. If impetigo is widespread, an oral antibiotic may be prescribed.

Skin Cancer

Skin cancer is a malignant growth on the skin, which usually develops in the epidermis and so is easily visible. The two most common types of skin cancer are basal cell carcinoma and squamous cell carcinoma and both these types are unlikely to spread to other parts of the body. The most dangerous type of skin cancer is malignant melanoma, which can be fatal if not treated early (Figure 18–3).

Basal cell carcinoma usually presents as a raised, smooth, pearly bump. It usually occurs on an area that has been exposed to the sun, such as the neck or shoulders. Small blood vessels may be seen in the tumour. Frequently, crusting and bleeding occur in

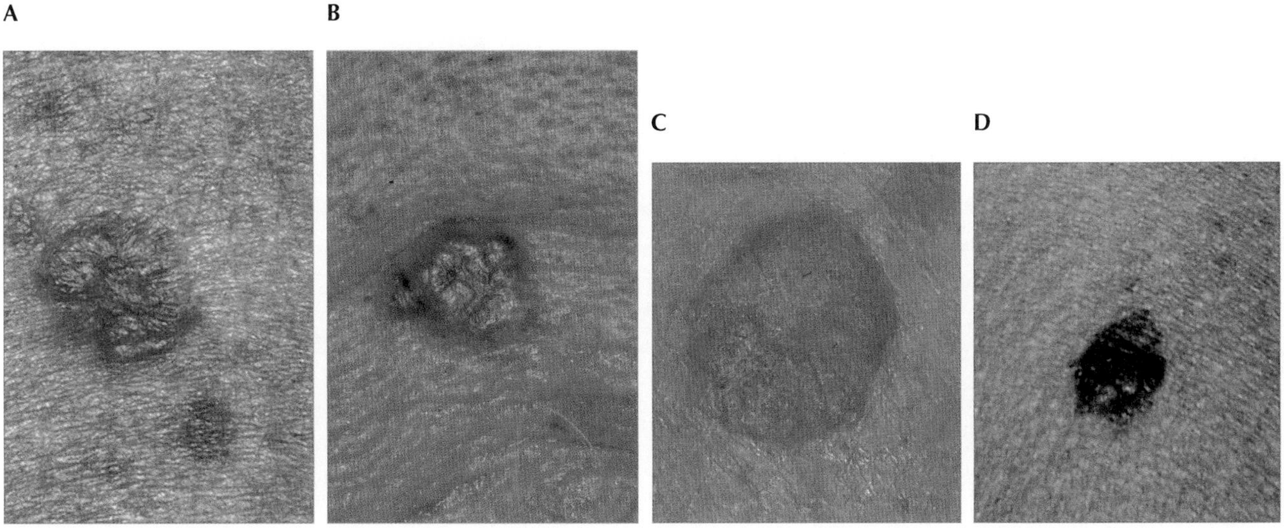

Figure 18–3 **A** and **B,** Two common presentations of basal cell carcinoma. **C,** squamous cell carcinoma. **D,** Malignant melanoma.
Source: Seidel, H.M., et al. (2003). *Mosby's Guide to physical examination* (5th ed., p. 209). St. Louis: Mosby.

the centre of the tumour, which can be mistaken for a sore that does not heal.

Squamous cell carcinoma presents as a red, scaling, thickened patch on sun-exposed skin. Bleeding and ulceration can occur. If it is not treated, it can increase in size.

Malignant melanomas are usually brown or black lesions. Any change in the size, shape, colour, or elevation of a mole can indicate a melanoma. Pain, itching, ulceration, or bleeding of an existing mole should be investigated. The appearance of a new mole during adulthood should be checked.

Treatment of skin cancer usually involves the removal of the lesion, ensuring that the edges are free of cancer cells. The lesion may be removed by surgery, radiation therapy, or cryotherapy (freezing off the lesion).

The most frequent cause of skin cancer is overexposure to the ultraviolet rays from the sun, so one should avoid excessive sun exposure. Using a broad-spectrum sunscreen will block out the harmful rays, and dermatologists recommend sunscreens with an SPF 15 or greater year-round for all skin types.

MUSCULO-SKELETAL DISORDERS

Musculo-skeletal disorders affect bones, joints, muscles, and the ability to move. Some disorders are caused by injury, and others result from aging or disease.

Fractures

A **fracture** is a break in the bone, and the tissues around the fracture, including muscles, blood vessels, nerves, and tendons, are usually injured. Fractures are open or closed (Figure 18–4). A *closed fracture* (*simple fracture*) means that the bone is broken but the skin is intact. An *open fracture* (*compound fracture*) means that the broken bone has come out through the skin.

Fractures are usually caused by falls and other accidents but can also result when bones are weakened by diseases such as cancer, alcoholism, and osteoporosis. Signs and symptoms of a fracture are:

- Limb appearing bent or out of position
- Pain
- Swelling
- Limited movement of limb or loss of function
- Bruising and colour changes in the skin at the fracture site
- Bleeding (internal or external)

To help the broken bone heal, the bone ends are brought into normal position—called *reduction*. *Closed reduction* involves moving the bone back into place, without opening the skin. *Open reduction* involves surgery—the bone is exposed and brought back into alignment. Nails, rods, pins, screws, plates, or wires are sometimes used to keep the bone in place (Figure 18–5). After reduction, the site of the fracture is immobilized, that is, movement of the bone ends is prevented by using a cast or traction (see the *Focus on Children: Fractures* box).

Cast Care. Casts are made of plaster, plastic, or fibreglass (Figure 18–6). Before applying the cast, the injured part is covered with a stockinette, which protects the skin. Casting material, which comes in rolls, is moistened and wrapped around the stockinette. Plastic and fibreglass casts dry

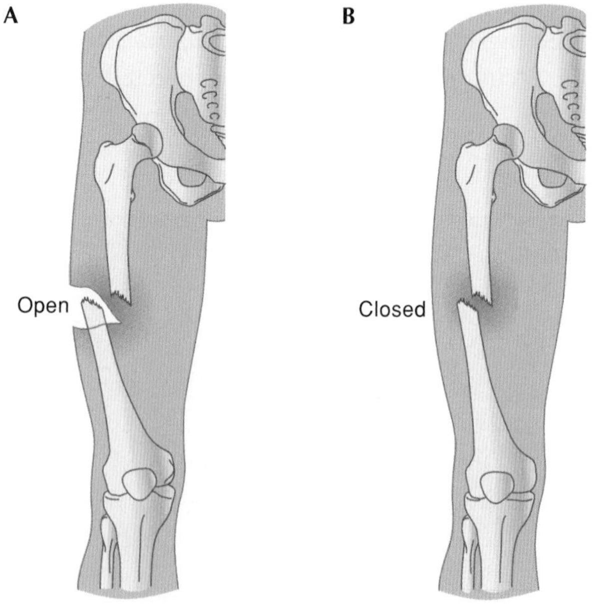

Figure 18–4 **A,** Open fracture. **B,** Closed fracture. **Source:** Thibodeau, G.A. & Patton, K.T. (2005). *The human body in health and disease* (4th ed.). St. Louis: Mosby.

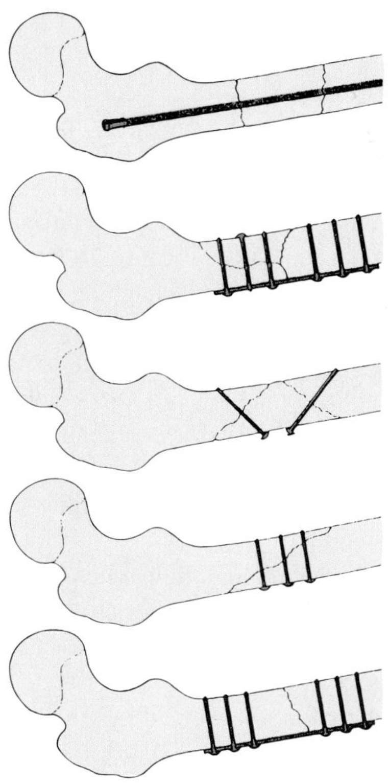

Figure 18–5 Devices used to reduce a fracture.
Source: Beare, P.G. & Myers, J.L. (1998). *Principles and practice of adult health nursing* (3rd ed.). St. Louis: Mosby.

quickly. A plaster cast dries in 24 to 48 hours. It is odourless, white, and shiny when dry. When wet, it is grey and cool and has a musty smell. Proper care

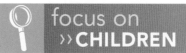

focus on
›› CHILDREN

Fractures

Falls and accidents involving motor vehicles, bicycles, skateboards, scooters, and rollerblades are common causes of fractures in children. Fractures in infants may be a sign of child abuse.

of a cast is important, and, as a support worker, you may assist with care of the cast (Box 18–3).

Traction. Traction reduces and immobilizes fractures. A steady pull from two directions keeps the bone in place. Traction is also used to prevent muscle spasms, correct or prevent deformities, and relieve pressure on a nerve. Traction is applied to the neck, arms, legs, or pelvis by using weights, ropes, and pulleys (Figure 18–10).

Skin traction is applied to the skin by using tape, a boot, or a splint an by attaching weights to the device (see Figure 18–10). *Skeletal traction* is applied directly to the bone by inserting wires or pins through the bone. For *cervical traction*, tongs are applied to the skull and weights are attached to the device.

Box 18–4 lists guidelines for caring for clients in traction.

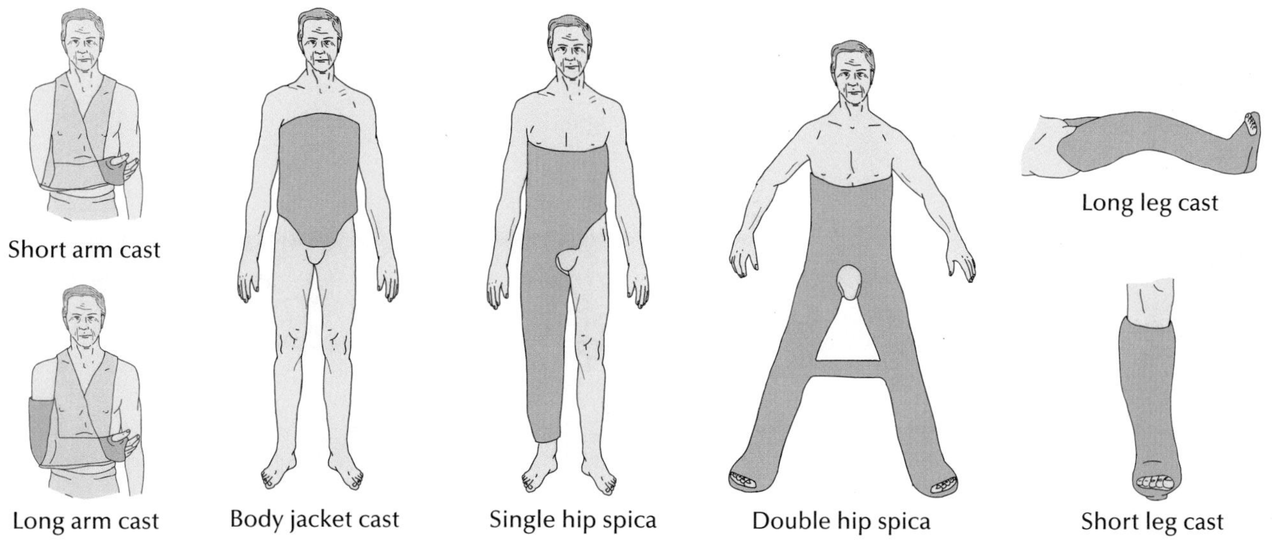

Figure 18–6 Common casts.

Box 18–3 Guidelines for Cast Care

- Do not cover the cast with blankets, plastic, or other material. A plaster cast gives off heat as it dries. Covers prevent the escape of heat. Burns can occur if the heat cannot escape.
- Turn the client periodically, as directed by the care plan. All cast surfaces are exposed to the air at one time or another. Turning promotes even drying.
- Do not place a wet cast on a hard surface because this will flatten the cast. The cast must keep its shape. Use pillows to support the entire length of the cast (Figure 18–7).
- Support a wet cast with your palms when turning and positioning the client (Figure 18–8), as fingertips can dent the cast, and the dents can cause pressure areas that can lead to skin breakdown.
- Protect the client from rough cast edges. *Petalling* involves covering the cast edges with tape (Figure 18–9). If a stockinette is used, the physician pulls it up over the cast, and secures it in place with a roll of cast material.
- Sometimes, with an open reduction, a window is cut in the cast so that the incision and healing process can be observed; the oxygen is allowed to reach the incision, which can assist in the promotion of healing. Also, demarking on the cast is often used with an open reduction to observe and assess the amount of fluid loss (bleeding) that is taking place postoperatively.
- Keep a plaster cast dry. A wet cast loses its shape. Some casts could be near the perineal area. The nurse may apply a waterproof material around the perineal area after the cast dries.
- Do not let the client insert anything into the cast. Itching under the cast will cause an intense desire to scratch. Items used for scratching (pencils, coat hangers, knitting needles, back scratchers, etc.) can open the skin, and an infection can develop. Items used for scratching can also wrinkle the stockinette or be lost in the cast, causing pressure and skin breakdown.
- Elevate the arm or leg in cast on pillows. This reduces swelling.
- Ensure you have enough help when turning and repositioning the client. Plaster casts can be heavy and awkward, and you could easily lose your balance.
- Position the client as directed by your supervisor and the care plan.
- Report these signs and symptoms immediately:
  - *Pain*—warns of a pressure ulcer, poor circulation, or nerve damage
  - *Swelling and a tight cast, numbness, pale skin, or cyanosis*—all signs of reduced blood flow to the area
  - *Numbness or inability to move fingers or toes*—a sign of pressure on a nerve
  - *Temperature changes on the skin*—cool skin means poor circulation; hot skin means inflammation
  - *Chills, fever, nausea, vomiting, odour, or drainage on or under the cast*—may signal an infection under the cast.

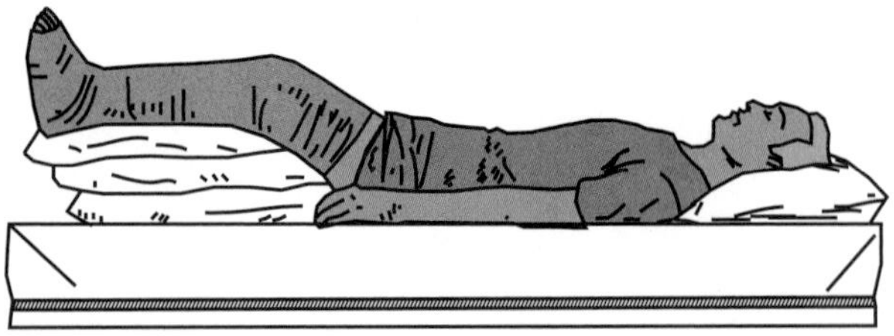

Figure 18–7 Pillows support the entire length of the wet cast. **Source:** Harkness, G.H., & Dincher, J.R. (1999). *Medical-surgical nursing: Total patient care* (10th ed.). St. Louis: Mosby.

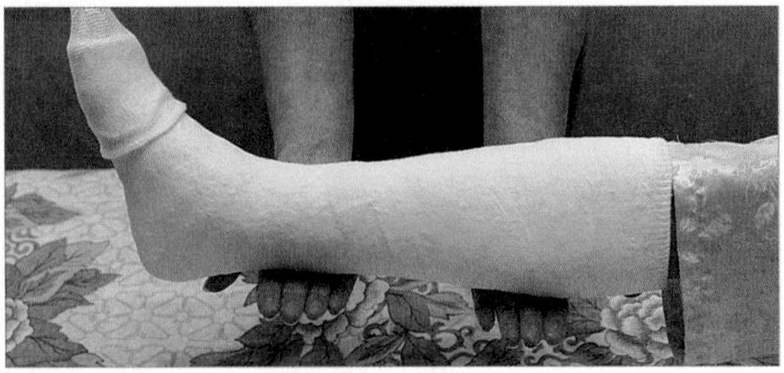

Figure 18–8 Support the cast with your palms during lifting.

A

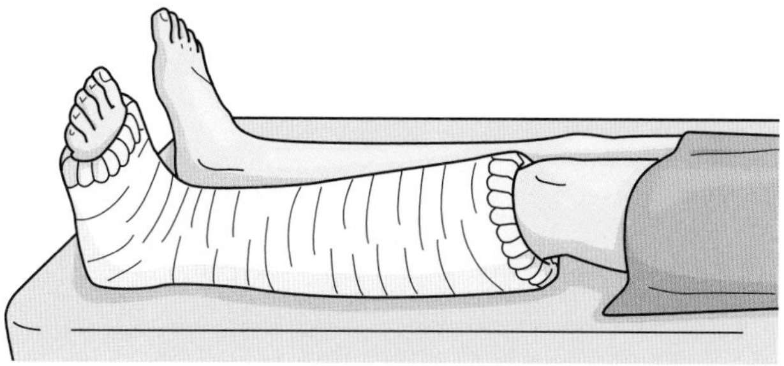

B

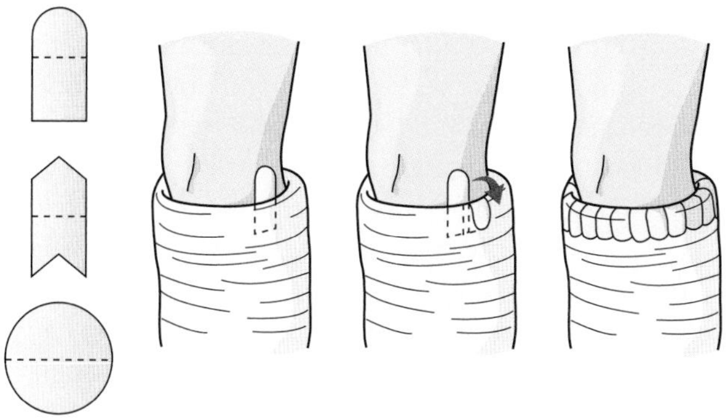

Figure 18–9 A, The edges of the cast are petalled. **B,** Pieces of tape are used to make petals. The petal is placed inside the cast and then brought over the edge.

Box 18–4 Caring for Clients in Traction

- Follow the guidelines for caring for clients confined to bed (see Box 18–1 on page 251).
- Keep the client in good alignment.
- Do not remove the traction.
- Do not touch the weights on the traction setup (Figure 18–10). You are not responsible for adding, removing, or maintaining the weights.
- Position the client as directed. Usually only the back-lying position is allowed. Slight turning is allowed with some types of traction. If the client is allowed to reposition, gently hold the weight up to allow the client to reposition and then gently allow the weight to return and hang freely without a sudden pull to the traction site, as this could result in injury to the client or to the surgical site.
- Provide the fracture pan for elimination.
- Put bottom linens on the bed from the top down. The client can use the trapeze to raise the body off the bed.
- Check pin, nail, wire, or tong sites for redness, drainage, or odours. Report any observations to your supervisor at once.
- Observe for the signs and symptoms listed under cast care (see Box 18–3 on page 258). Report these observations to your supervisor at once.

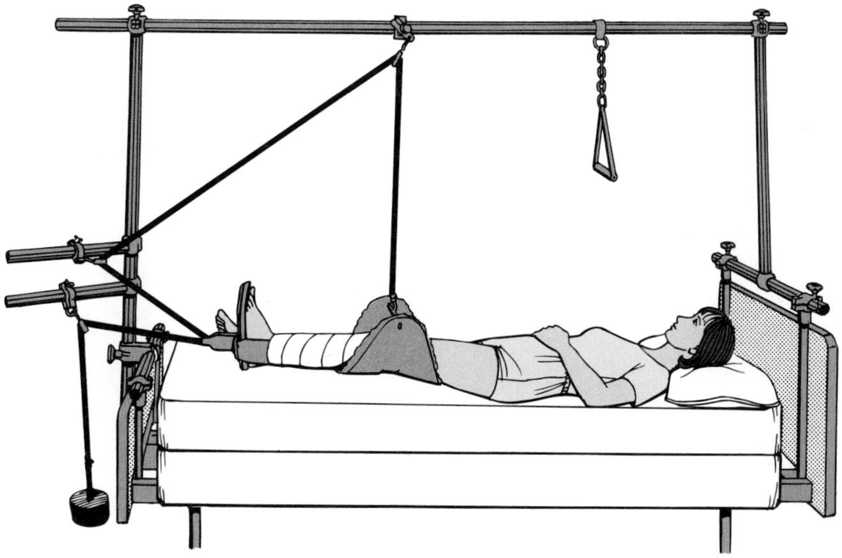

Figure 18–10 Traction setup. Note the weights, pulleys, and ropes. **Source:** Monahan, F.D. et al. (2007). *Phipps' medical-surgical nursing: Health and illness perspectives* (8th ed.). St. Louis: Mosby.

Hip Fractures. Fractured hips are common in older adults, especially in older women. They are serious because healing is slower in older people. The person is also at risk for life-threatening postoperative complications such as pneumonia, urinary tract infections, and thrombi in the leg veins, as well as pressure ulcers, constipation, and confusion.

The fractured hip is fixed in position with a pin, nail, plate, screw, or artificial hip joint. The client needs preoperative and postoperative care (see Chapter 46). Box 18–5 describes the support care required. Usually rehabilitation is needed after surgery. If home care is not possible, the client requires subacute or long-term care. Unless complications develop, the client usually returns home after successful rehabilitation (see the *Focus on Home Care: Clients Recovering From Hip Fractures* box.)

Box 18–5 Caring for Clients With Hip Fractures

- Follow the guidelines in Box 18–1 on page 251 if the client is confined to bed.
- Transfer, turn, and reposition the client, as directed. Turning and positioning depend on the type of fracture and the surgery performed. Usually the client is not positioned on the operative side.
- Keep the operated leg abducted at all times (**abduction** involves movement of a body part away from the median plane). The leg is abducted when the client is supine, being turned, or in a side-lying position (Figure 18–11, *A*). Use pillows or abductor splints, as directed (Figure 18–11, *B*).
- Prevent external rotation of the hip (turning outward). Use trochanter rolls, pillows, sandbags, or abductor splints, as directed (see Chapter 24).
- Provide range-of-motion exercises, as directed. Do not exercise the affected leg.
- Provide a straight-backed chair with armrests. The client will need a high, firm seat, so avoid placing the client in a low, soft chair.
- Position the chair on the client's unaffected side.
- Do not let the client stand on the affected leg unless allowed by the physician.
- Support and elevate the affected leg, as directed, when the client is in a chair.
- Apply elastic stockings, as directed (see Chapter 30).
- Remind the client to not cross his or her legs while seated.

focus on ››HOME CARE

Clients Recovering From Hip Fractures

The artificial hip joint can dislocate (move out of place) with **adduction**, internal rotation (turning inward), and severe hip flexion. Lying on the affected side, sitting in low seats, sitting with the legs crossed, bending from the waist, and putting on shoes and socks or stockings would involve these movements and should be avoided for 6 to 8 weeks after surgery.

An occupational therapist helps the client learn to do self-care activities, and the client uses self-help devices for dressing (see Chapter 33). The client needs a raised toilet seat for elimination and a shower chair for bathing. The client uses a pillow or abductor splint between the legs when in bed. A physiotherapist helps the client learn muscle-strengthening exercises. A walker is usually needed for walking.

A

B

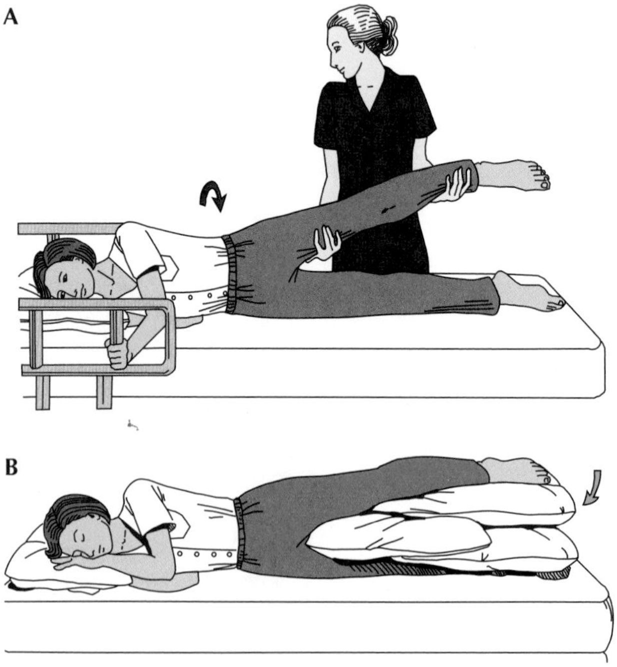

Figure 18–11 A, The hip is abducted when the client is turned. **B,** Pillows are used to maintain the hip in abduction. **Source:** Phipps, W.J., Sands, J.K., & Marek, J.F. (1999). *Medical-surgical nursing: Concepts and clinical practice* (6th ed.). St. Louis: Mosby.

Osteomyelitis

Osteomyelitis is the inflammation or infection of the bone marrow often caused by *Staphylococcus* bacteria. This can be a complication of a bone fracture or orthopedic surgery, and, if not recognized early, it can be very difficult to cure and can lead to chronic pain, loss of function, constant drainage, and even death. Osteomyelitis occurs often in the femur and tibia and more frequently in males, which could be related to a higher number of trauma injuries in them.

When working with a client with a recent fracture, you should report any acute localized pain, redness, drainage, fever, and malaise (tiredness) in the client. Treatment may include surgery to drain the area, followed by administration of antibiotics. As a support worker caring for a client with a recent fracture, you must report any symptoms which might indicate osteomyelitis.

Amputation of a Limb

An **amputation** is the removal of all or part of an extremity. While a *traumatic amputation* occurs by accident, *surgical amputation* is performed when an extremity has been so severely damaged due to a motor vehicle or other accident that it has to be removed. Amputation may also be necessary to treat or prevent disease (such as cancer) or if gangrene has occurred. **Gangrene**—a condition in which there is tissue death—is caused by infection, frostbite, burns, injuries, and circulatory disorders, all of which interfere with blood flow, thus depriving tissues of oxygen and nutrients. Poisonous substances and waste products build up in the tissues, and, as a result, the tissue dies and becomes black, cold, and shrivelled (Figure 18–12). If untreated, gangrene can spread through the body and cause death.

All or part of an upper extremity—including fingers, the hand, forearm, or entire arm—may be removed. Similarly, toes, the foot, lower leg below or above the knee or entire leg may be amputated. The client may feel that the limb is still there or may complain of pain in the amputated part. This is called *phantom limb pain*. The dominant theory for the cause of this pain is the irritation of the nerve endings in the stump, which is a normal reaction that may last only for a short time after surgery or for many years.

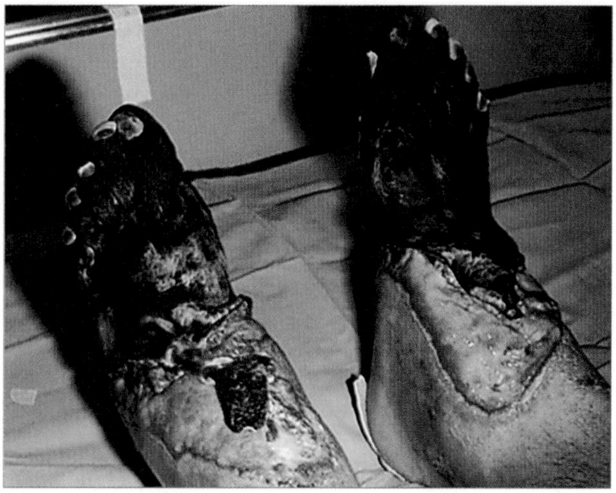

Figure 18–12 Gangrene. **Source:** Auerbach, P.S. (1995). *Wilderness medicine: Management of wilderness and environmental emergencies* (3rd ed.). St. Louis: Mosby.

The client who has undergone an amputation needs a lot of support care, since the amputation affects the client's whole life, including body image, daily activities, and work.

Prostheses. Most clients with amputations are fitted with prostheses (prosthetic devices; singular: *prosthesis*)—artificial replacements for missing body parts (Figure 18–13). A prosthesis can be made for any body part, including hand, arm, leg, eye, and breast.

For arm and leg prostheses, in order to fit the prosthesis, the stump (remaining part of the limb) is conditioned, which involves shrinking and shaping the stump into a cone shape using an elastic stocking or bandage (Figure 18–14). It is important

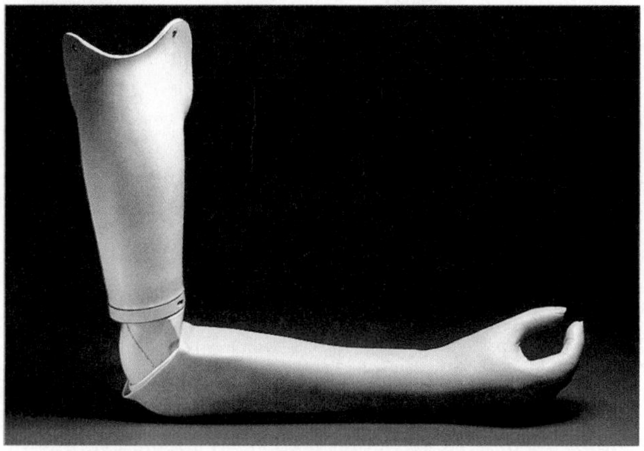

Figure 18–13 Arm prosthesis. **Courtesy:** Motion Control, Subsidiary of Fillauer, Salt Lake City, UT.

to wash the elastic stocking, as normal moisture could accumulate and cause the stocking to break down, which, in turn, would increase the possibility of breakdown of the skin or healed incision.

The client needs to exercise to strengthen the other limbs, and physiotherapists and occupational therapists help the client learn how to use the prosthesis.

Prostheses and Skin Care. Proper skin care is important for clients who have prostheses. For clients with leg or arm prostheses, the stump is confined in the prosthesis. Since the skin is not exposed to air, it may become hot and moist, and irritation, blisters, and skin infections can occur.

Follow the client's care plan. The skin at the prosthesis site requires daily skin care. Damp skin inside a prosthesis can become irritated, so usually the skin is cleaned at the end of the day to keep it thoroughly dry.

Wash the skin with warm water and soap—sometimes with medicated soaps, depending on the client's needs. Rinse the skin thoroughly with warm water to remove any soap residue, and towel dry gently. The client's care plan may call for skin lotion or cream to be applied to the entire stump area, as this keeps the skin soft and prevents skin damage.

Notify your supervisor at once if the client complains of pain at the prosthesis site. Also, report any signs of redness, swelling, or drainage at the site.

Most prostheses are washed every day with warm soapy water, rinsed well, and towel dried. Prostheses are very valuable, so do not handle them unless instructed in the care plan. Keep the prosthesis in its box or container when not in use.

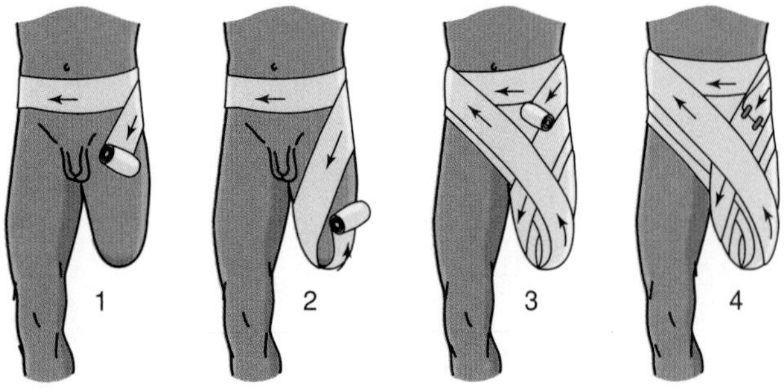

Figure 18–14 A midthigh amputation is bandaged to shrink and shape the stump. **Source:** Monahan, F.D. et al. (2007). *Phipps' medical-surgical nursing: Health and illness perspectives* (8th ed.). St. Louis: Mosby.

Osteoporosis

Osteoporosis is a bone (*osteo*) disorder in which the bone becomes porous and brittle (*porosis*) and breaks easily. Bones of the spine, hips, and wrists are affected most often, and this is common in older adults and in postmenopausal women. After menopause, the ovaries stop producing the hormone *estrogen,* which results in bone changes. Lack of dietary calcium is also a major cause of osteoporosis.

Smoking, high alcohol intake, lack of exercise, prolonged bedrest, and immobility are risk factors for osteoporosis. For bone to form properly, it must continually bear weight. If not, calcium is not absorbed, and the bone becomes porous and brittle. Back pain, gradual loss of height, and a stooped posture occur. Fractures are a great risk if the client falls or has an accident. Sometimes, bones are so brittle that the slightest activity, for example, turning in bed or getting up from a chair, can cause a fracture.

Because there is no cure for osteoporosis, prevention is important. The diet must contain enough calcium and vitamins. Estrogen is prescribed for some women after menopause. Weight-bearing exercises, for example, strength training (lifting weights), walking, jogging, dancing, and stair climbing, may also prevent osteoporosis.

Some clients with osteoporosis wear a back brace or corset or use walking aids. While you provide support care to a client, protect the client from falls and accidents. Transfer, turn, and reposition the client gently.

Arthritis

Arthritis—which means joint (*arthr*) inflammation (*itis*)—is the most common joint disease. *Inflammation* means swelling, redness, heat, and pain. Pain and decreased mobility occur in the affected joints. Clients with severe arthritis may require **arthroplasty**—surgical replacement (*plasty*) of a joint (*arthro*) to relieve pain and restore joint motion. Ankle, knee, hip, shoulder, wrist, finger, and toe joints can be removed and replaced with an artificial joint.

There are many different types of arthritis. The two most common are osteoarthritis and rheumatoid arthritis.

Osteoarthritis. *Osteoarthritis* (OA) is the most common form of arthritis, which tends to occur in people after 40 and becomes more common with increasing age. Approximately 80% of Canadians are affected by osteoarthritis by age 75.[2]

OA usually affects the weight-bearing joints—the hips, knees, ankles, and spine. However, joints in the fingers and thumbs can also be affected. In OA, cartilage (the material that cushions the ends of the bones) gradually breaks down, and eventually, the involved bones rub together, causing pain, especially when the joint is moved. In OA, joints become swollen, stiff, and painful.

Pain is often less severe in the morning and worsens during the day. Pain occurs with weight-bearing and joint motion, and severe pain can interfere with rest and sleep. The joints become stiff after the client has not moved for a period, and cold weather and dampness can also increase the symptoms.

Bones can also thicken and form growths called spurs, which change the shape of the bone and joint. Spurs called *Heberden's nodes* are common in the fingers (Figure 18–15).

OA has no cure. Treatment involves relieving pain and stiffness, and physicians often prescribe Tylenol or special arthritic medications as well as heat or cold applications. In the treatment for obese clients, weight loss and a low-fat, low-calorie diet are often advised. During the advanced stage of OA, the client may need a cane or walker. Measures to prevent falls are important, and assistance with activities of daily living is given as needed. Elevated toilet seats are helpful when there is limited range of motion in the hips and knees.

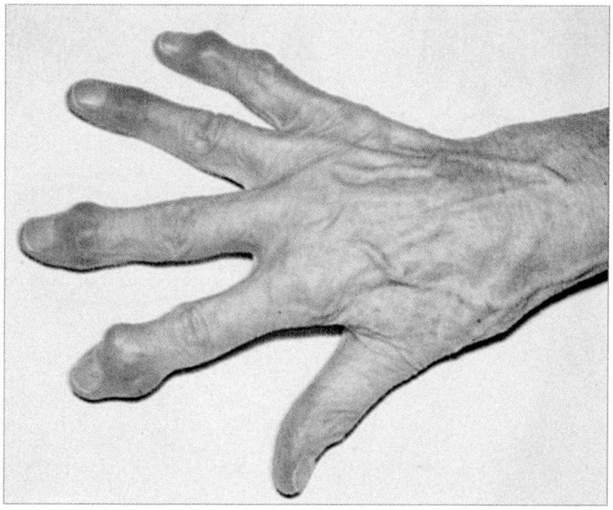

Figure 18–15 Spurs that occur in the end joints of fingers are called Heberden's nodes. **Source:** Kamal A., & Brocklehurst, J.C. (1991). *A color atlas of geriatric medicine* (2nd ed.). St. Louis: Mosby.

Rheumatoid Arthritis. *Rheumatoid arthritis* (RA) is a chronic and progressive disease that affects 1 in 100 Canadians.[3] It usually occurs in people between the ages of 25 and 50. However, RA can affect people of all ages, from toddlers to older adults, and is found to be more common in women than in men (see *Focus on Children: Arthritis* box.)

In RA, connective tissue throughout the body is affected. The immune system does not recognize the connective tissue as "normal" and attacks and destroys it. The disease can destroy connective tissue of the heart, lungs, eyes, kidneys, and skin, but it mainly affects the joints, which become painful, swollen, and stiff. RA usually starts with the smaller joints in the fingers, hands, and feet and moves on to the larger joints (wrists, elbows, and shoulders; ankles, knees, and hips). Eventually, the organs in the body also become affected by RA.

RA occurs on both sides of the body. For example, if the right wrist is involved, so is the left wrist. Fatigue and fever are common.

Pain and stiffness are usually worst when the client wakes in the morning but gradually decrease during the day. Eventually, the normal tissue is replaced by scar tissue, and deformities in the joints can develop (Figure 18–16).

Treatment goals are to maintain joint motion, control pain, and prevent deformities. Rest is

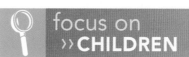

focus on
›› CHILDREN

Arthritis

When RA occurs in children, it is called *juvenile rheumatoid arthritis (JRA)*. JRA can affect the child's growth and development. Eye inflammation is another complication.

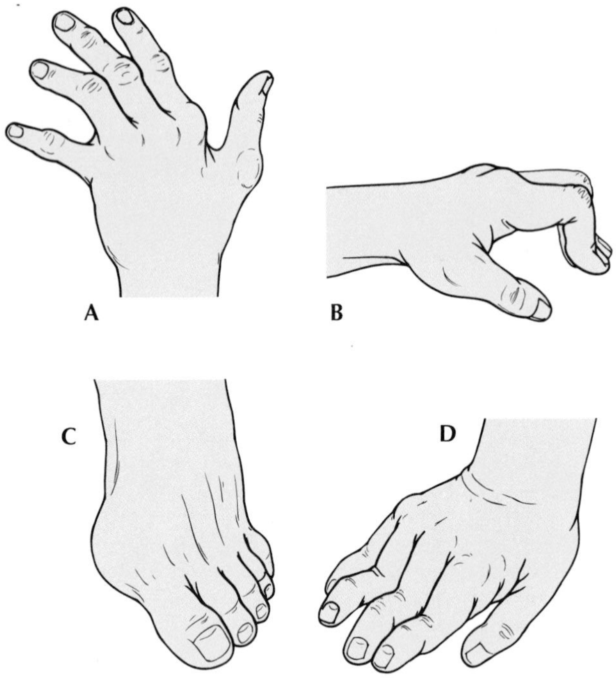

Figure 18–16 Deformities caused by rheumatoid arthritis. **Source:** Lewis, S.M., Heitkemper, M.M., & Dirkson, S.R. (2000). *Medical-surgical nursing: Assessment and management of clinical problems* (5th ed.). St. Louis: Mosby.

balanced with exercise. Adequate sleep—8 to 10 hours—is necessary each night, along with morning and afternoon rest periods. Bed rest is needed if several joints are involved and if fever is present (see Box 18–1 on page 251).

The client has to do range-of-motion (ROM) exercises. Walking aids may be needed, and splints may be applied to the affected body parts. Safety measures to prevent falls are practised. The physician prescribes medications as well as heat or cold applications for relief of pain and inflammation. Some clients may need joint replacement surgery.

Fibromyalgia. **Fibromyalgia** is a condition associated with aching, stiffness, and fatigue in muscles, ligaments, and tendons and often affects the neck, shoulders, upper back, lower back, and hips as well as the legs, knees, and feet. Because of the pain and stiffness in the affected parts, the client commonly experiences fatigue and sleep disturbances. Persistent fatigue makes even simple tasks difficult. Clients diagnosed with fibromyalgia have usually gone through many tests to rule our other disorders, and it can be very frustrating for them as there are as yet no specific tests to identify this condition. As the support worker, you need to empathize with your client and encourage them to accept the treatments indicated on the care plan.

There is no cure for fibromyalgia. Heat and cold applications, massage, and regular stretching and ROM exercises are helpful. Occupational therapy may be required, along with prescribed medications to relieve pain, relax muscles, and promote sleep.

Scleroderma. **Scleroderma** is a rare chronic disease caused by excessive deposits of collagen in the skin or other organs. There are two main types of scleroderma: (1) *Localized scleroderma* is less severe and usually affects the skin. Muscles and bones may be affected, but internal organs are not. The lesions on the skin can appear either as hard, oval, white lesions with a purple ring around them or as hard, reddish scales. (2) *Generalized scleroderma* affects the skin as well as internal organs and can cause damage to the organs. There is no cure for scleroderma, and treatment usually involves medications to soften the skin and reduce inflammation. Clients may be self-conscious because of the appearance of their skin. As the support worker, you must treat them with respect. Treatment for the affected internal organs varies depending on the damage.

Gout. **Gout,** also called metabolic arthritis, is a disease caused by the accumulation of uric acid in the cartilage of a joint, especially in the tendons. It usually affects the big toe first but can affect other joints as well. The signs and symptoms of gout include severe and sudden pain, swelling, redness, warmness, and stiffness of the joint and possibly a low-grade fever. Even simply placing a blanket over the affected area may cause severe pain to the client with gout. Treatment involves pain medication and anti-inflammatory drugs. Applying ice packs may help relieve pain. Follow the care plan.

Lupus. Lupus is a chronic autoimmune disease that can affect any part of the body. It is potentially fatal, as the body's immune system attacks healthy cells and tissues, causing inflammation and tissue damage. This can be a difficult disease to diagnose as client's symptoms can vary and be mistaken for other illnesses. One common sign is the classic butterfly rash. Other signs and symptoms will vary depending on the organs involved. Clients with lupus may have periods of illness alternating with periods of remission. Follow the care plan carefully, as each client's treatment will be different.

NERVOUS SYSTEM DISORDERS

The nervous system communicates signals between the brain and the body, so nervous system disorders affect physical and cognitive functions. *Physical functions* include tasks such as moving, touching, seeing, hearing, and controlling the bowel and bladder. *Cognitive functions* include tasks controlled by the mind (the word *cognitive* is related to knowledge), such as thinking, reasoning, understanding, remembering, learning, reading, and problem solving.

Epilepsy

Epilepsy is a chronic disorder involving recurring seizures. Temporary changes occur in the brain because of a burst of electrical energy, which results in a seizure, affecting awareness, movement, or sensations. A *seizure* (or *convulsion*) involves violent and sudden contractions or tremors of muscle groups and causes uncontrolled movements and loss of consciousness. Seizures can occur in one part of the brain or involve the whole brain. Some clients have an aura, or warning, of a seizure before it starts.

Some infants can have a single seizure caused by a very high fever. A single seizure does not mean epilepsy; seizures recur in epilepsy. Known causes of epilepsy include:

- Brain injury before, during, or after birth
- Lack of oxygen before, during, or after birth
- Problems with brain development before birth
- The mother having an injury or infection during pregnancy
- Head trauma (accidents, gun shot wounds, sports injuries, falls, blows to the head)
- Chemical imbalance
- Poor nutrition
- Brain tumour
- Childhood fevers
- Poisons, such as lead and alcohol
- Infections, such as meningitis and encephalitis
- Stroke

Children and young adults are commonly affected, but epilepsy can develop at any time during a client's life. It can occur because of any problem affecting the brain, for example, cerebral palsy, mental retardation, autism, Alzheimer's disease.

There is no cure at this time for epilepsy, but medication can control the seizures for many clients. Surgery has been used for clients suffering from severe, uncontrolled seizures. When controlled, epilepsy usually does not affect learning and activities of daily living. Activity and job limits occur only in severe cases. For example, if there are chances of a client having a seizure at any time, job choices and activities such as driving may be limited. Each province has regulations regarding driver's licenses for clients with epilepsy.

Support care of a client experiencing an epileptic seizure is simply to prevent them from self-injury. Lower the client to the floor, if possible, and move objects away from the client. You should move the client away from sharp edges, place something soft under the head, and, if possible, move the client onto the side to avoid asphyxiation (choking on vomit). If it is not possible to move the client during the seizure, put him or her in the recovery position as soon as the seizure is over. If the seizure lasts longer than 5 minutes or more seizures follow one after another, you should immediately call 911.

Never place anything in the client's mouth. It can cause injury to you or your client. Clients will not swallow their tongues but may bite them during the seizure.

After a seizure, the client may be exhausted and confused and may not be aware that a seizure has occurred. Stay with the client until he or she returns to the normal condition. You may need to help the client wash and change clothes, as some clients may vomit, void, or soil themselves during or after the seizure. Some clients will fall into a deep sleep, and some will experience a headache after a seizure.

You should record your observations—duration of the seizure, parts of the body involved, any mannerisms noted, and your client's behaviour after the seizure has stopped.

Stroke

Stroke, or **cerebral vascular accident (CVA)**, is the fourth leading cause of death in Canada and also the leading cause of nervous system disabilities in adults.

The Heart and Stroke Foundation of Canada defines **stroke** as a sudden loss of brain function. Stroke is caused by one of the following:

- An interruption of blood flow to the brain, often caused by a blood clot
- The rupture of a blood vessel in the brain

When a vessel to the brain is blocked or bursts, blood supply to a part of the brain is suddenly obstructed, and the brain cells in the affected area do not get oxygen and nutrients. This results in brain injury, and the functions controlled by that part of the brain are lost or impaired.

Temporary interruption of blood flow to the brain is called a **transient ischemic attack (TIA)**. Even though there is no permanent brain injury with TIA, it is an important warning sign, as sometimes a TIA occurs before a stroke. So a client having a TIA needs immediate medical attention.

The risk of stroke increases with age—most strokes affect people aged 65 or older. Men are at slightly higher risk than women, but more women die from stroke than do men. Risk factors other than gender include high blood pressure, smoking, diabetes, heart disease, high blood cholesterol, lack of exercise, and high alcohol intake.

Common warning signs of a stroke are listed in Box 18–6. Stroke is a medical emergency, so the client needs immediate medical attention.

If the client survives the stroke, some brain injury is likely. The injured area in the brain cannot send messages to control certain parts of the body, so normal function is affected, depending on the area of brain injury (Figure 18–17). The effects of stroke include:

- ***Hemiplegia***—paralysis (*plegia*) of one side (*hemi*) of the body; the right arm and leg or the left arm and leg could be affected
- Weakness on one side of the body
- Loss of facial muscle control
- Changing emotions (the person may cry easily, sometimes for no apparent reason)
- Difficulty swallowing (dysphagia)
- Dimmed vision or loss of vision
- Loss of ability to speak or understand others (see Chapter 36)
- Changes in sight, touch, movement, and thought
- Impaired memory
- Urinary frequency, urgency, or incontinence
- *Aphasia*—loss of speech

Box 18–6 Warning Signs of a Stroke

- Sudden weakness, numbness, or tingling in the face, arm, or leg
- Sudden loss of speech or trouble understanding speech
- Sudden vision problems, particularly in one eye
- Sudden, severe headache with no known cause
- Sudden, unexplained dizziness

Source: Heart and Stroke Foundation of Canada. *Stroke warning signs*. Retrieved on February 15, 2008, from http://ww2.heartandstroke.ca/Page.asp?ArticleID=4988&From=SubCategory&PageID=1965&Src=stroke

Following a stroke, the client's behaviour is affected. The client may forget about or ignore the weaker side due to loss of movement and feeling on that side. If vision is affected, the client may not see one side of the visual field, and this can cause the client to eat food from only one side of the plate or to read only one side of a page.

After a stroke, clients may no longer recognize familiar objects or know how to use them. Telling time may be hard for these clients, and they may not recognize people. Memory problems or difficulty learning and remembering new information are common. Clients may forget what to do or how to do it, or if they do know, their bodies may not be able to act. This makes it difficult for them to carry out activities of daily living (see Chapter 35).

Depression is common after a stroke as a result of the brain injury and also often due to illness and disability. As the support worker, encourage your

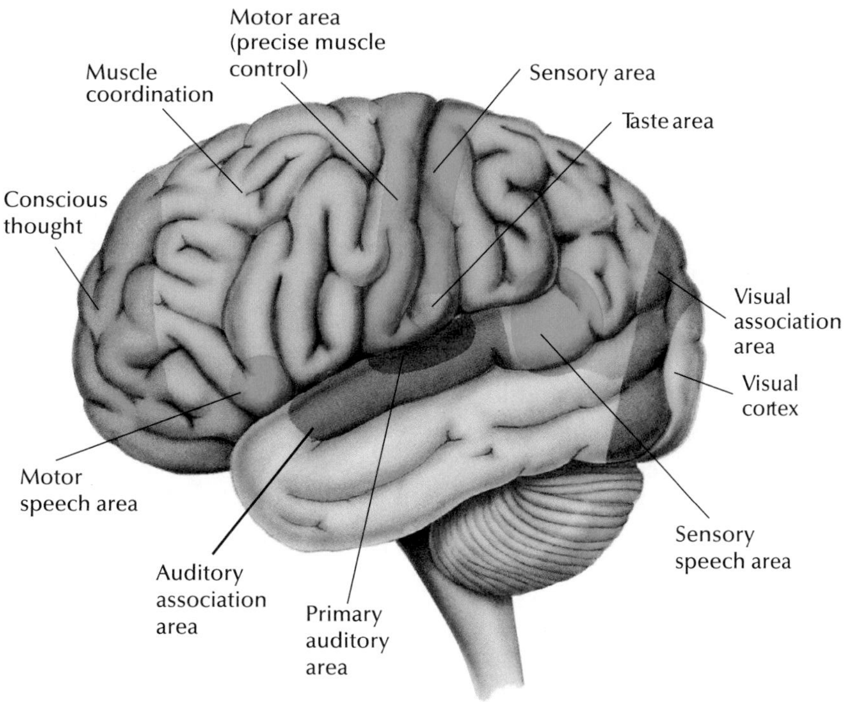

Figure 18–17 Functions lost due to a stroke depend on the area of brain injury. **Source:** Thibodeau., G.A., & Patton, K.T. (1997). *The human body in health and disease* (2nd ed.). St. Louis: Mosby.

clients to share their feelings during this difficult period. Sometimes their emotional responses may seem exaggerated or inappropriate. Outbursts of anger, moaning, laughing, or crying for little or no reason are common. Remember, these reactions are beyond the client's control, so be patient and kind with them. Report to your supervisor any changes in the client's behaviour or mood.

Rehabilitation usually starts immediately after a stroke, and many clients are able to regain or improve lost functions. Speech, physical, and occupational therapies are usually ordered by the physician. Self-help devices may be necessary (see Chapter 33), and the client may depend partially or totally on others for care. While many stroke survivors return home and require home care, some may need subacute or long-term care depending on the client's needs and condition. Many clients require assistance with activities of daily living, but they are encouraged to do as much as possible for themselves. Clients who are immobile need good skin care to prevent pressure ulcers, and they also may require a bladder or bowel control training program and range-of-motion exercises. Communication methods are established for clients with language impairments (see Chapter 36).

Acquired Brain Injuries

Acquired brain injury is damage to brain tissue caused by disease, medical condition, accident, or violence. When the head is subjected to violent forces, the brain is bashed against the skull, resulting in bleeding, swelling, and bruising of brain tissue. Brain injury can be permanent. Most acquired brain injuries are caused by motor vehicle accidents. Other common causes are falls, sports and recreational injuries, acts of violence, work-related accidents, and other nervous system injuries, for example, spinal cord injuries. Brain injury can also occur without any outward signs of physical damage, for example, when babies are shaken violently.

Some acquired brain injuries are caused by lack of oxygen to the brain due to accidents, diseases, and conditions. Lack of oxygen destroys brain cells and can cause permanent brain injury. Conditions during birth, near drowning, choking, suffocation, and stroke can cause acquired brain injury.

Signs and symptoms depend on the severity and location of the injury. Confusion, poor coordination, personality changes, headache, dizziness, fatigue, problems with vision, sensitivity to noise or light, or problems with sleep may occur. Behavioural changes include moodiness, irritability, or an inability to sit still. Cognitive problems include difficulty making decisions, problems with attention or concentration, or problems recalling simple words. Severe brain injury can result in intellectual disability, speech problems, breathing difficulties, and loss of bowel and bladder control. Rehabilitation is required (see Chapter 33) for these clients, and support care depends on their needs and abilities.

Parkinson's Disease

Parkinson's disease is a neurological disorder in which cells in certain parts of the brain are gradually destroyed. It is progressive, and as yet there is no cure. The disease is usually seen in people over 50 years of age. Signs and symptoms become worse over time. They include:

- ***Tremors***—often start in one finger and spread to the whole arm. Pill-rolling movements (rubbing of the thumb and index finger) may occur, and this may progress to tremors in the legs, jaws, and face.
- ***Stiff muscles***—stiffness in the arms, legs, neck, and trunk
- ***Masklike expression***—inability to blink or smile. A fixed stare is common.
- ***Slow movement***—a slow, shuffling walk and inability to lift up the feet.
- ***Stooped posture and impaired balance***—inability to walk, with increased risk of falls.

Other signs and symptoms that can develop over time include swallowing and chewing problems, constipation, and bowel and bladder problems. Sleep problems and depression as well as dementia—memory loss, slow thinking, and emotional changes (see Chapter 35)—can also occur. Speech changes include slurred speech, monotone, and soft speech. Some clients may talk too fast or repeat what they say.

Medications specific for Parkinson's disease along with exercise and physiotherapy are prescribed to help improve or maintain strength, posture, balance, and mobility. The client needs to have regular rest periods and avoid stress, as tiredness and stress can make the symptoms worse. The client may need help with activities of daily living. Measures to promote normal elimination are practised, and safety practices to prevent falls and choking are followed. As the support worker, treat the client with dignity and respect. Remember, the client's masklike facial expression does not show the person's true feelings.

Huntington's Disease

Huntington's disease is an inherited neurological disorder. It destroys brain cells and causes uncontrolled movements, emotional disturbances, and cognitive losses. Signs and symptoms may appear any time between the ages of 20 and 60. They begin with twitching, fidgeting, and clumsiness, and over time, the client's arms and legs constantly move, making walking impossible. The client may have difficulty eating and swallowing and is unable to perform many activities of daily living.

Clients with Huntington's disease also may have slurred speech, depression, irritability, and apathy. Cognitive losses include loss of intellectual speed, attention, and short-term memory. Concentration on intellectual tasks becomes increasingly difficult as the disease progresses. Currently, there is no cure, and there are no treatments to prevent or control the disease.

Support care depends on the client's needs. Safety practices should be followed to prevent falls, choking, and other accidents.

Multiple Sclerosis

Multiple sclerosis (MS) is a progressive neurological disease in which nerve impulses are not sent to and from the brain in a normal manner, so functions are impaired or lost.

Canadians have one of the highest rates of MS in the world, and it is the most common neurological disease affecting young adults in Canada.[4] Symptoms usually start between the ages of 20 and 40 years, with women being affected more often than men. The onset is gradual, and symptoms vary greatly from client to client. A client can also have different symptoms at different times, with conditions improving during periods of remission. Common symptoms of MS are:

- Blurred vision, double vision, or blindness
- Extreme fatigue
- Loss of balance, dizziness, difficulty walking, and clumsiness
- Muscle weakness and stiffness
- Tingling, numbness, or a burning feeling in one area of the body
- Sensitivity to heat
- Difficulty speaking
- Difficulty swallowing
- Bladder and bowel problems
- Impotence or diminished sexual arousal
- Short-term memory loss
- Difficulties concentrating
- Impaired judgement or reasoning

There is no cure as yet for MS. Support care depends on the client's needs and condition. At first, the client may need home care, especially with housekeeping, to prevent fatigue. As mobility decreases, the client depends more on others, and measures have to be taken to prevent injury and to promote bowel and bladder elimination. Eventually, the client may require long-term care. If the client is confined to bed, follow the measures in Box 18–1 on page 251.

Amyotrophic Lateral Sclerosis

Amyotrophic lateral sclerosis (**ALS**), also known as **Lou Gehrig's disease,** is a neurological disorder that leads to loss of all muscle control but does not affect intelligence. In Canada, about 3000 people are currently living with this disease,[5] which occurs most commonly between the ages of 40 and 70. ALS is a progressive disease, in which nerve cells in the brain and spinal cord are gradually destroyed.

Usually, the first sign of the disease is difficulty using the fingers and hands. The client may not be able to pick up a cup, lace shoes, pull up zippers, or do buttons. The client then has difficulty walking, and stumbling and falling are common. Eventually, all muscle control is lost, and the client is unable to speak, swallow, move, or breathe independently. Eventually death occurs.

The client is alert and can think clearly through the course of the disease. Even if your client cannot speak, remember that he or she can still understand what you and others say. The speech therapist may recommend new communication methods. Follow the care plan.

The client eventually becomes confined to bed and is usually placed in a side-lying position. Follow the guidelines for caring for clients who are confined to bed (see Box 18–1 on page 251).

Spinal Cord Injuries

The spinal cord is a pathway that allows communication between the brain and the rest of the body, so when it is damaged, the nerves cannot send messages between the brain and parts of the body, and partial or total paralysis may occur. **Paralysis** is the complete or partial loss of ability to move a body part or muscle group. Often, spinal cord injuries, most of which are permanent, are caused by motor vehicle accidents (MVAs).

Which parts of the body are paralyzed depends on where the spinal cord was injured. The higher up the spine the injury occurs, the greater is the loss of function (Figure 18–18). Spinal cord injuries at the thoracic level (chest area) or lower may cause

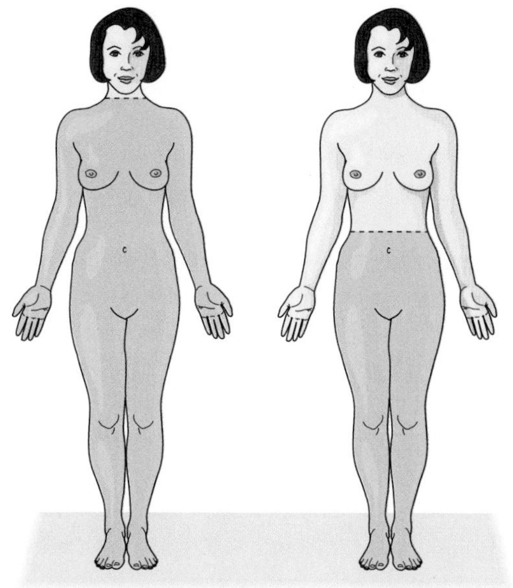

Figure 18–18 The shaded areas indicate the areas of paralysis.

paraplegia—paralysis (*plegia*) from the waist down. Injuries in the cervical region (neck) may cause **quadriplegia**—paralysis (*plegia*) of all four (*quad*) limbs and the trunk; the client is paralyzed from the neck down. Cervical traction is often necessary for these clients, and clients have a special bed that keeps the spine straight at all times.

Clients who have had recent spinal cord injuries require rehabilitation (see Chapter 33), and the rehabilitation program depends on the client's needs and remaining abilities. Paralyzed clients usually need care as listed in Box 18–7.

CARDIOVASCULAR DISORDERS

The cardiovascular system involves the heart and blood vessels. The heart pumps blood continuously through the vessels, and blood delivers oxygen, nutrients, and other substances to the body's cells and removes waste products. Cardiovascular disorders involve problems in the heart or in the blood vessels and are the leading causes of death in Canada.[6]

Box 18–7 Care of Clients With Paralysis

- Assist with activities of daily living and home management tasks. Follow the care plan.
- Prevent falls. Follow the care plan for safety measures and the use of bed rails.
- Keep the call bell within reach (in facilities). Check the client often if he or she is not able to use the call bell.
- Prevent burns by checking the temperature of the bath water, heat applications, and food.
- Turn and reposition the client at least every 2 hours. Follow the care plan.
- Maintain good alignment. Use supportive devices according to the care plan.
- Prevent pressure ulcers. Follow the care plan.
- Assist with transfers.
- Follow bowel and bladder training programs.
- Assist with range-of-motion and other exercises, as ordered by the physician.
- Assist with food and fluids, as needed. Provide self-help devices, as ordered. Feed the client, if necessary.
- Follow the client's rehabilitation plan.
- Give emotional support.

Phlebitis

Phlebitis is an inflammation of a vein. It occurs most often in the legs. Phlebitis can be caused by a bacterial infection, a chemical irritation, trauma, lupus, or a genetic condition. Signs and symptoms include redness and warmth in the area, pain, burning, and swelling. Provide support care according to the care plan.

Thrombus

A **thrombus** is a blood clot that forms in a blood vessel. If it occurs in a large blood vessel, it will decrease the blood flow through the blood vessel. If it occurs in a small blood vessel, it may completely stop the blood flow, which can result in the death of the tissue below the blockage. A thrombus can form as a result of a stroke, heart attack, deficiencies in the blood's clotting ability, or extended periods of inactivity, such as following surgery (see Chapter 46). A thrombus or a part of it may dislodge and travel through the body until it lodges in another blood vessel. A travelling blood clot is called an *embolus*, which can eventually move to the lungs and cause severe respiratory problems and death.

Encouraging your clients to keep active is very important to avoid the formation of blood clots. It is especially important to encourage leg exercises if your client is confined to bed. Follow the care plan.

Hypertension

Hypertension is abnormally high blood pressure. The systolic pressure is 140 mm Hg or higher, or the diastolic pressure is 90 mm Hg or higher (see Chapter 41). Elevated measurements must occur on two consecutive occasions to consider a diagnosis of hypertension. Risk factors identified by the Heart and Stroke Foundation of Canada are listed in Box 18–8.

Narrowed blood vessels are a common cause of hypertension because when vessels narrow, the heart has to pump with more force to move blood through the vessels. Other causes of hypertension include underlying medical problems, such as kidney disorders, head injuries, complications of pregnancy, and tumours.

Hypertension can damage other body organs. The heart may enlarge so that it can pump with more force. Blood vessels in the brain may burst and cause a stroke, and blood vessels in the eyes, kidneys, and other organs may be damaged.

At first, hypertension may not cause signs or symptoms, so many people with hypertension do not even know they have it. Usually, it is discovered when blood pressure is measured during routine checkups. Signs and symptoms develop as the disorder progresses. Headache, blurred vision, and dizziness may be reported. Complications of hypertension include stroke, heart attack, kidney (renal) failure, and blindness.

Certain medications can lower blood pressure. The client with hypertension needs to quit smoking and get enough exercise and rest. A sodium-restricted diet (low-salt diet) and, if the client is overweight, a low-calorie diet are ordered by the physician.

Box 18–8 Risk Factors for Hypertension

- *Age*—blood pressure tends to rise with age, beginning at about age 35
- *Ethnicity*—the incidence of hypertension is higher among Canadians of South Asian, Aboriginal, or African descent
- *Family history*—if a parent has hypertension, the adult child has a greater chance of also developing it. The risk increases if both parents have hypertension
- *Obesity*—the risk increases if the excess weight is stored around the abdomen
- *Diabetes*—people with diabetes are at increased risk for hypertension
- *Stress*—repeated exposure to stress may raise blood pressure levels
- *Alcohol*—excessive alcohol consumption increases blood pressure
- *Smoking*—cigarette smoking may contribute to hypertension in some people

Coronary Artery Disease

The coronary arteries are in the heart and supply the heart with oxygen- and nutrient-rich blood. **Coronary artery disease (CAD)** is a condition in which the coronary arteries are narrowed or blocked by thickening and narrowing of the artery walls—called *atherosclerosis*. This is caused by a buildup of cholesterol (a soft, waxy substance) and other fatty substances along the inside walls of the arteries (Figure 18–19). When the coronary arteries are narrowed or blocked, blood flow to the heart is slowed or stopped. The heart muscle does not get enough oxygen and nutrients and cannot work properly, which leads to chest pain and heart attack.

Risk factors for CAD include:

- Hypertension
- High blood cholesterol
- Lifestyle factors (lack of exercise, obesity, smoking, excessive alcohol, stress)
- Uncontrolled diabetes
- Age (more common in older adults)
- Gender (more common in men)
- Family history of CAD

Treatment for CAD involves reducing risk factors. Nothing can be done about the person's gender, age, and family history. However, efforts are directed at weight loss, regular exercise, quitting smoking, and a healthy diet. Controlling blood pressure and diabetes also is important.

Angina Pectoris. **Angina pectoris** means chest (*pectoris*) pain (*angina*) due to coronary artery disease. It occurs when the heart muscle does not get enough oxygen. Clients with angina are at risk for

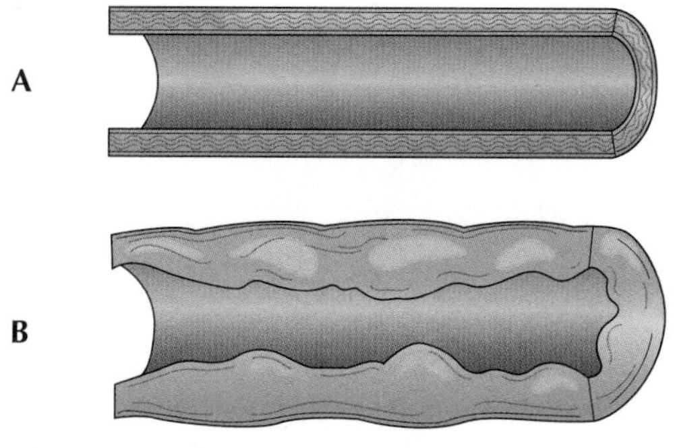

Figure 18–19 **A,** Normal artery. **B,** Fatty deposits on the walls of arteries with atherosclerosis.

a heart attack. Physical exertion is the most common trigger for angina. Other triggers include emotional stress, extreme cold or heat, heavy meals, alcohol, and smoking.

The chest pain associated with angina has been described as a feeling of heaviness, tightness, or pressure. Usually the pain occurs on the left side, and some clients feel severe pain that lasts 2 to 15 minutes. Pain may travel (radiate) to the jaw, neck, shoulders, back, and arms (Figure 18–20). Sometimes, angina is mistaken for indigestion or heartburn when felt in the upper abdominal area. Besides pain, the client may have shortness of breath, nausea, sweating, dizziness or light-headedness, fatigue, or palpitations (quick heartbeats). These signs and symptoms cause the client to stop the activity and rest. Rest often relieves the symptoms in 3 to 15 minutes, as it reduces the heart's need for oxygen. Therefore, normal blood flow is achieved and heart damage is prevented.

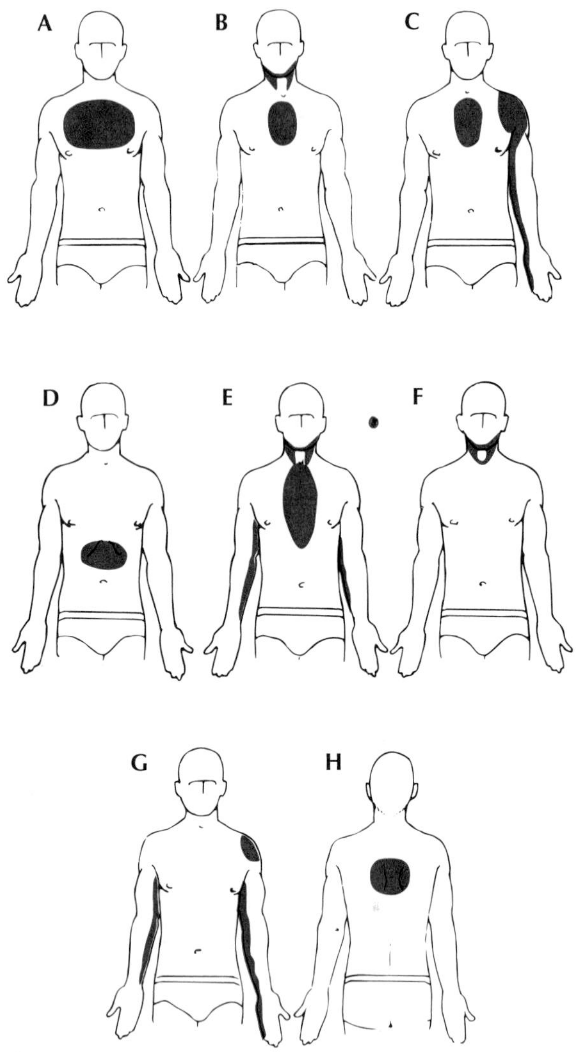

Figure 18–20 Shaded areas show where the pain of angina pectoris is located. **Source:** Phipps, W.J., Cassmeyer, V.L., Sands, J.K., & Lehman, M.K. (1995). *Medical-surgical nursing: Concepts and clinical practice* (5th ed.). St. Louis: Mosby.

Besides resting and avoiding common triggers, *nitroglycerin,* in tablet, ointment, patch, or spray form, often is prescribed to relieve angina. The client carries the medication with him or her at all times and takes a dose whenever an angina attack occurs. If a client has taken the maximum amount of nitroglycerin and there is no pain relief, call 9-1-1 and your supervisor.

Some clients need coronary artery bypass surgery. The surgery creates a bypass around the diseased part of the artery and thus increases blood flow to the heart. Many clients with angina eventually have heart attacks (myocardial infarctions).

Myocardial Infarction. A **myocardial infarction (MI)** is death (*infarction*) of heart tissue (*myocardium*) caused by lack of oxygen to the heart due to sudden interruption of blood flow to the heart. Atherosclerosis or a thrombus (blood clot) obstructs blood flow through an artery, and sudden cardiac death (*cardiac arrest*) can occur as a result. The area of damage may be small or large (Figure 18–21). Common terms for MI are **heart attack**, *coronary, coronary thrombosis,* and *coronary occlusion.*

The client has one or more of the signs and symptoms listed in Box 18–9. Often, the client denies that he or she is having an MI. The average client waits almost 5 hours before getting help; however, it must be remembered that an MI is an emergency. Efforts are directed at relieving pain, stabilizing vital signs, giving oxygen, and calming the client. Many medications need to be given as well. The client is treated in a hospital coronary care unit (CCU), which has emergency equipment and medications needed to prevent life-threatening complications.

The client is kept in the CCU for 2 to 3 days, and when stable, the client is transferred to another nursing unit. The client is allowed to increase the level of activity gradually. Medications and measures to prevent complications are continued. Rehabilitation is provided in hospital and is continued when the

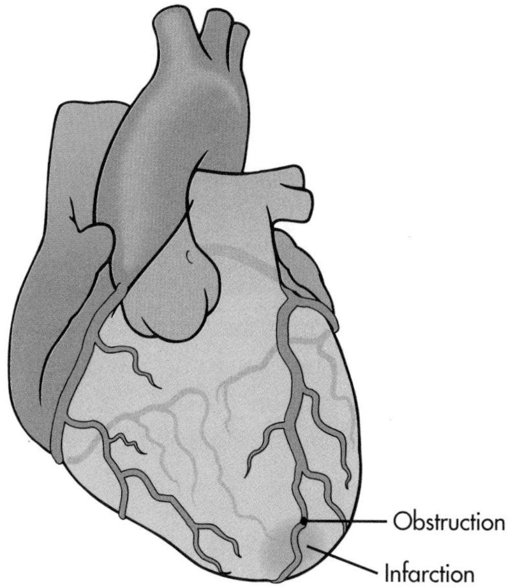

Figure 18–21 Myocardial infarction. **Source:** Lewis, S.M., Heitkemper, M.M., & Dirkson, S.R. (2000). *Medical-surgical nursing: Assessment and management of clinical problems* (5th ed.). St. Louis: Mosby.

client returns home with the goal to prevent another heart attack. The rehabilitation program includes an exercise program and teaching about medications, dietary changes, activity, and lifestyle modifications. Normal activities, including sexual activity, are increased slowly, and the client can return to work when advised by the physician.

Congestive Heart Failure

Congestive heart failure (CHF), or heart failure, occurs when the heart cannot pump blood normally. Blood backs up and causes an abnormal amount (congestion) of fluid in the tissues. CHF may affect the right side, left side, or both sides of the heart.

The right side of the heart receives blood from body tissues and pumps it into the lungs to get oxygen. With right-sided heart failure, blood backs up into the veins. Fluid collection in the body produces weight gain. The feet and ankles become swollen, and the neck veins become enlarged. The liver becomes engorged, impairing liver function. Congestion in the abdomen may cause digestive problems, including loss of appetite, abdominal pain, and (eventually) loss of weight.

The left side of the heart receives blood from the lungs and pumps it into the rest of the body. With left-sided heart failure, blood collects in the lung tissue. This results in difficulty breathing (dyspnea), increased sputum (mucus in the lungs), cough, and gurgling sounds in the lungs. Dyspnea is worse during activity and when the client is lying down, which disrupts sleep. The client may wake up with a feeling of suffocation. Fatigue and weakness in the limbs are common.

In advanced CHF, the brain may not get enough oxygen, causing confusion and behaviour changes. Poor blood flow to the kidneys results in impaired kidney function and low urine output.

CHF can be treated and controlled by medications that can strengthen the heart and reduce the amount of fluid in the body. Treatment also includes a sodium-restricted diet and administration of oxygen. Weight is measured daily to check for weight gain, an early sign of fluid buildup. Most clients with CHF prefer semi-Fowler's or Fowler's position for breathing. As a support worker, you may be involved in:

- Maintaining bed rest (see Box 18–1 on page 251)
- Measuring intake and output

Box 18–9 Signs and Symptoms of Myocardial Infarction

- Sudden, severe chest pain, usually on the left side
- Pain described as crushing, stabbing, or squeezing; most people complain of feelings of tightness, heaviness, pressure, fullness, or burning in the chest
- Pain that radiates to the neck and jaw, and down the arm or to other sites
- Pain that is more severe and lasts longer than angina
- Pain that is not relieved by rest and nitroglycerine
- Indigestion
- Shortness of breath
- Nausea or vomiting
- Dizziness
- Perspiration
- Cyanosis (bluish lips and nail beds from lack of oxygen in the blood)
- Cold and clammy skin
- Low blood pressure
- Weak and irregular pulse
- Fear and anxiety; a feeling of doom

- Measuring daily weight
- Restricting fluids, as ordered by the physician
- Assisting with transfers or ambulation
- Assisting with self-care activities
- Maintaining good positioning and body alignment according to the care plan
- Applying elastic stockings to reduce leg swelling

See *Focus on Children: CHF* and *Focus on Older Adults: CHF* boxes.

Arrhythmias

Arrhythmias are abnormal (*a*) heart rhythms (*rhythmias*). They happen when the heart's electrical system malfunctions. Sometimes heartbeats are skipped, or there are extra beats. Usually, the client's health is not affected, but some arrhythmias are more serious. They can cause dizziness, shortness of breath, fainting, or death. Sometimes, avoiding caffeine (coffee, tea, colas, and chocolate) and alcohol may prevent arrhythmias. Medications are needed for severe arrhythmias.

Pacemakers—medical devices that are implanted in the client's body—are used to treat some arrhythmias. They monitor heart rates, and when necessary, they give small electric shocks to stimulate heartbeats. Pacemakers can run on batteries for several years. Clients with pacemakers should avoid any areas or equipment that have strong electrical or magnetic fields.

focus on ›› CHILDREN

CHF

Congenital heart defects can cause congestive heart failure in children. (Congenital comes from the Latin word *congenitus,* meaning *to be born with.*)

focus on ›› OLDER ADULTS

CHF

Many older adults who have CHF may need home care or long-term care. The older adult is at risk for skin breakdown. Tissue swelling, poor circulation, and fragile skin combine to increase the risk of pressure ulcers. Good skin care and regular position changes are essential.

RESPIRATORY DISORDERS

The respiratory system is made up of the lungs and their airways. The airways bring oxygen into the lungs and remove carbon dioxide from the body. Respiratory disorders interfere with this function and threaten life.

Asthma

In **asthma,** a respiratory disease characterized by narrowed air passages, sudden episodes of breathing difficulties (asthma attacks) occur. The client becomes short of breath, produces wheezing sounds, and may be very frightened. The client may also have a rapid pulse, perspiration, and cyanosis. Allergies, exercise, cold air, and emotional stress are common causes of asthma attacks.

Medications are used to treat asthma, but sometimes emergency room treatment may be necessary for severe attacks. The client and family are taught how to prevent asthma attacks, as repeated attacks can damage the respiratory system.

Pneumonia

Pneumonia is an infection of the lung tissue. Alveoli (tiny air sacs within the lungs) in the affected area fill with pus, mucus, and other liquid, and oxygen and carbon dioxide are not exchanged properly, causing insufficient oxygen in the blood.

Bacteria and viruses cause pneumonia, and clients who are immobile or who aspirate are at higher risk for developing it. The onset can be gradual or sudden. Signs and symptoms include: shaking, chills, severe chest pain, a cough that produces rust-coloured or greenish sputum, high temperature, rapid breathing and pulse rate, cyanosis, and confusion. While providing support care, follow Standard Practices. Isolation Precautions may also be ordered by the physician to prevent the spread of pneumonia.

Bronchitis

Acute *bronchitis* is inflammation of the bronchi caused by bacteria or viruses and can last for several days or weeks. Chronic bronchitis is not generally caused by a virus (see COPD below).

A client with acute bronchitis usually has a cough that produces sputum (phlegm). The colour of the sputum will tell if the infection is viral or bacterial. Fever, fatigue, shortness of breath, and chest pain may accompany the cough. Antibiotics are used to treat bacterial bronchitis, and viral bronchitis will usually disappear on its own. While providing support care to a client, if you observe blood-tinged sputum, report it immediately to your supervisor.

Chronic Obstructive Pulmonary Disease

Chronic obstructive pulmonary disease (COPD) is the fourth leading cause of death among Canadian men and the seventh among Canadian women.[7] It is a chronic lung disorder that obstructs (blocks) the airways and makes breathing difficult. COPD refers to chronic bronchitis and emphysema, which often occur together. COPD is a progressive disease, gradually worsening over time.

Smoking is the most common cause of COPD. Long-time exposure to chemical fumes and to certain dusts is another cause.

COPD cannot be cured but can be controlled. The client must quit smoking and avoid second-hand smoke. Medications to open the airways are usually delivered by metered dose inhalers, or "puffers" (see Chapter 40). Breathing exercises and oxygen therapy may also be ordered. Fluid intake is encouraged to decrease the thickness of secretions, and efforts are made to prevent respiratory tract infections. If one occurs, prompt treatment is necessary.

Chronic Bronchitis. Chronic bronchitis is a chronic inflammation of the bronchi, the large airway passages entering the lungs. Large amounts of mucus are produced in the bronchi, and the bronchial walls swell. The mucus is thick and difficult to cough up, so it cannot be cleared completely and thus obstructs the airways. This makes airflow into and out of the lungs difficult. Therefore, the body cannot get normal amounts of oxygen. The excess mucus also provides a place for the growth of microbes, so infection is a risk. Coughing is the first and most common symptom of chronic bronchitis. The client also has difficulty breathing and tires easily. Eventually, breathing becomes difficult even when the client is resting.

Emphysema. Emphysema occurs when the walls of the alveoli are damaged and become less elastic than normal. They do not expand and shrink normally when the client inhales and exhales, and as a result, when the client breathes out, air is trapped in some of the alveoli and not exhaled. As the disease progresses, more alveoli become involved and more air is trapped. The normal exchange of oxygen and carbon dioxide cannot occur in affected alveoli. As more air is trapped in the lungs, the person develops a *barrel chest* (Figure 18–22).

Breathing is very difficult for people with emphysema. Sometimes they lose weight because eating is difficult when they are out of breath. Clients with emphysema usually prefer to sit upright and slightly forward, as breathing is easier in this position.

Treatments include:

- Antibiotics to fight infection
- Medications to ease chest pain, cough, and fever
- Proper diet
- Proper fluid and hydration
- Fowler's or semi-Fowler's position to make breathing easier
- Oxygen therapy

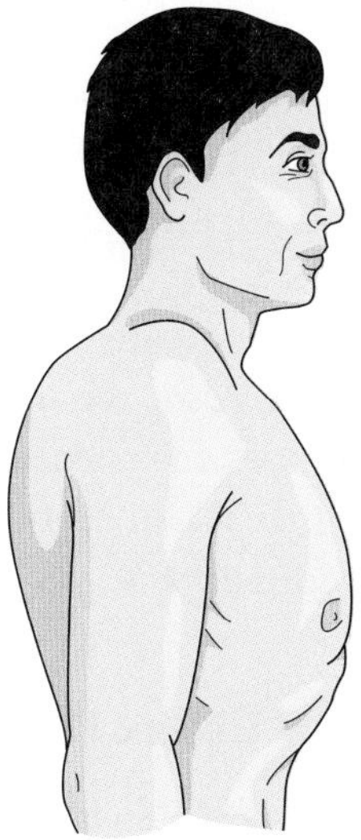

Figure 18–22 Barrel chest due to emphysema.

DIGESTIVE DISORDERS

The digestive system breaks down food for absorption by the body and also eliminates solid wastes. See Chapter 32 for a discussion on some digestive disorders—diarrhea, constipation, flatulence, and fecal incontinence—and the support care for clients with ostomy pouches.

Vomiting

Vomiting is the act of expelling stomach contents through the mouth and signals illness or injury that can be life-threatening. The vomitus (material vomited) can be aspirated (inhaled into the lungs) and obstruct the airway. Vomiting large amounts of blood can lead to shock. The following measures are practised when a client vomits:

- Follow Standard Precautions.
- Turn the client's head well to one side. This prevents aspiration.
- Place a kidney basin or other container under the client's chin.
- Remove the vomitus from the client's immediate environment.
- Provide oral hygiene. This helps remove the taste of vomitus.
- Eliminate odours.
- Change linens or client's clothing, as necessary.
- Observe vomitus for colour, odour, and undigested food. Vomitus that looks like coffee grounds contains digested blood. This indicates internal bleeding and must be reported immediately.
- Estimate the amount of vomitus. For example, is it about a cupful or a plateful? Some facilities may require you to measure and record the amount of vomitus.
- Report immediately to your supervisor that the client has vomited. Also, report your observations. Some facilities may require you to save the vomitus so that it can be observed or sent to a laboratory for analysis.

Gastro-esophageal Reflux Disease (GERD)

GERD is a common disorder of unknown cause. The muscle band at the end of the esophagus and the start of the stomach relaxes at inappropriate times, and this allows the stomach acids to go up the esophagus. Clients refer to this as "heart burn," which is the most common symptom of GERD. Other symptoms include a sour taste in the mouth, bad breath, belching, and difficulty or pain when swallowing. Treatment usually involves medication.

Gallbladder Disease

The *gallbladder* is a pear-shaped sac that stores bile (see Chapter 14). For reasons not known yet, the components of bile often form stones in the gallbladder, which can cause inflammation, called **cholecystitis.** Stones can obstruct the flow of bile into the digestive system. Symptoms of cholecystitis include severe pain in the abdomen, nausea, vomiting, and, in some cases, jaundice. Treatment may include surgery and a low-fat diet.

Liver Disease

The liver plays an important part in carbohydrate and protein metabolism and produces bile. Two of the most common disorders of the liver are **hepatitis** and **cirrhosis.**

Hepatitis is inflammation of the liver caused by a group of viruses—hepatitis A to hepatitis G—that are responsible for most of the liver damage. Hepatitis can also be caused by toxins such as alcohol or drugs, other infections, or a metabolic disorder (see pages 282–283 for a discussion on communicable hepatitis diseases).

Cirrhosis occurs as a result of chronic liver disease. Liver tissue is gradually replaced by scar tissue, which affects liver function. This is most commonly caused by alcoholism and hepatitis C virus. There is no cure for cirrhosis, but treatment can halt further damage. Some signs and symptoms are weight loss, jaundice, enlarged liver, fatigue, and accumulation of fluid in the abdomen.

Celiac Disease

Celiac disease is a disorder of the small intestine caused by a reaction to gluten protein found in wheat. This disorder can occur in all ages, after early infancy. Symptoms can included diarrhea, failure to thrive (in children), weight loss, and fatigue. Diarrhea is usually large in volume, foul smelling, and pale in colour. The only effective treatment is a gluten-free diet. As the support worker, you must ensure that you follow the care plan regarding your client's diet. Since many foods can contain small traces of gluten, accurate reporting of foods that cause symptoms can help identify foods to be avoided by the client.

Irritable Bowel Syndrome (IBS)

Irritable bowel syndrome (IBS) is a disorder of the bowel characterized by abdominal pain and changes in bowel habits. The two main types of IBS are (1) IBS with diarrhea, and (2) IBS with constipation. A client suffering from IBS with diarrhea often has abdominal bloating, urgency, and frequent loose and watery stools that sometimes contain mucus. IBS with constipation can also cause abdominal bloating. The client's stools are hard or lumpy, and clients frequently need to strain during bowel movement and have the feeling of incomplete bowel emptying. Abdominal pain, which can be quite severe, is usually relieved after bowel movement.

The cause of IBS is not known as yet. Stress is thought to trigger episodes. Treatment will vary depending on which type of IBS the client is diagnosed with. Medication for IBS with diarrhea would consist of antidiarrheals, and medications for IBS with constipation would consist of stool softeners or laxatives. For some clients, avoiding nonsoluble fibrous foods can help control episodes.

Compassion is required when caring for a client with IBS, since the disease can be quite stressful and embarrassing. You may be asked to record the dietary intake of your client in order to determine which foods trigger episodes.

Colitis

Colitis is inflammation of the colon. Signs and symptoms of colitis include fever, pain, abdominal tenderness, rectal bleeding, and ulcerations in the colon. Treatment may include antibiotics and anti-inflammatory drugs. A reduction in the intake of carbohydrates has helped some clients. Surgery may be required to remove the affected part of the colon.

Crohn's Disease

Crohn's disease is a chronic, inflammatory condition of the gastro-intestinal tract, characterized by flare-ups and periods of remission. It can affect all age groups, as there is no exact cause for this disorder. Any part of the gastro-intestinal system can be affected, but it most commonly affects the last part of the small intestine and the large intestine. Symptoms can vary depending on the area affected. The most common symptoms are abdominal pain, diarrhea, and weight loss. Some clients have episodes of bloody diarrhea and can have as many as 20 bowel movements in a day. Bowel obstructions can occur due to the narrowing of the intestines from the chronic inflammation.

Crohn's disease can affect other body systems, and some of these complications include skin rashes, arthritis, eye inflammation, mouth ulcers, and anemia.

Treatment for a flare-up usually involves medications to reduce inflammation and infection if present. During remission, the goal of treatment is to build up the client's physical and mental ability to cope with the next flare-up when it occurs. There is no cure for Crohn's disease, which is difficult for clients to accept.

Crohn's disease affects each client differently, depending on the areas of the bowel and other body systems affected. Your observations, recording, and reporting are very important to help your client during a flare-up. For example, if your client vomits, it could mean a bowel obstruction; if your client complains of pain around the anus, it could indicate an inflammation or start of an abscess; and if there is joint pain, it could be the start of the arthritis associated with Crohn's disease.

It is very important to record the colour and approximate volume of each bowel movement and to describe if blood is visible. During flare-ups clients can lose weight because of decreased food intake and malabsorption. They may hesitate to eat, fearful of more bouts of diarrhea. Follow the care plan for dietary intake.

Diverticular Disease

In many clients, small pouches develop and bulge outward through weak spots in the colon (Figure 18–23). Each pouch is called a *diverticulum.* (*Diverticulare* means *to turn inside out.*) The condition of having these pouches is called **diverticulosis.** (*Osis* means *condition of.*)

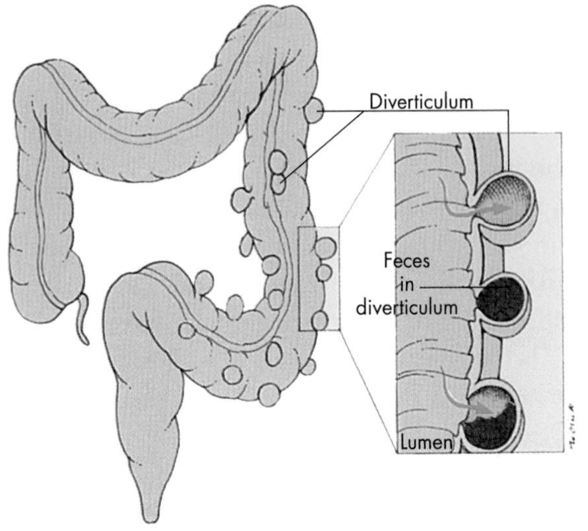

Figure 18–23 Diverticular disease.

Diverticular disease is very common in older adults. A low-fibre diet and constipation are risk factors.

When feces enter the pouches, the pouches can become inflamed and infected—which is called *diverticulitis* (*itis* means *inflammation*). The client has abdominal pain and tenderness on the lower left side of the abdomen. Fever, nausea and vomiting, chills, cramping, and constipation are likely. Bloating, rectal bleeding, frequent urination, and pain while urinating can also occur.

In case of a ruptured pouch, which is a rare complication, feces spill out into the abdomen, leading to a severe, life-threatening infection. A pouch also can cause a block in the intestine (intestinal obstruction), and feces and gas cannot move past the blocked part. These problems require surgery.

The physician orders dietary changes as well as antibiotics in some cases. Surgery is needed for severe disease, obstruction, and ruptured pouches, and the diseased part of the bowel is removed. Sometimes a colostomy is necessary (see Chapter 32).

URINARY DISORDERS

The kidneys, ureters, bladder, and urethra are the major structures of the urinary system. Disorders can occur in one or more of these structures.

Urinary Tract Infections

Urinary tract infections (UTIs) are common, and infection in one area of the urinary system can lead to infection of the entire urinary system.

Normally, the urinary system is sterile and has no microbes. However, microbes can enter the system through the urethra. Catheterization, urological examinations, sexual intercourse, poor perineal hygiene, incomplete bladder emptying, and poor fluid intake are common causes of UTIs. UTI is frequently acquired in health care settings.

Women are at high risk because microbes can easily enter the short urethra. Prostate gland secretions help protect men from UTIs. However, an enlarged prostate increases the risk of a UTI, so older men are at risk.

Cystitis is inflammation (*itis*) of the bladder (*cyst*). **Pyelonephritis** is inflammation (*itis*) of the pelvis (*pyelo*) or kidney (*nephr*). Infection is the most common cause of the inflammation. Signs and symptoms are:

- Urinary frequency and urgency
- Oliguria—scant (*olig*) urine (*uria*)
- Dysuria—difficult or painful (*dys*) urination (*uria*)
- Pain or burning during urination
- Foul-smelling urine
- Hematuria—blood (*hemat*) in the urine (*uria*)
- Pyria—pus (*py*) in the urine (*uria*)
- Fever and chills
- Pain in the lower abdomen or back

Treatment includes antibiotics and increased fluid intake—usually 2000 mL/day.

Renal Calculi

Renal calculi are kidney (*renal*) stones (*calculi*). Caucasian (white) men between the ages of 20 and 40 years are at greatest risk. Prolonged bed rest, immobility, and poor fluid intake are risk factors. Stones vary in size. Signs and symptoms include:

- Severe, cramping pain in the back and side, just below the ribs
- Pain in the abdomen, thigh, and urethra
- Nausea and vomiting

- Fever and chills
- Urinary frequency and urgency
- Oliguria—scant (*olig*) urine (*uria*)
- Dysuria—difficult or painful (*dys*) urination (*uria*)
- Hematuria—blood (*hemat*) in the urine (*uria*)
- Foul-smelling urine

Treatment involves providing pain relief and encouraging increased intake of fluids. The client needs to drink about 2000 to 3000 mL of fluid a day. Increased fluids cause stones to pass through excretion of the urine, and all urine is strained (see Chapter 31). Surgical removal of the stones may be necessary. Some dietary changes can prevent further formation of stones.

Renal Failure

Renal failure (kidney failure) occurs when the kidneys do not function or are severely impaired. Waste products are not removed from the blood, and the body retains fluids. As fluids build up in the bloodstream, the client may have puffy and swollen face, hands, and feet, and hypertension and congestive heart failure can result. Renal failure can be acute or chronic.

Acute Renal Failure. *Acute renal failure* occurs suddenly after severely decreased blood flow to the kidneys caused by severe bleeding, heart attack, congestive heart failure, burns, infections, or severe allergic reactions.

Acute renal failure is usually a temporary condition. With treatment, the client can be cured with no permanent damage to the kidneys. However, this is a very serious condition, as it can result in death.

Acute renal failure occurs in phases. At first *oliguria* (scant amount of urine) occurs, when urine output is less than 400 mL in 24 hours. This phase lasts a few days to 2 weeks. Then *diuresis*—the process (*esis*) of passing (*di*) urine (*uria*)—occurs, when large amounts of urine are produced, about 1000 to 5000 mL/day. Kidney function improves and returns to normal during the recovery phase. This can take from 1 month to 1 year. However, some people do not recover and develop chronic renal failure.

The physician orders medications, restricted fluids, and diet therapy. The care plan will likely include:

- Measuring and recording urine output every hour; an output of less than 30 mL/hr should be reported immediately
- Measuring and recording intake and output of fluid
- Restricting fluid intake
- Daily weight measurements using the same scale
- Frequent oral hygiene
- Measures to take if the client is confined to bed (see Box 18–1 on page 251)
- Measures to prevent infection

Chronic Renal Failure. In *chronic renal failure*, the kidneys cannot meet the body's needs. Nephrons of the kidneys are destroyed over many years. Hypertension and diabetes are common causes; some others are infections, urinary tract obstructions, and tumours.

Signs and symptoms appear when 80 to 90% of kidney function has been lost. A few of the many signs and symptoms are yellow skin; dry, itchy, or brittle skin; inflammation of the mouth; bruises and bleeding; hypertension; and a burning sensation in the legs and feet.

Every body system is affected as waste products build up in the blood. There is no cure; in the early stages, however, diet therapy, fluid restriction, and medications may slow kidney damage. The general care required for clients in chronic renal failure is described in Box 18–10.

Once the client has lost considerable kidney function, dialysis is needed. *Dialysis* is the process of removing wastes and excess water from the blood. Only specially trained nurses can perform this procedure. Initially, it is done in a dialysis unit, but eventually, some clients may be able to have home dialysis and you may be the caregiver. Your supervisor will ensure that you are aware of your responsibilities and scope of practice when giving care. Some clients may require kidney transplants.

Box 18–10 Care of Clients With Chronic Renal Failure

- Limit fluids.
- Measure the client's blood pressure in the supine, sitting, and standing positions.
- Measure weight daily with the same scale.
- Measure and record intake and output of fluids.
- Use bath oils, lotions, and creams on the skin to prevent itching. Follow the care plan.
- Provide frequent oral hygiene.
- Encourage rest.
- Prevent complications of bed rest if the client is confined to bed (see Box 18–1 on page 251).

ENDOCRINE DISORDERS

The endocrine system is made of glands that secrete chemical messengers called *hormones*. Hormones affect other organs and glands and are essential for body function. Endocrine disorders result in hormone levels that are too high or too low. The most common endocrine disorder is diabetes.

Diabetes

Diabetes is a disorder in which the body cannot produce or use insulin properly. *Insulin* is a hormone secreted by the pancreas. It is needed for the proper use of sugar (*glucose*) by helping the sugar obtained from foods to get into the cells. Without enough insulin in the body, sugar builds up in the blood—referred to as *hypergylcemia*, which means high (*hyper*) sugar (*glyc*) in the blood (*emia*). When cells do not have sugar for energy, they cannot perform their functions. Left untreated, mild hypergylcemia can lead to long-term complications. Severe hyperglycemia can be life-threatening.

Over two million Canadians have diabetes, and one third of them are unaware of it. Diabetes can develop in children and adults. Risk factors include obesity and a family history of diabetes. The risk increases after age 40. In Canada, people of Aboriginal descent are more likely than others to have diabetes.[8]

There are three types of diabetes:

- *Type 1 diabetes*—occurs most often in children and young adults. The pancreas does not produce insulin, which leads to severe hyperglycemia. These clients develop symptoms early in the disease and need treatment with daily insulin injections.
- *Type 2 diabetes*—usually develops in adulthood but can occur in children as well. This is the most common type of diabetes. The pancreas does not produce enough insulin, or the body does not effectively use the insulin that is produced. Obesity is a risk factor. The hyperglycemia is often mild, and the client may not notice symptoms. Treatment often consists of diet and exercise or oral medications. Insulin is sometimes required.
- *Gestational diabetes*—develops during pregnancy. It usually disappears after the baby is born. However, the woman is at risk for developing type 2 diabetes later in life.

A client with diabetes may experience clear symptoms, but remember that people with type 2 diabetes sometimes have symptoms that are so mild they do not notice them. Common signs and symptoms are:

- Increased thirst
- Frequent urination
- Constant hunger
- Unusual weight loss
- Extreme fatigue
- Dry, itchy skin
- Blurred eyesight

It is important that diabetes is controlled. If left untreated or poorly managed (as often happens with type 2 diabetes), the high levels of blood sugar slowly damage both the small and large blood vessels in the body. This causes many complications, including blindness, kidney disease, nerve damage, sexual dysfunction, and circulatory disorders. Circulatory disorders can lead to stroke, heart attack, and slow wound healing. Foot and leg wounds have very serious consequences for people with diabetes, as infection and gangrene can occur and sometimes lead to amputation.

There is no cure for diabetes, but the disease can be managed to reduce or prevent long-term complications. All clients with diabetes must follow a careful diet, and overweight clients need to lose weight. Exercise is included as part of the treatment plan, as regular exercise helps lower blood sugar levels, promotes weight loss, and reduces stress. Oral medications may also be necessary. Regular and proper foot and nail care provided by a professional is extremely important, as corns, blisters, and calluses on the feet can lead to infection and amputation.

Diabetes requires blood sugar monitoring—through finger-prick blood tests that determine the levels of sugar in the blood. Clients with type 1 diabetes need to test their blood sugar before each insulin dose, and those with type 2 diabetes usually need to monitor their levels once daily.

Clients with type 1 diabetes require insulin injections, usually one to four times daily, and some clients with type 2 diabetes also need insulin. Most clients monitor their sugar levels and administer their insulin themselves. The exact type and dose of insulin must be taken as ordered by the physician, in order to prevent complications from insulin therapy. If too much insulin is taken, hypoglycemia occurs. *Hypoglycemia* means low (*hypo*) sugar (*glyc*) in the blood (*emia*). If not corrected (by intake of sugar), it can lead to coma or death (Table 18–1).

Immediately report signs and symptoms of hyperglycemia and hypoglycemia. As the support worker, you may prepare meals for adults and children with diabetes. Diet is a very important part of managing diabetes. Follow the client's diet plan carefully, and serve meals and snacks on time.

Hyperthyroidism

Hyperthyroidism is caused by an overactive thyroid gland, resulting in too much thyroid hormone being produced. All of the body's processes are regulated by the thyroid hormone, so all of the body's functions speed up due to the excess thyroid. Since all body functions are affected, there can be many different signs and symptoms, including weight loss with increased hunger, hyperactivity, palpitations, nausea, vomiting, irritability, and depression. Treatment may be the surgical removal of some or all of the thyroid gland, administration of one dose of radioactive iodine to destroy some of the thyroid cells or medications that inhibit the production of the thyroid hormone.

Hypothyroidism

Hypothyroidism is caused by an underactive thyroid gland, and with decreased production of thyroid hormone, all of the body processes are slowed down. Signs and symptoms present are opposite from the signs and symptoms of hyperthyroidism. Some of the many signs and symptoms are weight gain, impaired memory, fatigue, sluggishness, irritability, constipation, and slower heart rate. Treatment consists of a thyroid supplement.

COMMUNICABLE DISEASES

A **communicable disease** is caused by microbes that spread easily, and can be transmitted from one person to another. Communicable diseases are spread in different ways (see Chapter 20):

- *Direct contact*—with the infected person
- *Indirect contact*—with contaminated dressings, linens, or surfaces
- *Airborne transmission*—occurs when the client sneezes and coughs
- *Vehicle transmission*—occurs through blood transfusions or by ingesting contaminated food, fluids, or drugs
- *Vector transmission*—occurs via animals, fleas, ticks, mites, and mosquitoes

There are many communicable diseases, for example, colds, influenza, measles, mumps, and chickenpox. Table 18–2 outlines common childhood communicable diseases; however, adults can also contract these diseases. This section discusses sexually transmitted infections (STIs), hepatitis, and acquired immune deficiency syndrome (AIDS).

While providing support care, you often cannot tell by looking at clients if they have a communicable disease. Sometimes, even clients with the communicable disease themselves may not know that they have it. Therefore, you must follow Standard Precautions when working with all clients. Standard Precautions prevent the spread of communicable diseases. You may also have to follow Transmission-Based Precautions with certain clients if so ordered by a physician (see Chapter 20). Follow the care plan.

Table 18–1 Hyperglycemia and Hypoglycemia

	Causes	Warning signs and symptoms
Hyperglycemia (High blood sugar)	Undiagnosed diabetes Not enough insulin or diabetes medication Overeating, or eating the wrong kind of food Too little exercise Stress—physical or emotional	Tiredness or fatigue Hunger Thirst Frequent urination Leg cramps Blurred vision Dry, itchy skin Flulike achiness Headache Flushed face Rapid, weak pulse Low blood pressure Sweet breath odour Slow, deep, and laboured breathing Confusion Nausea and vomiting Convulsions Loss of consciousness
Hypoglycemia (Low blood sugar)	Too much insulin or diabetes medication Omitting or delaying a meal or snack Eating too little food Too much exercise Vomiting	Hunger Weakness Trembling, shakiness Sweating Headache Dizziness Faintness Irritability, anxiety Confusion, disorientation Rapid pulse Low blood pressure Rapid, shallow breathing Changes in vision Cold, clammy skin Unconsciousness Convulsions

Hepatitis

Hepatitis is inflammation (*itis*) of the liver (*hepat*). It is often caused by an infection of the liver by certain viruses. When the viral infection of the liver first occurs, it is called *acute hepatitis,* which may or may not cause symptoms that are recognized by the infected person. Acute hepatitis often lasts less than 1 or 2 months. Signs and symptoms of acute hepatitis include nausea, vomiting, and pain in the abdomen. After about 2 weeks, dark urine and jaundice (a yellowish colour in the skin and whites of the eyes) develop in some, but not all, clients. Some clients with hepatitis have light-coloured stools, muscle pain, drowsiness, irritability, and itching, as well as diarrhea and general aching in the joints accompanied by redness and swelling.

For mild cases of acute viral hepatitis, no medication or other treatment is available or necessary. The disease runs its course and resolves by itself.

Table 18–2 Common Communicable Childhood Diseases

Disease	Transmission	Signs and Symptoms
Chickenpox (varicella)	Direct contact or airborne contact with respiratory secretions; direct contact with skin lesions	Fever, rash, and skin lesions
Measles (rubeola)	Direct or indirect contact with nasal secretions	Fever, cough, rash, inflammation of the mucous membranes of the nose, nasal discharge, bronchitis
Mumps	Direct contact with saliva droplets	Fever, headache, swollen salivary glands, earache
Pertussis (whooping cough)	Airborne or direct contact with droplets from the respiratory tract	Fever, sneezing, severe cough at night; coughs are short and rapid followed by a "whoop" or crowing sound with inhalation
Rubella (German measles)	Airborne or direct contact with secretions from the nose and pharynx	Fever, headache, loss of appetite, nasal inflammation, sore throat, cough, rash
Scarlet fever	Airborne or direct contact with nasal and pharyngeal secretions	Fever, chills, headache, vomiting, abdominal pain, red and swollen tonsils and pharynx, rash

The primary goals for managing acute viral hepatitis are providing good nutrition, preventing additional damage to the liver, and preventing transmission to others.

Some cases of acute hepatitis do not resolve. If hepatitis lasts longer than 6 months, it is called *chronic hepatitis*. Chronic hepatitis causes liver damage over a long period of time. The normal cells of the liver are eventually replaced with scar tissue—a condition known as *cirrhosis*, which can cause complete liver failure. When the liver fails, the client will need life-saving liver transplantation.

There are three major viruses that cause hepatitis in Canada: hepatitis viruses A, B, and C. All can be passed from one person to another.

- ***Hepatitis A virus***—is spread by the fecal–oral route; that is, the virus is transmitted when traces of feces are ingested. Food, water, and drinking and eating vessels (cups, bowls, cutlery) can be contaminated with feces. The virus is ingested when contaminated food or water is consumed. It can also be ingested when a person eats or drinks from a contaminated vessel. Risk factors include crowded living conditions and poor sanitation and hygiene. While providing support care, always wear gloves when assisting with perineal care, cleaning incontinent clients, and handling bed pans and rectal thermometers. Clients with fecal incontinence, confusion, or dementia can cause contamination. Carefully look for contaminated items and areas. Good hand washing is essential for everyone. Assist the client with hand washing, if necessary. Hepatitis A does not cause chronic hepatitis (see *Focus on Children: Hepatitis* box).

- ***Hepatitis B and C viruses***—are in an infected person's blood and certain body fluids (semen and vaginal secretions) and can be spread through intercourse or by sharing needles with an infected person. These viruses can also be spread during blood transfusions and childbirth (from the mother to the child) and also by needle stick injuries and by direct contact between open skin and infected blood or body fluids (see Chapter 20). Therefore, follow Standard Precautions when contact with blood or body fluids is likely. Transmission-Based Precautions are ordered as necessary. Hepatitis B (in 10 to 15% of the cases) and hepatitis C (in 70 to 85% of the cases) can cause chronic hepatitis.

focus on
››CHILDREN

Hepatitis

Hepatitis A is more common among preschool and school-age children than among adults because the virus is easily spread among children. Poor hygiene practices after defecation lead to contamination of eating and drinking vessels, toys, and other surfaces. Also, young children often put their hands, toys, and other items in their mouths.

Acquired Immune Deficiency Syndrome

Acquired immune deficiency syndrome (AIDS) is a disease of the immune system caused by the *human immunodeficiency virus* (*HIV*). AIDS affects the person's ability to fight infections. Clients with AIDS may get infections such as pneumonia and tuberculosis (TB) and are also at increased risk for cancers. Sometimes they experience central nervous system damage, which may cause memory loss, loss of coordination, paralysis, mental health disorders, and dementia.

A person may be infected with HIV but not have signs and symptoms of AIDS. This person is a carrier and can transmit the virus to others. There is no cure for HIV infection; however, several medications have been developed recently that slow its progress to full-blown AIDS. With current treatment, infected persons can remain AIDS-free for many years.

HIV is spread from an infected person to someone else when there is an exchange of certain body fluids—blood, semen, vaginal secretions, or breast milk. HIV is transmitted mainly by:

- Unprotected intercourse with an infected person ("unprotected" means without a condom). The virus enters the bloodstream through small breaks in the mucous membranes of the rectum, vagina, penis, or mouth
- Needle-sharing among intravenous (IV) drug users
- HIV-infected mothers to their babies at birth or during breastfeeding
- ***Infection can also be spread when infected body fluids come in direct contact with broken skin.*** Needle stick injuries can thus spread HIV (see Chapter 20).

HIV is *not* spread by saliva, tears, urine, sweat, sneezing, coughing, and insects or through casual contact, including hugging, touching, or shaking hands with an infected person.

AIDS is the last stage of HIV infection. If HIV infection is not treated, AIDS develops in about 10 years after the initial infection. The following are possible warning signs of HIV infection:

- Rapid weight loss
- Dry cough
- Fever or night sweats
- Fatigue
- Swollen glands in the armpits, groin, or neck
- Diarrhea that lasts for more than a week
- White spots or unusual blemishes on the tongue, in the mouth, or in the throat
- Pneumonia
- Red, brown, pink, or purplish blotches on the skin or inside the mouth, nose, or eyelids
- Memory loss, confusion, or dementia

You may be providing support care to clients who have AIDS or who are HIV carriers. In some of the procedures, you may be in contact with the client's blood. Standard Precautions are important to protect yourself and others from being infected by the HIV virus. ***These precautions apply when you are caring for all clients.*** Remember, you may care for a client who has the HIV virus but shows no symptoms, or you may care for a client who has undiagnosed HIV infection. As long as you strictly follow all Standard Precautions, you need not fear working with clients with HIV infection or AIDS (see the *Focus on Older Adults: HIV and AIDS* box.)

Sexually Transmitted Infections

Sexually transmitted infections (STIs) are spread through sexual contact (Table 18–3 on page 285). Some clients may not be aware that they are infected, while some others may know and still not seek treatment, commonly due to embarrassment.

STIs are usually associated with the genital area, but other areas, such as the rectum, ears, mouth, nipples, throat, tongue, eyes, and nose, may also be involved. Most STIs are spread only through sexual contact. The use of condoms helps prevent the spread of STIs and is also very important for preventing the spread of HIV and AIDS. Some

focus on
»OLDER ADULTS

HIV and AIDS

AIDS is often considered a young person's disease. Also, people often think that older adults are not sexually active and are therefore not at risk for AIDS. Older adults get and spread HIV in the same ways as younger adults, the exceptions being through childbirth and breastfeeding. Consider every client as potentially infectious. Follow Standard Practices with all clients.

STIs can be spread through a break in the skin, contact with infected body fluids (blood, semen, saliva), or contaminated blood or needles. Following Standard Practices is therefore necessary at all times.

Influenza

Influenza ("the flu") is a respiratory tract infection caused by a virus. In Canada, the flu season is from November or December through April or May. Millions of people suffer from the flu. Influenza is

Table 18–3 Sexually Transmitted Infections

Disease	Signs and Symptoms	Treatment
Genital herpes	Recurrent, painful, fluid-filled sores on or near the genitalia (Figure 18–24) The sores may have a watery discharge Itching, burning, and tingling in the genital area Fever Swollen glands	No known cure Medication can be given to control discomfort
Venereal warts	*Males*—Warts appear on the penis, anus, or genitalia *Females*—Warts appear near the vagina, cervix, and labia	Application of special ointment that causes the warts to dry up and fall off Surgical removal may be necessary if the ointment is not effective
Gonorrhea	Burning on urination Urinary frequency and urgency Vaginal discharge (females) Urethral discharge (males)	Antibiotic medications
Syphilis	*Primary syphilis*—appears 10 to 90 days after exposure Painless chancre (a type of sore) on the penis, in the vagina, or on genitalia; chancres may also be present elsewhere on the body *Secondary syphilis*—appears about 2 months after the chancre, lasting up to 1 year Rash, general fatigue, loss of appetite, nausea, fever, bone and joint pain, hair loss, lesions on the lips and genitalia *Tertiary syphilis*—appears 3 to 15 years after infection Damage to the cardiovascular system and central nervous system; blindness; dementia	Antibiotic medications

highly contagious and spreads when an infected person coughs or sneezes. It can also be spread by indirect contact—for example, by touching an object, such as a doorknob or a telephone, that was recently handled by an infected person.

Onset is usually sudden, with headache, chills, and cough, followed by fever, loss of appetite, muscle aches, and tiredness. Coldlike symptoms, including runny nose, sneezing, watery eyes, and throat irritation, occur, as well as nausea, vomiting, or diarrhea, especially in children. Recovery is usually complete in 1 to 2 weeks. However, some people develop serious and life-threatening complications, for example, pneumonia.

During support care, good hygiene and Standard Precautions reduce the risk of infection. Washing your hands before and after client contact is essential. The most effective method of prevention is the flu vaccine. People at high risk need yearly flu vaccinations. At-risk people include:

- People 65 years of age and older
- Residents of long-term care facilities
- People who have chronic diseases
- Caregivers and people who live with someone in a high-risk group

Your employer may request or require that you get a yearly flu vaccination, as it protects you and your clients.

Tuberculosis

Tuberculosis (TB) is a bacterial infection, usually affecting the lungs. However, TB can also occur in the brain, kidneys, bones, lymph nodes, and urinary and digestive systems.

TB was a major cause of death in the early 1900s. When TB medications were introduced in the 1940s, a dramatic decline in the number of TB cases resulted. However, TB still occurs and is a major health problem in many parts of the world. In the late 1980s, the number of cases began to increase.

The bacteria causing TB are spread by airborne droplets (see Chapter 20) when the infected person coughs, sneezes, or speaks and others in the environment inhale the bacteria. Anyone who has close, frequent contact with an infected person is at risk. TB is more likely to occur in close, crowded areas, such as inner-city neighbourhoods. People with HIV infection are also at risk.

Sometimes bacteria can reside in a person and not cause an infection until many years later. The person may not have symptoms at first, and the disease may be found during a routine chest X-ray or a TB skin test. Early signs and symptoms are tiredness, loss of appetite, weight loss, fever, and night sweats. Coughing occurs and becomes more frequent as the disease progresses; increased sputum production and chest pain also occur.

Clients with active TB may need to be treated in a hospital, and when they return home, they must continue taking TB medications daily for several months.

Clients with TB need to cover their noses and mouths with tissues when coughing or sneezing and then flush the tissues down the toilet. In health care facilities, tissues used by clients with TB are placed in a biohazard bag and disposed of following facility policy. Standard Practices and Airborne Precautions must be practised during care of a client with TB (see Chapter 20).

A B

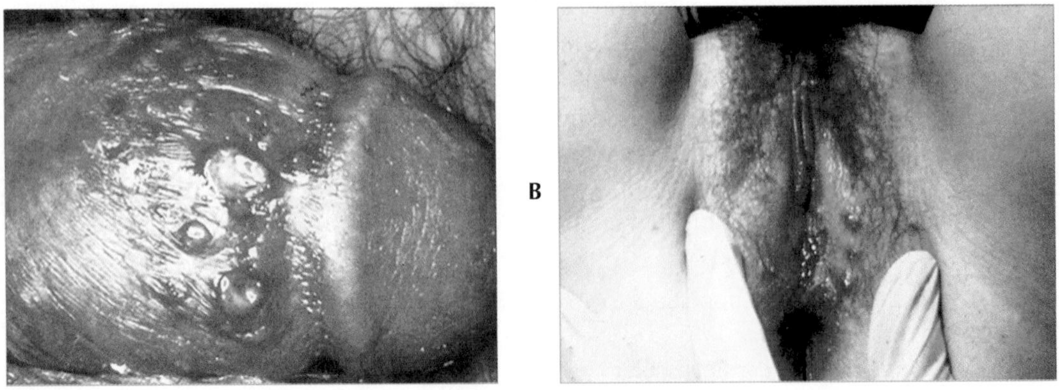

Figure 18–24 Genital herpes. **A,** Sores on the penis. **B,** Sores on the perineum. **Courtesy:** USPHS, Washington, DC.

REVIEW

Answers to these questions are at the bottom of page 288.

Circle T if the answer is true or circle F if the answer is false.

1. T F A sore that does not heal is a warning sign of cancer.
2. T F Stroke is a complication of hypertension.
3. T F A common treatment of hypertension is a high-sodium diet.
4. T F The pain of angina is relieved with rest and nitroglycerin.
5. T F Myocardial infarction means heart attack.
6. T F A pacemaker is a device used to treat renal failure.
7. T F Clients with congestive heart failure need to drink extra fluids.
8. T F Smoking is the most common cause of COPD.
9. T F The flu season in Canada is June through October.
10. T F Stroke often causes hemiplegia.
11. T F Clients with Parkinson's disease often have blank, expressionless faces.
12. T F Clients with Huntington's disease are not affected intellectually.
13. T F Canada has one of the lowest rates of MS in the world.
14. T F A client with advanced ALS cannot speak or move but can hear and understand.
15. T F Clients with brain or spinal cord injuries require amputations.
16. T F Arthritis usually affects bones and muscles.
17. T F Fibromyalgia is a respiratory disorder.
18. T F Clients with osteoporosis have an increased risk for fractures.
19. T F When lifting a cast, support it with your palms, not your fingertips.
20. T F When caring for a client in traction, remove the weights if he or she is uncomfortable.
21. T F After a hip pinning, the operated leg is abducted at all times.
22. T F Hyperglycemia means low sugar in the blood.
23. T F Diabetes can cause circulatory disorders.
24. T F Good foot care is especially important for people with diabetes.
25. T F Vomiting can cause aspiration.
26. T F Passing a kidney stone is called cystitis.
27. T F Clients with chronic renal failure need increased fluid intake.
28. T F Hepatitis B virus is spread by the fecal–oral route.
29. T F HIV is spread by infected urine.
30. T F The HIV virus remains in the infected person's body for life.
31. T F STIs are usually spread by sexual contact.
32. T F Hives are caused by an allergic reaction.
33. T F Eczema is a skin infection caused by a mite.
34. T F Psoriasis is caused by the infection of a hair follicle.
35. T F A cyst can contain air, fluids, or semi-solid material.
36. T F Impetigo is not contagious.
37. T F There is no cure for scleroderma.
38. T F Gout usually affects the big toe.
39. T F Lupus is a chronic autoimmune disease.
40. T F If your client is having an epileptic seizure, you should put something between the teeth so that he or she will not swallow the tongue.

REVIEW

Answers to these questions are at the bottom of the page.

41. T F GERD occurs when stomach acids go up the esophagus.

42. T F Cholecystitis is inflammation of the gallbladder.

43. T F Celiac disease is a disorder of the large intestine.

44. T F A client with IBS can suffer from diarrhea or constipation.

45. T F Crohn's disease is a chronic inflammatory condition of the bowel.

46. T F Hyperthyroidism is caused by an underactive thyroid gland.

Answers: 1.T, 2.T, 3.F, 4.T, 5.T, 6.F, 7.F, 8.T, 9.F, 10.T, 11.T, 12.F, 13.F, 14.T, 15.F, 16.F, 17.F, 18.T, 19.T, 20.F, 21.T, 22.F, 23.T, 24.T, 25.T, 26.F, 27.F, 28.F, 29.F, 30.T, 31.T, 32.T, 33.F, 34.F, 35.T, 36.F, 37.T, 38.T, 39.T, 40.F, 41.T, 42.T, 43.F, 44.T, 45.T, 46.F

CHAPTER 19

Safety

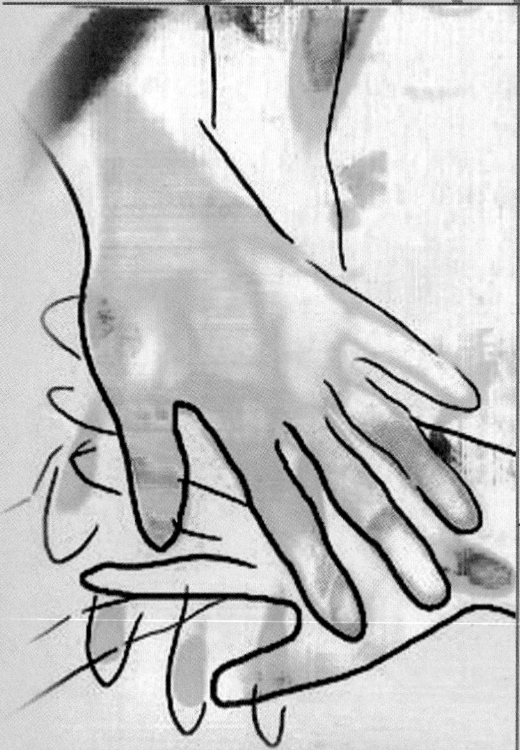

OBJECTIVES

- Define the key terms listed in this chapter.
- List risk factors for accidents.
- Describe how identifying the client, providing call bells, and using bed rails correctly promote client safety.
- Identify the safety measures to prevent falls.
- Describe how restraints can cause injury to clients and why they should be avoided.
- Identify how a client's quality of life can suffer as a result of being restrained.
- Identify the safety measures to prevent falls, poisoning, suffocation, and burns.
- Identify fire prevention measures.
- Describe what to do during a fire.
- Describe the causes of and emergency care for burns.
- Describe how to prevent equipment accidents.
- List the four steps to reporting a workplace injury, as identified by the Workplace Safety and Insurance Board.
- Apply the information provided in this chapter to protect yourself in the workplace.

key terms

assault Intentionally attempting or threatening to touch a person's body without the person's consent.

battery The touching of a person's body without the person's consent.

bed rails The metal or plastic sides of a hospital bed that are used to prevent a client from falling out of bed.

call bell A safety device for hospital patients and long-term care residents that enables them to call for assistance.

Canadian Charter of Rights and Freedoms The *Charter* is part of the Canadian Constitution and is a constitutional document. It applies at the federal and provincial/territorial levels. All other laws must be consistent with its rules. The *Charter* lists the basic rights and freedoms to which all Canadians are entitled.

chemical restraints Medication that is ordered by a doctor and given to a client to control unsafe, undesirable, or bizarre behaviour or movement. A chemical restraint is not given to cure a person's medical condition but merely to control behavioural symptoms.

environmental restraints Barriers, furniture, or devices that prevent a client from having free movement.

hazardous material Any substance that presents a physical hazard or a health hazard in the workplace.

incident report A report submitted whenever an accident, error, or unexpected problem arises in the workplace. Also known as an **occurrence report.**

mobility The ability to move around.

occurrence report See **incident report**.

OH&S (occupational health and safety) legislation Federal and provincial laws designed to protect employees from injuries and accidents in the workplace; these laws outline the rights and responsibilities of employers, supervisors, and workers.

physical restraints Garments or devices used to restrict movement of the whole body or parts of the body.

restraint Any device, garment, barrier, furniture, or medication that limits or restricts freedom of movement or access to one's body.

suffocation Occurs when breathing stops due to lack of oxygen.

Workplace Hazardous Materials Information System (WHMIS) A national system that provides safety information about hazardous materials; includes labelling, material safety data sheets (MSDS), and employee education.

workplace violence Any physical assault or threatening behaviour that occurs in a work setting that is directed toward the client and/or members of the health care team.

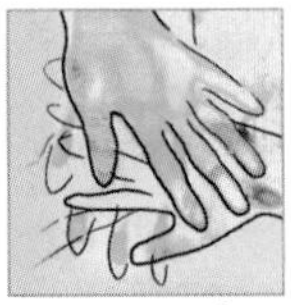

Safety is a basic need and right. You, as the support worker, your clients, and your co-workers have the right to safety, whether in a client's home or in the facility where you are employed. Promoting client safety is also one of the priorities of support work. Because of their age, or their physical or emotional health condition, many clients are at great risk for accidents and injuries, so facilities and community care agencies try to create and maintain a safe environment for their clients.

In the past, clients and residents were restrained in the hope that this would protect them from harm. In many circumstances, however, clients have been harmed *because* of their restraint. In this chapter, the topic of safety, including reasons for not using restraints, is discussed. In the section that addresses restraints, alternatives to restraint use are recommended.

In a safe environment, clients have little risk of accidents or injuries, and they feel safe and secure physically and emotionally. Both you and your employer share the responsibility to ensure client and worker safety. Your employer must ensure that workplace safety rules are followed and provide training to staff to update their knowledge about lifts, WHMIS, fire safety, smoking, and other safety-related topics. It is your responsibility to know and practise the basic safety measures that you have learned, to protect your clients, yourself, and others.

ACCIDENT RISK FACTORS

Anyone can be accidentally injured, but children, older adults, and people living with illnesses or disabilities are especially vulnerable to accidents. Factors that increase their risk of accidental injury are given below.

Impaired Awareness. People need to be aware of their surroundings in order to protect themselves from injury, and those who are unconscious are unaware of their surroundings and are unable to react or respond to danger. An unconscious person, therefore, relies on others for protection. Some people who have intellectual disabilities or who are confused or disoriented might not be able to recognize and avoid danger and could harm themselves. For example, a confused client may wander outside in the middle of winter without a coat, gloves, or boots.

Some people (including health care workers!) are more likely to get into accidents because they have a decreased sense of awareness regarding their surroundings, possibly because they are preoccupied with things other than what they are doing. Some may be just tired; according to newspaper reports, fatigue is often a factor in many motor vehicle accidents along Canada's highways.

Some prescribed medications can cause drowsiness and thus reduced awareness of surroundings as a side effect. So people should always follow the instructions provided by their health care providers.

Some people may be under the influence of drugs or alcohol (or both), and because of this, their reflexes, vision, balance, or coordination may be compromised. Some are overconfident and have what is sometimes called a sense of "invulnerability." They simply do not believe that they could ever get into an accident or be injured. These are the people that tend to speed while driving, do not wear their seatbelts, do not heed health warning signs, do not go to their doctors for medical checkups, and have unsafe habits, such as smoking or engaging in unprotected sex, and they learn about safety the hard way!

Impaired Vision. Poor vision can lead to falls. People may not be able to see the obstacles in their path (such as toys, small rugs, furniture, or electrical cords), or they may not be able to judge distances or depth correctly. They may also have problems reading labels on medicines, cleaners, and other containers, which can result in poisonings.

Some people who have decreased eyesight might require eyeglasses but refuse to wear them. Others might wear their eyeglasses all the time but not see clearly because they have not kept their prescriptions up to date. As a support worker, you should always ensure that your client's glasses are properly cleaned (see Chapter 37).

Impaired Hearing. People with impaired hearing have problems hearing explanations and instructions or may not hear warning signals or fire alarms. Since they are not alerted to danger, they do not know that they must move to safety. Chapter 37 deals with ways to communicate with people with hearing problems.

Impaired Taste, Smell, and Touch. Diminished senses of taste and smell may cause someone to eat spoiled food or not be aware of a gas leak. Diminished sense of touch may make a person unable to feel heat and cold, as well as pain and discomfort. For example, Mrs. Gagnon has poor circulation to her legs and feet, and because of that, she does not feel the presence of blisters on her feet caused by her new shoes. There is a risk of the blister becoming a serious wound.

Impaired Mobility. **Mobility** means the ability to move around. Aging, disease, and injury can affect mobility, so some people cannot walk or propel wheelchairs. Being unable to move oneself out of danger is a serious safety risk, and even minor changes in mobility increase accident risks. For example, a person with a sore knee may not be able to recover his or her balance from a stumble and end up having a fall.

Medications. Some medications have side effects such as loss of balance, drowsiness, lack of coordination, reduced awareness, confusion, and disorientation, among others. Some people on certain medications even become fearful and uncooperative. These side effects increase the risk of accidents, so they must be reported to your supervisor.

Age. Children and older adults are at risk for injuries (see Chapter 16 and Box 19–1 for a discussion on risk factors).

SAFETY MEASURES AT HOME AND IN THE WORKPLACE

Safety is something we take for granted until someone we know or love is injured. We need to be aware of safety hazards in our homes as well as in our workplaces, wherever that may be. As a support worker, it is your responsibility to ensure the safety of your clients and co-workers as well as your own, and this begins with the recognition of common safety hazards.

It is your responsibility to report any lapses in safety measures immediately to the proper authority, usually your supervisor. Use your common sense when you need to reach for items beyond your reach. Never use a chair, stool, or ladder for this unless you know for sure that you have health care coverage in case of a fall. Common sense and simple safety measures can prevent most accidents.

The safety measures listed in this chapter apply to both facility and community settings. Whatever the setting, your employer has safety policies to protect clients and staff. In the community, case managers, for example, check the client's home for safety hazards during the assessment phase. If there are any safety hazards, they are then corrected by the case manager, other professionals, or the client's

Box 19–1 Risk Factors for Accidents and Falls in Older Adults

One estimate suggests that approximately half of continuing care residents fall in any 1-year period. Ninety percent of hip fractures are caused by falls and even noninjurious falls can result in postfall anxieties that inhibit day-to-day activities.[1] Any injury may be serious for older adults because their bodies take longer to heal and recover. An injury that may be minor to a younger person (such as a broken bone) may be life-threatening to an older adult.

It is true that proper nutrition and lifestyle choices will enable many older adults to live longer and healthier lives than ever before. However, many of them will still experience age-related changes, which will increase their risk for falls and other accidents (see Chapter 17). These changes include the following:

- Weaker muscles
- Slower, less steady movements
- Slowed reaction time
- Balance problems
- Reduced sensitivity to heat
- Decreased vision
- Hearing problems
- Dulled senses of smell, taste, and touch
- Memory problems
- Joint pain and stiffness
- Low blood pressure

In addition to the above more common physical changes, other factors can predict the likelihood of an older adult for falling:

- A history of falls
- Foot problems
- Ill-fitting shoes
- Elimination problems—incontinence or frequent urination
- Dizziness and lightheadedness, especially on standing
- Depression
- Poor judgement or dementia
- Memory problems
- Unfamiliar surroundings
- Treatment equipment (IV poles, drainage tubes and bags, and others)
- Improper use of wheelchairs, walkers, canes, and crutches

family. In continuing care facilities, there are policies and procedures that are aimed at protecting the safety of clients and staff. Finally, all community and facility settings have individualized client care plans, which also list the safety measures needed by each client.

It is important to follow all safety policies and care plans. Despite careful planning and policies, avoidable accidents can still happen because employees may fail to follow the care plan and safety policies.

Preventing Falls and Injuries

Falls are the most common cause of accidental injuries in all settings, and children (see Chapter 16) and older adults are at greatest risk. ***While you should always supervise all of your clients, you should pay particular attention to children, clients in wheelchairs, clients with a history of injury, sedated clients, the elderly, and cognitively impaired clients, as they are at greatest risk of injuries related to falls.***

The risk for falls increases with age and illness (see Box 19–1). Falls may result in death, serious injuries, or changes in the older person's quality of life. For example, after a fall, an older adult may avoid leaving the house for fear of falling, and this may lead to feelings of isolation, anxiety, and depression. It may also lead to increased dependency on others.

Residents in long-term care facilities are at greater risk for falls than are older adults living at home.[1] Residents in facilities tend to be older, use more medications, and require more assistance with their activities of daily living. Many have impairments that affect their abilities to think, remember, communicate, or concentrate—for example, brain injuries, mental disabilities, dementia, and other conditions that cause confusion and disorientation—which increase residents' risk for falls.

Many facilities have fall prevention programs. Patients and residents are assessed to determine their risk for falls, and those who are at high risk are provided extra supervision and assistance. Methods used to identify them include a coloured bracelet worn by the client and a sign, sticker, or tag placed above the client's bed, at the nurses' station, or on the client's chart to indicate that the client is at greater risk for falling.

Most falls occur in bedrooms, bathrooms, and on stairs. Many occur when the client rushes to get to the bathroom or commode without help. Most falls in facilities occur in the evening, between 1800h (6:00 p.m.) and 2100h (9:00 p.m.). Falls also are more likely during shift change, when the majority of the staff are trying to listen to the shift report.

The safety measures listed in Box 19–2 help prevent falls in home and facility settings. Many are included in fall prevention programs and care plans. Always follow the client's care plan for specific safety measures.

RESTRAINTS AND HOW TO AVOID THEM

A **restraint** is any device, garment, barrier, furniture, or medication that limits or restricts freedom of movement or access to one's body. Restraints are rarely used now; only a small number of the many types of restraints that were allowed in the past are still allowed in Canada today. Only these will be discussed in this textbook.

It is important to know that every effort is made to protect clients without resorting to the use of restraints. In the past, there have been instances in Canada where clients were severely injured (and even died) as the result of restraint application, so many laws that prohibit their general use have been enacted since then. ***Restraints can cause emotional harm and serious physical injury. Restraints require a physician's order, after consultation with the client's family.***

In most provinces, the client or power of attorney (see Chapter 11) must sign a consent form that allows restraint to be used. ***Support workers never decide if restraints are to be used.*** Under our ***Canadian Charter of Rights and Freedoms,*** threatening a client with applying a restraint is considered an **assault**, and using a restraint on a client without doctor's orders is considered a **battery** (see Chapter 11).

Box 19–2 Safety Measures to Prevent Falls Among Older Adults and Others at Risk

- Report throw rugs and small mats that are not secure. They can be secured with carpet tape or nonskid backing. Make sure throw rugs and small mats are not in high-traffic areas or at the top of stairways.
- Report loose floor boards and tiles. Report frayed, torn, or bumpy rugs and carpets.
- Keep traffic areas free of telephone and electrical cords. Cords and wires can be taped next to the wall so the client will not trip over them.
- Keep the floors and stairways free of clutter. Never leave items on the stairs.
- Use only nonglare and nonslip floor wax.
- Clean up water and other spills immediately.
- Ensure lighting is good, especially near stairways and bathrooms. Offer to replace burned-out light bulbs.
- Turn on night-lights in the halls, especially near the bathroom, in case the client has to get up in the middle of the night.
- Keep a clear path from the bedroom to the bathroom.
- Do not rearrange the client's furniture.
- Use nonslip rubber bath mats or nonslip strips in bathtubs and showers.
- Make sure the client's footwear and clothing fit properly. Shoes and slippers must have nonskid soles. Long shoelaces should be avoided. Clothing should not be loose or drag on the floor. Belts must be tied or secured in place.
- Ensure crutches, canes, and walkers have nonskid tips. Make sure the client uses these devices correctly.
- Check wheelchair brakes. Make sure they can be locked and unlocked. Remind the client to keep the brakes locked when not moving the wheelchair, as the brakes prevent the chair from moving when the client transfers to or from the chair. Lock both brakes before you transfer the client to or from the wheelchair. Do not let the client stand on the footrests. Make sure front wheels point forward. This keeps the wheelchair balanced and stable. Remove the armrests and footrests (if removable) when the client transfers to or from the wheelchair (see Chapters 23 and 24).
- Encourage the client to wear their glasses or hearing aids, as needed. Reading glasses should not be worn when the client is up and about.
- Position the client in bed, chair, or wheelchair properly. Use pillows, wedge pads, or seats, as directed by the care plan.
- Check the client often. Careful and frequent observation is important, especially for those with risk factors.
- Electronic warning devices may be used. Weight-sensitive alarms placed on beds or wheelchairs detect movement or absence of weight and sound an alarm (Figure 19–1).
- Respond to all alarms at once.
- Clients at risk for falls can wear hip or coccyx protectors to minimize the risk for injury if a fall occurs. ***But they do NOT replace frequent monitoring!***
- Place the call bell within the client's reach. Ask the client to call for assistance when getting out of bed or a chair or when walking. Answer calls as soon as possible, before the client tries to get up without help.
- Offer assistance often to clients who need help with elimination. Help them to the bathroom as soon as requested, or offer a bedpan, urinal, or commode at regular times.
- Keep the bedpan or urinal within easy reach of those able to use these devices without help.
- Keep beds in the lowest position, except when giving bedside care.
- Never leave the client alone when the bed is raised.
- Use bed rails strictly according to the care plan. If a client tends to get up without calling for assistance, the care plan may state that bed rails be left down. For other clients, the care plan may call for raised bed rails. Know your employer's rules for using bed rails. Bed rails can be unsafe if used incorrectly. Follow the care plan for more safety rules regarding bed rails.
- Floor cushions (Figure 19–2) provide a soft landing spot if the client does fall out of bed. The bed should always be left at its lowest level.
- Roll guards can prevent a client from rolling out of bed (Figure 19–3).

(continued on page 295)

Box 19–2 Safety Measures to Prevent Falls Among Older Adults and Others at Risk (cont'd)

- Encourage clients to use handrails and grab bars. Facilities provide them in hallways, bathrooms, and on both sides of stairways to provide support for those who are unsteady when walking (Figure 19–4).
- Barriers are used to prevent wandering (Figure 19–5).
- Lock the wheels on bed legs when giving bedside care and transferring the client.
- In facilities, be careful when turning corners, entering corridor intersections, and going through doors. A person coming from another direction could be injured in a collision.
- In both facilities and homes, do a safety check of the room after visitors leave. They may have lowered a bed rail, removed the call bell, or moved a walker out of reach. They also may have brought an item that could harm the client.
- In facilities, family and friends are usually allowed to visit during busy times or during the evening and night shifts. A warm drink, soft lights, or a back massage may be used to calm the client who is agitated after visits. Companions are provided to sit with the client who is agitated or restless.

A

B

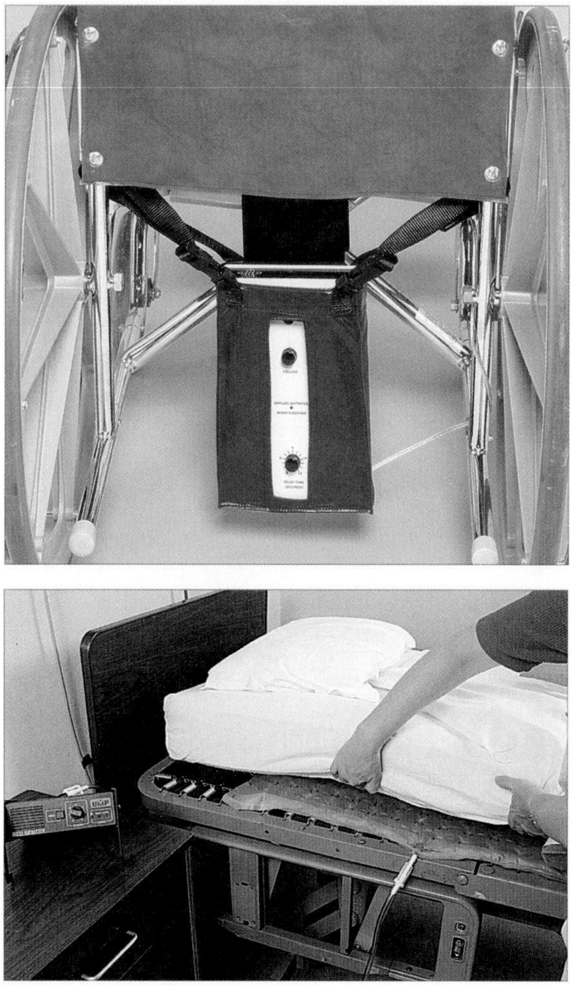

Figure 19–1 Weight-sensitive alarms may be used on wheelchairs or beds. **Courtesy:** J.T. Posey Company, Arcadia, CA.

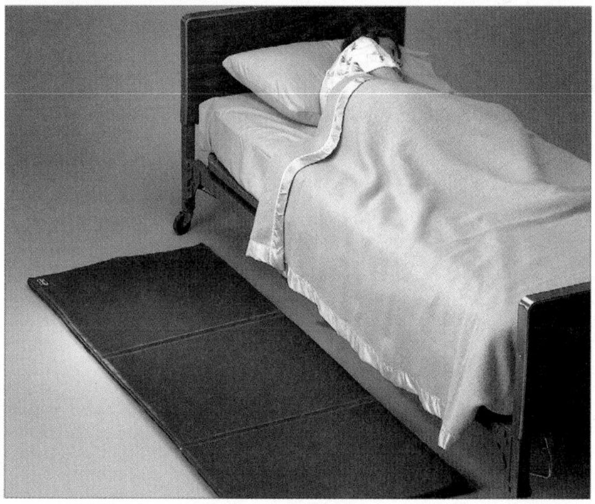

Figure 19–2 Floor cushion. **Courtesy:** J. T. Posey Company, Arcadia, CA.

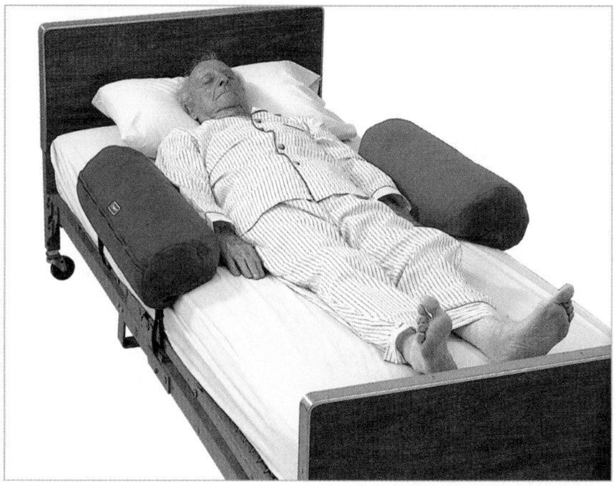

Figure 19–3 Roll guard. **Courtesy:** J. T. Posey Company, Arcadia, CA.

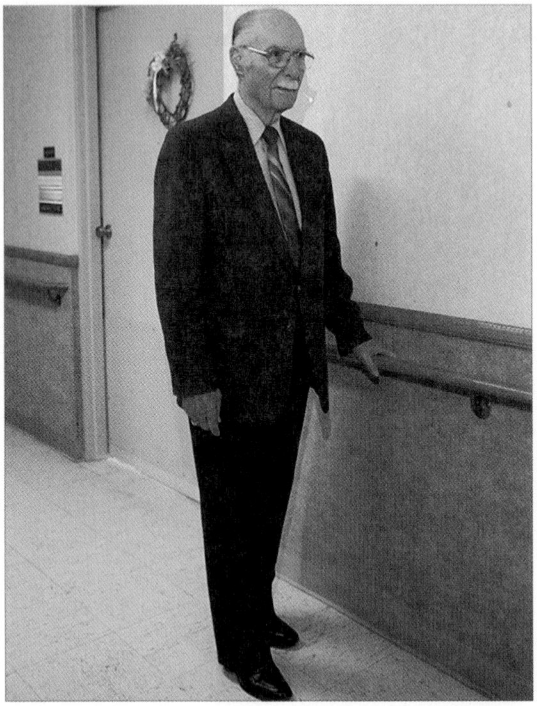

Figure 19–4 Handrails provide support to clients when walking. **Courtesy:** J.T. Posey Company, Arcadia, CA.

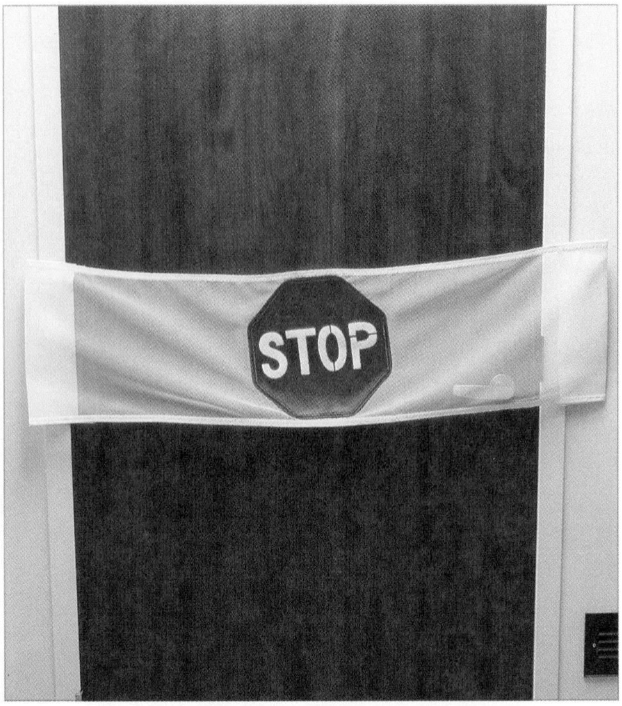

Figure 19–5 Barriers safely prevent clients from wandering. **Courtesy:** J.T. Posey Company, Arcadia, CA.

supporting MRS. GERHLBARDT

Maria Gerhlbardt is an 80-year-old widow who lives alone in her own home, a small, clean, comfortable two-storey house. Her bedroom is on the main floor, but the house's only bathroom is on the second floor. Mrs. Gerhlbardt and her husband bought this home 50 years ago when they first came to Canada from Europe. She is very proud of her house, and it is easy to see that she is a very neat and tidy person.

Mrs. Gerhlbardt is able to care for herself in most ways, although she does need some assistance in the winter to go out for banking, shopping, and doctor's appointments. As her support worker, you have arranged to visit her for 45 minutes a day, 5 days a week, to assist her with dressing and cooking. She hired you directly after you answered her personal ad for a support worker in the newspaper and is paying you privately.

Mrs. Gerhlbardt is a very friendly, mentally alert woman. However, she has such severe osteoarthritis and osteoporosis that she is bent over whenever she stands up. To avoid going up and down the stairs to use the bathroom, Mrs. Gerhlbardt has placed an old china bowl on a chair next to her bed and uses it as a bedside commode. She also has such severe arthritis in her hands and feet that she often has difficulty getting dressed. Her kitchen is very clean and always smells of cooking, but you have noticed that the light bulbs in her kitchen are either burned out or very dim, leaving it very dark. Mrs. Gerhlbardt, however, seems to know where everything is in her kitchen.

You have also noticed that Mrs. Gerhlbardt has many throw rugs, which cover her gleaming floors. She has told you that they were the last purchase she and her husband made together before he died of a heart attack 20 years ago and that she will "never get rid of them." She is particularly fond of the rug at the top of her stairs.

How would you go about providing support care for Mrs. Gerhlbardt?

Guidelines Regarding the Use of Restraints

All support workers need to keep in mind the guidelines discussed in this book regarding restraints. Remember that:

- ***Unnecessary restraint is false imprisonment*** (see Chapter 11). ***There must be a written consent in the client's chart for using the restraint.***
- ***Restraints are never used to discipline a client.*** Discipline is any action that punishes or penalizes.
- ***Restraints are never used for staff convenience.*** They should not be used to make the staff's job easier. If a restraint *must* be used, the least restrictive method is chosen by the physician. If clients are in danger of harming themselves or others, physicians usually advise them to enter a facility, where safe care can be provided.
- ***Always try to determine the cause of the client's agitation or behaviour.*** Staff should try to determine and understand the causes and reasons for a client's harmful behaviour (see Managing Challenging Behaviours in Chapter 35). By knowing and treating the causes, the need for restraints can usually be prevented. When determining the causes of harmful behaviour, health care professionals consider some of the following questions:
  - Is the client injured or in pain? Clients who are "out of sorts" may react in an agitated, and even aggressive manner.
  - Is the client afraid?
  - Is the client seeing, hearing, or feeling things that are not real?
  - Is the client confused or disoriented?
  - Are medications causing the behaviour? ***If the client's medications were recently changed, this can cause a change in behaviour. This should be reported immediately to the supervisor!***
  - Is the behaviour occurring because the client has not taken the medication?
  - Does the client need to urinate or defecate?
  - Is clothing or a dressing tight or causing other discomfort?
  - Is the client's position uncomfortable?
  - Is the client too hot, too cold, hungry, or thirsty?
  - Are body fluids, secretions, or excretions causing skin irritation?
- ***Restraint use should always be avoided.*** The health care professionals caring for the client identify restraint alternatives (Box 19–3), and these should become part of the care plan. As the support worker, it is your responsibility to follow the care plan, along with the rest of the health care team. Changes to the care plan may be made, as needed. If restraint alternatives do not protect the client, the physician may, as a last resort, order a restraint to be applied.
- ***Informed consent is required.*** Restraints cannot be used without informed consent. The client must understand the reason for the restraint. He or she is told how the restraint will help the planned treatment and what the risks of restraint use are. The client has the choice to give or withhold consent. If the client is not capable of giving informed consent, a family member or substitute decision maker is given the information, and this person must decide whether or not to give consent. Only the physician or nurse can provide the necessary information and obtain informed consent.
- ***Restraints are used only in extreme cases and when necessary to prevent harm.*** Restraints can hurt a person's dignity, so they are used only after other measures fail to protect the client or others. Some clients with physical, emotional, or behavioural problems may act in ways that are harmful to themselves or others. The following are examples of harmful behaviour:
  - Mr. Gorsky, 22, suffers from a severe mental illness. He tries to strangle a staff member, putting her life in danger.
  - Nicole Black, 3, tries to rip out the stitches in her chest. The wound could become infected, putting her life in danger.
  - Mr. Whyte has dementia. He constantly scratches his thighs, and unfortunately, his doctors have never been able to determine why he does this, and no medication seems to help. In the past, Mr. Whyte had

scratched himself so hard that he had deep, bleeding wounds on his thighs, which caused a severe skin infection requiring hospitalization. Also, Mr. Whyte frequently tries to undress himself.

- ***Restraints require a physician's order.*** If restraints are needed, a physician's order is required. The physician explains why the restraint is needed, which one to use, and how long to use it. This information is on the care plan and on your assignment sheet.
- ***The <u>least</u> restrictive method is used.*** For example, most environmental restraints are less restrictive than physical restraints.
- ***The manufacturer's instructions must be followed.*** The manufacturer of the restraining device has instructions on applying and securing it, and failure to follow them could harm the client. You could be found negligent if you improperly apply or secure a restraint. ***You are never allowed to use items such as bed sheets that are not standard restraints to restrain a client.***
- ***Restraints are applied by knowledgeable workers. You must receive proper training and instruction before applying restraints.*** Some facilities require you to obtain certification to apply restraints. Make sure you know what is required of you (Box 19–4).
- ***The client's basic needs are met.*** The restraint must be snug and firm but not tight. Tight restraints affect circulation and breathing. The client must be comfortable and able to move the restrained part to a limited and safe extent. ***The person must be checked at least every 15 minutes or as often as required.*** Food, fluid, comfort, exercise, and elimination needs must

Box 19–3 Alternatives to Restraints

- If the client is living at home, he or she may be moved to a facility.
- Diversion is provided to calm or distract the client. This includes TV, videos, music, games, books, relaxation tapes, back massages, exercise programs, outdoor time, and simple tasks.
- Lifelong habits and routines are encouraged: for example, showers before breakfast; walks before lunch; TV after lunch.
- Provide activities that occupy the client's time and energies (such as gardening or bird watching), according to the client's care plan, their needs, and abilities. Sometimes, a client who has dementia may try to do something that he or she "used to do" in the past and will become agitated if confined or not allowed to do it (see *Supporting Mr. Lee* on page 301 for an example of a solution).
- Attention and companionship are provided by support workers, family, friends, and volunteers visiting with the client. Visits and observations are made every 15 minutes.
- A calm, quiet setting is provided; noise levels are reduced.
- Staff members provide consistent care; they explain procedures and care measures.
- The client spends time in supervised areas, for example, in the lounge or near the nurses' station.
- The client is allowed to walk around in safe areas, and the entire staff is kept informed of this.
- Confused clients are helped to orient themselves to people, time, and place. Calendars and clocks are placed such that they are easily seen by the client.
- The call bell is placed within reach of the client.
- Food, fluid, and elimination needs are met; the bedpan, urinal, or commode is kept within reach.
- Clients who must be toileted may demonstrate agitated behaviours; it will help to toilet them at regular intervals.
- Lighting is adjusted to meet the client's needs and preferences.
- Uninterrupted sleep is promoted.
- Rooms and furniture meet safety and comfort needs (e.g., lower bed, reclining chair, cushioned walls and furniture). Warning devices are used on beds, chairs, and doors; doors have knob guards.
- Pillows, wedge cushions, posture, and positioning aids are used to prevent the client from falling out of bed.

be met. Ensure that the client has adequate support even while staff members are taking breaks.

- ***More than one staff member may be needed to safely apply the restraint.*** Clients in immediate danger of harming themselves or others are restrained quickly. Combative and agitated clients can hurt themselves and the health care worker when restraints are being applied. Two or more workers may be needed to complete the task safely and quickly.
- ***The client's quality of life is protected.*** Restraints are used for as short a time as possible. The care plan must show how to reduce restraint use. The goal is always to meet the client's needs with as little restraint as possible. Visit with the client, and offer reassurance.

Box 19–4 Safety Measures for Using Restraints

- Use the restraint specified in the care plan. The least restrictive device is used.
- Follow employer policies and procedures.
- Use only restraints that have manufacturer instructions and warning labels.
- Follow the manufacturer's instructions. Some restraints are safe for use with beds, chairs, and wheelchairs, while some others are used only with certain equipment.
- Do not use sheets, towels, tape, rope, straps, bandages, or other items to restrain a client.
- Use only intact restraints. Check for tears, cuts, or frayed fabric or straps.
- Do not use restraints to position a client on the toilet.
- Do not use restraints to position a client on furniture that does not allow for correct application. Follow the manufacturer's instructions.
- Position the client in good body alignment before applying the restraint (see Chapter 23).
- For mitt restraints, you should be able to slide one or two fingers under the restraint (Figure 19–6).
- Follow the manufacturer's instructions regarding checking for snug fitting.
- Use a belt restraint with chairs or wheelchairs. Position the client in the chair so that his or her hips are well to the back of the chair. Apply the belt restraint at a 45-degree angle over the hips (Figure 19–7).
- Bed rails are one type of environmental restraint. Use them only if indicated in the care plan. Check with your supervisor and the care plan for instructions on when to raise or lower bed rails. According to your supervisor's instructions, use bed rail covers or gap protectors, which prevent the client from getting trapped between the rails or the bed rail bars.
- If mitt restraints are applied, check the client's circulation every 15 minutes. You should feel a pulse at a pulse site below the restraint. Fingers or toes should be warm and pink. Tell the nurse at once if:
  - You cannot feel a pulse
  - Fingers are cold, pale, or blue in colour
  - The client complains of pain, numbness, or tingling in the restrained hand
  - The skin is red or damaged
- If a belt restraint is used, check the client at least every 15 minutes. The client should be able to breathe easily.
- Check the client at least every 15 minutes for safety and comfort. For example, clients can often easily slip down in Geri-Chairs and become injured.
- Remove the restraint and reposition the client every 2 hours. Meet the client's basic needs during this time and whenever necessary:
  - Meet elimination needs.
  - Give skin care.
  - Perform range-of-motion exercises or help the client ambulate (see Chapter 24). Follow the care plan.
  - Offer food and fluids.
  - Record what was done, the care given, your observations, and the time and details of what you reported to the nurse. Follow your employer policy for recording.
- Keep the call bell within the client's reach.
- Report to the nurse every time you checked the client and released the restraint. Report your observations and the care given. Follow your employer policy for reporting.

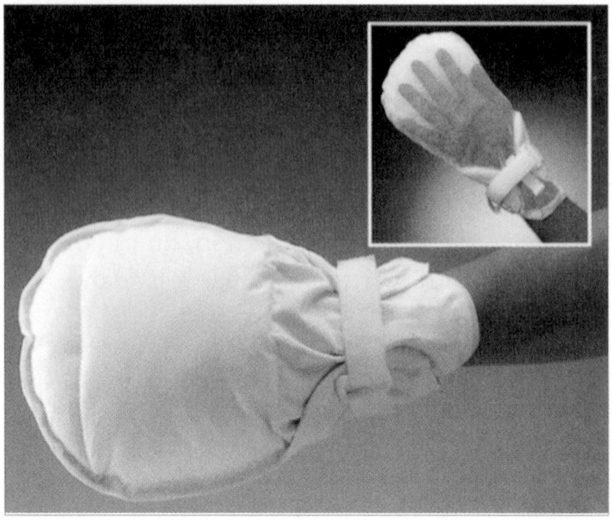

Figure 19–6 Mitt restraint. **Courtesy:** J. T. Posey Company, Arcadia, CA.

- ***The client is observed at least every 15 minutes or more often, as required by the care plan.*** Restraints can be dangerous, and injuries and deaths can occur from improper use and poor observation. Frequent observation alerts the staff to complications such as breathing and circulation problems. Practise the safety measures listed in Box 19–4.

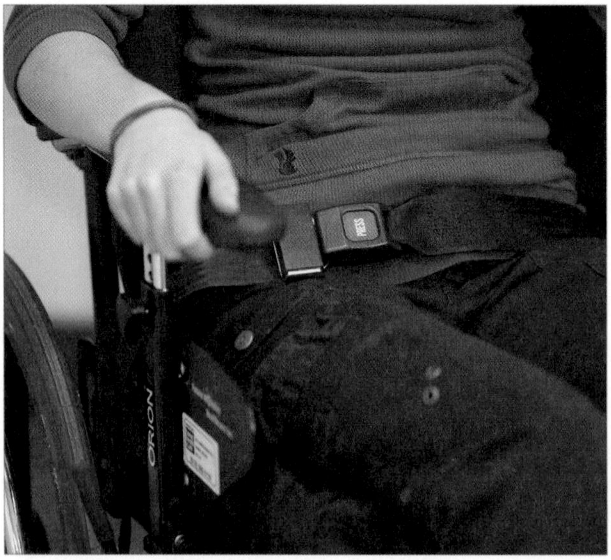

Figure 19–7 A belt restraint. Note that it must be secure enough to avoid sliding, but never applied too tightly. **Courtesy:** Brian Hillier.

- ***The restraint is removed, the client is repositioned, and basic needs are met at least every 2 hours.*** These needs include food, fluid, elimination, skin care, and range-of-motion exercises. The client is helped to ambulate (walk) according to the care plan.
- ***Information about restraints must be recorded in the client's chart.*** When caring for restrained clients, give verbal reports to your supervisor. If you are allowed to chart, include this information:
  - The type of restraint applied
  - The reason for the application
  - Safety measures taken, as listed in the care plan (e.g., bed rails padded and up)
  - The time you applied the restraint
  - The time you removed the restraint
  - The care given when the restraint was removed
  - Client's skin colour and condition
  - The pulse rate in the restrained part
  - Complaints of a tight restraint, difficulty breathing, and pain, numbness, or tingling in the restrained part (report these complaints to your supervisor at once)

Types of Restraints

There are three types of restraints:

1. **Physical restraints**—garments or devices used to restrict movement of the whole body or parts of the body. They are attached to a body part (e.g., a mitt restraint) or go around the client's waist and wheelchair (e.g., a belt restraint) (Figure 19–8).
2. **Environmental restraints**—barriers, furniture, or devices that prevent free movement. Environmental restraints are near the body, but not directly attached to it. They confine the client to a specific place, such as a bed, chair, or room. Examples of environmental restraints include:
   - Geriatric chairs (Geri-Chairs) or chairs with attached trays (Figure 19–9). These are used for people who need support to sit up
   - Any chair placed close to a wall so that a client cannot move
   - Bed rails
   - Locked rooms, seclusion areas

supporting MR. LEE

Won Lee, a 76-year-old man, is a client in a continuing care facility. He has dementia, and did not remember his wife or daughters at their last visit. Lately, he has also seemed unable to speak or understand English.

The staff members at the facility where Mr. Lee resides have noticed that he becomes very agitated in the early mornings. He has fallen several times trying to get out of bed, and more recently, before his bath, he tries to pull the linens away from the staff. He has scratched several of the support workers who have tried to remove the linens from his hands.

Support workers have tried toileting him more frequently, but nothing they have tried seems to decrease Mr. Lee's agitation. Mr. Lee has become so agitated that the staff members are afraid that he will hurt himself or others, so they suggest holding a client conference to discuss ways to safely care for Mr. Lee.

Mr. Lee's family members, his doctor, the occupational therapist, and some of the nurses and support workers who care for him attend the family conference. Mr. Lee's family is very concerned after hearing of his increasing agitation and wish to discuss the routines he kept while he was younger. Mrs. Lee tell the staff that waking up very early to get to work had been part of her husband's routine his entire adult life. She also informs them that they used to own a large laundry company, where he had worked for over 50 years.

Mrs. Lee says that when her husband was stressed at work, he would always do something physical, such as folding linens or ironing shirts. At Mrs. Lee's suggestion, it is agreed that when he wakes up the next morning, the night staff will help Mr. Lee to get out of bed and sit by the nursing station, where he will be allowed to fold linens. It is hoped that this will "settle" him.

The next morning, when Mr. Lee begins to become agitated in his bed, the staff quickly toilet him and assist him to a chair by the nursing station, where a large laundry basket of freshly laundered towels and facecloths has been placed. Mr. Lee sits quietly and folds the linens. He is neither agitated nor aggressive any more, and he smiles while he is "working." Before lunchtime, he is given the opportunity to fold clients' clothing protectors and linen napkins in the dining room. The staff members are surprised at Mr. Lee's change in disposition and decide that they will maintain this new routine the next day as well in order to see if it continues to reduce Mr. Lee's agitation.

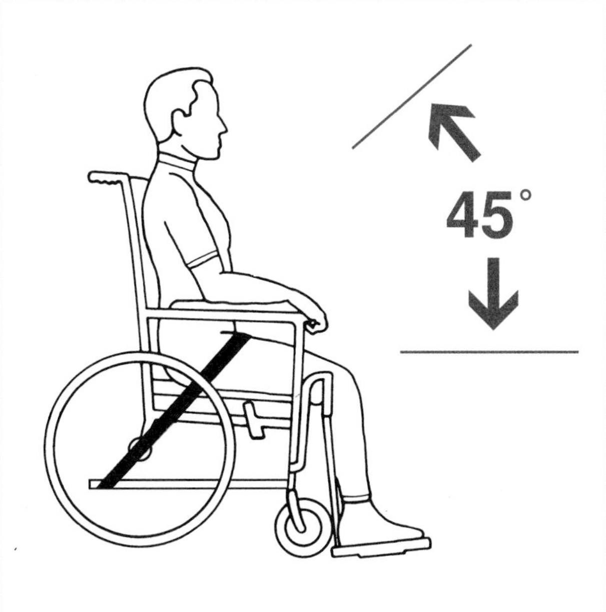

Figure 19–8 The safety belt is at a 45-degree angle over the hips. **Courtesy:** J. T. Posey Company, Arcadia, CA.

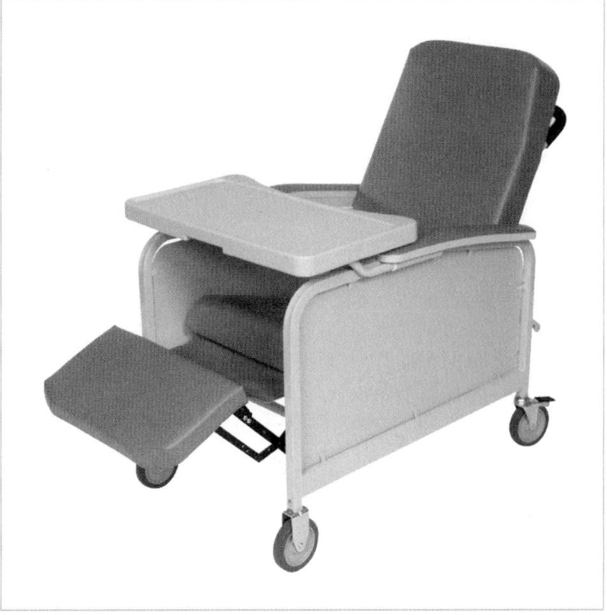

Figure 19–9 A Geri-Chair. **Courtesy:** Winco, Ocala, FL.

PROVIDING COMPASSIONATE CARE

Caring for Clients Who Are Restrained

A common misunderstanding is that restraints will decrease agitated behaviour. In fact, restraints often make people more agitated, confused, or combative. People who are restrained may not understand what is happening to them and may try to get out of the restraint. They may beg anyone who passes by to free them.

Try to put yourself in the client's situation to better understand how he or she might be feeling. Imagine what it would be like to have your hands and arms restrained:

- Your nose itches, but you cannot scratch it.
- You need to use the bathroom, but you cannot get up, so you soil yourself.
- You are thirsty, but you cannot reach for your glass of water.
- You are not wearing your eyeglasses, so you cannot identify people coming in and out of your room.
- You are lying in an uncomfortable position, but you cannot turn or move in bed.
- You hear the fire alarm, but you cannot get up and move to a safe place. You must wait until someone rescues you.

What would you do? Would you calmly lie or sit there? Would you try to get free from the restraint? Would you cry out for help? What would the staff think? Would they think that you are agitated and uncooperative or just uncomfortable?

Treat a restrained client like you would want to be treated in a similar situation—with kindness, caring, respect, and dignity. Meet the client's food, fluid, and elimination needs, and make sure the he or she is as comfortable as possible. Restrained clients need repeated explanations and reassurance. Visit with the client often, and be a good listener. Spending time with the client may have a calming effect.

3. **Chemical restraints**—medications used only to control behaviour or movement; they are not otherwise required for the client's medical condition. Sometimes confused and disoriented clients become anxious, agitated, or aggressive, and the physician may order medications to control these behaviours without making the client sleepy or impairing function. Like all restraints, chemical restraints *must not be used for discipline or staff convenience.* They must not be used if they impair physical or mental function and should only be used for as long as indicated. Using chemical restraints is out of your scope of practice, as support workers are never permitted to administer medications. Only a physician or nurse can administer chemical restraints.

Using Bed Rails

An important part of safe client care is using the **bed rails** on hospital beds correctly. Bed rails are raised and lowered according to the care plan. Bed rails are half, three-quarters, or the full length of the bed and lock in place with levers, latches, or buttons. When half-length rails are used, each side may have two rails—one for the upper part of the bed and the other for the lower part.

When to Use Bed Rails. Your supervisor and the care plan will tell you when to raise the bed rails. For example, clients who are unconscious or sedated, as well as those who are confused or disoriented, need the bed rails raised. Some clients just feel safer with the bed rails up, and some others use them to change positions in bed. If the care plan calls for raised bed rails, keep them up at all times, except when giving bedside care.

In the past, health care providers were taught that bed rails should always be placed up on a bed. However, having the bed rails up all the time can cause some clients to become restless. Check the client's care plan, and report any observations of increased restlessness to your supervisor.

Hazards Associated With Bed Rail Use. Bed rails present certain hazards (Figure 19–10). The client can fall when trying to climb over them. Another risk is entrapment; that is, a client can get caught,

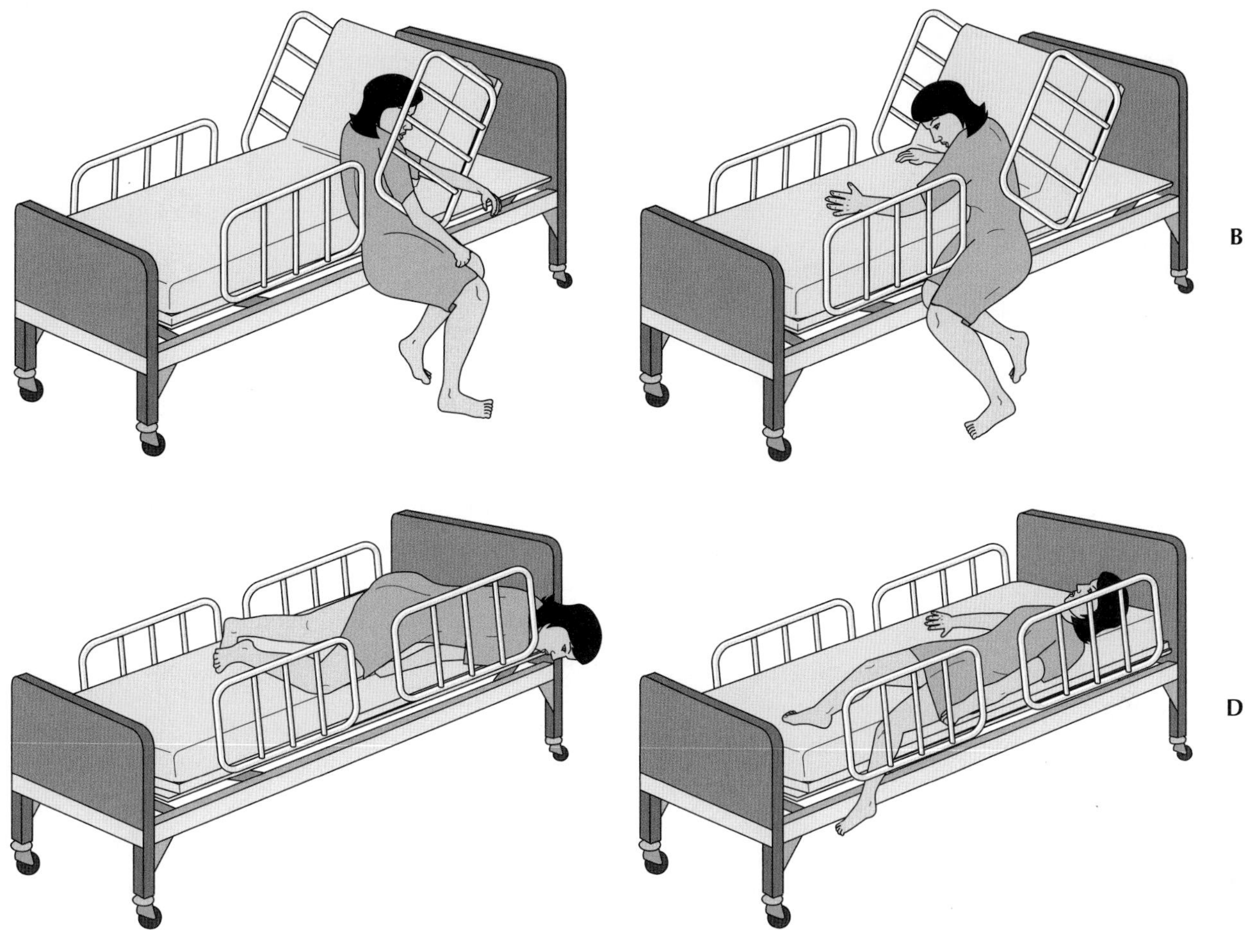

Figure 19–10 Bed rail hazards. **A,** The client is trapped between the bed rail bars. **B,** The client is trapped between two half-length rails. **C,** The client is trapped between the bed rail and the headboard. **D,** The client is trapped between the bed rail and the mattress. **Source:** Adapted from Sorrentino, S.A. & Gorek, B. (2003). *Mosby's textbook for long-term care assistants* (4th ed., p. 149). St. Louis: Mosby.

trapped, or entangled in the gaps in bed rails, which can occur between:

- The bars of the bed rail
- The two half-length rails
- The bed rail and the headboard or footboard
- The bed rail and mattress

Injury or death can occur if the client's head, neck, chest, arm, or leg becomes trapped in these gaps.

Who Is at Greatest Risk of Injury With Bed Rails? Clients at greatest risk are those who are:

- Confused or disoriented
- Restrained
- Small in size
- Have poor muscle control or tend to have seizures

For an adult client's safety, all bed rail gaps should be no more than 10 cm (4 in.). Sometimes padding is placed over the bed rails to cover the gaps in the rails (Figure 19–11). Gap protectors may also be used for split bed rails (Figure 19–12). Follow the manufacturer's instructions and employer policy for the use of gap protectors or padded bed rails.

Because bed rails prevent the client from getting out of bed, they are considered environmental restraints. They cannot be used unless they are needed to treat the client's medical symptoms. The client or the substitute decision maker must give consent for use of raised bed rails. The need for bed rails must be carefully noted in the client's chart and care plan.

Check clients often when raised bed rails are used. You should always adjust the bed height to its

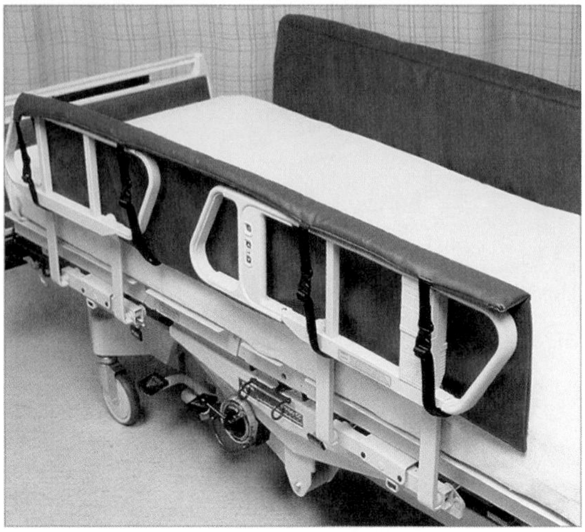

Figure 19–11 Padded bed rails. **Courtesy:** J.T. Posey Company, Arcadia, CA.

lowest position whenever bed rails are in use and whenever the client is not directly supervised by the staff. In some instances, instead of using bed rails, a client's mattress could be placed on a lower bed frame or placed directly on the floor during the night. This ensures that the client has less risk of injury because he or she will not fall out of bed. The mattress that is placed on the floor during the night would be returned to the bed in the morning in order to preserve the client's dignity and privacy.

How to Use Bed Rails. Many of the procedures described in this book include using bed rails, and this will help you learn how to use them correctly. However, remember that not all beds have bed rails and not all clients who have beds equipped with bed rails use them. Your supervisor, the care plan, and your assignment sheet will tell you which clients will need the use of bed rails. To give care when bed rails are used, lower the rail that is near you, and leave the bed rail raised on the opposite side. Keep both bed rails raised if you need to leave the bedside for any reason. Remember to raise the rail again after completing the procedure.

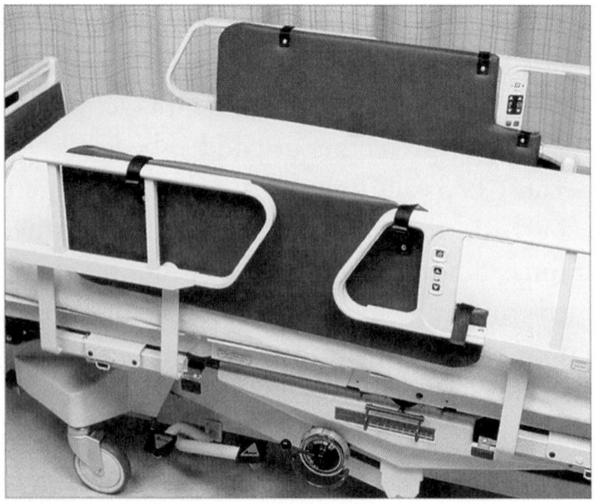

Figure 19–12 Gap protectors. **Courtesy:** J.T. Posey Company, Arcadia, CA.

PREVENTING POISONING

The most common ways adults are poisoned are by eating or drinking contaminated food and water and by overdosing on medications. Carelessness, confusion, and difficulty reading medication labels can lead to accidental overdose. Sometimes poisoning occurs as a suicide attempt. Confused or disoriented adults may eat poisonous substances. Follow the same safety measures for children listed in Chapter 16 for adults as well (Figure 19-13). Common harmful substances include:

- Medications and vitamins
- Household cleaners—such as bleach, drain cleaner, floor wax, furniture polish, soaps, detergents, and toilet, window, and oven cleaners
- Personal care products—such as aftershave, rubbing alcohol, nail polish and remover, shampoo and conditioner, bath oil, bubble bath, cosmetics, perfumes, deodorant, mouthwash, diaper wipes, and baby oils and powders
- Houseplants
- Insecticides, fertilizers, and insect sprays
- Alcohol and tobacco products, including nicotine gum, patches, and sprays

What to Do If You Suspect Poisoning. In community settings, the phone number for the local poison control centre should always be posted near the telephone or carried in your bag. You might suspect poisoning if you find empty pill bottles or hazardous products lying around. You might also suspect poisoning if the client suddenly collapses, vomits, or has difficulty breathing. If you suspect poisoning:

- Contact the emergency medical services (EMS) for your area by dialing 9-1-1 on the

A 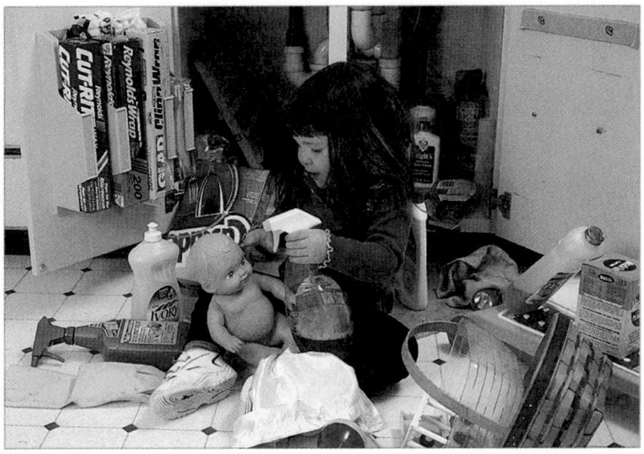 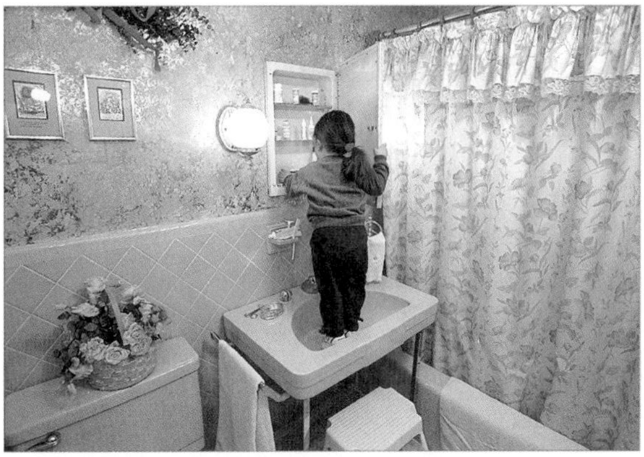 B

Figure 19–13 Harmful substances must be kept in locked areas, out of the reach of children and confused adults. **A,** Household cleaners are within reach when placed in low cabinets. **B,** The bathroom medicine chest holds many hazardous substances.

telephone. The EMS operator will give you clear instructions.

- Gather any empty pill bottles or other evidence of poisoning to determine what has been ingested and how much.
- Stay with your client. Be sure to remain calm.

PREVENTING BURNS

Many burns to older adults occur in the kitchen, for example, while cooking in clothes with loose-fitting sleeves, which might dangle over the burner and catch fire. Bath water and heating pads that are too hot can cause burns. Accidental burns from careless smoking or unattended cigarette butts in ashtrays are also common causes of burns. Box 19–5 lists safety measures aimed at preventing burns.

Care of the Client With Burns

Burns can severely disfigure and disable a person (Figure 19–14) and can even cause death. Most burn injuries occur in the home. Infants and children as well as older adults are at highest risk. Burns are caused by:

- Dry heat—fire, stoves, space heaters
- Moist heat—hot liquids, steam
- Chemicals—oven cleaner, drain cleaner, rust remover, and so on
- Electricity—faulty electrical equipment, live wires, or lightning (Figure 19–15)
- Radiation—sunlight

Burns can be minor or severe. ***Burns are more severe and require emergency help when:***

- They are located on the head, face, neck, hands, feet, or genitals
- They are spread over a large area of the body
- The burned person is under 2 or over 50 years of age or has a pre-existing medical condition (such as diabetes or hypertension)

The size and depth of the burn also affect its severity.

First Aid for Minor Burns. For minor burns that are limited to a small area, do the following:

- Immediately cool the injured area to reduce pain, swelling, blistering, and tissue damage. Immerse the area of the burn in a sink of cool water, run cool water over it, or cover it with a clean, wet, cool cloth.
- Once pain is reduced, gently pat the skin dry and cover it with dry, lint-free, clean cloth or gauze. Secure the dressing with tape, being careful not to touch the burn with the tape.
- *Do not* apply oil, butter, salve, or ointments on a burn.
- Report the burn to your supervisor. Seek medical attention, if necessary.

What to Do if the Burn Appears Serious. Emergency care of severe burns includes the following:

- This includes activating the EMS system for your area, usually by dialing 9-1-1 by telephone.

- For *chemical burns*, carefully and quickly brush off any loose chemical powder with a cloth. Flush the area with large amounts of cool water (such as in a shower) for 15 to 20 minutes. Carefully remove contaminated clothing while flushing the area.

Box 19–5 Safety Measures to Prevent Burns

Protecting Older Adults and Others at Risk

- Educate clients about the dangers of wearing clothes with loose-fitting sleeves while cooking.
- In facilities, ensure that clients smoke only in designated smoking areas, if at all. Many facilities no longer allow smoking to take place on their premises. Clients who smoke must be a designated distance away from the doors of the facility.
- Supervise clients who smoke and who cannot protect themselves. Some facilities insist that some or all of the clients who do smoke wear "smoking jackets," which are made up of nonflammable material, to prevent burns in the case of a dropped cigarette.
- Do not allow clients to smoke in bed. The client could fall asleep and drop the cigarette into the bed sheets or on his or her clothing and start a fire.
- Follow safety guidelines when applying heat and cold (see Chapter 43).
- Before feeding a client who cannot feed himself of herself, test the temperature of the food by dipping a clean spoon into the food and touching the inner aspect of your lower arm with the spoon. Remember to place the spoon into the used cutlery container after doing this.
- Always test the temperature of the water in the tub, shower, or basin, with either a water thermometer or your wrist or elbow, before bathing an adult client or helping him or her bathe. Check for "hot spots" in the water, and mix the water well by moving your hand back and forth in the water.
- Water temperature in a tub should be checked even if the tub has an electronic temperature sensor, in case it is not working properly.
- Assist with eating and drinking, as needed. Spilled hot foods and fluids can cause burns.

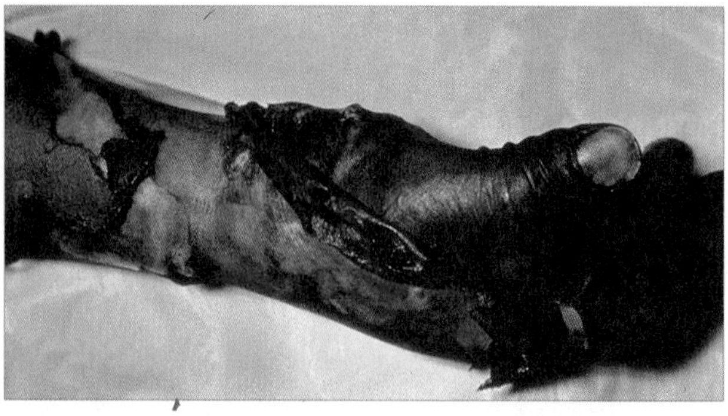

Figure 19–14 An example of a severe burn. **Source:** Ignatavicius, D.D., & Workman, M.L. (2002). *Medical-surgical nursing: Critical thinking and collaborative care* (4th ed.). Philadelphia: Saunders.

- For *electrical burns*, secure your safety first. Do not touch the person if he or she is still in contact with the electrical source. Have the power source turned off, or remove the electrical source first. Use an object that does not conduct electricity (rope or wood) to remove the electrical source. Do not apply water on the burn, as water may increase the risk of shock.

A

B

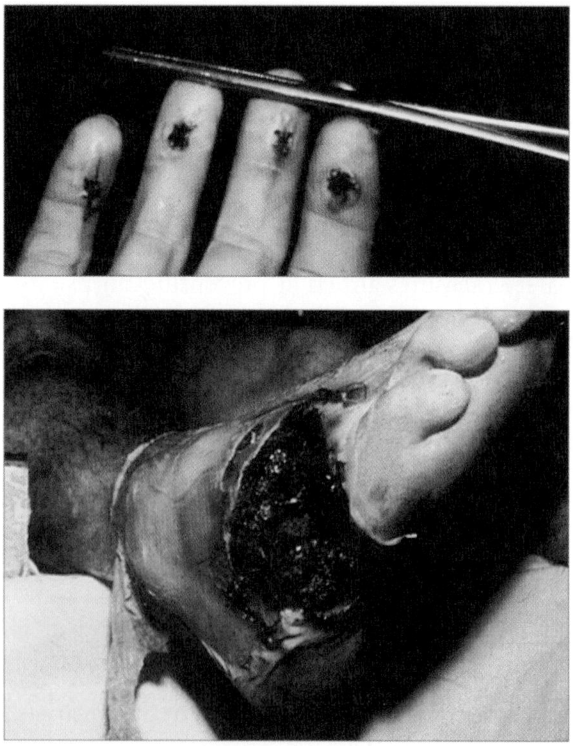

Figure 19–15 An electrical burn. **A,** The electrical current enters through the hand. **B,** The electrical current exits through the foot. **Source:** Sanders, M. (1994). *Mosby's paramedic textbook*. St. Louis: Mosby.

- For *heat source burns*, stop the burning process. Protect yourself from the source of the burn. Extinguish flames with water, or roll the person in a blanket, coat, sheet, or towel.
- Remove burned clothing that is not sticking to the skin. Do not pull at clothing if it is sticking to the burn. Remove any jewellery, tight clothing, or belts before the injured area swells.
- Administer rescue breathing and CPR, as needed.
- Cool the burned skin with cool water, not ice. Do not use cold water on large, third-degree burns. Do not immerse the burn in ice water. Cover the burn with a clean, cool, moist compress. (Use towels, sheets, or any other clean cloth.) Re-apply the cool compress for up to 20 minutes (for burns on the hands, feet, or face) or up to 1 hour (for second-degree burns). Pat the area dry.
- Loosely cover the burn wounds with a clean, dry covering. Thick, sterile gauze is preferable, but you can use towels, sheets, or any other clean cloth. Tape the covering in place, being careful not to touch the burn with the tape.
- Do not put oil, butter, salve, or ointments on the burn.
- Do not break the blisters.
- Cover the client with a blanket or coat to prevent heat loss.
- Watch for signs of shock. Stay with the client until help arrives.

PREVENTING SUFFOCATION

Suffocation occurs when breathing stops due to lack of oxygen. Brain damage or death may occur depending on how long the person has been deprived of oxygen, sometimes within 3 to 4 minutes. Common causes include choking, drowning, inhaling gas or smoke, strangulation, and electrical shock. Children under 1 year, clients who have difficulties chewing and swallowing, and clients with serious mobility or mental impairments are at risk of suffocation (see Box 19–6).

Carbon Monoxide Poisoning

Carbon monoxide (CO), also known as the "silent killer," is a colourless, odourless, tasteless gas, produced by burning of material containing carbon, such as in common household appliances or fireplaces. When these appliances or fireplaces are not properly ventilated, carbon monoxide can build up in the air and enter the bloodstream of the

Box 19–6 Safety Measures to Prevent Suffocation in Adults

- When feeding adult clients, do not rush them. Cut food into small, bite-sized pieces for those who cannot do so themselves.
- Observe and report any indication that the client is having difficulty swallowing, such as drooling, pocketing food, or coughing (see Chapter 27).
- If the client has had any of the above signs of swallowing difficulties, choose foods that they can easily swallow. Foods such as canned peaches might easily become lodged in the client's throat while eating.
- Make sure the client's dentures fit properly and are in place. Report any loose teeth or dentures.
- Before serving any food or fluids, check the care plan about dealing with the client's swallowing problems. The client may ask for something that he or she cannot swallow.
- Tell your supervisor at once if the client has problems swallowing.
- Do not give food or fluids orally to clients with feeding tubes, unless it is stated in their care plan. Remember that all clients who are NPO (not by mouth) for any reason must not receive foods or fluids orally.
- Open doors and windows if you notice gas odours. Immediately report gas odours to your supervisor, or dial 9-1-1 if the odour is strong. Assist your client to move out of the area.
- Position the client in bed properly (see Chapter 23).
- Use bed rails properly (see pages 302–304).

unsuspecting people or animals that inhale the air. They have no idea about what is happening to them—that this gas, instead of oxygen, is quickly binding to their red blood cells, which can be fatal (see Chapter 14).

Early symptoms of carbon monoxide poisoning—such as headaches, nausea, and fatigue—are often mistaken for flu symptoms because this deadly gas goes undetected in a home. Prolonged exposure can lead to brain damage and even death. As in suffocation, the person dies from a lack of oxygen to the brain.

Carbon Monoxide Detectors. Carbon monoxide detectors are strongly recommended for all homes, especially in areas of the home where the family members gather and spend the most time, such as kitchens and bedrooms. It is important that manufacturer's instructions are followed and that the devices are checked periodically to ensure that they work properly. Some are connected to household electricity (they may be hard wired or plugged in), and some work on batteries. Batteries must be replaced routinely, such as every month. Carbon monoxide detectors are inexpensive, but they can save lives!

PREVENTING ACCIDENTS WITH EQUIPMENT

As a support worker, you will be required to use equipment, such as household appliances, mechanical lifting devices, wheelchairs, and walkers in clients' homes as well as in facilities. All equipment is unsafe if broken, not used correctly, or not working properly.

When using any type of equipment, you must know what you are doing. You also must make sure that the equipment is in safe working order. Follow the safety measures in Box 19–7 to prevent equipment accidents.

Box 19–7 Safety Measures to Prevent Equipment Accidents

- Follow your employer policies and procedures.
- Follow the manufacturer's instructions.
- Read all cautions and warning labels.
- Do not use unfamiliar equipment. Ask for needed training. Ask for supervision the first time you use the item.
- Use equipment only for its intended purpose.
- Inspect all equipment before use. Check for broken or damaged parts. Check for cracks, chips, rough or sharp edges, or loose bolts and screws. These can cause cuts, stabs, or scratches. Do not use or give damaged items to clients.
- Notify your supervisor immediately about the broken equipment. Follow your employer's policies for reporting equipment in need of repair or equipment-related accidents.
- Do not try to repair broken equipment yourself.
- Make sure electrical cords are not frayed or damaged in any way (Figure 19–16). Make sure that not too many cords are plugged into one electrical outlet (Figure 19–17). Frayed cords and overloaded electrical outlets can cause electric shocks.
- Make sure all electrical equipment has three-pronged plugs (Figure 19–18). Two prongs carry electrical current, and the third prong grounds the current and carries leaking electricity to the earth and away from the item, thus preventing electric shocks.
- Stop using any electrical equipment and ***immediately report it*** to your supervisor if:
  - It gives you a shock
  - It produces sparks, buzzing sounds, or a burning odour
  - Lights dim or flicker
  - The power shuts down
- Immediately report any shock received while using a piece of equipment.
- Keep electrical equipment away from water (water conducts electricity).
- Hold on to the plug (not the cord) when removing it from an outlet.
- Turn off equipment when you are finished using the item.

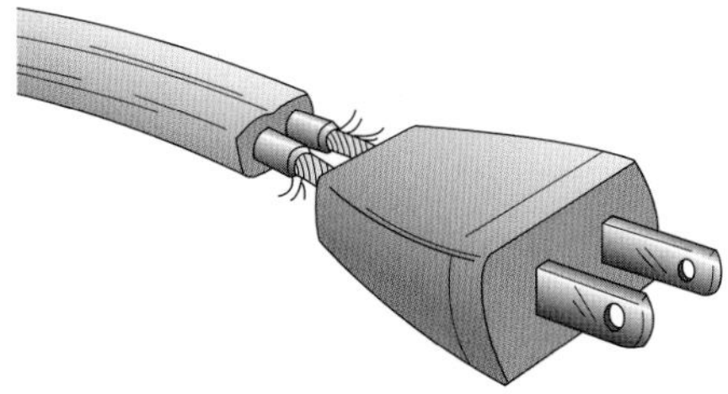

Figure 19–16 A frayed electrical cord.

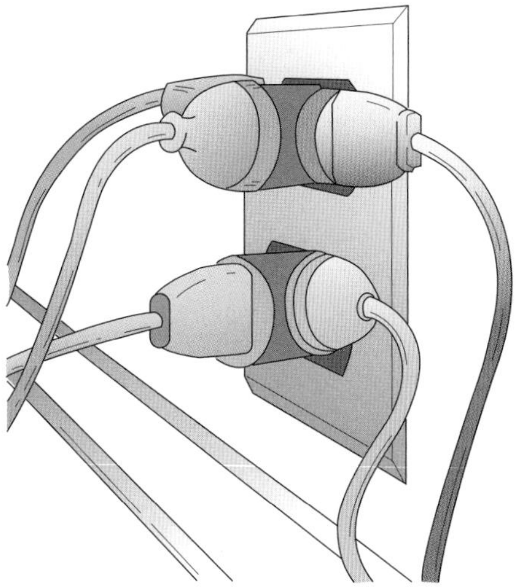

Figure 19–17 An overloaded electrical outlet.

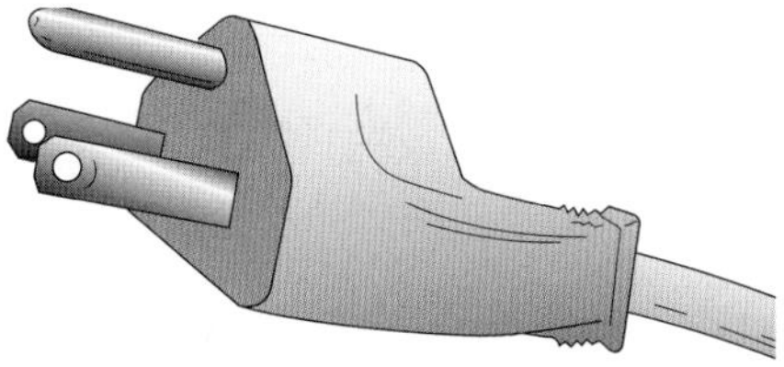

Figure 19–18 A three-pronged plug.

PREVENTING FIRES

Fires are a constant danger in homes and facilities. Unsafe smoking, cooking accidents, faulty electrical equipment and wiring, and heating equipment are major causes. The entire health care team must be vigilant to prevent fires. Box 19–8 lists fire prevention measures (see also the *Focus on Home Care: Fire Safety* box).

Fires and the Use of Oxygen. Some clients have difficulty breathing or do not receive enough oxygen from the air, so oxygen therapy is prescribed by physicians. This means they receive additional oxygen through a nasal tube or face-mask. The oxygen is supplied through portable oxygen tanks, wall outlets, or oxygen concentrators (see Chapter 44).

Oxygen systems are widely used in facilities and in home care. However, oxygen is a serious fire hazard, as it supports combustion. Therefore you should ensure that combustible items (such as petroleum jelly on the client's lips, or clothing, towels, and sheets that are static-charged) are kept away from the source of the oxygen, to reduce the risk of a fire. Special safety measures are needed where oxygen is used and stored (see Box 19–9).

What to Do During a Fire. The health care team must act quickly and responsibly during a fire. The key to surviving a fire is to be prepared before one starts. Know your employer's policies and procedures for fire emergencies. Know where to find fire alarms, fire extinguishers, and emergency exits. Facilities conduct fire drills to practise emergency fire procedures (see the *Focus on Home Care: Being Prepared for a Fire* box).

focus on
›› HOME CARE

Fire Safety

It is essential to have working smoke detectors on every floor of the home and ideally outside each sleeping area. Always identify all smoke detectors in clients' homes, and make sure they are working. Notify your supervisor and the family if you find a smoke detector that is not working.

focus on
›› HOME CARE

Being Prepared for a Fire

Plan what to do in each client's home even before a fire occurs. The first time you enter a client's home, plan two fire escape routes from every room. If the client lives in an apartment building, identify the fire alarms in the hallways in case you ever need to use them.

Box 19–8 Safety Measures to Prevent Fires

- Smoke only in areas where it is allowed. Do not smoke in the client's home.
- Supervise clients who smoke. This is very important for clients who are confused, disoriented, or sedated.
- Provide ashtrays for clients who are allowed to smoke.
- Check smoking areas, especially furniture, for dropped cigarettes and ashes.
- Be sure all ashes, cigars, and cigarettes are put out before emptying ashtrays.
- Empty ashtrays into a metal container partially filled with sand or water. Do not empty them into plastic containers or wastebaskets lined with paper or plastic bags.
- Do not allow clients to smoke in bed or while lying down; they could fall asleep and drop a lit cigarette onto the sheets or cushion, starting a fire.
- Do not light matches or lighters or smoke around flammable liquids or materials.
- Keep matches and lighters out of the reach of children.
- Avoid deep frying in oil, since oil is highly flammable. If you must deep fry, use a deep-fryer rather than a shallow pan.
- Do not drape tea towels or other material over the oven door.
- Use potholders to remove hot items from the oven. Do not use tea towels.
- Follow the manufacturer's instructions when using space heaters. Keep them at least 1 m (3 ft) away from curtains, drapes, and furniture, and do not leave them unattended.
- Keep flammable liquids and materials away from fireplaces, radiators, heat registers, and other sources of heat or flame.
- Store flammable liquids in their original containers.
- Do not run electrical cords under carpets.
- Use extension cords only as a temporary measure.
- Prevent equipment accidents. Follow the measures listed in Box 19–7.
- Follow the safety measures for oxygen use (see Box 19–9 and Chapter 44).

Box 19–9 Safety Measures for Using Oxygen

- Never smoke around oxygen equipment. Remove all items related to smoking (such as ashtrays and lighters) from the room.
- "No Smoking" and "Oxygen in Use" signs should be placed on the front door of the client's home, apartment, or room and near the area where the oxygen is being directly used. Some people ignore such rules; however, be sure to remind the client, family, and visitors to never smoke around oxygen equipment.
- Keep oxygen tanks away from open flames (such as pilot lights, candles, and incense) and heat sources (such as stoves, heating ducts, radiators, and space heaters).
- Remove from the room materials that can ignite easily, for example, alcohol, nail polish remover, oils, and greases.
- Make sure the client does not use toiletry items that are flammable, such as perfume, petroleum jelly, hairspray, and after-shave lotion, when receiving oxygen.
- Turn off electrical items before unplugging them. Sparks can occur when electrical items are unplugged while still on.
- Use electrical equipment, including shavers, hair dryers, radios, and stereo equipment, only if it has a three-pronged plug and is in good working order.
- The oxygen source should be shut off and removed from the client prior to shaving the client with an electric shaver, when drying a client's hair with a blow dryer, and when using a curling iron on the client's hair because of the risk of sparks from such equipment.
- Remove all wool and synthetic fabrics from the room because they could create static electricity. Wear cotton uniforms, and use cotton blankets and clothing for the client.

The acronym RACE will help you remember what to do if you discover a fire in a home or a facility:

- **R**—for **Rescue**. Rescue people in immediate danger. Move them to a safe place.
- **A**—for **Alarm**. Sound the nearest fire alarm. Notify the switchboard operator. Or call 9-1-1 if in a client's home.
- **C**—for **Confine**. Close doors and windows to confine the fire. Turn off oxygen or electrical equipment in use in the general area of the fire.
- **E**—for **Extinguish** or **Evacuate**. Use a fire extinguisher on a small fire that has not spread to a larger area. If the fire cannot be easily extinguished, evacuation will be necessary.

Always keep equipment away from all exits.

Using a Fire Extinguisher. In many facilities, only supervisory or registered staff are allowed to use a fire extinguisher, while in some all employees are required to demonstrate use of a fire extinguisher. It is your responsibility to know the rules of your agency in this regard and to receive the proper training regarding the use of a fire extinguisher. Fire extinguishers are readily available in facilities; however, home care clients should also have them available. If the client has a fire extinguisher in the home, identify it and make sure that (a) the pin is intact, with (b) the plastic seal secured to the body of the extinguisher, and (c) the pressure dial reads "full." Notify your supervisor and the family if the fire extinguisher does not have any of these components.

Never attempt to fight a large or spreading fire with an extinguisher. Fire extinguishers are only useful against small fires that have not spread from where they started, for example, a wastebasket or a cushion. Do not use a fire extinguisher on a fire that is fed by gas or flammable liquid.

Types of Fire Extinguishers. Different extinguishers are used for different kinds of fires. Use the ABCs to remember the types of extinguishers:

- Class A: **Ash**. Materials that burn and leave ash, such as paper and wood.
- Class B: **Burn/Boil**. Materials that can burn or boil, such as oil and grease.
- Class C: **Current**. Materials that have an electric current, causing electrical fires.

Using the wrong extinguisher on a fire makes the fire worse. Many extinguishers are multipurpose ones, designed to fight all types of fires. Learn how to use a fire extinguisher *before* an emergency, and when you must use a fire extinguisher, remember the acronym "PASS" (Figures 19–19 and 19–20).

P—**P**ull the pin out.
A—**A**im at the base of the fire.
S—**S**queeze the handle.
S—**S**weep from side to side, spraying the contents of the extinguisher.

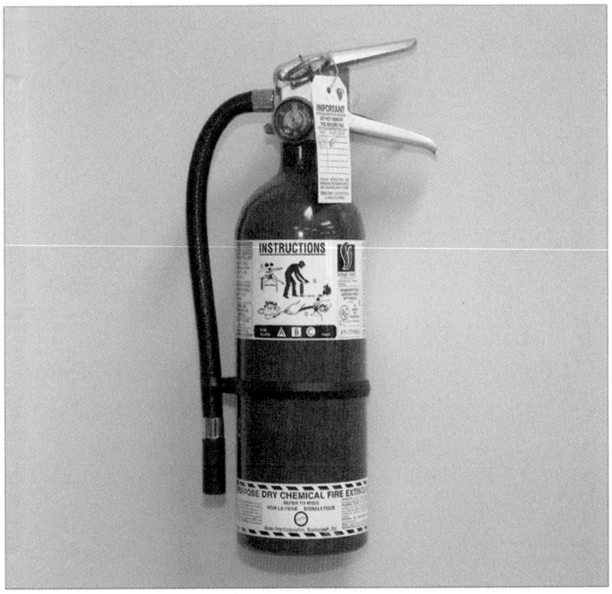

Figure 19–19 A typical fire extinguisher. **Courtesy:** Brian Hillier.

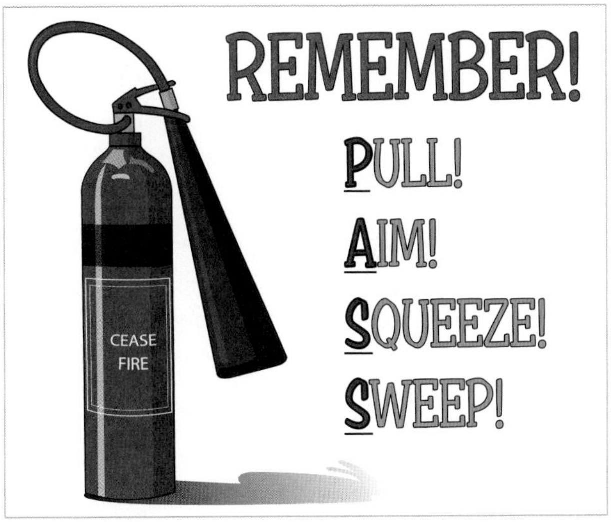

Figure 19–20 P.A.S.S.

Evacuating. When evacuating a facility or a home, several safety measures apply (see Box 19–10). Facilities have evacuation policies and procedures. If evacuation is necessary, clients closest to the danger are taken out first. Those who can walk are given blankets to wrap around themselves, and a staff member escorts them to a safe place. Figure 19–21 and Figure 19–22 show how to rescue people who cannot walk. ***Remember that these procedures are for emergency evacuation only and are not intended to be used routinely to move a client.*** Once firefighters arrive, they direct rescue efforts.

Box 19–10 Safety Measures for Evacuating a Building

- Never use elevators in a building on fire.
- Touch doors before opening them. Do not open a hot door. Use another way out. If the door is cool, open it carefully. If heat and smoke rush in, shut the door again.
- If smoke is present, look for another escape route that is smoke-free. If you must exit through smoke, cover your nose and mouth with a damp cloth. Do the same for the client and family. Have everyone crawl to the nearest exit to stay below the smoke.
- If your clothes catch on fire, do not run. Drop to the ground, cover your face, and roll to smother the flames. If possible, wrap a rug or blanket around yourself. If a client's clothing is on fire, get him or her to roll on the floor until the fire is out. Alternatively, cover the person with a blanket or coat; start by protecting the client's head and neck, and then lay out the blanket or coat over the burning area. Pat the burning area until the fire goes out.
- Once you and your client get out of the burning building, never go back in.
- If you get trapped by fire or smoke in a room, shut the door and block any gaps, such as under a door, with blankets or other thick material that will keep smoke from entering the room. If possible, call 9-1-1 or the fire department and tell them exactly where you are in the building. Go to the window and shout for help, and hang a large piece of material, such as a towel, sheet, or clothing, from the window, which will attract the firefighters' attention.

Identifying the Client

As a support worker, you will be required to care for many people, each having different treatments, therapies, and activity limits. Before performing a procedure, make sure you are giving the right care to the right person. Follow employer policies and procedures for identifying clients. Life and health are threatened if you give wrong care to a client.

In home care settings, identifying the client is easy, as there is usually only one client per home. Make sure you bring the right assignment sheet for the right home. In other community settings, such as group homes and assisted-living facilities, you might have more than one client in the home. Always make sure you are giving the right care to the right person. Read the name on the care plan for each client carefully.

In continuing care facilities, many residents receive care in the same place, and you will often care for the same residents over an extended period of time. You will get to know these residents very well and will easily recognize them. Be careful to give the right care to the right person. Check the resident's name and room number on the assignment sheet carefully. Do not confuse one resident's care plan with another's. Some continuing care facilities have a photograph identification system. The resident's picture is taken on admission and the photo placed in the person's medical record. Other facilities post identifying information in the resident's room. Learn about your employer's policies and procedures for identifying residents.

In hospitals, patients usually are admitted and discharged within a short period of time, and it may not be easy to identify every client on sight. Therefore hospitals usually assign identification (ID) bracelets to patients (Figure 19–23) containing information, including the patient's name, room number and bed number, age, gender, and physician.

Use the ID bracelet to identify the client before giving care. Treatment cards or assignment sheets specify the care to be given. To identify a client in a hospital:

- Compare identifying information on the treatment card or assignment sheet with that on the ID bracelet (Figure 19–24). Carefully check the client's full name. Some people share the

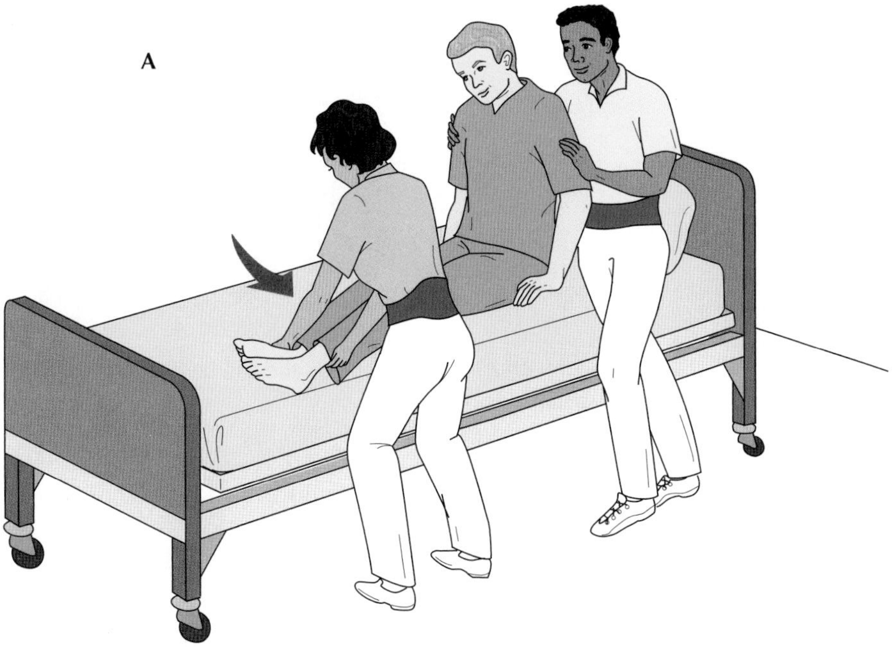

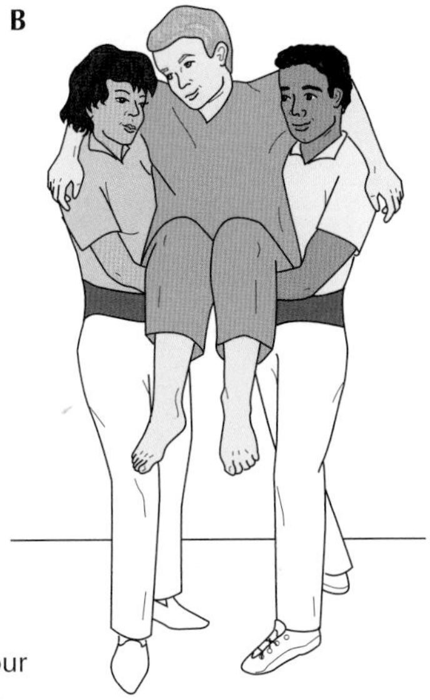

Figure 19–21 Swing carry technique. **A,** Assist the client to a sitting position. A co-worker grasps the client's ankles as you both turn the client so that he sits on the side of the bed. **B,** Pull the client's arm over your shoulder. With one arm, reach across the client's back to your co-worker's shoulder. Reach under the client's knees and grasp your co-worker's arm. Your co-worker does the same.

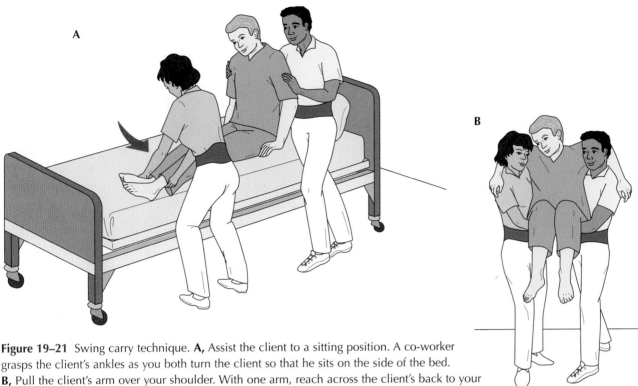

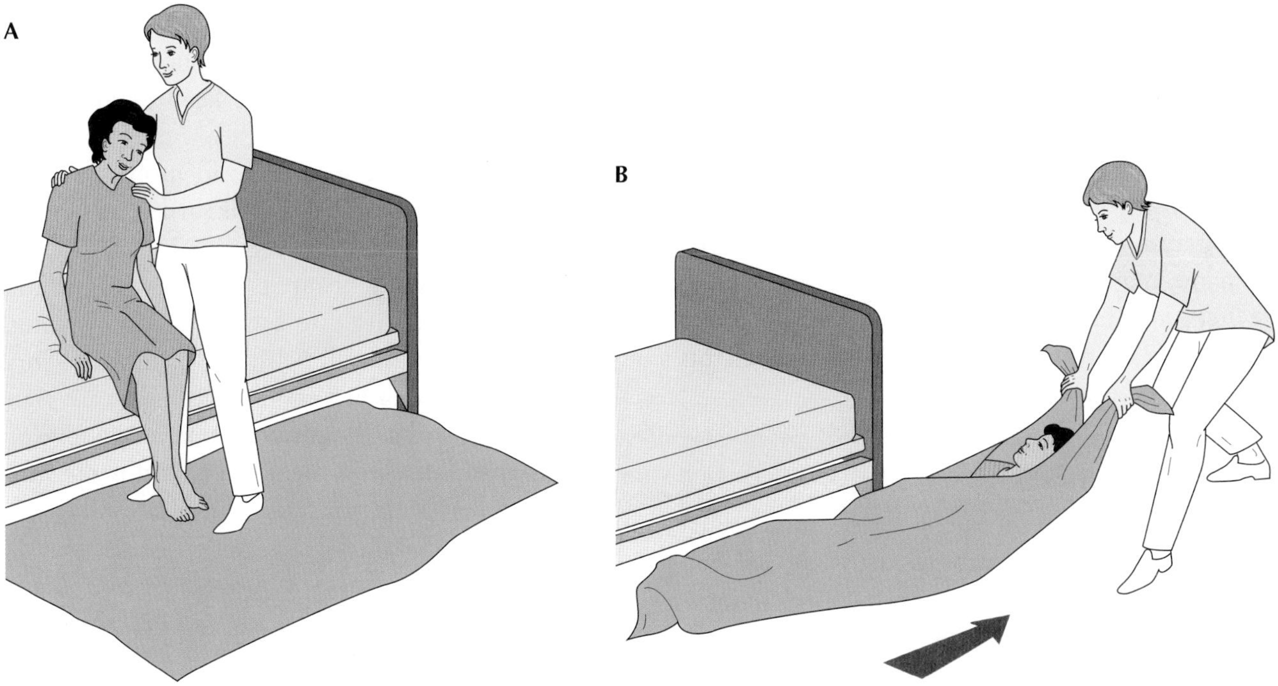

Figure 19-22 One-rescuer carry. **A,** Spread a blanket on the floor. Make sure the blanket will extend beyond the client's head. Help the client sit on the side of the bed. Place one of your knees on the bed near the client's side. From behind the client's back, grasp the client under the arms with both of your arms, and cross your hands over her chest. Lower the client to the floor by sliding her down one of your legs. **B,** Wrap the blanket around the client. Grasp the blanket over the head area. Pull the client to a safe area.

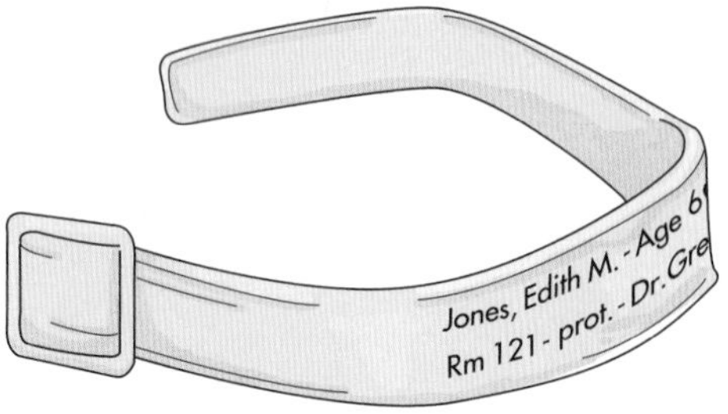

Figure 19–23 ID bracelet.

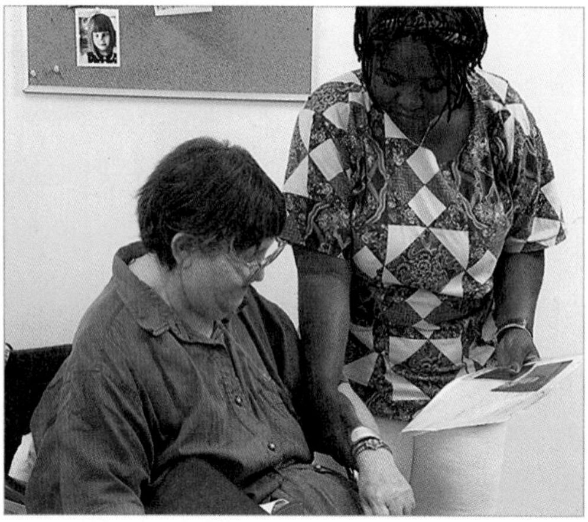

Figure 19–24 In hospitals, compare the ID bracelet against the assignment sheet to accurately identify the client.

same first and last names, for example, common names such as John Smith.

- Call the client by name when checking the ID bracelet. This is a courtesy you extend to the client as you touch him or her and before giving care. However, just calling the client by name may not be enough to identify him or her accurately, as confused, disoriented, drowsy, hearing-impaired, or distracted clients may answer to any name.

Using the Call Bell

Call bells are important safety devices for hospital patients and long-term care residents. A **call bell** enables a client to call for assistance. Different facilities use different call systems. The term "call bell" is used in this book when referring to any one of a number of call systems that a facility may use. Most systems consist of a cord that is attached to the bed or a chair. A button is at the end of the cord (Figure 19–25). To get help, the client presses the button, which causes a signal to ring at the nurses'

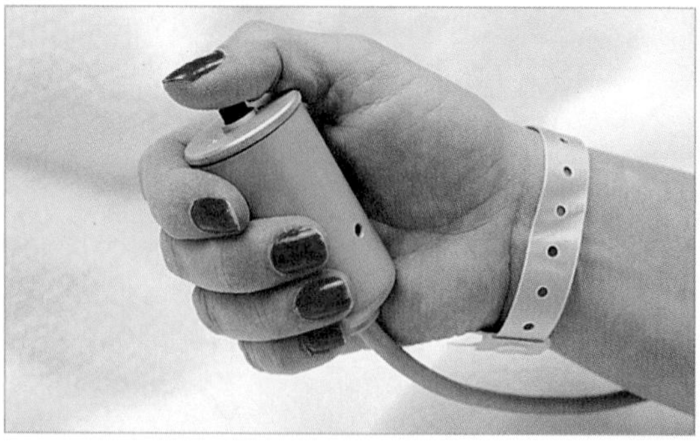

Figure 19–25 A client presses the call bell button when assistance is needed.

station. Or pressing the button may turn on a light above the client's door and at the nurses' station (Figure 19-26, *A*). These alert the health care team that the client needs assistance.

Some call bells are also connected to an intercom at the nurses' station (Figure 19–26, *B*). Using the intercom, a support worker or a nurse can talk with the client who has called for help. In newer facilities, the call bell system may be directly connected to cordless phones carried by the staff. As the support worker in the facility, you would respond directly to the client by phone, and the client can tell you what he or she needs. However, be careful when using an intercom or a cell phone, as people nearby can hear what you say; keep in mind the client's right to confidentiality.

Some clients have limited hand mobility. They may need a special call bell that is turned on by tapping it with a hand or fist (Figure 19–27).

Patients and residents are taught how to use the call bell when admitted to a facility. Some clients, however, cannot use call bells, for example, clients who are confused or in a coma. Check the care plan carefully for special communication methods for these clients. Check on them often, and make sure that their needs are met (see the *Focus on Home Care: Call Bells* box).

Whenever you finish a procedure and leave the client's room, make sure the call bell is within the client's reach. You must:

- Keep the call bell within the client's reach in the room, bathroom, and shower or tub room. Even if the client cannot use the call bell, keep it within reach of visitors and staff, as they may need to call for help.

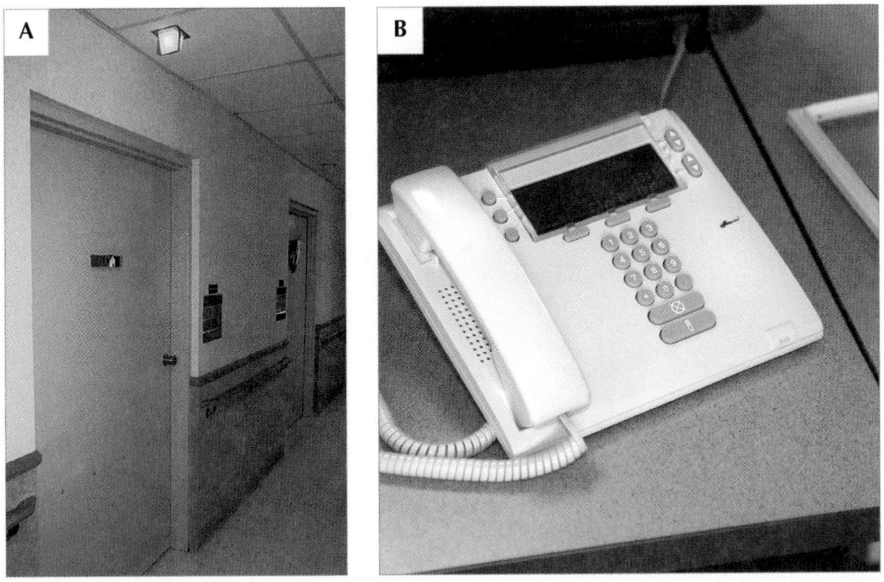

Figure 19–26 **A,** The light above the door of the client's room. **B,** Light panel of intercom system at the nurses' station. In newer facilities, the call bell may be directly connected to a cordless phone carried by the staff. The support worker would then respond to the client by phone. **Courtesy:** Brian Hillier.

- Place the call bell on the client's strong (unaffected) side.
- Remind the client to use the call bell when help is needed.
- Answer call bells promptly. The client may have an urgent need to use the bathroom. You can prevent embarrassment by promptly helping the client to the bathroom. A prompt response also helps prevent infection, skin breakdown, pressure ulcers, and falls.

Leaving a client without a call bell can be regarded as negligence or punishment. In either case, it is certainly regarded as emotional abuse (see Chapter 21).

focus on
›› **HOME CARE**

Call Bells

Some home care clients are confined in the bed or in a particular part of the home, and they need a way to call for help. Tap bells, dinner bells (Figure 19–28), baby monitors, and other devices are all useful in home care settings. Or you can give the client a small can with a few coins inside so that it can be rattled to get attention. Children's toys with bells, horns, and whistles may also be useful. Whatever the client decides to use, keep the calling device within his or her easy reach.

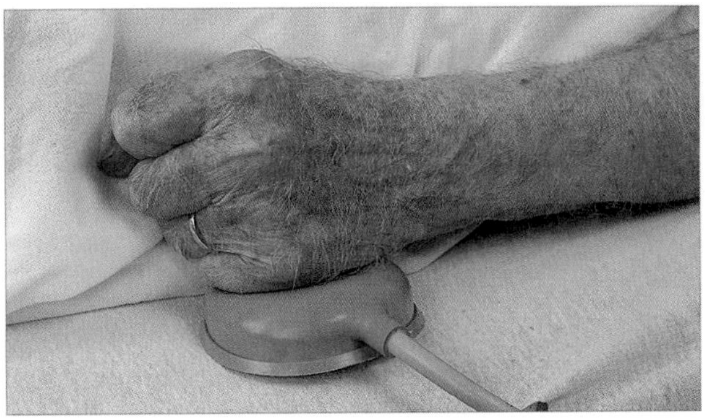

Figure 19–27 Call bell for a client with limited hand mobility.

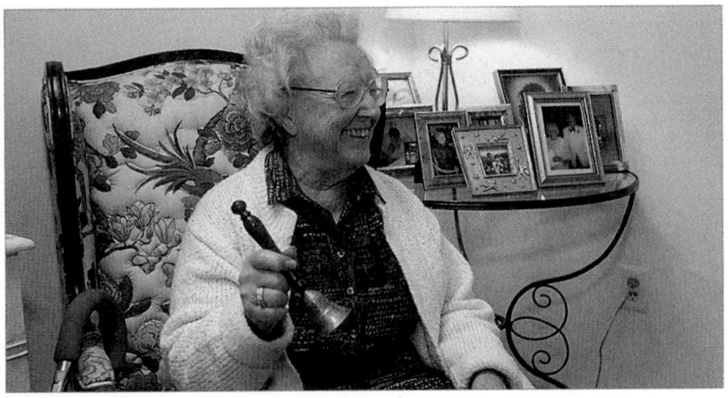

Figure 19–28 This woman rings a dinner bell when she needs assistance.

PROMOTING YOUR PERSONAL SAFETY

As a support worker, you are sometimes exposed to safety hazards on the job. You could have an accident if your workplace environment is not safe. You could be injured when working with hazardous materials. You might also be at risk for workplace violence.

Creating a Safe Workplace

In Canada, each province and territory has occupational health and safety (OH&S) legislation. **OH&S legislation** is designed to protect employees from injuries and accidents in the workplace. In most places, this legislation is called the *Occupational Health and Safety Act* (http://www.canoshweb.org/en/legislation.html). It is revised regularly to reflect changes in policies. The name of this Act varies across the country.

The details of the legislation also vary from one place to another, but the basic elements are similar. In general, the legislation assumes that all people in the workplace—employers, supervisors, and workers—are responsible for their own health and safety and also have certain rights and duties.

Employers' and Supervisors' Responsibilities. According to OH&S legislation, your employer and supervisor must take every reasonable precaution to protect your health and safety (see the *Focus on Home Care: OH&S Legislation* box).

Your employer is responsible for:

- Having written policies that promote safety
- Training and educating you about these policies
- Creating a health and safety committee to identify hazards in the workplace and investigate accidents
- Responding to reports of workplace hazards
- Warning you about safety hazards and correcting these hazards, whenever possible
- Reporting all accidents promptly to the government department responsible for occupational health and safety

> focus on
> ››HOME CARE
>
> **OH&S Legislation**
>
> When you are providing services to a home care client, the client's home is considered a workplace, and the home care agency is considered your employer. Therefore, agencies have the same obligations to their employees as do facilities.

- Making sure that all necessary equipment is available (including personal protective equipment, such as gloves and masks) and is kept in good working order

Employees' Responsibilities. You are responsible for:

- Following all safety policies and procedures
- Using all recommended protective equipment and clothing
- Reporting all safety hazards and concerns immediately to your supervisor or a representative of your health and safety committee
- Completing an **incident report** (also known as an **occurrence report**) (Figure 19–29). This is a report submitted to your employer whenever an accident, error, or unexpected problem arises in the workplace. Figure 19–29 shows an example of a generic incident report. Your agency's incident reports may differ slightly.

According to the OH&S legislation, you have the right to refuse to do unsafe work. This applies whether you are working in a facility or a community setting. However, you cannot refuse to work if:

- The danger is a normal part of the job
- Your refusal would endanger the client

For example, you could not refuse to provide care to a client with a communicable disease because you are afraid of contracting the disease. However, you could refuse to provide care to a client with a communicable disease if protective gloves, masks, and gowns are not available.

REPORT OF INCIDENT AND INJURY

PLEASE PRINT IN INK To be completed by Employee

Employer ____________________ Location ____________________

Name of Client ____________________ Identification No. ____________________

Birth Date ____________________ Sex ☐ Male ☐ Female Telephone ( ) ____________________

Name of employee (if incident included them) ____________________ Shift ____________________

Occupation ____________________ Department ____________________

If you did see incident occur:

Date of incident ____________________ Time of incident ____________________ ☐ am ☐ pm

Describe what caused the injury/symptoms, what you were doing just before the incident, and what you did after the incident (if you need more space, write on the back of this form). Be specific – name any objects or substances involved:

____

____

____

Describe what you saw:

____

____

____

Did anyone else see the incident? ☐ Yes ☐ No If yes, who? ____________________

Did you report this incident to anyone? ☐ Yes ☐ No If not, why not? ____________________

If yes, to whom did you report it? ____________________ Title/Position ____________________ When? ____

What part(s) of the body was/were affected? (BE SPECIFIC: for example, right elbow, left knee, right index finger)

____

What type of injury resulted? (BE SPECIFIC: for example, bruise, scrape, laceration, pull)

____

Was any first aid provided at the scene? ☐ Yes ☐ No If yes, describe: ____________________

Was other medical treatment sought? ☐ Yes ☐ No If yes, when? ____________________

Where? ____________________ If treatment was not sought immediately, explain why:

____

If this injury happened to you: Is this an aggravation of a previous injury/symptom? ☐ Yes ☐ No If yes, when were you last treated for the previous injury? ____________________ By whom or where? ____________________

Have you ever had a similar injury? ☐ Yes ☐ No If yes, describe other injury: ____________________

____

Figure 19–29 A sample incident report. **Courtesy:** St. Joseph's at Fleming, Peterborough, ON.

Handling Hazardous Materials

A **hazardous material** is any substance that presents a physical hazard or a health hazard in the workplace. Physical hazards can cause fires or explosions. Health hazards are chemicals that can cause acute or chronic health problems, for example, kidney or lung damage, cancer, or burns.

OH&S legislation requires that health care employees understand the risk of hazardous materials and know how to safely handle them. In order to provide this information, the Canadian government created the **Workplace Hazardous Materials Information System (WHMIS)**.

WHMIS is a national system that provides safety information about hazardous materials. It includes labelling, material safety data sheets (MSDS), and employee education. WHMIS applies to hazardous materials that meet certain criteria, known as *controlled products,* which include compressed gases and products that are poisonous, corrosive, reactive, or that can catch fire or explode. You may work with or around controlled products; for example:

- Drugs used in cancer therapy (chemotherapy, anticancer drugs)
- Gases used to sterilize equipment
- Oxygen used in oxygen therapy
- Certain disinfectants and cleaning solutions
- Mercury (found in some thermometers and blood pressure devices)

The following are the three components of WHMIS:

1. ***Labels***—WHMIS labels provide the essential information needed to safely handle a controlled product (Figure 19–30). The supplier applies the label, but if the product is made at the workplace, the employer designs and applies the label. Warning labels provide the following information:
   - Product information—the brand, code, or chemical name of the product
   - Supplier information—the name and address of the supplier
   - Hazard symbols—pictures that show the kind of hazard the product presents (Figure 19–31).
   - Risk phrases—short phrases that describe the physical and health hazards; for example, "Spray may catch fire if used near an open flame."
   - Precautionary statements—safety measures to be taken when using or handling the product; for example, "Keep in a cool place." They also list necessary personal protective equipment; for example, "Wear gloves if skin contact may occur."
   - First aid measures—measures that are necessary in case of an accident or emergency
   - Reference to the MSDS—statement that tells that an MSDS is available

   Read and follow all warning labels. A container must have a label, and this label must not be removed or damaged in any way. If a warning label is removed or damaged, do not use the product. Take the container to your supervisor and explain the problem. Do not leave the container unattended.
2. ***Material Safety Data Sheets (MSDS)***—these provide detailed information about each hazardous material. They are obtained from suppliers or developed by employers. Each MSDS provides information about the product, specifies if it can cause a fire or explosion, and describes its health hazards. The MSDS also tells how to safely handle, use, store, and dispose of the product and also lists first aid measures.
3. ***Worker education***—employers must provide WHMIS education to employees who work

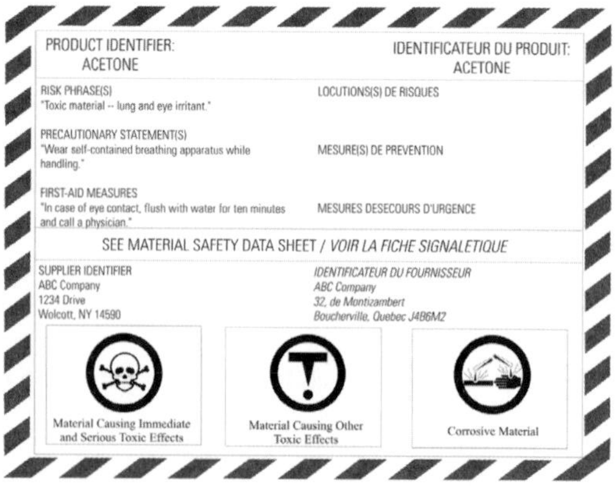

Figure 19–30 Sample WHMIS hazard label.

	Flammable and Combustible Material	Product may catch fire or burst into flames if exposed to heat, sparks, or flame.
	Oxidizing Material	Product may cause a fire or explosion if it is exposed to combustible material.
	Compressed Gas	Product is under high pressure. May explode or burst when heated, dropped, or damaged.
	Corrosive Material	Product can cause burns to eyes, skin, or respiratory system.
	Dangerously Reactive Material	Product may react with light, heat, extreme temperatures, or vibration, causing an explosion, fire, or release of poisonous gases.
	Poisonous and Infectious Material: Immediate and Serious Toxic Effects	Product may be fatal or cause serious or permanent damage to health if exposed to even once.
	Poisonous and Infectious Material: Other Toxic Effects	Product may cause cancer, birth defects, or other permanent damage if exposed to repeatedly.
	Poisonous and Infectious Material: Biohazardous and Infectious Material	Product may cause disease, serious illness, or death.

Figure 19–31 WHMIS Symbols. **Source:** The Canadian Centre for Occupational Health and Safety, Hamilton, Ontario. (2008). Retrieved October 27, 2007, from http://www.ccohs.ca/oshanswers/legisl/msds_lab.html?print.

with controlled products. Information is given about WHMIS labels, MSDS, and hazard information. The employees also learn how to safely handle, use, store, and dispose of controlled products.

Reducing Personal Security Risks

Workplace violence is any physical assault or threatening behaviour that occurs in a work setting. It includes:

- Psychological trauma—threat, obscene phone call, and harassment of any nature (being followed, sworn at, or shouted at)
- Robbery
- Rape
- Kidnapping
- Beating, stabbing, and shooting
- Murder

Workplace violence can occur in any place where an employee is carrying out a work-related task.

This includes buildings, parking lots, field locations, homes, and travel to and from work assignments.

Home care workers, especially, have personal security risks. They work alone in an unknown, uncontrolled environment and often work early or late hours. Clients, family members, or any person in the home could act violently toward them.

You can expect your employer to make your workplace as safe as possible. However, you must also protect yourself from harm. Box 19–12 lists personal safety measures. Follow them all the time. Most of the rules presented apply to support workers working in facilities and in the community.

Box 19–12 Personal Safety Measures

Driving to and From Work

- Familiarize yourself with the area where you will be driving. Plan your route in advance, keeping to well-travelled streets and routes that you know. Note the locations of nearby police stations, public telephones, gas stations, and other public buildings that may be of help in an emergency.
- Let your supervisor and a member of your family know the route you will take.
- Keep with you the phone number of a reliable tow truck company.
- Keep maps in the car.
- Maintain your car in good working order at all times.
- Always use a seat belt.
- Be prepared for winter driving conditions. Keep a survival kit in the car—booster cables, shovel, extra clothing, sand, and road flares.
- Keep cash with you for gas or to make a phone call.
- Have a cellular phone for emergencies on the road. Do not use one while driving. Pull off the road if you need to make an emergency call.
- Pull over to a safe spot away from traffic if you have car trouble. Put on your emergency lights, and call for help if you have a cellular phone. Keep your doors locked and windows rolled up until help arrives. Never leave the car and walk off alone for help.
- Check for places to park. Choose a well-lit, busy area. If using a parking garage, park near entrances, exits, and on a lower level. Try to stay close to the parking attendant if possible. Be aware of passengers sitting in parked cars, and avoid parking by these cars if possible. Lock your car doors as you leave.
- Ask for an escort to walk you back to your car after work. Many facilities provide this service. In a home setting, ask a family member to escort you.
- Have your car key ready so you can get into the car quickly. Do not fumble for keys on the way to or at the car. If necessary, you can use your car keys as a weapon. Carry them in your strong hand. Have one key extended (Figure 19–32). If you are attacked, slash at the attacker's face with the key.
- Check for a possible intruder in the front and back seats before getting into your car.
- If you think someone is following you, cross the street or change directions. Head toward a public building or a lighted house. If you are scared, yell for help.
- Lock car doors when you get in the car. Keep windows rolled up.
- Keep purses, backpacks, and other valuables under the seat or near your side. Do not leave them on the seat. They are easy targets for robberies.
- Do not carry valuables. Do not bring your purse or valuables into clients' homes. Leave them at home or in the car trunk. If an attacker demands something you have, give it. The only thing of value is *you*. Report the crime to the police.
- Carry a whistle or shriek alarm. Carry a travel size can of aerosol hair spray. Go for the attacker's face. If someone tries to force you into a vehicle, do whatever you can to resist being pulled in. Fight back even if you see a weapon (yell, kick, push your thumbs into the attacker's eyes). You are at much greater risk if you are forced into the vehicle.

(continued on page 321)

Box 19–12 **Personal Safety Measures** (cont'd)

Visiting Clients

- Call your supervisor when you arrive and leave a client's home.
- Be cautious in hallways, elevators, and stairwells in apartment buildings. Do not get on an elevator with a stranger who makes you anxious.
- Stay in the centre of the hallways and avoid hidden corners in apartment buildings. If someone threatens you, knock on as many doors as possible and yell to get attention. If you are attacked, pull the fire alarm.
- Pause for a few seconds when entering someone's home. Assess the environment. Check any threats to your safety. This includes used syringes, strange odours, clutter, unfamiliar people, or household items that could be used as weapons. Note the location of the phone. Note any obstacles blocking exits.
- Keep your shoes on. In an emergency, you may need to leave in a hurry. In the winter, bring a pair of shoes for indoor use.
- Leave if a client or anyone else is abusive or makes sexual comments or suggestions.
- If you feel uncomfortable or threatened in any way, go to a safe place and immediately call your supervisor.
- Let the client lead the way down corridors, up staircases, and so on.
- Leave an exit route or place yourself between the exit and the client. Never allow yourself to be cornered. Decide if you should leave a door open or unlocked. Tell the client not to shut or lock a door if the action makes you uncomfortable.
- Sit in a hard-backed chair. You can get up faster from a firm chair than from a soft chair or sofa.
- Sit with your strong leg back and your other leg forward. This position lets you get out of your seat quickly without using your hands.
- Ask that pets be restrained or kept out of the room, if you are nervous about them.
- If a client or family member becomes angry and begins to scream, stay calm. (Refer to the section entitled, "Managing Disruptive Behaviours" in Chapter 35).
- Report any unusual incidents to your supervisor as soon as possible.

Source: Health Care Health and Safety Association of Ontario (HCHSA) & Workplace Safety and Insurance Board (WSIB) of Ontario. (2000). *Health and safety in the home care environment,* pp. 13–24, 43–47. Toronto: HCHSA.

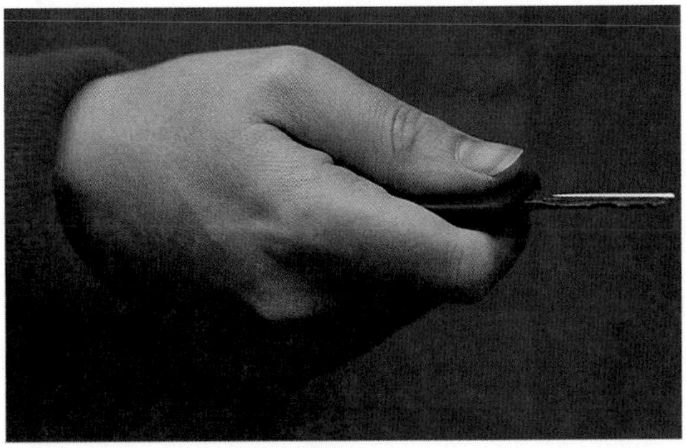

Figure 19–32 Car keys can be used as a weapon.

REVIEW

Answers to these questions are at the bottom of page 324.

Circle T if the answer is true or circle F if the answer is false.

1. T F **Older adults are at risk for accidents because of changes in the body.**
2. T F **The use of medications may increase a client's risk for accidents.**
3. T F **Restraints can be used for staff convenience.**
4. T F **A device is a restraint only if it is attached to the person's body.**
5. T F **Bed rails are restraints.**
6. T F **Restraints can be used to protect the client from harming others.**
7. T F **Unnecessary restraint is false imprisonment.**
8. T F **Informed consent is needed for restraint use.**
9. T F **You can apply restraints when you think they are needed.**
10. T F **You should remove restraints every 2 hours to reposition the client and give skin care.**
11. T F **Some medications are restraints.**
12. T F **Children are not at increased risk for accidents during times of stress or change.**
13. T F **Middle-aged women have the greatest risk for falling.**
14. T F **Falls in facilities are more likely to occur during the evening.**
15. T F **Rushing to get to a bathroom or commode is a major cause of falls.**
16. T F **Socks and bedroom slippers help prevent falls.**
17. T F **Childproof caps should be kept on medications and harmful products.**
18. T F **Medicines and harmful products can be stored in food containers out of the reach of children.**
19. T F **Do not carry or drink hot liquids while holding a child.**
20. T F **You are not responsible for reporting if any equipment is broken or damaged.**
21. T F **To correctly identify a hospital patient, call him or her by name.**
22. T F **Smoking is allowed where oxygen is used.**
23. T F **Hazardous materials must have warning labels.**

Circle the BEST answer.

24. **What is the most common accident in all settings?**
    - A. Burns
    - B. Suffocation
    - C. Falls
    - D. Poisoning
25. **You are caring for Rani, a 6-week-old infant. Which is safe?**
    - A. Checking her in her crib often
    - B. Laying her on her stomach with her head to the side for sleep
    - C. Propping her baby bottle on a rolled towel when feeding her
    - D. Tasting her bottle after warming it
26. **Mr. Higgins is 86 years old. Which of the following are *unsafe* for him?**
    - A. Nonglare, waxed floors
    - B. Electrical cords and other items on the floor in high-traffic areas
    - C. Safety rails and grab bars in the bathroom
    - D. Nonskid shoes
27. **To prevent falls, you should do the following:**
    - A. Wipe up spills right away
    - B. Avoid night-lights, as they cause glare
    - C. Discourage the use of hand rails and grab bars
    - D. Keep the bed in the highest position

REVIEW

Answers to these questions are at the bottom of page 324.

28. **Which action best prevents falls?**
   A. Assisting the client to the washroom once each shift
   B. Answering calls for assistance promptly
   C. Keeping the bed in the highest position
   D. Always using bed rails on residents in continuing care facilities

29. **Mrs. Carrera often tries to get up without help. You should do the following:**
   A. Remind her to call for assistance
   B. Check on her twice per shift
   C. Allow her to go to the washroom on her own
   D. Decide on your own to keep the bed rails up

30. **Which is a common cause of burns?**
   A. Hot bathwater and heating pads
   B. Spilling of cold liquids
   C. Using a microwave oven
   D. Suffocation

31. **You are caring for an infant and young children. Which measure is the safest to use?**
   A. Using an old tie as a belt when putting a child in a highchair
   B. Ironing the clothes while the children play at your feet
   C. Removing stuffed animals and toys from the crib at naptime
   D. Not placing a seat belt on a child in a car if it upsets him or her

32. **To prevent equipment accidents, you should do the following:**
   A. Fix broken or cracked equipment with duct tape
   B. Fix broken items yourself
   C. Stop using electrical equipment if it produces a burning odour
   D. Remove the third prong on plugs if you have only two-prong outlets

33. **You are using certain equipment. Which of the following is *unsafe?***
   A. Following the manufacturer's instructions
   B. Keeping electrical items away from water and spills
   C. Pulling on the cord to remove a plug from an outlet
   D. Turning off electrical items after using them

34. **A fire alarm sounds. Which of the following is *unsafe*?**
   A. Turning off oxygen
   B. Moving clients to a safe place
   C. Using elevators for a quick exit
   D. Closing doors and windows

35. **Your clothing is on fire. Which is the best thing you should do?**
   A. Pour the first thing you can grab on your burning clothes
   B. Run outside
   C. Dial 9-1-1 and wait for help
   D. Roll on the ground to smother the flames

36. **Bed rails are raised when:**
   A. The client tries to get up without assistance
   B. Your supervisor and the care plan tells you to raise them
   C. The client has a seizure
   D. You decide they should be

37. **Which of the following is a common hazard of bed rails?**
   A. Burns
   B. Strangulation
   C. Infections
   D. Pressure sores

38. **According to occupational health and safety legislation, employers are responsible for:**
   A. Expecting employees will educate themselves about safety policies
   B. Doing the unsafe work themselves
   C. Warning employees of any potential and existing safety hazards
   D. Forcing employees to do unsafe work

REVIEW

Answers to these questions are at the bottom of the page.

39. **You gave Mr. Ford the wrong treatment. What should you do?**
    - A. Report the error at the end of the shift
    - B. Take action only if Mr. Ford was harmed
    - C. Ask Mr. Ford what to do
    - D. Complete an incident report as soon as you realize the error

40. **You are working with a WHMIS-controlled product. You should:**
    - A. Use a liquid even though you can no longer read the label
    - B. Wear any needed personal protective equipment
    - C. Remove the label after using the product
    - D. Review instructions on the Material Safety Data Sheet after using the material

41. **You work the night shift. Which of the following is *unsafe*?**
    - A. Parking in a well-lit area
    - B. Locking your car
    - C. Looking for your keys while at the car
    - D. Checking the back seat before entering your car

Answers: 1.T, 2.T, 3.F, 4.F, 5.T, 6.T, 7.T, 8.T, 9.F, 10.T, 11.T, 12.F, 13.F, 14.T, 15.T, 16.F, 17.T, 18.F, 19.T, 20.F, 21.F, 22.F, 23.T, 24.C, 25.A, 26.B, 27.A, 28.B, 29.A, 30.A, 31.C, 32.C, 33.C, 34.C, 35.D, 36.B, 37.B, 38.C, 39.D, 40.B, 41.C

CHAPTER 20

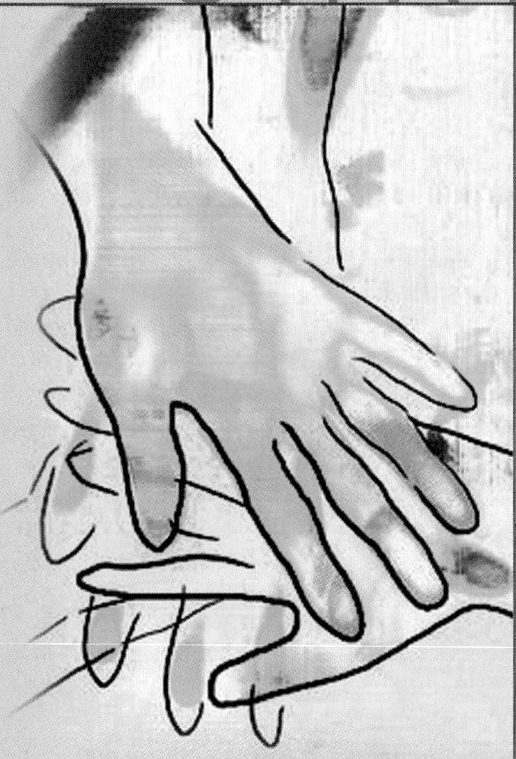

Preventing Infection

OBJECTIVES

- Define the key terms listed in this chapter.
- Distinguish between pathogens and nonpathogens.
- Summarize what microbes require in order to live and grow.
- List the signs and symptoms of infection.
- Describe the chain of infection.
- List ways in which microbes are transmitted.
- List risk factors for infection.
- Describe common aseptic practices.
- Explain why hand washing is important.
- Describe when to wash your hands and general guidelines for hand washing.
- Describe cleaning, disinfection, and sterilization methods.
- Compare and contrast the principles and practices of Standard Practices and Transmission-Based Precautions.
- Summarize how to use personal protective equipment (PPE).
- Describe the principles and practices of surgical asepsis.
- Apply the procedures described in this chapter to your clinical practice properly.

key terms

acquired immune deficiency syndrome (AIDS) **AIDS** is caused by the human immunodeficiency virus **(HIV)**. HIV damages the immune system and makes a person susceptible to opportunistic infections.

asepsis The practice of reducing or eliminating potential pathogens (bacteria, viruses, fungi, and parasites). There are two levels of asepsis: (a) **medical asepsis,** for which the goal is the exclusion of all *pathogenic micro-organisms* through medical aseptic technique, and (b) **surgical asepsis,** which aims to exclude *all micro-organisms and their spores* through surgical aseptic technique.

biohazardous waste Items that may be harmful to others because they are contaminated with blood, body fluids, secretions, or excretions; *bio* means life and *hazardous* means dangerous or harmful.

***C. difficile* (*Clostridium difficile*)** A bacterium that causes diarrhea and colitis. It is the most common cause of infectious diarrhea in hospitalized patients in the industrialized world and one of the most common infections in hospitals and long-term care facilities.

carrier A person who is able to transfer a pathogen to others without getting an active infection himself of herself because the pathogen has become part of that person's **normal flora.**

clean technique A method of giving care using proper hand washing and clean equipment in order to reduce the risk of spreading pathogens. Also known as **medical asepsis** or "no touch" technique.

colonization A process during which bacteria live on or in the body and survive as part of that person's **normal flora.**

communicable disease A disease caused by microbes that spread easily. Also known as **contagious disease.**

communicable phase The period when a person is infectious and can spread pathogens on to others.

contagious disease A disease that is very likely to spread to others.

contamination The process of being exposed to micro-organisms, including pathogens.

disinfection The process of destroying pathogens.

droplet A drop of liquid.

febrile respiratory illness (FRI) is a term used to describe a wide range of respiratory infections, such as colds, influenza, influenza-like illness (ILI) and pneumonia, spread through droplets. People with FRI may have a fever of greater than 38°C and new or worsening cough or shortness of breath. *Note*: Some elderly people or people with immune problems may *not* have a high fever.

fomite Any nonliving object that is capable of carrying infectious organisms and may serve as a mode of transmission.

hand hygiene The process of removing soil and excess microbes from the hands. Hand hygiene may be accomplished by either **hand washing** or the use of **waterless hand rubs** that sanitize the hands. Hand hygiene should always be practised before and after client contact or when in contact with any soiled material. Wearing latex or vinyl gloves should never take the place of hand hygiene. Hand hygiene should always be performed after removing the gloves.

hand washing The process of removing soil and excess microbes from the hands, using soap and running water. It is one form of **hand hygiene**.

health care associated infection (HAI) An infection acquired while a person is a patient, client, or resident in a health care facility or while receiving care from a health care provider. This term has replaced the term "**nosocomial infection.**"

HIV (human immunodeficiency virus) The virus that causes **AIDS**. HIV damages the immune system and makes a person susceptible to opportunistic infections.

incubation period The time between exposure to a pathogenic organism, and when signs and symptoms first appear.

infection A disease state resulting from the invasion and growth of microbes in the body.

infection control Policies and procedures to prevent the spread of infection within health care settings.

influenza A highly contagious infection of the respiratory tract by the causative virus in airborne droplets. Symptoms include sore throat, cough, fever, muscular pains, and weakness.

key terms

isolation precautions Guidelines for preventing the spread of pathogens; includes **Standard Practices** and **Transmission-Based Precautions**.

medical asepsis Practices that reduce the number of pathogens and prevent their spread. Also known as **clean technique.**

metabolism The body's physical and chemical processes that create and use energy. It is also associated with the breaking down of chemicals for excretion.

methicillin-resistant *Staphylococcus aureus* (MRSA) A type of multidrug-resistant organism (MRO) that is resistant to the antibiotic called methicillin.

microbe See **micro-organism**.

micro-organism A form of life (*organism*) that is so small (*micro*) it can be seen only with a microscope. Also known as a **microbe**.

multidrug-resistant organism (MRO) A strain of bacteria that is very difficult to treat with common antibiotics; examples are MRSA and VRE.

nonpathogen A microbe that does not usually cause infection or disease and is not harmful to humans.

normal flora The mixture of different environmental organisms usually found on the surface of the skin and mucous membranes.

nosocomial infection See **health care associated infection (HAI).**

pandemic An epidemic that has spread over a large region or even worldwide.

pathogen A microbe that can cause harm, such as an infection or a disease.

personal protective equipment (PPE) Special clothing and equipment that act as a barrier between microbes and a person's hands, eyes, nose, mouth, and clothes; includes gloves, gowns, masks, and eye protection.

reservoir The environment in which microbes live and grow; host.

Routine Practices See **Standard Practices**.

sharps Equipment or item that may pierce the skin; includes needles, razor blades, and broken glass.

spore coat The protective shell that surrounds dormant bacteria and viruses, which protects them from external harm.

Standard Practices Guidelines to prevent the spread of infection from blood, body fluids, secretions, excretions, nonintact skin, and mucous membranes. Also known as **Routine Practices** or **Standard Precautions**.

Standard Precautions See **Standard Practices**.

sterile Free of all microbes, both pathogens and nonpathogens as well as their spores.

sterile field A work area free of all microbes, both pathogens and nonpathogens.

sterile technique See **surgical asepsis**.

sterilization The process of destroying *all* microbes.

surgical asepsis Practices that keep equipment and supplies free of *all* microbes. Also known as **sterile technique**.

Transmission-Based Precautions Guidelines to contain pathogens within a certain area, usually the client's room.

tuberculosis (TB) A chronic infection caused by the bacterium *Mycobacterium tuberculosis*, usually transmitted through airborne droplets reaching a person's respiratory system.

vector An organism that spreads infection by transmitting pathogens from one host to another but is not the cause of the infection.

VRE (vancomycin-resistant *Enterococcus*) A type of multidrug-resistant organism (MRO).

waterless alcohol-based hand rubs (waterless antiseptic hand-wash) Hand hygiene products containing 60 to 90% alcohol that are rubbed into the hands, and then allowed to dry completely. These rubs are used before and after direct contact with a client, bedding, or any object which may be contaminated with pathogens.

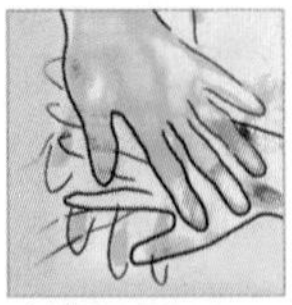

Infection can be a serious safety and health hazard. Some infections cause only minor symptoms, while others are much more serious. They may delay a person's recovery, create long-term health problems, or even cause death in some situations. Older adults, people with health challenges, and people with disabilities are at increased risk for developing infections. Infections can easily spread from worker to client, from client to client, or from client to worker.

All members of the health care team must take every precaution to protect clients and themselves from infection. As a support worker, in order to prevent infection, you must understand how infections spread and also must follow your employer's infection control policies. **Infection control** refers to policies and procedures to prevent the spread of infection within health care settings. ***Proper hand hygiene is the easiest way to reduce the risk of infection spread to yourself and others, and should always accompany any other infection control efforts.***[1]

MICRO-ORGANISMS

A **micro-organism** (**microbe**), sometimes called a "germ" or "bug," is a form of life (*organism*) that is so small (*micro*) it can be seen only with a microscope. Microbes live and grow everywhere—in water, air, food, soil, plants, and animals and on inanimate (nonliving) objects such as clothing, furniture, medical equipment, and personal care items. Microbes also live and grow on and in people—on the skin and in the mouth, nose, respiratory tract, stomach, and intestines.

Most microbes usually do not cause infection or disease, and these are called **nonpathogens**. Some microbes that are harmful and can cause infection or disease are called **pathogens.**

Types of Micro-organisms

Within health care settings, the three types of microbes that cause the greatest risk for infection are bacteria, viruses, and fungi.

1. ***Bacteria***—single-celled microbes that naturally occur on living, dead, or inanimate objects. They can multiply rapidly or, if necessary, can remain dormant (nonactive), surrounded by a protective shell called a **spore coat.** This spore coat can make it difficult to kill bacteria, so they may live for a long time. In the right conditions, bacteria can become active again and resume multiplying rapidly. They can be nonpathogenic, or they can cause serious infections in any body system. Infections caused by bacteria are usually treated with antibiotics.
2. ***Viruses***—microbes that are much smaller than bacteria and invade living cells in order to grow and multiply. They take over the cells' machinery to produce new virus particles. Like bacteria, viruses can also remain dormant (nonactive) surrounded by a protective shell called a *spore coat,* making it difficult to kill the virus for an indefinite period of time. **AIDS,** hepatitis, influenza, and the common cold are examples of infections caused by viruses. Antibiotics are not effective against viruses, but a few antiviral medications that can kill specific viruses are available. Some viral diseases (such as measles, polio, and many types of influenza) can be prevented by vaccination.
3. ***Fungi***—microbes that live only on organic matter, such as plants and animals. Certain types of yeasts and moulds are common fungi that can be pathogenic. In humans, fungi can infect the mouth, vagina, skin, feet, and other body areas. Many fungal infections, such as athlete's foot, are mild, but fungi can also cause life-threatening infections, especially in susceptible people.

All three types of microbes require certain conditions to live and grow. The **reservoir** (host) is the environment where the microbe lives and grows. Microbes grow in reservoirs that are *warm* and *dark* and need *water* and *nourishment.* Most microbes also need *oxygen,* although some can thrive without it. Many microbes in living organisms grow best at body temperature but are destroyed by heat and light.

Normal Flora

Normal flora contain microbes that naturally live and grow in certain locations on or in the human body. Certain microbes, for example, are found on the skin, in the respiratory tract, or in the intestines.

These microbes are harmless (nonpathogens) or even beneficial to the body ("good bacteria") because they survive by consuming potentially harmful bacteria that try to invade the body. When a nonpathogen is transmitted from its natural site to another site or host, it becomes a pathogen. For example, *Escherichia coli* is a bacterium normally found in the colon and assists with food **metabolism**. If *E. coli* enters a different body system (for example, the urinary system), it can cause a serious infection.

The numbers of microbes that make up the normal flora of a body surface are constantly controlled by microbes that consume them. Maintenance of healthy normal flora, therefore, is a delicate number balance of all types of beneficial bacteria that share the same body area. When a person is ill or on medications (such as antibiotics) some of the normal flora can be killed, and this balance is disrupted. The person can then develop a potentially harmful infection.

Antibacterial soaps—intended to be used for hand washing or for washing contaminated substances from skin—have been blamed for certain illnesses in some people because their *overuse* (using them for bathing, for example) can destroy the delicate balance of a person's normal flora.

Multidrug-Resistant Organisms

Bacteria reproduce very quickly and in large numbers and can quickly make a person ill if there are not enough "good bacteria" or normal flora to stop them from multiplying. Misuse and over-prescribing of antibiotics in the past have led certain strains of bacteria to mutate (change) their spore coats to make them more resistant to either a person's normal flora or most antibiotics. This means that some people now have infections that are resistant to most antibiotics.

These resistant bacteria are known as **multidrug-resistant organisms (MROs),** sometimes called "super bugs." Infections with MROs are becoming increasingly common and are easily spread among people at risk for infection (such as babies, older adults, and people with a serious medical condition or a weakened immune system). Since they are difficult to treat, they can be fatal if the infection is severe. Because of this, MROs pose a serious threat to patients and residents in health care facilities.

The two most common MROs are **MRSA** (methicillin-resistant *Staphylococcus aureus*) and **VRE** (vancomycin-resistant *Enterococcus*). Box 20–1 describes these organisms. As a support worker, you will be trained to take special precautions when you are in contact with clients infected, or suspected of being infected, with MROs.

THE SPREAD OF PATHOGENS

An **infection** is an illness or disease state resulting from the invasion and growth of pathogens in the body. These pathogens may have been introduced into the body from an inanimate object (such as a soiled sheet) or from another person who has a **communicable** or **contagious disease**. A communicable (contagious) disease is caused by pathogens that spread easily—for example, the common cold, influenza, chickenpox, hepatitis, pneumonia, tuberculosis, and AIDS.

A *local infection* is an infection that occurs in one body part, such as an infected cut on the arm. A *systemic infection* involves the whole body, and the affected person would have *generalized* (entire body) signs and symptoms of infection. Some or all of the signs and symptoms of infection are listed in Box 20–2 (also see the *Focus on Older Adults: Signs and Symptoms of Infection* box).

Being exposed to pathogens *does not always* result in an infection, as the body can protect itself from infection. There are three possible outcomes of exposure to a pathogen:

1. ***The immune system destroys the pathogen.*** The pathogen does not live and grow within the body, so an infection does not occur (see Chapter 14 to review the discussion on the immune system).
2. ***The immune system does not destroy the pathogen, and yet an infection does not develop.*** Even though the person remains healthy, the pathogen is still present within the body and can be transmitted to others. In this case, the person is colonized with the pathogen. **Colonization** occurs when bacteria live on or in the body and survive as part of

that person's normal flora. They are not harmful to that person but might be harmful to another person who does not have *those* bacteria as part of their normal flora. The person is considered a **carrier** of the pathogen and can transfer the pathogen to others.

3. ***An infection develops sometime after exposure to the pathogen.*** The period between exposure to the pathogen and the onset of illness is called the **incubation period,** which may be relatively short or last for years. During the incubation period, the person can transfer the pathogen to others. The time during which a person is at risk of transferring pathogens to others (putting people at risk of "catching" the illness) is known as the **communicable phase**. The incubation period and length of time for the communicable phase vary from pathogen to pathogen.

Box 20-1 Multidrug-Resistant Organisms: MRSA and VRE

MRSA

MRSA (methicillin-resistant *Staphylococcus aureus*) is a type of common germ that is not killed by most antibiotics. The symptoms of MRSA depend on which body system is infected. Most people with MRSA do not have signs or symptoms of an infection but instead carry the bacteria on the skin, in the nose, or in the gastrointestinal tract. These people are known as *carriers.* A person who is a carrier of the MRSA bacteria may not carry these bacteria forever, as they can be treated with certain powerful antibiotics, or the problem may resolve itself.

Patients in hospitals who have incisions, wounds, or tubes that make it possible for the germs to enter their bodies are prone to develop MRSA infection, which is most likely spread in hospital or long-term care settings through person-to-person contact, through contact with infected wound discharge or urine, or through health care workers who fail to practise hand hygiene.

If the MRSA germ is suspected, a test is done to confirm its presence. If the test proves positive for MRSA, an antibiotic is prescribed. When a person is found to be a carrier of MRSA on the skin or in the nose, ointments, special antiseptic soaps, and sometimes antibiotics in pill form are used to destroy the MRSA bacteria.

VRE

Enterococci are bacteria that are normally found in the digestive tract and are not dangerous in healthy people with strong immune systems, as the balance of healthy flora in their digestive tract helps keep the bacteria from getting out of control. Because of overuse of antibiotics, however, a strain of *Enterococcus* has become resistant to all antibiotics, including vancomycin, and is called vancomycin-resistant *Enterococcus* (VRE). It is most commonly spread from the hands of health care workers who acquired VRE after contact with clients colonized or infected by the bacteria or from handling contaminated material or equipment.

VRE is dangerous because it cannot be controlled with antibiotics, and it causes life-threatening infections in people with compromised immune systems—the very young, the very old, and the very ill. Also, it can easily pass on the resistance gene to other, more dangerous bacteria, such as *Staphalococcus* and *Streptococcus.*

There are other ways that VRE can be spread, for example, from contact with surfaces such as call bells, bed rails, blood pressure cuffs, and other equipment. Contamination of the environment with VRE is more likely when a client has diarrhea.

Both MRSA and VRE can cause serious infections. The best way to stop the spread of both the MRSA and VRE bacteria is by careful hand washing with an antibacterial soap. This is especially important for health care workers and visitors. The number of people visiting a very sick person should be limited to one. Residents in long-term care facilities who have recently been admitted to a large hospital are usually tested for MROs before they are transferred back to their facilities. If they are found to have drug-resistant bacteria, they are then isolated from other residents.

Sources: Government of Ontario, Ministry of Health and Long Term Care, Provincial Infectious Diseases Advisory Committee. (March 2007). *Best practices for infection prevention and control of resistant Staphyloccoccus aureus and Enterococci.* Toronto, Ontario (ISBN 1-4249-2320-4); Ronnie Falcao, Mountain View, CA. Retrieved June 23, 2007, from http://www.gentlebirth.org/vre/vremain.html#What.

Box 20–2 Signs and Symptoms of Infection

- Fever and chills
- Increased pulse and respiratory rates
- Aches, pain, or tenderness
- Fatigue and loss of energy
- Loss of appetite
- Nausea
- Vomiting
- Diarrhea
- Rash
- Sores on mucous membranes
- Redness and swelling of a body part
- Discharge or drainage from the infected area that may have a foul odour
- New or increased cough, sore throat, or runny or stuffy nose
- Burning pain when urinating, or the need to urinate more often or with increased urgency

focus on ›› OLDER ADULTS

Signs and Symptoms of Infection

Older adults are especially at risk for infections because of the normal age-related changes occurring in their bodies. If they had a serious health concern before they were infected, they are also more likely than younger adults to become seriously ill or to die from an infection. This is why, for example, pneumonia and influenza are often life-threatening illnesses in older adults.

Older adults often do not show the usual signs of infection. Fever, pain, and swelling, for instance, are usually absent in older adults because they tend to have lower body temperatures, decreased pain sensation, and less immune response to infection.

Sometimes the only sign of infection in older adults is a change in behaviour. If an older client displays any of the following, report it to your supervisor:

- New or increased confusion or delirium
- New or increased incontinence
- Loss of appetite
- Decreased ability to perform activities of daily living
- Falls
- Changes in mood—for example, a client who is usually talkative, cheerful, and cooperative becomes unusually quiet, moody, and uncooperative

A **pandemic** occurs when a communicable illness or infection spreads throughout the population of a country or even throughout the world. The Canadian government, for example, is preparing for an influenza (the "flu") pandemic. Normally, people are exposed to different strains of the influenza virus many times during their lives, so even though the virus may change (or mutate), previous exposures to influenza may offer them some protection against infection. However, for unknown reasons, three to four times in a century, a radical change takes place in the influenza A virus, causing a new strain to emerge.[2] In the past, this has resulted in widespread illness and many deaths, especially among the young, ill, or the elderly. The Canadian government is involved in attempts to prevent such a disaster from happening through widespread public health teaching and influenza vaccinations.

The Chain of Infection

Many factors work together for an infection to develop. The spread of infection involves a process known as the chain of infection (Figure 20–1). The links in the chain are as follows:

- ***Pathogen***—a microbe capable of causing disease.
- ***Reservoir***—the environment where the pathogen lives before it infects a person. Remember, a pathogen can live on or in a person or animal (a *host*), food, water, soil, or inanimate objects.
- ***Portal of exit***—the path by which the pathogen leaves the reservoir. Portals of exit in the human body are the body openings (mouth; nose; and rectal, vaginal, and urethral openings), breaks in the skin (a scrape, cut, or other wound), and breaks in the mucous membranes (in the mouth, eyes, nose, vagina, and rectum). Pathogens are carried through the portals of exit by blood, body fluids, excretions, or secretions.

These include urine, stool, vomitus, saliva, mucus, pus, vaginal discharge, semen, wound drainage, and sputum (respiratory secretions).

- ***Mode of transmission***—how the pathogen travels from the portal of exit to the next reservoir or host. Microbes can be transmitted by physical contact (direct and indirect), droplets in the air, air currents, an infected vehicle or **vector** (such as a mosquito), or a **fomite** (any nonliving material, such as bed linen). The mode of transmission depends on the type of microbe. Some microbes are transmitted in more than one way (Table 20–1 on the next page).
- ***Portal of entry***—where the pathogen enters the new host's body. Portals of entry are the same as the portals of exit—body openings and breaks in the skin or mucous membranes.
- ***Susceptible host***—a person at risk for infection. Whether or not the pathogen grows and multiplies in the new host depends on the state of the person's immune system. Remember, the immune system protects the body from infection. A person whose immune system is weakened is *immunocompromised*. (*Immuno* comes from *immunity*, which means protection against a certain disease. *Compromised* means weakened.) He or she is more likely to acquire the infection. There are many factors that increase the risk of infection (see Box 20–3).

Infections in Health Care Settings

A **health care associated infection (HAI)** is an infection acquired while the person was a patient, client, or resident in a health care facility or from any type of health care provider. In the past, HAIs were called "**nosocomial infections,**" and you might hear this term used by some of the older staff members you work with. Infections can also be acquired in home care and other community settings. People in health care settings are usually at high risk for infection. They might also have some or all of the risk factors for infection listed in Box 20–3.

Microbes can enter the body through equipment used in treatments, therapies, and tests, so it is important that all equipment be kept free of pathogens. Workers can transfer microbes from client to client and from themselves to clients.

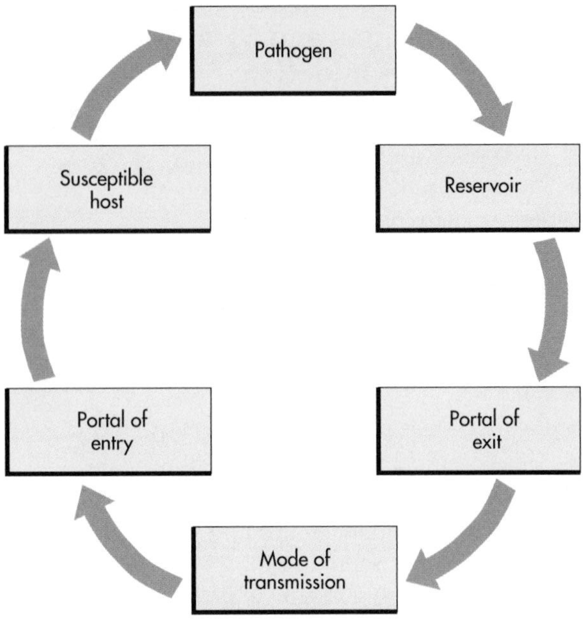

Figure 20–1 The chain of infection. **Source:** Redrawn from Potter, P.A., Perry, A.G., Ross-Kerr, J.C., & Wood, M.J. (2006). *Canadian fundamentals of nursing* (3rd ed., p. 785). Toronto: Elsevier Canada.

Box 20–4 lists ways the support worker can reduce the risk of spreading infections to others, or even to themselves and their families.

Box 20–3 Factors That Increase the Risk of Infection

- Extremes of age (the very young and the very old are at risk)
- Poor nutrition
- Stress
- Lack of sleep
- The presence of disease or illness. Many diseases or their treatments weaken the immune system, for example, AIDS, cancer (especially if the person is receiving chemotherapy or radiation therapy), organ transplants, and kidney failure.
- Certain medications
- Invasive procedures—for example, intubations and surgeries
- Invasive devices—for example, intravenous lines (IVs) and urinary catheters
- Open wounds
- Living in close contact with people who have communicable diseases
- Having contact with multiple caregivers

Table 20–1 Modes of Transmission of Micro-organisms

Mode of Transmission and Examples of Infectious Diseases	Description	
1. Contact transmission Multidrug-resistant organisms Gastrointestinal (GI, enteric) organisms Skin infections Wound infections	Occurs by transfer of microbes through physical touch. Contact transmission is by direct or indirect contact.	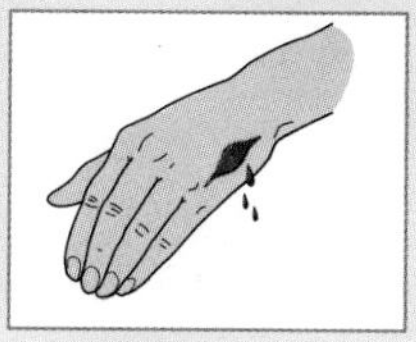
Direct contact transmission	Occurs by touching an infected or colonized person. Skin-to-skin contact is required. Many personal care activities require direct contact, such as bathing or turning a client in bed. Even shaking hands transmits microbes.	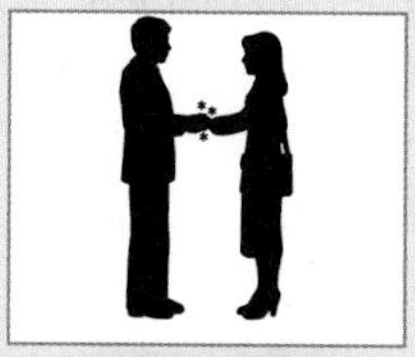
Indirect contact transmission	Occurs by touching a contaminated object such as transmission soiled linen, tissue, eating and drinking utensils, dressings, equipment, and surfaces in the client's room.	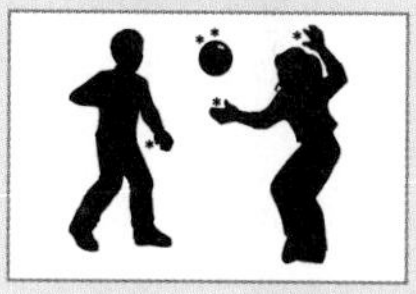
2. Droplet transmission Meningitis Pneumonia Influenza Mumps	Occurs when microbes are spread across short distances (less than 1 m) in the air by **droplets**. Coughing, sneezing, and talking propel droplets that carry microbes from the respiratory system through the air (Figure 20–2), and the droplets settle on another person or object in the environment.	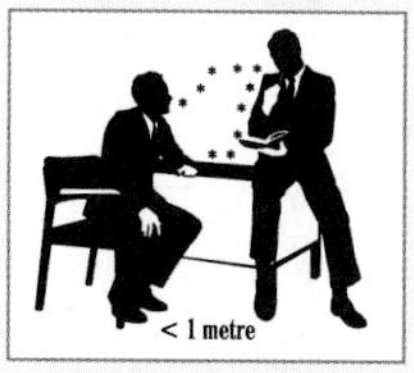
3. Airborne transmission Measles Chickenpox Tuberculosis (TB) SARS (severe acute respiratory syndrome) FRI (febrile respiratory illness)	Occurs when microbes are transmitted across long distances (farther than 1 m) by air currents. These microbes are contained in dust particles (acting as **fomites**) or evaporated droplets in the air. Microbes carried in this manner can travel across a room or even farther. People may then inhale the microbes or have contact with them if they are deposited on the skin.	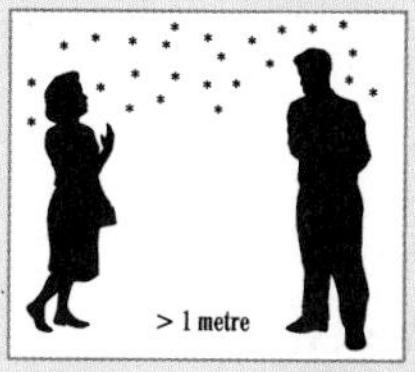
4. Vehicle transmission Hepatitis A, B, & C HIV/AIDS	Occurs when microbes are transmitted by a contaminated source (vehicle). Common vehicles of transmission include food, water, medication, and invasive medical equipment, as well as bodily fluids. One vehicle can transmit microbes to many people, resulting in an outbreak.	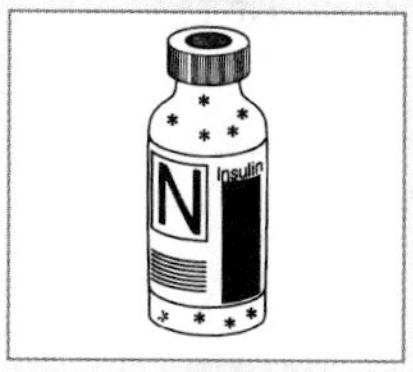
5. Vectorborne transmission West Nile virus Lyme disease	Occurs when insects (fleas, ticks, mites, mosquitoes) or pests (mice) transmit microbes to humans. These are known as **vectors**. This type of transmission is rare in health care settings.	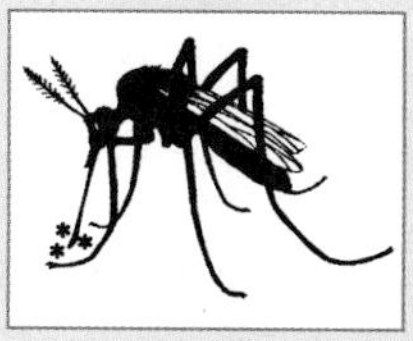

Source: Health Canada. (1999). *Infection control guidelines: Routine practices and additional precautions for preventing the transmission of infection in health care* (p. 26, Figure 1). Reproduced with permission of the Minister of Public Works and Government Services Canada, 2003. Retrieved September 2007 from http://www.phac-aspc.gc.ca/publicat/ccdr-rmtc/99pdf/cdr25s4e.pdf

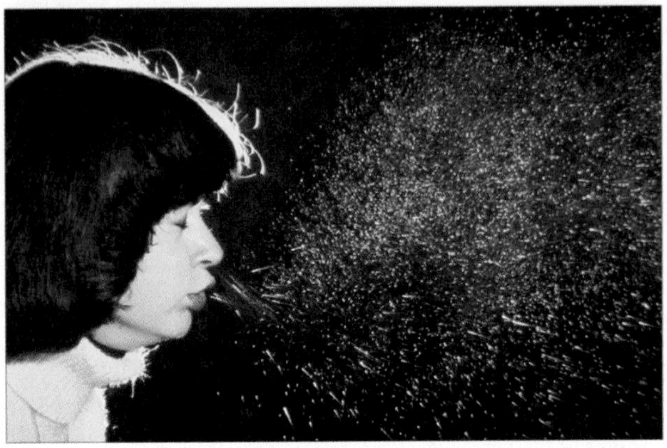

Figure 20–2 Droplets propelled into the air by a sneeze. During a common cold, most of the droplets contain virus particles. **Source:** Lester V. Bergman/Corbis/Magma.

The most common infections that occur within health care settings include respiratory tract infections (colds, pneumonia, bronchitis, and influenza), urinary tract infections, gastrointestinal tract infections (causing nausea or diarrhea), and skin infections (such as wound or IV site infections).

Sick, frail, and older clients have a hard time fighting infections, so it is up to the health care team to prevent the spread of infection. In health care settings, three practices that help prevent infections are:

1. Medical asepsis
2. Isolation precautions
3. Surgical asepsis

Vaccinations

Table 20–2 presents a chart listing the routine vaccinations and the recommended ages for receiving them. Health care agencies require workers to have their routine vaccinations up to date before they start work.

In addition to these vaccinations, the *hepatitis B* vaccination (comprising three injections over 6 months) is recommended for all those working in health care settings. This vaccination protects against acquiring hepatitis B from clients (see Chapter 18). The antibody levels can be checked periodically after vaccination to ensure immunity to hepatitis B. Some health care facilities suggest that their employees be vaccinated for *hepatitis A* (usually given along with hepatitis B vaccine), especially if they handle food. Check with your local health unit (or employer) for more information about this vaccine.

A yearly **influenza** vaccination is also highly recommended (and sometimes required) for anyone working in the health care field. This vaccine is very important to protect both the health care worker and clients from influenza, which can be very dangerous to older adults and people with weakened immune systems.

Box 20–4 Ten Ways the Support Worker Can Break the Chain of Infection

1. Take care of yourself. Get enough rest, and eat nutritious food. Do not smoke. Box 20–3 lists other factors that increase the risk for infection.
2. Bathe frequently, and ensure your hair, teeth, and nails are clean and pathogen-free. You should never wear artificial nails when providing care! Wear a clean uniform, socks, and underwear daily.
3. Practise proper hand hygiene between contacts with clients (follow the steps listed in this box and in Boxes 20–5, 20–6, and 20–7).
4. Practise proper hand hygiene after removing used gloves and before putting clean gloves on.
5. Never take "shortcuts" when it comes to hand hygiene, such as using waterless hand sanitizer on your gloved hands to avoid changing gloves! This is poor technique!
6. Avoid touching your face, hair, or clothing after completing hand hygiene.
7. Avoid coming to work if you have a fever. Some agencies provide masks to wear if either you or someone you are caring for has a cough or runny nose (see Figure 20–2 for an illustration of how a sneeze can spread infection!).
8. Never place linens—clean or soiled—on the floor. This is a sure way to infect others!
9. If you are in a client's home, practise the points outlined in the "Focus on Home Care" sections in this chapter.
10. Always use personal protective equipment (PPE) properly. Refer to Boxes 20–10 and 20–11 on pages 349 and 350.

Tuberculosis (TB) is a highly infectious bacterial disease that many of the older adults now living in long-term care facilities might have been exposed to in their youth when TB was much more common. TB is still a global health concern—more common among people with immune problems (such as **HIV** and AIDS), in places where people live in extreme closeness to each other (such as group homes, prisons, and long-term care facilities), and in developing countries that lack adequate health care. New staff and residents of long-term care facilities are required to have a two-

Table 20–2 Communicable Illnesses and Diseases: Care and Immunization

Illness	How Contracted	Signs and Symptoms	Care	Immunization
Chickenpox (shingles)	airborne	Fever, painful vesicles (with shingles, the vesicles are usually along a nerve root on one section of the body)	Rest; do not scratch or irritate the vesicles. In the case of shingles, see the doctor for medication/treatment; isolate from people who have not had chickenpox	Chickenpox immunization may be given
C. difficile (*Clostridium difficile*)	Airborne, direct contact	Severe diarrhea and abdominal cramping	Rest, fluids, treating the symptoms. The person should be under a doctor's care. Hand hygiene very important. Isolate from others	None
Febrile respiratory illness (FRI)	Droplet-spread respiratory infections, such as colds, influenza, influenza-like illness (ILI) and pneumonia.	Fever greater than 38°C and new or worsening cough or shortness of breath. *Note*: Some elderly people or people with immune problems may *not* have a high fever	Rest, fluids, treating the symptoms. The person should be under a doctor's care. Airborne isolation precautions	Influenza vaccine (for certain viral strains)
Measles	Airborne; direct droplet transmission of virus	Fever and rash	Rest, isolation, cool sponge baths	Immunization given with that for mumps and rubella (MMR)
Rubella	Droplet, airborne	Begins with symptoms of upper respiratory infection, fine raised rash	Rest; isolate from people who have not had vaccine	Vaccine (MMR); Never give vaccine to women who are pregnant or trying to get pregnant

(continued on page 336)

Table 20–2 Communicable Illnesses and Diseases: Care and Immunization (cont'd)

Illness	How Contracted	Signs and Symptoms	Care	Immunization
Hepatitis (A, B, & C)	Hepatitis A is spread through direct contact through fecal-contaminated water or food. Hepatitis B & C are spread by direct contact with contaminated blood or body fluids	Jaundice, swollen liver, loss of appetite, changes in urine or stool colours	Must consult a doctor for medical treatment; if Hepatitis B & C, avoid contact with blood or body fluids	Vaccine available for Hepatitis A, B, but not for Hepatitis C.
HIV and AIDS	Spread by direct contact with contaminated blood or body fluids	Chills, fever, cough, tiredness, confusion, stiff neck, oral lesions, nausea, vomiting, etc.	Must consult a doctor for medical treatment; avoid contact with blood or body fluids	No vaccine currently available
HPV (Human papilloma virus)	More than 50 types of HPV; some spread through sexual contact	May have visible warts on hands and feet, oral, anal and genital cavities	Must consult a doctor for medical treatment; avoid contact with infected areas, blood or body fluids	No vaccine currently available
MRSA (see Box 20–1, p. 330)	Direct contact with people who have MRSA	Same symptoms as any other skin infection	Avoid contact with infected items or people; infections require medical care	No vaccine currently available
VRE (see Box 20–1, p. 330)	Direct contact with people who have VRE	Same symptoms as any other skin infection	Avoid contact with infected items or people; infections require medical care	No vaccine currently available

step TB skin test (or a chest X-ray, if the doctor thinks it is necessary) so that they do not risk spreading or contracting TB. As a support worker, it is very important that you inform your doctor if you think you have been exposed to a client or family member who is suspected of having TB.

MEDICAL ASEPSIS

Asepsis is the practice of reducing or eliminating potential pathogens (bacteria, viruses, fungi, and parasites). There are two levels of asepsis: (a) **medical asepsis**, for which the goal is to exclude *all pathogenic micro-organisms* through medical aseptic technique, and (b) **surgical asepsis**, which aims to exclude *all micro-organisms* and their spores through surgical aseptic technique.[3]

Medical asepsis (or **clean technique**) refers to the practices that:

- Reduce the number of pathogens
- Prevent the spread of pathogens from person-to-person or place-to-place

Medical asepsis is the most common technique, and it should be practised by *all* health care workers because they have an important role in preventing the spread of infection to others.

In most health care units, the term *clean* is used to refer to anything that has no visible contaminants. For example, after we have washed our hands or our clothing, we refer to them as being "clean." We use clean gloves (not sterile surgical gloves), and we change them between clients. We use the word *contaminated* (unclean) to describe anything that has been exposed to pathogens whether or not the contamination is visible (such as soiled bed linen). **Contamination** is the process of exposure to pathogens.

A *clean* environment is different from a *sterile* environment. **Sterile** means free from *all* microbes, including pathogens, nonpathogens, and their spores. Because infection is a risk, microbes cannot be present during surgery or invasive procedures, so operating rooms and instruments inserted into the body must be sterile. **Surgical asepsis** (also called **sterile technique**) refers to the practices that keep equipment and supplies free of *all* microbes and their spores. **Sterilization** is the process of destroying *all* microbes, both pathogens and nonpathogens, and their spores.

HAND HYGIENE

Applying waterless, alcohol-based hand sanitizers or hand washing with soap and running water is the easiest and most important way to prevent the spread of infection. You use your hands in almost every task you perform as a support worker. They can easily pick up microbes from any client, place, or thing, and then transmit them to other clients, places, or things. If you touch your eyes, nose, or mouth with your contaminated hands, you can also transfer microbes into your own body. **Hand hygiene** should therefore be practised before and after client contact of any kind, since hand hygiene removes most microbes from the skin.

Because hands are contaminated very easily, you need to practise hand hygiene often and properly. Although hand hygiene is a simple procedure, many health care workers do it incorrectly. You should remember that ***gloves never take the place of hand hygiene***. Your skin will breed microbes in the dark, warm, moist environment of your gloved hands. You should always wash or sanitize your hands after removing your gloves and before putting new ones on. Box 20–5 lists guidelines for proper hand hygiene.

Wearing Gloves

Disposable gloves provide a protective barrier between your hands and the client's blood, body fluids, secretions, excretions, nonintact skin, and mucous membranes. Gloves protect you from acquiring microbes from the client, and the client from acquiring microbes that are on your hands. However, gloves are used as additional protection and not as a substitute for **hand washing**.

Box 20–5 When to Practise Hand Hygiene

- ***Immediately before and after giving care.*** This means cleaning your hands before caring for a client, after caring for the client, and then again immediately before you care for the next client
- Whenever your hands are visibly soiled
- After contact with your own or another person's blood, body fluids, secretions, or excretions
- After touching objects that are contaminated, such as soiled linens, tissues, toilet paper, garbage bags, bed pans, or diapers
- Before and after preparing, handling, and eating food
- Before and after feeding a client
- Before putting on disposable gloves and after removing them
- After personal body functions, such as urinating or defecating; changing tampons or sanitary pads; and sneezing, coughing, or blowing your nose

Note: If you have touched any object that has been contaminated with pathogens (such as feces), or you can see visible contamination on your hands, you should thoroughly wash your hands with soap and running water instead of using the waterless hand sanitizer to clean your hands.

1 2 3 USING WATERLESS ALCOHOL-BASED HAND RUBS

Procedure

Waterless alcohol-based hand rubs clean hands effectively and are convenient to use. Some manufacturers of these hand rubs recommend that you wash your hands with water and soap after a maximum of 10 applications of their product to remove accumulated dead skin and bacteria on your hands. Your hands must be dry before you apply a hand rub because moisture dilutes the alcohol in the rub and makes it less effective. The hand rub is also not effective if your hands are visibly soiled. Apply liquid hand cleansers as follows:

1. Pour about 3 to 5 mL ($^1/_2$ to 1 teaspoon) of waterless, alcohol-based hand rub onto both hands.
2. Rub hands together. Make sure that all areas of the hands are covered, including areas between the fingers. Rub hands together for about 15 seconds to properly spread the waterless, alcohol-based hand rub.
3. Clean under the fingernails by rubbing fingertips on the wet palms.
4. Rub hands until they are dry, between 30 seconds and 1 minute.

1 2 3 HAND WASHING

Procedure

1. Make sure you have soap, paper towels, a wastebasket, and an orange stick, nail file, or soft nail brush.
2. Push your watch and sleeves up well over your wrists. Remove rings.
3. Stand away from the sink. Do not let your hands, body, or uniform touch the sink, as the sink is contaminated. Stand so the soap and faucet are easy to reach (Figure 20–3).
4. Turn on and adjust the water until it feels warm. Always wash your hands under warm running water.
5. Wet your wrists and hands thoroughly under running water. Keep your hands at a level lower than your elbows (see Figure 20–3). Your hands are often dirtier than your elbows and forearms. If you hold your hands and forearms up, dirty water runs from hands to elbows, and those areas become contaminated as well. Soap should never be applied to dry skin because it can irritate it, so it is important to first wet the areas that you plan on washing!
6. Apply about 5 mL (1 teaspoon) of liquid soap to your hands. If using bar soap, do not touch the soap dish when you pick up the soap. Rinse the bar soap well before you use it. Do not touch the soap dish as you put the soap back.
7. Rub your palms together and interlace your fingers to work up a good lather (Figure 20–4). This step should last at least 15 seconds. The rubbing action helps remove microbes and dirt. Pay attention to areas often missed during hand washing: thumbs, knuckles, sides of the hands, little fingers, and under the nails.
8. Wash each hand and wrist thoroughly. Clean well between the fingers.
9. Clean fingernails by rubbing the fingertips of one hand against the palm of the other hand (Figure 20–5). Clean under the fingernails with a nail file, orange stick, or soft nail brush (Figure 20–6), since microbes can grow easily under fingernails. This step is very important for the first hand washing of the day and when your hands are highly soiled.

(continued on page 339)

1 2 3 HAND WASHING

Procedure (cont'd)

10 Rinse your wrists and hands well, keeping your hands and forearms down. Water should flow from the arms to the hands.

11 Spend enough time lathering and rinsing. The duration of the hand wash is as important as the technique. Check your employer's policy regarding the duration required. At least 15 to 20 seconds will be needed to remove most microbes on the skin. Wash your hands longer if they are dirty or soiled with blood, body fluids, secretions, or excretions.

12 Repeat steps 6 through 11, if needed.

13 Pat dry by starting at your fingertips and working up to your forearms. You will thus dry the cleanest area first.

14 Turn off the faucet using the paper towel that you dried your hands with (Figure 20–7). Remember that faucets are contaminated, and using paper towels prevents clean hands from becoming contaminated again.

15 Apply hand lotion or cream after washing your hands. This prevents skin chapping and drying. Skin breaks can occur in chapped and dry skin. Remember, skin breaks are portals of entry for microbes.

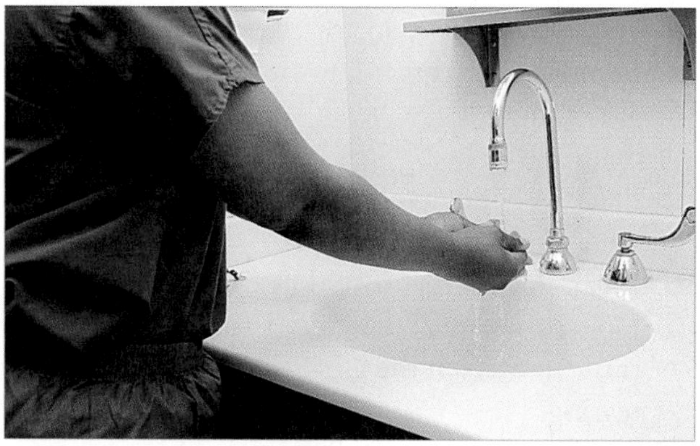

Figure 20–3 Do not touch the sink with your uniform. Keep your hands lower than your elbows.

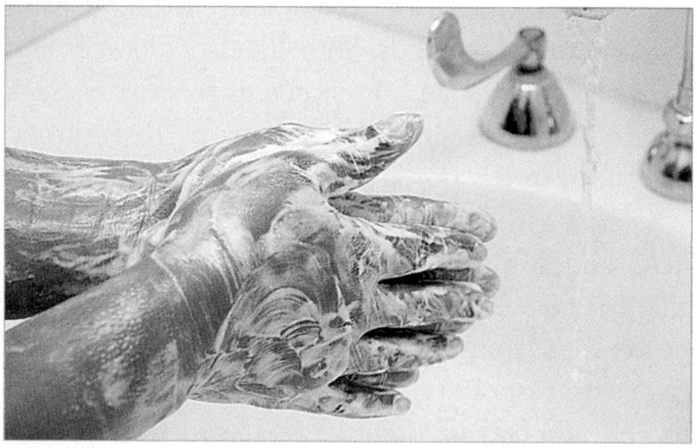

Figure 20–4 Rub your palms together to work up a good lather.

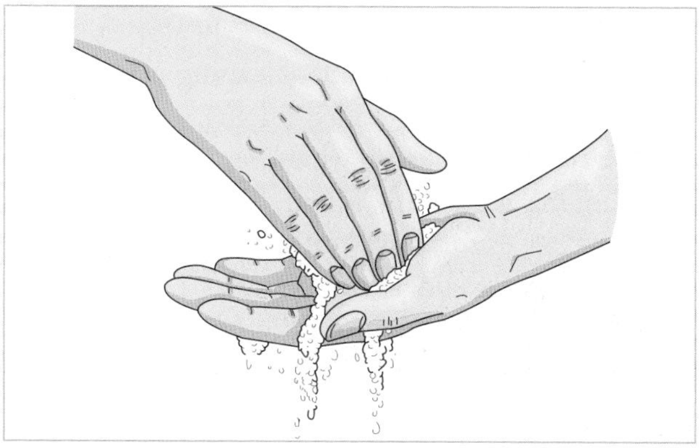

Figure 20–5 Rub your fingertips against your palm to clean under the nails.

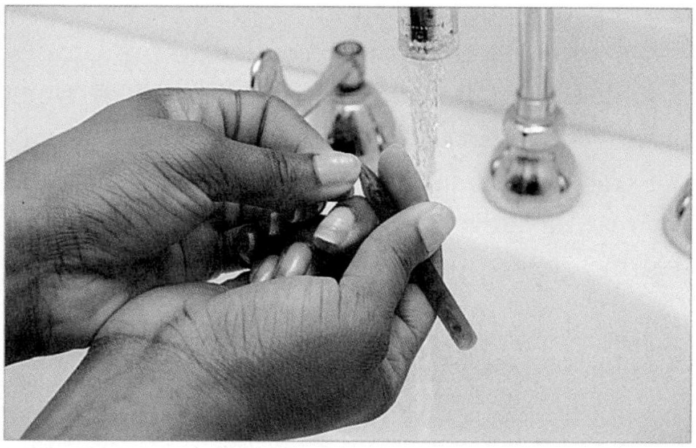

Figure 20–6 Use a nail file to clean under your fingernails.

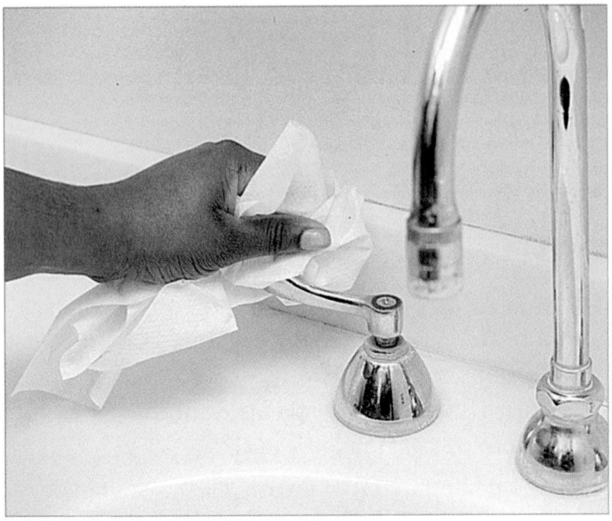

Figure 20–7 Use a paper towel to turn off the faucet.

focus on
»HOME CARE

Focus on Hand Hygiene When Giving Home Care

A client's home might not have everything you need for proper hand washing, such as soap or paper towels. Do not use the client's cloth towels for drying your hands, but use paper towels instead. Check with your supervisor before visiting the client. Most agencies provide workers with needed basic supplies to take with them on visits. Bring paper towels with you for home visits. You should always carry waterless alcohol-based hand rub when you go on home visits, in case the home lacks available hand hygiene supplies.

Gloves are not required for most routine support care activities where contact is limited to a client's intact skin. Do not wear gloves when they are not needed. Continuous wear will cause breakdown of the skin on your hands. Your hands will sweat and then become dry, and the skin will eventually crack if gloves are worn continuously. Remember, cracked skin is a portal of entry for microbes.

Gloves are often made of latex (a rubber product), and some people are allergic to latex. This allergy can cause skin rashes, as well as more serious problems such as asthma and shock. If you experience skin rashes and difficulty breathing, report it to your supervisor right away. If you have a latex allergy, you need to wear latex-free gloves. Some clients may be allergic to latex, so you cannot wear latex gloves when caring for them. Check their care plan for this information.

No special technique is required to put on disposable gloves. Be careful not to tear them when putting them on, as pathogens can enter through the tear. Carelessness, long fingernails, and rings can tear the gloves. Remember the following about wearing gloves:

- Wear gloves if you have cuts, abrasions on your hands, or bitten fingernails.
- Wash and dry your hands before putting on gloves.
- You need a new pair for every client.
- Remove and discard torn, cut, or punctured gloves right away. Wash your hands. Then put on a new pair.
- Practise hand hygiene each time you remove your gloves.
- Wear gloves only once. Discard them after use.
- Do not use waterless hand rubs on gloves, as this can weaken the glove, increasing its risk for tearing.
- Put on clean gloves before touching mucous membranes or broken (nonintact) skin.
- Wear gloves when contact with surfaces or items contaminated by blood, body fluids, secretions, or excretions is likely (for example, when handling bedpans, cleaning a bathroom floor, or removing soiled linens).
- Put on new gloves whenever gloves become contaminated with blood, body fluids, secretions, or excretions. You may need more than one pair of gloves for a task. This prevents cross-contamination of different body sites.
- Replace gloves if you touch an unclean surface.

1 2 3 REMOVING GLOVES

Procedure

1. Make sure that gloves only touch gloves. Do not let gloves touch the skin on your wrists or arms.
2. Grasp a glove just below the cuff with the gloved fingers of your opposite hand. Grasp it on the outside (Figure 20–8, *A*).
3. Pull the glove down over your hand so it is turned inside out (Figure 20–8, *B*).
4. Hold the removed glove with your other gloved hand.
5. Insert two fingers of your bare hand inside the cuff of the remaining glove (Figure 20–8, *C*).
6. Pull the glove down (inside out) over your hand and the already removed glove (Figure 20–8, *D*).
7. Drop both gloves together into the appropriate container. Follow employer policy.
8. Practise hand hygiene.

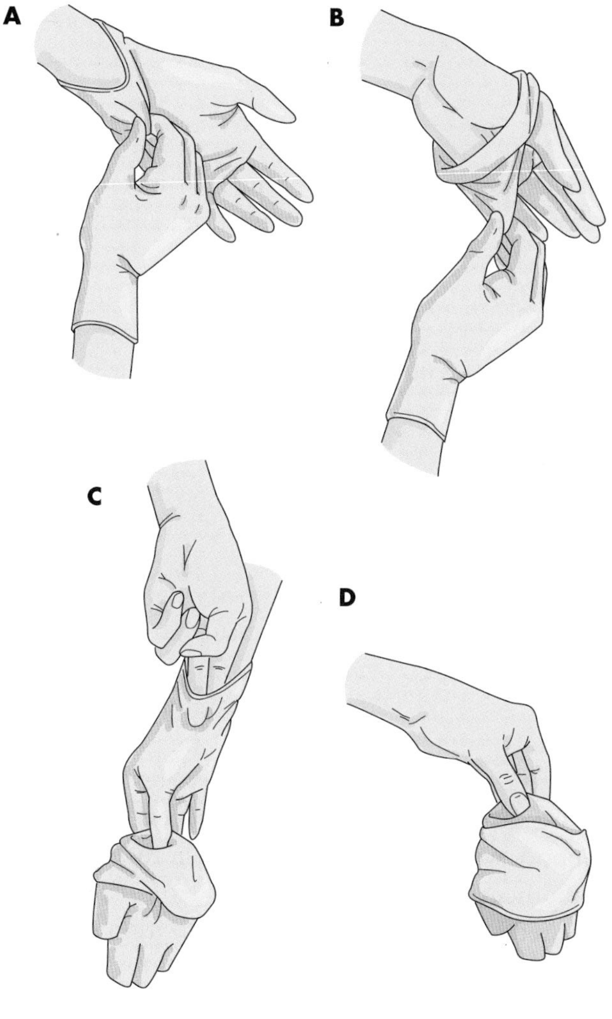

Figure 20–8 Removing gloves. **A,** Grasp the glove below the cuff. **B,** Pull the glove down over the hand. The glove is inside out. **C,** Insert the fingers of your ungloved hand inside the other glove. **D,** Pull the glove down over your hand and the other glove. The glove is inside out.

Care of Supplies and Equipment

Remember, microbes live on people and on objects. Contaminated equipment and supplies can easily become a source of infection.

Many items used in facilities and home care are disposable, which means they are used only once and then discarded. In these cases, cleaning them is not an issue. Some items, however, *are* reused, such as bedpans, urinals, washbasins, water pitchers, and drinking cups. In facilities where reusable items are used, they are labelled with the client's name, room, and bed number. They are never used or "borrowed" for another client.

Reusable items must be decontaminated. There are three levels of decontamination: *cleaning, disinfection*, and *sterilization.*

Cleaning. Cleaning reduces the number of microbes present on an item. It also removes any visible organic material, such as dirt, blood, body fluids, secretions, and excretions. For some equipment, periodic cleaning is all that is required. For example, items like crutches and blood pressure cuffs need to be cleaned only when visibly soiled and between use on different clients. Follow employer policy about when and how to clean items. The following guidelines apply when cleaning equipment:

- Wear personal protective equipment when cleaning items that may be contaminated with blood, body fluids, secretions, or excretions. **Personal protective equipment (PPE)** comprises special clothing and equipment that act as a barrier between microbes and your hands, eyes, nose, mouth, and clothes, such as gloves, gowns, masks, and eye protection (goggles or face shields) (see page 349). Follow your employer's policies about the use of PPE when cleaning equipment.

- Rinse the item first in cold water to remove any organic material. Warm or hot water makes the protein in organic material thick, sticky, and hard to remove, much like the way the protein in an egg will permanently change texture when it is heated.
- Wash the item with soap and hot water.
- Scrub the item thoroughly. Use a brush, if necessary.
- Rinse the item in warm water.
- Dry the item.
- Disinfect or sterilize the item.
- Disinfect equipment and the sink used in the cleaning procedure.
- Discard gloves and other PPE.
- Practise hand hygiene.

Disinfection. **Disinfection** is the process of destroying all pathogens, except their spores. Spores can be destroyed only by the sterilization process. An item must be thoroughly cleaned before it is disinfected.

Reusable items are disinfected with chemicals such as alcohols or chlorines (*chemical disinfectants*). Such items include:

- Metal bedpans
- Glass thermometers
- Commodes
- Countertops
- Tubs
- Room furniture

Follow your employer's policies regarding when and how to disinfect equipment and supplies (see the *Focus on Home Care: Disinfectants* box.)

Chemical disinfectants can burn and irritate the skin. Wear utility gloves or rubber household gloves that are waterproof to prevent skin irritation. Do not wear disposable gloves when using disinfectants. Some chemical disinfectants have special measures for use and storage. Check the material safety data sheet (MSDS) before handling a disinfectant (see Chapter 19). Follow your employer's policies.

Sterilization. Sterilizing destroys all nonpathogens and pathogens, including spores. Very high temperatures are used because most microbes can only be destroyed by heat.

Boiling water, radiation, liquid or gas chemicals, dry heat, and steam under pressure are sterilization methods. Items that enter the body or are used during surgery, for example, IV catheters, urinary catheters, and needles, have to be sterilized. In facilities, specially trained workers are responsible for carrying out the sterilization process. Therefore, support workers are *not* responsible for sterilizing equipment. However, you may be required to clean the items in preparation for sterilization (see the *Focus on Home Care: Sterilization* box.)

See Box 20–6 for guidelines on how to follow medical asepsis measures.

focus on
›› HOME CARE

Disinfectants

Detergent and hot water are common disinfectants for utensils, linens, and clothes. Many commercial products are available for household surfaces, including sinks, countertops, floors, toilets, tubs, and showers. In home care settings, use the products preferred by the client's family or as instructed by your supervisor.

Vinegar is an effective and cheap disinfectant. You can use it to clean bedpans, urinals, commodes, and toilets. To make a vinegar solution, mix 250 mL (1 cup) of white vinegar and 750 mL (3 cups) of water. Make sure you label the container properly as "vinegar solution." Also, put the date and your name on the container.

focus on ››HOME CARE

Sterilization

In home care, almost all medical items that must be sterile are commercially prepared and are disposable. However, you may be required to sterilize noninvasive items, such as cloth diapers or glass baby bottles.

Cloth diapers and other colour-fast linens can be sterilized by soaking them in a solution of 1 part household bleach and 10 parts water. One cup of bleach can be added to the wash when laundering items soiled with blood and body fluids. Always check with your client and your supervisor for direction before using bleach. Some linens cannot be bleached, so check the labels on clothes before using bleach to wash them (see Chapter 25).

Glass baby bottles and other such items can be sterilized in boiling water. Place the items in a large pot filled with cold water. Cover the pot and bring the water to a full boil. Boil the items for at least 15 minutes, then turn off the heat, and allow the water and the items to cool. Use tongs to remove the items, and let them air dry on a clean towel. Although boiling water is a convenient and inexpensive method of sterilization in the home, it does not always kill all the spores and viruses. Therefore, facilities do not use boiling water for sterilizing items.

Box 20–6 Medical Asepsis Measures You Should Follow

Controlling Reservoirs

- Maintain your personal hygiene. Bathe, shampoo your hair, brush your teeth, and change clothes daily.
- Never wear artificial nails when providing care. They trap many micro-organisms (including pathogens), can scratch your client, and can tear your gloves if they are worn.
- Make sure your vaccinations are up to date (see Table 20–2).
- Dispose of or store soiled tissues, linens, and other materials in leak-proof plastic bags.
- Empty garbage at least once a day.
- Keep tables, countertops, wheelchair trays, and other surfaces clean and dry.
- Wash contaminated areas with soap and water. Stool, urine, and blood contain microbes. So do other body fluids, secretions, and excretions.
- Clean work surfaces after completing a task, when they are dirty, and after blood or other potentially infectious material is spilled. Follow employer policies.
- Provide for the client's hygiene (see Chapter 29).
- Keep drainage containers below the drainage site (see Chapter 31).
- Cook meats and poultry adequately. Wash fruits and raw vegetables before eating or serving them. Handle and store all foods safely (see Chapter 27).
- Wash all cooking and eating utensils with soap and water after use.

Controlling Portals of Exit

- Cover your nose and mouth when coughing or sneezing. Wash your hands afterward.
- Give tissues to clients to use when coughing or sneezing.
- Wear personal protective equipment, as needed.
- Check your hands frequently for cuts, scrapes, or other breaks in the skin. Report any to your supervisor.

Controlling Transmission

- Wash your hands properly and at appropriate times (see Boxes 20–4 and 20–5).
- Assist clients with hand hygiene:
  - Before and after handling or eating food
  - After elimination
  - After coughing, sneezing, or blowing the nose
  - After changing tampons, sanitary pads, incontinence products, or other personal hygiene products
  - After contact with blood, body fluids, secretions, or excretions
  - Any time their hands are soiled

(continued on page 344)

Box 20–6 **Medical Asepsis Measures You Should Follow** (cont'd)

- Make sure all clients have their own care equipment, including washbasins, bedpans, urinals, commodes, and glass thermometers. Make sure all clients have their own toothbrush, drinking glass, towels, washcloths, eating and drinking utensils, and other personal care items. Do not share these items among clients or among the client's family members.
- Do not take equipment and supplies from one client's room to use for another client. Even if the item is unused, do not take it from one room to another.
- Hold equipment and linens (clean or contaminated) away from your uniform. This prevents the transfer of microbes from the equipment to your uniform and from your uniform to the equipment (Figure 20–9).
- Prevent dust movement, as dust carries microbes. Do not shake linens. Use a damp cloth for dusting.
- Remove soiled linens by folding them with the dirtiest areas in the centre.
- Clean from the cleanest area to the dirtiest. This prevents soiling a clean area.
- Clean away from your body. Do not dust, brush, or wipe toward yourself. Otherwise you transmit microbes to your skin, hair, and clothing.
- Flush urine and stool down the toilet. Avoid splatters and splashes. Cover bedpans and commodes with a lid when transporting them in order to contain microbes as well as odours.
- Pour contaminated liquids directly into sinks or toilets. Avoid splashing them onto other areas. Clean and disinfect the sink and contaminated areas afterward.
- Avoid sitting on a client's bed. You will pick up microbes and transfer them to the next surface that you sit on, possibly another client's bed.
- Do not use items that have touched the floor, as the floor is contaminated. Do not let linens (clean or soiled) touch the floor.
- Disinfect tubs, showers, shower chairs, bedpans, urinals, and commodes after each use. Follow your employer's disinfection procedures.
- Report pests in the room—ants, spiders, mice, and so on.

Controlling Portals of Entry

- Provide good skin care and oral hygiene according to the care plan (see Chapter 29). This promotes intact skin and mucous membranes. Damaged skin and mucous membranes provide portals of entry.
- Do not let the client lie on tubes or other items in order to protect their skin from injury.
- Make sure linens are dry and wrinkle-free (see Chapter 26). This protects the client's skin from injury.
- Turn and reposition the client as directed in the care plan (see Chapter 23). This protects the client's skin from injury.
- Assist with or clean the client's genital area after elimination, as needed (see Chapter 29). This is called perineal care. Wipe and clean from the urethra (the cleanest area) to the rectum (the dirtiest area). This helps prevent urinary tract infections.
- Make sure drainage tubes are properly connected. Otherwise microbes can enter the drainage system.

Protecting the Susceptible Host

- Follow the care plan to meet hygiene needs. This protects the skin and mucous membranes of the client.
- Follow the care plan to meet nutrition and fluid needs. This helps prevent infection.
- Assist with coughing and deep-breathing exercises, as directed. This helps prevent respiratory infections.

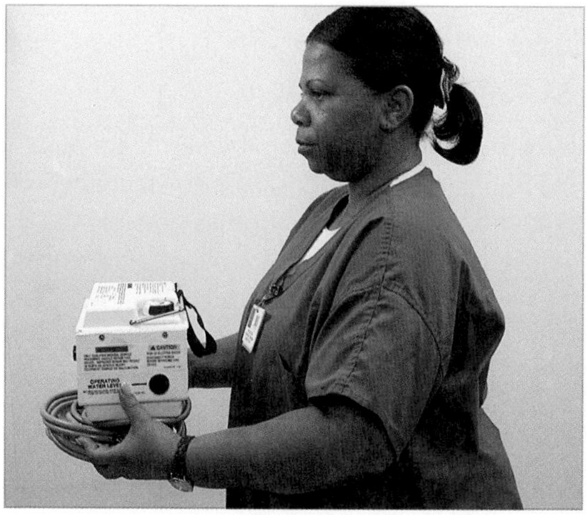

Figure 20–9 Hold equipment away from your uniform.

ISOLATION PRECAUTIONS

Along with medical asepsis, infection control policies also use isolation precautions to reduce the risk of infection. **Isolation precautions** are guidelines for preventing the spread of pathogens. The most recent isolation precautions were developed in 1996 in the United States by the Centers for Disease Control and Prevention (CDC). These precautions have been accepted by Health Canada and are currently used in most Canadian health care facilities and community care agencies.

There are two types of isolation precautions: **Standard Practices** (also known as **Routine Practices**) and **Transmission-Based Practices.** Both types of precautions provide guidelines on how to contain microbes. Standard Practices are practised at all times (discussed earlier in this chapter). Transmission-Based Precautions are practised when caring for clients with certain communicable diseases. There are three types of Transmission-Based Precautions: (a) Airborne Precautions, (b) Droplet Precautions, and (c) Contact Precautions. The choice of precautions depends on how a particular pathogen is spread, so you should understand how infections are spread.

Standard Practices

Standard Practices (sometimes also known as Routine Practices or Standard Precautions, depending on the province you live in) are guidelines to prevent the spread of infection from:

- Blood
- All body fluids, secretions, and excretions (except sweat), whether or not blood is visible
- Nonintact skin (skin with open sores, wounds, cuts, scrapes, or other breaks)
- Mucous membranes (including the membranes in the nose, eyes, mouth, vagina, and rectum)

Box 20–7 summarizes the Standard Practices. Because you cannot tell by looking at someone whether or not they carry pathogens, everyone must be considered a potential source of infection. Therefore, ***Standard Practices should be used when caring for all clients in all settings.***

Standard Practices stress the following:

- Hand washing
- Appropriate use of PPE (gloves, gowns, masks, and goggles or face shield)
- Proper care and cleaning of equipment, environmental surfaces, and linen
- Safe management of sharps. A **sharp** is a piece of equipment or an item that may pierce the skin. These include needles, scalpels, razors, and broken glass.

Transmission-Based Precautions

Some clients have (or are suspected of having) communicable diseases, which are highly contagious. In certain cases, additional isolation precautions are required to protect staff, visitors, and other clients from the infection.

Transmission-Based Precautions are guidelines to contain pathogens within one area, usually the client's room. Only clients infected or colonized with certain pathogens are placed under Transmission-Based Precautions. These precautions are followed in addition to Standard Practices. You will be told when Transmission-Based Precautions are ordered for a client.

When a client in a facility is under Transmission-Based Precautions, he or she is usually placed in a private or semi-private room in order to isolate his or her germs from infecting others. The isolation

Box 20–7 Standard Practices

Hand Hygiene

- Wash your hands after touching blood, body fluids, secretions, excretions, nonintact skin, mucous membranes, and contaminated items. Wash your hands even if you wore gloves.
- Practise hand hygiene immediately before putting on gloves and immediately after removing gloves.
- Practise hand hygiene between client contacts.
- Practise hand hygiene, whenever necessary, to avoid transferring microbes to other people or areas.
- Practise hand hygiene between tasks and procedures on the same client. This prevents cross-contamination of different body sites.
- Use plain soap for routine hand washing. Your supervisor will tell you when other types of soap or agents are needed.

Gloves

- Wear gloves when touching blood, body fluids, secretions, excretions, nonintact skin, mucous membranes, and contaminated items. Clean, disposable, nonsterile gloves are adequate.
- Change gloves between tasks and procedures on the same client.
- Change gloves after contact with material that may be highly contaminated.
- Remove gloves promptly after use.
- Remove gloves before touching uncontaminated items and surfaces.
- Remove gloves before going to another client.
- Practise hand hygiene immediately after removing gloves. This prevents the transfer of microbes to other clients or areas.

Masks and Eye Protection

- Wear a mask and eye protection (goggles or a face shield) during procedures and tasks that are likely to cause splashes or sprays of blood, body fluids, secretions, or excretions to protect your eyes, nose, and mouth from contact with splashes or sprays (see Figure 20–11 on page 351).

Gowns

- Wear a gown during procedures and tasks that are likely to cause splashes or sprays of blood, body fluids, secretions, or excretions. The gown protects the skin and also prevents contamination of clothing. A clean, nonsterile gown is adequate.
- Remove a used gown as soon as possible.
- Practise hand hygiene after removing the gown. This prevents transfer of microbes to other clients or areas.

Care of Equipment

- Handle used care equipment carefully. Equipment may be contaminated with blood, body fluids, secretions, or excretions. Do not let the equipment touch your skin, mucous membranes, or clothing. Also, prevent the transfer of microbes to other clients or areas.
- Do not use one client's reusable items for another client. The item must be cleaned and disinfected or sterilized before it is used again.
- Discard disposable (single-use) items properly.

Environmental Control

- Follow employer procedures for the routine care, cleaning, and disinfection of surfaces. This includes environmental surfaces, bed rails, bedside equipment, and other frequently touched surfaces.

Linen

- Follow employer policy for linen that is soiled with blood, body fluids, secretions, or excretions. The policy describes how to handle, transport, and process soiled linen.
- Do not touch soiled linen to your skin, mucous membranes, or clothing.
- Prevent the transfer of microbes to other clients and areas when handling linens.

Occupational Health and Bloodborne Pathogens

- Use extreme care when handling needles, scalpels, razor blades, and other sharp instruments or devices.
- Use extreme care when handling sharp instruments after procedures.
- Use extreme care when cleaning used instruments.
- Use extreme care when disposing of used needles.

(continued on page 347)

Box 20–7 Standard Practices (cont'd)

- Never recap used needles. Do not handle them with both hands. Never direct the needle point toward any body part. Use a one-handed "scoop" technique or a mechanical device that holds the needle sheath.
- Do not remove used needles from disposable syringes by hand.
- Do not bend, break, or otherwise handle used needles by hand.
- Place used disposable syringes and needles, scalpel blades, and other sharp items in puncture-resistant containers.
- Place reusable syringes and needles in a puncture-resistant container for transport to the reprocessing area.
- Use barrier devices for rescue breathing.

Client Placement

- A private room is used if the client:
  - Contaminates the area
  - Does not or cannot assist in maintaining hygiene or environmental control
- Follow your supervisor's instructions if a private room is not available.

room must have hand washing and toilet facilities. It also must have wastebaskets and laundry and garbage containers lined with plastic bags. An isolation sign that states that precautions are in place is usually displayed on the outside of the room door.

Sometimes Transmission-Based Precautions are necessary for home care clients to protect other household members and home care workers. For example, if a client is infected with a multidrug-resistant organism, Transmission-Based Precautions might be required. As a member of the home care team, you will be told of the need for these precautions. An isolation sign is not needed in the home.

The rules in Box 20–8 are a guide for giving safe care when Transmission-Based Precautions are used (see Box 20–9). Your employer may have these or other guidelines. Know your employer's policies about isolation precautions.

Box 20–8 General Rules for Transmission-Based Precautions

- Wear personal protective equipment, as required.
- Collect all needed equipment before entering the room. Limit the number of trips in and out of the room.
- Prevent contamination of equipment and supplies. If you drop anything on the floor, consider the item contaminated, and do not use it.
- Use mops wetted with a disinfectant solution to clean floors. Floor dust is contaminated.
- Prevent drafts. Pathogens are carried in the air by drafts.
- Use paper towels to handle contaminated items.
- Remove items from the room in sturdy, leak proof plastic bags.
- Double bag items if the outer part of the bag is or can be contaminated (see page 352–353).
- Follow employer policy for removing and transporting disposable and reusable items.
- Return reusable dishes, eating utensils, and trays to the food service department or kitchen. Discard disposable dishes, eating utensils, and trays in the waste container in the client's room.
- Do not touch your hair, nose, mouth, eyes, or other body parts when providing care.
- Do not touch any clean area or object if your hands are contaminated.
- Place clean items or objects that you bring into the room on paper towels.
- Do not shake linen.
- Use paper towels to turn faucets on and off.
- Tell your supervisor if you have fever, cuts, open skins areas, vomiting, diarrhea, a sore throat, or a cough.

Box 20–9 Types of Transmission-Based Precautions

Airborne Precautions

For known or suspected infections caused by microbes transmitted by airborne droplets.

Examples: Measles, chickenpox, TB (tuberculosis), FRI (febrile respiratory illness,) and SARS (severe acute respiratory syndrome)

Practices:

- Follow Standard Practices.
- A private room is required.
- Keep the room door closed and the client in the room.
- Wear respiratory protection (such as an N-95 respirator) when entering the room of a client with known or suspected tuberculosis or SARS (see Box 20–11). A disposable surgical mask does not provide enough protection. Follow employer policy for care of clients with tuberculosis.
- Do not enter the room of a client with known or suspected measles or chickenpox if you are susceptible to the disease. If you are susceptible but must enter the room, wear respiratory protection. A disposable surgical mask does not provide enough protection. Respiratory protection is not needed if you are immune to measles or chickenpox.
- Limit moving and transporting the client from the room. The client must be made to wear a mask if moving or transporting him or her from the room is necessary.
- For home care clients, revise these precautions, as necessary. For example, wear respiratory protection when in the client's home. Check with your supervisor and the care plan before entering the home.

Droplet Precautions

For known or suspected infections caused by microbes transmitted by droplets produced by coughing, sneezing, or talking

Examples: Meningitis, pneumonia, influenza, and mumps

Practices:

- Follow Standard Practices.
- A private room is preferred.
- The room door can be open if the bed is more than 1 m (3 ft) from the door. Otherwise, keep the room door closed.
- Wear a disposable surgical mask when working within 1 m (3 ft) of the client. (Wear a mask on entering the room if required by employer policy.)
- Limit moving and transporting the client from the room. The client should wear a mask if it is necessary to move or transport the client from he room.
- For home care clients, revise these precautions, as necessary. Household members should avoid sharing common articles or eating utensils. Check with your supervisor and the care plan before entering the home.

Contact Precautions

For known or suspected infections caused by microbes transmitted by:

- Direct contact with the client (skin-to-skin contact that occurs during care)
- Indirect contact (touching surfaces or care items in the client's room)

Examples: Multidrug-resistant organisms and gastrointestinal, respiratory, skin, or wound infections

Practices:

- Follow Standard Practices.
- A private room is preferred.
- The room door can be left open.
- Wear gloves when entering the room.
- Wear a gown when entering the room if the client is incontinent or has diarrhea, an ileostomy, a colostomy, or wound drainage not contained by a dressing.
- Make sure gloves cover your wrists and the cuff of your sleeve or gown (Figure 20–12).
- Change gloves after touching anything that might have high concentrations of microbes (for example, fecal material or wound discharge).
- Remove gloves before leaving the client's room (see the Procedure box "Removing Gloves" on page 340).
- Remove gloves so that the inside part is on the outside. The inside is *clean*.
- Discard gloves in a container for contaminated waste (see page XXX). Follow employer policy.

(continued on page 349)

Box 20–9 Types of Transmission-Based Precautions (cont'd)

- Practise hand hygiene immediately after removing gloves. Your supervisor will tell you what agent to use (usually an antimicrobial agent or a waterless alcohol-based hand sanitizer).
- Do not touch potentially contaminated surfaces or items after removing gloves and washing hands.
- When opening the door, use a paper towel to touch the doorknob. Discard the paper towel in the garbage pail inside the room as you leave.
- Remove the gown before leaving the client's room. Make sure your clothing does not touch potentially contaminated surfaces in the client's room.
- Limit moving or transporting the client from the room. Maintain precautions if moving or transporting the client is necessary.
- For home care clients, revise these precautions, as necessary. Check with your supervisor and the care plan before entering the home.

Protective Measures

Standard Practices and Transmission-Based Practices involve wearing personal protective equipment (gloves, mask, gown, and eye protection). Your supervisor and employer policy will guide you about when to use PPE. Box 20–10 lists the proper order for putting on and taking off a full set of PPE. Standard Precautions also involve careful handling of sharps. Transmission-Based Precautions involve extra measures when removing linens, garbage, and equipment from the room. Special measures are also needed when transporting clients.

Box 20–10 Order for Putting on and Taking off a Full Set of PPE

Put on PPE in the following order (wash hands first):

- Mask
- Goggles or face shield
- Gown
- Gloves

Take off PPE in the following order:

- Gloves
- Gown

(Perform hand hygiene.)

- Goggles or face shield
- Mask

(Perform hand hygiene.)

Wearing Masks and Respiratory Protection. Masks (also called surgical masks), which are disposable, prevent pathogens from entering your mouth and nose, protect you from splashes or sprays of blood, body fluids, secretions, or excretions, and prevent the spread of microbes from your respiratory tract. Breathing can cause masks to become wet or moist. A wet or moist mask is considered to be contaminated, so you must apply a new mask when this happens (see the Procedure box "Wearing a Mask" on page 350).

There are different types of masks for different situations. If you are required to wear *respiratory protection*, a special face mask that filters the air must be worn, for example, the N-95 respirator used for clients under airborne isolation precautions (Figure 20–10). Box 20–11 discusses different types of masks. It is *your responsibility* to be fitted for the correct type of mask and to wear it properly, following employer policy. When used for Airborne and Droplet Precautions, everyone—staff, clients, and visitors—needs to wear them.

Wearing Protective Apparel. Gowns, plastic aprons, shoe covers, boots, and leg coverings prevent the spread of microbes by protecting your clothes, wrists, and arms from contact with blood, body fluid, secretions, and excretions. They also protect against splashes and sprays.

Gowns must completely cover your clothing. The sleeves are long with tight cuffs. The gown opens at the back and is tied at the neck and waist. The inside and neck are *clean*, and the outside and waist strings

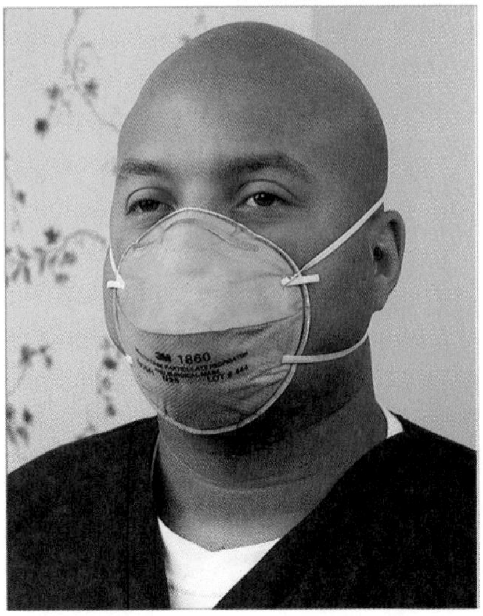

Figure 20–10 The N-95 respirator. Respiratory protection is used when caring for clients with tuberculosis and other infections requiring Airborne Precautions.

Box 20–11 Particulate Respirator Masks

Special masks (such as the N-95 mask in Figure 20–10) are designed to provide respiratory protection against certain airborne infections, such as tuberculosis and SARS. The N-95 is the most common size of mask, that is, it fits most people, but it is not intended to be used by people with beards.

If the N-95 mask does not fit, you need to be "fit-tested" with any of the other available mask sizes. It is your responsibility to make sure that you have been fit-tested. Under specific conditions, a trained mask-fit tester will spray a special solution of either a very sweet or bitter substance toward you to find out if you can taste them through your mask.

If you *do* taste the sweet or bitter solutions through your mask, it means that the mask does not have the proper seal around your nose and mouth. Without a good seal, you should not enter the isolation or treatment room, and you should inform your supervisor about this. If you are exposed to an airborne pathogen because you have on a mask that does not fit properly, you will not be able to prevent the pathogen from entering your body.

1 2 3 WEARING A MASK

Procedure

1. Practise hand hygiene.
2. Pick up the mask by its upper ties. Do not touch the part that will cover your face.
3. Place the mask over your nose and mouth (Figure 20–11, *A*).
4. Place the upper strings over your ears. Tie the strings in the back toward the top of your head (Figure 20–11, *B*).
5. Tie the lower strings at the back of your neck (Figure 20–11, *C*). The lower part is under your chin.
6. Pinch the metal band around your nose. The top of the mask must be snug over your nose. If you wear glasses or protective eye-wear, the top of the mask must be snug over your nose and under the bottom edge of the eyewear.
7. Practise hand hygiene.
8. Put on gloves if needed.
9. Provide care to the client. Avoid coughing, sneezing, and unnecessary talking.
10. Change the mask if it becomes moist or contaminated.
11. When the task has been finished, remove and discard the gloves. Wash your hands.
12. Remove the mask:
    - a Untie the lower strings.
    - b Untie the top strings.
    - c Hold the top strings. Remove the mask.
    - d Bring the strings together. The inside of the mask folds together (Figure 20–11, *D*). Do not touch the inside of the mask.
13. Discard the mask. Follow employer policy.
14. Practise hand hygiene.

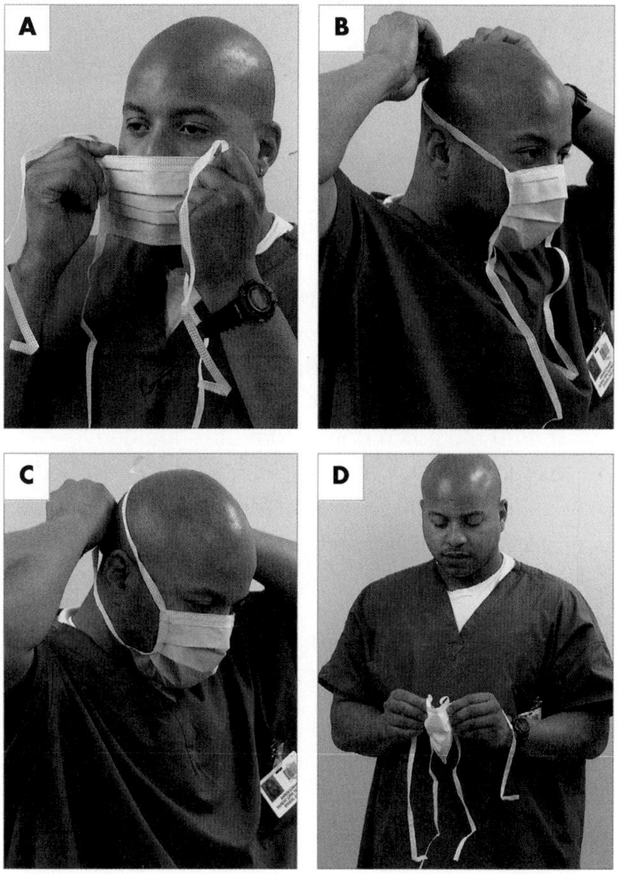

Figure 20–11 Donning a mask. A, Cover your nose and mouth with the mask. B, Tie upper strings at the back of your head. C, Tie lower strings at the back of your neck. D, Fold the inside of the mask together after removing it.

are *contaminated.* Gloves should be worn so that they cover the cuffs of the gown (Figure 20–12).

Gowns are used only once. A wet gown is contaminated and must be replaced with a dry one. Disposable gowns are made of paper and should be discarded after one use. Reusable gowns are made of cloth and must be laundered before reuse.

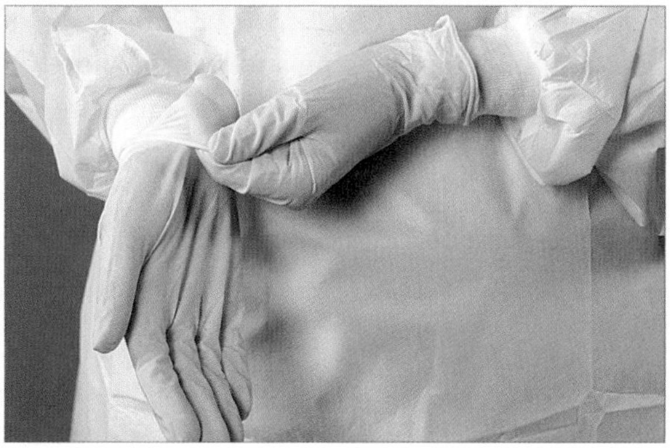

Figure 20–12 The gloves cover the cuffs of the gown.

Wearing Eye Protection and Face Shields. Goggles and face shields protect your eyes, mouth, and nose from splashing or spraying of blood, body fluids, secretions, or excretions (see Figure 20–11). You may need such protection when giving care to clients, cleaning instruments, or disposing of contaminated fluids.

Discard disposable eye protection after use. Reusable eye protection should be cleaned with soap and water and then disinfected before reuse.

Disposing of Sharps. Although you do not administer injections, you may come across needles that are improperly disposed of. This is especially common in home care. For example, while changing sheets for a client who has diabetes, you may find a forgotten needle in the bed. Or while emptying the garbage can, you could find an IV device that was mistakenly tossed into it. You must always watch out for stray sharps, especially if you know the client frequently uses needles.

Standard Precautions say that used needles must not be bent or broken. Place them and other sharps into a container that is:

- Tightly capped
- Puncture-resistant
- Leak proof

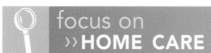

focus on
›› HOME CARE

Sharps Containers

Home care agencies often use sharps containers that are different from those used in facilities. Safe sharps containers used in home care include empty bleach bottles, coffee cans with the plastic lids taped closed, and plastic milk bottles. Glass or clear plastic containers should not be used. The home care agency is responsible for collecting the containers and disposing of them according to agency policy and local laws.

1 2 3 DONNING AND REMOVING A GOWN

Procedure

1 Remove your watch and all jewellery.
2 Roll up uniform sleeves.
3 Practise proper hand hygiene.
4 Pick up a clean gown. Hold it out in front of you and let it unfold. Do not shake the gown.
5 Put your hands and arms through the sleeves (Figure 20–13, *A*).
6 Make sure the gown covers the front of your uniform and is snug at the neck.
7 Tie the strings at the back of the neck (Figure 20–13, *B*).
8 Overlap the back of the gown. Make sure the gown covers your uniform. The gown should be snug, not loose (Figure 20–13, *C*).
9 Tie the waist strings at the back.
10 Put on gloves. Ensure they cover the cuffs of the gown (see Figure 20–12).
11 Provide care to the client.
12 Remove and discard the gloves.
13 Remove the gown:
  a Untie the waist strings.
  b Practise proper hand hygiene.
  c Untie the neck strings. Do not touch the outside of the gown.
  d Pull the gown down from the shoulder.
  e Turn the gown inside out as it is removed. Hold it at the inside shoulder seams and bring your hands together (Figure 20–13, *D*).
14 Roll up the gown away from you. Keep it inside out.
15 Discard the gown. Follow employer policy.
16 Practise hand hygiene.

This container may be made of steel or heavy plastic and provided by your employer. The container should be labelled. Other containers can be used as long as they follow the criteria (see the *Focus on Home Care: Sharps Containers* box.)

If your skin is pierced by a needle stick or another sharp, you must report the incident at once. You are at risk for infections, including HIV, hepatitis B, and hepatitis C. Assume that all clients are potential carriers of these viruses. ***Never ignore a sharps injury***.

Immediately after being poked by a sharp, encourage bleeding from the site of your injury and flush the area with large amounts of water for about 5 minutes. You should then seek prompt medical attention according to employer policy. Your client may be asked to consent to testing for the above-mentioned viruses to help with managing your exposure. Confidentiality is important through this process. You will be told of evaluation results and also of any medical conditions that may need treatment.

Bagging Items. Items contaminated with blood, body fluids, secretions, or excretions are called **biohazardous waste** and may be harmful to others. (*Bio* means life, and *hazardous* means dangerous or harmful.) These items are considered infectious and must be disposed of in specially marked containers, according to employer policy. Biohazardous waste includes used gloves, dressings, incontinence products, and soiled linen. Containers for these items are lined with sturdy, leak proof plastic bags that may be colour-coded. The containers are labelled with the universal *BIOHAZARD* symbol (Figure 20–14).

Contaminated waste is placed in a container labelled with the *BIOHAZARD* symbol. Follow employer policy for bagging and transporting. One bag is usually adequate. Double-bagging involves two bags and is not needed unless the contaminated waste touches the outside of the first bag. Two staff members are needed for double-bagging in isolation rooms:

- One worker is inside the room.
- The other worker is at the doorway outside the room.
- The worker in the room places contaminated items into a bag. Then the bag is sealed.

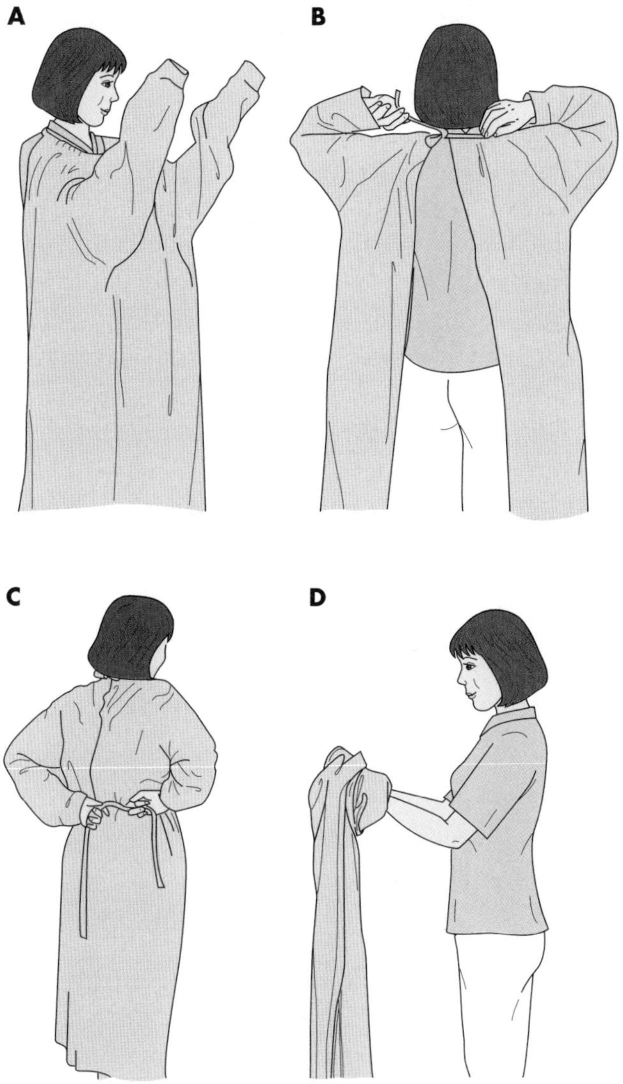

Figure 20–13 Gowning technique. **A,** Put your arms and hands through the sleeves. **B,** Tie the strings at the back of your neck. **C,** Overlap the gown in the back to cover your entire uniform. **D,** Turn the gown inside out as you remove it.

- The worker outside the room holds open another bag. This bag is clean. A wide cuff is made on the clean bag to protect the hands from contamination (Figure 20–15).
- The contaminated bag is placed in the clean bag at the doorway.

Bag and transport linens according to employer policy. All linen bags must have a *BIOHAZARD* symbol. Bag soiled linen in the room where it was used. Handle soiled linen as little as possible. It should not be sorted or rinsed in client care areas. Do not overfill the bag with linen. Tie the bag securely. Linen that is very wet or soiled should be double-bagged to prevent leakage. Place the linen bag in a laundry hamper lined with a biohazard plastic bag.

Transporting Clients on Transmission-Based Precautions. When on Transmission-Based Precautions, clients usually do not leave their rooms. However, they may have to go to another area of the facility for special treatments or tests.

Transporting procedures vary among facilities. Some require transport by bed, which prevents contaminating wheelchairs and stretchers. Other facilities use wheelchairs and stretchers.

A safe transport means that other residents or patients, staff, and visitors are protected from

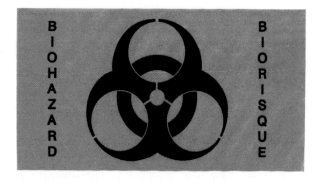

Figure 20–14 *BIOHAZARD* symbol.

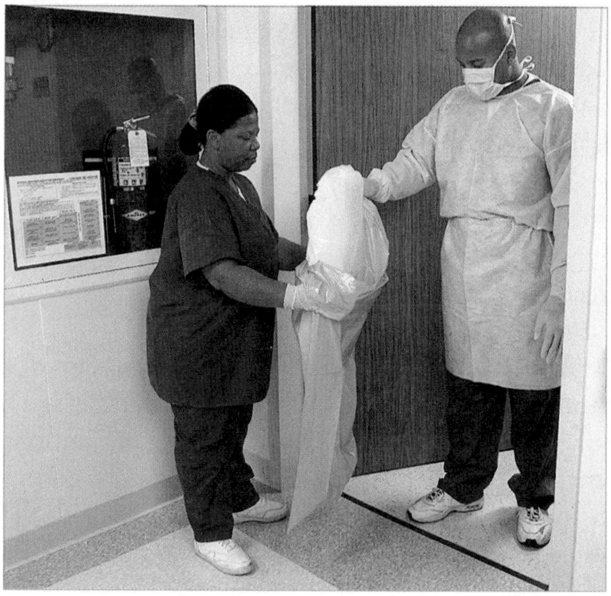

Figure 20–15 Double-bagging. One worker is in the room inside the doorway. The other is outside the room. The contaminated bag is placed inside the clean bag.

infection. Follow employer policies and these guidelines to safely transport clients:

- The client wears a clean gown or pyjamas and an isolation gown.
- The client wears a mask if on Airborne or Droplet Precautions.
- Cover any draining wounds.
- Give the client tissues and a leak proof bag. Used tissues are placed in the bag.
- Wear a gown, mask, and gloves, as required by the isolation precaution.
- Place an extra layer of sheets and absorbent pads on the stretcher or wheelchair. This protects against draining fluids.
- Do not allow anyone else into the elevator. This reduces exposure to the infection.
- Alert staff in the receiving area about the isolation precautions. They should wear gowns, masks, protective eyewear, and gloves, as needed.
- Disinfect the stretcher or wheelchair after use.

Basic Needs and Transmission-Based Precautions

All clients have love, belonging, and self-esteem needs, but often care is not taken to meet them when Transmission-Based Precautions are used. Visitors and staff tend to avoid the client, as the extra effort required to put on personal protective equipment may discourage them from visiting. Some visitors may be afraid of getting the disease and are anxious during the visit and unsure about what they can touch safely.

Without intending to, visitors and staff can make the client feel ashamed and guilty about having a contagious disease. As a result, he or she can feel lonely, unloved, and rejected. Self-esteem easily suffers, and depression is a risk.

It is important to understand the reasons for using Transmission-Based Precautions. Do not be afraid of the client. Remember, the precautions enable you to interact safely with the client and help meet the client's need for belonging and self-esteem. The following actions are helpful:

- Remember that it is the pathogen that is undesirable, not the client.
- Treat the client with respect, kindness, and dignity.
- Allow the client to make choices and decisions, whenever possible.
- Provide newspapers, magazines, and other reading material.
- Provide hobby materials, if possible.
- Place a clock or radio in the room.
- Encourage the client to telephone family and friends.
- Provide a current television schedule.
- Organize your work so that you can stay to visit with the client.
- Say hello from the doorway often, if the door can be left open.

Young children and clients with dementia do not understand the need for isolation precautions. Personal protective equipment may frighten children. It also may increase confusion and cause fear and agitation in adults with dementia. The following measures can help in such situations:

- Let the client see your face before putting on a mask or protective eyewear.
- Tell the client who you are and what you are going to do.
- Use a calm, soothing voice.
- Do not hurry the client.
- Follow the care plan and your supervisor's instructions for individual approaches.
- Report signs of increased confusion or changes in behaviour to your supervisor.

SURGICAL ASEPSIS

As was previously stated in this chapter, there are two levels of asepsis: (a) medical asepsis, for which the goal is exclusion of *all* ***pathogenic*** *micro-organisms* through medical aseptic technique, and (b) surgical asepsis, which aims to exclude *all micro-organisms* through surgical aseptic technique. **Surgical asepsis** (**sterile technique**) refers to practices that keep equipment and supplies free of *all* microbes—pathogens and nonpathogens. The goal of surgical asepsis is the same one of maintaining sterility, which is keeping things free of *all* microbes, including spores. Surgical asepsis is required any time the skin or sterile tissues are penetrated.

Some procedures require surgical asepsis, for example, catheterizations, IV administrations, suctioning, sterile dressing changes, and blood collection. Support workers are not normally authorized to do these procedures. However, you could be delegated to do them, or you might assist with these procedures. You should therefore understand the principles of surgical asepsis.

Principles of Surgical Asepsis

In order to prevent introducing microbes into the client, sterile procedures require the use of sterile gloves and sterile equipment. If an item is contaminated, the client is at risk for infection, so a sterile field is needed. A **sterile field** is a work area free of pathogens and nonpathogens (including spores). Remember that *clean* is different from *sterile!* All items in contact with the client are kept sterile. Box 20–12 lists the principles and practices of surgical asepsis. Follow them to maintain a sterile field when assisting with a sterile procedure.

You must also wear personal protective equipment to prevent contact with blood, body fluids, secretions, and excretions.

Box 20–12 Principles and Practices for Surgical Asepsis

- A sterile item can touch only another sterile item.
- If a sterile item touches a clean item, the sterile item is contaminated.
  - A sterile package that is open, torn, punctured, wet, or moist is contaminated.
  - A sterile package is contaminated after the expiration date on the package.
  - Place only sterile items on a sterile field.
  - Use sterile gloves or sterile forceps to handle other sterile items (Figure 20–16).
  - Consider any item to be contaminated if you are unsure of its sterility.
  - Do not use contaminated items. They are discarded or resterilized.
- Sterile items or a sterile field are always kept within your vision and above the level of your waist.
  - If you cannot see an item, the item is contaminated.
  - If the item is below the level of your waist, the item is contaminated.
  - Keep sterile gloved hands above the level of your waist and within your sight.
  - Do not leave a sterile field unattended.
  - Do not turn your back on a sterile field.
- Airborne microbes can contaminate sterile items or a sterile field.
  - Prevent drafts. Close the door and avoid extra movements.
  - Ask other staff in the room to avoid extra movements.
  - Avoid coughing, sneezing, talking, or laughing over a sterile field. Turn your head away from the sterile field if you must talk.
  - Wear a mask if you need to talk during the procedure.
  - Do not assist with sterile procedures if you have a respiratory infection.
  - Do not reach over a sterile field.
- Fluids flow downward, in the direction of gravity.
  - Hold wet items down (see Figure 20–16). If held up, fluid flows down into a contaminated area. The contaminated fluid flows back into the sterile field when the item is held up.
- The sterile field is kept dry, unless the area below it is sterile.
  - The sterile field is contaminated if it gets wet and the area below it is not sterile.
  - Avoid spilling and splashing when pouring sterile fluids into sterile containers.
- The edges of a sterile field are contaminated.
  - A 2.5 cm (1 in.) margin around the sterile field is contaminated (Figure 20–17).
  - Place all sterile items inside the 2.5 cm margin of the sterile field.
  - Items outside the 2.5 cm margin are contaminated.
- Honesty is essential to sterile technique.
  - You know when you have contaminated an item or sterile field. Be honest with yourself even if no other staff members are present.
  - Remove the contaminated item and correct the situation. If necessary, start over with sterile supplies.
  - Report the contamination to your supervisor.

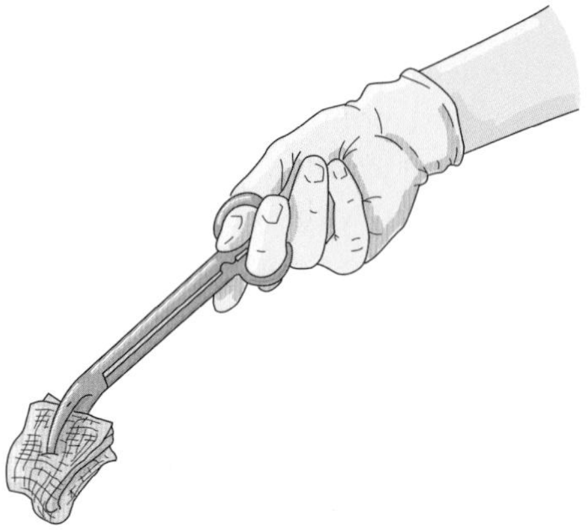

Figure 20–16 Sterile forceps are used to handle sterile items.

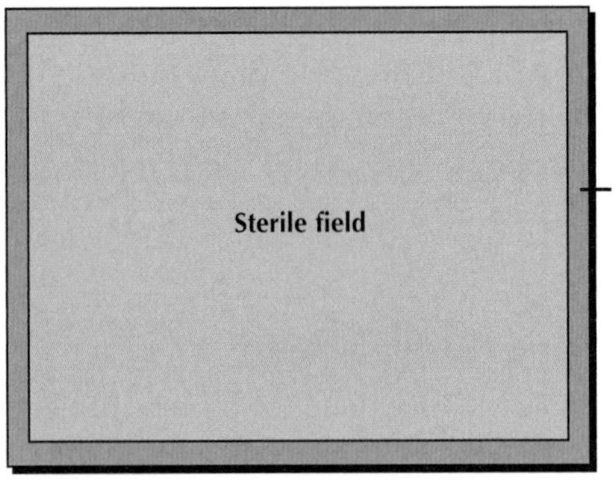

Figure 20–17 The 2.5 cm (1 in.) margin around a sterile field is considered contaminated.

Donning and Removing Sterile Gloves

You might need sterile gloves when assisting with a sterile procedure. You put them on after the sterile field has been set up. After sterile gloves are on, you can handle sterile items within the sterile field, but you cannot touch anything outside the sterile field.

Sterile gloves are disposable and come in peel-back packaging. They come in many sizes so that they will fit snugly. The insides are powdered for ease in donning the gloves. Also, the right and left gloves are marked on the package.

Always keep sterile gloved hands above your waist level and within your vision. Only touch items within the sterile field. If your gloves become contaminated, remove the gloves and put on a new pair. Also, replace gloves that are torn, cut, or punctured.

1 2 3 DONNING AND REMOVING STERILE GLOVES

Procedure

1 Inspect the package for sterility.
- **a** Check the expiration date.
- **b** See if the package is dry.
- **c** Check for tears, holes, punctures, and watermarks.

2 Arrange a work surface.
- **a** Make sure you have enough room.
- **b** Arrange the work surface at waist level and within your vision.
- **c** Clean and dry the work surface.
- **d** Practise proper hand hygiene.
- **e** Do not reach over or turn your back on the work surface.

3 Open the package. Grasp the flaps. Gently peel the flaps back.

4 Remove the inner package. Place it on your work surface.

5 Read the manufacturer's instructions on the inner package. It may be labelled with left, right, up, and down.

6 Arrange the inner package for left, right, up, and down. The left glove is placed on your left side and the right glove on your right. Place the cuffs near you with the fingers pointing away.

7 Use the thumb and index finger of each hand to grasp the folded edges of the inner package.

8 Fold back the inner package to expose the gloves (Figure 20–18, *A*). Do not touch or otherwise contaminate the inside of the package or the gloves. The inside of the inner package is a sterile field.

9 Note that each glove has a 5 to 7.5 cm (2 to 3 in.) cuff. The cuffs and insides of the gloves are not sterile.

(continued on page 357)

1 2 3 DONNING AND REMOVING STERILE GLOVES

Procedure (cont'd)

10 Put on the right glove if you are right-handed and the left if you are left-handed.

- **a** Pick up the glove with your other hand. Use your thumb and index and middle fingers (Figure 20–18, *B*).
- **b** Touch only the cuff and inside of the glove.
- **c** Turn the hand to be gloved palm side up.
- **d** Lift the cuff up. Slide your fingers and hand into the glove (Figure 20–18, *C*).
- **e** Pull the glove up over your hand. If some fingers get stuck, leave them that way until the other glove is on. ***Do not use your ungloved hand to straighten the glove. Do not let the outside of the glove touch any nonsterile surface.***
- **f** Leave the cuff turned down.

11 Put on the other glove with your gloved hand.

- **a** Reach under the cuff of the second glove. Use the four fingers of your gloved hand (Figure 20–18, D). Keep your gloved thumb close to your gloved palm.
- **b** Pull on the second glove (Figure 20–18, *E*). Your gloved hand cannot touch the cuff or any other surface. Hold the thumb of your first gloved hand away from your gloved palm.

12 Adjust each glove with the other hand. The gloves should be smooth and comfortable (Figure 20–18, *F*).

13 Slide your fingers under the cuffs to pull them up (Figure 20–18, *G*).

14 Touch only sterile items.

15 Remove the gloves as in Figure 20–8 on page 341.

16 Practise hand hygiene.

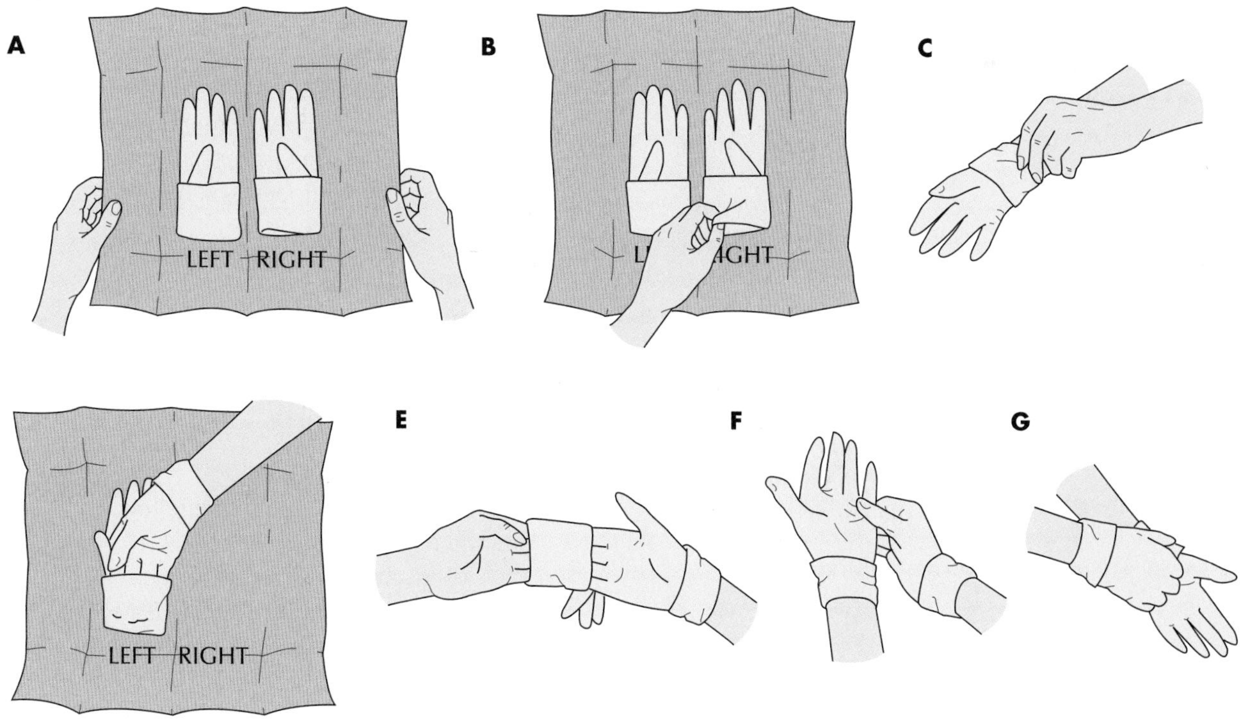

Figure 20–18 Donning sterile gloves. **A,** Open the inner wrapper to expose the gloves. **B,** Pick up the glove at the cuff with your thumb and index finger. **C,** Slide your fingers and hand into the glove. **D,** Reach under the cuff of the other glove with your fingers. **E,** Pull on the glove. **F,** Adjust each glove for comfort. **G,** Slide your fingers under the cuffs to pull them up.

REVIEW

Answers to these questions are at the bottom of page 359.

Circle T if the answer is true or circle F if the answer is false.

1. T F **A pathogen can cause an infection.**
2. T F **Multidrug-resistant organisms are easily treated with antibiotics and are not a risk in facilities.**
3. T F **Older adults often do not show the usual signs of infection.**
4. T F **A person who is colonized by a pathogen cannot transfer the pathogen to others.**
5. T F **The presence of illness and the use of invasive devices increase the risk of infection.**
6. T F **Wash your hands before *or* after giving care.**
7. T F **You should hold your hands and forearms up during the hand washing procedure.**
8. T F **The duration of the hand wash is not important.**
9. T F **Disinfecting items usually involves chemicals.**
10. T F **Unused items in a client's room can be used for another client.**
11. T F **Isolation precautions include Standard Precautions *and* Transmission-Based Precautions.**
12. T F **Standard Precautions are used only when the client has a specific contagious disease.**
13. T F **Transmission-Based Precautions are guidelines that help keep pathogens within one area, usually the client's room.**
14. T F **Gloves are worn at all times.**
15. T F **A mask is contaminated when moist.**
16. T F **Goggles, masks, and gowns are worn when there is a risk of splashing blood or body fluids.**
17. T F **You do not need to report a sharps injury if the bleeding is not severe.**
18. T F **Double-bagging of contaminated items is always required.**
19. T F **An item is sterile if nonpathogens are present.**
20. T F **A sterile item can touch only another sterile item.**
21. T F **The 2.5 cm edge around a sterile field is considered contaminated.**

Circle the BEST answer.

22. **Most pathogens are destroyed by:**
    - A. Water
    - B. High heat
    - C. Oxygen
    - D. Nourishment
23. **Aseptic practices:**
    - A. Destroy spores
    - B. Reduce the number of microbes
    - C. Are a link in the chain of infection
    - D. Destroy all microbes—pathogens and nonpathogens
24. **Standard Practices:**
    - A. Are used for all clients
    - B. Involve surgical asepsis
    - C. Prevent the spread of airborne pathogens
    - D. Are not necessary for children or older clients
25. **Gloves are always worn in the following situations:**
    - A. When washing a person's face
    - B. When the client has a cold
    - C. While washing spilled juice from the floor
    - D. If you bite your fingernails

REVIEW

Answers to these questions are at the bottom of the page.

26. **Proper use of personal protective equipment involves the following:**
    - A. Reusing your face mask after your break
    - B. Using waterless hand sanitizer on disposable gloves for reuse
    - C. Removing protective equipment after leaving the work area
    - D. Wearing gloves when touching contaminated items or surfaces

27. **Circle the words that indicate signs of infection:**
    fever, vomiting, pain, tenderness, constipation, hunger, redness, fatigue, bluish skin around the mouth, a change in behaviour, bleeding, swelling, loss of appetite.

Answers: 1.T, 2.F, 3.T, 4.F, 5.T, 6.F, 7.F, 8.F, 9.T, 10.F, 11.T, 12.F, 13.T, 14.F, 15.T, 16.T, 17.F, 18.T, 19.F, 20.T, 21.T, 22.B, 23.B, 24.A, 25.D, 26.D, 27. Fever, vomiting, pain, tenderness, redness, fatigue, a change in behaviour, swelling, loss of appetite.

CHAPTER 21

Abuse

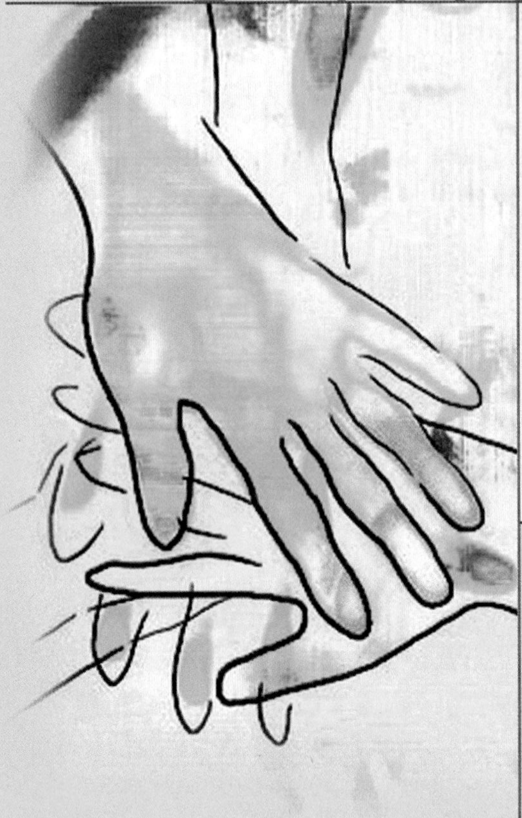

OBJECTIVES

- Define the key terms listed in this chapter.
- Identify the legal act that is meant to protect all Canadians, new immigrants, and visitors from abuse.
- Describe the types of abuse.
- Describe the cycle of abuse.
- Describe spousal abuse, child abuse, and abuse of older adults.
- Describe how clients and health care workers can be abused.
- Explain what to do if you have an abusive client.
- Identify signs of abuse.
- Explain your legal responsibilities when reporting abuse.
- Describe what to do if a client tells you that he or she is being abused.
- Apply the information in this chapter to your clinical practice properly.

key terms

abuse Physical or mental harm caused by someone in a position of trust—such as a family member, partner, or caregiver.

ageism Bias and discrimination against older adults.

Canadian Charter of Rights and Freedoms (1982) A law which states that Canada values equality and diversity and that no one should be abused or has the right to treat others unfairly.

child neglect When a child's parents or other caregivers are not meeting the essential needs for emotional, psychological, and physical development.

emotional abuse An attack on a person's self-esteem, such as constantly insulting, humiliating, or rejecting him or her, or saying that he or she is "stupid" or "bad." All of these can harm the person's sense of worth and self-confidence. People at any age could be emotionally abused.

emotional neglect Occurs when a person's need to feel loved, wanted, safe, and worthy is not met. Emotional neglect can range from the context of the abuser simply being unavailable to that in which the abuser openly rejects the person. People at any age could be emotionally neglected.

failure to thrive A term to describe infants, babies, or children who are below the norms for body weight, growth, or cognitive development.

financial abuse The misuse of a person's money or property.

marginalization Preventing a person from having any power or control over his or her life or health care because of language, life circumstances, or role in society, resulting in the person being shunned from mainstream society. For example, people addicted to drugs or alcohol and sex-trade workers are often **marginalized** from society.

physical abuse Force or violence that causes pain, injury, and sometimes death.

psychological abuse See **emotional abuse.**

right The entitlement of a person or persons to something. For example, Canadians have a **right** to safety and security.

sexual abuse Unwanted sexual activity.

sexual harassment Any conduct, comment, gesture, threat, or suggestion that is sexual in nature; a form of sexual abuse.

spousal abuse Abuse of a partner by a partner in an intimate relationship, such as a marriage or common-law relationship. The abuse may be physical, sexual, emotional, or financial, or any combination of these.

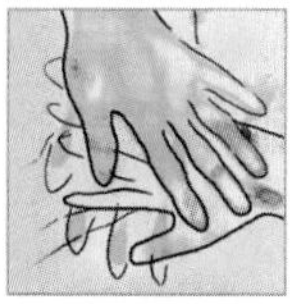

The Canadian government has enacted laws to protect people from abuse and discrimination of any kind. In Chapter 12, we discussed each person's right to be treated with respect and the need to accept people's differences at all times. This is especially true for the clients that we, as support workers, care for. It is unfortunate, however, that some workers do not recognize that ***all clients have the right to safe, respectful treatment.*** When clients' rights are ignored, they become victims of abuse.

Abuse results when physical or mental harm is caused by someone in a position of trust, such as a family member, partner, or caregiver. Unlike random acts of violence, which take place in all societies, abuse implies a relationship between the abuser and the abused. The abuser has power and control over the abused, and often, the victim is physically, emotionally, or financially dependent on the abuser. Abuse occurs in all age groups, at all social levels, in all cultures, and in all races. It can occur in community settings and in health care facilities. As a support worker, you must know how to recognize and report suspected abuse.

In this chapter, we will discuss the ***Canadian Charter of Rights and Freedoms,*** which is the foundation for all of the country's laws that make abuse illegal. We will also discuss (a) the types of abuses that exist, (b) persons who are at highest risk for abuse, and (c) ways to recognize and to report abuse.

CANADIAN CHARTER OF RIGHTS AND FREEDOMS

The basic human **rights** of Canadians, immigrants, and even visitors to Canada are protected by law. Since 1982, the most important protection is the *Canadian Charter of Rights and Freedoms,* which states Canada values equality and diversity and that no one should be abused or has the right to treat others unfairly. Knowingly failing to comply with any of these statements can be considered **abuse** (refer to http://www.charterofrights.ca/en/02_00_01).

Respect for All. The charter also requires everyone to respect the basic human rights of others. This means government, the police, the courts, and other Canadians are legally obligated to respect your rights and the rights of others.

Guaranteed Freedoms. Because of the *Charter*, people living in Canada have many basic rights and freedoms (see Box 21–1).

TYPES OF ABUSE

There are many ways in which people can abuse others, and more than one type of abuse can occur at the same time. The different types of abuse are as follows:

- ***Physical abuse***—force or violence that causes pain, injury, and sometimes death. Physical abuse includes pinching, hair pulling, pushing, slapping, hitting, shaking, choking, biting, or kicking. It also includes burning, poisoning, using weapons, or throwing things (like a chair or a hammer) at someone.
- ***Sexual abuse***—unwanted sexual activity, such as rape and attempted rape. Unwanted touching, fondling, kissing, and exposure (when the abuser shows his or her genitals to the victim) are also considered sexual abuse. **Sexual harassment**—another form of sexual abuse—is any conduct, comment, gesture, threat, or suggestion that is sexual in nature.
- ***Emotional abuse (psychological abuse)***—words or actions that cause mental harm. It usually involves an attack on a person's self-esteem, for example, constantly insulting, humiliating, or rejecting a person, or saying that he or she is "stupid"' or "bad." All of these can harm the person's sense of worth and self-confidence. Emotional abuse can happen to infants, children, teens, adults, and seniors.

Emotional abuse lessens the victim's dignity and self-worth because he or she is called names, yelled at, insulted, mocked, threatened, or sworn at. The victim may be ignored for long periods of time or may not be allowed to do preferred activities or visit with family, friends, or others. Threatening to harm someone or something that the victim loves (such as a child or a pet) is another example of emotional abuse.

- ***Financial abuse***—the misuse of a person's money or property, usually for the abuser's financial gain. Financial abuse includes stealing; forging signatures; selling property or possessions without permission; and persuading or tricking victims to change their wills or give up control of their finances. Some abusers do not allow their victims access to their own money.
- ***Neglect***—failing to meet the basic needs of a dependent person. Victims of neglect are usually children, people with disabilities, and frail older adults. Neglect occurs when a clean, comfortable, and safe environment is not provided. In some cases, the caregiver may even withhold or deny basic needs such as food, water, or clothing. Personal care, medical care, education, and attention and love may also be denied or withheld. The caregiver may knowingly neglect the victim or unintentionally neglect the person because he or she is unable to provide adequate care.

THE CYCLE OF ABUSE

Abuse usually occurs over and over again, as the abuser tries to dominate the victim with power and control. It often follows a pattern, known as the cycle of abuse (Figure 21–1). There are three phases in the cycle.

1. ***The tension-building phase***—Tension starts to build between the abuser and the victim. Everyday events and comments irritate and

anger the abuser. As the abuser becomes more angry and stressed, he or she grows more aggressive. The victim may try to calm, soothe, and please the abuser, stay out of the abuser's way, or try not to say or do anything that might anger or upset the abuser.

Box 21–1 The Rights and Freedoms of All Canadians

The *Canadian Charter of Rights and Freedoms* (1982) ensures that all Canadians, new immigrants, and visitors to Canada have the following rights:

- ***Fundamental Freedoms:*** This section includes the rights to: freedom of conscience and religion; freedom of thought, belief, opinion and expression, including freedom of the press and other media of communications; and freedom of peaceful assembly and association.

  This means that Canadians, new immigrants, and visitors to Canada have the right to practise the religions of their choice and that they can express their views without fear of being punished in any way. This also means that they can voice their opinions in print (in a newspaper or pamphlet, for example), in person, or on the Internet, radio, or TV. We all have the right to choose who we want to communicate with (or not), and we can join together in a *peaceful* manner to voice our opinions (for example, to go on strike, or to demonstrate in front of a building by holding up placards).
- ***Equality Rights:*** This section includes the rights to equal treatment before and under the law and equal benefit and protection of the law without discrimination based on race, national or ethnic origin, colour, religion, sex, age, and mental or physical disability. Other grounds of discrimination that were not specifically set out in the *Charter,* such as sexual orientation and marital status, were recognized in 1985.

  This means that we are all considered equal, and nobody can get poorer (or special) treatment because of their ethnic background, colour, religion, sex, age, or disability of any kind.
- ***Democratic Rights:*** These sections contain the right to vote, the right to run for public office, and the maximum duration and sitting of legislative bodies.
- ***Mobility:*** This section ensures the right to move from place to place within Canada and ensures that Canadian citizens are free to enter and leave Canada as they please. It also gives citizens and permanent residents the right to move to and live in any province.
- ***Legal Rights:*** These sections set out the rights that protect us in our dealings with the justice system. These rights ensure that individuals who are involved in legal proceedings are treated fairly, especially those charged with criminal offences, and include the rights:
  - To life, liberty, and security of the person
  - To be secure from unreasonable search and seizure
  - To be free from unnecessary detention or imprisonment
  - To be informed promptly for reasons for any arrest or detention
  - To retain and instruct counsel on arrest or detention
  - To trial within a reasonable time by an impartial tribunal
  - To the presumption of innocence
  - To protection against self-incrimination
  - To freedom from cruel and unusual treatment or punishment
  - To the assistance of an interpreter
- ***Language Rights:*** These sections confirm that English and French are the official languages of Canada and assert the equality of the French and English languages in particular situations. The language rights include the right to use English or French in Parliament and in any court established by Parliament, including the Supreme Court of Canada. Federal laws must be published in both English and French.
- ***Minority Language Education Rights:*** This section establishes that provincial governments must provide certain English or French language minority rights. Minority language education applies when there is a sufficient number of eligible children to justify providing schooling in that language.

2. ***The abusive phase***—Tension explodes into an abusive event. The abuse may involve neglect or physical, sexual, emotional, or financial abuse. Often, the abuse is triggered by an event unrelated to the victim's behaviour.
3. ***The honeymoon phase***—The abuser feels ashamed or sorry. He or she apologizes and promises never to do it again. He or she may offer gifts or be very loving and attentive. At this stage, the abuser and victim may both believe that the abuser can change.

If specific measures are not taken to stop the cycle of abuse, it continues. There may be days, weeks, months, or years between abusive events. Usually, the time between episodes gradually shortens, and the abuse becomes more frequent and more intense. It is important for the victim and abuser to recognize the problem and get help in order to stop the cycle.

RECOGNIZING SIGNS OF ABUSE

As a support worker, you are responsible for recognizing signs of abuse (see Box 21–2 for a list of signs of various kinds of abuse). These signs generally apply to all abusive relationships in all settings.

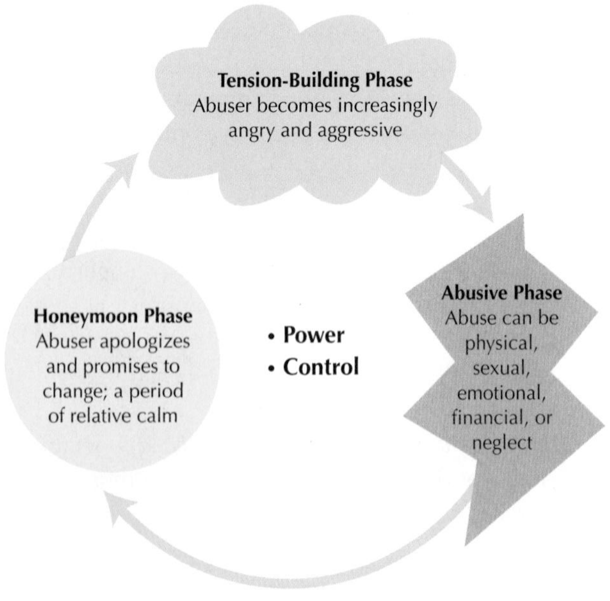

Figure 21–1 The cycle of abuse.

However, you are not qualified to judge whether or not your client is being abused. You may think you recognize one or some of the signs listed in Box 21–2, but it may not mean that abuse has occurred. These signs might, however, suggest that abuse could be a possibility.

Watch for signs of abuse or neglect in the course of your daily work with your clients. Immediately report any suspicions or observations to your supervisor. Your supervisor will ensure that the situation is investigated. Know your employer's procedures on reporting observations or suspicions.

ABUSIVE RELATIONSHIPS

Abuse can occur in many different kinds of relationships. Both women and men can be abused by their spouses or partners; children can be abused by their parents; older adults can be abused by their adult children; clients can be abused by health care workers; and health care workers can be abused by their clients (see Box 21–3 on page 367).

Abusive relationships are complex, and there is usually no single cause for the abuse. However, in all relationships, a person is more likely to be abusive if he or she:

- Has problems with alcohol or drugs
- Has a mental illness (for example, major depression) or severe personality flaws (for example, an explosive temper, inability to control impulses, or lack of empathy for others)
- Has been abused as a child
- Is going through a period of high stress, such as divorce, unemployment, poverty, or illness

SPOUSAL ABUSE

Spousal abuse is abuse that occurs between intimate partners in a marriage or common-law relationship and may be physical, sexual, emotional, or financial. Usually more than one type of abuse is present in the relationship.

Both women and men can be abused by their partners. One Canadian study found that similar

Box 21–2 Signs and Symptoms of Abuse

Physical Abuse

- Physical injuries (such as burns, bumps, bruises, scratches, cuts, or fractures) that occur frequently, are left untreated, and either are unexplained or have unlikely explanations
- New injuries that appear while older injuries are still healing
- Frequent injuries (such as burns, bruises, welts, or cuts) on the face, neck, inner arms, back, upper arms and inner thighs; people who are abused often try to hide their injuries under clothing or makeup
- Welts, bruises, or burns that have the shape of the object that caused the injury; for example, the shape may be of a handprint, belt, or wooden spoon
- Unexplained missing or loose teeth
- A very groggy or overly sedated client

Sexual Abuse

- Irritation, injury (such as cuts and bruises or scarring) of the thighs, perineum, or breasts
- Intense fear of bathing or perineal care
- Torn, stained, or bloody underwear
- Vaginal discharge, genital odour, and painful urination
- Difficulty walking or sitting
- Avoidance of touching

Emotional Abuse

- A change in behaviour, especially if the client seems depressed or unusually quiet or withdrawn
- Fearful behaviour, especially in the presence of the suspected abuser; for example, the client cowers, avoids eye contact, or trembles
- Unwillingness to talk or answer questions
- Change in behaviour when the suspected abuser enters and leaves the room
- Withholding of permission to socialize with family or friends or client's withdrawal from contacts
- Private conversations not allowed—the suspected abuser insists on being present or within hearing distance of all conversations
- Change in the behaviour of the suspected abuser (who may be the caregiver)—on one occasion he or she is pleasant and cooperative and is defensive or hostile on another occasion
- Caregiver's failure to show any affection toward the person in his or her care; or the affection displayed seems strained or "put on for show"
- Frequent statements by the caregiver that the person in his or her care is difficult or demanding

Financial Abuse

- The caregiver refuses to spend money on caring for the person
- The client has many unpaid bills (such as utilities, telephone, or rent) or bounced cheques, even though he or she has money
- There is lack of adequate food, clothing, personal care items, or furnishings, even though the client can afford them
- The suspected abuser seems more concerned about the cost, rather than the quality, of the care
- Personal belongings are missing, and there is no explanation
- The suspected abuser does not have a job and is secretive about his or her source of income
- The client has to ask for permission to write cheques or spend money

Neglect

- Unsafe, unclean, or inadequate living conditions
- Lack of personal hygiene. For example, a neglected client may have ingrown nails, decayed teeth, untreated sores, matted hair, body odour, or dirty clothing
- Signs of poor nutrition and fluid intake, such as weight loss, extreme thirst, a thin, bony appearance, and sunken eyes or cheeks; dehydration may make the skin feel dry and papery
- Pressure sores
- Medications not purchased
- Lack of supervision or attention for prolonged periods of time

(continued on page 366)

Box 21–2 **Signs and Symptoms of Abuse** (cont'd)

Infants and Children

All of the above as well as the following are signs of abuse or neglect in children and infants:

- Sudden behaviour changes—for example, bedwetting, loss of bladder or bowel control during the day, or loss of appetite
- Prolonged vomiting or diarrhea
- Developmental delays, such as not gaining weight or not reaching developmental milestones (for example, sitting or standing)
- Lack of energy in infants, shown by lack of interest in the surroundings, infrequent crying, and generally an undemanding disposition

Sources: Boyack, V. (1997). *Golden years—hidden fears: Elder abuse. A handbook for front-line helpers working with seniors,* p. 7. Calgary: Kerby Centre; Quinn, M.J., & Tomita, S.K. (1997). *Elder abuse and neglect: Causes, diagnosis, and intervention strategies* (2nd ed.), pp. 55, 76. New York: Springer; Government of Canada, Department of Justice. (2007). *Abuse of older adults: A fact sheet from the Department of Justice Canada.* Retrieved May 21, 2007, from http://www.justice.gc.ca/en/ps/fm/adultsfs.html

numbers of women and men reported being abused by their partners.[1] However, women are usually more severely injured than are men. Domestic violence rates among intimate couples usually increase when the woman is pregnant or caring for an infant.[2]

Why Do They Stay? People who are abused by their partner often deny the abuse. They also often choose to stay with their partners, in spite of serious physical violence. Some victims may stay because they are afraid of leaving their abuser, as the abuser may threaten them with harm, death, or denial of child custody. In some circumstances, the victim may stay so that the children can continue to have the financial and other comforts of a two-parent home. Some victims stay because they do not know where to go or how to get help. Some others may believe that they are responsible for the abuse, that no one will believe them, or that the abuser will change and the relationship will work.

CHILD ABUSE

Child abuse occurs when a parent, guardian, or caregiver mistreats or neglects a child, which may result in:

- injury
- significant emotional or psychological harm
- serious risk of harm to the child

Child abuse is a gross misuse of a caregiver's position of trust and authority over a child. Children who are abused tend to experience more social problems and perform less well in school than other children, and this can have lasting effects on their social adjustment and success in life. Victims of childhood abuse are at greater risk of themselves becoming violent abusers and criminals.

Child abuse can take many different forms:

- ***Physical abuse***—is the deliberate application of force on any part of a child's body, which may result in a nonaccidental injury. Physical abuse also includes behaviours such as shaking, choking, biting, kicking, burning or poisoning a child, holding a child under water, or any other harmful or dangerous use of force or restraint. Some people confuse punishment with physical abuse.

  Children who are both emotionally and physically abused exhibit the greatest degree of aggression, delinquency, and interpersonal problems. Women who were abused in childhood are more likely to suffer from depression, low self-esteem, and suicidal thoughts. While physical abuse will put a child in immediate danger of injury, psychological or emotional abuse can have even more negative and long-term consequences for the child than physical abuse.
- ***Emotional abuse***—(see general description of Emotional Abuse on page 362). Emotional

Box 21–3 Persons at Highest Risk for Abuse

Even though potentially anybody could be abused (or, for that matter, be an abuser, given the right circumstances), there are certain groups of people that are *especially* at risk for being abused. Abuse may damage a person's sense of self-worth and dignity and increase his or her social isolation, which makes them even more vulnerable to abuse. Also, abused persons may be unable to access (or not be knowledgeable about) support systems that are available. These people include:

- ***Marginalized persons (especially women):*** Thosewho (a) do not speak an official language, (b) belong to a visible minority group, (c) are geographically isolated, (d) have a physical or intellectual disability, (e) have a mental health disorder, (f) are (or were) a substance abuser, or (g) work in the sex-trade industry. People who fall in this category are considered to be **marginalized**, meaning they are prevented from having any power or control—due to their language (they speak a language other than English or French as their main language), their life circumstances (including poverty), or their role in society—and are shunned by mainstream society because of it.

  People who are marginalized are usually treated as though they were "invisible," and they often feel powerless to report abuse, or they may not be understood or believed, in which case authorities may not give as much attention to their reports as to other people's reports.
- ***Children:*** Children are usually dependent on the person who is caring for them. They are too young to know how to defend or protect themselves. Some parents or caregivers think that they have the right to "discipline" their children using abusive force or words. Others are overwhelmed with the stress and responsibilities of being a parent or guardian, or they very likely were abused themselves in their childhood.
- ***Older adults:*** Older adults may not know how to escape from an abuser or may lack the strength to seek safety and shelter.
- ***Socially or geographically isolated seniors:*** Seniors who cannot get out of the places where they live may not have an opportunity to tell anyone that they are abused. Bruises and other obvious physical signs might also go unnoticed if these older seniors are prevented from having contact with others.
- ***Seniors with reduced cognitive capacity:*** These seniors may not know or remember that they have been abused. They may no longer have control over their finances, so they may not know that their money or belongings are being taken.
- ***Dependent seniors with disabilities:*** These seniors may not have opportunities to interact with others, so abuses can often go unrecognized. In the case of physical abuse, bruises are often explained away by the abuser as being caused by the disability, age, or general health condition of the senior.
- ***Seniors cared for by people with substance abuse problems:*** People with substance abuse problems may lack impulse control—that is, the ability to control their angry outbursts or to deal with the senior's own challenging behaviours in a nonviolent manner. Others may have financial problems and steal from the senior they care for in order to support their substance addiction.

Source: Government of Canada, Department of Justice. (2006). *Family violence publications.* Retrieved July 25, 2007, from http://www.justice.gc.ca/en/ps/fm/publi.html

abuse is often part of a pattern of family stress and dysfunctional parenting.

- ***Child sexual abuse***—occurs when a child is used for sexual purposes by an adult or adolescent. It involves exposing a child to any sexual activity or behaviour. Sexual abuse involves fondling, inviting a child to touch or be touched sexually, or even sexual intercourse, juvenile prostitution, and sexual exploitation through pornography. Sexual abuse is also considered to be a form of emotional abuse.
- ***Child neglect***—occurs when a child's parents or other caregivers fail to meet the essential needs for a child's emotional, psychological and physical development. **Physical neglect** occurs when a child's needs for food, clothing, shelter,

cleanliness, medical care, and protection from harm are not adequately met. **Emotional neglect** occurs when a child's need to feel loved, wanted, safe, and worthy is not met. Emotional neglect can range from the context of the abuser simply being unavailable to that in which the abuser openly rejects the child. Physical assaults are more likely to be reported, but neglect can have equally serious consequences for a child.

- ***Other forms of emotionally abusive treatment***—include forcing a child into social isolation, intimidating, exploiting, terrorizing, or routinely making unreasonable demands on a child. Some provinces in Canada now include exposure of a child to violence between the parents as a form of emotional abuse.[3] A recent study of wife assault found that children witness violence against their mothers in almost 40% of violent marriages.[4]

Situations That Increase the Risk of Child Abuse

- ***Family crisis.*** Divorce, unemployment, moving, poverty, and crowded living conditions all cause stress. Stress can lead to abuse.
- ***Single-parenting.*** A recent study found that almost half of all cases of child abuse involved children living in a single-parent family.[1] Possibly this is because some single parents are under great stress. This can also mean that they may be more likely to abuse a vulnerable parent under their care.
- ***Isolation.*** Many abusive people do not have close relationships with their extended family, friends, or community.[1] As a result, they do not understand normal child development and behaviour, so they may have unrealistic expectations of the child. For example, they may think a crying baby is being bad. They may believe hitting or slapping are appropriate forms of discipline.
- ***Caring for children with special needs.*** Children with physical or mental disabilities or chronic illness are especially at risk for being abused. Children with personalities or behaviours that the abuser considers "different" or unacceptable are also at greater risk.

"Failure to Thrive"

"Failure to thrive" is a term that describes infants, babies, or children who are below the norms for body weight, growth, or cognitive development. One of the many known causes is that children with "failure to thrive" have been subjected to caregiver neglect. In extreme cases, it can lead to permanent developmental delays and even the death of the child. Many of the mothers of these infants were themselves likely abused as children.

What Can Be Done to Prevent Child Abuse?

Most abusive parents do not consciously set out to harm their children. If there are more and better efforts to assist troubled families, parents at risk of abusing may be reached and helped before they resort to violence. Prevention is a good investment, in terms of both the personal and social costs that can be saved. There are many ways to prevent abuse, including:[5]

- ***Parenting education.*** This can help parents to better understand normal child development and to have a more nurturing and enjoyable relationship with their children. Positive approaches to parenting can help parents deal with children of any age.
- ***Child abuse prevention programs.*** Abused children tend to repeat the pattern of abuse later when they become adults, so identification of potential abusers and prevention are the most effective means to stop the cycle of violence.
- ***Being supportive.*** If a child tells you, as the support worker, about an abusive situation or experience, you need to show the child that you believe him or her and ensure that the information is promptly reported to the appropriate authorities.
- ***Teaching children.*** Children should know how to recognize and say no to abusive or exploitative behaviour and that they have the right to be free from abuse. As a support worker, you can help children and adults find information and assistance to prevent an abusive or neglectful pattern from developing.

supporting TAYLOR

Taylor is a 6-year-old boy who was born with fetal alcohol syndrome (see Chapter 38). His weight is below the average for a child his age, and he has hearing and vision difficulties as well as behavioural problems. You have been assigned to Taylor as his support worker, to assist him with bathing, toileting, and eating. Because of Taylor's frequent verbal outbursts and his tendency to bite, kick, and scratch, his mother has decided to home-school Taylor. This is your first visit with Taylor in his home.

Taylor's mother, a nicely dressed woman, greets you at the door. The house is clean, neat, and stylishly furnished. In the course of your conversation, Taylor's mother tells you that she is a lawyer, and because of Taylor's situation, she plans on practising law from her home. During this initial visit, while she is showing you around the house, she repeatedly blames her ex-husband for Taylor's condition; she says her ex-husband had a "terrible drinking problem."

When you meet Taylor, he gives you a big hug and asks you if you can stay all day. He then turns on the television; because of his hearing and vision difficulties, he needs to sit very close to it, with the sound turned up. Taylor's mother yells at Taylor, telling him, "Turn the (*uses a swear word*) TV down!" Taylor does so but begins to cry. Taylor's mother then asks you to make sure that Taylor keeps quiet while you are with him.

ABUSE OF OLDER ADULTS

Older adults are at risk for all types of abuse—physical, sexual, emotional, and financial—as well as neglect. Financial and emotional abuses are most commonly reported by older adults. Abusers are usually family members, such as an adult child or grandchild. Often, the abuser is the older adult's primary caregiver. Most abusers of older adults depend on their victims for financial help or housing, for example, an adult son who moves in with his parent after losing his job.[6]

Abused older adults sometimes choose not to complain about the abuse. Like abused spouses, they may fear the abuser or may not know where or how to get help. They may fear being forced to move into a long-term care facility if they report their caregiver. Some older adults are not able to report abuse, as they may have physical or mental disabilities. Victims of neglect especially are often unable to report their situation (see Box 21–2).

In addition to the factors that have been identified earlier in this chapter, some other factors that might increase an older person's risk for being abused include:

- ***Stress.*** Family caregivers are more likely to be abusive when they resent their role. Taking care of an older adult can be extremely stressful, especially when the person receiving care is physically or mentally disabled. If the caregiver is unprepared or unable to fulfill the duties, he or she can feel overwhelmed.
- ***Ageism.*** Ageism is another cause of abuse (see Chapter 17). **Ageism** is bias and discrimination against older adults. Caregivers who do not respect the dignity or abilities of older adults are more likely to be abusive. For example, a caregiver who thinks that older adults are incapable of managing money may take control of the person's finances without permission (financial abuse).
- ***Vulnerability.*** Many of the factors that increase older adults' vulnerability to abuse may also compound the effects of the abuse. According to the Department of Justice for the Government of Canada, older adults are vulnerable to abuse because of the following factors:[7]
  a. Living conditions (inadequate housing, geographical isolation)
  b. Unemployment (not employed or retired from an employer)
  c. Dislocation (new to the area)
  d. Racism (prejudice because of skin colour)
  e. Homophobia (prejudice because of sexual orientation)
  f. Disability (physical, mental, or developmental limitations)
  g. Economic vulnerability (few financial assistances or poverty)
  h. Social isolation, language or literacy skills (isolated because of geographical location, inability to speak, read, or write the local language)

i. Lack of access to community and health services
j. Lack of access to housing, or long-term care facilities
k. Lack of access to the justice system.

ABUSE OF CLIENTS IN A FACILITY OR HOME SETTING

Abuse of clients can happen in a facility or home care setting, and clients can be abused by any member of the health care team. In facilities, they can be abused by visitors or a member of the staff.

Clients are at risk for all types of abuse—physical, sexual, emotional, and financial—as well as neglect. Abusive situations include: using restraints inappropriately, handling the client roughly, isolating the client in his or her room, stealing from the client, not reviewing the care plan regularly, not responding to a call for help, not checking on the client for long periods of time, and leaving the client lying in soiled linen or clothes. ***Violating a client's rights*** is another form of abuse, for example, providing care against the person's wishes, failing to provide privacy, failing to keep personal or medical information confidential, and not letting residents visit or use the phone in private.

Abuse can be very obvious, such as roughly handling or force-feeding a client. Or it can be very subtle (not obvious), for example, staff can demean or belittle clients by calling them "grandma" or "slugger" or by referring to their incontinence briefs as "diapers." These are embarrassing for the client and violate the "DIPPS" principles.

Stress Can Trigger Client Abuse. As with all abusive relationships, stress sometimes leads to or triggers the abuse of clients (see *Supporting Mrs. Finnie*). Some workers may not have received enough training or education to cope with the situations; or too much work and too few workers may contribute to

supporting MRS. FINNIE

Evelyn Finnie is a 65-year-old woman who is a resident in an extended care facility. She has periods of confusion, but she is reasonably coherent most days. She has been confined to a wheelchair ever since she suffered a severe stroke 15 years ago and is dependant on supportive care for all of her basic needs. She is often described as being "demanding" and "manipulative" by the staff that you work with, and you have noticed that she does have specific preferences for how she is bathed, dressed, or fed.

This is your first time working evenings at this very busy agency. While the nurse in charge seems nice and has asked you to talk to her whenever you have any questions, you are expected to be busy assisting the other support workers. You are told by the other support workers that h.s. (bedtime) care begins at 1830h (6:30 pm). You are shocked that it begins at such an early hour but decide to go along with the staff. Your co-worker, Jane, whom you have been partnered with, has been working on evening shifts for the past 25 years. She tells you that Mrs. Finnie should be the first resident prepared for bed, so she can "get out of your hair." Jane tells you that she is just waiting to retire from her job and that she likes to get everyone in bed early so she can have a "decent break."

Jane advises you to put an incontinence brief on Mrs. Finnie instead of assisting her with toileting (this would require a mechanical lift). Mrs. Finnie gets very upset because of this and says loudly that she wants to "go in the toilet." Jane steps in and completes putting the brief on Mrs. Finnie, telling her that she could just "let it go in her diaper all night." When Mrs. Finnie tries to wiggle during the application of her incontinence brief, Jane holds her down and says in a loud voice, "Who do you think you are? I am so tired of your acting like a queen. Now stay still, or this will really hurt!"

All the other residents who would normally be toileted by mechanical lifts have incontinence briefs applied to them as well, although none of the other residents complains. Jane is nice to some of the residents but seems impatient with some others. When you ask her about this, she says, "I remember who gave me a hard time and who didn't!"

You are shocked and very disturbed by the evening's events, but really do not know what to do. What should you have done? What would you do differently next time?

a high level of stress. Some clients can be uncooperative or abusive toward the staff, for example, they may hit or yell at the worker. Some workers respond to abusive clients by being abusive to them in return.

However, there is no excuse for abusive behaviour from a support worker. Sometimes you will work with difficult clients in stressful situations, and you must recognize when you are feeling stressed. Take time out if you begin to lose your temper. Always treat your clients gently and with respect, even when they resist your care.

To prevent your behaviour from becoming abusive, immediately discuss difficult or aggressive clients with your supervisor. Your supervisor will help you decide how to handle them. If necessary, you can ask for a change of assignment (see Chapter 9 for a discussion on how to manage stress).

REPORTING ABUSE

Every Canadian province and territory has legislation that imposes a duty on members of the public and professional organizations to report cases where they have reasonable grounds to suspect that a child, a person with physical or mental challenges, or an older adult is being abused by a parent, adult child, caregiver, or guardian. As a support worker, you have this obligation as well.

All of the victims can be subjected to physical, emotional, and sexual abuse, and usually the caregiver—a parent, child, grandparent, step-parent, or relative—is the abuser. Sometimes the abuser is a nonrelative who is close to the person, such as a family friend or a parent's or adult child's partner.

Boys and girls as well as men and women are equally likely to be victims, so all age groups are at risk. Abuse occurs in all types of families: rich and poor, educated and uneducated. Whether the caregiver of a child—a physically or mentally challenged son or daughter—or of a parent, most abusers do not feel that they have any help during times of stress.

Some people think that abuse is a private family matter, and it should remain behind closed doors. Others believe that they cannot do anything about it, so they should not even try. This is not true. If you have reasonable grounds to suspect that someone is being abused or neglected, promptly report your concerns to the child welfare agency, the provincial or territorial Social Services department, or the police force in your community. If necessary, the report can be made anonymously.

Reporting is not difficult or time consuming. In all cases, the person reporting is protected from any kind of legal action, provided the report is not falsely made, motivated by malice.

Where to Go for Services. Contact these local organizations when abuse is suspected or recognized:

- Child welfare agency
- Social service agency
- Police department
- Hospital
- Mental health centre
- Distress centre
- Other community service organization that provides counselling and support to children and families

Many of these organizations are listed among the emergency telephone numbers on or near the first page of your local telephone directory.

Children who want help can also directly ***call the Kids' Help Phone at 1-800-668-6868.***

ABUSE OF HEALTH CARE WORKERS

Sometimes health care workers, including support workers, are abused while on the job. You are at risk for physical or verbal abuse from your clients, your clients' family members, or other members of the health care team.

Health care workers are especially at risk for abuse when they work with clients who have a mental illness or a condition that affects behaviour, such as schizophrenia and dementia (see Chapters 34 and 35). Clients who are addicted to drugs or alcohol, who have a history of abusive behaviour, or who are being placed in restraints are also more likely to be abusive toward you.

Staff abuse should never be ignored or accepted as "part of the job." Examples of abusive behaviours by the cognitively aware client or from a co-worker or supervisor include:

- Threatening to harm you or trying to scare you
- Denying meal breaks, drinking water, bathroom use, or hand-washing facilities
- Swearing, name calling, and using racial or cultural slurs
- Hitting, pushing, kicking, spitting, biting, pinching, or other physical attacks
- Inappropriate touching
- Sexually assaulting or harassing
- Following you home or finding out your home phone number and calling you at home

All agencies have policies about what to do in the case of co-worker abuse. Your employer will have policies on dealing with abusive clients. Box 21–4 lists general safety measures to follow when dealing with abusive clients.

The Sexually Aggressive Client. Some clients want the health care team members to help meet their sexual needs, so they may flirt or make sexual advances or comments. Some may even expose themselves, masturbate, or inappropriately touch health care workers. Often there are reasons for such behaviours; they may be more common when the client is cognitively impaired. Understanding this helps you deal with the problem (see Chapter 35).

Changes in a client's mental condition can reduce the social "filtering" that usually stops a person from acting on their sexual urges in public. Sexual behaviour in a client is usually not intended to be abusive, but it still must be dealt with, and you must notify your supervisor if a client makes sexual advances toward you.

If the client (or co-worker) is cognitively aware, however, these behaviours can anger or embarrass

Box 21–4 **What to Do When a Client Is Abusive**

- Stay calm.
- Stand up so that the client is not in a dominant position. Stand far enough away from the client, about 2 m (6 ft) so that he or she cannot hit or kick you.
- Position yourself close to a door in case you have to escape quickly.
- Note the locations of call bells, alarms, closed-circuit monitors, and other security devices.
- Keep your hands free. Do not touch the client.
- Listen to the client. Restate what he or she says in your own words.
- Talk to the client calmly. Do not raise your voice or argue, scold, or interrupt the client. Be polite and positive. Avoid such comments as "Calm down" or "You have no reason to be mad at me." Instead, acknowledge the client's frustrations, and tell the client you will get your supervisor to speak to him or her.
- Watch the client's body language, including shaking or clenching fists or a change in posture. This may be a sign that the client is ready to hit or push.
- If you are in a facility, tell the client that you will get a nurse to speak to him or her. Make sure that the client is safe, and quickly leave the room. Tell the nurse or the security officer about the situation. If you cannot leave and you suspect the client is going to lose control, sound a call bell, alarm, or other security device.
- If you are in a client's home, leave the house if you think you are in danger. Go to a safe place and immediately call your supervisor. If you cannot leave the house and you feel threatened, call the police by dialling 9-1-1.
- Complete an incident report after an abusive encounter (see Chapter 19 for an example of an incident report). In Chapter 35, the section Managing Disruptive Behaviours has examples of different types of disruptive behaviours and ways to de-escalate most situations.

the worker, which is normal. Sometimes clients do not have any mental or physical problems that cause sexual aggression but behave aggressively for other reasons. They may touch their health care workers because they have unmet needs for love and belonging or self-esteem and are feeling lonely or unloved. For example, a divorced client may behave sexually toward you because he wants to prove that he is attractive and can perform sexually. Remember that you must be professional in these situations:

- Ask the client not to touch you, telling him or her where you were touched.
- Tell the client that you will not do what he or she wants.
- Tell the client that his or her behaviour makes you uncomfortable. Politely ask the client not to act in that way.
- If you feel your safety is at risk, leave the client's room or house. Call your supervisor.
- Tell your supervisor about what happened. She or he can help you decide if further action is necessary. If you are uncomfortable being with the client, you have the right to ask to be assigned to another client.

Sexual Harassment. Sexual harassment—a form of sexual abuse—happens in the workplace when clients, their families, or co-workers make sexual comments, gestures, threats, or suggestions to you. If their behaviour offends you or makes you uncomfortable, it is harassment.

Remember that it is your responsibility to ***firmly but politely explain to the person that his or her conduct is unwelcome and unacceptable. Never assume that the person knows that you do not approve this behaviour.*** Be assertive, but never rude. Most people will stop the harassing behaviour when they realize it is unacceptable.

Try to have a reliable witness when you make your objections, and always make a note of the details—when and where it happened and what was said. Keep this documentation in a safe place, so if this ever happens again, you will have a record of this. If the harassment continues, tell your supervisor about it. In Canada, employers are legally required to prevent sexual harassment at work. All employers have policies on how to deal with sexual aggression and harassment.

Your Legal Responsibilities

You are legally required to report child abuse. If you witness or even suspect child abuse, you must report it. Each province and territory has rules about what must be reported and to whom. However, *all* require that witnessed and suspected child abuse be reported directly to child protection authorities. (Look up your local child welfare agency or social service agency in the phone book.) Do not rely on your supervisor to make the report for you. However, consult with your supervisor before making your report and get his or her advice.

As long as you have reasonable grounds for reporting, no legal action can be taken against you if your suspicions are eventually proved wrong. Your name will be kept confidential. In some provinces, ***failing to report child abuse can result in fines or imprisonment***.

Several provinces and territories also have laws that require health care workers to report witnessed or suspected abuse of the elderly or the disabled within facilities. In these provinces, workers must report abuse directly to a public authority. Even if your province or territory does not require public reporting, inform your supervisor about any cases or suspicions of abuse. Be sure to write down your observations, including as many details as you can, and keep this information in a safe place. It will help you remember details, if needed, in the future. Know your employer's policy and provincial or territorial law concerning the reporting of abuse within a facility.

In Canada, the Department of Justice has a fact sheet that describes what constitutes abuse of the elderly. It is understood that mentally capable adults can make their own choices and decisions about seeking help. Therefore, in home care settings, you do not need to report abuse of older adults or spouses to a public authority. However, immediately report your suspicions to your supervisor, according to your employer's policies.

How to Report Abuse

Your employer will have specific rules regarding how to report your observations. It is very important to record all your observations and make your reports in writing. Keep all your notes, in case you are asked to remember details later on. In general, when you report abuse—whether to your supervisor or to a public authority—you should record the following:

- The alleged victim's name, address, phone number, age, and sex
- The alleged abuser's name, address, phone number, and relationship to the victim
- Description of abuse or neglect, suspicions, and evidence obtained to date; record the date, time, and place; only state the facts that you know or were told by the victim; do not make assumptions

Whenever you report your suspicions, it is essential that you respect and protect your client's right to privacy. Only tell those who need to know. Do not gossip, or tell anyone who is not directly involved.

When Clients Speak of Abuse

You should be prepared for the possibility that a client or child may tell you that he or she is being abused. In such situations, it is important that you support the person and know how to offer help immediately. Follow your employer's guidelines and policies. The following are some general guidelines on how to be supportive:

- Listen attentively. Let the person tell you what happened in his or her own words. Recognize the person's feelings.
- Reassure the person that you believe what he or she has said. Stay calm and do not show anger or disgust. Do not deny or ignore the problem. Do not ask what the person did to make the abuser angry. This will only make the victim think that the abuse was his or her fault.
- Assure the person that you will do what you can to help. Notify your supervisor at once. Your employer's guidelines and policies will say what should be provided to people who are living with abuse. Helpful community resources include the police, women's shelters, counselling services, telephone help lines, and legal clinics.
- Provide emotional support to the person whatever he or she decides to do. Remember, you cannot force an adult to make a certain decision or take a particular action. People who are capable of making their own informed decisions have the right to decide for themselves whether to live with the abuse or to accept help. Some people choose not to accept help; this is their right, and you must accept their decision. People who are not capable of making informed decisions must get the help of a professional.

REVIEW

Answers to these questions are at the bottom of page 376.

Circle the **BEST** answer.

1. **The *Canadian Charter of Rights and Freedoms* applies to:**
   A. Citizens of Canada
   B. Visitors to Canada
   C. New immigrants
   D. All of the above

2. **The *Canadian Charter of Rights and Freedoms* states that:**
   A. Canada values equality and diversity
   B. No one should be abused or has the right to treat others unfairly
   C. People who are in jail have no rights
   D. A and B only

3. **Which example of abuse is considered to be *physical* abuse?**
   A. Calling the person worthless
   B. Taking bankbooks away
   C. Not allowing the thermostat to be turned up on very cold days
   D. Withholding affection

4. **In which phase during the cycle of abuse does the abuser seem loving and attentive?**
   A. Honeymoon phase
   B. Resolution phase
   C. Tension-building phase
   D. Abusive incident

5. **Who are more likely to be abusive?**
   A. Women
   B. Men
   C. People who have a problem with alcohol or drugs
   D. Parents with close family and social relationships

6. **Which statement about spousal abuse is true?**
   A. You are obligated to press charges against your abusive spouse.
   B. Abuse only involves violence.
   C. Women and men can be abused.
   D. Only one type of abuse is usually present.

7. **Which statement about child abuse is true?**
   A. You must have proof that abuse has occurred before you report it.
   B. All victims of child abuse are girls.
   C. You must report any suspicions of child abuse directly to the child protection authorities.
   D. Infants are not at risk for child abuse.

8. **Children who are both physically and emotionally abused exhibit:**
   A. More delinquency
   B. Greater resilience with their problems
   C. Fewer emotional problems
   D. Better grades and school attendance

9. **When a parent does not provide adequate medical or dental care, this is called:**
   A. Emotional abuse
   B. Emotional neglect
   C. Physical abuse
   D. Physical neglect

10. **You suspect that a child client is being abused. What should you do?**
    A. Report your concerns to your supervisor
    B. Tell your best friend
    C. Tell the child's parents
    D. Report your concerns to the Kids Help Phone

11. **Which of the following is an example of abuse of a client?**
    A. Inappropriate use of restraints
    B. Reviewing the care plan regularly
    C. Responding to a call bell before taking a coffee break
    D. Asking a client to try to wash his own face

12. **When confronted by an abusive client, you should:**
    A. Stand next to the person
    B. Stand about 1 m (3 ft) away from the person
    C. Sharply tell the person to stop
    D. Quickly leave the room or house if you think you are in danger

REVIEW

Answers to these questions are at the bottom of the page.

13. **Which is a sign of physical abuse?**
    A. Stiff and sore joints
    B. Old bruises and new bruises
    C. Fresh fruit in the fridge
    D. Confusion and dementia

14. **Intense fear of bathing or perineal care may be a sign of:**
    A. Physical abuse
    B. Emotional abuse
    C. Sexual abuse
    D. Neglect

15. **Which is a sign of emotional abuse?**
    A. Isolation from family and friends
    B. Bills that are not paid
    C. Taking the older adult to the doctor
    D. Pressure sores

16. **Mr. Deol states, "My daughter won't give me food until I give her my pension cheque." This is a sign of:**
    A. Financial abuse
    B. Emotional abuse
    C. Neglect
    D. Physical abuse

17. **You suspect an adult client is being abused. What should you do?**
    A. Call the police
    B. Tell the family
    C. Tell your supervisor
    D. Ask the person if he or she was abused

Answers: 1.D, 2.D, 3.C, 4.A, 5.C, 6.C, 7.C, 8.A, 9.D, 10.A, 11.A, 12.D, 13.B, 14.C, 15.A, 16.A, 17.C

CHAPTER 22

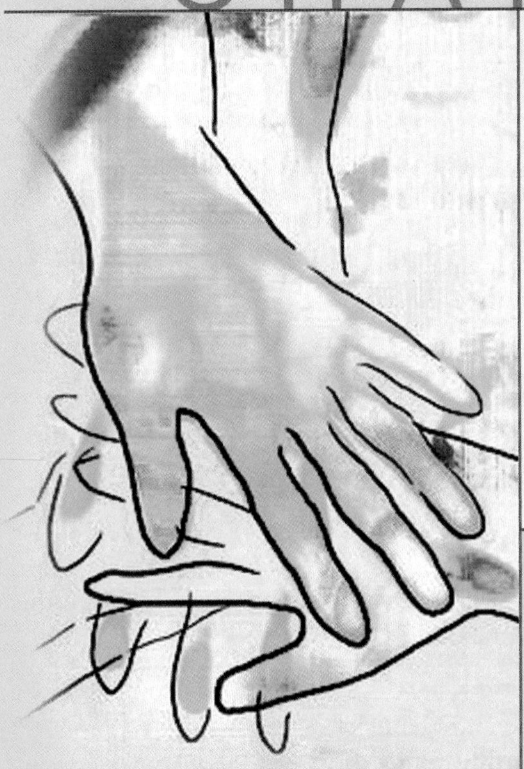

Promoting Client Well-Being

OBJECTIVES

- Define the key terms listed in this chapter.
- Describe how to promote well-being during the admission, transfer, and discharge procedures.
- Describe why comfort is important.
- Describe four types of pain.
- List the signs and symptoms of pain.
- List the care plan measures that relieve pain.
- Describe why rest and sleep are important.
- Describe the factors that affect sleep.
- Describe common sleep disorders.
- List care plan measures that promote sleep.
- Perform the procedures described in this chapter.

key terms

acute pain Sudden pain due to injury, disease, trauma, or surgery; it generally lasts less than 6 months.

admission Official entry of a client into a hospital or other health care facility.

chronic pain Pain that lasts longer than 6 months; it may be constant or occur off and on.

discharge Official departure of a client from a hospital or other health care facility.

insomnia A chronic condition in which the client cannot go to sleep or stay asleep throughout the night.

nocturia The need to urinate during the night.

phantom limb pain Pain felt in a body part that is no longer there.

radiating pain Pain that is felt not just at the site of tissue damage but extends to nearby areas.

transfer Moving a client from one room or unit to another or to another facility.

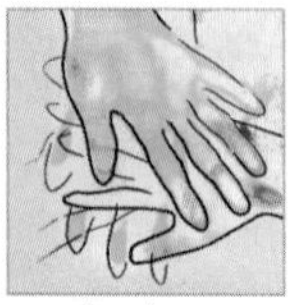

Clients should feel safe, comfortable, and relaxed in their environment, which may be any of the settings described in Chapter 3. These include private homes, assisted-living dwellings, apartments, units in long-term care facilities, and hospital rooms. Consider these examples:

- Mr. Kremer, 88, moves from his home to a long-term care facility, but he feels like a stranger there. Each time you approach him, you introduce yourself to him, explain your role, and what you will be doing. You make his room feel more like home by helping arrange his possessions he has brought with him. You introduce him to other staff and clients. He begins to feel more secure and comfortable.
- Jose Cruz, 17, is admitted to hospital following a car accident. He has some pain and is also anxious and fearful. A nurse gives him medication to control his pain. She explains what to expect during surgery and afterward. He feels better knowing what will happen next.
- Ms. Lalonde, 35, has a disorder that has caused paralysis. You help her to bathe and dress. You change her bed, do her laundry, and clean her house. She feels more relaxed and comfortable in fresh clothes and a clean environment.

Feeling safe, comfortable, and relaxed contributes to well-being. Support workers play a key role in promoting the well-being of their clients.

WELL-BEING DURING TRANSITIONS

Clients often need to move from one environment to another, for example:

- Into and out of facilities (admissions and discharges)
- From one room or unit in a facility to another (transfers)

Transitions are difficult for most people. Do you remember how you felt the last time you moved? You probably felt sad if you had to leave friends and family behind. You might have felt strange and disoriented in your new environment.

For clients who are elderly or unwell, moving from one environment to another can be very difficult. Many clients feel anxious, unsettled, and alone. Moving can even cause or increase signs of confusion in some clients. You can promote clients' emotional well-being during transitions when you help them with the admission, transfer, and discharge processes.

Admitting a Client to a Facility

Admission is the official entry of a client into a health care facility, and the process can cause uncertainty, anxiety, and fear. Clients often worry about medical tests, treatment, and surgery. They may fear pain and serious health problems. Clients moving to a long-term care facility often feel sad about leaving home. The facility is strange and unfamiliar—they do not know what to expect and where to go for meals or who to approach if they have questions. They worry about getting meals, finding the bathroom, and getting help.

The admission processes in long-term facilities and hospitals are similar but there are some differences as well.

Long-Term Care Facilities. The admission process in long-term care facilities usually starts several days before the new client enters the facility. Many facilities have admissions coordinators who make the process as simple and easy as possible for the client. If the client is able, he or she is taken on a tour of the facility before admission; the various services and recreational activities available are discussed and visiting policies and the client's rights explained. Details are handled before the client arrives, so the client is not bothered on arrival with forms and procedures.

The staff members are informed of the admission and room assignment. The room is prepared according to facility policy and the wishes of the new client and family. Most facilities provide a bed, a bedside stand, and a chair, although the client can use his or her own, if desired.

Clients are encouraged to make their rooms as homelike as possible. Long-term care legislation in some provinces as well as the Bill of Resident's Rights in some facilities state that clients have the right to choose their furnishings and display personal items in their rooms (see Chapter 11). Furniture is delivered in advance. Families are often involved in preparing the room—they arrange the items, hang pictures, and install curtains or blinds from the client's home. Some may even put up wallpaper.

As a support worker in the facility, when the new client arrives, you might help with the admission process. The process may become routine for you, but remember that it is *not* routine for the client. It is a major life event. Try to imagine how you would feel if you had to leave your home and enter a facility. Long-term care clients have often left behind their homes, family, friends, neighbours, and pets. Some facilities allow clients to bring their pets with them, and some have pets belonging to the facility. Clients now have to live in a strange place, and they may have to share a room with a stranger. Their health is probably declining, and they may have little hope for the future. Understandably, therefore, the new client feels anxious and out of place. Rarely, a couple may be admitted into the facility at the same time. If it is their wish, facilities will place them together in a room.

First impressions of the facility are important. A cold and uncaring reception would make the new client feel unwanted, whereas a warm welcome will help reassure and comfort the person (see the *Providing Compassionate Care: Welcoming a New Client to a Long-Term Care Facility* box.) The procedure described on page 380 can be used in both long-term care facilities and hospitals.

Hospitals. Except in emergencies, the hospital admission process starts in the admissions office. A member of the admitting staff gives the new client an ID number and a bracelet. The client signs a consent-for-treatment form and the nursing unit is notified that a client is being admitted. As a support worker, you may be asked to prepare the room for the client. A porter, a support worker, or an admitting office staff member brings the client to the nursing unit, sometimes by wheelchair or stretcher.

At the nursing unit, a nurse usually greets and admits the client. If the client is not in pain or distress, you may be asked to greet the client and assist with admission procedures. Introduce yourself by name and title. Call the client by his or her name in the proper manner. Remember that the client and family may be feeling anxious, so accompany them to the room. Be friendly and gentle, and do not rush them. Admission procedures involve:

- Weighing and measuring the client (see Chapter 41)
- Obtaining a urine specimen, if ordered (see Chapter 31)
- Orienting the client to the room, nursing unit, and hospital

Transfers

A **transfer** occurs when a client is moved from one room or nursing unit to another or to another facility. Transfers usually occur when a client's condition changes. Some clients are transferred for rehabilita-

PROVIDING COMPASSIONATE CARE

Welcoming a New Client to a Long-Term Care Facility

- **Dignity.** Treat the new client and his or her belongings with respect. Greet the client by name. Ask the client what name he or she would like the staff to use. Introduce yourself by name and title to the client and family (Figure 22–1). Do not rush into admission procedures. Treat the client and family as if they are guests in your home. Offer them refreshments, and tell them about the many good things about the facility. Listen to their concerns or questions, and do not overload them with information. Explain details about routines, recreation facilities, and other matters only if the new client seems eager to hear them. Reassure clients that they do not need to remember everything. Remind them that they can ask questions and talk to the staff at any time.
- **Independence.** A homelike setting is important to a client's independence and control. Help new clients feel at home. Show them their room, and explain how to use the various equipment in the room. Offer to help unpack and arrange their belongings (unless this has been done by the family). Make sure the client can reach the phone, TV, and light controls.
- **Preferences.** Some new clients want to arrange their own rooms, and they should always have the choice in arranging personal items. The health care team makes sure that the client's choices are safe, will not cause falls or other accidents, and do not interfere with the rights of others.
- **Privacy.** Show the new client how to draw the privacy curtains. Explain that the health care team respects all clients' right to privacy. Explain how you maintain privacy during personal care and other procedures.
- **Safety.** Explain how to use the call bell (see Chapter 19), and ensure that it is within easy reach. Show the client around the bathroom, and point out safety features, such as grab bars. Review safety and emergency procedures according to facility policy.

tion, and some request a room change when roommates do not get along. A client may or may not welcome a transfer, and the client's physician, nurse, or social worker usually explains the reason for the transfer. You may assist with the transfer or carry out the entire procedure. Clients are usually transported by wheelchair or stretcher or on their beds.

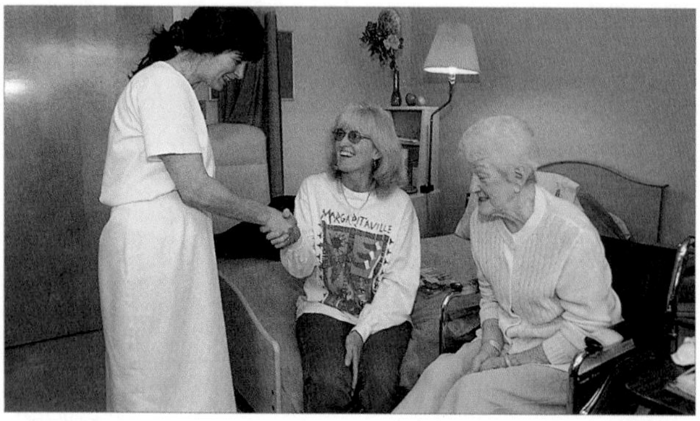

Figure 22–1 A support worker introduces herself to a new client and family member. **Source**: Sorrentino, S.A. (2000). *Mosby's textbook for nursing assistants* (5th ed., p. 552). St. Louis: Mosby.

Be sensitive and compassionate as you carry out this procedure, as clients need support and reassurance. The new client does not know the staff on the new unit, so introduce the client to the staff and the new roommate. Wish the client well as you leave.

Discharges

Discharge is the official departure of a client from a hospital or other health care facility. Some clients have recovered enough to go home, while some need home care. Others are discharged to another hospital, to a long-term care facility, or to a hospice. The physician, nurse, dietician, social worker, and other health care team members plan the client's discharge. They teach the client and family about diet, exercise, medications, treatments, and dressing changes if the client is going home. The case manager arranges for home care, rehabilitation, special therapy, and equipment, if required.

You may help clients pack their belongings and get ready to leave and then transport them out of the facility. In a hospital, the physician must write a discharge order before a client is allowed to leave. In a long-term care facility, permission must be obtained from the nurse. In some facilities, the chart contains instructions as to when the client may leave and with whom.

Always use good communication skills when assisting with a client's discharge. Wish the client and family well as they leave the facility.

Sometimes, a client may want to leave without permission. If a client tells you that he or she wants or intends to leave, notify the nurse immediately.

COMFORT

Comfort is a feeling of contentment. The client is not in any physical or emotional pain, and is calm and at peace. Age, illness, pain, and inactivity, as well as factors such as temperature, ventilation, odours, noise, and lighting affect comfort.

- ***Temperature.*** Most people are comfortable when the room temperature is between 20 and 23°C (68–74°F). Infants, older adults, and ill people generally need higher room temperatures for comfort. Government legislation dictates minimum comfortable temperatures in long-term care facilities. In home care settings, clients set the temperature they want. Some clients may be concerned with the cost of heating. You can help these clients keep warm by providing them with extra clothing or blankets.
- ***Ventilation.*** Stale room air affects comfort. Facilities have ventilation systems that ensure fresh air. In home care settings, you can open windows and doors and turn on fans, as the client desires. Protect clients from drafts by making sure they are dressed warmly, covered with blankets, and away from drafty areas.
- ***Odours.*** Many bodily substances and fluids have unpleasant odours that can embarrass clients. Body, breath, and smoking odours may also offend some. Clients can experience great discomfort from perfumes worn by a caregiver. Do not wear perfumes or any scented products when you are at work. If you smoke, wash your hands and brush your teeth after you have smoked. If you do not have time to brush your teeth, use mouthwash or suck on a breath mint. A clean fresh uniform must be used for every shift. Good hygiene, housekeeping practices, and ventilation help eliminate odours. To reduce odours:
  - Empty and clean bedpans, urinals, commodes, and kidney basins promptly
  - Change and dispose of soiled linens and clothing promptly
  - Clean clients who are wet or soiled by urine, feces, vomitus, or wound drainage
  - Dispose of incontinence and ostomy products promptly
  - Keep laundry containers closed
  - Assist clients to maintain good personal hygiene
- ***Noise.*** Ill clients are sensitive to noise. Health care facilities can be noisy places. The clanging of bedpans, the clatter of dishes, phones ringing, loud talking, and television sounds can disturb people. Answer phones promptly. Households, too, can be noisy, particularly when young children and teenagers live at home. Help control noise levels by talking quietly and handling equipment carefully. Some noises in facilities can be frightening, especially for new clients. Explain the source of the noise to help the client feel secure.
- ***Lighting.*** Glares, shadows, and dull lighting can cause falls, headaches, and eyestrain. Dim light often helps clients rest better. Bright light is helpful when giving care, and it also helps clients feel cheerful and stimulated. Before adjusting lights, ask clients about their preferences. Make sure light switches are within reach. Some clients may request a night light or that the TV is left on all night.

Room Furniture and Equipment

Clients' rooms are furnished and equipped for comfort and safety:

- ***Bathrooms.*** Most facility bathrooms have a sink, call bell, mirror, and toilet with handrails (Figure 22–2), and some have showers. Toilets in some facilities are higher than regular toilets, which makes moving to and from wheelchairs easier for clients, especially for clients with

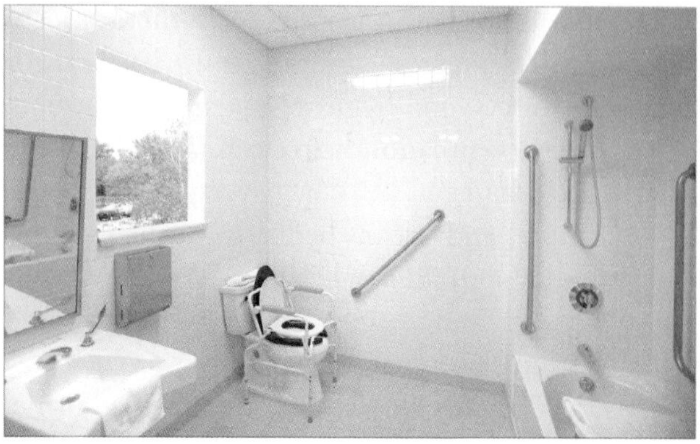

Figure 22–2 A facility bathroom. **Source**: Brian Hillier.

joint problems. Some bathrooms are private, while others are shared. Most bathrooms in private homes do not have elevated toilets and handrails. In such cases, you must make sure the client's bathroom is clean and safe.

- ***Beds.*** For those who are confined to bed, comfort is especially important. Hospital beds have electrical or manual controls that allow clients to sit up and lie down without effort. Many home care clients have regular beds. Use pillows to help clients sit comfortably in a regular bed (see Chapter 26).
- ***Overbed tables.*** Hospitals and many long-term care facilities have overbed tables. These tables can be positioned over the bed and the height adjusted for a client in bed or in a chair. The overbed table is used for placing meal trays, eating, reading, writing, and other activities. It is also used as a work area for bedside procedures. Never place bedpans, urinals, or soiled linens on an overbed table. Always clean the table carefully after each use.
- ***Bedside furniture.*** Most hospitals and long-term care facilities have bedside stands for personal items (Figure 22–3). In private homes, bedside furniture varies—it could be a bedside stand, a small table, or nothing at the bedside.
- ***Chairs.*** A hospital room usually has one or two chairs. Long-term care clients may bring their own chairs from home (Figure 22–4). Home care clients often have a favourite chair. Make sure that the chair is kept clean and free of food particles. Plump cushions regularly.
- ***Privacy curtains and screens.*** Privacy curtains are standard in hospitals and long-term care facilities (Figure 22–5). These are suspended from the ceiling and pulled around the bed before care. Privacy curtains prevent others from seeing the client, but they do not block sound or prevent conversations from being overheard. In home care settings, portable screens can be used for privacy (Figure 22–6).
- ***Closet and drawer space.*** Hospitals and long-term care facilities provide closet and drawer space for the client's clothing. Government legislation in some provinces states that long-term care clients must have easy access to the closet and its contents.
- ***Medical equipment.*** Most hospital rooms have blood pressure equipment mounted on the wall. An IV pole (IV standard) is used to hang an IV

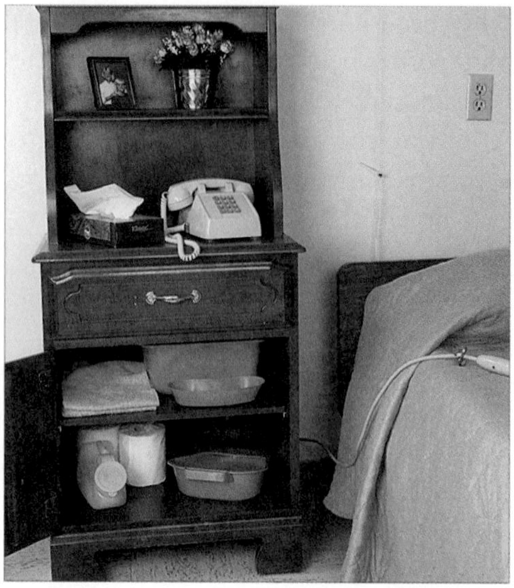

Figure 22–3 A bedside stand in a long-term care facility is used to store personal care items.

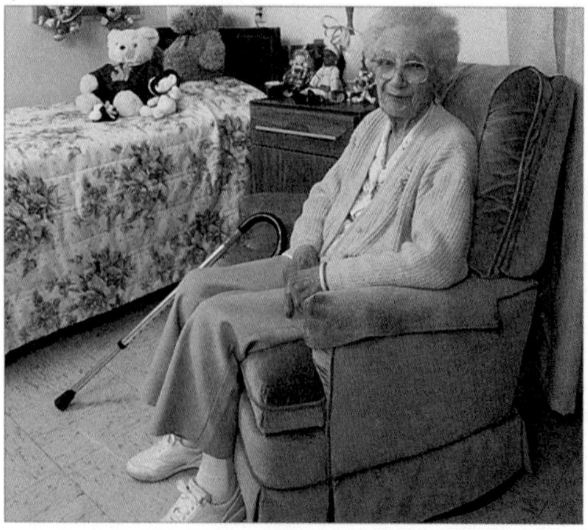

Figure 22–4 A client's chair from home.

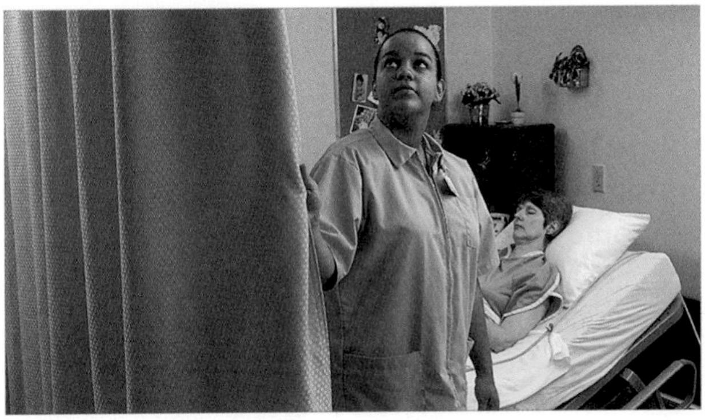

Figure 22–5 Curtains around the bed provide privacy in hospitals and long-term care facilities. **Source**: Sorrentino, S.A. (2000). *Mosby's textbook for nursing assistants* (5th ed., p. 28). St. Louis: Mosby.

infusion bag or a feeding bag. Some hospital beds have an IV pole stored in the bed frame. The IV pole may be a separate piece of equipment that is brought to the bedside when needed. Hospital rooms also have wall outlets for oxygen and suction (Figure 22–7). Oxygen tanks, oxygen concentrators and portable suction equipment are common in both long-term care and home care settings. Only medically necessary equipment is kept in the client's room.

Pain

To have discomfort or pain means to ache, hurt, or be sore. Discomfort and pain are subjective. You cannot see, hear, touch, or smell a client's discomfort or pain. You must rely on what the client and the client's body language tell you. Report complaints and observations to your supervisor.

Pain is personal and differs for each client. What may be *hurt* to one client may be *ache* to another.

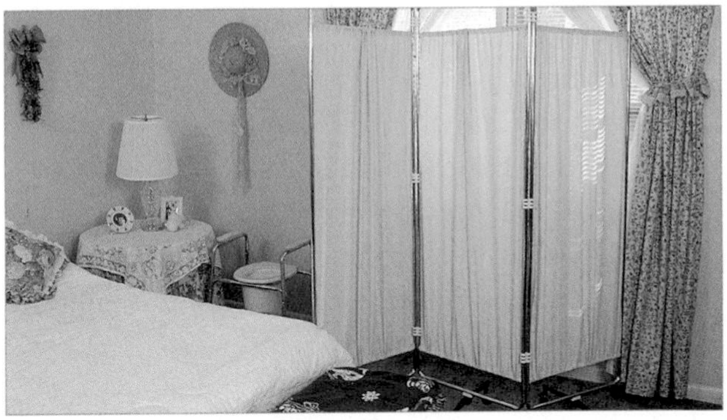

Figure 22–6 Portable screens provide privacy in the home.

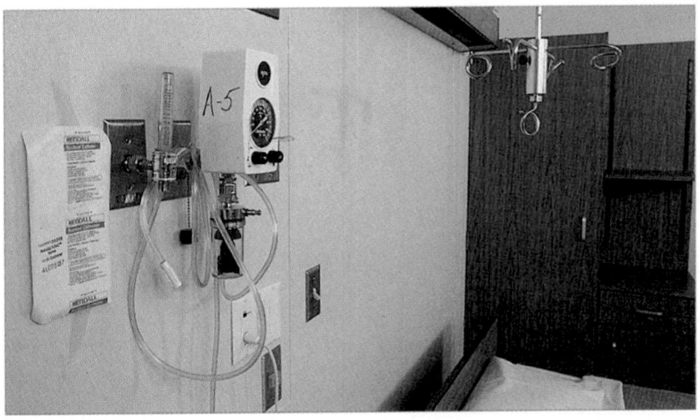

Figure 22–7 This hospital room has blood pressure equipment, an IV pole, and oxygen and suction outlets.

What one client calls *sore*, another may call *burning*. If a client complains of pain or discomfort, the client *has* pain or discomfort, and you must believe the client. Remember, you cannot see, hear, feel, or smell the pain. Pain may signal tissue damage.

Pain is not only physical. Clients also feel emotional, social, and spiritual pain. When a person is suffering, the whole self feels the pain. Clients in pain may be sad, impatient, irritable, or angry. As a support worker, you must be especially kind and empathetic.

Some clients have impairments that may affect their ability to recognize pain (e.g., Alzheimer's disease) or to report pain (e.g., aphasia).

Types of Pain. There are different types of pain.

- **Acute pain** is felt suddenly from injury, disease, trauma, or surgery, when tissue is damaged; it usually lasts less than 6 months and decreases with healing.
- **Chronic pain** lasts longer than 6 months. Pain is constant or occurs off and on. Arthritis and cancer are common causes of chronic pain.
- **Radiating pain** is felt not just at the site of tissue damage but extends to nearby areas as well. Pain from a heart attack is often felt on the left side of the chest, left jaw, left shoulder, and left arm. A diseased gallbladder can cause pain in the right upper abdomen, the back, and the right shoulder (Figure 22–8).
- **Phantom limb pain** is felt in a body part that is no longer there; this is due to the disruption of nerve endings in the stump. A client who has had a leg amputated may still feel leg pain.

Factors Affecting Pain. Pain does not always affect all clients the same way. Many factors affect reactions to pain.

- ***Past experience.*** A client may have had pain before. The severity of pain, its cause, how long it lasted, and whether relief occurred all affect the client's current response to pain. Knowing what to expect can help or hinder a client in handling pain. Clients who have never experienced pain may be fearful because they do not know what to expect.
- ***Anxiety.*** An anxious client feels troubled or threatened. Pain and anxiety are related—pain can cause anxiety, and anxiety can make the pain feel worse. Lessening anxiety therefore helps reduce pain. For example, the nurse explains to Mr. Schett that he will have pain after surgery and that he will receive medication for pain relief. When Mr. Schett feels pain after surgery, he knows what to expect—that medication will relieve it. This helps reduce his anxiety and therefore the amount of pain he feels.
- ***Rest and sleep.*** Rest and sleep restore energy and help the body to repair itself. Ill and injured clients need more sleep than usual. Lack of rest and sleep affects how a client copes with pain. Pain seems worse when a client is tired or restless.
- ***Attention.*** The more a client thinks about the pain, the worse it can seem. Sometimes pain is so severe that it is all a client thinks about. However, even mild pain can seem worse if a client dwells on it too much. Pain often seems worse at night when there are no distractions.
- ***The meaning of pain.*** Pain means different things to different people. Some see it as a sign of serious weakness or of a serious illness. Some clients ignore or deny their pain. Some clients may use their pain to avoid certain people or things, while some others use it to get attention.
- ***Support from others.*** Pain is easier to deal with when family and friends offer comfort and support. The presence of a friend or loved one can be very comforting. Clients who do not have caring family and friends must deal with their pain alone, and this can increase their fear, anxiety, and suffering. Be especially sensitive to clients who are suffering alone.
- ***Culture.*** Culture affects how a client responds to pain (see the *Respecting Diversity: Pain Reactions* box). In some cultures, clients in pain show no reaction at all, while in other cultures, clients in pain display strong verbal and nonverbal reactions.
- ***Age.*** See the *Focus on Children: Pain Reactions* and *Focus on Older Adults: Pain Reactions* boxes.

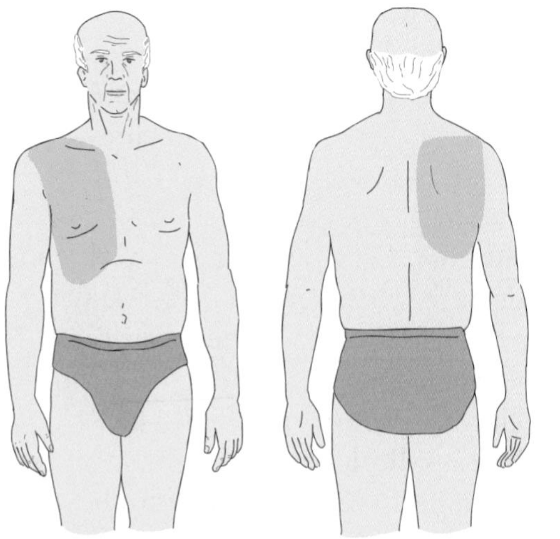

Figure 22–8 Gallbladder pain radiates to the right upper abdomen, the back, and the right shoulder.

Signs and Symptoms of Pain. Your client may tell you about his or her pain, or body language and behaviour may indicate the pain. For example, Ms. Raj grimaces when she moves but denies having any pain. Report any information and observations about the client's pain to your supervisor. Always use the client's exact words when you report and record. Report the following:

- ***Location.*** Where is the pain? Ask the client to point to the area of pain (Figure 22–9). Remember, pain can radiate. Ask the person if the pain is anywhere else and to point to those areas.
- ***Onset and duration.*** When did the pain start? How long has the pain lasted?
- ***Intensity.*** Does the client complain of mild, moderate, or severe pain? Examples of tools that can be used by clients to describe the intensity of pain are illustrated in Figures 22–10, 22–11, and 22–12.
- ***Description.*** Ask the client to describe the pain. Box 22–1 on page 387 lists some words

RESPECTING DIVERSITY

Pain Reactions

In the Philippines, pain is viewed as the will of God, and it is believed that God will give the person the strength to bear the pain. In Vietnam, pain relief may not be requested until the pain becomes severe. The people of India accept pain quietly but will accept some relief measures. In China, showing emotion is seen as weakness of character, so pain is often not reported, and pain relief measures must be offered more than once before they are accepted. The Chinese consider it impolite to accept something the first time it is offered.

Remember, individuals may not follow every belief and practice of their culture and religion. Each client is unique. Also, do not judge the client by your own standards.

Adapted from: Geissler, E.M. (1998). *Pocket guide to cultural assessment* (2nd ed.). St. Louis: Mosby.

used to describe pain. Write down what the client says, and use the client's exact words.

- ***Factors causing pain.*** Factors causing pain may include moving or turning in bed, coughing or deep breathing, and exercise. Ask what the client was doing before the pain started and when it started.
- ***Vital signs.*** What are the client's pulse, respirations, and blood pressure? With the occurrence of pain, often there are increases in the readings of these vital signs.
- ***Other signs and symptoms.*** Does the client have other symptoms: dizziness, nausea, vomiting, weakness, numbness, tingling, or others? Box 22–2 lists the signs and symptoms that often occur with pain.

Measures to Relieve Pain. Nurses and case managers use the care planning process to promote comfort and relieve pain. Box 22–3 lists measures that are often part of the care plan. Medications ordered by the physician provide pain relief, but medications can cause drowsiness, dizziness, and coordination problems. Clients on pain relief medications must be protected from injury. Follow the care plan for safety practices.

focus on ››CHILDREN

Pain Reactions

Many children do not understand pain, as they have had few experiences with pain. They do not know what to expect or how to deal with pain and therefore must rely on adults for help.

Caregivers, however, do not always know when children are in pain, since toddlers and preschool children may not know words that express pain. Crying and fussing infants and toddlers can mean many different problems, not just pain. Caregivers must therefore be alert for behaviours and situations that signal pain. One tool that can be used to assess pain in children is the Wong-Baker Pain Rating Scale (see Figure 22–12 on page 386), which uses six different faces ranging from a smiling, happy face to a very sad face and the children point to the face that indicates how much pain they are having.

focus on ››OLDER ADULTS

Pain Reactions

Some older adults have multiple health problems that cause pain, and they may think that a new pain is related to an existing health problem; also, chronic pain may mask the new pain, or older adults may deny or ignore pain because of what it might mean.

Older adults may also have conditions (e.g., dementia) that affect their pain perception, or they may be unable to reliably recognize and report that they are in pain. This places them at greater risk for undetected disease or injury. Pain alerts a client to illness or injury, so if pain is not felt, the client may not realize he or she has a problem and seek health care.

Some older adults have disorders that affect their thinking and reasoning, and some cannot communicate verbally. The only indication of pain in such cases will be changes in behaviour, so report any changes in a client's behaviour to your supervisor.

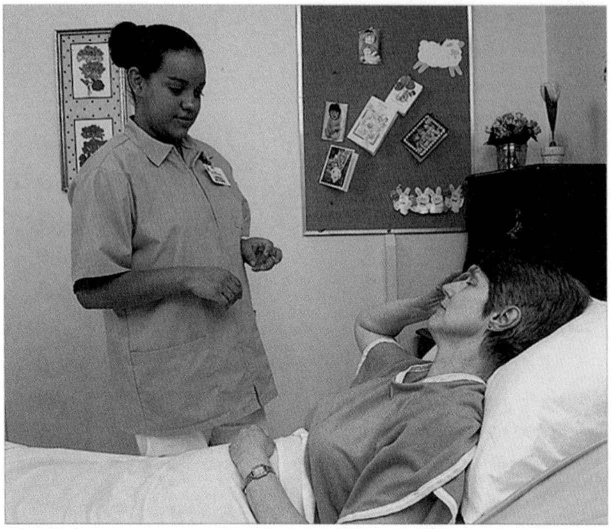

Figure 22–9 A client points to the area of pain.

Measures other than medications that control pain include distraction, relaxation, and guided imagery. Nurses and therapists teach clients these measures, and you may be trained to assist with some of them.

- ***Distraction*** involves a change in a client's focus of attention. Attention is directed away from the pain through distractions such as conversation, music, television, games, and needlepoint.
- ***Relaxation*** means absence of mental or physical stress. A relaxed state reduces pain and anxiety. The nurse or therapist teaches the client to breathe deeply and slowly and to contract and relax muscle groups. A comfortable position and a quiet room are important to achieve relaxation.

Present Pain Intensity/Verbal Descriptor Scale (PPI)
The PPI is a pain assessment tool that may be used with clients who find a numeric rating scale difficult to use. The PPI is a 6 point, fixed interval scale that measures pain intensity. Clients should be asked to listen to the anchor words and indicate which word best describes their pain, at rest ("R") and with activity ("A"). Document the score corresponding to the descriptor.

Present Pain Intensity/Verbal Descriptor Scale

Anchor Word	Documentation
No Pain	0
Mild	2
Discomforting	4
Distressing	6
Horrible	8
Excruciating	10

Figure 22–10 Present Pain Intensity/Verbal Descriptor Scale. **Source:** Melzack, R., & Torgerson, W.S. (1971). On the language of pain. *Anesthesiology*, 34(1), 50–61.

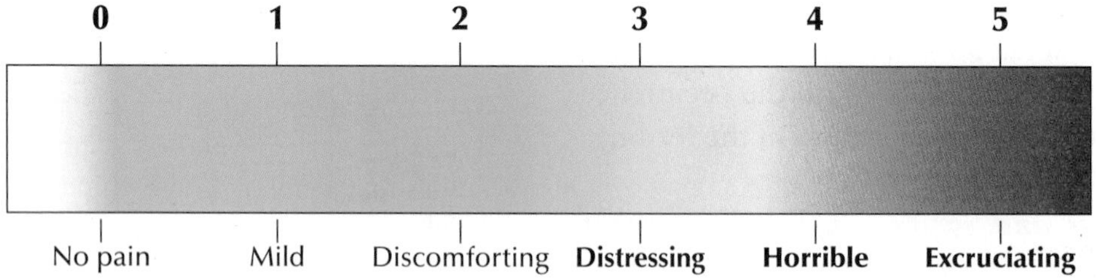

Figure 22–11 Colour Visual Analogue Scale.

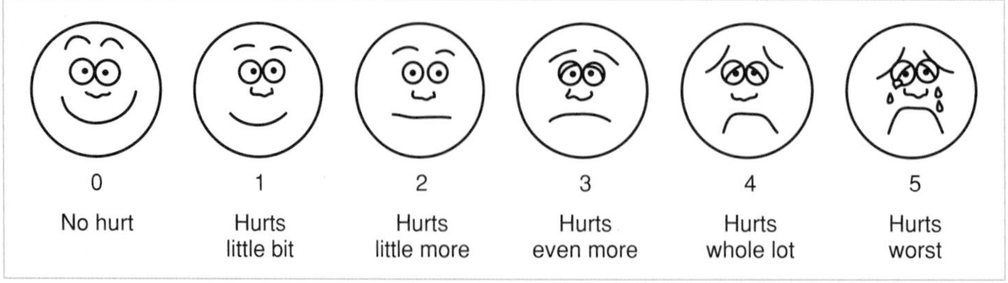

Figure 22–12 Wong-Baker FACES Pain Rating Scale. **Source:** Wong, D.L., Hockenberry-Eaton, M., Wilson, D., Winkelstein, M. L., & Schwartz, P. (2001). *Wong's essentials of pediatric nursing* (6th ed., p. 1301). St Louis: Mosby. Reprinted by permission.

Box 22–1 Words Used to Describe Pain

- Aching
- Burning
- Cramping
- Crushing
- Dull
- Gnawing
- Knifelike
- Piercing
- Pressing
- Sharp
- Sore
- Squeezing
- Stabbing
- Throbbing
- Viselike

- ***Guided imagery*** involves creating an image in the mind and focusing on it. The client is asked to think of a pleasant scene, for example, a warm, sunny beach. The nurse uses a calm, soft voice when helping the client focus on the mental picture of the scene and also coaches the client to do relaxation exercises. Soft music, a blanket for warmth, and a darkened room may help.

Box 22–2 Signs and Symptoms of Pain

Body Responses

- Increased pulse, respirations, and blood pressure
- Nausea
- Pale skin (pallor)
- Sweating (diaphoresis)
- Vomiting

Behaviours

- Changes in speech; slow or rapid, loud or quiet
- Crying
- Gasping
- Grimacing
- Groaning
- Grunting
- Holding the affected body part (splinting)
- Being irritable
- Maintaining one position; refusing to move
- Moaning
- Being quiet
- Being restless
- Rubbing
- Screaming
- Rocking back and forth

Box 22–3 Measures to Promote Comfort and Relieve Pain

Wait 30 minutes after administration of pain medication before giving care.

- Position the client in good body alignment. Use pillows for support.
- Keep bed linens tight and wrinkle-free.
- Make sure the client is not lying on drainage tubes.
- Assist with elimination needs.
- Provide blankets for warmth and to prevent chilling.
- Use correct lifting, moving, and turning procedures.
- Provide extra support for painful areas during movement. Use your hands or a pillow, if appropriate.
- Give a back massage.
- Provide soft music to distract the client.
- Use touch to provide comfort.
- Allow family and friends to visit, if requested by the client.
- Avoid sudden or jarring movements.
- Handle the client gently.
- Practise safety measures if the client is receiving strong pain medication or sedatives:
  - If the client is in a hospital bed, keep the bed in the lowest position.
  - Follow the care plan for bed rail use.
  - Check on the client every 10 to 15 minutes.
  - Provide assistance when the client is up.
  - Provide heat or cold applications, as directed.
  - Provide a calm, quiet, darkened environment.

REST AND SLEEP

To be rested means to be calm, at ease, relaxed, and free from anxiety and stress. Rest involves physical inactivity, but some people choose to do calming or relaxing activities while resting, for example, reading, listening to music, and watching television.

A comfortable position and good body alignment are important for rest, and a quiet setting and a clean, dry, and wrinkle-free bed promote rest as well. Many clients spend a great deal of time in bed, so it is important for a support worker to know the different types of beds and how to position them for the client's comfort (see Chapter 26). Some clients rest easier in a clean, neat, and uncluttered room. Clients sleep in very different ways. Some clients may not have slept in a bed for most of their lives, perhaps for cultural reasons—for example, Aboriginal clients may not want to sleep on mattresses. Some clients may want to sleep sitting in a chair for ease of breathing; for example, a client with COPD would find it easier to breathe in the sitting position. The client's personal preference is very important when promoting rest and sleep; for example, every client will have his or her own preference for the number of blankets they want on the bed.

Basic needs must be met for clients to rest. Thirst, hunger, elimination needs, pain, discomfort, anxiety, and fear, as well as unmet needs for love and belonging, can affect rest. You can promote rest by meeting clients' needs. For clients in a facility or living alone, visits or telephone calls from family and friends may promote relaxation. (See the *Providing Compassionate Care: Helping Clients to Rest* box.)

You must plan and organize care so that clients can rest without interruptions. Some clients feel refreshed after resting for 15 or 20 minutes, while others need more time. Health care routines usually allow time for an afternoon rest.

Ill or injured clients need to rest often. Some need to rest during or after care. For example, a bath tires Mr. Rajan, so to gather the energy to dress, he must rest in a chair. Some clients need up to a few hours to complete oral hygiene, bathing, grooming, and dressing. Others need to rest after meals. Do not rush clients. Allow rest periods, as needed.

The physician may order bed rest for a client (see Chapter 24 for a discussion on bed rest, its complications, and advice on preventing complications).

Sleep is a basic physical need. It saves the body energy, lets the mind and body rest, and allows body functions to slow. During sleep, vital signs fall, and tissue heals and repairs itself. Sleep lowers stress, tension, and anxiety. After sleep, a person usually feels refreshed, more energetic, and mentally alert. During sleep, the normal adult passes through four to six cycles of *NREM* and *REM* phases—four levels of nonrapid eye movement (NREM) and one level of rapid eye movement (REM) in each cycle (Table 22–1). Children and infants have more deep sleep, while the elderly have more light sleep.

The amount of sleep required varies for each age group and declines with age (Table 22–2). Clients may require more sleep when they are sick or recovering from illness or injury (see the *Focus on Older Adults: Sleep* box on page 390).

Several factors affect the amount and quality of sleep. Quality relates to how well a person sleeps. Does the person sleep soundly and feel refreshed in

PROVIDING COMPASSIONATE CARE

Helping Clients to Rest

- **Dignity.** Protecting a client's dignity can promote rest. Some clients may find hospital gowns embarrassing and may rest better wearing their own gowns or pyjamas. Many clients feel better about themselves when they are clean and well-groomed. Help clients with their personal hygiene and grooming before rest.
- **Independence.** Many clients follow rituals or routines before resting—for example, going to the bathroom, brushing teeth, having a snack or beverage, praying, locking doors, and making sure loved ones are safe at home. Some clients have a favourite blanket. Ask clients about their preferences, and help them follow their rituals and routines, when possible.
- **Preferences.** Allow clients to do as much as possible without assistance. The client decides when and where he or she wants to rest. Provide a restful environment according to the client's wishes.
- **Privacy.** Lack of privacy can make rest impossible, so close doors and privacy curtains, if the client so desires.
- **Safety.** The client's safety needs must be met (see Chapter 19) to achieve a good rest. Clients trying to rest must feel that they are safe from falls or other injuries. In facilities, the call bell must be within reach. Understanding the reasons for their treatments and knowing how procedures are done can also help clients feel safe, so make sure you explain procedures before they are performed.

the morning? Or is the person restless and wakeful during sleep?

- ***Illness.*** Discomfort, pain, nausea, and coughing can affect sleep. Also, clients may be awakened frequently for treatment or medication.
- ***Nutrition.*** Certain foods and drinks can affect sleep, for example, those containing caffeine, such as coffee, chocolate, tea, and colas. A protein found in milk, cheese, and beef can promote sleep.
- ***Exercise.*** Exercise makes people tired and helps them sleep. However, it is also a stimulant. Exercising before bed may disrupt sleep. Allow at least 2 hours between exercise and bedtime.
- ***Environment.*** Most people sleep better in their own beds and in familiar surroundings. Any change in the environment, as well as noise and light, can affect sleep. Promote a quiet environment with the right amount of light preferred by the client.
- ***Medications.*** Sleeping pills promote sleep. Medications for anxiety, depression, and pain can cause drowsiness and can also interfere with sleep. The person may not feel mentally alert or refreshed the next day.
- ***Alcohol.*** Alcohol disrupts normal sleep patterns. The person may wake up and have difficulty falling asleep again.
- ***Change and stress.*** Change disrupts sleep. This can range from small changes in routine, such as staying up late to watch a game on television, to stressful life events, such as a new job or a divorce.
- ***Emotional problems.*** Fear, worry, anxiety, and depression affect sleep. People in emotional distress may have difficulty falling asleep, or they may wake up often and have problems falling asleep again.

Table 22–1 Stages of the Sleep Cycle

Stage 1: NREM	**Stage 4: NREM**
Includes lightest level of sleep Stage lasts a few minutes Decreased physiological activity begins with gradual fall in vital signs and metabolism Person is easily aroused by sensory stimuli such as noise Awakened, person feels as though daydreaming has occurred	Deepest stage of sleep Very difficult to arouse sleeper If sleep loss has occurred, sleeper will spend considerable portion of night in this stage Vital signs are significantly lower than during waking hours Stage lasts approximately 15 to 30 minutes Sleepwalking and enuresis may occur
Stage 2: NREM	**REM Sleep**
Period of sound sleep Relaxation progresses Arousal remains relatively easy Stage lasts 10 to 20 minutes Body functions continue to slow down	Vivid, full-colour dreaming may occur Less vivid dreaming may occur in other stages Stage usually begins about 90 minutes after sleep has begun Typified by autonomic response of rapidly moving eyes, fluctuating heart and respiratory rates, and increased or fluctuating blood pressure Loss of skeletal muscle tone occurs Gastric secretions increase Very difficult to arouse sleeper Duration of REM sleep increases with each cycle and averages 20 minutes
Stage 3: NREM	
Involves initial stages of deep sleep Sleeper is difficult to arouse and rarely moves Muscles are completely relaxed Vital signs decline but remain regular Stage lasts 15 to 30 minutes	

Source: Potter, P.A., Perry, A., Ross-Kerr, J.C., & Wood, M.J. (2001). *Canadian fundamentals of nursing* (3rd ed., p. 1212), Box 37–1. Toronto: Harcourt Canada.

- ***Nocturia.*** The need to urinate during the night disrupts sleep. With advancing age, there is reduced bladder tone, which increases the need to void frequently.

Sleep Disorders

Sleep disorders are chronic problems that affect the amount and quality of sleep and can cause fatigue, irritability, poor judgement, and other problems. Signs and symptoms of sleep disorders are listed in Box 22–4. Routines in many facilities do not accommodate residents' individual sleep and awake cycles. Frequent sleep interruptions during the night or being awakened early in the morning can cause sleep deprivation. Some facilities have adopted the GentleCare philosophy, part of which is allowing clients to awaken themselves in the morning. Better incontinence products and mattresses in some facilities make it possible for clients to sleep better.

Insomnia. **Insomnia** is a chronic condition in which the person cannot go to sleep or stay asleep throughout the night. The person is unable to fall asleep or stay asleep, or he or she wakes early and is unable to fall asleep again. Ill or injured clients often suffer from insomnia because they may be depressed or anxious, pain and discomfort may keep them awake, or they may be afraid of dying during sleep.

Sleep Deprivation. In sleep-deprived people, the amount and quality of sleep declines. Illness and hospital care are common causes of sleep deprivation in clients. The light and sound during night-time care can interfere with sleep. Health care providers also often suffer from sleep deprivation because of rotating shifts. There can be both physiological symptoms and psychological symptoms (see Box 22–5).

Sleepwalking. Sleepwalkers walk about while they are sleeping, often for several minutes. The person is not aware that he or she is sleepwalking and has no memory of doing so on awakening. Children sleepwalk more than adults do. Stress, fatigue, and some medications can cause sleepwalking. The risk of falling during sleepwalking is great. Ill clients may trip or pull out tubes and catheters. Guide sleepwalking clients back to their beds. Awaken them gently, as they can startle easily.

Your Role in Promoting Rest and Sleep

If required, measures to promote sleep are included in the client's care plan (see Box 22–6). Check the

Table 22–2 Average Sleep Requirements

Age Group	Hours per Day
Newborns (birth to 4 weeks)	14–18
Infants (4 weeks to 1 year)	12–14
Toddlers/preschoolers (1 to 6 years)	11–12
Middle/late childhood (6 to 12 years)	10–11
Adolescents (12 to 18 years)	8–9
Young adults (18 to 40 years)	7–8
Middle-aged adults (40 to 65 years)	7
Late adulthood (65 years and older)	5–7

Source: Potter, P.A., Perry, A.G., Ross-Kerr, J.C., & Wood, M.J. (2006). *Canadian fundamentals of nursing* (3rd ed., p. 1216–1217). Toronto: Elsevier Canada.

focus on ››OLDER ADULTS

Sleep

Older adults have less energy than do younger people. They may nap at certain times or on and off during the day. Organize care so that naps are not disturbed. Avoid waking an older client from a nap.

Long-term care clients are allowed to choose when they nap and sleep. They also have the right to choose what measures help promote comfort, rest, and sleep. Follow the care plan and the client's wishes.

Clients are sometimes prepared for bed as early as 6:00 p.m. They may not be ready to sleep at this time but may want to watch television, listen to the radio, or read.

Source: Potter, P.A., Perry, A.G., Ross-Kerr, J.C., & Wood, M.J. (2006). *Canadian fundamentals of nursing* (3rd ed., p. 1216). Toronto: Elsevier Canada.

Box 22–4 Signs and Symptoms of Sleep Disorders

- Hand tremors
- Slowed response to questions, conversations, or situations
- Difficulty finding the right word
- Decreased attention
- Decreased reasoning and judgement
- Irregular pulse
- Red, puffy eyes with dark circles
- Moodiness; mood swings
- Disorientation
- Fatigue and/or sleepiness
- Restlessness and/or agitation
- Irritability
- Hallucinations (see Chapter 34)
- Coordination problems
- Slurred speech

Source: Potter, P.A., Perry, A.G., Ross-Kerr, J.C., & Wood, M.J. (2006). *Canadian fundamentals of nursing* (3rd ed., p. 1212). Toronto: Elsevier Canada.

care plan to make sure you are giving correct care. Observe the client closely, and report any of the signs and symptoms listed in Box 22–5.

Box 22–5 Sleep Deprivation Symptoms

Physiological Symptoms

- Ptosis, blurred vision
- Fine motor clumsiness
- Decreased reflexes
- Slowed response time
- Decreased reasoning and judgement
- Decreased auditory and visual alertness
- Cardiac arrhythmias

Psychological Symptoms

- Confusion and disorientation
- Increased sensitivity to pain
- Being irritable, withdrawn, apathetic
- Excessive sleepiness
- Agitation
- Hyperactivity
- Decreased motivation

Source: Potter, P.A., Perry, A., Ross-Kerr, J.C., & Wood, M.J. (2001). *Canadian fundamentals of nursing* (3rd ed., p. 1216). Toronto: Harcourt Canada.

As mentioned earlier, many clients have rituals and routines before bedtime—such as having a bedtime snack, watching a television program, or reading a book. Some long-term care clients may like to check on friends and loved ones before going to bed. Whatever the routine, it is important to the client, and you must help him or her with it, as much as possible.

Sleep disturbances are common in some types of dementia. In clients with dementia, confusion and restlessness often increase at night, and night wandering is common. Night wandering in a safe and supervised setting can be helpful for some clients (see Chapter 35). The measures listed in Box 22–6 may help.

Box 22–6 Measures to Promote Sleep

- Organize care to allow for uninterrupted rest.
- Encourage the client to avoid physical activity before bedtime.
- Discourage the client from tending to business or family matters before bedtime.
- Allow flexible bedtimes. Bedtime is whenever the client is ready to sleep.
- Ensure a comfortable room temperature.
- Help the client take a warm bath or shower.
- Provide a bedtime snack, if needed.
- Have the client avoid caffeine and alcohol.
- Have the client void before going to bed. Make sure incontinent clients are clean and dry.
- Follow the client's bedtime rituals.
- Make sure the client wears loose-fitting nightwear.
- Provide for warmth (blankets, socks).
- Make sure linens are clean, dry, and wrinkle-free.
- Allow the client to read, listen to music, or watch television, if they so desire.
- Stay and talk with the client.
- Reduce noise.
- Darken the room: close shades, blinds, and curtains. Shut off or dim lights in the room and hallway.
- Position the client in good body alignment. Support body parts, as ordered.
- Implement measures to relieve pain.
- Give a back massage, if ordered.
- Assist with relaxation exercises, as ordered.

REVIEW

Answers to these questions are at the bottom of the page.

Circle T if the answer is true or circle F if the answer is false.

1. T F **A client is greeted by name when being admitted to a nursing unit in a hospital or long-term care facility.**
2. T F **Transfers are usually related to changes in a client's condition.**
3. T F **A physician must write the discharge order before a patient can leave a hospital.**
4. T F **Pain affects all people in the same way.**
5. T F **Moderate exercise, such as walking, is considered rest.**

Circle the BEST answer.

6. **Most long-term care facilities:**
   - A. Discourage clients from bringing personal items from home
   - B. Have strict rules about the appearance of residents' rooms
   - C. Encourage residents to make their rooms homelike
   - D. Allow residents to bring only one piece of furniture from home
7. **A client complains of pain on the left side of the chest, up into the left jaw, and down to the left shoulder and left arm. This is:**
   - A. Acute pain
   - B. Chronic pain
   - C. Radiating pain
   - D. Phantom pain
8. **The nurse gives Mr. Smith a medication for pain. A procedure is scheduled for this time. You should:**
   - A. Perform the procedure before the medication is given
   - B. Perform the procedure right after the medication is given
   - C. Wait 30 minutes to let the medication take effect
   - D. Omit the procedure for the day
9. **You must protect Mr. Smith from injury after he is given medication. You should do the following:**
   - A. Keep the bed in the lowest position
   - B. Follow the care plan for bed rail use
   - C. Check on him every 30 to 45 minutes
   - D. Let him get out of bed on his own
10. **Which measure is an example of a distraction?**
    - A. Avoiding talking with the client
    - B. Keeping the room dark
    - C. Turning off the radio
    - D. Giving a back massage
11. **Mr. Smith tires very easily. His morning care includes a bath, hair care, and getting dressed. His bed is made after he is dressed. When should he rest?**
    - A. After morning care is completed
    - B. After his bath and before hair care
    - C. After you make the bed
    - D. Whenever he needs to

Answers: 1.T, 2.T, 3.T, 4.F, 5.F, 6.C, 7.C, 8.C, 9.A, 10.D, 11.D

CHAPTER 23

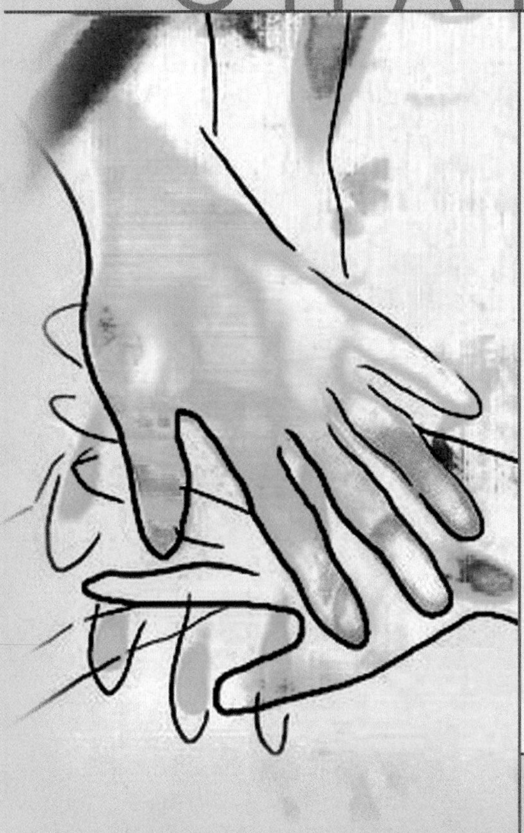

Body Mechanics: Moving, Positioning, Transferring, and Lifting the Client

OBJECTIVES

- Define the key terms listed in this chapter.
- List the purpose and rules of using good body mechanics.
- Describe how good body alignment and position changes are important for the client.
- Identify the comfort and safety measures for positioning clients in bed.
- Describe how to position a client in the basic bed positions and in a chair.
- Describe comfort and safety measures for moving, turning, and lifting clients in bed.
- Differentiate between a transfer and a lift.
- Identify safety measures used when transferring clients.
- Identify the purpose of a transfer belt and a transfer board.
- Demonstrate how to move a client in bed.
- Apply the information provided in this chapter in your practice by performing the procedures described.

key terms

base of support The area on which an object rests. If the base of support is adequate, this will prevent the object from tipping.

body alignment The way in which body parts (head, trunk, arms, and legs) are positioned in relation to one another, whether lying, sitting, or standing. Also known as **posture**.

body mechanics The movement of the body. Proper body mechanics ensures the body moves in an efficient and careful way.

centre of gravity The horizontal midpoint of a person's body. Also known as **line of gravity**.

fanfold A method of folding sheets, in which the sheet is folded back and forth, in a form that resembles a fan.

friction The rubbing of one surface against another.

high-Fowler's position A semi-sitting position in bed; the head of the bed is elevated 45 to 60 degrees or the person is propped up with a backrest or pillows.

lateral position A side-lying position that uses pillows to support the back and separate the lower legs.

lift Moving a person from one place to another, without his or her weight-bearing or assistance.

lift sheets See **turning sheets**.

line of gravity The line dividing the body where the collection of the person's mass and all the weight of the object can be considered to be concentrated. Also known as **centre of gravity**.

log-rolling Turning the person as a unit, in alignment, with one motion. The client's knee may be bent if necessary, but his or her neck and spine should be turned in one step and never twisted.

low-Fowler's position A semi-sitting position in bed; the head of the bed is elevated 15 to 30 degrees, or the person is propped up with a backrest or pillows.

lunge (or stride) stance A position whereby you place one foot in front of the other foot, keeping both feet about a shoulder width apart. This stance will enable you to keep your balance while performing the various tasks necessary in this chapter.

manual lift Physically moving a client who cannot weight-bear without the assistance of a mechanical lift.

mechanical lift A device that can elevate and move the person while in a special body sling. This device reduces the risk for injury to the support worker.

"no-lift" policy Agency regulations that prohibit you from manually lifting clients over a certain weight. You need to use a mechanical lifting device instead. In some agencies, "no-lift" policies extend to include situations where the client is agitated or uncooperative.

pelvic tilt A standing position whereby your pelvis is tilted by tightening the stomach muscles and flattening out the small of the back. It is used prior to lifting an object or transferring a resident in order to reduce the risk of back injury.

posture Body alignment.

prone position A front-lying position on the abdomen, with the head turned to one side.

shearing The process in which skin sticks to a surface and the muscles under the skin slide in the direction the body is moving. Shearing can result in skin tearing.

Sims' position A left side-lying position; the right leg is sharply flexed so that it is not on the left leg, and the left arm is positioned along the client's back.

slider board A friction-reduced board with handles, which is placed under a person, is grasped by the handles, and then slid (with the client on the board) from one bed to another.

stroke A stroke is the sudden death of some of the brain cells due to a lack of oxygen. A stroke occurs when blood flow to the brain is affected, by blockage or rupture of an artery to the brain, resulting in abnormal function of brain. Also known as **cerebral vascular accident (CVA)**.

supine position A back-lying position.

transfer To move a person from one place to another, using the client's assistance with partial to full weight-bearing.

transfer belt A strong strap that is secured around the client's/resident's waist, to help and support the client to stand, sit, and walk. It is removed after the activity is completed.

key terms

transfer board A smooth board placed between two surfaces (for example, a chair and a wheelchair) that allows the client to slide over more easily. Transfer boards are usually used when the client cannot weight-bear but can assist by using her or his upper body.

turning sheets Turning sheets are used to safely move a client up in bed, and they give support workers a more secure grasp. These sheets can be made of a variety of waterproofed material, or even folded sheets. Turning sheets prevent pain, skin damage, and bone and joint damage by protecting the client's skin from friction and **shearing** when the client is moved in bed. Also known as **slider sheets**, **lift sheets**.

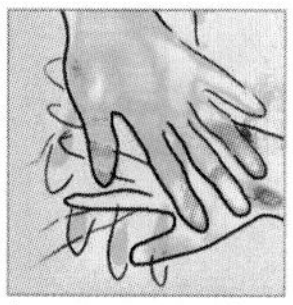

As a support worker, you will find that your daily activities often include lifting, moving, and carrying items—for example, lifting grocery bags, pushing wheelchairs, moving the client's bed, or carrying garbage and laundry bags. You also move, turn, reposition, and lift clients when you help them move in their beds or into chairs or wheelchairs and back again.

You must protect yourself and the client during the moving, positioning, and transferring activities. Back injuries and muscle and joint strains are serious and common injuries among health care workers and support workers. Use your body correctly. Knowing the proper techniques will help protect you and your client from injury.

BODY MECHANICS

Body mechanics refers to the movement of the body in an efficient and careful way and involves good posture and balance, as well as using the strongest and largest muscles for work. (Review the structure and function of the musculo-skeletal system in Chapter 14.) Good body mechanics reduce the risk of injury. Fatigue, muscle strain, and injury can result from the improper use and positioning of the body during activity or rest, so you must focus on both your client's and your own body mechanics during all activities.

Body alignment (or posture) is the way the body parts (head, trunk, arms, and legs) are positioned in relation to one another. Good body alignment enables the body to move and function with strength and efficiency, reduces strain on the muscles and joints, and prevents injury. For people with limited mobility, correct body alignment helps prevent disabling complications such as muscle atrophy and contractures (see Chapter 24).

Figure 23–1 shows a person standing with good body alignment. Note that both sides of the body are in line with each other—this is called the **line of gravity**. Body balance is achieved when a relatively low **centre of gravity** (the horizontal midpoint of a person's body) is balanced over a wide, stable base of support and a vertical line falls from the centre of

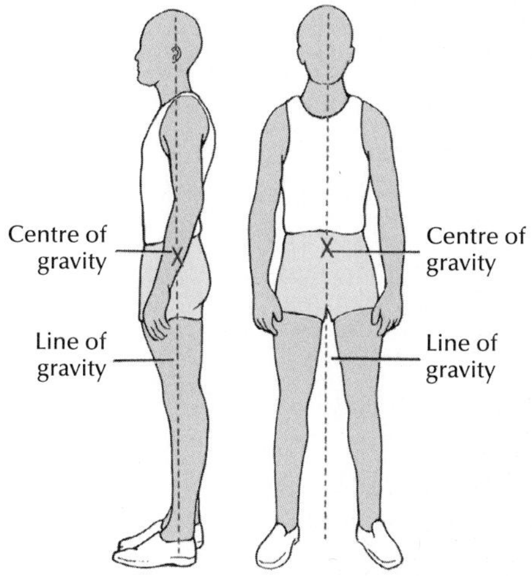

Figure 23–1 Proper body alignment when standing. Note how feet are placed apart for a wide base of support. Note where the lines and centres of gravity are. **Source:** Potter, P.A., Perry, A., Ross-Kerr, J.C., & Wood, M.J. (2001). *Canadian fundamentals of nursing* (3rd ed., p. 950). Toronto: Harcourt Canada.

gravity and through the base of support. The midpoint of the person's body, from both front and back, is known as the person's centre of gravity.

When a person is standing with good posture:

- Head and neck are erect and straight
- Shoulders and hips are parallel to each other
- Shoulders are back
- Chest is out
- Spine maintains natural lumbar curve
- Abdomen is tucked in and the pelvis tilted in (also known as a "**pelvic tilt**"). This helps improve the posture, strengthen the lower spine, and reduce the risk of back injury.
- Knees are slightly flexed
- Arms are hanging comfortably at the sides
- Feet are about shoulder-width apart.
- Toes are pointing forward; one foot is slightly forward

Lying down and sitting also require good alignment.

The position of the feet is especially important for good body mechanics because feet provide the base of support. A **base of support** is the area on which an object rests. A wide base of support provides more stability and balance than a narrow base of support. You should stand with your feet and legs apart for a wide base of support, especially when moving, lifting, or transferring weight. A **lunge (or stride) stance** describes placing one foot in front of the other foot, keeping the two feet about a shoulder width apart. This stance will enable you to keep your balance while performing the various tasks necessary as described in this chapter.

The strongest and largest muscles are in the shoulders, upper arms, hips, and thighs, and you should use these muscles for lifting and moving. Using smaller and weaker muscles, such as those in the lower back, will place strain and exertion on your back and lead to back fatigue and injury. Follow the guidelines in Box 23–1 to safely and efficiently move clients and objects.

Box 23–1 Guidelines for Good Body Mechanics

- Assess the situation before you begin any attempt to move the client. Get help if you think the weight is more than you can safely turn or transfer. Many employers have a **"no-lift" policy**, and if this is the case, workers are not allowed to lift or move clients without mechanical aid. ***Always check the care plan and know employer policy before moving a client.***
- Face your work area. This prevents unnecessary twisting. Remember to stand with a wide base of support.
- Bend at your knees and hips and squat when lifting or setting down objects below your waist. Do not bend forward from your waist or you will strain your small back muscles (Figure 23–2).
- Tighten your stomach muscles and tuck in your pelvis as you lift. Keep your back straight. Use your leg and thigh muscles as you lift the item to waist level. You legs should be bearing the weight, not your back.
- Hold objects *close* to your body when lifting, moving, or carrying them, which would involve the upper arm and shoulder muscles (see Figure 23–2). Holding objects *away* from your body would place a strain on the small muscles in your lower arms. Do not lift objects higher than chest level. Use both hands and arms to lift, move, or carry heavy objects.
- Avoid unnecessary bending and reaching. If your client is on a hospital bed, raise the bed so that it is close to your waist. Adjust the overbed table so that it is at your waist level. Arrange all equipment and supplies in a convenient, easy-to-reach location before you begin a task. If necessary, move a chair next to the bedside and arrange your supplies on it. If an object is higher than chest level, use a step stool to reach it.
- Turn your whole body as one unit when changing the direction of your movement. Do not twist your body. Move your feet in the direction of the turn. Work with smooth and even movements. Avoid sudden or jerky motions. Take your time.
- Push, slide, or pull heavy objects whenever you can, rather than lifting them. Pushing with your body weight is easier than pulling. Widen your base of support when pushing or pulling. Move your front leg forward when pushing. Move your rear leg back when pulling (Figure 23–3).

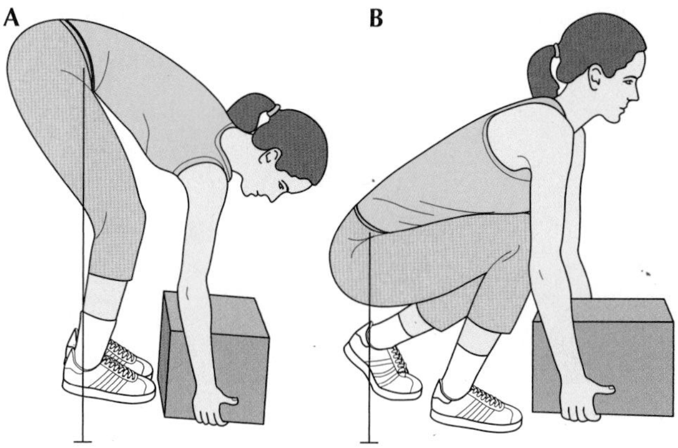

Figure 23–2 Picking up a box using incorrect (A) and good (B) body mechanics. **Source:** Adapted from Potter, P.A., Perry, A., Ross-Kerr, J.C., & Wood, M.J. (2001). *Canadian fundamentals of nursing* (3rd ed., p. 957). Toronto: Harcourt Canada.

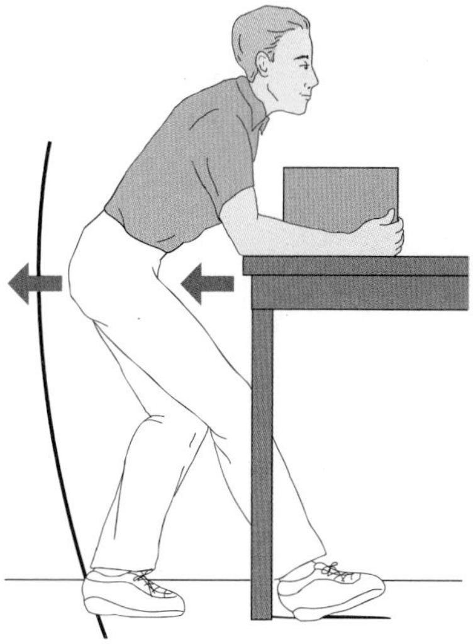

Figure 23–3 Move your rear leg back when pulling an item.

MOVING CLIENTS IN BED

Some clients can move and turn in bed themselves, while some others may need some help. They cannot move independently, but they can often work with you as you move them. Some clients are unable to move at all or even help when others move them, as they may be unconscious, paralyzed, or very weak. When moving some clients, assistive devices may be necessary. For example, a turning sheet (see page 399) or a mechanical lift (see page 423) may be required. Sometimes two or three workers may be needed to move a client.

Check with the care plan, your supervisor, and the client to find out if the client can help with moving. Always make sure that you can safely move the client on your own. ***Do not attempt a move a client by yourself if you think you may not be able to do it safely.*** If your agency has a "no-lift" policy, you should never attempt moving or lifting the client without checking first with your supervisor. You must consider the client's safety and your own safety (see the *Focus on Long-Term Care: Transferring and Lifting Safety Precautions* on page 415 and the *Focus on Home Care: Getting Help With Moving and Repositioning a Client* box).

Comfort and Safety Measures

The client's skin must be protected when you are moving and repositioning them. Otherwise, friction and shearing will injure the skin and cause infection and pressure ulcers (see Chapter 24). **Friction** is the rubbing of one surface against another. When a client is moved in bed, skin rubs against the sheet. **Shearing** occurs when the skin sticks to a surface and muscles slide in the direction the body is moving (Figure 23–4). Shearing can happen when a client slides down in bed or is moved in bed. Shearing can be very painful to the client and can lead to serious skin and health problems.

Reduce friction and shearing by rolling or lifting the client. A cotton drawsheet (see Chapter 26) serves as a turning sheet to move the client in bed and reduce friction. Some employers use turning pads for this purpose (see the *Focus on Older Adults: Shearing* box). A **slider board** is used to slide a client from one bed to another. A slider board is a friction-reduced board with handles that is placed under a person, is grasped by the handles and then slid (with the client on the board) from one bed to another.

Follow these comfort and safety measures when moving clients in bed:

- Check with your supervisor and the care plan about limits or restrictions in positioning or moving the client. For example, clients with severe arthritis and osteoporosis (see Chapter 24) may experience pain or injury when being moved. Your supervisor will tell you what measures to take when moving these clients.
- Decide how to move the client and how much help you need *before* attempting the move.
- Ask for help *before* starting the move.

focus on ››HOME CARE

Getting Help With Moving and Repositioning a Client

Some clients you care for may have mechanical lifting devices in their home. However, usually you will not have a co-worker to help you move home care clients. In that case, plan your duties ahead of time with your supervisor.

A nurse or physiotherapist is responsible for teaching the client's family or primary caregiver about body mechanics and moving, positioning, and transferring the client.

Remember, a helper in a facility is a co-worker. A helper in a home care setting is usually a trained family member or primary caregiver. In home care settings, it is common for a client's family members, the primary caregiver, or another person in the home to want to assist you in moving their loved one. It is your responsibility to make sure that anyone who helps you has received training.

- Communicate directions to your helper. Count 1-2-3 and then move together. ***Decide BEFORE you attempt this whether you both should move at the count of three or immediately after.***
- Move the client in small steps. Several small movements may be easier than one large movement.
- Cover and screen the client to protect privacy rights.

focus on ››OLDER ADULTS

Shearing

Older adults are at great risk for shearing. Their skin is fragile and easily torn. ***Always*** use a lift, a turning sheet, or a turning pad when lifting and moving older adults. Remember that older clients usually have less body fat, which means that they have more pronounced bony areas and the skin over bony areas is more likely to shear (tear and scrape) than that over other parts of the body.

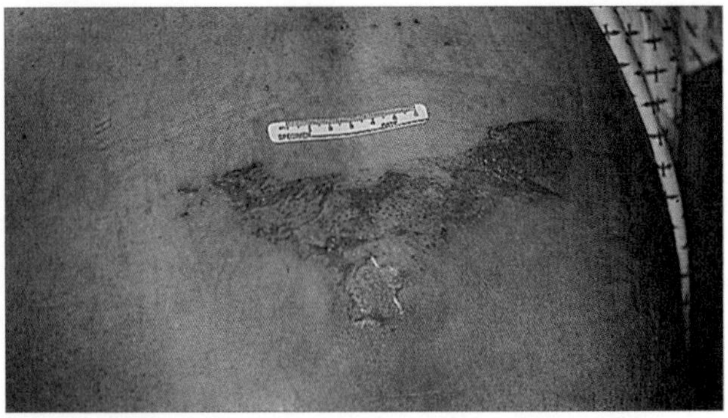

Figure 23–4 Shearing often occurs over the coccyx bone, just above the buttocks. When the head of the bed is raised for the sitting position, the skin on the client's buttocks stays in place, but internal structures move forward as the client slides down in bed. Skin that is pinched between the mattress and the hip bones can become scraped or even torn. To prevent shearing when moving a client up in bed, always use lift sheets. **Source:** Potter, P.A., Perry, A., Ross-Kerr, J.C., & Wood, M.J. (2001). *Canadian fundamentals of nursing* (3rd ed., p. 1503). Toronto: Harcourt Canada.

- Protect tubes or drainage containers connected to the client. Make sure that the tubing is not pulled, tangled, or pinched during the move.
- Position clients in good body alignment after lifting or moving them.
- Make sure linens are wrinkle-free after moving the client. Straighten the linens, as needed.

Moving the Client up in Bed

When sitting up in bed, it is easy for the client to slide down toward the middle or foot of the bed (Figure 23–5). The client is then moved up in bed

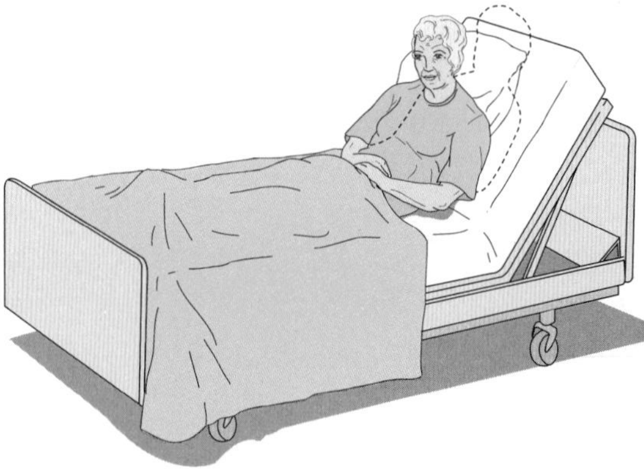

Figure 23–5 A client in poor alignment after sliding down in bed—shoulders are slouched, head and neck are forward, and the spine is curved.

to maintain good body alignment and comfort. Moving the client up in bed is also usually done before providing bedside care.

You can move children and lightweight adults up in bed by yourself if they are able to help. The client helps by pushing with his or her hands or feet to move up in bed. Or the client may have a *trapeze* (Figure 23–6) to aid with moving. A trapeze is a device that attaches to the bed or to a frame over the bed, and the client grasps the bars of the trapeze and pulls.

Clients who are very heavy or weak need two people to move them. Remember to check with your supervisor or the client's care plan before attempting to move a client. Having someone help you protects you and the client from injury.

Turning sheets (also known as **lift sheets** or **slider sheets**) should be used to easily and safely move a client up in bed (Figures 23–7 and 23–8). Using a turning sheet prevents pain, skin damage, and bone and joint injuries because the client is lifted more evenly. The turning sheet prevents the client's skin from friction and shearing when he or she is being moved in bed, and it makes it easier for the support workers to have a secure grasp. The turning sheet is used to move older adults, clients with arthritis or spinal cord injuries, and clients who are unconscious or paralyzed, who do not require a mechanical lift.

The turning sheet can be a waterproof material or even a folded sheet (see Chapter 26). It is placed under the client from above the head to above the

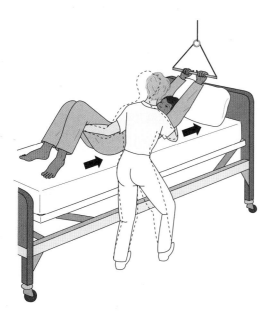

Figure 23–6 The client grasps a trapeze and flexes his or her knees. Shift your body weight from the rear leg to the front leg as you move the client up in bed. Make sure the client does not shear his or her buttocks when moving this way.

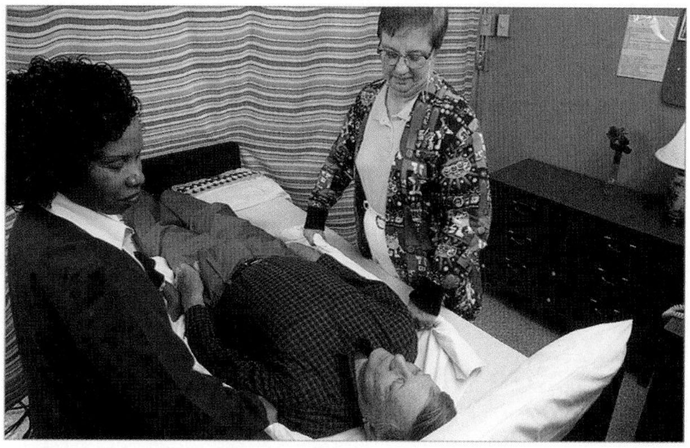

Figure 23–7 A turning sheet is used to move the client up in bed. The turning sheet extends from the client's head to above his or her knees and is held close to the client near the shoulders and buttocks.

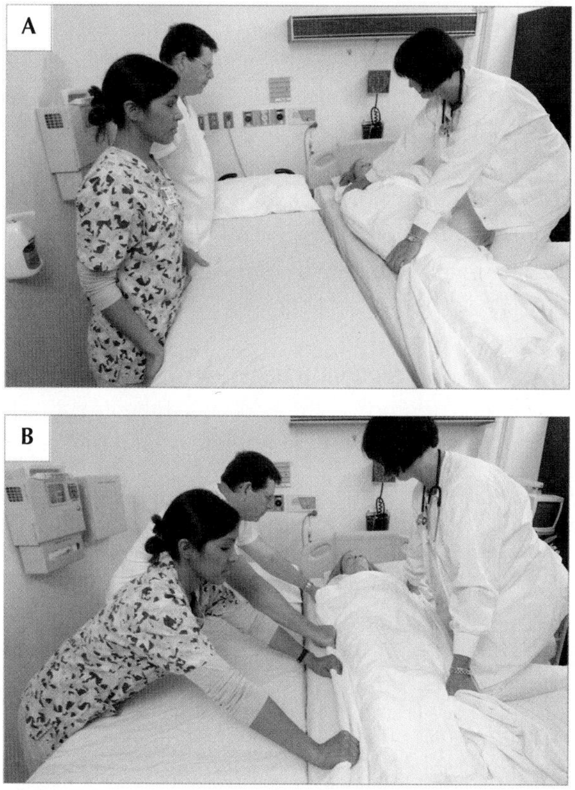

Figure 23–8 Transferring the person to a stretcher with a helper. **A,** The stretcher is against the bed and is held in place. **B,** A drawsheet is used to transfer the person from the bed to a stretcher.

knees. You and your helper should roll the turning sheet closely to the client's body and grasp the sheet firmly, with palms up. Check with your supervisor and the care plan to see if a turning sheet is required. Using a turning sheet will reduce possible injuries to the client.

1 2 3 MOVING THE CLIENT UP IN BED

Remember to promote:

- **D**ignity • **I**ndependence • **P**references • **P**rivacy • **S**afety

Pre-Procedure

1 Identify the client according to employer policy.
2 Ask someone to help you.
3 Perform hand hygiene.
4 Explain the procedure to the client.
5 Provide for privacy.
6 Raise bed to a comfortable working height. Make sure bed wheels are locked. Follow the care plan for bed rail use. Lower the head of the bed to a level appropriate for the client. It should be as flat as possible.*

Procedure

7 You and your helper should stand on either side of the bed. Lower one of the bed rails.
8 Log-roll the client to one side (see the box *Log-Rolling the Client*) so that the client is facing the bed rail that is up.
9 The worker on the side facing the client should hold and support the client. Ensure that the client is in proper body alignment and safely positioned. Some clients feel better if they can hold onto the bed rail, and if this is the case, keep the bed rail up.
10 The other support worker should **fanfold** a turning sheet and place it behind the client from the back of the head to the thighs. The fanfolded sheet should be tucked as close to the client's body as possible.
11 Instruct the client that he or she will be rolling over a "bump" in the bed. Assist the client to log-roll over to the opposite side. Place the bed rail facing the client in the "up" position to allow the client to grasp it.
12 Lower the bed rail on the opposite side, grasp the turning sheet and straighten it out.
13 Assist the client to log-roll onto his or her back. Lower the raised bedrail.
14 Roll the sides of the turning sheet up close to the client.
15 Grasp the rolled up turning sheet firmly near the person (see Figure 23–7). Ensure that the client's head is supported.
16 Place the client's pillow against the headboard, if the client can do without the pillow.
17 Move the client up in bed on the count of three. Each worker should shift their weight from the rear leg to the front leg.
18 If it is more comfortable for both of you, place your knees closest to the client's head on the bed when performing steps 15 and 16 above.
19 Unroll the turning sheet.
20 Provide for safety and comfort. Position the client in good body alignment according to the care plan. Straighten linens.
21 If the client is *lying in a hospital bed*, the easiest and safest method to raise the client's head and shoulders is to raise the head of the bed. Use the electronic control to raise the head of the bed.

Post-Procedure

22 Put the pillow under the client's head and shoulders. Tidy up the bed linens. Place the call bell within reach.*
23 Provide for safety and comfort. Position the client in good body alignment. Raise the head of the bed to an appropriate level for the client.
24 Return bed to lowest position, if necessary. Follow the care plan for bed rail use.*
25 Remove privacy measures.
26 Perform hand hygiene.
27 Report and record your actions and observations according to employer policy.

*Steps marked with an asterisk may not apply in community settings.

When moving a client in bed, it is also very important that you pay close attention to your own body alignment and posture. You can reduce your risk for injury if you do a few simple stretching exercises before beginning. To reduce your risk of back injury, you should either raise the level of the client's bed or place your knee (the one that is closest to the head of the client) on the bed (not applicable to community settings). By placing your knees on the bed, you will reduce your risk of bending and hurting your back. While moving your client, you should avoid twisting or bending your back. Lastly, remember that it safer for both you and your client when you move the client by grasping the turning sheet instead of the client.

Turning the Client

Turning clients onto their sides helps prevent complications from bed rest. Certain care procedures require the side-lying position when the clients are turned toward you or away from you. The direction depends on the client's condition and on the situation. If you are going to turn someone over in bed, it is usually safer and easier to try to log-roll them. **Log-rolling** turns a person over from their back or side to their other side. One of the client's knees (the one opposite from the side the client is being turned onto) may be bent, if necessary (if this is stated in the client's care plan), ***but you must always make sure the client is in good body alignment. You must always turn the client's neck and spine in one step making sure they are never twisted.***

Many clients have certain conditions, such as arthritis in the spine or knees, that make turning painful for them. When turning these clients, it is best to log-roll them using a turning sheet. Remember to check with your supervisor and the care plan to determine the correct procedure to use for each client.

Some clients will need a minimum of two people to log-roll them, and maybe even three people if the client is tall or heavy. Clients who will need at least two people to log-roll them include:

- Clients with arthritic spines or knees (common in older adults)
- Clients recovering from hip fractures
- Clients with spinal cord injuries (the spine must be kept straight at all times following spinal cord injury)
- Clients recovering from spinal surgery (the spine must be kept straight at all times following spinal cord surgery)

1 2 3 LOG-ROLLING THE CLIENT

Remember to promote:

• Dignity • Independence • Preferences • Privacy • Safety

Pre-Procedure

1 Identify the client according to employer policy.
2 Ask someone to help you if you need assistance.
3 Perform hand hygiene.
4 Explain the procedure to the client.
5 Provide for privacy.
6 Raise the bed to a comfortable working height. Make sure the bed wheels are locked. Follow the care plan for bed rail use. Lower the head of the bed to a level appropriate for the client. It should be as flat as possible.*

Procedure

7 Stand on the side of the bed opposite to where you will turn the client.
8 Lower the bed rail near you if it is up. The far bed rail is left up if used.
9 Move the client to the side near you (see the *Moving the Client to the Side of the Bed* box, page 406.)
10 Cross the client's arms over his or her chest. Cross the leg near you over the far leg. If the client cannot cross the leg, you can simply bend their leg. Place a pillow between the client's knees before turning them.

(continued on page 402)

1 2 3 LOG-ROLLING THE CLIENT

Procedure (cont'd)

11 ***Method 1: Log-rolling the client away from you***
- **a** Stand with a wide base of support. Flex your knees.
- **b** Place one hand on the person's shoulder and the other on the client's buttock that is near you.
- **c** Roll the client in one step gently toward the other side of the bed (Figure 23-9), making sure that the client's neck and spine are not twisting. Shift your weight from your rear leg to your front leg.
- **d** If stated in the client's care plan, some clients can be log-rolled more easily by bending the knee opposite to the side they are going to turn onto. Again, ensure the client's neck and spine do not twist.

12 ***Method 2: Log-rolling the client toward you***
- **a** Lower the bed rail if it is up.
- **b** Go to the other side. Lower the bed rail if it is up.
- **c** Stand with a wide base of support. Flex your knees.
- **d** Place one hand on the client's far shoulder and the other on the far hip.
- **e** Roll the client toward you gently in one step making sure that his or her neck and spine do not twist (Figure 23–10).
- **f** If stated in the client's care plan, some clients can be log-rolled more easily by bending the knee opposite to the side they are going to turn onto. Again, ensure the client's neck and spine do not twist.

13 ***Method 3: Log-rolling the client with two helpers***
- **a** Stand on the side of the bed opposite to where you will turn the client. Your helper stands on the other side.
- **b** Lower the bed rails if they are up.
- **c** Move the client as a unit to the side of the bed near you. Use the turning sheet.
- **d** Place the client's arms across his or her chest. Place a pillow between the knees.
- **e** Raise the bed rail if used.
- **f** Go to the other side of the bed next to your helper.
- **g** Stand near the client's shoulders and chest. Your helper stands near the client's buttocks and thighs.
- **h** Stand with a broad base of support, one foot in front of the other.
- **i** Ask the client to hold his or her body rigid.
- **j** Roll the client in one step (Figure 23–11, *A*) or by using a turning sheet (Figure 23–11, *B*) gently toward the other side of the bed, making sure that the client's neck and spine are not twisting. Shift your weight from your rear leg to your front leg.
- **k** If stated in the client's care plan, some clients can be log-rolled more easily by bending the knee opposite to the side they are going to turn onto. Again, ensure the client's neck and spine do not twist.

14 Position the client. Follow the care plan and your supervisor's directions. The following position is common:
- **a** Place a pillow under the head and neck.
- **b** Adjust the shoulder. The client should not lie on an arm.
- **c** Flex the upper knee. Position the upper leg in front of the lower leg.
- **d** Support the upper leg and thigh with pillows.
- **e** Place a small pillow under the upper hand and arm.
- **f** Position a pillow against the back.

Post-Procedure

15 Provide for safety and comfort.
16 Place the call bell within reach.*
17 Return the bed to its lowest position. Raise or lower the bed rails according to the care plan.*
18 Remove privacy measures.
19 Perform hand hygiene.
20 Report and record your actions and observations according to employer policy.

*Steps marked with an asterisk may not apply in community settings.

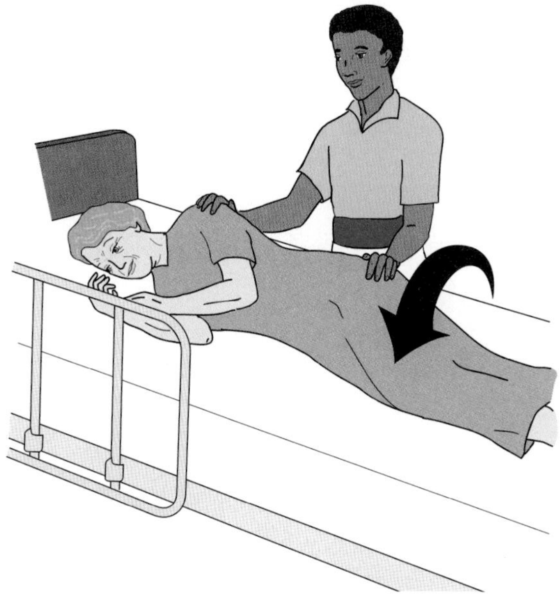

Figure 23–9 Log-rolling the client away from you.

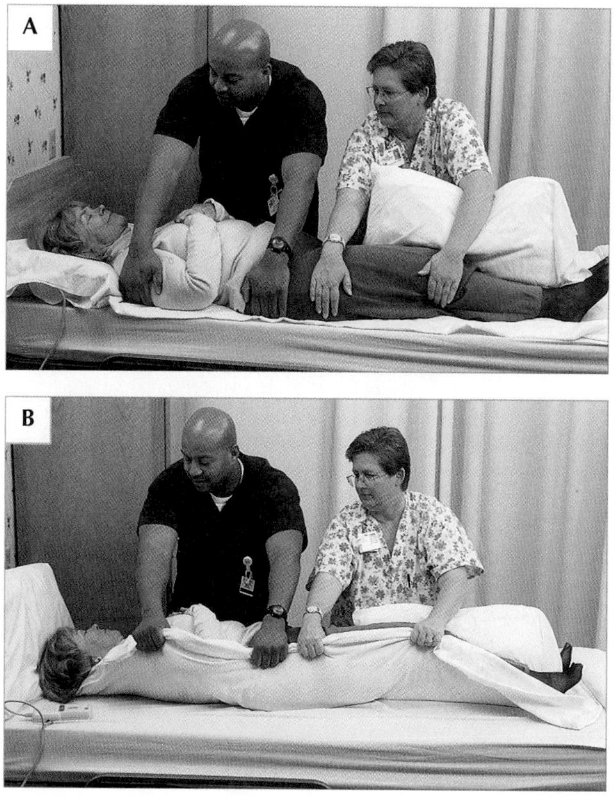

Figure 23–11 Log-rolling a client with assistance. **A,** A pillow is placed between the client's legs, and the arms are crossed on the chest. The client is on the far side of the bed. **B,** A turning sheet is used to log-roll the client. *Note:* If you plan on moving the client up in bed after log-rolling him or her, place the pillow against the headboard. **Source**: Sorrentino, S.A. & Gorek, B. (2003). *Mosby's textbook for long-term care assistants* (4th ed., p. 234). St Louis: Mosby.

Moving the Client from a Bed to a Stretcher

Stretchers are sometimes used to transport clients to other areas in a facility. They are used for clients who:

- Cannot sit up
- Must stay in a lying position
- Are seriously ill
- Are waiting for or returning from surgery

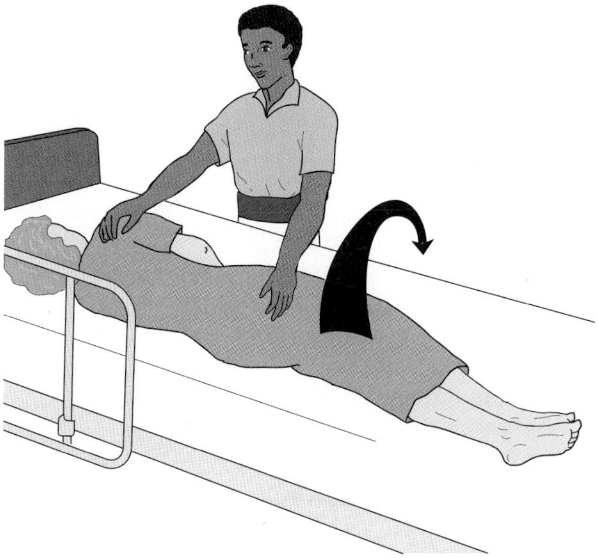

Figure 23–10 Log-rolling the client toward you.

The stretcher is covered with a folded flat sheet or bath blanket. A pillow and extra blankets are kept at hand. With your supervisor's permission, raise the head of the stretcher for Fowler's position. This increases the client's comfort.

A *slider board* is used to assist in moving the client. A slider board is a slippery board that is placed between the bed and the sheet underneath the client to allow the staff to move the client with less friction. It usually has handles on the sides to allow the support workers and other staff to grasp it easily. At least three staff members are needed to safely move a client. Remember, keep the client in good body alignment, and use good body mechanics.

After the client has been moved to the stretcher, put on the safety straps across the client's chest. The stretcher's side rails are kept up during transport of the client. The client should be moved feet first in the stretcher so that he or she can observe where they are going. As you push the stretcher, you should observe the client's breathing and colour during the transport. Never leave a client unattended on a stretcher.

1 2 3 MOVING THE CLIENT FROM A BED TO A STRETCHER

Remember to promote:

• Dignity • Independence • Preferences • Privacy • Safety

Pre-Procedure

1 Identify the client according to employer policy.
2 Ask two co-workers to help you.
3 Explain the procedure to the client.
4 Collect:
- Stretcher covered with a sheet or bath blanket
- Bath blanket
- Slider board
- Pillow(s), if needed

5 Perform hand hygiene.
6 Provide for privacy.
7 Raise the bed to a height equal to the height of the stretcher.

Procedure

8 You and your co-workers should position yourselves properly. Two workers stand on the side of the bed where the stretcher will be. The third worker stands on the other side of the bed.
9 Cover the client with a bath blanket. Fanfold top linens to the foot of the bed.
10 Loosen the cotton drawsheet on each side.
11 Lower the head of bed so that it is as flat as possible.
12 Lower bed rails, if used.
13 Being careful to secure the client's safety, log-roll the client onto one side. Place the slider board underneath the client, between the bed and the bottom sheet. Do not place the slider board directly next to the client's skin.
14 Log-roll the client onto his or her back. Position the client in good body alignment. Place the pillow under the client's head, and ensure that he or she is comfortable. The client's top sheet may remain on the client, if the client so desires.
15 Ask your co-workers to help move the client to the side of the bed by grasping the handles of the slider board.
16 Protect the client from falling, and have your co-workers position the stretcher next to the bed. They should stand behind the stretcher (Figure 23–12, *A*).
17 Lock the bed and stretcher wheels.
18 Roll up and grasp the slider board as shown in Figure 23–12, *B*. This supports the entire length of the client's body. (*Note*: In order to prevent back injuries to themselves, staff may have to kneel on the bed).
19 Transfer the client to the stretcher on the count of three by lifting and pulling him or her. Make sure the client is centred on the stretcher.
20 Place a pillow or pillows under the person's head and shoulders, if allowed.
21 Provide for safety and comfort.
22 Fasten safety straps. Raise the stretcher side rails.
23 Unlock the stretcher's wheels. Transport the client.

Post-Procedure

24 Perform hand hygiene.
25 According to employer policy, report and record the following:
- The time of the transport
- Where the person was transported
- Who went with him or her
- How the transfer was tolerated

26 Reverse the procedure to return the client to bed.

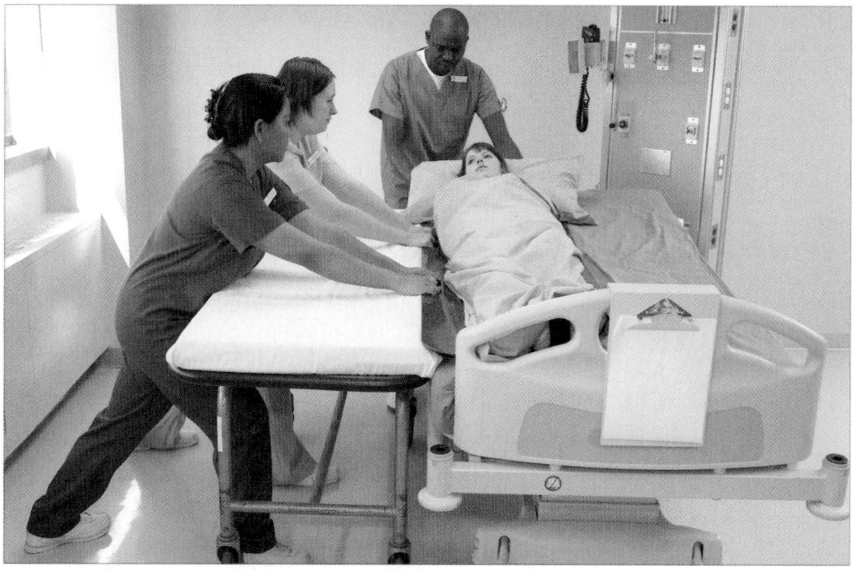

Figure 23–12 Moving the client to a stretcher. Making sure that the stretcher is in place against the bed, use a slider board to smoothly move the client from the bed to the stretcher. **Source:** Brian Hillier.

Moving the Client to the Side of the Bed

Many care procedures, for example, a bed bath, require moving the client to the side of the bed. When you move the client to the side of the bed, he or she is close to you, so you do not have to reach or stretch too much when doing the procedure. Also, you usually move clients to the side of the bed before repositioning or turning (log-rolling) them.

One method involves moving the client in segments. You can usually do this method by yourself. Some clients, such as older adults, people with arthritis, and people with spinal cord injuries, cannot be moved in segments. For these clients, using a turning sheet helps prevent pain, skin damage, as well as injury to the bones, joints, and spinal cord. When using a lift sheet to move a client to the side of the bed, it is best to have some help. Check with your supervisor for the correct procedure to use with each client.

Helping the Client to Sit on the Side of the Bed (Dangle the Legs)

Clients need to sit on the side of the bed (*dangle their legs*) for many reasons. Many older adults become dizzy or faint if they get out of bed too fast. They need to sit on the side of the bed for 1 to 5 minutes before walking or transferring. Some clients need to increase activity in stages. They progress from resting in bed to sitting on the side of the bed and then to sitting in a chair. Walking is the next step.

Some clients sit on the side of the bed when they need to perform their exercises. While dangling their legs, they cough and deep breathe. They also move their legs back and forth and in circles to stimulate circulation. The procedure is also part of preparing clients to walk or transferring them to a chair or wheelchair.

You might need a helper when assisting a client to sit on the side of the bed. Support the client if he or she has problems with balance or coordination by standing in front of them and placing your hands on their shoulders. For example, people recovering from a stroke often have problems with balance when sitting up. They must be always supported when dangling their legs to prevent falls and injuries. Check with your supervisor and the care plan for safety precautions necessary for each client.

After helping a client dangle the legs, report and record the following:

- Pulse and respirations (if instructed to measure)
- Pale or bluish skin colour (cyanosis)
- Complaints of dizziness, light-headedness, or difficulty breathing
- How well the activity was tolerated
- The length of time the client dangled the legs
- The amount of help needed
- Other observations or complaints

1 2 3 MOVING THE CLIENT TO THE SIDE OF THE BED

Remember to promote:

• Dignity • Independence • Preferences • Privacy • Safety

Pre-Procedure

1 Identify the client according to employer policy.
2 Ask someone to help you, if you need assistance.
3 Perform hand hygiene.
4 Explain the procedure to the client.
5 Provide for privacy.
6 Raise the bed to a comfortable working height. Make sure the bed wheels are locked. Follow the care plan for bed rail use. Lower the head of the bed to a level appropriate for the client. It should be as flat as possible.

Procedure

7 Stand on the side of the bed to which you will move the client.
8 Lower the bed rail near you if it is up.
9 Stand with your feet about 30 cm (12 in.) apart and one foot in front of the other. Flex your knees.
10 Cross the client's arms over his or her chest.
11 ***Method 1: Moving the client without a helper (in segments)***
   a Place your arm under the client's neck and shoulders.
   b Place your other arm under the middle of the client's back.
   c Rock backward and shift your weight to your rear leg. This moves the upper part of the client's body toward the edge of the bed (Figure 23–13, *A*).
   d Place one arm under the client's waist and one under the thighs.
   e Rock backward, moving the middle part of the client to the edge of the bed (Figure 23–13, *B*).
   f Place one arm under the client's thighs and one under the calves.
   g Rock backward, moving the client's legs to edge of the bed (Figure 23–13, *C*).
   h Repeat steps a through g, as necessary.
12 ***Method 2: Moving the client with a lift sheet***
   a Roll the lift sheet up close to the client. Your helper does the same.
   b Grasp the rolled-up lift sheet near the client's shoulders and buttocks. Your helper does the same. Make sure you support the client's head.
   c Rock backward on the count of three, moving the client toward you. Your helper rocks backward slightly and then forward toward you while keeping the arms straight. Repeat, if necessary.
   d Unroll the lift sheet.
13 Reposition the pillow under the client's head and shoulders.

Post-Procedure

14 Follow steps 15 through 20 in the *Log-Rolling the Client* box, page 402

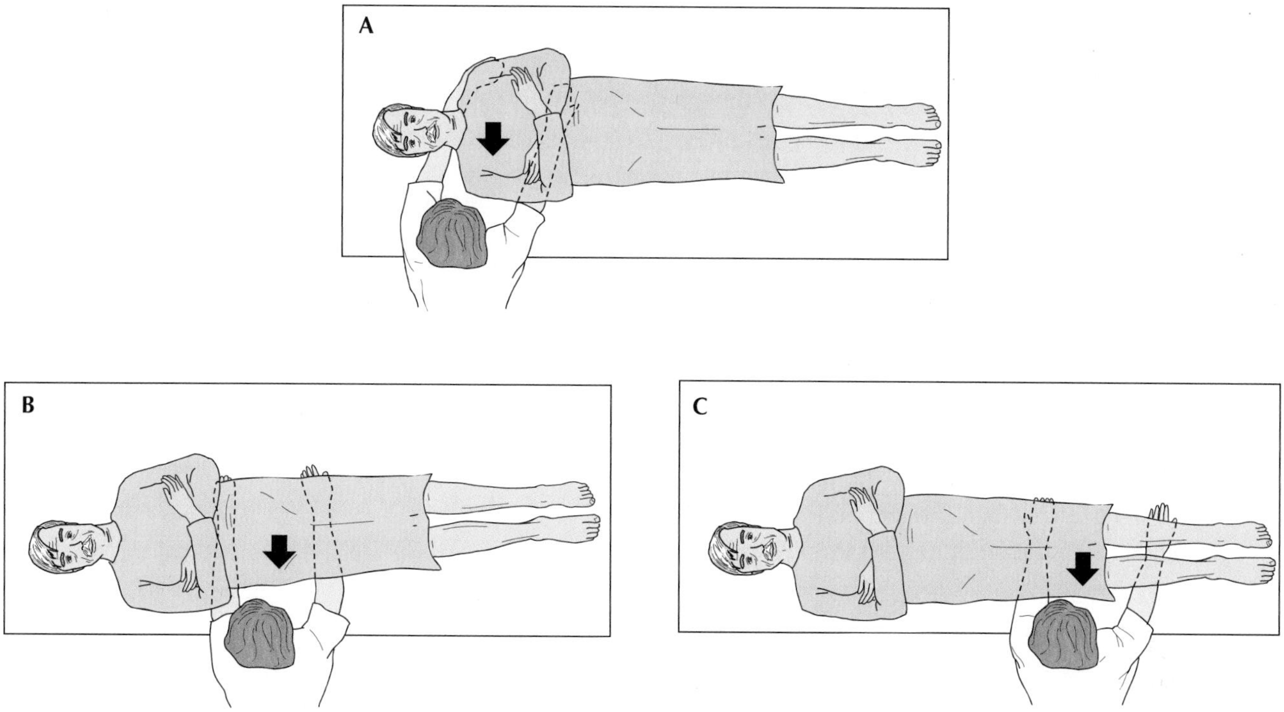

Figure 23–13 Move the client to the side of the bed in segments, always starting with the client's head and shoulders (A), then the torso and hips **(B)**, and lastly the legs **(C)**.

1 2 3 HELPING THE CLIENT SIT ON THE SIDE OF THE BED (DANGLE THE LEGS)

Remember to promote:

• **D**ignity • **I**ndependence • **P**references • **P**rivacy • **S**afety

Pre-Procedure

1 Identify the client according to employer policy.
2 Explain the procedure to the client.
3 Perform hand hygiene.
4 Decide what side of the bed to use.
5 Move furniture away to provide space to move.
6 Provide for privacy.
7 Position the client in a side-lying position facing you.
8 Make sure bed is in its lowest position and bed wheels are locked. Follow the care plan for bed rail use.*

Procedure

9 Help the client to a sitting position. (Raise the head of the bed or use pillows or a backrest.)
10 Stand near the client's waist on the side of the bed on which the client will be sitting.
11 Lower the bed rail if it is up.
12 Turn so that you face the client. Stand with a broad base of support.
13 Slide one arm under the client's neck and shoulders. Grasp the far shoulder. Place your other arm over the client's thighs near the knees. Grasp under the thighs (Figure 23–14, *A*).
14 Pivot back toward the head of the bed while pulling the client's feet, and lower the client's legs over the edge of the bed.

(continued on page 408)

1 2 3 HELPING THE CLIENT SIT ON THE SIDE OF THE BED (DANGLE THE LEGS)

Procedure (cont'd)

15 Help the client sit upright. Do not pull the client too close to the edge of the bed. Only the client's knees should be at the edge, not the thighs or buttocks (Figure 23–14, *B*).

16 Ask the client to hold on to the edge of the mattress. This supports the client in the sitting position. Allow the client to have his or her feet touch the floor.

17 Do not leave the client alone. Remain in front of the client. Place both hands on the client's shoulders for support, if necessary.

18 Check the client's condition:

- **a** Ask how he or she feels. Also, ask if the client feels dizzy or light-headed.
- **b** Check pulse and respirations.
- **c** Check for difficulty breathing, pale skin, or *cyanosis* (bluish skin colour).

19 Help the client lie down, if necessary.

20 Reverse the procedure to return the client to bed.

Post-Procedure

21 Provide for safety and comfort. Help the client move to the centre of the bed. Position the client in good body alignment according to the care plan.

22 Place the call bell within reach.*

23 Follow the care plan for bed rail use.*

24 Return furniture to its proper location.

25 Remove privacy measures.

26 Perform hand hygiene.

27 Report and record your actions and observations according to employer policy.

*Steps marked with an asterisk may not apply in community settings.

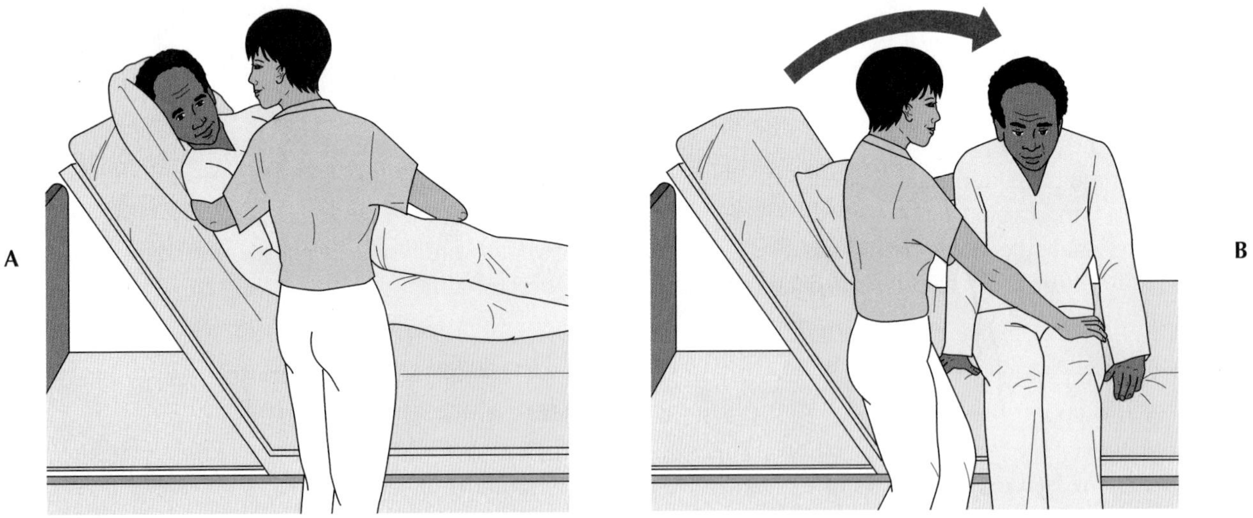

Figure 23–14 Helping the client sit on the side of the bed. **A,** Support the client under the shoulders and under the thighs. **B,** Pivot toward the foot of the bed while pulling the client's legs and feet over the edge of the bed. This brings the client to a sitting position.

POSITIONING THE CLIENT

The client must be properly positioned at all times. Regular position changes and good body alignment promote comfort and well-being, make breathing easier, and promote circulation. Proper positioning also helps prevent many complications, such as pressure ulcers (see Chapter 42) and contractures (see Chapter 24).

Most clients can move and reposition themselves. Some need reminding to adjust their position, while others need help or depend entirely on the health care team for position changes.

Comfort and Safety Measures

Whether in a bed or a chair, clients are repositioned at least every 2 hours and some more often. Follow your supervisor's instructions and the care plan.

The physician may order certain positions or position limits. Every time you position a client, check the skin for signs of redness, paleness, or discoloration. Report any of these observations immediately.

To safely position a client, follow these guidelines:

- Check with your supervisor and the care plan about the best positions for each client.
- Follow the scheduled times for repositioning the client.
- Use good body mechanics.
- Ask for help *before* beginning, if necessary.
- Explain the procedure to the client.
- Be gentle when moving the client.
- Provide for privacy.
- Leave the client in good body alignment; use pillows as directed in the care plan for comfort and support.
- Make sure linens are wrinkle-free; change or straighten them, as needed.
- Place the call bell (in facilities) within the client's reach.

Fowler's Position

Fowler's position is a semi-sitting position (Figure 23–15)—either high-Fowler's or low-Fowler's positions, depending on how high the head of the bed is up. To place a client in **high-Fowler's position**, raise the head of the bed to an angle of 45 to 60 degrees. To place a client in **low-Fowler's position**, raise the head of the bed to an angle of 15 to 30 degrees. Clients confined in bed often use either of these positions when eating, visiting with others, taking medications, reading, and watching TV. People with heart and respiratory disorders usually breathe better in a high-Fowler's position.

Important points about this position include:

- If the bed is not adjustable, use pillows for support. You can use a back rest, a foam wedge pillow, or sofa pillows. If using pillows for support, make sure the headboard is sturdy or the bed is pushed against the wall (see Chapter 26).
- Make sure the client is positioned in good alignment. The spine should be straight and the hips should be directly against the bend in the bed or the pillows.
- Place a small pillow behind the head and neck.
- Place small pillows under the arms and hands.
- Place a small pillow under the client's knees to keep them flexed. This can reduce back strain.
- Place small pillows under the lower back, thighs, and ankles if your supervisor tells you to do so.

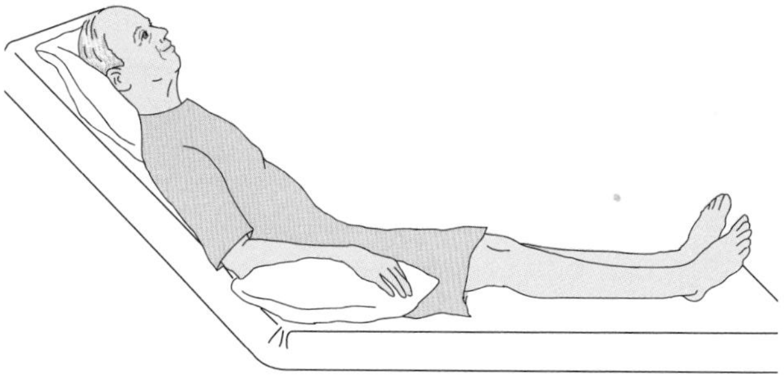

Figure 23–15 Fowler's position.

Supine Position

The **supine position** is a back-lying position (Figure 23–16), used for sleeping and resting.

To place a client in the supine position:

- Make sure the bed is flat. Lower the head of the bed, if necessary.
- Place a small pillow under the head and shoulders.
- Place the person's arms along the person's sides, palms facing down.
- Place a small pillow under his or her arms and hands.
- Place a small pillow under the client's knees to keep them flexed. This can reduce back strain.
- Place small pillows or rolled towels under the lower back, thighs, and ankles if your supervisor tells you to do so.

Lateral Position

The **lateral position** is a side-lying position (Figure 23–17). The client can lie on one side or the other. Check the client often to make sure he or she is not experiencing pain, numbness, or discomfort in this position.

To place a client in the lateral position:

- Make sure the bed is flat. Lower the head of the bed, if necessary.
- Position the client onto his or her side (see the box *Log-Rolling the Client*, page 401.)
- Bend the upper leg at the knee. Position the upper leg in front of the lower leg.
- Place a small pillow under the head and neck.
- Place small pillows under the upper leg and thigh.
- Place small pillows under the upper hand and arm.
- Position a small pillow against the client's back.

Sims' Position

Sims' position is a left side-lying position in which the right leg is sharply flexed so that it is not resting on the left leg. The left arm is positioned along the client's back. This position, in which the client is lying partly on the abdomen (Figure 23–18), is used for administering enemas and other procedures. It can also be used for resting if the client is comfortable in this position. It is, however, usually *not comfortable* for older adults, so if you must put them in this position, position them well with plenty of pillows. Check with your supervisor before positioning an older adult in Sims' position. Check the client frequently for good comfort and circulation in the lower arm and hand.

To place a client in Sims' position:

- Make sure the bed is flat. Lower the head of the bed, if necessary.
- Position the client onto his or her left side (see the box *Log-Rolling the Client*, page 401).
- Bend the upper (right) leg, and position it such that it does not lie on the lower (left) leg.

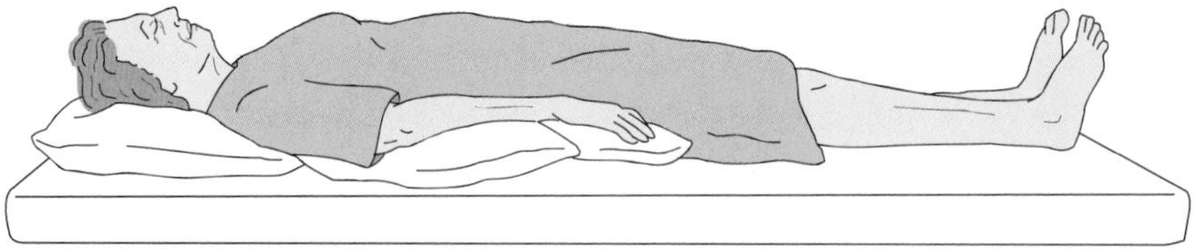

Figure 23–16 Supine position.

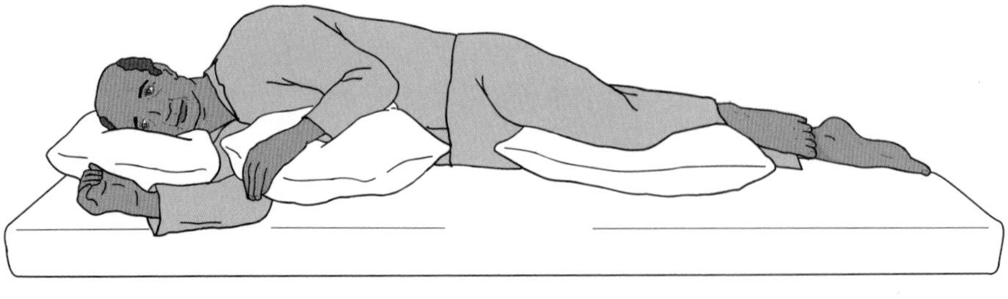

Figure 23–17 Lateral position.

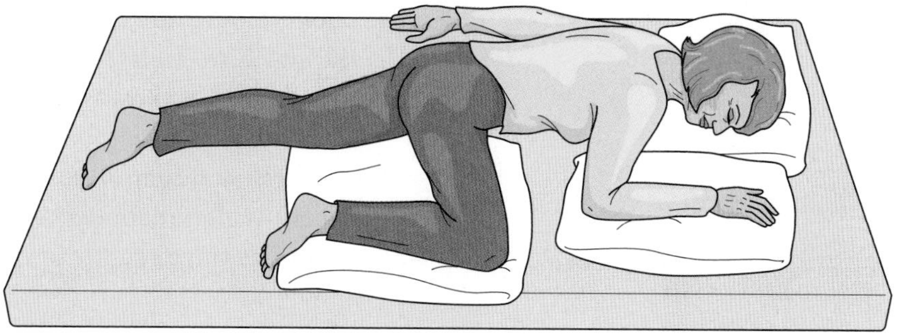

Figure 23–18 Sims' position.

- Bend the upper (right) arm, and position the hand, palm down, near the head.
- Place the lower (left) arm behind the client, palm facing up. If the client cannot tolerate this position, move this arm to a more comfortable position.
- Place a small pillow under the head and neck.
- Place small pillows under the upper arm and hand and under the upper leg.

Prone Position

The **prone position** is a front-lying position on the abdomen, with the head turned to one side (Figure 23–19). Many clients, including clients with limited range of motion in their necks, cannot tolerate the prone position. It is usually used, if at all, for a short period at a time. The prone position is used mainly to prevent shortening (contractures) of the thigh muscle, in clients who have had leg amputations and sit in a wheelchair for long periods of time. The prone position will help keep the thigh muscles in the amputated leg stretched. Use the prone position only if it is called for in the care plan.

To place a client in the prone position:

- Make sure the bed is flat. Lower the head of the bed, if necessary.
- Remove the pillows. Carefully turn the client onto the side and then onto the abdomen.
- Turn the client's head to one side.
- Bend the arms at the elbows, and place the hands near the head.
- Place small pillows under the client's head, abdomen, and lower legs (see Figure 23–19). If the client is positioned with the feet hanging over the end of the mattress, do not place a pillow under the lower legs.

Sitting Position

Clients in chairs or wheelchairs must hold the upper body and head erect to avoid poor alignment (Figure 23–20). Some require postural supports if they cannot keep the upper body erect (Figure 23–21), as supports help maintain good alignment. The health care team selects the best product for the client's needs, with consideration for the client's dignity, independence, preferences, and safety. Assist with providing postural supports, as needed.

To position a client in a chair or wheelchair:

- Position the client's back and buttocks against the back of the chair.
- Make sure the back is straight. The client should not be leaning to the side.

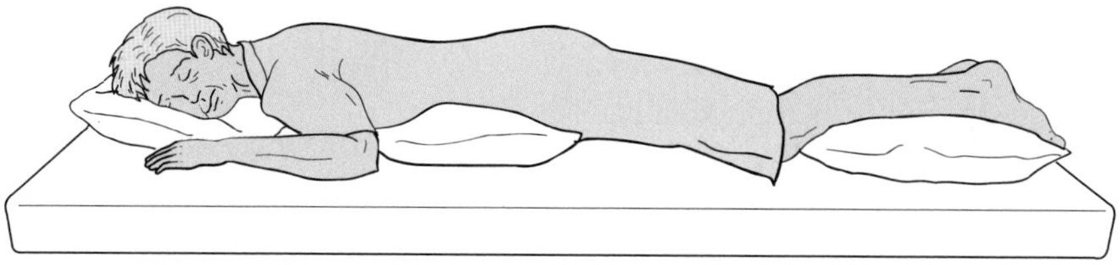

Figure 23–19 Prone position. If the client is tall, you may choose to dangle their toes over the end of the mattress.

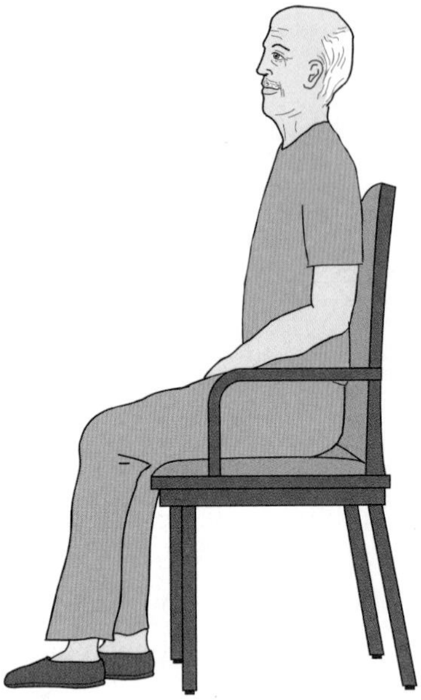

Figure 23–20 Client positioned in a chair. The client's feet are flat on the floor; the calves do not touch the chair; and the back is straight and against the back of the chair.

- Place the client's feet flat on the floor or on wheelchair foot rests.
- Place the backs of the knees and calves slightly away from the edge of the seat.
- Support the paralyzed (affected) arms on pillows. Follow the care plan. Some clients have special foam positioners (see Figure 23–21). Ask you supervisor about their proper use.

  These may be considered a restraint in some agencies. You must never apply these unless they are in the client's care plan.
- Position the client's wrists at a slightly flexed angle. Elevated wheelchair arm rests (Figure 23–22) are suitable for some clients who have the tendency to lean towards their paralyzed (affected) side.
- Place a small pillow between the client's lower back and the chair, if your supervisor tells you to do so.

Repositioning the Client in a Chair or Wheelchair. Clients can sometimes slide down in their chairs. For good body alignment and safety, they must be repositioned so that their back and buttocks are against the back of the chair. Although transfer belts are recommended to facilitate repositioning the client, some agencies do not carry them. ***Always check to see if this type of safety equipment is available at your agency.***

Some clients can help with repositioning, while some others need help. Use the following method if the client is alert, cooperative, can follow instructions, and has the strength to help:

- Lock the wheelchair wheels.
- Stand in front of the client. Block his or her knees and feet with your knees and feet.

A

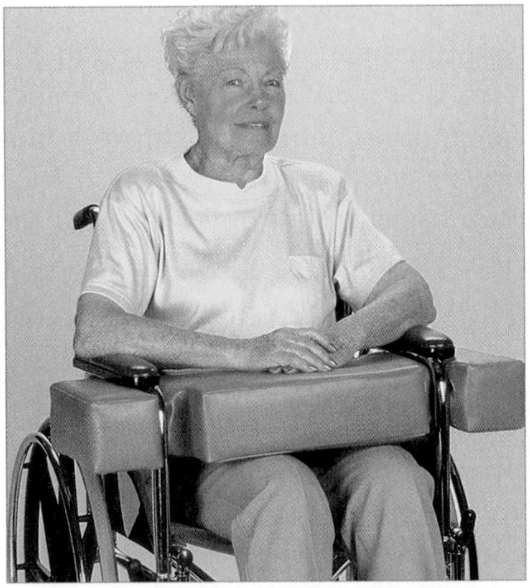

B

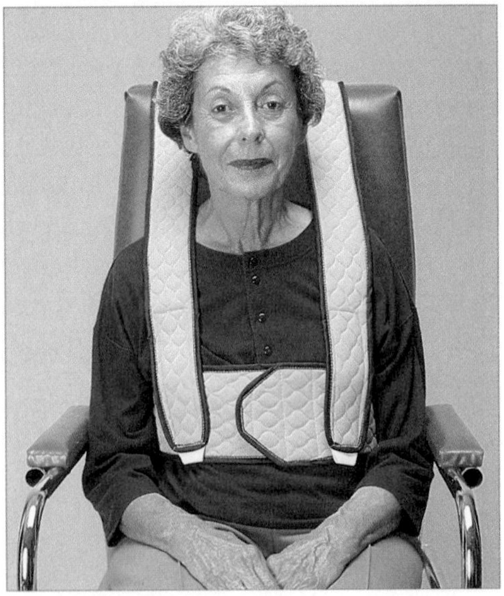

Figure 23–21 Postural supports. **A,** Pelvic holder. **B,** Torso support. These must be ordered by the client's doctor. It is your responsibility to check the client's skin under the supports every hour to watch for friction and irritation. **Courtesy:** J.T. Posey Company, Arcadia, CA.

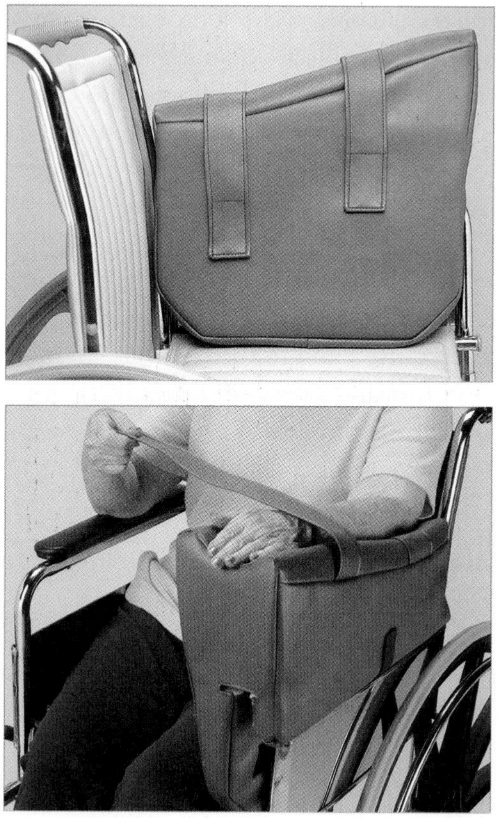

Figure 23–22 Elevated armrest. Note how the client's arm would be positioned with the Velcro strap. **Courtesy:** J.T. Posey Company, Arcadia, CA

- Place your knees in front of their knees.
- Apply a transfer belt (see page 414), if they are used at your agency.
- Position the client's feet flat on the floor.
- Position the client's arms on the armrests.
- Grasp the transfer belt on each side while the client leans forward. Or if a transfer belt is not available, put your arms under the client's arms and place your hands around the client's shoulder blades.
- Ask the client to push with his or her feet and arms on the count of three.
- Lift the client back into the chair on the count of three. ***Ensure that your back maintains its natural curve, as otherwise this can cause back injury.***
- As the client pushes with his or her feet and arms (Figure 23–23), push their knees with your knees. The client will be naturally repositioned back into the wheelchair.

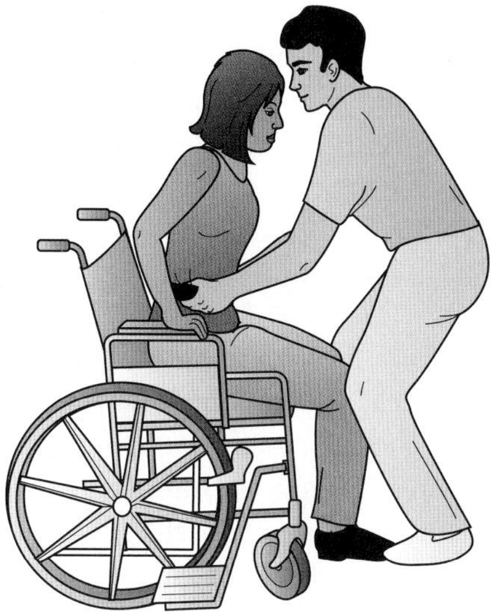

Figure 23–23 Repositioning the client in a wheelchair. Use a transfer belt to lift the client to the back of the chair.

TRANSFERRING THE CLIENT

The term **transfer** means helping a client move from one place to another. See Box 23–2 for the difference between a *lift* and a *transfer*. The client must be able to weight-bear to any degree. Clients are often moved from their beds to chairs, wheelchairs, commodes, toilets, or stretchers. Some clients need only minimal help with transferring, but some others need two (or occasionally three)

Box 23–2 The Difference Between a "Lift" and a "Transfer"

It is important that you know the difference between a "transfer" and a "lift." A transfer is the method used to move a client who can weight-bear to any degree. If the client cannot assist you by weight-bearing, a *lift* is used. Most times, health care workers cannot lift clients to transfer them. Occasionally, clients can be *manually lifted*, but most clients require a **mechanical lift**, especially if they are large, heavy, or restless. Because of the serious risk of back injury to the workers, most long-term care agencies no longer allow staff to manually lift clients, and have a strict "no-lift" policy. It is your responsibility to check to see if your agency has a "no-lift" policy *before* providing care to your clients.

people to help them. Your supervisor and the care plan will tell you how much help a client needs.

You should always remember to help the client out of the bed on his or her strong side. Place the chair or wheelchair with its back aligned with the head of the bed. Lock the bed and wheelchair wheels, and raise the footrests.

Know the Client. Never attempt a transfer without assistance if the client cannot help. Always make sure that you have enough room for a safe transfer. Clear the area of potential hazards. You may have to move furniture to make room for a chair, wheelchair, or stretcher. Before transferring a client, check the care plan or ask your supervisor if the client has a weaker side (or *affected side*), which is the side affected by disease or disability. The strong side (or *unaffected side*) is the side not affected by disease or disability and pulls the weak side along.

Transfers from the weak side are awkward and unsafe. The weak arm and leg may not be able to bear the client's weight. For example, a client's left side is weak from a **stroke**, and her right side is the stronger side. Plan to move the client so that her right side moves first.

Follow Principles of Safety and Good Body Mechanics. The number of people needed for a transfer depends on the client's physical capabilities, condition, and size. You should always check the client's care plan to see how many people are required to transfer him or her. Many long-term care facilities require the use of transfer belts when residents are transferred to or from chairs or wheelchairs. Check with your supervisor and the care plan for instructions on how much assistance is needed.

The rules of good body mechanics apply to transfers also. They will help you reduce the risk of injury to yourself and to the client. Also, follow the same comfort and safety measures listed for lifting and moving clients.

After transferring a client, report and record the following:

- Pulse rate (if it is to be measured, as directed) before and at the transfer
- Complaints of lightheadedness, pain, discomfort, difficulty breathing, weakness, or fatigue
- The amount of help needed to transfer the client
- How the client helped with the transfer

Applying Transfer Belts

A **transfer belt** is used in some agencies to transfer unsteady and disabled clients, and it helps prevent falls and other injuries. In many agencies, the belt goes around the client's waist, although some

1 2 3 APPLYING A TRANSFER BELT

Remember to promote:

• Dignity • Independence • Preferences • Privacy • Safety

Procedure

1. Identify the client, according to employer policy.
2. Explain the procedure to the client.
3. Perform hand hygiene.
4. Provide for privacy.
5. Assist the client to the sitting position.
6. Apply the belt around the client's waist over clothing. Do not apply it over bare skin. (*Note*: Some agencies require you to place the transfer belt around the client's hips.)
7. Tighten the belt so that it is snug. It should not cause discomfort or impair breathing. You should be able to slide your fingers under the belt.
8. Make sure that a woman's breasts are not caught under the belt.
9. Place the buckle off centre in the front or in the back for the client's comfort (Figure 23-24). The buckle should not be over the spine.
10. Grasp the transfer belt from underneath when using it to transfer a client.

A 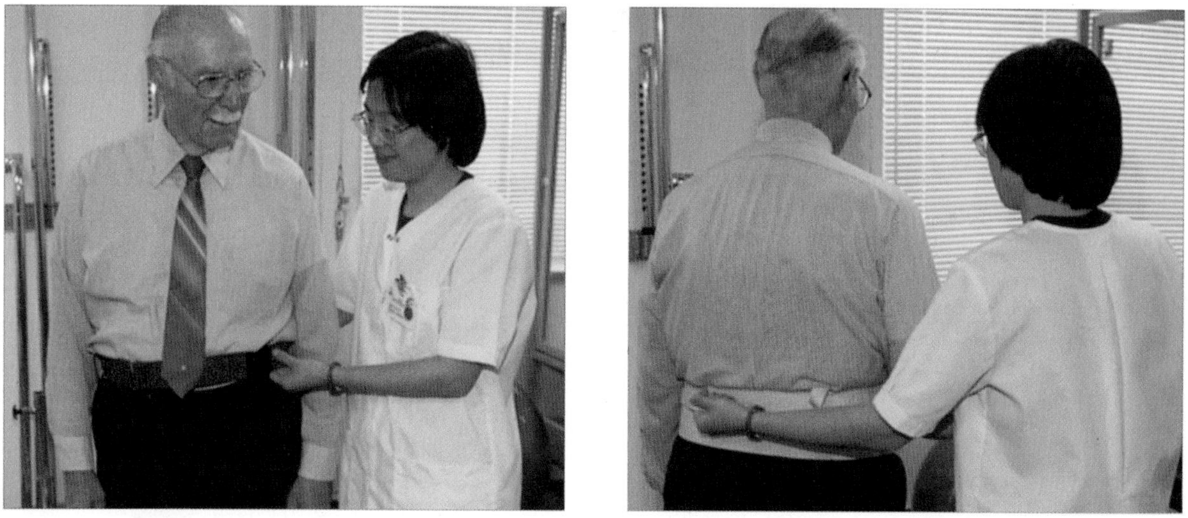 B

Figure 23–24 Transfer belt (gait belt). Note the different types of transfer belts. **A,** Position the belt buckle off centre in the front. **B,** Position the belt buckle off centre at the back. Grasp under the belt, with your fingers pointing up.

agencies require you to place the transfer belt around the client's hips. You should be aware of your agency's policies for placement before using a transfer belt.

Grasp the belt, with your fingers pointing up, to support the client during the transfer. The belt is called a *transfer belt* when used for walking with a client. Many facilities require staff to use these belts when transferring or walking a client. Always check the client's care plan before using a transfer belt.

Transferring a Client From the Bed to a Chair or Wheelchair

It is important to ensure safety during chair and wheelchair transfers. You must prevent falls in clients and protect your back from injury. Always hold the client securely during the procedure. Make sure the client wears nonskid footwear to prevent sliding or slipping. The chair or wheelchair must be able to support the client's weight.

Some agencies use **transfer boards** to assist certain clients to slide from their bed or chair to a wheelchair. Transfer boards are mostly used when the client is able to assist the staff. The client must have adequate padding on his or her buttocks, and the staff must ensure that shearing does not occur while sliding the client.

Most bedside chairs and wheelchairs have vinyl seats and backs, and because vinyl holds in body heat and can stick to the client, you should cover the back and seat with a folded blanket to promote comfort. Place small pillows or cushions behind the client's back, as instructed by your supervisor. As a support worker, it is important that you take necessary steps to promote comfort, prevent pressure ulcers, and maintain proper posture in the client.

focus on ›› LONG-TERM CARE

Transferring and Lifting Safety Precautions

In many long-term care facilities, residents have signs in their rooms that say how much assistance is needed to move them. The signs state whether the resident requires:

- Independent with No Assistance (or "No Assistance")
- Stand by (or "Observe and Supervise")
- One-person transfer
- Two-person transfer
- One-person lift*
- Two or more people to lift*
- Mechanical lift (or "MediLift/Argo**/Ground-Based Lift")
- Ceiling Lift
- Standing Lift (or "Sit–Stand")

* Not used in agencies that have a "no-lift" policy
** This is an example of a specific name brand. Your agency may use another name.

1 2 3 TRANSFERRING THE CLIENT TO A CHAIR OR WHEELCHAIR

Remember to promote:

• Dignity • Independence • Preferences • Privacy • Safety

Pre-Procedure

1 Identify the client, according to employer policy.
2 Explain the procedure to the client.
3 Collect:
- Wheelchair or arm chair
- One or two bath blankets
- Robe and nonskid footwear
- Paper or sheet
- Transfer belt, if needed
- Transfer board (if your agency uses them)
- Seat cushion, if used by the client

4 Perform hand hygiene.
5 Provide for privacy.
6 Decide which side of the bed to use. Move furniture away to provide space to move.

Procedure

7 Place the back of the chair aligned with the headboard.
8 Place a folded bath blanket or cushion on the seat, if needed.
9 Lock wheelchair wheels. Raise the foot rests or swing them out of the way.
10 Lower the bed to its lowest position. Lock the bed wheels. Lower the bed rail near you, if it is up.
11 Fanfold top linens to the foot of the bed.
12 Put nonskid footwear on the client.
13 Help the client dangle the legs (see *Helping the Client Sit on the Side of the Bed*, page 407.) Make sure his or her feet touch the floor.
14 Apply the transfer belt, if it will be used.
15 ***Method 1: Using a transfer belt***
- **a** Stand in front of the client. Stand with your feet apart. Flex your hips and knees. Align your knees with the client's knees.
- **b** Have the client hold onto the mattress. Or ask the client to place his or her fists on the bed by the thighs.
- **c** Make sure the client's feet are flat on the floor.
- **d** Have the client lean forward.
- **e** Grasp the transfer belt at each side.
- **f** Brace your knees against the client's knees. Block his or her feet with your feet (Figure 23–25, *A*).
- **g** Tell the client to push down on the mattress and to stand on the count of three. Pull the client into a standing position as you straighten your hips and legs. Keep your knees slightly flexed (Figure 23–25, *B*).

16 ***Method 2: Without using a transfer belt***
- **a** Follow steps 16 a–c.
- **b** Place your hands under the client's arms. Your hands are around the client's shoulder blades (Figure 23–26 *A*).
- **c** Have the client lean forward.
- **d** Brace your knees against the client's knees. Block his or her feet with your feet.
- **e** Tell the client to push down on the mattress and to stand on the count of three. Pull the client up into a standing position as you straighten your hips and legs. Keep your knees slightly flexed.

17 Support the client in the standing position. Hold the transfer belt, or keep your hands around the person's shoulder blades. Continue to block the client's feet and knees with your feet and knees.
18 Pivot on your foot and turn the client so that he or she can grasp the far arm of the chair. The client's legs will touch the edge of the chair (Figure 23–26, *B*).
19 Continue to turn the client until he or she grasps the other arm rest.
20 Lower the client into the chair as you bend your hips and knees. Keep your back straight, with your lumbar area curved. The client assists by leaning forward and bending the elbows and knees (Figure 23–26, *C*).
21 Make sure the client's buttocks are to the back of the seat. Position the client in good alignment.
22 Position the client's feet on the wheelchair foot rests.
23 Cover the client's lap and legs with a bath blanket. Keep the blanket off the floor and the wheels.
24 Remove the transfer belt, if it was used.
25 Position the chair as the client prefers. Lock the wheelchair wheels.

(continued on page 417)

1 2 3 TRANSFERRING THE CLIENT TO A CHAIR OR WHEELCHAIR

Post-Procedure

26 Provide for safety and comfort.
27 Place the call bell within reach.*
28 Remove privacy measures.
29 Perform hand hygiene.
30 Report and record your actions and observations, according to employer policy.
31 Reverse the procedure to return the client to bed.

*Steps marked with an asterisk may not apply in community settings.

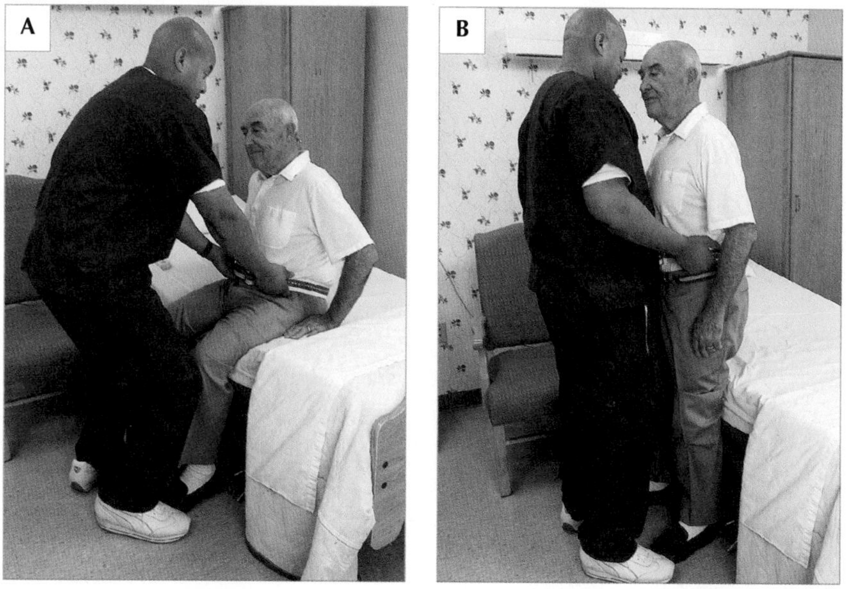

Figure 23–25 Transferring a client to a chair (or wheelchair) using a transfer belt. Position the chair next to and aligned with the headboard. **A,** Prevent the client from sliding or falling by blocking the client's knees and feet with your knees and feet. **B,** Pull the client up to a standing position. Support the client by holding the transfer belt and blocking the client's knees and feet.

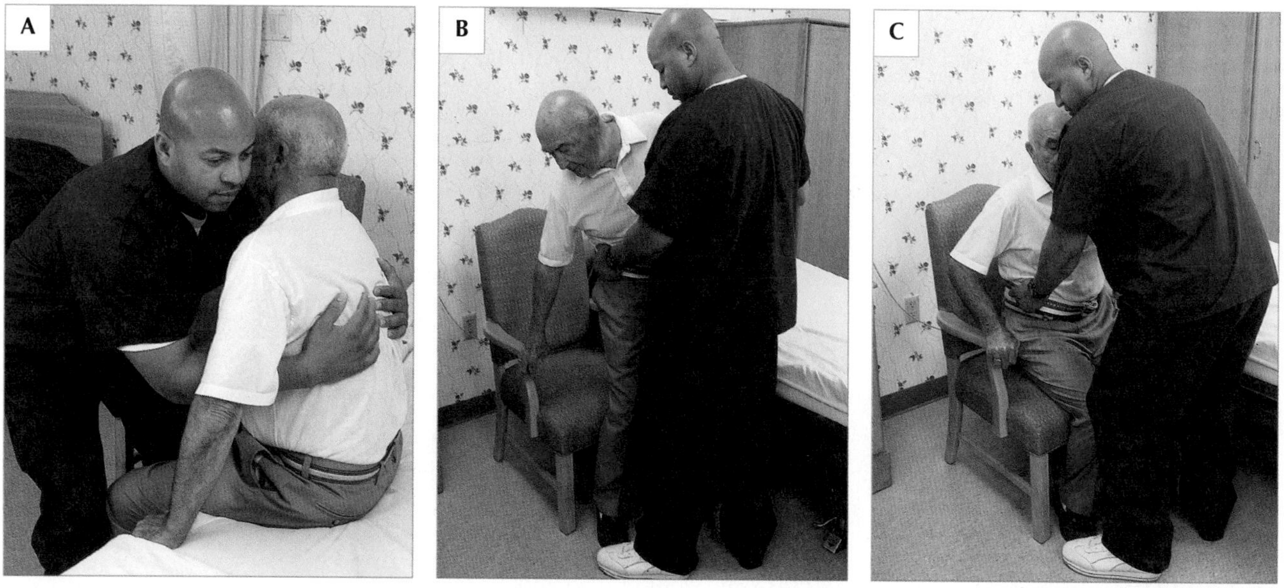

Figure 23–26 Transferring a client to a chair (or wheelchair) without a transfer belt. **A,** Place your hands under the client's arms and around the shoulder blades. Bend carefully, using your knees and maintaining your lumbar curve in your back. **B,** Support the client as he or she grasps the far arm of the chair. The client's legs are against the chair. **C,** Lower the client into the chair while the client holds onto the arm rests, leans forward, and bends the elbows and knees.

Other Transfers

The basic transfer from a bed to a chair or wheelchair can be modified for other situations. You can transfer a client from a wheelchair to a shower or bath chair. You can also transfer a client to and from a toilet. Carefully consider how to proceed. It is your responsibility to check first with your supervisor and the care plan to determine the client's physical abilities and limitations. Also, consider the client's environment. How much space do you have to move about? Are there assistive devices, such as grab bars or slider boards? Use good body mechanics, and apply the general safety and comfort rules.

1 2 3 TRANSFERRING THE CLIENT FROM A WHEELCHAIR TO A SHOWER (OR BATH) CHAIR

Remember to promote:

• Dignity • Independence • Preferences • Privacy • Safety

Pre-Procedure

1 Identify the client, according to employer policy.
2 Explain the procedure to the client.
3 Collect the necessary equipment, such as:
- Shower or bath chair
- Bath blanket
- Towel
- Transfer belt, if used

4 Perform hand hygiene.
5 Provide for privacy.
6 Check that the shower chair is securely positioned and locked in place. Do not transfer the client if the shower chair is not secure.
7 Check the grab bars near the shower. If they are loose, report it to your supervisor. Do not transfer the client if the grab bars are not secure.

Procedure

8 Position the wheelchair at a 90-degree angle to the shower chair. The client's strong side is near the shower chair.
9 Lock the wheelchair wheels.
10 Raise the foot rests. Remove or swing them out of the way.
11 Prepare the water.
12 Apply the transfer belt, if used.
13 Help the client stand and turn to the shower chair (see *Transferring the Client to a Chair or Wheelchair*, page 416, steps 16 and 17.) The client uses the grab bars or shower chair arm rests for support.
14 Support the client while he or she undresses. Hold the transfer belt, or keep your hands around the client's shoulder blades. Continue to block the client's feet and knees with your feet and knees. Instruct the client to hold onto the grab bars or arm rests for support. Undress the client.
15 Lower the client onto the shower chair.
16 Remove the transfer belt, if it was used.

Post-Procedure

17 Help the client dry off after the shower. Cover the client with a bath blanket.
18 Reverse the procedure to transfer the client from the shower chair to the wheelchair.
19 Help the client put on clean clothing.
20 Perform hand hygiene.
21 Report and record your actions and observations, according to employer policy.

*Steps marked with an asterisk may not apply in community settings.

1 2 3 **TRANSFERRING THE CLIENT TO AND FROM THE TOILET SEAT**

Remember to promote:

• Dignity • Independence • Preferences • Privacy • Safety

Pre-Procedure

1 Explain the procedure to the client.
2 Perform hand hygiene.
3 Provide for privacy.
4 Make sure the client has an elevated toilet seat so that the toilet seat and wheelchair are at the same level.
5 Check the grab bars near the toilet. If they are loose, tell your supervisor. Do not transfer the client to the toilet if the grab bars are not secure.

Procedure

6 Have the client wear nonskid footwear.
7 Position the wheelchair next to the toilet if there is enough room. If not, position the wheelchair at a right angle to the toilet (Figure 23–27). It is best if the client's strong side is near the toilet.
8 Lock the wheelchair wheels.
9 Raise the foot rests. Remove or swing them out of the way.
10 Apply the transfer belt, if used.
11 Help the client unfasten clothing.
12 Help the client stand and turn to the toilet (see *Transferring the Client to a Chair or Wheelchair,* page 416, steps 16 and 17). Have the client use the grab bars to turn toward the toilet.
13 Support the client while he or she lowers clothing. Hold the transfer belt, or keep your hands around the client's shoulder blades. Continue to block the client's feet and knees with your feet and knees. Have the client hold onto the grab bars for support. Lower the client's pants and undergarments.
14 Lower the client onto the toilet seat.
15 Remove the transfer belt, if used.
16 Tell the client that you will stay close by and to use the call bell (in facilities) or to call for you when help is needed. ***(Because of their increased risk for falling, some clients must have someone stay right by their side while they are toileting. Check with your supervisor if you are unsure!)***
17 Close the bathroom door to provide for privacy.
18 Stay near the bathroom. In the meanwhile, you may complete other tasks in the client's room.
19 Knock on the bathroom door when the client calls for you.
20 Help with wiping, perineal care, flushing, and hand washing, as needed. Wear gloves for this step.
21 Apply the transfer belt, if used.
22 Help the client stand, and support the client in the standing position. Hold the transfer belt, or keep your hands around the client's shoulder blades. Continue to block the client's feet and knees with your feet and knees.
23 Help the client pull up and secure his or her clothing.
24 Transfer the client to the wheelchair (see *Transferring the Client to a Chair or Wheelchair,* page 416, steps 19 through 26.)

Post-Procedure

25 Provide for safety and comfort.
26 Place the call bell within reach.*
27 Perform hand hygiene.
28 Report and record your actions and observations, according to employer policy.

*Steps marked with an asterisk may not apply in community settings.

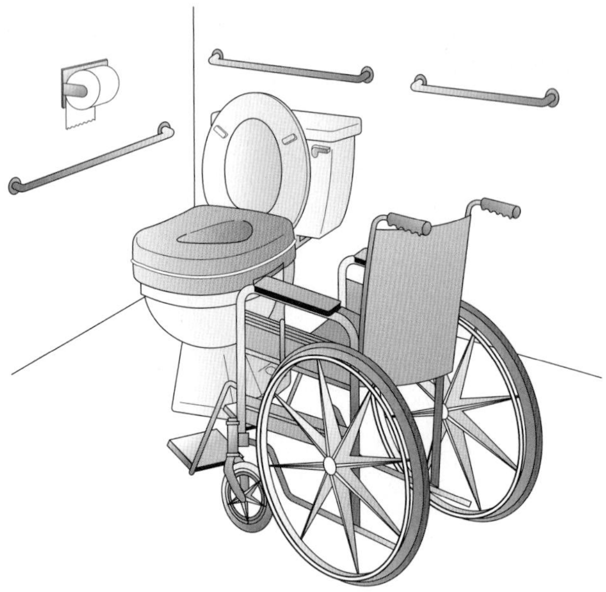

Figure 23–27 Position the wheelchair at right angle to the toilet.

LIFTING A CLIENT

Some clients need to be lifted when they cannot help with a transfer by weight-bearing. **Lifts** are used to physically move a client from one place to another, such as for moving them to chairs, stretchers, tubs, shower chairs, toilets, whirlpools, and vehicles. Because of the serious risk of back injury to the staff, most long-term care agencies no longer allow them to manually lift clients and have a strict "no-lift" policy.

Manual Lifts

When working in the home care sector, you might be responsible for lifting a client (**manual lift**), with the assistance of a family member. You must always check your agency's policies regarding lifts *before* going into a client's home. Before assisting with manual lifts, be certain that you do not have on any jewellery that might injure yourself or the client, that your shoelaces are tied, and you have done back-stretching exercises in order to reduce your risk for injury.

There are many reasons why clients may need to be lifted manually. With children, because of their small size, a mechanical lift may not be necessary. Other client's homes are too small for a mechanical lift to be manoeuvred around safely. In other situations, the client and his or her family may not be able to afford to rent or purchase a mechanical lift.

It is your responsibility to review the methods to manually or mechanically lift a client. By following these procedures—and following the guidelines of your agency—you can avoid injuring yourself or your client.

Mechanically Lifting a Client

There are many different kinds of mechanical lifts—mechanical and electric. Knowing how to use one type of lift does not mean that you know how to use others. Always follow the manufacturer's instructions. Employers usually provide special training for the use of mechanical lifts. You may also be required to take yearly refresher courses to keep your skills current. If you have questions, ask your supervisor. ***If you have not used a certain type of lift before, it is your responsibility to ask your supervisor to show you how to use it safely.***

Before using a lift:

- Make sure you are trained in its use.
- Make sure the lift works.
- Compare the client's weight and the lift's weight limit. Do not use the lift if a client's weight exceeds the lift's capacity.
- At least two people are usually needed to work a mechanical lift. Get a co-worker or a trained family member to help you.

1 2 3 MANUALLY LIFTING AND REPOSITIONING A CLIENT INTO A WHEELCHAIR WITH ASSISTANCE

These steps are lifts and should never be attempted if you work at an agency that has a "no-lift" policy. It is always preferred that you use a lift if there is ever a risk of injuring yourself or the client!

Remember to promote:

- Dignity • Independence • Preferences • Privacy • Safety

Pre-Procedure

1 Identify the client, according to employer policy.
2 Ask someone to help you.
3 Explain the procedure to the client.
4 Collect:
- Wheelchair with removable arm rests
- Bath blankets
- Footwear
- Cushion, if used

5 Perform hand hygiene.
6 Provide for privacy.
7 Decide which side of the bed to use. Move furniture away to provide space to move.

Procedure

8 ***Lifting into a wheelchair***
- **a** Ask for a trained family member or co-worker to help you. Decide who is taller, you or your helper. The taller person will stand behind the wheelchair and the other in front of the client.
- **b** Place the wheelchair at the side of the bed, aligned with the client's hips. Place a folded bath blanket or cushion on the seat.
- **c** Remove the wheelchair's arm rest that is near the bed.
- **d** Lock wheelchair wheels, and raise or remove the foot rest.
- **e** Make sure the bed is in its lowest position and bed wheels are locked. Lower the bed rail, if it is up.*
- **f** Fanfold top linens to the foot of the bed.
- **g** Help the client to the side of the bed near you. Help him or her to a sitting position by raising the head of the bed or using pillows for support.
- **h** Stand behind wheelchair, facing the client. Stand so your feet are shoulder-width apart. Flex your knees. Put your arms under the client's arms and grasp the client's forearms (Figure 23–28, *A*).
- **i** Have your helper grasp the client's thighs and calves (Figure 23–28, *B*).
- **j** Bring the client toward the chair on the count of three. Lower him or her into the chair (Figure 23–28, *C*).
- **k** Make sure the client's buttocks are to the back of the seat. Position the client in good alignment.

9 ***Lifting and repositioning the client in a wheelchair*** (Figure 23–29).
Use this method if the client cannot assist with repositioning and a helper is needed:
- **a** Lock the wheelchair wheels.
- **b** Apply a transfer belt.
- **c** Ask the client to place folded hands in his or her lap.
- **d** The taller person stands behind the wheelchair and grasps the transfer belt on each side.
- **e** The other person stands in front of the client. The hands and arms are placed under the client's knees.
- **f** On the count of three, lift the client to the back of the chair. The person in front supports the legs, while the person at the back uses the transfer belt.

10 Put the arm rest and foot rest back on the wheelchair.
11 Put the footwear on the client. Position the client's feet on the foot rest.
12 Cover the client's lap and legs with a blanket. Keep the blanket off the floor and wheels.
13 Position the chair as the client prefers. Lock the wheelchair wheels.

Post-Procedure

14 Follow steps 27 through 32 of *Transferring the Client to a Chair or Wheelchair*, page 416.

*Steps marked with an asterisk may not apply in community settings.

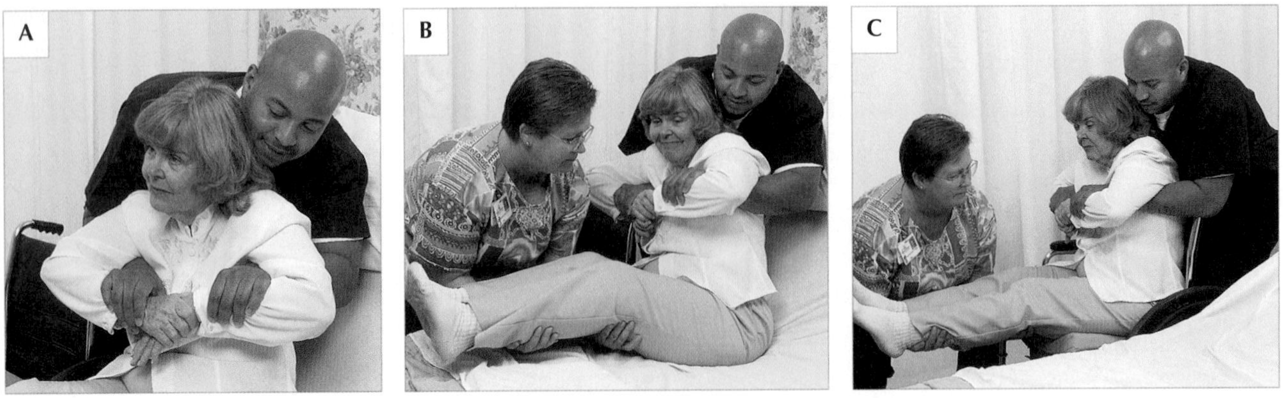

Figure 23–28 Transferring a client to a wheelchair, with assistance. **A,** Put your arms under the client's arms and grasp the client's forearms. **B,** Your helper holds the client's thighs and calves to support the legs during the transfer. **C,** Lower the client into the chair. *Note:* This procedure involves lifting the client. Make sure the person does not weigh more than you can safely lift. Some employers have a "no lift" policy. Know your employer policy before attempting this transfer.

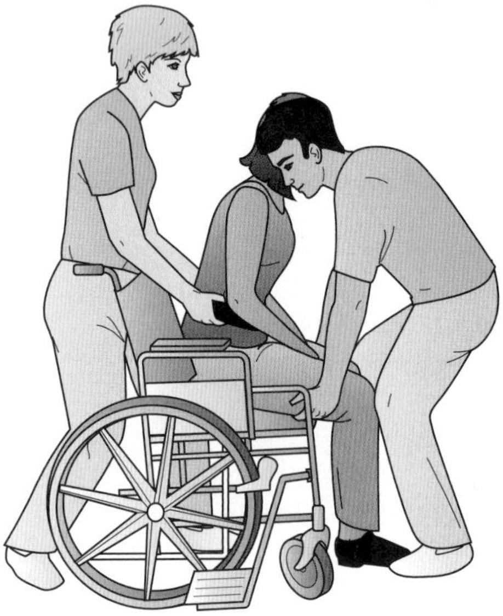

Figure 23–29 Two people (the support worker and a helper) lifting the client to reposition her in a wheelchair. The taller person stands behind the chair and lifts with the transfer belt. The other person stands in front of the client. Hands and arms are under the client's knees to support the legs during repositioning. Back should maintain its natural lumbar curve. *Note:* This procedure involves lifting the client. Make sure the person does not weigh more than you can safely lift. Some employers have a "no-lift" policy. Know your employer policy before attempting this transfer.

supporting MRS. QUOUONG

You have recently been hired as a support worker, and today is your first full day working alongside the staff. You have learned in your orientation that there are signs posted over each client's bed, stating the type of lift or transfer that they require. This agency has a strict "no-lift" policy. You have been told that at this agency, you should never manually lift anybody or anything over 23 kg (50.6 lb). During your morning care rounds, you and Rosie, the support worker you are working with, enter the room of Mrs. Quouong.

Mrs. Quouong, a 90-year-old resident, is very small, weighing only 36 kg (80 lb), and has very swollen ankles. Over her bed is a sign that indicates that she must be moved using a mechanical lift. Rosie closes the door to Mrs. Quouong's room and tells you to help her manually lift Mrs. Quouong. Rosie explains that it is easier and faster to manually move Mrs. Quouong than it is to move her mechanically. Besides, she explains, Mrs. Quouong is so small that if the two of you lifted her together, each of you would only be lifting 18 kg. Rosie tells you that for these reasons all the staff usually manually lift Mrs. Quouong. You are unsure about what you should do.

1 2 3 USING A MECHANICAL LIFT TO MOVE A CLIENT

The following procedure is a general guideline only. The mechanical lift that you are using may be different and may require different actions. Check with your employer to see what your responsibilities are.

Remember to promote:

- Dignity • Independence • Preferences • Privacy • Safety

Pre-Procedure

1 Identify the client, according to employer policy.
2 Ask someone to help you.
3 Explain the procedure to the client.
4 Collect:
- Mechanical lift
- Arm chair or wheelchair
- Footwear
- Bath blanket or cushion

5 Perform hand hygiene.
6 Provide for privacy.

Procedure

7 Put the footwear on the client. Centre the sling under the client (Figure 23–30, *A*). Turn the client from side to side—as if making an occupied bed—to position the sling (see Chapter 26). Position the sling according to the manufacturer's instructions.
8 Place the chair at the head of the bed. It should be aligned with the headboard and about 30 cm (1 ft) away from the bed. Place a folded bath blanket or cushion in the chair, if needed.
9 Lock the bed wheels, and lower the bed to its lowest position.*
10 Raise the lift so that it can be positioned over the client.
11 Position the lift over the client (Figure 23–30, *B*).
12 Lock the lift wheels in position.
13 Attach the sling to the swivel bar (Figure 23–30, *C*).
14 Assist the client to the sitting position. Raise the head of the bed or use pillows for support.
15 Cross the client's arms over the chest. Let him or her hold onto the straps or chains, but not to the swivel bar.
16 Raise the lift high enough until the client and sling are free of the bed (Figure 23–30, *D*).
17 Ask your helper to support the client's legs as you move the lift and client away from the bed (Figure 23–30, *E*).
18 Position the lift so that the client's back is toward the chair.
19 Position the chair so that you can lower the client into it.
20 Lower the client into the chair (follow manufacturer's instructions). Guide the client into the chair (Figure 23–30, *F*).
21 Lower the swivel bar to unhook the sling. Remove the sling from under the client, unless instructed otherwise.
22 Position the client's feet on the wheelchair foot rest.
23 Cover the client's lap and legs with a blanket. Keep the blanket off the floor and wheels.
24 Position the chair as the client prefers. Lock the wheelchair wheels.

Post-Procedure

25 Provide for safety and comfort.
26 Place the call bell within reach.*
27 Perform hand hygiene.
28 Report and record your actions and observations, according to employer policy.
29 Reverse the procedure to return the client to bed.

*Steps marked with an asterisk may not apply in community settings.

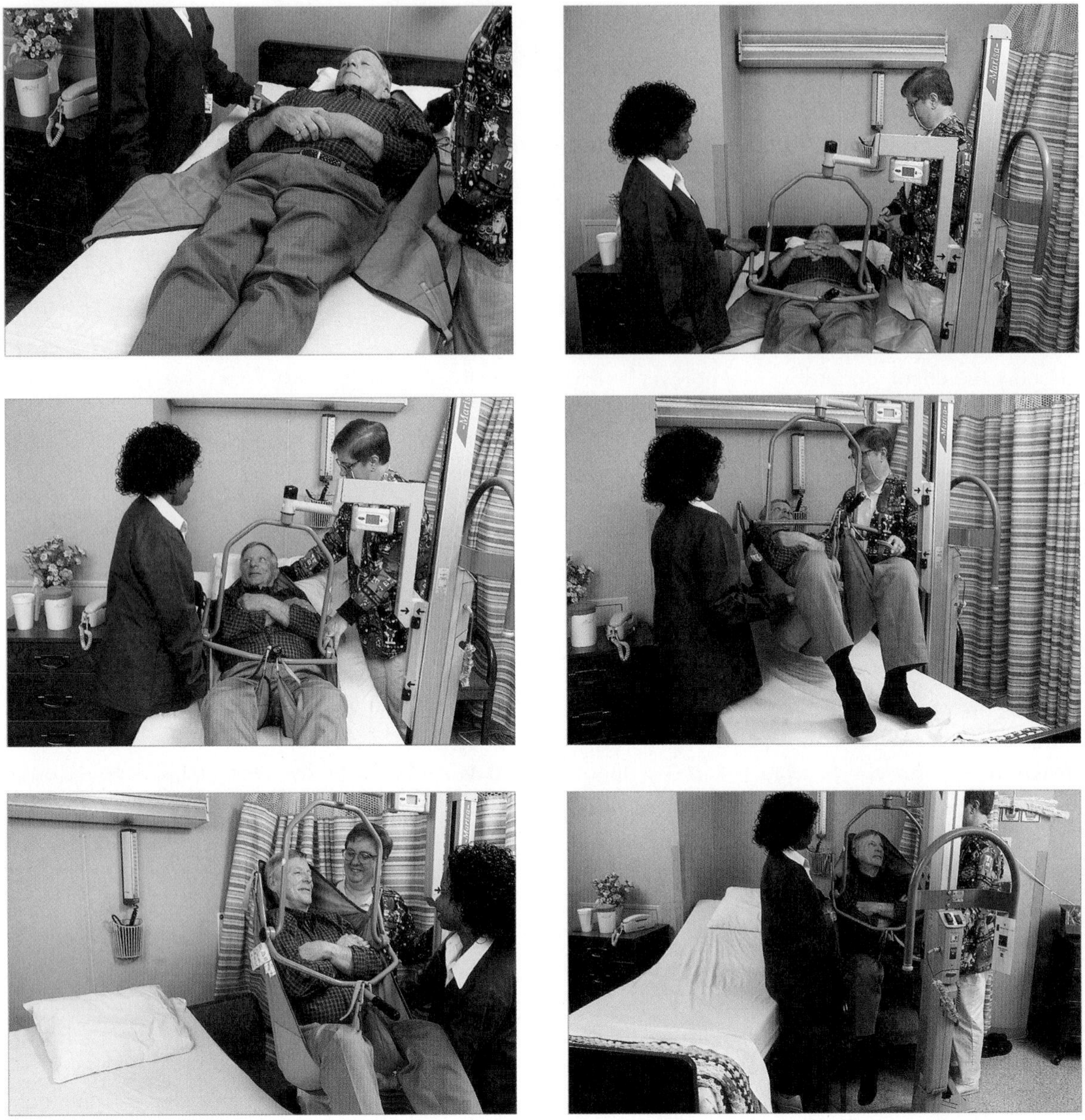

A B C D E F

Figure 23–30 Using a mechanical lift. **A,** Position the sling under the client according to manufacturer's instructions. **B,** Position the lift over the client. The lift's legs are spread to widen the base of support. **C,** Attach the sling to the swivel bar. **D,** Raise the lift until the sling and client are off the bed. **E,** Your helper supports the client's legs as you move the lift and client away from the bed. **F,** Guide the client into the chair.

REVIEW

Answers to these questions are at the bottom of page 426.

Circle T if the answer is true or circle F if the answer is false.

1. T F **Body mechanics refer to the way in which body parts are positioned in relation to one another.**
2. T F **Good body mechanics help protect you and the client from injury.**
3. T F **Body mechanics involve the use of small muscles.**
4. T F **Base of support is the area on which an object rests.**
5. T F **You should keep objects far away from the body when lifting, moving, or carrying them.**
6. T F **You should face the direction you are working in to prevent unnecessary twisting.**
7. T F **You should push, slide, or pull heavy objects rather than lift them.**
8. T F **Sliding the client reduces friction and shearing.**
9. T F **You should ask your supervisor about limits or restrictions in positioning or moving a client.**
10. T F **The right to privacy should be protected when you are moving, lifting, or transferring clients.**
11. T F **A lift sheet should extend from below the shoulders to above the knees.**
12. T F **A client should be moved to the side of the bed before being turned to the side-lying position.**
13. T F **Log-rolling is rolling the client in segments.**
14. T F **Clients with spinal cord injuries are log-rolled.**
15. T F **Repositioning prevents deformities and pressure on body parts.**
16. T F **The head of the bed is elevated 45 to 60 degrees for the supine position.**
17. T F **The Sims' position is the left side-lying position.**
18. T F **A transfer belt is part of a mechanical lift.**
19. T F **A client is being transferred from the bed to a chair. He needs nonskid footwear.**
20. T F **You are going to transfer a client from the bed to a chair. You should move her from the direction of the weak side of her body.**

Circle the BEST answer.

21. **Good body alignment means:**
    - A. The area on which an object rests
    - B. Having the head, trunk, arms, and legs aligned with one another
    - C. Using muscles, tendons, ligaments, joints, and cartilage correctly
    - D. The back-lying or supine position
22. **Support workers are at great risk for:**
    - A. Friction and shearing
    - B. Arm and hand injuries
    - C. Back injuries
    - D. Falls
23. **A client's skin rubs against the sheet. This is called:**
    - A. Shearing
    - B. Friction
    - C. Transferring
    - D. Posture
24. **Clients who are immobile must be repositioned at least every:**
    - A. 30 minutes
    - B. 1 hour
    - C. 2 hours
    - D. 3 hours

REVIEW

Answers to these questions are at the bottom of the page.

25. **The back-lying position is called:**
   - A. Fowler's position
   - B. The supine position
   - C. The prone position
   - D. Sims' position

26. **A client is positioned in a chair. The feet:**
   - A. Must be flat on the floor
   - B. Are crossed
   - C. Dangle
   - D. Must be positioned on pillows

27. **When transferring a client to bed, a chair, or the toilet:**
   - A. The client's strong side is moved first
   - B. The weak side is moved first
   - C. Pillows are used for support
   - D. The transfer belt cannot be used

28. **These statements are about transfers to and from a toilet. Which is *false*?**
   - A. The client wears nonskid footwear.
   - B. Wheelchair brakes must be locked.
   - C. The wheelchair is positioned so that the client's strong side is near the toilet.
   - D. The client uses the towel bars for support.

Answers: 1.F, 2.T, 3.F, 4.T, 5.F, 6.T, 7.T, 8.F, 9.T, 10.T, 11.F, 12.T, 13.F, 14.T, 15.T, 16.F, 17.T, 18.F, 19.T, 20.F, 21.B, 22.C, 23.B, 24.C, 25.B, 26.A, 27.A, 28.D

CHAPTER 24

Exercise and Activity

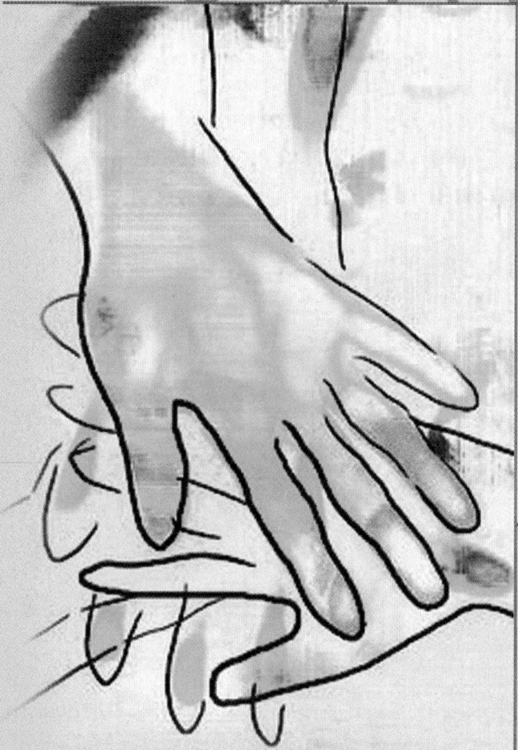

OBJECTIVES

- Define the key terms listed in this chapter.
- Describe bed rest.
- Describe the complications of bed rest and how to prevent them.
- Describe the devices used to support and maintain body alignment.
- Describe the purpose of a trapeze.
- Describe range-of-motion exercises.
- Describe how to help a falling client.
- Describe four walking aids.
- Perform the procedures described in this chapter.

key terms

abduction Moving a body part away from the midline of the body.

adduction Moving a body part toward the midline of the body.

ambulation The act of walking.

atrophy A decrease in size or a wasting away of tissue.

brace An apparatus worn to support or align weak body parts or to prevent or correct problems with the musculo-skeletal system; **orthosis**.

contracture The lack of joint mobility caused by abnormal shortening of a muscle.

deconditioning The loss of muscle strength from inactivity.

dorsiflexion Bending the toes and foot up at the ankle.

extension Straightening a body part.

external rotation Turning the joint outward.

flexion Bending a body part.

footdrop The foot falls down at the ankle (permanent **plantar flexion**).

hyperextension Excessive straightening of a body part.

internal rotation Turning the joint inward.

muscle atrophy A decrease in size or a wasting away of muscle.

orthosis A brace.

orthostatic hypotension A drop in (*hypo*) blood pressure when the client stands up (*ortho* and *static*). Also known as **postural hypotension**.

plantar flexion The foot (*plantar*) is bent (*flexion*) with the toes pointed away from the leg.

postural hypotension See **orthostatic hypotension**.

pronation Turning downward.

range of motion (ROM) Moving a joint to the extent possible without causing pain.

rotation Turning the joint.

supination Turning upward.

syncope A brief loss of consciousness; fainting.

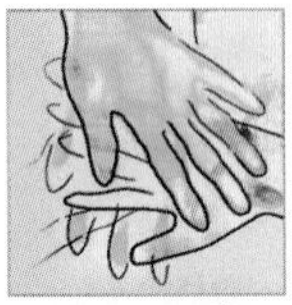

Being active is important for physical and mental well-being. Most people move about and function without help, but illnesses, surgery, injuries, pain, and aging can cause weakness and limit some activity. Some clients are weakened by chronic illnesses, and some others are confined to their beds for a long time. Some clients have permanent paralysis. Some disorders are progressive, causing decreases in activity, for example, multiple sclerosis, Parkinson's disease, arthritis, and muscular disorders (see Chapter 18). Inactivity, whether mild or severe, affects not only the normal functions of all body systems but also the client's mental well-being.

Deconditioning is the loss of muscle strength from inactivity. Whoever your clients may be—infants to older adults—deconditioning can occur at any age; however, older clients become deconditioned more quickly. So each client must be encouraged to be as active as possible. The care plan tells you about the client's activity level and what exercises to perform. Always check with your supervisor what bed rest means for each client.

To help promote exercise and activity, you need to understand:

- Bed rest
- How to prevent complications from bed rest
- How to help clients exercise

BED REST

Bed rest is ordered by the physician to treat a health problem and often to:

- Reduce physical activity
- Reduce pain
- Encourage rest
- Regain strength
- Promote healing

You must know what activities are allowed for each client, as specified in the care plan. Check with your supervisor if you have questions. The following types of bed rest are common:

- *Bed rest*—some activities of daily living (ADLs) are allowed—such as self-feeding, oral hygiene, bathing, shaving, and hair care
- *Strict bed rest*—everything is done for the client. No ADLs are allowed, except use of the bed pan/urinal, if client is continent
- *Bed rest with commode privileges*—the client can use the bedside commode for elimination needs
- *Bed rest with bathroom privileges (bed rest with BRP)*—the client can use the bathroom for elimination needs

Always ask your supervisor what bed rest means for each client.

Complications of Bed Rest

Long-term bed rest and lack of exercise and activity can cause serious complications, affecting every system in the body. Pressure ulcers, constipation, fecal impaction, urinary tract infections, renal calculi (kidney stones), blood clots (thrombi), and pneumonia (infection of the lung) can occur (see Chapter 18).

Contractures and muscle atrophy occur in the musculo-skeletal system. A **contracture** is the lack of joint mobility caused by the abnormal shortening of a muscle. The contracted muscle is fixed into position, is deformed, and cannot stretch (Figure 24–1). Common sites are the fingers, wrists, elbows, toes, ankles, knees, and hips. Contractures can also occur in the neck and spine. The person with a contracture is permanently deformed and disabled. **Atrophy** is the decrease in size or the wasting away of tissue. **Muscle atrophy** is a decrease in size or a wasting away of muscle (Figure 24–2). These complications from lack of activity must be prevented to maintain normal body movement.

Orthostatic hypotension and blood clots (see Chapter 46) occur in the cardiovascular system. **Orthostatic hypotension** (or **postural hypotension**) is a drop in (*hypo*) blood pressure when the client stands up (*ortho* and *static*). When he or she moves from lying or sitting to a standing position, the blood pressure drops, and the client experiences dizziness, weakness, and spots before the eyes, followed by **syncope** (fainting), which is a brief loss of consciousness. Box 24–1 lists the measures that prevent orthostatic hypotension, such as changing positions slowly.

You can help prevent complications from bed rest by providing good care. Make sure the client is in good body alignment. Reposition the client at least once every 2 hours, following the care plan (see Chapter 23). Also, help with range-of-motion (ROM) exercises, according to the care plan (see page 432).

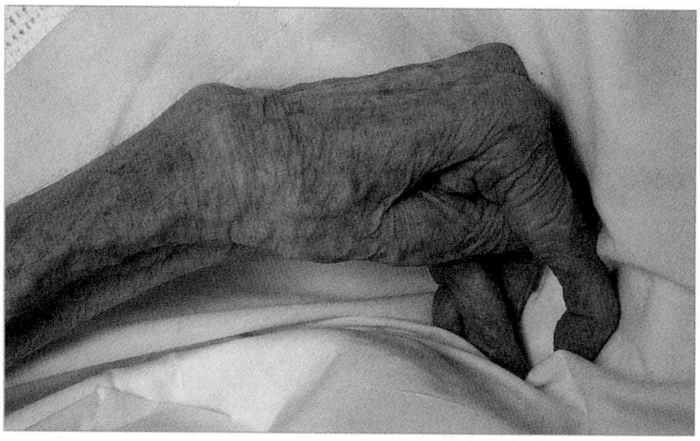

Figure 24–1 A contracture.

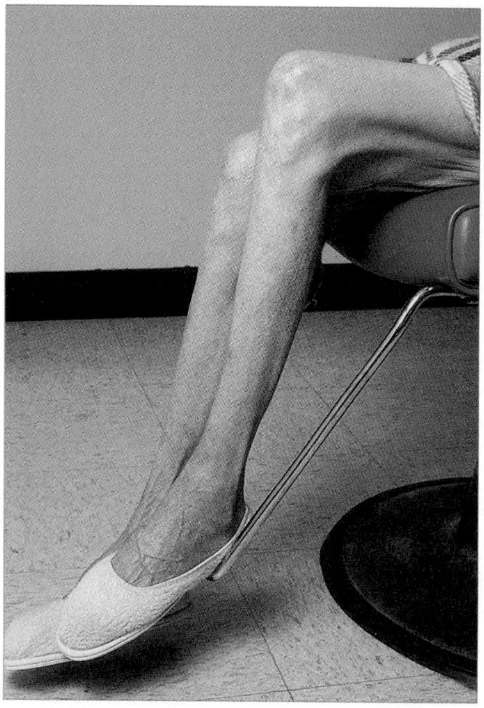

Figure 24–2 Muscle atrophy.

Box 24–1 Preventing Orthostatic Hypotension When Helping a Client From a Lying Position to a Standing Position

- Measure blood pressure, pulse, and respirations when the client is supine.*
- Position the client in Fowler's position. Raise the head of the bed slowly. If the bed cannot be raised, use pillows and backrests for positioning.
  - Ask the client if there is any weakness, dizziness, or spots before the eyes. Lower the head of the bed back to a flat position or remove the backrest if these symptoms occur.
  - Measure blood pressure, pulse, and respirations.*
  - Keep the client in Fowler's position for a short while. Ask the client if there is any weakness, dizziness, or spots before the eyes.
- Help the client to sit on the side of the bed with feet dangling over the edge (see Chapter 23).
  - Ask the client if there is any weakness, dizziness, or spots before the eyes. Assist the client to Fowler's position if any of these symptoms occur.
  - Measure blood pressure, pulse, and respirations.*
  - Have the client continue to sit on the side of the bed for a short while.
- Help the client to stand up. Stay close to the client, and use good body mechanics.
  - Ask the client if there is any weakness, dizziness, or spots before the eyes. Help the client sit on the side of the bed if any of these symptoms occur.
  - Measure blood pressure, pulse, and respirations.*
- Help the client sit in a chair or walk, as directed by the care plan.
  - Ask the client if there is any weakness, dizziness, or spots before the eyes. If the client is walking, help the client sit down if symptoms occur.
  - Measure blood pressure, pulse, and respirations.*
- Report measurements of blood pressure, pulse, and respirations to your supervisor.* Report other observations or complaints as well.

*Measure blood pressure, pulse, and respirations only if instructed (and allowed) to do so. Know your scope of practice and employer policy.

Positioning

Body alignment and positioning are discussed in detail in Chapter 23. Supportive devices are often used to support and maintain the client in a certain position:

- ***Bed boards***—are placed under the mattress (Figure 24–3) to prevent the mattress from sagging. They are usually made of plywood and are covered with canvas or other material. The two sections of the bed boards help raise the head of the bed and the foot of the bed.
- ***Foot boards***—are placed at the foot of mattresses (Figure 24–4) to prevent plantar flexion that can lead to footdrop. In **plantar flexion,** the foot *(plantar)* is bent *(flexion)* with the toes pointed away from the leg. **Footdrop** occurs when the foot falls down at the ankle (permanent plantar flexion). The foot board is placed in such a way that the soles of the feet are flush against it, and the feet are in good alignment as in the standing position. Foot boards also serve as bed cradles and keep top linens off the feet.
- ***Trochanter rolls***—prevent the hips and legs from turning outward (external rotation) (Figure 24–5). They are made by folding bath blankets to the desired length and rolling them up. The loose end is placed under the client, from hip to knee, and the roll is tucked alongside the body. Pillows or sandbags also are used to keep the hips and knees in alignment.
- ***Hand rolls or hand grips***—prevent contractures of the thumb, fingers, and wrist. Commercial hand rolls are commonly available (Figure 24–6). Foam rubber sponges, rubber balls, and finger cushions (Figure 24–7) also are used.
- ***Splints***—keep the wrist, thumb, and fingers in normal position. They are usually secured in place with Velcro. Some have foam padding (Figure 24–8).
- ***Bed cradles***—keep the weight of top linens off the feet (see Figures 42–5 and 42–6 on page 805). The weight of top linens can cause footdrop and pressure ulcers.

A

B

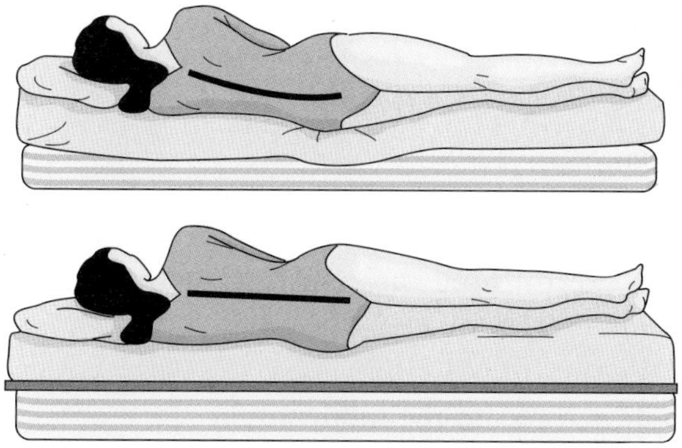

Figure 24–3 A, Mattress is sagging without bed boards. **B,** Bed boards are placed under the mattress, and there is no sagging.

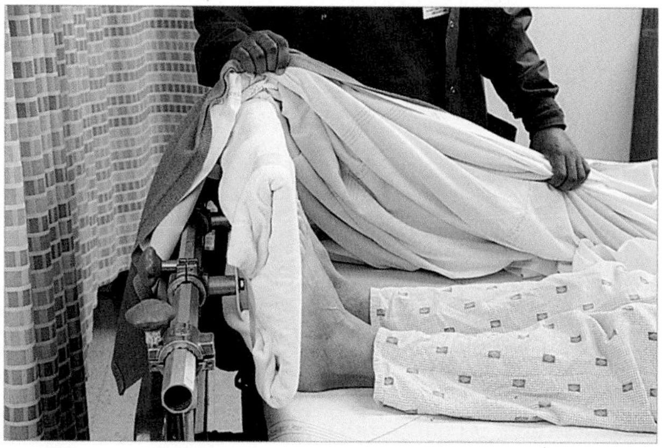

Figure 24–4 Foot board. Feet are flush against the board to keep them in normal alignment.

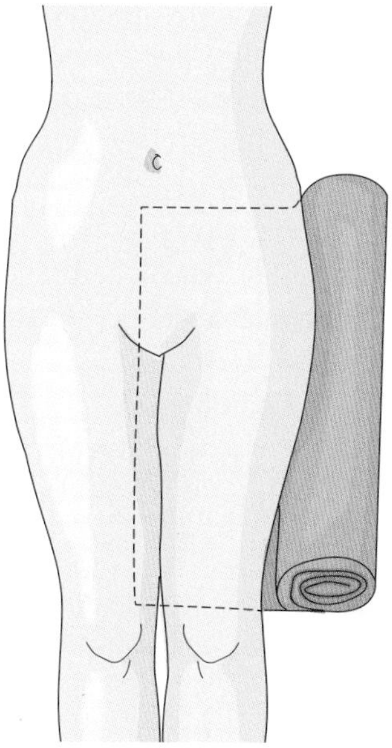

Figure 24–5 Trochanter roll made using a bath blanket. It extends from the client's hip to the knee.

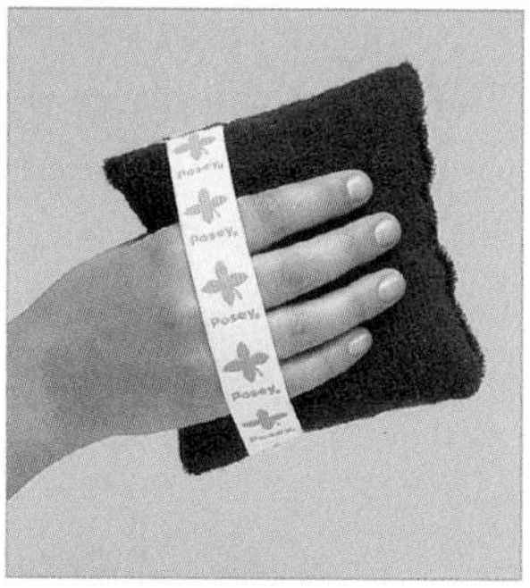

Figure 24–6 Hand grip. **Courtesy:** J.T. Posey Company, Arcadia, CA.

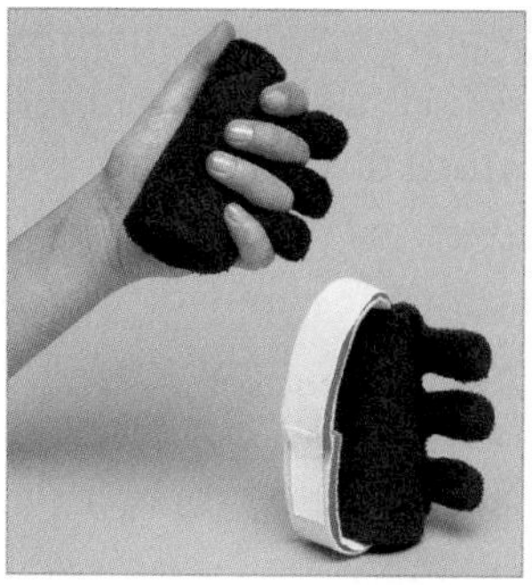

Figure 24–7 Finger cushion. **Courtesy:** J.T. Posey Company, Arcadia, CA.

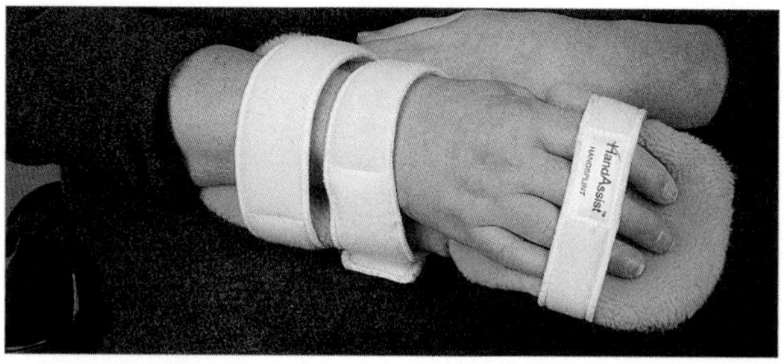

Figure 24–8 Splint.

Exercise

Exercise helps prevent contractures, muscle atrophy, and other complications of bed rest. Some exercise occurs with activities of daily living and from turning and moving in bed without assistance. However, additional exercises are needed for muscles and joints.

A trapeze is used for exercises to strengthen arm muscles. The trapeze is suspended from an overbed frame (Figure 24–9). The client grasps the bar with both hands to lift the trunk off the bed. The client can also use the trapeze to move up and turn in bed (see Chapter 23).

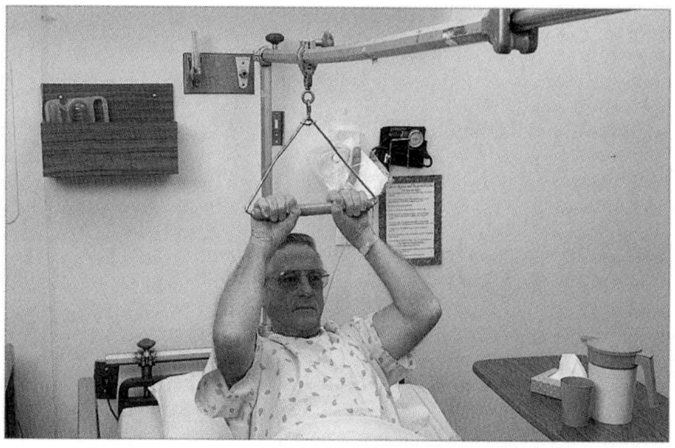

Figure 24–9 A trapeze is used to strengthen the arm muscles.

Range-of-Motion Exercises. Moving a joint to the extent possible without causing pain is the **range of motion (ROM)** of that joint. Range-of-motion exercises involve exercising the joints through their complete range of motion (see Box 24–2). Clients who need these exercises usually do them at least twice a day. Range-of-motion exercises are active, passive, or active-assistive:

- ***Active*** **ROM** exercises are done by the client independently.
- ***Passive*** **ROM** exercises involve having another person move the joints of the client through their range of motion.
- ***Active-assistive*** **ROM** exercises are done by the client with some help from another person.

Range-of-motion exercises occur naturally during activities of daily living—such as bathing, hair care, eating, reaching, and walking—all of which involve joint movements. Clients on bed rest and clients who have mobility loss from illness or injury, however, get very little activity. Therefore, their care plans usually call for ROM exercises. The care plan tells you which joints to exercise and whether the exercises are to be active, passive, or active-assistive. If you have questions, ask your supervisor (see the *Focus on Children: Play* and *Focus on Long-Term Care: Activity Programs* boxes.)

Range-of-motion exercises can cause injury, such as muscle strain, joint injury, and pain, if not done properly. Follow the guidelines in Box 24–3 when performing or assisting with range-of-motion exercises.

After performing ROM exercises with the client, report and record the following:

- The time the exercises were performed
- The joints exercised
- The number of times the exercises were performed on each joint
- Complaints of pain or signs of stiffness or spasm
- The degree to which the client took part in the exercises

Box 24–2 Joint Movements

Abduction—moving a body part away from the midline of the body
Adduction—moving a body part toward the midline of the body
Extension—straightening a body part
Flexion—bending a body part
Hyperextension—excessive straightening of a body part
Dorsiflexion—bending the toes and foot up at the ankle
Rotation—turning the joint
Internal rotation—turning the joint inward
External rotation—turning the joint outward
Plantar flexion—bending the foot down at the ankle
Pronation—turning downward
Supination—turning upward

focus on ›› CHILDREN

Play

Depending on the child's activity limits, any play activity promotes active ROM exercises in children. Some examples are:

- Kicking a Mylar balloon or foam rubber ball
- Playing "pat-a-cake" and having the child clap, kick, jump, or do other motions
- Playing basketball using a wastebasket and a foam rubber ball or wadded paper
- Playing video games for finger and hand movements
- Playing with finger paints, clay, or play dough
- Having tricycle or wheelchair races
- Playing "hide and seek" by hiding a toy in the bed or room
- Colouring and painting

Always check the care plan for the child's activity limits. If you are still unsure, check with your supervisor.

Adapted from: Hockenberry, M.J., et al. (2007). *Wong's nursing care of infants and children* (8th ed.). St. Louis: Mosby.

focus on »LONG-TERM CARE

Activity Programs

Provincial and territorial long-term care legislation requires that long-term care facilities have an assessment and care planning process to prevent unnecessary reduction in a client's range of motion. Prevention involves active, active-assistive, or passive ROM exercises. Splints and braces are used, if needed.

Long-term care legislation also requires activity programs for clients, as recreational activities are important for the physical and mental well-being of older adults. During recreational activities, joints and muscles are exercised, and circulation is stimulated. Recreational activities also provide social opportunities and are mentally stimulating.

The activities must meet the interests and physical and psychosocial needs of each client. Facilities often arrange for bingo, movies, dances, exercise groups, shopping trips, museum trips, concerts, and guest speakers, as well as gardening activities.

The right to personal choice is protected in all arrangements, so the client chooses which activities to take part in. Activities should promote physical, intellectual, social, spiritual, and emotional well-being, which is promoted when the client attends activities of personal choice. The client must not be forced to take part in an activity that has no interest for him or her.

Clients may need help getting to an activity and in participating. You must provide assistance as necessary.

Activity ideas are always welcome from anybody. Clients may share ideas with you or tell you about favourite pastimes, or you may have your own ideas. Share these with the health care team so that they are given to the team that plans activities.

Box 24–3 Guidelines for Performing Range-of-Motion Exercises

- Exercise only the joints you are instructed to exercise.
- Expose only the body part being exercised.
- Use good body mechanics.
- Support the part being exercised.
- Move the joint slowly, smoothly, and gently.
- Do not force a joint beyond its present range of motion or to the point of pain.
- ***Perform range-of-motion exercises to the neck only if allowed by employer policy.*** In some facilities and agencies, only physical or occupational therapists do neck exercises because of the danger of neck injuries.

1 2 3 PERFORMING RANGE-OF-MOTION EXERCISES

Remember to promote:

• **D**ignity • **I**ndependence • **P**references • **P**rivacy • **S**afety

Pre-Procedure

1 Identify the client, according to employer policy.
2 Explain the procedure to the client.
3 Perform hand hygiene.
4 Obtain a bath blanket.
5 Provide for privacy.
6 Raise the bed to a comfortable working height. Follow the care plan for bed rail use.*

Procedure

7 Lower the bed rail closer to you if it is up.
8 Place the client in the supine position.
9 Cover the client with a bath blanket. Fanfold top linens to the foot of the bed.
10 Exercise the neck, ***if allowed by your employer and if your supervisor instructs you to do so*** (Figure 24–10):
- **a** Place your hands over the client's ears to support the head. Support the jaws with your fingers.
- **b** *Flexion*—bring the head forward so that the chin touches the chest.
- **c** *Extension*—straighten the head.
- **d** *Hyperextension*—bring the head backward until the chin points up.
- **e** *Rotation*—turn the head from side to side.
- **f** *Lateral flexion*—move the head to the right and to the left.
- **g** Repeat b through f five times—or the number of times stated on the care plan.

11 Exercise the shoulder (Figure 24–11):
- **a** Grasp the wrist with one hand. Grasp the elbow with your other hand.
- **b** *Flexion*—raise the arm straight in front and over the head.
- **c** *Extension*—bring the arm down to the side.
- **d** *Hyperextension*—move the arm behind the body. (Do this if the client sits in a straight-backed chair or is standing.)
- **e** *Abduction*—move the straight arm away from the side of the body.
- **f** *Adduction*—move the straight arm to the side of the body.
- **g** *Internal rotation*—bend the arm at the elbow. Place it at the same level as the shoulder. Move the forearm down toward the body.
- **h** *External rotation*—Move the forearm toward the head.
- **i** Repeat b through h five times—or the number of times stated on the care plan.

12 Exercise the elbow (Figure 24–12):
- **a** Grasp the client's wrist with one hand. Grasp the elbow with your other hand.
- **b** *Flexion*—bend the arm so the hand touches the same-side shoulder.
- **c** *Extension*—Straighten the arm.
- **d** Repeat b and c five times—or the number of times stated on the care plan.

13 Exercise the forearm (Figure 24–13):
- **a** *Pronation*—turn the hand so that the palm is down.
- **b** *Supination*—turn the hand so that the palm is up.
- **c** Repeat a and b five times—or the number of times stated on the care plan.

14 Exercise the wrist (Figure 24–14):
- **a** Hold the wrist with both hands.
- **b** *Flexion*—bend the hand down.
- **c** *Extension*—straighten the hand.
- **d** *Hyperextension*—bend the hand back.
- **e** *Radial flexion*—turn the hand toward the thumb.
- **f** *Ulnar flexion*—turn the hand toward the little finger.
- **g** Repeat b through f five times—or the number of times stated on the care plan.

(continued on page 435)

1 2 3 PERFORMING RANGE-OF-MOTION EXERCISES

Procedure (cont'd)

15 Exercise the thumb (Figure 24–15):
- **a** Hold the client's hand with one hand. Hold the thumb with your other hand.
- **b** *Abduction*—move the thumb out from the inner part of the index finger.
- **c** *Adduction*—move the thumb back next to the index finger.
- **d** *Opposition*—touch each fingertip with the thumb.
- **e** *Flexion*—bend the thumb into the hand.
- **f** *Extension*—move the thumb out to the side of the fingers.
- **g** Repeat b through f five times—or the number of times stated on the care plan.

16 Exercise the fingers (Figure 24–16):
- **a** *Abduction*—spread the fingers and thumb apart.
- **b** *Adduction*—bring the fingers and thumb together.
- **c** *Extension*—straighten the fingers so that the fingers, hand, and arm are straight.
- **d** *Flexion*—make a fist.
- **e** Repeat a through d five times—or the number of times stated on the care plan.

17 Exercise the hip (Figure 24–17):
- **a** Support the leg. Place one hand under the knee. Place your other hand under the ankle.
- **b** *Flexion*—raise the leg.
- **c** *Extension*—straighten the leg.
- **d** *Abduction*—move the leg away from the body.
- **e** *Adduction*—move the leg toward the other leg.
- **f** *Internal rotation*—turn the leg inward.
- **g** *External rotation*—turn the leg outward.
- **h** Repeat b through g five times—or the number of times stated on the care plan.

18 Exercise the knee (Figure 24–18):
- **a** Support the knee. Place one hand under the knee. Place your other hand under the ankle.
- **b** *Flexion*—bend the leg.
- **c** *Extension*—straighten the leg.
- **d** Repeat b and c five times—or the number of times stated on the care plan.

19 Exercise the ankle (Figure 24–19):
- **a** Support the foot and ankle. Place one hand under the foot. Place your other hand under the ankle.
- **b** *Dorsiflexion*—pull the foot forward. Push down on the heel at the same time.
- **c** *Plantar flexion*—turn the foot down. Or point the toes.
- **d** Repeat b and c five times—or the number of times stated on the care plan.

20 Exercise the foot (Figure 24–20):
- **a** Continue to support the foot and ankle.
- **b** *Pronation*—turn the outside of the foot up and the inside down.
- **c** *Supination*—turn the inside of the foot up and the outside down.
- **d** Repeat b and c five times—or the number of times stated on the care plan.

21 Exercise the toes (Figure 24–21):
- **a** *Flexion*—curl the toes.
- **b** *Extension*—straighten the toes.
- **c** *Abduction*—spread the toes apart.
- **d** *Adduction*—pull the toes together.
- **e** Repeat a through d five times—or the number of times stated on the care plan.

22 Cover the leg.

23 Raise the bed rail, if used. Go to the other side. Lower the bed rail near you if it is up.

24 Repeat steps 11 through 21.

Post-Procedure

25 Cover the client. Remove the bath blanket.

26 Provide for safety and comfort.

27 Place the call bell within reach.*

28 Return the bed to its lowest position. Follow the care plan for bed rail use.*

29 Remove privacy measures.

30 Return the bath blanket to its proper place.

31 Perform hand hygiene.

32 Report and record your actions and observations according to employer policy.

*Steps marked with an asterisk may not apply in community settings.

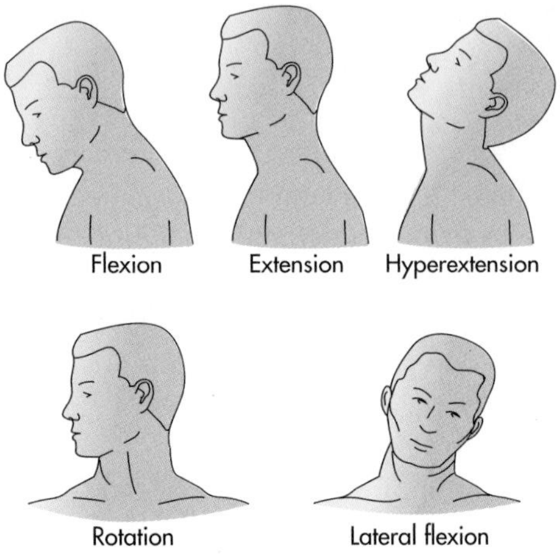

Figure 24–10 Range-of-motion exercises for the neck.

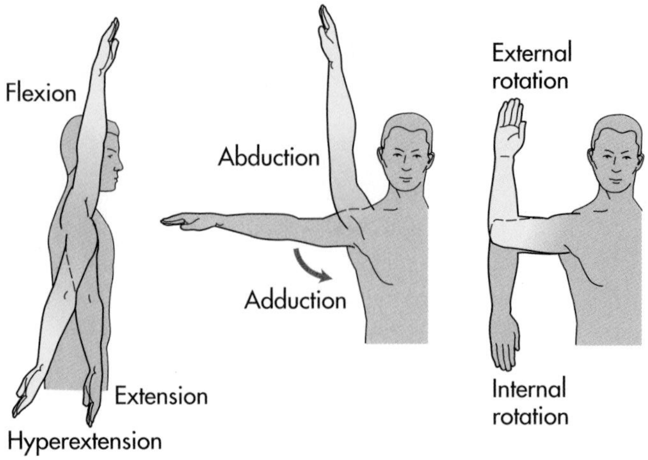

Figure 24–11 Range-of-motion exercises for the shoulder.

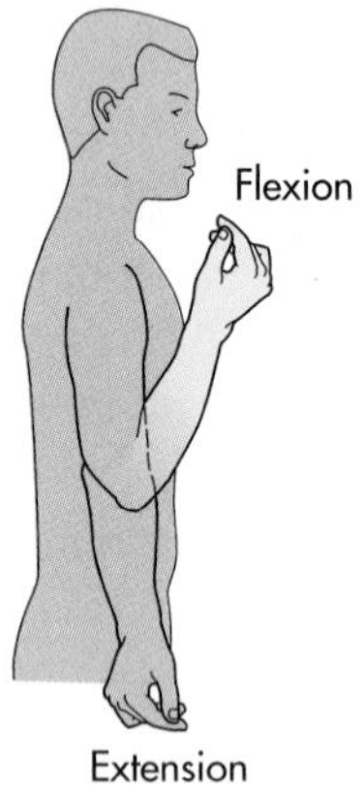

Figure 24–12 Range-of-motion exercises for the elbow.

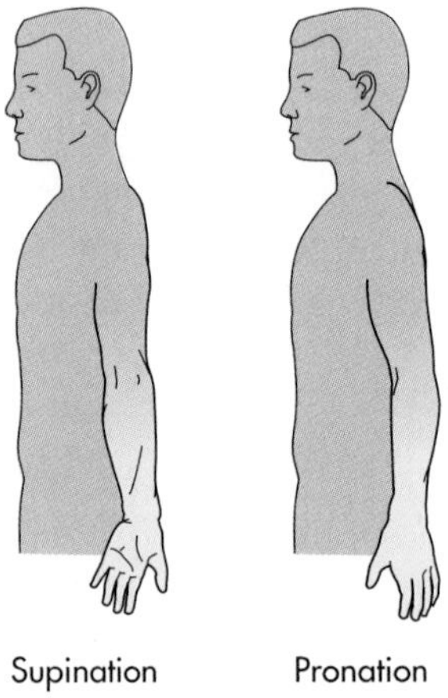

Figure 24–13 Range-of-motion exercises for the forearm.

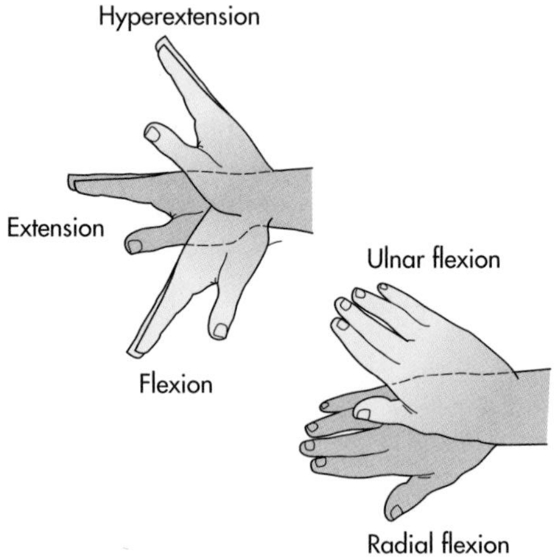

Figure 24–14 Range-of-motion exercises for the wrist.

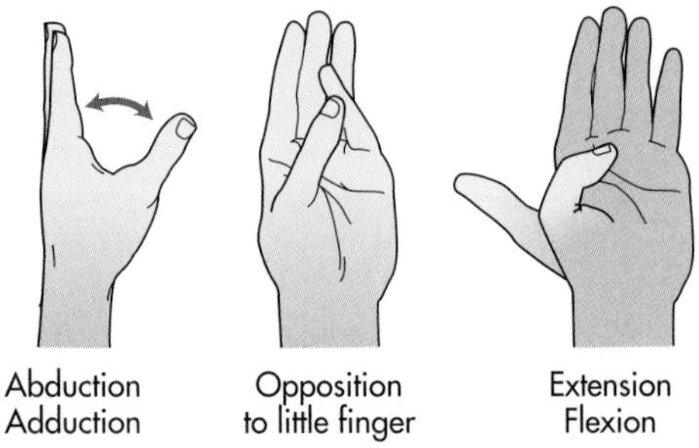

Figure 24–15 Range-of-motion exercises for the thumb.

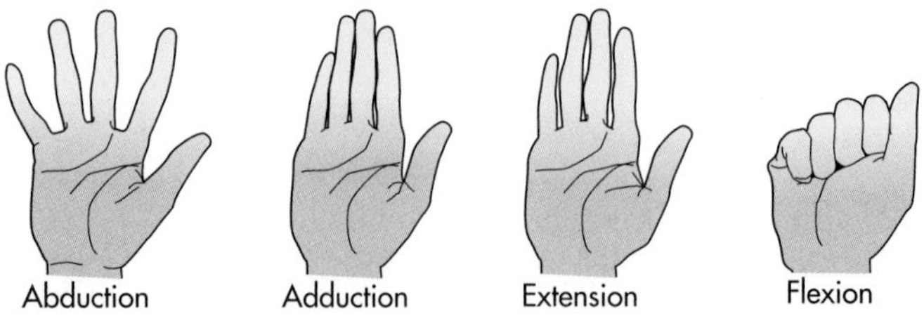

Figure 24–16 Range-of-motion exercises for the fingers.

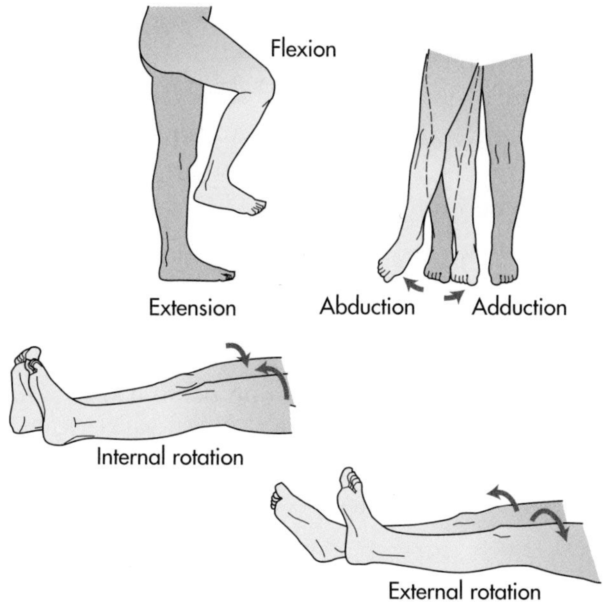

Figure 24–17 Range-of-motion exercises for the hip.

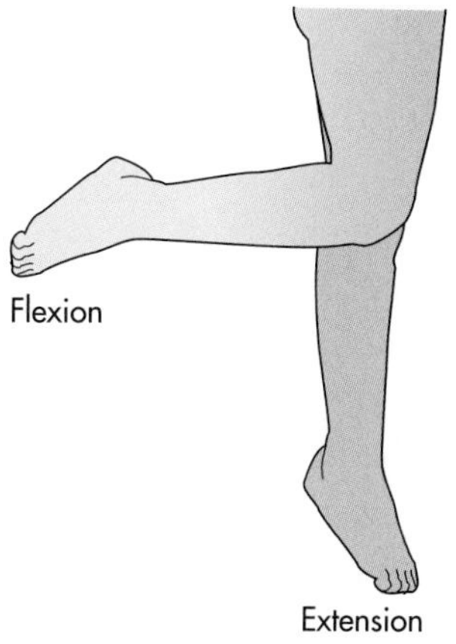

Figure 24–18 Range-of-motion exercises for the knee.

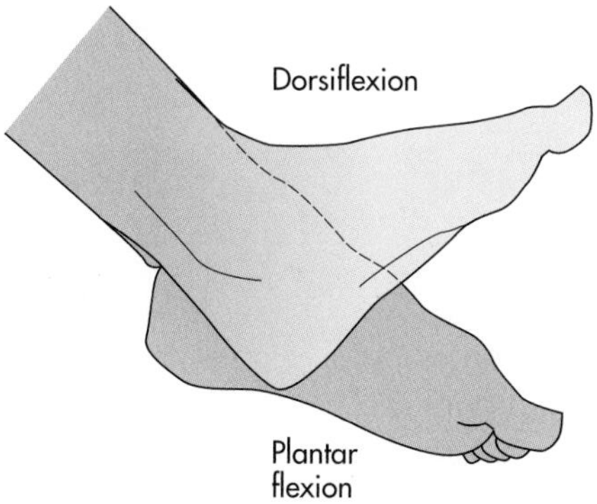

Figure 24–19 Range-of-motion exercises for the ankle.

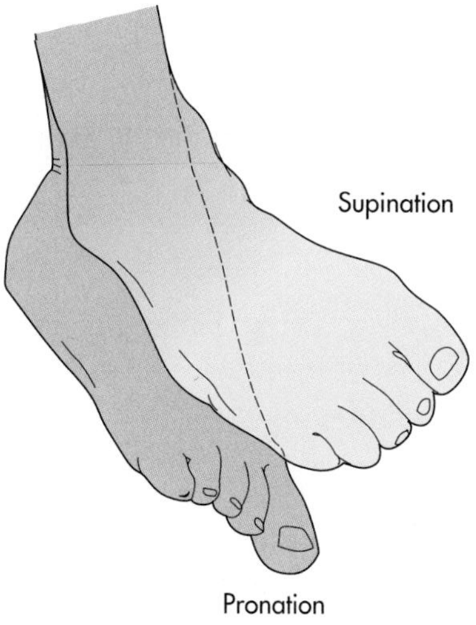

Figure 24–20 Range-of-motion exercises for the foot.

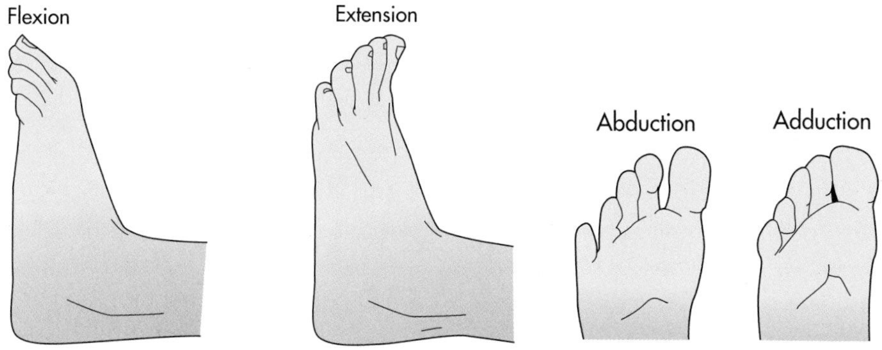

Figure 24–21 Range-of-motion exercises for the toes.

AMBULATION

Walking regularly helps prevent deconditioning. Many clients need help walking. Some clients become strong enough to walk independently, but many continue to need help, some even permanently.

After bed rest, activity is usually increased slowly and in steps. First, the client dangles the legs (sits on the side of the bed). The next step is to sit in a bedside chair, followed by walking about in the room and then in the hallway. **Ambulation**, the act of walking, is not a problem if complications (such as contractures and muscle atrophy) have been prevented by proper positioning and exercise.

For clients who are weak and unsteady, use a gait (transfer) belt when helping them walk (see box below and Chapter 23). Encourage the client to use hand rails along the wall for additional support. Always check the client for orthostatic hypotension.

Before beginning the walk, remove any obstacles in the path. If necessary, place a chair nearby in case the client needs to rest. Make sure the client is wearing nonskid footwear.

Encourage personal choices in walking. The client may want to walk outside and may prefer to walk at a particular time of day. The client may want to wait until a visitor arrives or leaves. Allow such choices, whenever safe and possible. However, be sure to get your supervisor's approval.

After helping the client with ambulation, report and record the following:

- How well the client tolerated the activity
- Any complaints of pain or discomfort
- The distance walked

1 2 3 HELPING THE CLIENT TO WALK

Remember to promote:

• Dignity • Independence • Preferences • Privacy • Safety

Pre-Procedure

1 Identify the client, according to employer policy.
2 Explain the procedure to the client.
3 Perform hand hygiene.
4 Gather the following:
- Robe and nonskid shoes
- Paper or sheet to protect bottom linens
- Gait (transfer) belt

5 Provide for privacy.

Procedure

6 Lower the bed to its lowest position. Lock the bed wheels. Lower the bed rail if used.*
7 Fanfold top linens to the foot of the bed.
8 Place paper or sheet under the client's feet. This protects the bottom sheet from the shoes. Put the shoes on the client.
9 Help the client to dangle the legs (see *Helping the Client Sit on the Side of the Bed (Dangle the Legs)*, page 407 in Chapter 23.)
10 Help the client put on the robe.
11 Apply the gait belt (see *Applying a Transfer Belt*, page 414.)
12 Help the client stand up (see *Transferring the Client to a Chair or Wheelchair*, page 416 in Chapter 23.) Grasp the gait belt on each side, or place your arms under the client's arms around to the shoulder blades.
13 Stand at the client's side while he or she gains balance. Hold the belt at the side and back, or have one arm around the back to support the client.
14 Encourage the client to stand erect with the head up and back straight.
15 Help the client walk. Walk to the side and slightly behind the client. Provide support with the gait belt (Figure 24–22), or have one arm around the back to support the client.

(continued on page 439)

1 2 3 HELPING THE CLIENT TO WALK

Procedure (cont'd)

16 Encourage the client to walk normally. The heel should strike the floor first. Discourage shuffling, sliding, or walking on tiptoes.
17 Walk the required distance if the client can tolerate the activity. Do not rush the client.
18 Help the client return to bed:
- **a** Have the client stand at the side of the bed.
- **b** Pivot him or her a quarter turn. The backs of the knees should touch the bed.
- **c** Grasp the sides of the gait belt.
- **d** Lower the client onto the bed as you bend your knees. Remove gait belt and robe.
- **e** Help the client lie down (see *Helping the Client Sit on the Side of the Bed (Dangle the Legs)*, page 407 in Chapter 23.)

19 Help the client to the centre of the bed.
20 Remove footwear. Remove the paper or sheet over the bottom sheet.

Post-Procedure

21 Provide for safety and comfort.
22 Place the call bell within reach.*
23 Follow the care plan for bed rail use.*
24 Remove privacy measures.
25 Return the robe and shoes to their proper place.
26 Perform hand hygiene.
27 Report and record your actions and observations according to employer policy.

*Steps marked with an asterisk may not apply in community settings.

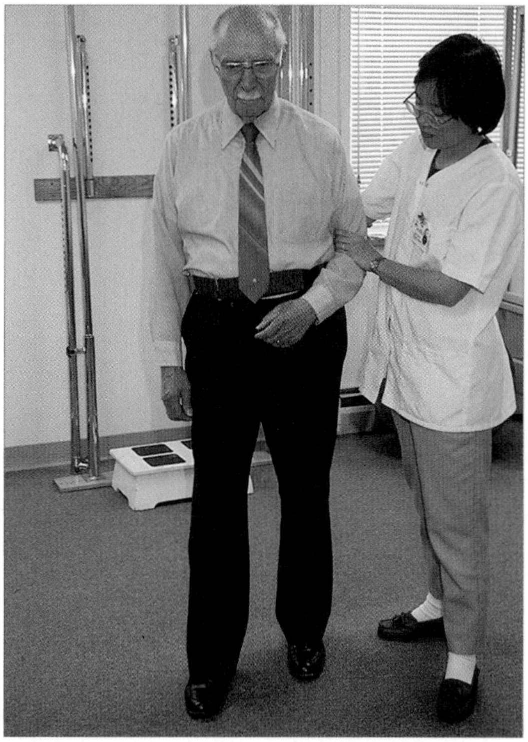

Figure 24–22 Assist with ambulation by walking slightly behind the client's side. Use a gait belt for the client's safety.

Falls

A client may start to fall when standing or walking. The client may be weak, lightheaded, or dizzy. Fainting may occur. Falling may be caused by slipping or sliding on spills, waxed floors, or throw rugs or by wearing improper shoes (see Chapter 19).

When a client is falling, the tendency is to try to prevent the fall. However, trying to prevent a fall could cause greater harm. You could injure yourself and the client as you twist and strain to stop the fall. Or you could lose your balance, and both you and the client could fall, causing head, hip, and knee injuries to occur.

If a client starts to fall, ease him or her to the floor. This lets you control the direction of the fall and also protect the client's head.

Your response after the fall will depend on whether you work in a facility with help readily available or in a private home where you will likely be working alone (see the *Focus on Home Care: When a Client Falls* box on page 441).

If a client falls in a facility, do not move the client or allow him or her to get up. Remain calm, and reassure the client. Call for a nurse to check the client for injuries, and later, complete an incident report, as required by facility policy.

1 2 3 HELPING THE FALLING CLIENT

Remember to promote:

• Dignity • Independence • Preferences • Privacy • Safety

Procedure

1. Stand with your feet apart. Keep your back straight.
2. Bring the client close to your body as quickly as possible. Use the gait belt if the client is wearing one. If not, wrap your arms around the client's waist. You can also hold the client under the arms (Figure 24–23, *A*).
3. Move your leg so the client's buttocks rest on it (Figure 24–23, *B*). Move your leg near the client.
4. Lower the client to the floor. Let him or her slide down your leg to the floor (Figure 24–23, *C*). Bend at your hips and knees as you lower the client.
5. After the fall:
   - **a** If you are in a facility, call for a nurse. Stay with the client.
   - **b** If you are in a home care setting, check for obvious signs of injury. ***If you suspect injury, do not move the client.*** Call your supervisor. Keep the client warm and calm until help arrives. If the client is not injured and can assist, help the client up.
6. Report and record the following, according to employer policy:
   - How the fall occurred
   - How far the client walked
   - How activity was tolerated before the fall
   - Any complaints before the fall
   - The amount of assistance needed by the client while walking
7. Complete an incident report and the actions you took.

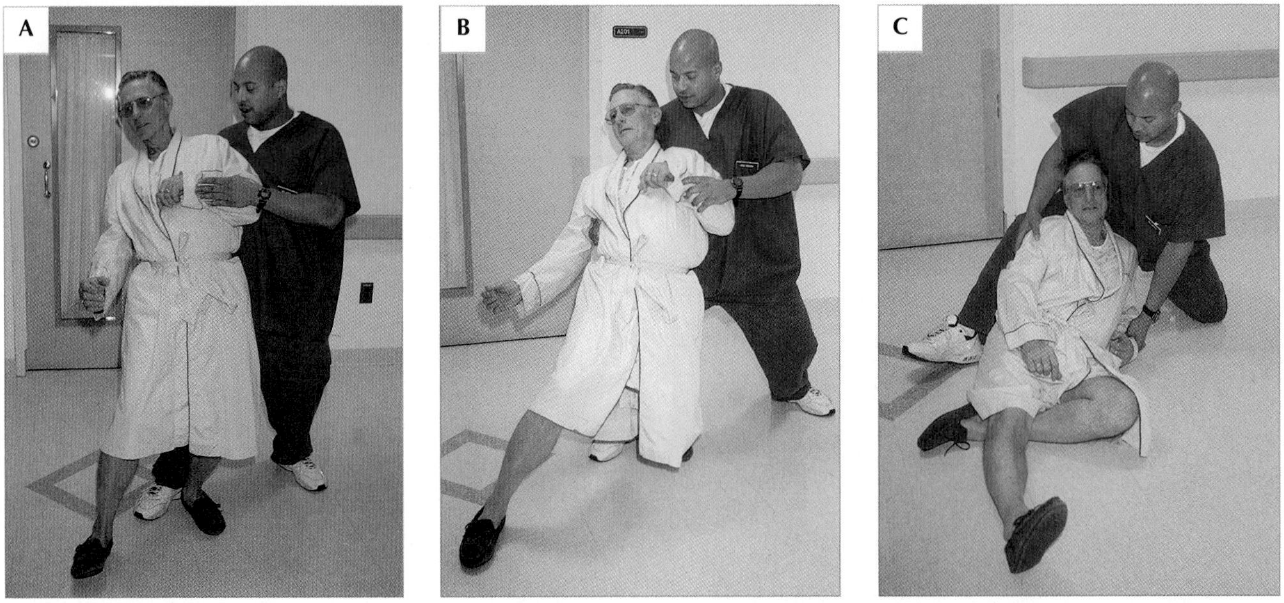

Figure 24–23 Helping a client who is falling. **A,** Hold the client close to your body. **B,** Move your leg to support the client's buttocks. **C,** Slide the client down your leg to the floor.

focus on
›› HOME CARE

When a Client Falls

When working in a private home, you will not have a nurse present to help if a client falls. Be aware of any procedures required by your employer before a fall occurs. Use the following as a guide.

If a client starts to fall, ease him or her to the floor (see *Helping the Falling Client*). After the fall, check for the following signs:

- Pain or tenderness
- Swelling or bruising
- Inability to move a limb or difficulty moving a limb
- Bleeding
- Client report of having felt or heard a bone snap or pop

If you observe any of the above, or if you suspect the client has a head, neck, or back injury, ***do not move the client***. Call your supervisor for help. Keep the client warm and calm, and stay with him or her until help arrives.

If the client is unhurt and is able to assist, help him or her up. Follow these steps:

- Place a chair beside the client. Have the client use the armrests for support.
- Support the client's hips and assist him or her into a kneeling position, facing the chair.
- Have the client rest his or her forearms on the chair.
- Tell the client to lift one knee and place the foot on the floor. Assist as required.
- On the count of three, help the client push up, stand, and pivot into the chair, while holding onto the armrests.
- Once in the chair, let the client rest before assisting him or her up again.

Report the fall to your supervisor. Complete an incident report, according to employer policy.

Walking Aids

Walking aids support the body and are ordered by the physician, nurse, or physical therapist. The type ordered depends on the client's physical condition, the amount of support needed, and the type of disability.

Crutches. Crutches are used when the client cannot use one leg or when one or both legs need to gain strength. Some clients with permanent leg weakness use crutches, usually Lofstrand crutches (Figure 24–24), which are made of metal. A metal band fits around the forearm. Axillary crutches, made of wood or metal, extend from the underarm (*axilla*) to the ground (Figure 24–25). A regulated health care professional teaches the client to safely use crutches.

The client learns to walk using crutches, climb up and downstairs (Figures 24–26 and 24–27), and sit and stand. Safety is important, as the client using crutches is at risk for falls. Follow these safety measures:

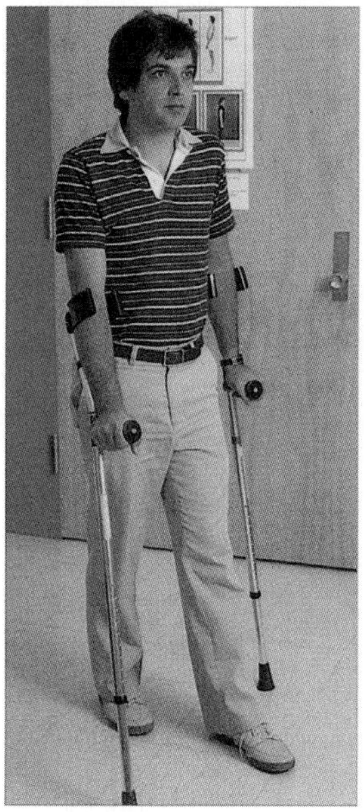

Figure 24–24 Lofstrand, or Canadian, crutches. **Source:** Elkin, M.K., Perry, A.G., & Potter, P.A. (2000). *Nursing interventions and clinical skills.* St. Louis: Mosby.

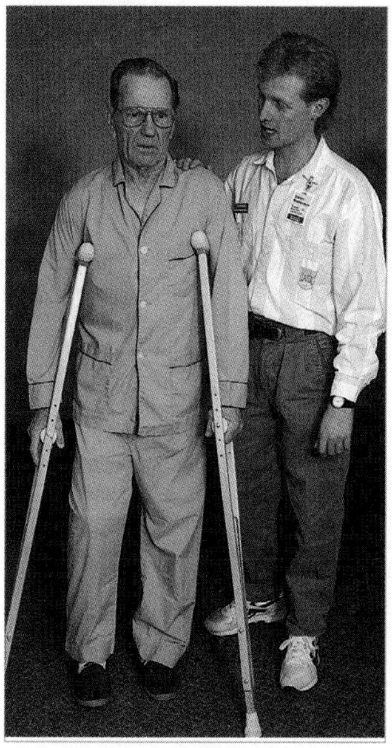

Figure 24–25 Axillary crutches. **Source:** Elkin, M.K., Perry, A.G., & Potter, P.A. (2000). *Nursing interventions and clinical skills.* St. Louis: Mosby.

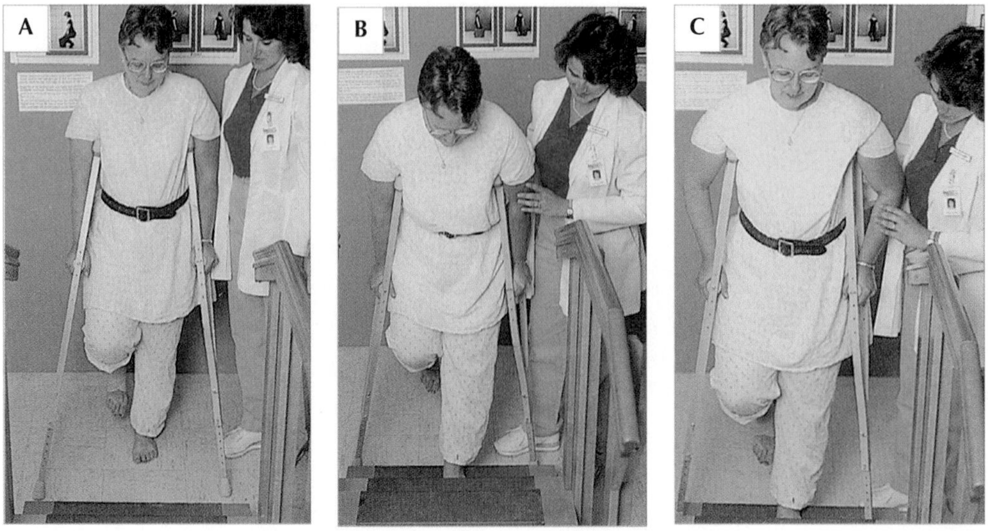

Figure 24–26 Ascending stairs. **Source**: Potter, P.A., Perry, A.G., Ross-Kerr, J.C., & Wood, M.J. (2006). *Canadian fundamentals of nursing* (3rd ed., p. 963). Toronto: Elsevier Canada.

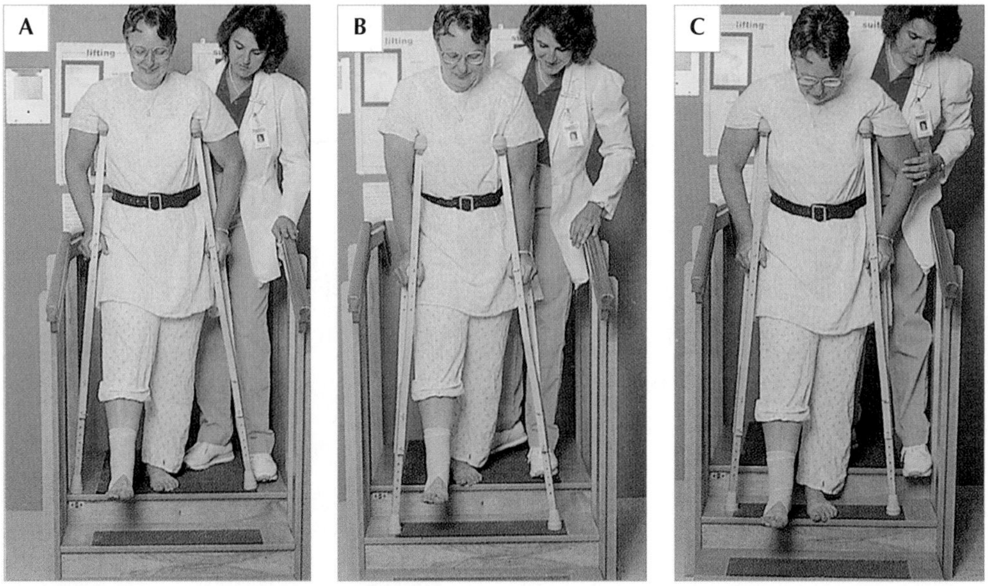

Figure 24–27 Descending stairs. **Source**: Potter, P.A., Perry, A.G., Ross-Kerr, J.C., & Wood, M.J. (2006). *Canadian fundamentals of nursing* (3rd ed., p. 964). Toronto: Elsevier Canada.

- Check the crutch tips. Report worn or torn crutch tips to your supervisor, and replace them according to policy. Inform your supervisor. If the tips are wet, dry them with a towel or paper towels.
- Check crutches for flaws—wooden crutches for cracks and metal crutches for bends. All bolts must be tight.
- Make sure the client wears well-fitted, flat, nonskid street shoes.
- Ensure the client's clothing fits well. Loose clothing may get caught between the crutches and underarms. Loose clothing can also hang forward and block the person's view of the feet and crutch tips.
- Practise safety measures to prevent falls (see Chapter 19).
- Keep crutches within reach of the client when not in use.

Canes. Canes are used to help support a weak side of the body and to provide balance. Single-tip and four-point (quad) canes (Figure 24–28) are available. A cane is held on the *strong (unaffected) side* of the body. (If the left leg is weak, the cane is held in the right hand.) Four-point canes give more support than do single-tip canes but are harder to move.

The cane tip is about 15 to 25 cm (6 to 10 in.) to the side of the foot and about 15 to 25 cm (6 to 10 in.) in front of the foot on the strong side. The grip is level with the hip.

The person walks as follows:

Step A: The cane is moved forward 15 to 25 cm (6 to 10 in.) (see Figure 24–29, *A*).

Step B: The weak leg (opposite the cane) is moved forward even with the cane (see Figure 24–29, *B*).

Step C: The strong leg is brought forward and ahead of the cane and the weak leg (Figure 24–29, *C*).

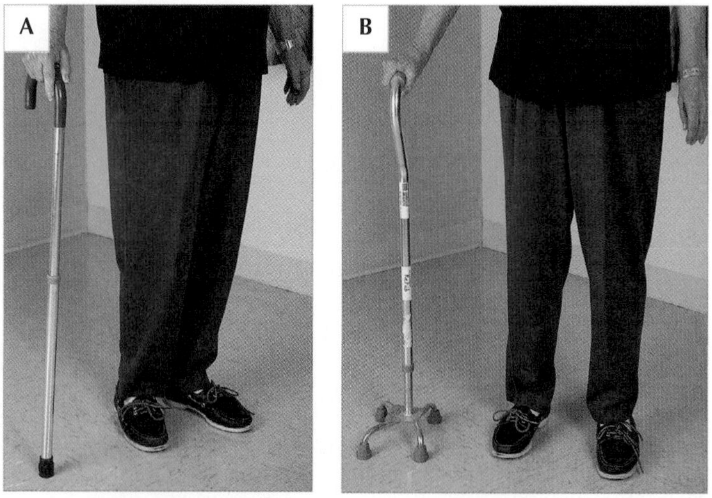

Figure 24–28 **A,** Single-tip cane. **B,** Four-point (quad) cane.

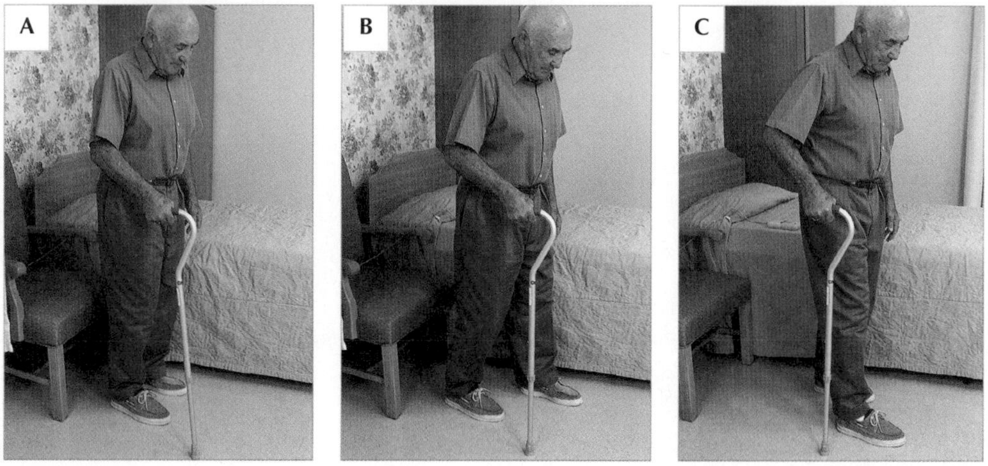

Figure 24–29 Walking with a cane. **A,** The cane is moved forward about 15 to 25 cm (6 to 10 in.). **B,** The leg opposite the cane (weak leg) is brought forward even with the cane. **C,** The leg on the cane side (strong leg) is moved ahead of the cane and the weak leg.

Walkers. A walker is a four-point walking aid (Figure 24–30). It gives more support than does a cane. Many people feel safer and more secure with a walker than with a cane. There are many kinds of walkers. The standard walker is picked up and moved about 15 to 20 cm (6 to 8 in.) in front of the client. The client then moves the weak leg and foot and then the strong leg and foot up to the walker (Figure 24–31).

A wheeled walker has wheels on the front legs and rubber tips on the back legs (Figure 24–32). The client pushes the walker ahead about 15 to 20 cm (6 to 8 in.) and then walks up to it. The rubber tips on the back legs prevent the walker from moving while the client is walking or standing.

Baskets, pouches, and trays can be attached to walkers (see Figure 24–30). The attachment is used to carry needed items. The client is more independent and does not have to rely on others. The attachment also keeps the hands free to grip the walker.

The client uses the walker for support when moving from a standing to a sitting position. Assist clients with walkers, as needed (see Box 24–4).

A

B

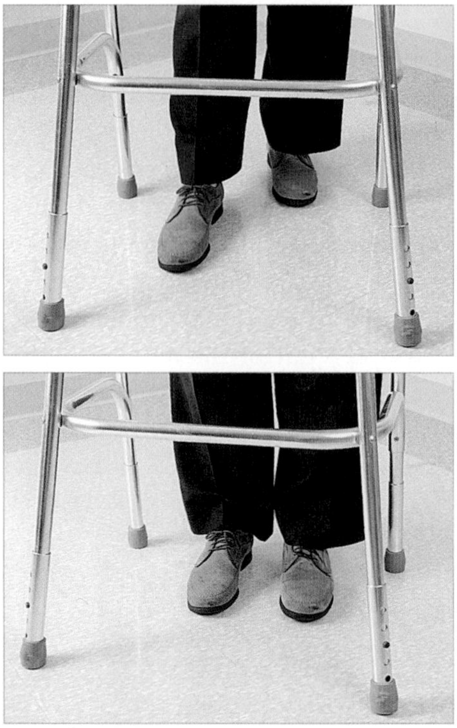

Figure 24–31 Walking with a walker. **A,** The walker is moved about 15 cm (6 in.) in front of the person. **B,** Both feet are moved up to the walker.

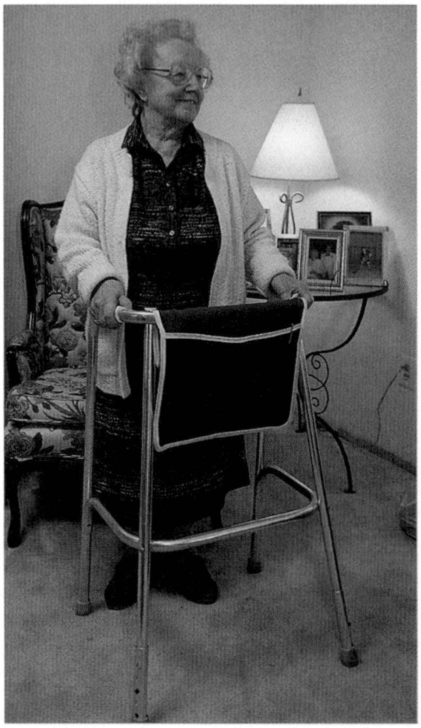

Figure 24–30 A walker.

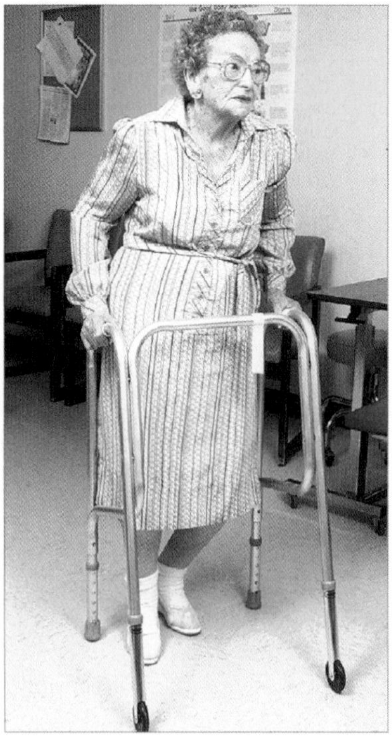

Figure 24–32 A woman using a wheeled walker. **Source**: Sorrentino, S.A. & Gorek, B. (2003). *Mosby's textbook for long-term care assistants* (4th ed., p. 467). St Louis: Mosby.

Box 24–4 Helping Clients With Walkers to Sit and Stand

Helping the Client Sit on a Chair, Wheelchair, or Toilet

- Lock the wheels of the wheelchair.
- Ask the client to stand with his or her back to the chair, wheelchair, or toilet.
- Ask the client to back up with the walker until his or her knees touch the seat.
- Ask the client to take one hand off the walker and to use that hand to reach and grasp the armrest or grab bar.
- Help the client slowly sit down. His or her buttocks should be at the back of the seat.
- If armrests or grab bars are not available, support the client as he or she sits down. (Use a transfer belt if the client is weak or unsteady.)
- Move the walker away from the client.
- Support the client in the standing position.
- Place your hands under the client's arms and over the shoulder blades.
- Block the client's feet and knees with your feet and knees.
- Lower the client onto the seat slowly.

Helping the Client Sit on a Bed

- Use a transfer belt if the client is weak or unsteady.
- Raise the head of the bed to a sitting position.
- Ask the client to stand with his or her back to the bed. He or she should be near the middle of the bed.
- Ask the client to back up with the walker until his or her knees touch the bed.
- Ask the client to reach for the bed with one hand. Assist as necessary.
- Help the client sit down slowly.
- Provide for comfort.

Helping the Client Move From Sitting to Standing

- Place the walker so that the client can reach it with ease.
- Let the client position the walker.
- Ask the client to move to the edge of the seat or bed.
- Help the client rise to a standing position, as needed.
- Do not let your client pull himself or herself up with the walker. He or she should push on the mattress or chair armrests and then transfer hands to the walker.

Braces. A **brace** (**orthosis**) is an apparatus—metal, plastic, or leather—worn to support or align weak body parts or to prevent or correct problems with the musculo-skeletal system (see Chapter 33). A brace is applied over the ankle, knee, or back (Figure 24–33). An ankle–foot orthosis (AFO) is positioned in the shoe (Figure 24–34); then the foot is inserted, and the device is secured in place with a Velcro strap.

Skin and bony points under the braces should be kept clean and dry to prevent skin breakdown. Report redness or signs of skin breakdown (see Chapter 42) and any complaints of pain or discomfort. In facilities, the nurse assesses the skin under braces during every shift. The care plan tells you when to apply and remove a brace.

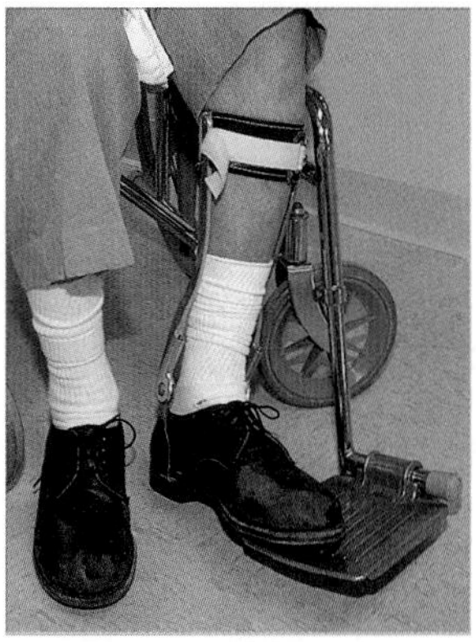

Figure 24–33 Leg brace.

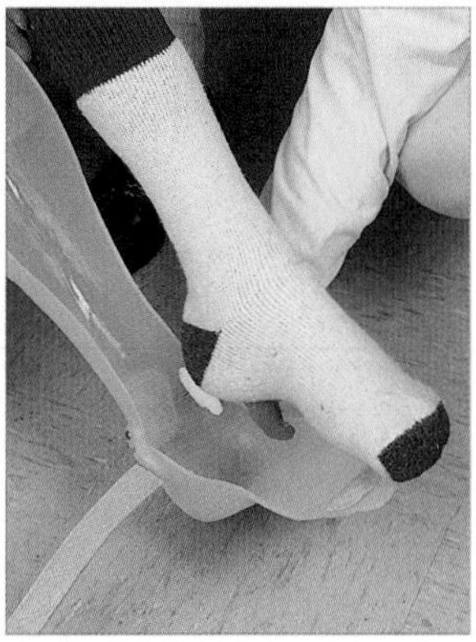

Figure 24–34 Ankle–foot orthosis.

REVIEW

Answers to these questions are at the bottom of the page.

Circle the **BEST** answer.

1. **Ms. Porter is in bed rest. Which statement is *true?***
   - A. She has orthostatic hypotension.
   - B. Bed rest helps reduce pain and promotes healing.
   - C. Everything will be done for her.
   - D. Bed rest is not the cause of contractures.
2. **Which helps prevent permanent plantar flexion?**
   - A. Bed boards
   - B. A foot board
   - C. Trochanter rolls
   - D. Hand rolls
3. **Which prevents the hip from turning outward?**
   - A. Bed boards
   - B. A foot board
   - C. Trochanter roll
   - D. A leg brace
4. **A contracture is:**
   - A. The loss of muscle strength as a result of inactivity
   - B. The lack of joint mobility caused by the shortening of a muscle
   - C. A decrease in the size of a muscle
   - D. A blood clot
5. **Passive range-of-motion exercises are performed by:**
   - A. The client
   - B. A health care team member
   - C. The client with the assistance of someone else
   - D. The client with the use of a trapeze
6. **ROM exercises are ordered for Ms. Porter. You should avoid doing one of the following:**
   - A. Support the body part being exercised
   - B. Move the joint slowly, smoothly, and gently
   - C. Force the joint through full range of motion
   - D. Exercise only the joints indicated by your supervisor
7. **Flexion involves:**
   - A. Bending the body part
   - B. Straightening the body part
   - C. Moving the body part toward the body
   - D. Moving the body part away from the body
8. **You are getting a client ready to crutch walk. You should do the following:**
   - A. Ensure the client wears loose clothing
   - B. Have the client wear slippers
   - C. Get any pair of crutches from physical therapy
   - D. Tighten the bolts on the crutches
9. **A single-tip cane is used:**
   - A. At waist level
   - B. On the strong side
   - C. On the weak side
   - D. On either side

Circle **T** if the answer is true or circle **F** if the answer is false.

10. T F **A single-tip cane and a four-point cane give equal support.**
11. T F **When a cane is used, the feet are moved first.**
12. T F **Mr. Jameel uses a walker. First, he moves the walker in front of him. Then, he moves his feet forward.**
13. T F **Mr. Jameel starts to fall. You should try to prevent the fall.**
14. T F **A client has a brace. Bony areas need protection from skin breakdown.**

Answers: 1.B, 2.B, 3.C, 4.B, 5.B, 6.C, 7.A, 8.D, 9.B, 10.F, 11.F, 12.T, 13.F, 14.T

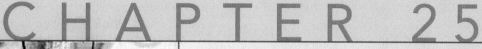

CHAPTER 25

Home Management

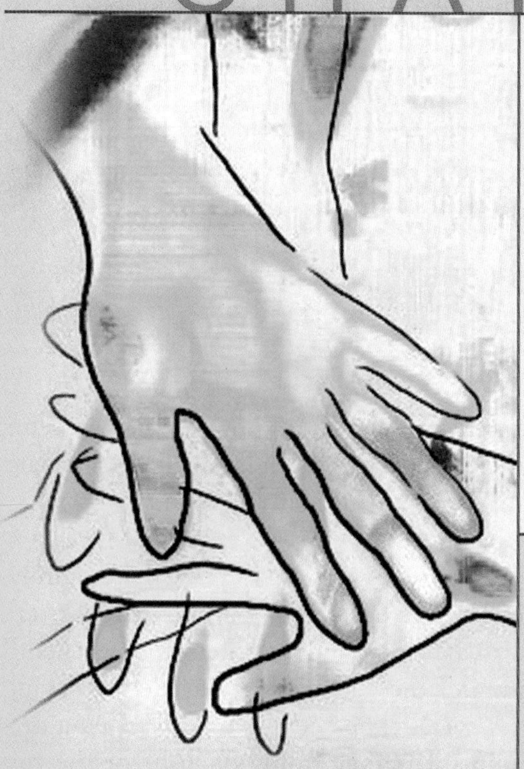

OBJECTIVES

- Define the key terms listed in this chapter.
- Describe why home management is important.
- Explain your role in home management.
- Describe your role in handling your client's money.
- Explain how to use cleaning supplies safely.
- Describe how to clean bedrooms, living rooms, bathrooms, and kitchens.
- Describe how to do laundry properly.
- Differentiate between the various laundry care symbols.
- Apply the procedures described in this chapter to your clinical practice properly.

key terms

dignity The state of feeling worthy, valued, and respected.

home management The cleaning and organizing of a home.

independence The state of not depending on others for control or authority.

laundry care symbols Symbols on garment tags that indicate how to launder or care for specific garments.

mildew A microscopic, fungal parasite that is responsible for the black discoloration that is often visible over bathroom surfaces and causes a foul odour in bathrooms.

preferences The right to or the act of selecting someone or something over another or others.

privacy Privacy is the state of being free from unsanctioned intrusion, as well as the degree to which an individual can determine which personal information is to be shared with whom and for what purpose. It is one of the most important and comprehensive of all human rights, and yet it is one of the hardest to protect.

safety The state of being free from actual, threatened, or imagined danger, risk, or injury.

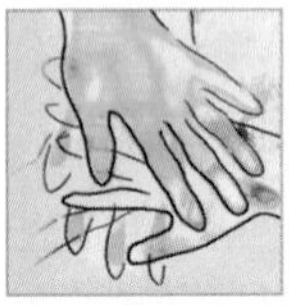

Some clients need help keeping their living environment clean, orderly, healthy, and safe. You might be assigned to **home management**—the cleaning and organizing of a home—involving light housekeeping tasks, such as straightening and cleaning parts of rooms, vacuuming, dusting, washing dishes, making beds, and doing laundry. Occasionally, you may be also required to take care of your clients' pets, such as walking their dog if they are unable to do this. Whatever your tasks are, they will be specified on each client's care plan. You will not be assigned heavy housecleaning tasks, such as washing windows or cleaning carpets.

You might do basic housekeeping tasks in a hospital or long-term facility as well. However, most facilities have a housekeeping staff. This chapter discusses home management in community care settings.

YOUR ROLE IN HOME MANAGEMENT

A clean and orderly setting is important for health and safety. Dust, dirt, and damp areas promote the growth of microbes, and clutter can cause falls and serious injury. Some people cannot do regular housekeeping—people who are ill, disabled, and recovering from surgery or injuries; new parents and caregivers tending to sick family members; and older adults.

Who Pays for What Services? The client, family, and case manager decide what household tasks are required to be done and list them in the client's care plan, and the client is responsible for paying for these services. The client is usually given a certain amount of money from which he or she can pay for these services. In some circumstances and in some provinces, however, the funding agency is billed directly by the agency providing the services, without the client's involvement. Some of these tasks, such as regular cleaning and laundry, are funded by home care services. Some tasks—such as pet care—are not funded for the client but are paid for separately by the client or family.

You must complete the tasks listed in the care plan, but you need to be flexible. For example, your task is to straighten and clean the bathroom after you have helped Mrs. Jacob with personal care. However, since Mrs. Jacob is incontinent of urine, you need to provide skin care and help her change into clean clothes. The client's immediate personal care needs take priority.

Whatever the household task, remember the priorities of support work (see the *Providing Compassionate Care: Home Management* box.)

Handling Your Client's Money. As a support worker, you may be occasionally required to assist your client with his or her personal banking, buying groceries for the client, or paying bills. In order to assist your client with this task, you should keep the following points in mind:

- This duty must be clearly written in the client's care plan, and it should specify *exactly* what your responsibilities are. Some clients with severe arthritis, for example, may just need assistance with handling their money because they cannot hold it without dropping it. Others may need you to pick up some groceries, and provide an account of the purchases.
- Your supervisor should be able to answer any questions that you might have about your agency's policies when it comes to financial responsibilities. Notify your supervisor promptly if you are asked to do something that is not specified in the client's care plan.
- You should not agree to anything that is not specified on your client's care plan. If you have any concerns or questions, you should consult your supervisor.

PROVIDING COMPASSIONATE CARE

Home Management

- **Dignity** is the state of feeling worthy, valued, and respected. All people deserve a neat, clean, peaceful setting. Illness, disability, surgery, or injury may limit a person's ability to clean. Helping with home management promotes comfort, emotional well-being, and dignity. Treat your client's home and belongings with respect and care.
- **Independence** is the state of not depending on others for control or authority. For some clients, accepting help means a loss of control. Respect your client's wishes for independence and control. As they recover, some clients gradually assume responsibility for home management. Occupational therapists help some clients learn new ways to perform household tasks. For example, Mr. Ho, who had an arm amputated, is trying to make his bed using techniques he learned in occupational therapy, but his progress is slow. Do not make the bed for him. Be patient, and praise him for trying and for the amount of work he has done.
- **Preferences** are the rights to or the act of selecting someone or something over another or others. Follow your client's preferred methods for household tasks. These will be listed in the care plan. Respect that all people have different preferences and standards. For example, Mrs. Neal may not show any interest in having a neat bedroom, but she may not tolerate even a tiny stain on her blouse.
- **Privacy** is the state of being free from unsanctioned intrusion, as well as the degree to which an individual can determine which personal information is to be shared with whom and for what purpose. It is one of the most important and comprehensive of all human rights, and yet it is one of the hardest to protect.

  Some people may view your presence as an intrusion. Find out if there are any areas that the client considers private or "off limits" for you. If there may be rooms, parts of rooms, or items that a client does not want touched or cleaned, respect these wishes. Never judge or criticize a client's housekeeping standards. Never talk to others about the cleanliness of a client's house. This would be unprofessional and unethical.
- **Safety** is the state of being free from actual, threatened, or imagined danger, risk, or injury. Some cleaning solutions have WHMIS labels (see Chapter 19). Read these and other product labels carefully. Follow all use and storage instructions. Do not let people walk on mopped floors, which may be slippery and cause a fall. Put away buckets and cleaning solutions when you are finished with them. Store cleaning solutions out of reach of children and from adults with dementia. Clear away clutter. If the client's safety is at risk, talk to your supervisor.

- All money that you handle should be recorded in the appropriate manner. Some agencies, for example, record all transactions on a page to which the support worker is required to attach receipts. When you are given money to purchase an item, you will be responsible to record how much cash was given to you and the amount of change that you were returning. You should be aware of your particular responsibilities in this matter.
- Always provide receipts for any transaction that you did on your client's behalf. If your agency's policy is to notify your supervisor before and after banking, you should do so promptly.
- Remember that the client's personal identification number (PIN) and banking account numbers are private and you should NOT have access to them. If the client has difficulty typing in his or her numbers, for example, a banking associate should be asked to do this. You should step away far enough so that you do not hear the numbers.

Dealing with Conflicting Demands

Many people have set routines and want things done in certain ways. Because of time constraints or for health and safety reasons, it may not be possible for you to follow them. You may have to deal with conflicting demands because the care plan says one thing but the client wants something different (see the boxes *Support Workers Solving Problems: Conflicting Home Management Demands* and *Supporting Mrs. Washington*). Listen to your client. Discuss complaints, if any, with your supervisor.

GETTING ORGANIZED

Usually, home management tasks are assigned in addition to personal care and other tasks. The key to completing home management tasks as well as your other duties is to use your time wisely. Review the time management skills described in Chapter 9. Follow the guidelines in Box 25–1 and these general points:

- ***Set priorities.*** Follow the care plan. Do the most important tasks first.
- ***Set a routine.*** Discuss the routine with your client. Agreeing about the routine will help you manage your time.
- ***Use your time well.*** Start with tasks that have waiting periods or that run automatically. For example, laundry and personal care activities are on your list. Start the laundry first. Leave soiled linens to soak while you help your client with his or her bath.
- ***Finish tasks, and put items away.*** Finish tasks that you have started. After finishing, put all items away in their proper places.
- ***Set time limits for each task.*** This helps you stay organized and finish on time.
- ***Focus on the task.*** Do not let your mind wander. For example, do not carelessly wipe a counter while talking to your client. Focus on the person. Then clean the counter properly.
- ***Put the client's needs first.*** Remember your first priority is to promote the client's comfort, well-being, and safety. Follow the care plan.

SUPPORT WORKERS SOLVING PROBLEMS

Conflicting Home Management Demands

<< Scenario >>

Rosa's client, Mrs. Yeung, 67, is recovering from heart surgery. Mrs. Yeung asks Rosa to wash the bathroom floor. Rosa explains that the care plan does not specify washing the floor, but Mrs. Yeung is upset because she wants the floor washed.

<< Discussion >>

Mrs. Yeung tells Rosa that she feels too ill to clean her house and wants Rosa to do it for her. Rosa explains that she must be on time for her next appointment and suggests that Mrs. Yeung talk to the case manager. Rosa shows that she cares by listening to Mrs. Yeung, who regains her composure. Rosa reports the matter to her supervisor.

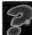

supporting ▸ MRS. WASHINGTON: PART 1

Ida Washington is an 82-year-old woman who lives alone in her own home. Last month, Mrs. Washington fell down her front steps and broke her hip. She requires weekly support worker assistance with her bath, as well as grocery shopping, laundry, and light housework, as she does not have anybody else who can help her. You are the support worker who was assigned to Mrs. Washington.

Mrs. Washington is very happy to have assistance with bathing, shopping, and housecleaning, but she is very particular about how her laundry is done. She uses an old-fashioned type of washing machine called a "wringer washer" to wash her clothes, and she hangs her wet laundry outside to dry on a clothesline. She does have an electric clothes dryer, but she only uses it in the wintertime.

On your first day, Mrs. Washington explains that she wants her clothing separated by colour and washed in her wringer washer. You do notice that her instructions differ from those on the care symbol labels on the clothing. You have never seen or operated a wringer washer, and you are nervous about operating it safely. For example, you do not know how to put clothing through the wringer to squeeze out the water. You do not know what to do in this situation, as it is your first assignment since being hired.

Box 25–1 Cleaning Guidelines

- ***Clear away clutter.*** Put items in their proper places. Nothing should be on the floor or counter unless it belongs there. Do not leave items on stairs or in high traffic areas. Ask the client where to put away things. If the client does not know, place items neatly out of the way. Tell the client where you put the things. Check with the client before throwing anything away, as even a scrap of paper may be important to him or her.
- ***Work from higher to lower.*** Begin in higher areas and work your way to the bottom. Dust and dirt from higher surfaces fall on lower surfaces. For example, when vacuuming stairs, start at the top of the stairs and work down to the bottom.
- ***Work from far to near.*** For example, when wiping a kitchen counter, make brisk strokes from the back to the front. When washing a floor, start at the far end of the room and work toward the door.
- ***Work from dry to wet.*** Begin with rooms and areas without sinks, tubs, showers, and toilets, and then clean bathrooms and kitchens. Sweep the floors before washing them.
- ***Work from cleanest to dirtiest.*** This helps avoid contaminating clean areas with microbes from a dirtier area. For example, wipe the cleanest part of the counter first. Clean the area used for food preparation last.
- ***Change cleaning cloths and water frequently.*** Do not wait for these to become visibly dirty before changing them. Use fresh cloths for each task. For example, use one cloth for dusting and another for wiping counters.
- ***Use a damp cloth for dusting.*** The moisture in a damp cloth picks up dust, whereas a dry cloth simply stirs the dust around.
- ***Rinse and dry washed surfaces.*** This removes soapy residue and dampness.
- ***Avoid soiling a clean area.*** For example, do not walk on a washed floor until it is dry.

EQUIPMENT AND SUPPLIES

Some homes have enough cleaning equipment and supplies and others do not. The following items are needed for cleaning. Clean and store items, as appropriate, after use.

Equipment

- ***Clean rags, sponges, cloths, or paper towels.*** After use, wash rags, sponges, and cloths in hot, soapy water. Hang them to air dry, or dry them in a dryer.
- ***Broom, dustpan, and brush.*** After use, shake the broom and brush into a large, moistened bag. Wipe the dustpan with a damp cloth.
- ***Mop and bucket.*** Wash and rinse both after use.
- ***Toilet brush.*** Rinse in a bucket of cold water. Flush water down the toilet.
- ***Utility gloves.*** Wash in hot, soapy water, and hang to dry.
- ***Vacuum cleaner.*** Use the right attachments to clean carpets and upholstery. Follow manufacturer's instructions. Replace filter bags, as needed. Make sure the cord and plug are in good repair.
- ***Dish washing materials.*** After use, clean all the cloths, sponges, scouring pads, and brushes.

Supplies

- ***Detergents***—for laundry and dish washing
- ***All-purpose cleaners***—for counters, floors, and other surfaces
- ***Glass cleaners***—for mirrors
- ***Special cleaners***—for bathrooms, toilets, mirrors, ovens, etc.
- ***Cleansers and scouring powders***—for scrubbing
- ***Disinfectants***—cleaners that destroy pathogens. Bleach can be used as a disinfectant, but must be used with caution because it can damage fabrics.
- ***Baking soda***—to eliminate refrigerator odours, counter stains, etc.
- ***White vinegar***—can be used as a disinfectant to clean toilets and commodes. Also can be used to clean mirrors. (Mix one part white vinegar to three parts water.)

If supplies and equipment are lacking, you may have to clean with what the client has on hand. Use your problem-solving skills (see *Supporting Mrs. Washington: Part 2).*

supporting MRS. WASHINGTON: PART 2

You arrive at Mrs. Washington's house, ready to assist with her bathing and to clean her bathroom afterward. While gathering your necessary equipment, you notice that Mrs. Washington has cloths and paper towels but no cleaners. She also does not have a mop for mopping the floor. At most agencies (including your new agency), the policy is to try to find cleaning substitutes before calling the office.

You are able to locate a bottle of white vinegar in the kitchen and make a cleaning solution with water and vinegar in a bucket. You use this to clean the bathroom. You decide that because Mrs. Washington's bathroom is small, you can wash her floor using a cloth, with the vinegar-and-water solution. You learned in school that a paste made of baking soda and water makes a good cleaner for the tub and sink surfaces as well. You are able to locate a box of baking soda in her cupboard.

Later, you report your actions to your supervisor, and you identify what supplies are needed at Mrs. Washington's house. Your supervisor tells you that she is pleased that you used your resourcefulness in finding alternative cleaning solutions, and that you did not skip cleaning Mrs. Washington's bathroom just because she did not have name-brand cleaning solutions. Your supervisor then asks if you can think of another way to make your own "mop," in case of a similar situation in the future.

USING CLEANING PRODUCTS SAFELY

Cleaning products can cause harm if not used and stored properly. Remember the following points:

- ***Read all labels carefully.*** Follow manufacturers' instructions. Be familiar with WHMIS hazard labels (see Chapter 19).
- ***Never mix cleaning products.*** Some products contain chemicals that create poisonous fumes when mixed. Mixing anything containing bleach and ammonia, for example, produces a deadly gas called chlorine. Remember to read product labels and to follow the instructions on the container.
- ***Wear utility gloves when using cleaning products.*** Do not use disposable gloves. They are too thin and can easily puncture; therefore, they would not provide you with protection from these harsh chemicals.
- ***Never use products in unlabelled containers.***
- ***Store products in their original containers.***
- ***Keep cleaning products away from food.***
- ***Be careful to ensure that you never splash bleach or any other chemical.*** If any chemical does splash and land on your skin (or in your eye) you should know how to treat it, and you should always read the product label BEFORE you use it.
- ***Keep cleaning products out of reach of children and adults with dementia.***
- ***Use products only for their intended purpose.*** Some products can harm the surfaces you are trying to clean!
- ***Keep aerosol cans away from heat sources.***
- ***Ask the client before using a strong cleaner on a surface.***
- ***Rinse strong, abrasive cleaners immediately after use.***
- ***Do not scrub vigorously.*** You could damage a delicate surface.

CLEANING BEDROOMS

Some clients spend very little time in bed, while some others spend most or all of their time in bed. They may even eat their meals in their bedroom, so the bedroom should be clean, orderly, and comfortable (Box 25–2). You need to:

- Make the bed
- Straighten bedding, as needed
- Change the linens, as needed

Box 25–2 Cleaning Bedrooms

Task	Supplies and Equipment	Process
Making the bed/ straightening linens		See Chapter 26
Changing the linens	Sheets Pillowcases Protective sheets or pads Blankets Comforter or bedspread	See Chapter 26
Straightening the room		Straighten items on bedside table Remove old magazines and newspapers, used tissues, drinking glasses, etc. (with permission from the client) Place reading material and glasses within reach Put away clothing, shoes, and other items (with permission from the client) Look for items under and behind the bed Empty the wastebasket

(continued on page 454)

Box 25–2 Cleaning Bedrooms (cont'd)

Task	Supplies and Equipment	Process
Replenishing supplies	Pitcher and glass Tissues and toilet paper Other supplies as necessary	Discard stale water; wash pitcher and glass; and refill pitcher and glass Replenish supplies, as needed
Wiping surfaces	Two cloths Hot, soapy water	Wipe doors, door knobs, and light switches Dry with dry cloth
Dusting	Damp cloth	Dust all surfaces, including dressers, bookshelves, windowsills, bedside tables, lamps, etc.
Cleaning commodes	Toilet bowl cleaner or disinfectant Bucket of hot water Utility gloves Toilet brush or sponge Fresh cloths or paper towels	Wear gloves Flush contents in the toilet; do not splash Clean the commode bowl, under the bowl, and under and behind the seat (Figure 25–1) Clean and dry commode surfaces with fresh cloths or paper towels
Cleaning floors	Vacuum Broom, dustpan, and brush Mop and bucket of hot, soapy water Damp mop	Vacuum rugs Sweep and damp mop floor Use dry mop for hardwood Shake and vacuum area rugs

Adapted from: Birchenall, J., & Streight, E. (1997). *Mosby's textbook for the home care aide* (pp. 93–94). St. Louis: Mosby.

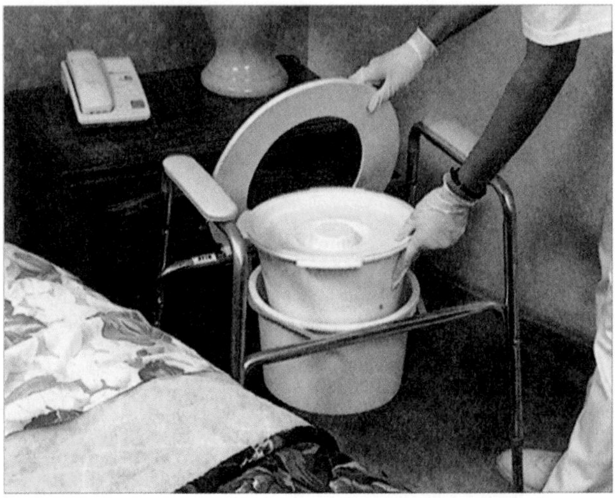

Figure 25–1 Clean commode surfaces thoroughly. **Source**: Birchenall, J., & Streight, E. (2003). *Mosby's textbook for the home care aide* (2nd ed., p. 295). St. Louis: Mosby.

CLEANING LIVING ROOMS

Some people use their living rooms infrequently; for some others, the living room is the main living area—they may eat and sleep in their living room. Whatever the situation, living rooms should be kept clean and comfortable (Box 25–3).

CLEANING KITCHENS

A clean kitchen is critical to preventing the spread of foodborne illnesses (see Chapter 27). Box 25–4 (on pages 456–457) describes how to clean the kitchen. When cleaning kitchens, remember the following:

Box 25–3 Cleaning Living Rooms

Task	Supplies and Equipment	Process
Straightening the room		Remove clutter and items that could cause falls (with permission from the client) Open windows (if possible) while you are cleaning, to rid the room of stale air and odours Keep windows open while using cleaning supplies in the house Close windows after you have finished cleaning Remove dirty dishes and ashtrays Look under cushions and under furniture arms for food particles and other items Bundle up old newspapers and place them in the recycling box (or the appropriate place) Sweep or vacuum crumbs off furniture Plump cushions
Replenishing supplies	Tissues Other supplies	Provide fresh water, tissues, reading materials, and other supplies
Wiping surfaces	Two cloths Hot, soapy water	Wipe doors, door knobs, and light switches Dry with dry cloth
Dusting	Damp cloth	Dust all furniture, including the television, electronic equipment, etc.
Cleaning floors	Vacuum cleaner Broom, dustpan, and brush Mop and bucket of hot, soapy water Damp mop	Vacuum rug Sweep and damp mop floor Use dry mop for hardwood Shake and vacuum area rug

Adapted from: Birchenall, J., & Streight, E. (1997). *Mosby's textbook for the home care aide* (p. 143). St. Louis: Mosby.

- Do not pour dirty or contaminated liquids down the kitchen sink. Flush them down the toilet.
- Use one cloth for counters, another for wiping floors, and another for dishes.
- Use paper towels to dry your hands. Do not dry your hands on a towel used for dishes.
- Change cloths daily or as needed. Wash in bleach in hot water.
- Use paper towels, when possible.
- Clean the microwave after every use.
- Do not put soiled diapers into the kitchen garbage.

Recycling Items. Most municipalities in Canada encourage residents to recycle their waste cardboard and paper, cans, jars, and other items. You should be aware of the items that are allowed to be recycled in the client's area, as each municipality has its own rules and specifics regarded recycling.

Some areas specify that certain types of waste must be disposed of in a specific colour of container. For example, one municipality may insist that paper and cardboard be placed into a red container, cans and jars into a blue container, and wet waste that can be composted placed into a green container. If the client lives in an apart-

Box 25–4 Cleaning Kitchens

Task	Supplies and Equipment	Process
Cleaning surfaces (counters, stove top, table)	Hot, soapy water Boiling water Disinfectant	Wipe surfaces with cloth and hot, soapy water Rinse and dry Scrub with disinfectant and rinse with boiling water if the surfaces were in contact with raw poultry, meat, fish, or eggs; dry thoroughly with paper towels
	Baking soda Cloth or sponge Second cloth or paper towel to dry counter	Use baking soda to remove stubborn counter stains Wipe table (and mats) with cloth and hot soapy water
Cleaning toasters or toaster ovens		Unplug the toaster, turn it upside down and shake it gently to remove crumbs. Wipe up the crumbs. Remove crumb tray and wash, if necessary, in warm, soapy water. Dry carefully, and replace into toaster.
Microwave oven	Hot soapy water, or diluted vinegar solution on clean cloth or paper towel	Soften grease splatters inside the microwave by placing a cup of water into the microwave and microwaving it on "high" for 90 seconds Wash the interior thoroughly, and dry it with a clean cloth or paper towel (When cooking food in the microwave, remember to always cover the food with a dish or paper towel to prevent splatters)
Cleaning cutting boards	Hot, soapy water Boiling water Disinfectant Cloth and brush	Wash with hot, soapy water Rinse and pat dry with paper towels Scrub with disinfectant, and rinse with boiling water if the surfaces were in contact with raw poultry, meat, fish, or eggs; dry thoroughly with paper towels
Washing dishes	Liquid detergent and hot water Dish cloth, scouring pads, or brushes	Scrape food remnants from dishes Wash glassware and cups first, then utensils, plates, bowls, pots, and pans Soak pots and pans in hot water if food is stuck on them Rinse items well in hot water Place items in a drainer to dry; air drying is cleaner than towel drying
Using automatic dishwashers	Dishwasher detergent	Read instructions or ask family member to demonstrate use Scrape large food particles and rinse dishes before loading (Figure 25–2) Place glasses and cups in washer upside down

(continued on page 457)

Box 25–4 Cleaning Kitchens (cont'd)

Task	Supplies and Equipment	Process
		Do not stack items on top of one another, as they will not clean properly Do not put the following in a dishwasher: electrical appliances, delicate glasses, fine china, sharp knives, cast iron, wood, or most plastics Check with the client before putting pots and pans in the dishwasher Use only dishwasher detergent; other soaps or detergents will cause damage
Cleaning kitchen sinks	Hot, soapy water Scouring powder Boiling water Disinfectant Paper towels	Clean with hot, soapy water and scouring powder Clean with disinfectant and paper towels if sink has been used for the preparation of poultry, raw meat, fish, or eggs; pour boiling water down sink after the sink has been cleaned; dry with paper towel Wipe taps with hot, soapy water; dry with paper towel
Cleaning refrigerators	Hot, soapy water	Open all containers; discard food items that have expired, do not look fresh, or are more than 2 days old (check with client). See *Supporting Mrs. Washington: Part 3.*
	Baking soda	Remove items from shelves, one shelf at a time; remove shelves and wash with cloth and hot, soapy water; dry with paper towels or a clean cloth; replace items when shelf has been cleaned and dried
	Cloth or paper towels	Clean drawers and inside of door Clean interior (all surfaces) of the refrigerator Place a small bowl of baking soda in the refrigerator to absorb odours Wipe the door of refrigerator and handle
Disposing of waste	Garbage bags Utility gloves	Wear gloves Remove and discard garbage; place in garage or throw down apartment chute Whenever possible, place recyclable items in the proper container
	Paper towels Hot, soapy water	Wash garbage can using paper towels and hot, soapy water Place fresh bag in container Check with client on recycling of newspapers, cans, and glass Place items in appropriate recycling box
Cleaning kitchen floors	Broom and dustpan and brush Damp mop Hot, soapy water	Sweep kitchen floor Damp-mop kitchen floor

Adapted from: Birchenall, J., & Streight, E. (1997). *Mosby's textbook for the home care aide* (pp. 143–144). St. Louis: Mosby.

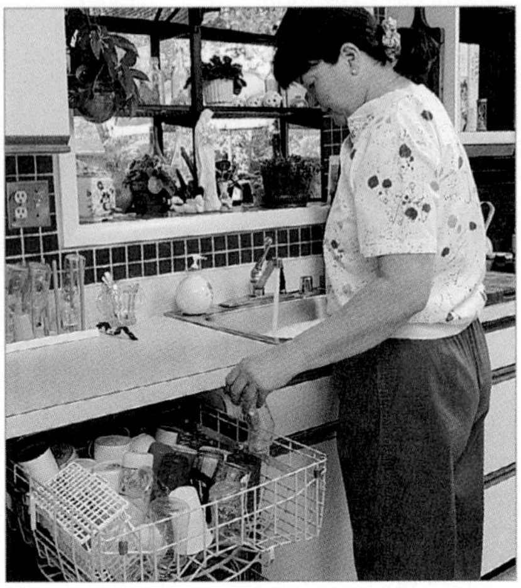

Figure 25–2 Rinse dishes before loading them into the dishwasher.

supporting MRS. WASHINGTON: PART 3

It is now time to clean Mrs. Washington's kitchen. You perform all of the steps in Box 25–4: *Cleaning Kitchens.* While you are cleaning Mrs. Washington's refrigerator, however, you notice that many of the items in her fridge, such as her processed salad dressings, barbeque sauce, and margarine, are past their expiry dates, some even by several months. Before you throw them out, however, you check with Mrs. Washington.

Mrs. Washington seems to be annoyed at your suggestion to throw away some of her food and instructs you to put the items back in her refrigerator. You comply with her instruction and proceed with your duties in a pleasant manner. She does not mention this again.

You report this concern to your supervisor, and your supervisor, who does not seem shocked by this, asks why you think Mrs. Washington is reluctant to throw away the outdated items from her fridge.

ment building, you may be responsible for bringing down the recycling items to the area where they are placed and putting them into their appropriate bins.

Recycling reduces the amount of waste that would eventually fill our dumpsites and landfills and is an environmentally responsible action all of us can participate in.

CLEANING BATHROOMS

Bathrooms need special attention because microbes easily grow and spread in damp places (Box 25–5), so family members must keep bathrooms clean. Toilets must be cleaned thoroughly with a disinfectant or toilet bowl cleaner. Wear utility gloves for cleaning toilets. Brushes or sponges used to clean the toilet must not be used for cleaning other areas in the house.

Surfaces in a bathroom should always be dried well to prevent **mildew** (a microscopic fungal parasite) growth, which is usually responsible for the black discoloration seen on bathroom surfaces and causes a foul odour in bathrooms.

Since some cleaners can scratch surfaces, use special cleaners for the bathroom. If they are not available, use laundry detergent (or a small amount of dish soap) and a cloth, or even a vinegar-and-water solution.

Practise the following hygiene measures:

- Rinse and dry bar soaps after use.
- Flush the toilet with the seat down to prevent splashing and the spread of microbes.
- Rinse the sink after it has been used for washing, shaving, or oral hygiene.
- Remove and dispose of hair from the sink, tub, or shower.
- Hang damp towels and bath mats out to dry, or place them in a hamper.
- Wash bath mats, the wastebasket, and the laundry hamper every week.
- Put out clean towels.
- Wipe up water spills.
- Wipe out the bathtub or shower immediately after use.
- Provide enough toilet paper and tissue.
- Open shower doors to prevent mildew from developing inside the shower.

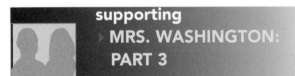

Box 25–5 Cleaning Bathrooms

Task	Supplies and Equipment	Process
Cleaning sinks	Cloths or sponge Utility gloves Hot, soapy water Disinfectant	Wipe sink with hot, soapy water and disinfectant Rinse and dry with dry cloth Wipe and dry taps
Cleaning bathtubs, showers, and shower curtains	Cloths or sponge Utility gloves Hot, soapy water Disinfectant	Wipe with hot, soapy water and disinfect showers and shower curtains Rinse and dry with dry cloth Wipe and dry taps
Replenishing supplies	Toilet paper Tissues Soap and shampoo Toothpaste Other supplies, as needed	Check and replenish supplies
Cleaning surfaces	Cloths or sponge Utility gloves Hot, soapy water Disinfectant	Wipe window sills, bathroom tiles, soap holders, and door handles with hot, soapy water and disinfectant Rinse and dry all surfaces
Cleaning mirrors	Glass cleaner or white vinegar and water Paper towels	Wipe with paper towels and cleaner Dry with paper towels
Cleaning toilets	Toilet bowl cleaner or disinfectant NEVER use bleach in the toilet bowl, as it could cause a toxic gas to be released Bucket of hot water Utility gloves Toilet brush or sponge Fresh cloths or paper towels	Wear gloves Clean toilet tank Clean the toilet bowl, outside and inside; clean under the bowl and under and behind the seat Clean and dry the toilet seat and outer surfaces with fresh cloths or paper towels Clean and dry toilet handle with fresh cloths or paper towels
Cleaning floors	Bucket of hot, soapy water Disinfectant Utility gloves Mop, cloths, or sponge	Clean floor last Dry floor to prevent falls Vacuum carpeted floors

Adapted from: Birchenall, J., & Streight, E. (1997). *Mosby's textbook for the home care aide* (p. 141). St. Louis: Mosby.

- Do not pour dirty or contaminated liquids in the sink. Flush them down the toilet.

Some clients are at high risk for infection—for example, clients recovering from surgery and those undergoing chemotherapy—so their bathrooms must be kept very clean. The care plan lists extra measures that are needed for these clients, such as:

- Clean the tub, shower, and sink with disinfectant before and after use.
- Use paper towels for hand drying.

DOING LAUNDRY

When doing laundry, your goal is to clean clothing items without damaging them. Many clients' houses and apartments will have laundry facilities. If not, a laundromat has to be used, and you will need the right amount of change to operate the washing and drying machines in the laundry facilities. Find out if the client keeps change for this purpose.

Ask your client (or family member) about which detergent, bleach, and fabric softener to use. Also, find out if there are any special laundry instructions. For instance, are garments air-dried or dried in a dryer? Follow your client's preferences. Box 25–6 describes how to do laundry properly.

Removing Stains. There many new stain treatment products on the market, which do remove stains effectively when their instructions are followed carefully. If the client does not have any stain-removing products and you are asked to remove stains from clothing, alternative cleaners (such as using a paste of baking soda and water on stains) might be useful. You should never attempt to remove stains without the client's permission. Also, apply the stain treatment on an area that is not readily seen (such as an inside seam) to ensure it will not damage that article of clothing.

Laundry Care Symbols. Most garments have **laundry care symbols** on inside labels that indicate how to care for the garment (Figure 25–3 on page 462). This is the new standard used in Canada (CAN/CGSB-86.1-2003), and it is consistent with American as well as international care symbols. In the new standard, five basic symbols identify care treatments for washing, bleaching, drying, ironing, and professional cleaning. The symbols are in black and white, replacing the previous edition's "traffic-light" colours of green, amber, and red.

The temperature of a treatment appears either in degrees Celsius or is defined by a series of dots (a hand iron symbol with one dot means that the garment can be safely ironed at a temperature of 110°C). Bars are used to help illustrate how aggressive you can be when washing the garment. For example, one bar below a wash tub means the garment should be machine washed using a mild treatment. Other symbols define techniques for professional cleaning, hand washing, and natural drying—dry flat, line dry, drip dry, dry in the shade.

Common symbols include the following:

- 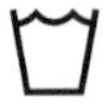 *The washtub symbol*—tells how to wash or not wash the garment. The water temperature is given in centigrade.
-  *The triangle symbol*—tells if bleach can be used. A "Cl" inside the triangle means chlorine bleach can be used.
-  *The square symbol*—tells how to dry items.
- 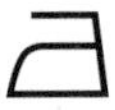 *The iron symbol*—tells if the garment can be ironed.
- 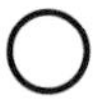 *The circle symbol*—tells if the garment needs to be dry cleaned.

When doing laundry, remember the following:

- Do not leave wet items in the washer. Moisture can cause mildew.
- If possible, dry items in a dryer rather than hanging them to dry. Quick drying helps eliminate microbes.
- Do not leave items in the dryer, as this can wrinkle or damage the fabric.
- Use the hottest water and the longest wash cycle allowed for the item (see Figure 25–3).

Laundry Soiled with Body Substances

Follow employer policy and Standard Practices (see Chapter 20) when handling laundry soiled with blood, body fluids, secretions, or excretions. The policy describes how to handle, transport, and process soiled laundry. Do the following when handling laundry soiled with body substances:

- Wear gloves.
- Place soiled laundry in leak-proof plastic bags. Secure bags to prevent spillage.
- Keep soiled laundry away from other laundry.
- Double bag laundry if the outside of the first bag becomes contaminated with body substances.

Box 25–6 Doing Laundry

Task	Process
Reading manufacturer's instructions	Read instructions on the washer, dryer, and laundry product Read garment's care label
Sorting items to be washed	Separate by fabric Separate heavily soiled or stained items Sort by colour: whites, darks, and coloured fabrics Close zippers, hooks, and buttons Check pockets for tissue, change, and other items If unsure about washing or dry cleaning, ask the client
Presoaking	Presoak heavily soiled and stained items Use the hottest water safe for the fabric Soak in bleach or borax for 30 minutes See Box 25–7 about removing blood, urine, and fecal stains
Prewashing	Prewash heavily soiled items after presoaking Use the recommended amount of detergent Use the hottest water safe for the fabric
Selecting the water temperature and the cycle	Use hot water (54–65°C / 130–150°F) and the regular cycle for heavily soiled clothes, cloth diapers, and whites Use warm water (38–43°C / 100–110°F) and the permanent press cycle for moderately soiled clothes and permanent press fabrics; for example, nylon, polyester, and acrylic Use cold water (26–38°C / 80–100°F) for bright colours, fabrics with colours that may run, fragile fabrics, and lightly soiled garments Use the gentle cycle when the label recommends it Wash garments with colours that may run (for example, bright reds) separately
Loading the machine	Use a high water level for a full machine Select the water level appropriate for wash size Do not overload the washer Wash large items separately Use a measuring cup for the detergent; follow directions on the package
Using the dryer	Remove lint from the filter Do not overload the dryer Use cooler temperatures, per instructions on garment labels Do not put woollen sweaters or garments that may shrink (see labels) in the dryer; lay these items flat to dry on a towel or clothes rack Use a sheet of fabric softener (with permission from the client) Remove garments soon after dryer stops to prevent wrinkling Remove lint from the filter
Ironing	Check garment labels before ironing Use a steam iron for heavily wrinkled clothing Make sure the iron is hot before using it After you have finished ironing, be sure to turn off the iron and unplug it Many older irons do not have an automatic shut-off. Ensure that the hot iron is not in a place where people or pets can accidentally burn themselves.

Adapted from: Birchenall, J., & Streight, E. (1997). *Mosby's textbook for the home care aide* (pp. 146–147). St. Louis: Mosby.

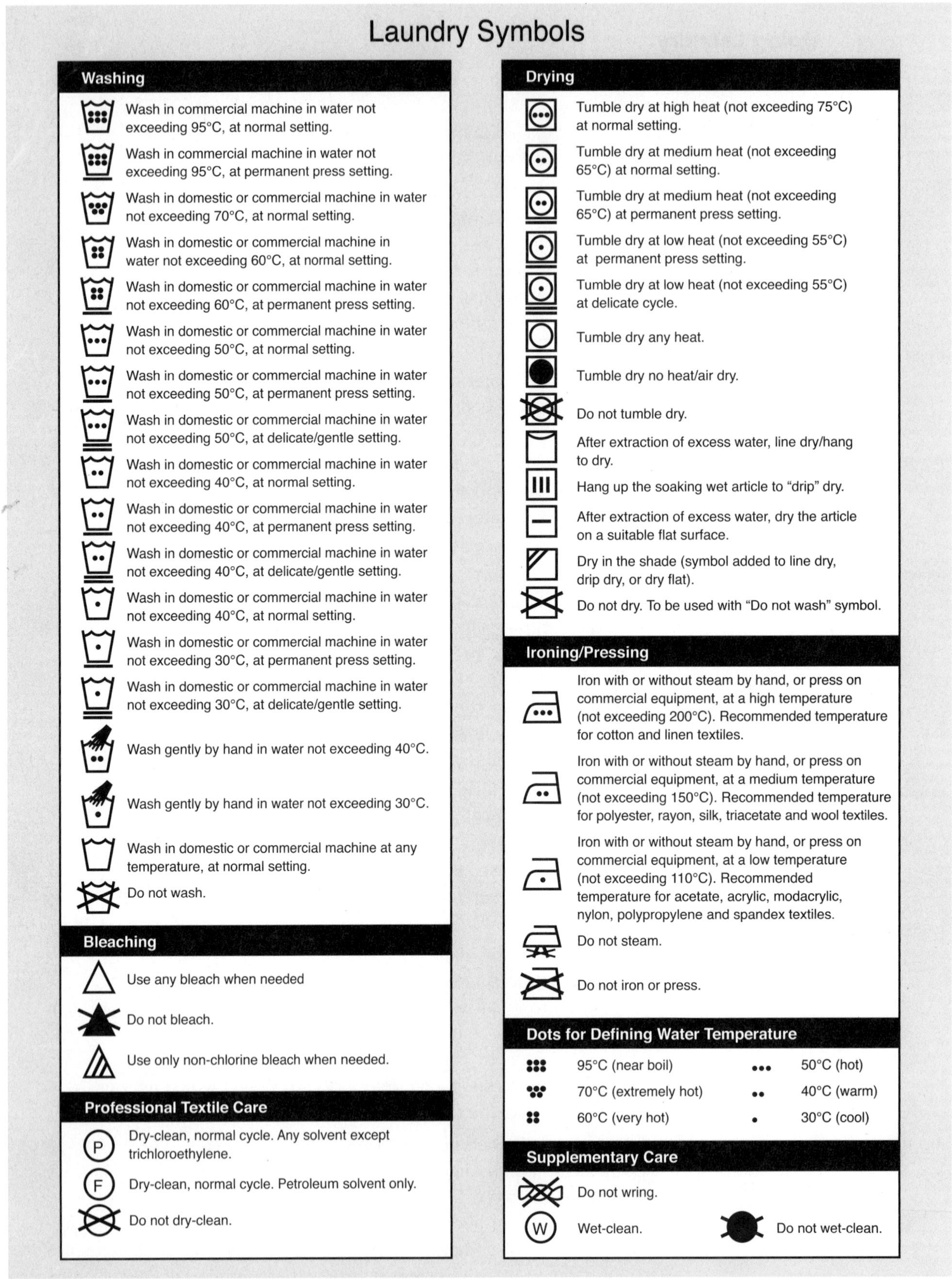
Laundry Symbols
Washing
Wash in commercial machine in water not exceeding 95°C, at normal setting.
Wash in commercial machine in water not exceeding 95°C, at permanent press setting.
Wash in domestic or commercial machine in water not exceeding 70°C, at normal setting.
Wash in domestic or commercial machine in water not exceeding 60°C, at normal setting.
Wash in domestic or commercial machine in water not exceeding 60°C, at permanent press setting.
Wash in domestic or commercial machine in water not exceeding 50°C, at normal setting.
Wash in domestic or commercial machine in water not exceeding 50°C, at permanent press setting.
Wash in domestic or commercial machine in water not exceeding 50°C, at delicate/gentle setting.
Wash in domestic or commercial machine in water not exceeding 40°C, at normal setting.
Wash in domestic or commercial machine in water not exceeding 40°C, at permanent press setting.
Wash in domestic or commercial machine in water not exceeding 40°C, at delicate/gentle setting.
Wash in domestic or commercial machine in water not exceeding 40°C, at normal setting.
Wash in domestic or commercial machine in water not exceeding 30°C, at permanent press setting.
Wash in domestic or commercial machine in water not exceeding 30°C, at delicate/gentle setting.
Wash gently by hand in water not exceeding 40°C.
Wash gently by hand in water not exceeding 30°C.
Wash in domestic or commercial machine at any temperature, at normal setting.
Do not wash.
Bleaching
Use any bleach when needed
Do not bleach.
Use only non-chlorine bleach when needed.
Professional Textile Care
P
Dry-clean, normal cycle. Any solvent except trichloroethylene.
F
Dry-clean, normal cycle. Petroleum solvent only.
Do not dry-clean.
Drying
Tumble dry at high heat (not exceeding 75°C) at normal setting.
Tumble dry at medium heat (not exceeding 65°C) at normal setting.
Tumble dry at medium heat (not exceeding 65°C) at permanent press setting.
Tumble dry at low heat (not exceeding 55°C) at permanent press setting.
Tumble dry at low heat (not exceeding 55°C) at delicate cycle.
Tumble dry any heat.
Tumble dry no heat/air dry.
Do not tumble dry.
After extraction of excess water, line dry/hang to dry.
Hang up the soaking wet article to "drip" dry.
After extraction of excess water, dry the article on a suitable flat surface.
Dry in the shade (symbol added to line dry, drip dry, or dry flat).
Do not dry. To be used with "Do not wash" symbol.
Ironing/Pressing
Iron with or without steam by hand, or press on commercial equipment, at a high temperature (not exceeding 200°C). Recommended temperature for cotton and linen textiles.
Iron with or without steam by hand, or press on commercial equipment, at a medium temperature (not exceeding 150°C). Recommended temperature for polyester, rayon, silk, triacetate and wool textiles.
Iron with or without steam by hand, or press on commercial equipment, at a low temperature (not exceeding 110°C). Recommended temperature for acetate, acrylic, modacrylic, nylon, polypropylene and spandex textiles.
Do not steam.
Do not iron or press.
Dots for Defining Water Temperature
95°C (near boil)
70°C (extremely hot)
60°C (very hot)
50°C (hot)
40°C (warm)
30°C (cool)
Supplementary Care
Do not wring.
W
Wet-clean.
Do not wet-clean.

Figure 25–3 Laundry symbols. **Source:** Industry Canada's Office of Consumer Affairs. *Guide to apparel and textile care symbols.* Retrieved July 16, 2007, from http://consumer.ic.gc.ca/epic/site/oca-bc.nsf/en/h_ca02221e.html

Removing Stains. Stains caused by bodily fluids (urine, vomitus, or blood) or solids (stool) should be always rinsed in cold water. Rinsing them in hot water causes the protein in the bodily fluid or solid to change, much like how an egg changes its appearance when it is cooked. Without soaking in cold water, stains will be almost impossible to remove in the future.

When removing stains, handle chemicals carefully (Box 25–7). Follow label instructions. Remember that both chlorine bleach and ammonia are poisonous. Each of them, by themselves, can burn or irritate the eyes and skin. Take care not to inhale ammonia fumes. Open a window when using ammonia. ***Remember to never mix chlorine bleach and ammonia because doing so creates a toxic gas.***

Make sure that clothes can be cleaned with bleach. Some people are allergic to chemicals in cleaning products. Check the care plan. If you are not sure, ask your supervisor.

The directions in Box 25–7 apply to both white and colour-fast clothes and linens. If possible, treat stains immediately before they become set in the fabric.

Box 25–7 **Removing Stains**

Urine Stains

- Rinse in cold water
- Soak in a solution of 1 L of warm water, 2 mL liquid (hand) dishwashing detergent, and 15 mL of ammonia for 30 minutes.
- Rinse in cool water.
- Soak in a solution of 1 L warm water and 15 mL of vinegar for 1 hour.
- Machine wash with chlorine bleach and detergent; dry as usual.

Blood Stains

- Rinse in cold water.
- Soak in a solution of 1 L warm water, 2 mL liquid (hand) dishwashing detergent, and 15 mL ammonia for 15 minutes.
- If fabric is strong, gently rub stain; continue as long as stain responds to treatment.
- Soak another 15 minutes in the solution used above.
- Soak in a solution of 1 L warm water and 15 mL enzyme product for 30 minutes.
- Wash in machine using chlorine bleach and detergent; dry as usual.

Fecal Stains

- Rinse in cold water.
- Soak in a solution of 1 L warm water, 2 mL liquid (hand) dishwashing detergent, and 15 mL ammonia for 30 minutes.
- Wash in machine using chlorine bleach and detergent; dry as usual.

Adapted from: Birchenall, J., & Streight, E. (1997). *Mosby's textbook for the home care aide* (p. 145). St. Louis: Mosby.

PERFORMING TASKS NOT INCLUDED ON THE CLIENT'S CARE PLAN

Occasionally, you might be asked to perform a task not included on the client's care plan. While some of the tasks might seem easy to do, others might not. For example, one client may ask you to make her a sandwich, even though meal preparation is not on that client's care plan. Another client may ask you to wash her windows, so she could clearly see the birds coming to her birdfeeder.

You should remember that you will not be paid for performing any tasks that are *not* on the client's care plan. Some employers frown on the support worker providing "free" services (that is, services that the client would normally be paying your agency for you to perform). Some agencies' insurance companies will not compensate you if you are injured while performing a task that is not on your client's care plan. You should also be aware that if you provide "free" services, the client will probably expect the same services from other support workers in the future!

Occasionally, the client (or their friends or family) will see you as a source of free services (see *Supporting Mrs. Washington: Part 4*). Be aware that when you are occasionally asked to perform a task that is not on your care plan, you should know how to respond to the client or others in each situation. Remember that you should always be professional, calm, and respectful if you must refuse someone's request for services that are not on your client's care plan.

Consult With Your Supervisor. Before performing a task that is not on the client's care plan, it is always a good idea to consult your supervisor about it. Your supervisor is aware of your agency's policies regarding such situations. Occasionally, your supervisor will say that it is "up to you," especially if the request is not time-consuming or does not require special skills. For example, your client may ask you to fill his birdfeeder while you are around his canary's cage. This is neither a complicated nor time-consuming task, so your supervisor might very well allow you to do this. Other favours can be time-consuming and may therefore put you behind in your schedule, especially if you have other clients to see that day.

Some favours are beyond your scope of practice, and you should ***never be persuaded to perform them.*** For example, since Mrs. Smith's arthritis is acting up and she cannot handle her insulin syringe, she asks you to help her with it. In this situation, it is important that you immediately call your supervisor and consult with her about what you should do, as there is considerable risk of harming the client. Your supervisor may send a nurse over to Mrs. Smith's house or go there herself or himself.

supporting MRS. WASHINGTON: PART 4

Mrs. Washington finally agrees to your supervisor's suggestion that she allow you to wash her laundry at her next-door neighbour's home. Mrs. Washington's neighbour, Sue Black, is a very pleasant 30-year-old woman, who happens to be the receptionist at your agency. Sue has been very nice to Mrs. Washington after her fall. She took care of her mail while she was in the hospital; she had suggested to Mrs. Washington that you could do her laundry at her house and had talked to your supervisor about it.

Because Sue is usually at work, she has given Mrs. Washington her house key so that you can use her washer and dryer while she is away. Today, Sue is home with a cold. She greets you at her door to let you into her house and asks that you do her a favour—that you fold the load of her clothing that is in her dryer and then do another load of her clothes before you leave Mrs. Washington's house for the day. This will, however, put you behind in time to see your next client.

You are not sure what to do, especially considering Sue has been kind enough to allow the use of her washer and dryer for your client. Because Sue works at the same agency as you do, you are uncertain about how to handle this situation. What should you do?

REVIEW

Answers to these questions are at the bottom of the page.

Circle the **BEST** answer.

1. **Home management duties include:**
   A. Personal care and hygiene tasks
   B. Organizing the garage
   C. Light housekeeping tasks
   D. Cleaning the attic

2. **Which of the following is a true statement?**
   A. The client, family, and case manager decide on required housekeeping tasks.
   B. Housekeeping tasks are never on the care plan.
   C. If you consult with the client, you can change the care plan at any time.
   D. The care plan is only a suggestion for what you should be doing.

3. **When cleaning a surface, you should:**
   A. Work from the bottom to the top
   B. Work from near to far
   C. Work from cleanest to dirtiest
   D. Work from wet to dry

4. **You need to do laundry, dust surfaces, and mop the floor. In which order should you do these tasks?**
   A. Do laundry, dust, and mop
   B. Dust, mop, do laundry
   C. Mop, do laundry, dust
   D. Do laundry, mop, dust

5. **When clearing clutter, you must:**
   A. Use your judgement about important and unimportant items
   B. Throw away all stray pieces of paper
   C. Gather things in one place so the client can put them away later
   D. Ask the client before throwing anything away

6. **You are not familiar with the client's cleaning products. You should:**
   A. Contact your supervisor
   B. Follow label directions
   C. Ask the client to buy new products
   D. Replace them with your favourite brand of products

7. **When are utility gloves necessary?**
   A. When loading the dishwasher
   B. When folding clean linens
   C. When cleaning the toilet
   D. When putting cleaning products away

8. **When working in a kitchen, you should:**
   A. Dry the dishes with a tea towel rather than let them air dry
   B. Use paper towels to dry your hands
   C. Use one cloth to wash surfaces, dishes, and floors
   D. Pour contaminated liquid down the kitchen sink

9. **When doing laundry, the hot water cycle is used for:**
   A. Diapers
   B. Lightly soiled clothes
   C. White lingerie
   D. Delicate fabrics

10. **Which of the following should you do when handling linens soiled with body substances?**
    A. Wash them with other garments in hot water
    B. Throw them away
    C. Ask the client to help you
    D. Follow Standard Practices

11. **Why should you never mix bleach with anything containing ammonia (including urine)?**
    A. The urine stains will become permanent
    B. When mixed, they will form a poisonous gas
    C. The bleach will not be as effective
    D. Nothing will happen

12. **Why are fecal stains always rinsed in cold water?**
    A. It is too wasteful to use hot water to rinse them out.
    B. Cold water is cheaper for the client.
    C. Using hot water will cause the item to shrink.
    D. Hot water can cause the protein in the fecal material to thicken.

Answers: 1.C, 2.A, 3.C, 4.A, 5.D, 6.B, 7.C, 8.B, 9.A, 10.D, 11.B, 12.D

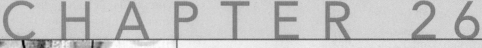

CHAPTER 26

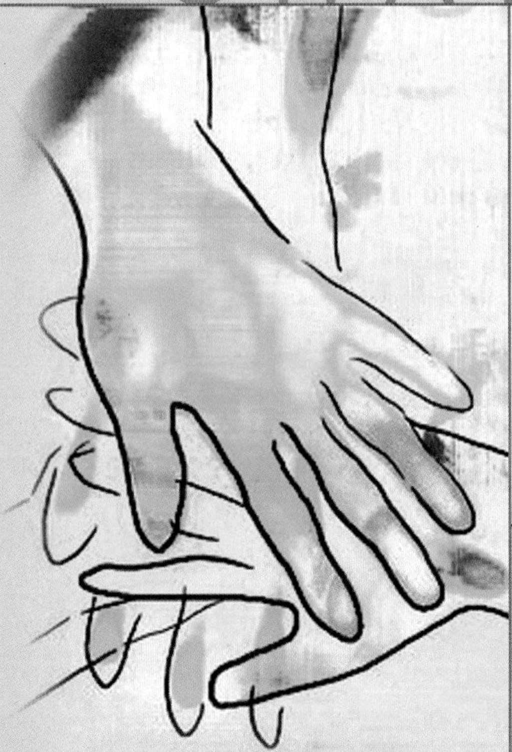

Beds and Bed Making

OBJECTIVES

- Define the key terms listed in this chapter.
- Identify the basic bed positions.
- Describe how to handle linens according to the rules of medical asepsis.
- List the purposes of cotton drawsheets and plastic drawsheets.
- Describe general rules for bed making.
- Describe the differences between open, closed, and occupied beds.
- Demonstrate the procedures described in this chapter.

key terms

drawsheet A small sheet placed over the middle of the bottom sheet; it helps keep the mattress and bottom linens clean and dry; can be used to turn and move the client in bed.

lift sheet See **turning sheet**.

plastic drawsheet A drawsheet placed between the bottom sheet and the cotton drawsheet to keep the mattress and bottom linens clean and dry.

turning sheet A sheet used to move a client up in bed. Also known as **lift sheet**.

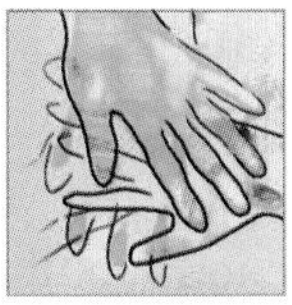

Different clients spend different amounts of time in bed—some are on complete bed rest and never get out of bed; some are on partial bed rest (getting up only to stretch or go to the bathroom); and some spend their waking hours out of bed, using the bed only to rest or sleep.

It is important to know the different types of beds, how to position them for the client's comfort, and how to make beds. A clean, dry, and wrinkle-free bed promotes the client's comfort and safety and helps prevent skin breakdown and pressure ulcers (see Chapter 42).

In facilities, beds are usually made in the morning after clients' baths or while they are taking a shower or out of the room. Clients usually like their beds made and rooms clean before visitors arrive. In private homes, beds are made according to the care plan and the client's preferences.

Linens must be straightened whenever they are loose or wrinkled and at bedtime. Check linens for crumbs after meals, and remove the crumbs. Linens are changed whenever they become wet, soiled, or damp. Follow Standard Practices when changing linens soiled with blood, body fluids, excretions, or secretions.

THE BED

Many home care clients use their regular beds. Hospital beds are used in hospitals and long-term care facilities, as well as in the homes by home care clients. Hospital beds usually have bed rails (see Chapter 19 for a discussion on bed rails and their use). Remember, bed rails have many safety hazards. Raise and lower them only as directed by your supervisor and the care plan.

Regular Beds

You will see twin-, double-, queen-, and king-sized beds, as well as waterbeds, sofa sleepers, cots, and recliners, in clients' homes. Also, a number of private homes have Craftmatic or Ultramatic beds. Clients in the community receiving palliative care often have hospital-type beds.

Regular beds cannot be raised. The lower the bed, the more you will have to bend and reach when giving care or making the bed, so use good body mechanics to protect your back (see Chapter 23).

A good mattress is neither too hard nor too soft. A poor-quality mattress may not provide needed support or comfort and could harm the client's back or skin. If you are concerned about the client's mattress, tell your supervisor.

Hospital Beds

Hospital beds have electrical or manual controls and can be raised horizontally to give care, which reduces bending and reaching. The lowest horizontal position lets the client get out of bed with ease (Figure 26–1) and may also be necessary as a safety measure for the client. The head of the bed can be kept flat or raised to varying degrees for the client's comfort.

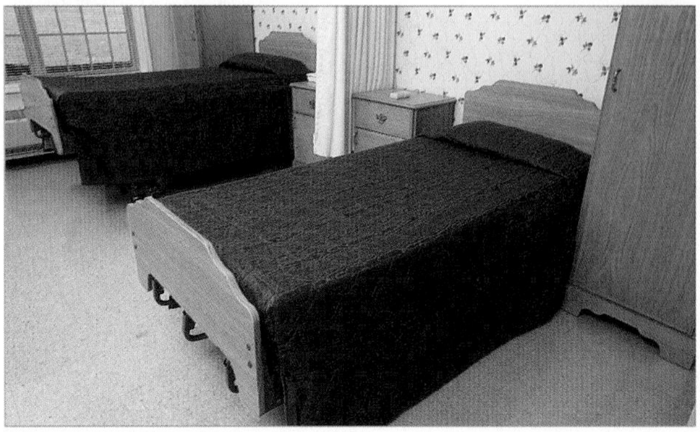

Figure 26–1 One bed is in the highest horizontal position and the other in the lowest horizontal position.

Most hospital beds are electrically controlled. Controls are on a side panel, bed rail, or panel at the foot of the bed (Figure 26–2), and clients are taught how to safely use the controls. Clients are warned not to raise the bed to the high position and not to adjust the bed to positions that could harm them. They are told of any position limits or restrictions.

Most electrically controlled beds can be "locked" into any position to prevent the client from raising or lowering the head or foot of the bed. Clients restricted to certain positions—for example, clients with dementia—may need to have their beds locked. You must also be alert to potential dangers if children, confused clients, or clients with impaired cognition or altered levels of consciousness have easy access to the controls. Follow the care plan, and check with your supervisor.

Manually operated beds are, however, still in use. They have cranks at the foot of the bed (Figure 26–3)—the left crank raises or lowers the head of the bed, the right crank adjusts the knee portion, and the centre crank raises or lowers the entire bed.

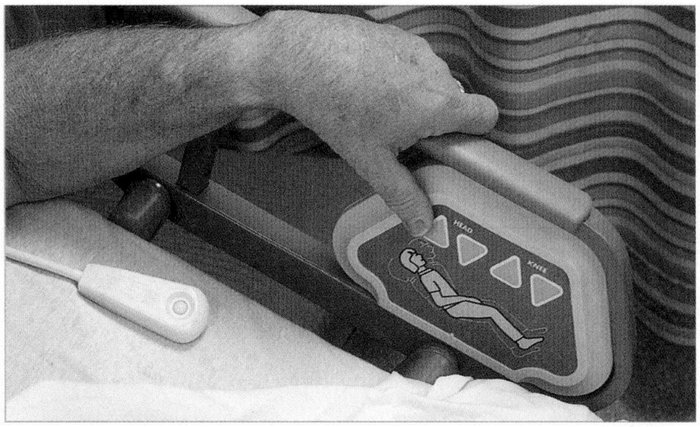

Figure 26–2 Controls for an electrically operated bed.

The cranks are pulled out and up for use, and after use they should be pushed in and turned down. Cranks in the "up" position are safety hazards, as anyone walking past could bump into them.

Hospital beds should always be left in their lowest position for the safety of the client. Only raise the bed immediately before giving care and when making the bed. As soon as you have finished, return the bed to its lowest position. Never leave the client alone when the bed is raised.

Hospital bed legs have wheels that let the bed move easily. Some beds have wheels that can be locked to prevent the bed from moving (Figure 26–4). Other beds have different locking mechanisms. Make sure bed wheels are locked when you are giving bedside care and when transferring a client to and from the bed. You or the client could be injured if the bed moves during the transfer.

Bed Positions

There are six basic bed positions:

1. ***Flat***—the usual sleeping position. The position is also used after a spinal cord injury or surgery for cervical traction and to deliver care.
2. ***Fowler's position***—a semi-sitting position. The head of the bed is elevated 45 to 60 degrees (Figure 26–5). The reasons for positioning a client in Fowler's position are described in Chapter 23.
3. ***High-Fowler's position***—the head of the bed is raised to a 90-degree angle. This position is used when feeding a client.

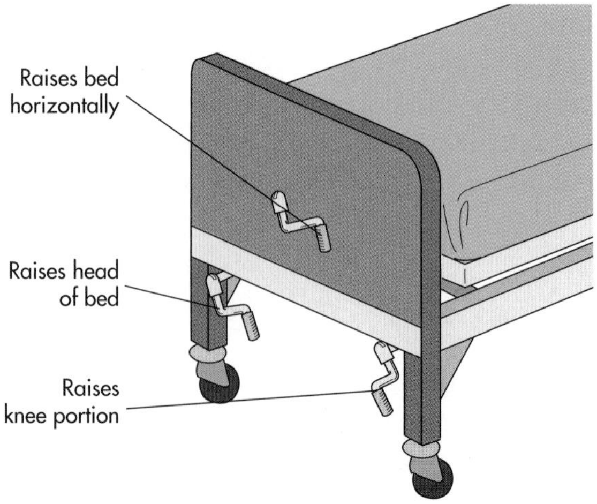

Figure 26–3 Manually operated hospital bed.

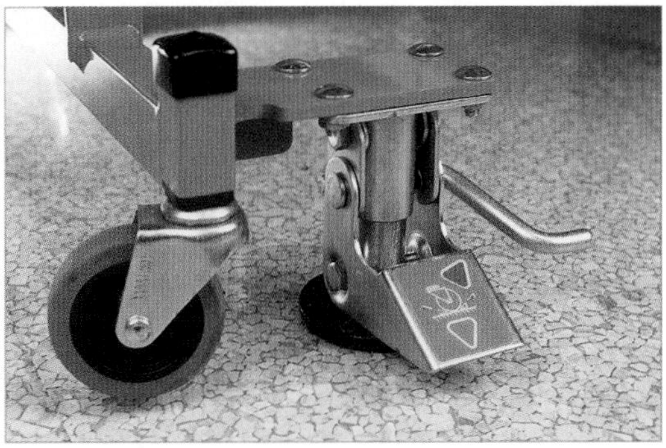

Figure 26–4 Lock on a bed wheel. **Source**: Sorrentino, S.A. (2004). *Assisting with patient care* (2nd ed., p. 148). St. Louis: Mosby.

4. ***Semi-Fowler's position***—the head of the bed is raised 30 degrees and the foot of the bed may be raised at the knee (Figure 26–6). This is a comfortable position. If the foot of the bed is raised, the client does not slide down in bed. However, raising the knee portion can interfere with leg circulation. Check with the care plan and your supervisor before positioning a client in semi-Fowler's position. This position is used when a client is receiving gastric feedings to reduce regurgitation and risk of aspiration (see the *Focus on Home Care: Fowler's and Semi-Fowler's Positions* box).
5. ***Trendelenburg position***—the head of the bed is lowered, and the foot of the bed is raised (Figure 26–7). A physician's order is required for this position. Blocks are placed under the client's legs at the foot of the bed. Some beds allow the entire bed frame to be tilted into Trendelenburg position. This position is used for postural drainage.
6. ***Reverse Trendelenburg position***—the opposite of Trendelenburg position. The head of the bed is raised, and the foot of the bed is lowered (Figure 26–8). Blocks are put under the client's legs at the head of the bed, or the bed frame is tilted. This position requires a physician's order and is used to promote gastric emptying.

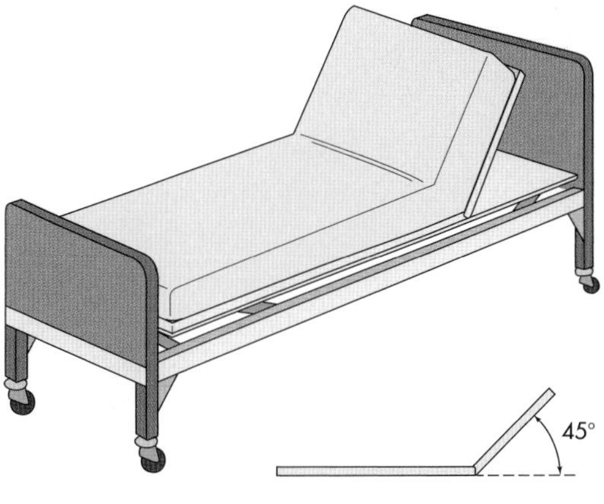

Figure 26–5 Fowler's position.

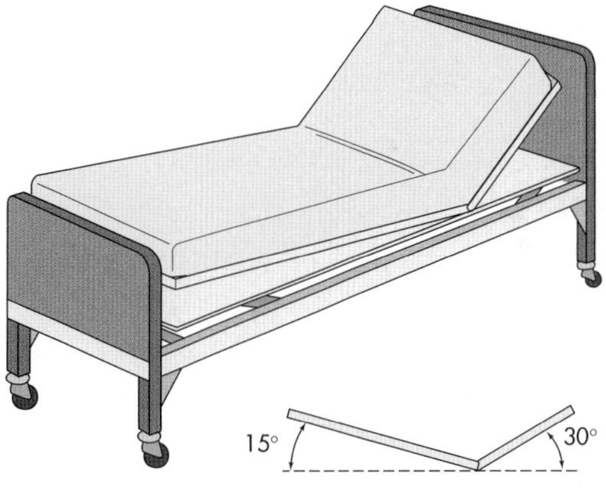

Figure 26–6 Semi-Fowler's position.

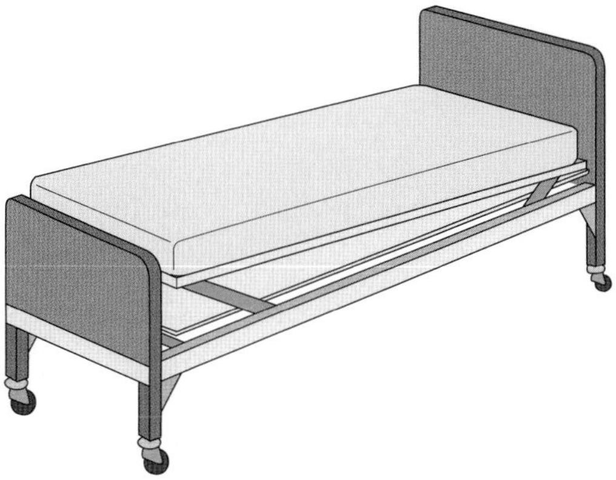

Figure 26–7 Trendelenburg position.

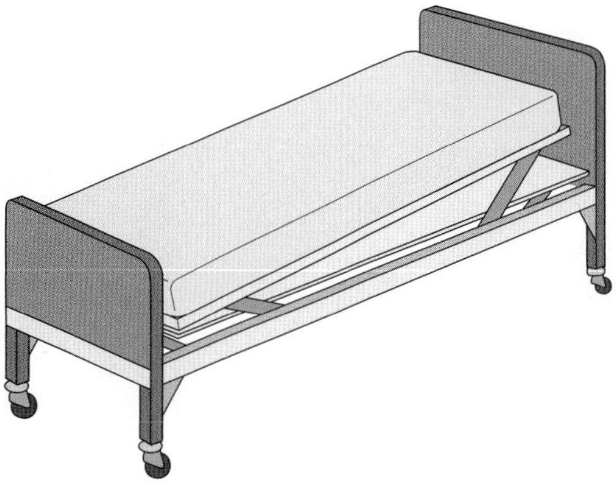

Figure 26–8 Reverse Trendelenburg position.

focus on
›› HOME CARE

Fowler's and Semi-Fowler's Positions

Fowler's and semi-Fowler's positions can be achieved with regular beds by using back rests or pillows (Figure 26–9). Check the headboard to make sure it is sturdy, as it needs to provide support when the client leans against it. Large, sturdy, sofa pillows are useful if a back rest is not available.

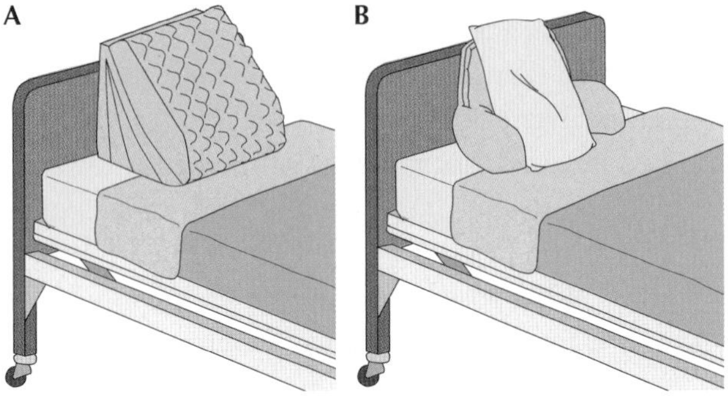

Figure 26–9 Back rests for regular beds. **A,** Wedge pillow. **B,** Study pillow with arm rests.

LINENS

When handling linens and making beds, follow the rules of medical asepsis. Perform hand hygiene before collecting clean linens. Your uniform is considered dirty, so you must always hold linens away from your body and uniform (Figure 26–10). Never shake linens in the air, as that spreads microbes. Clean linens should be placed on a clean surface. Never put clean or dirty linens on the floor. If clean linen accidentally touches the floor, put it in the laundry. If you are changing the linens in a semi-private room or a room with four beds, remember that linens for one client should be placed only on that client's furniture, not on another client's furniture. Take into the room only the linen you will need. If you find you have taken extra linen into the room, do not place it back in the linen room or on the linen cart but leave it in the client's room.

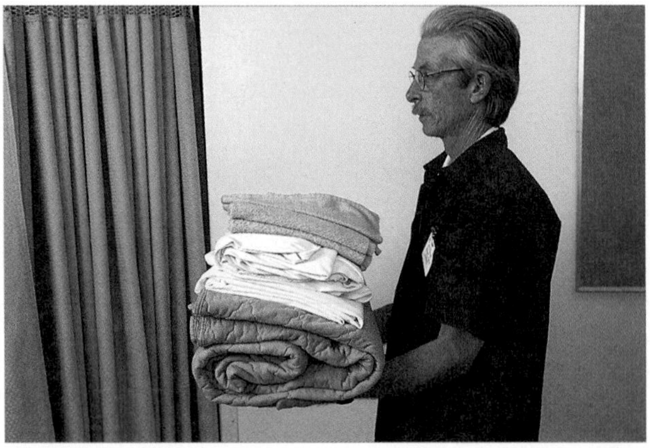

Figure 26–10 Hold linens away from your body and uniform.

Collect required linens in the order you will use them:

- Mattress pad
- Bottom sheet (flat sheet or fitted sheet)
- Plastic drawsheet or disposable bed protector (if used)
- Cotton drawsheet or lift sheet or turning sheet
- Top sheet (flat sheet)
- Blanket
- Bedspread
- Pillowcase(s)

Use one arm to hold the linens and the other hand to pick them up. Make sure the item you will use first is at the bottom of your stack. (You picked up the mattress pad first. It is at the bottom. The pillowcase is at the top.) You need the mattress pad first. To get it on top, place your arm over the pillowcase. Then, turn the stack over onto the arm with the pillow case (Figure 26–11). The arm that held the linens is now free. Place the clean linens on a clean surface.

Follow Standard Practices when removing linens. Used linen is considered dirty (contaminated with microbes). Wear gloves if the linens are soiled with blood, body fluids, secretions, or excretions. Also, check the linens for misplaced personal belongings—dentures, hearing aids, eyeglasses, watches, or jewellery—that clients may leave in their beds. Watch for stray needles in the linen, especially when clients self-medicate.

Remove each piece of linen separately. Roll the linen away from you. The side that touched the client will be inside the roll. The side that has not touched the client is outside (Figure 26–12).

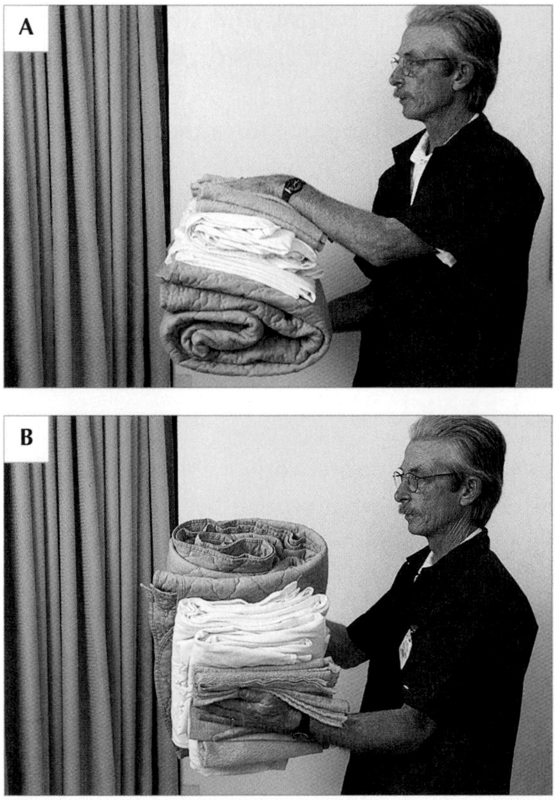

Figure 26–11 Collecting linens. **A,** Place your arm over the top of the linen stack. **B,** Turn the linen stack over onto your arm. Note that the linens are held away from the body.

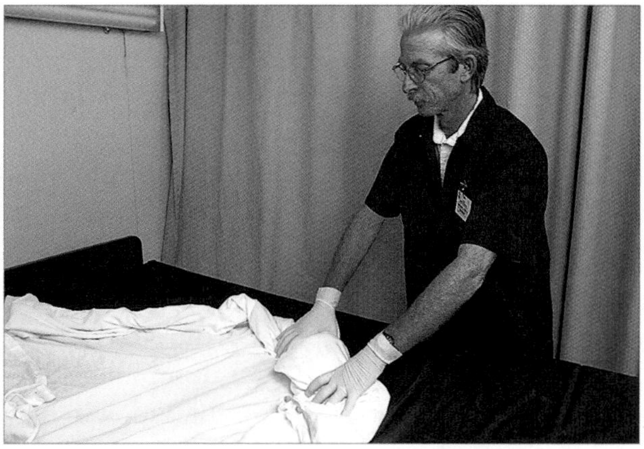

Figure 26–12 Roll dirty (used) linen away from you.

Immediately place used linens in a laundry container or a special linen bag. Remove the bag from the client's room. Soiled linens should never be placed on the floor as this will contribute to the spread of pathogens. Follow employer policy regarding soiled linen (see Chapter 20).

How often linen is changed varies among work settings (Table 26–1). Follow the care plan and employer policy. ***In all settings, linens are changed when wet, damp, or soiled.***

Table 26–1 Linen Changes in Different Settings

Setting	How Often	Special Considerations
Home care	Usually weekly When wet, damp, or soiled	Follow the client's preferences for linen choice. For example, some clients want extra blankets. Others do not want any blankets.
Long-term care	Usually weekly. Pillowcases, top and bottom sheets, and drawsheets (if used) may be changed twice a week. When wet, damp, or soiled	Some clients bring their own bedspreads, pillows, blankets, or quilts from home. Use them when making the bed. Remember, these items are the client's property. Handle with care. Make sure they are labelled with the client's name. If the facility uses coloured linens, let the client choose what colour to use. Also, let the client decide how many pillows or blankets to use. If possible, the client also chooses the time when you make the bed.
Hospitals	Daily When a client is discharged When wet, damp, or soiled	The mattress pad, plastic drawsheet, blanket, and bedspread are reused for the same client. They are not reused if wet, damp, soiled, or very wrinkled.

A **drawsheet** is a small sheet placed over the middle of the bottom sheet. It helps keep the mattress and bottom linens clean and dry. It is also called the cotton drawsheet because it is made of cotton. A **plastic drawsheet** is waterproof and protects the mattress and bottom linens from dampness and soiling. It is placed between the bottom sheet and cotton drawsheet.

The cotton drawsheet protects the client's body from contact with the plastic and absorbs moisture. However, discomfort and skin breakdown may occur. Plastic sheets retain heat and are hard to keep tight and wrinkle-free.

Many employers use waterproof pads/soaker pads instead of plastic drawsheets. Plastic drawsheets are usually used only for clients with bowel or bladder control problems or those with excessive wound drainage.

Cotton drawsheets are often used without plastic drawsheets. Plastic-covered mattresses cause some clients to perspire heavily, which increases their discomfort. A cotton drawsheet reduces heat retention and absorbs moisture; it is often used as a lift/turning sheet (see Chapter 23). When used for this purpose, it is not tucked in at the sides.

A turning sheet is used to safely move a client up in bed and give support workers a more secure grasp. These sheets can be made up of waterproof material or even by folding a sheet. Turning sheets prevent pain and skin damage by protecting the client's skin from friction and shearing when the client is being moved in bed. It is called a **lift sheet** in some agencies.

The bed making procedures that follow include plastic and cotton drawsheets to help you learn how to use them. Check with your supervisor if they can be used with your clients (see the *Focus on Home Care: Drawsheets* box.)

BED MAKING

Your job as a support worker will include making beds. No matter what type of bed you make, safety and medical asepsis are important. Follow Standard Practices. Box 26–1 lists the guidelines for bed making (also see the *Focus on Children: Crib Safety* box).

The Closed Bed

A *closed bed* is made when the bed is expected to be unoccupied for a certain period. Top linens are pulled up, and the bedspread is neatly pulled over the pillow (Figure 26–13). A closed bed is usually made when the client is up for most or all of the day. Clean linens are used, as needed.

In facilities, after a client is discharged, the bed frame and mattress are cleaned and disinfected. A closed bed is made and made ready for a new client.

focus on ››HOME CARE

Drawsheets

A flat sheet or flannel blanket folded in half can serve as a drawsheet. Usually a sheet the same size as the bed or a larger size is easier to use for this purpose. Your supervisor and the care plan will tell you what to use.

Medical supply stores sell plastic drawsheets and waterproof pads. The case manager discusses the need for these items with the client and family. Some clients place plastic mattress protectors on their beds, but these protectors do not protect the bottom linens (cotton drawsheet, bottom sheet, and mattress pad). Some clients prefer to place a small plastic sheet under the drawsheet. Again, your supervisor and the care plan will tell you what is safe to use for the client. Do not use plastic garbage bags or dry-cleaning bags, as these are not strong enough to protect the linens and mattress. They slide easily and can move out of place, and the danger of suffocation is great if the bag covers the client's nose and mouth.

Box 26–1 Guidelines for Bed Making

- Use good body mechanics at all times.
- Follow the rules of medical asepsis.
- Follow Standard Practices.
- Make the bed according to the client's wishes and the care plan. If the client's wishes are unsafe, tell your supervisor.
- Have a bag bin ready for disposal of soiled linen.
- Perform hand hygiene before handling clean linen and after handling dirty linen.
- Bring enough linen to the client's room.
- Do not use torn linen.
- Never shake linens in the air. Shaking linens spreads microbes, lint, and dust.
- Extra linen in a client's room is considered contaminated. Do not use it for other clients (in facilities) or family members (in home care settings). Put it in with the dirty laundry.
- Hold linens away from your uniform. Dirty linen as well as clean linen must not touch your uniform.
- Never put dirty linen on the floor or on clean linen. Handle and dispose of linen according to employer policy (see Chapter 20).
- Keep bottom linens tucked in and wrinkle-free.
- Completely cover a plastic drawsheet with a cotton drawsheet. A plastic drawsheet must not touch the client's body.
- Straighten and tighten loose sheets, blankets, and bedspreads, whenever necessary.
- Make one side of the bed, as much as possible, before going to the other side. This practice saves time and energy.
- Change wet, damp, and soiled linens right away.

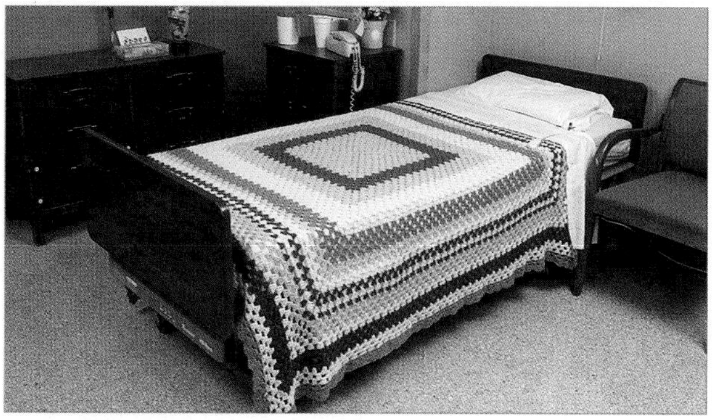

Figure 26–13 A closed bed. **Source**: Sorrentino, S.A. & Gorek, B. (2003). *Mosby's textbook for long-term care assistants* (4th ed., p. 277). St. Louis: Mosby.

focus on ›› CHILDREN

Crib Safety

Cribs, crib linens, mattresses, linens, and bumper pads all pose many dangers to infants, as they can lead to strangulation and suffocation. Report any safety hazard to your supervisor. Always follow these safety rules:

- The crib mattress must be firm. A soft mattress can cover the baby's nose and mouth causing suffocation.
- The mattress must fit snugly in the crib frame. The baby's head could get caught between the frame and the loose mattress and cause strangulation.
- The space between the mattress and crib sides should be no more than 3 cm. Only two adult fingers should fit in the space. If more than two fingers fit, the mattress is too small.
- The mattress must be at least 65 cm (26 in.) lower than the top of the crib rails to protect the baby from falling out of the crib. The mattress should be lowered even more when the baby can stand in the crib.
- Plastic garbage bags and dry-cleaning bags must not be used to protect the mattress.
- Bumper pads are no longer recommended for use in cribs, as they pose a risk of strangulation for the baby.
- Do not tuck blankets and top sheets under the mattress, as the baby can get caught in them.
- Do not place pillows, fluffy comforters, stuffed toys, or heavy blankets in the crib with the baby in it, as these items can cause suffocation.
- Check linens for loose threads, stitching, and trim, as these can cause strangulation.
- The space between the side bars should be no more than 6 cm.
- Cribs manufactured before 1986 do not meet regulations and must not be used.

1 2 3 MAKING A CLOSED BED

Remember to promote:

• **D**ignity • **I**ndependence • **P**references • **P**rivacy • **S**afety

Pre-Procedure

1 Perform hand hygiene.
2 Collect:
- Clean linen
- Mattress pad
- Bottom sheet (flat or fitted sheet)
- Plastic drawsheet (if needed)
- Cotton drawsheet, lift sheet, or turning sheet (if used)
- Top sheet
- Blanket
- Bedspread
- Two pillow cases
- Gloves
- Laundry bag

3 Place linen on a clean surface.
4 Place laundry bag near the bed.
5 Make sure linens have been removed and the bed and bed frame cleaned if the client has been discharged.*
6 Raise the bed to a comfortable working height.*

Procedure

7 Put on gloves if linens are soiled with blood, body fluids, secretions, or excretions.
8 Remove dirty linen. Roll each piece away from you and place it in the laundry bag.
9 Remove and discard gloves. Perform hand hygiene.
10 Move the mattress to the head of the bed.
11 Put the mattress pad on the mattress. Make sure the pad is even with the top of the mattress.
12 Place the bottom sheet on the mattress pad (Figure 26–14):
- **a** Unfold it lengthwise.
- **b** Place the centre crease in the middle of the bed.
- **c** Position the lower edge even with the bottom of the mattress.
- **d** Place the large hem at the top and the small hem at the bottom.
- **e** Face hem-stitching downward, away from the person.

13 Open the sheet. Fanfold it toward the other side of the bed (Figure 26–15).
14 Tuck the top of the sheet under the mattress. Make sure the sheet is tight and smooth.
15 Make a mitred corner if you are using a flat sheet (Figure 26–16).
16 Place the plastic drawsheet on the bed about 35 cm (14 in.) from the top of the mattress (if used).
17 Open the plastic drawsheet and fanfold it toward the other side of the bed.
18 Place a cotton drawsheet over the plastic drawsheet. It must cover the entire plastic drawsheet (Figure 26–17).
19 Open the cotton drawsheet. Fanfold it toward the other side of the bed.
20 Tuck both drawsheets under the mattress, or tuck each in separately.
21 Go to the other side of the bed.
22 Mitre the top corner of the bottom sheet.
23 Pull the bottom sheet tight so that there are no wrinkles, and tuck in the sheet.
24 Pull the drawsheets tight so that there are no wrinkles. Tuck both in together or separately (Figure 26–18).
25 Go to the other side of the bed.
26 Put the top sheet on the bed:
- **a** Unfold it lengthwise.
- **b** Place the centre crease in the middle.
- **c** Place the large hem even with the top of the mattress.
- **d** Open the sheet, and fanfold it to the other side.
- **e** Face hem stitching outward, away from the client.

27 Place the blanket on the bed:
- **a** Unfold it so that the centre crease is in the middle.
- **b** Put the upper hem about 15 to 20 cm (6 to 8 in.) from the top of the mattress.
- **c** Open the blanket. Fanfold it to the other side.

(continued on page 475)

1 2 3 MAKING A CLOSED BED

Procedure (cont'd)

- **d** If steps 33 and 34 are not done, turn the top sheet down over the blanket. Hem stitching should be facing down.

28 Place the bedspread on the bed:
- **a** Unfold it so that the centre crease is in the middle.
- **b** Place the upper hem even with the top of the mattress.
- **c** Open and fanfold the bedspread to the other side.
- **d** Make sure the bedspread facing the door is even and covers all the top linens.

29 Tuck in top linens together at the foot of the bed. They should be smooth and tight. Make a mitred corner.

30 Go to the other side.

31 Straighten all top linen. Work from the head of the bed to the foot.

32 Tuck in the top linens together. Make a mitred corner.

33 Turn the top hem of the bedspread under the blanket to make a cuff (Figure 26–19).

34 Turn the top sheet down over the spread. Hem stitching should be facing down. ***(Steps 33 and 34 are not done in some homes and facilities. If the bedspread covers the pillow, tuck the spread under the pillow.)***

35 Place the pillow on the bed.

36 Open the pillowcase so that it is flat on the bed.

37 Put the pillowcase on the pillow (Figure 26–20). Fold extra material under the pillow at the seam end of the pillowcase.

38 Place the pillow on the bed. The open end should be away from the door and the seam of the pillowcase toward the head of the bed.

Post-Procedure

39 Attach the call bell to the bed.*

40 Lower the bed to its lowest position. Lock the bed wheels.*

41 Put towels, wash cloth, pyjamas, and bath blanket on the bedside stand.*

42 Remove the laundry bag from the room. Follow employer policy for dirty linen.

43 Perform hand hygiene.

*Steps marked with an asterisk may not apply in community settings.

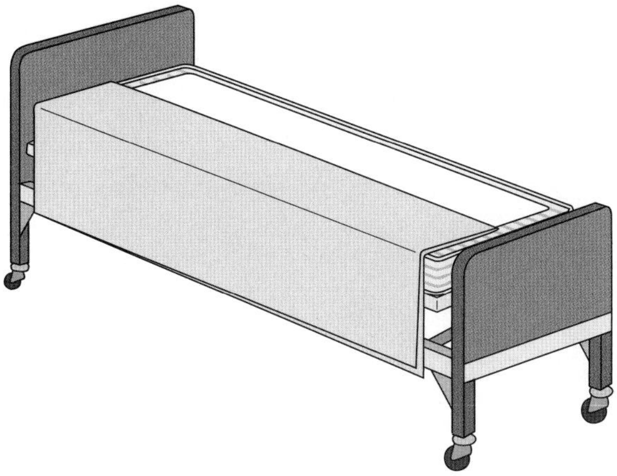

Figure 26–14 The bottom sheet is on the bed with the centre crease in the middle. The lower edge of the sheet is even with the bottom of the mattress.

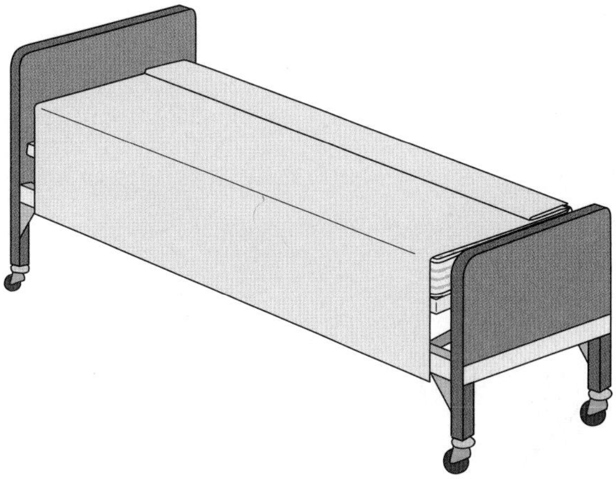

Figure 26–15 The bottom sheet is fanfolded to the other side of the bed.

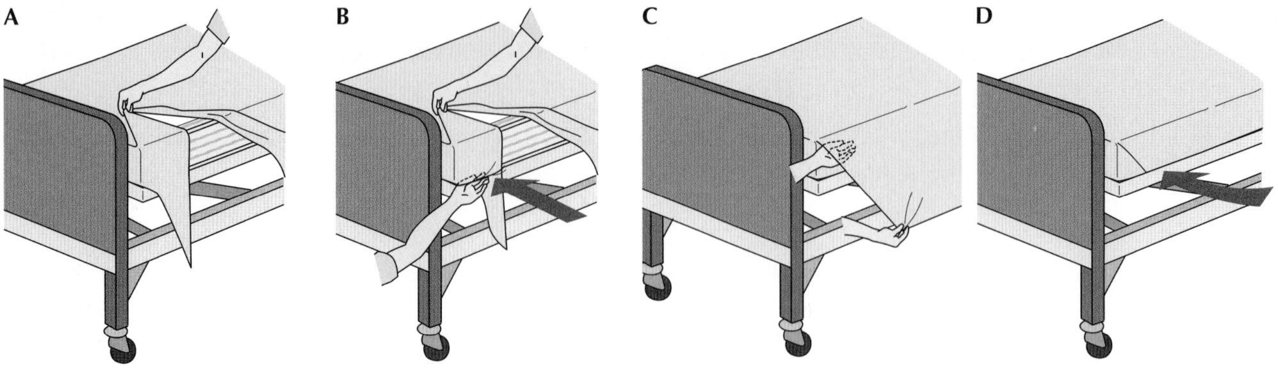

Figure 26–16 Making a mitred corner. **A,** Tuck the bottom sheet under the mattress. Raise the side of the sheet onto the mattress. **B,** Tuck the remaining portion of the sheet under the mattress. **C,** Bring the raised portion of the sheet off the mattress. **D,** Tuck the entire side of the sheet under the mattress.

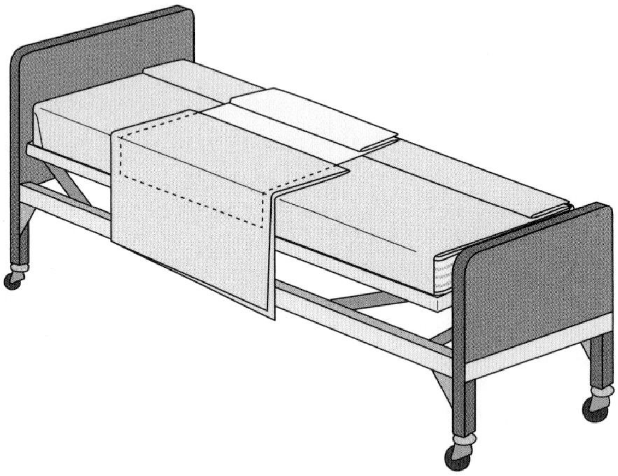

Figure 26–17 A cotton drawsheet completely covers the plastic drawsheet.

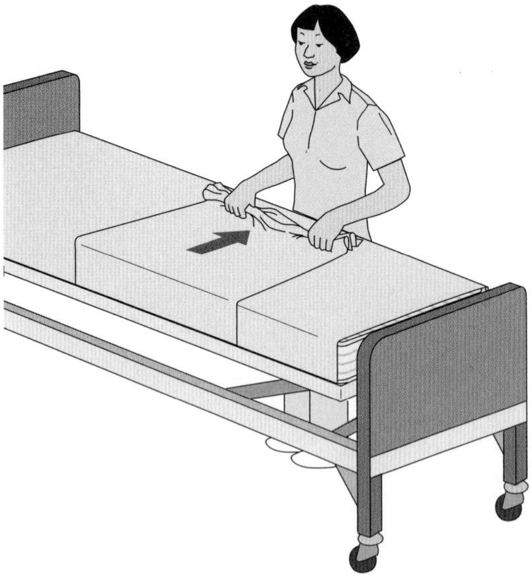

Figure 26–18 Pull the drawsheet tight to remove wrinkles.

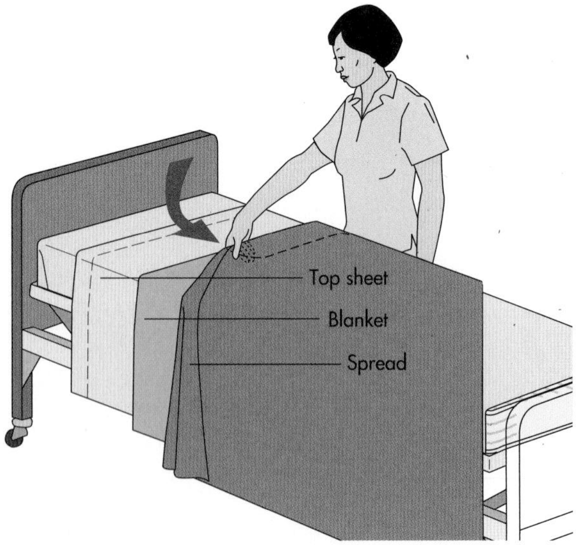

Figure 26–19 Turn the top hem of the bedspread under the top hem of the blanket to make a cuff.

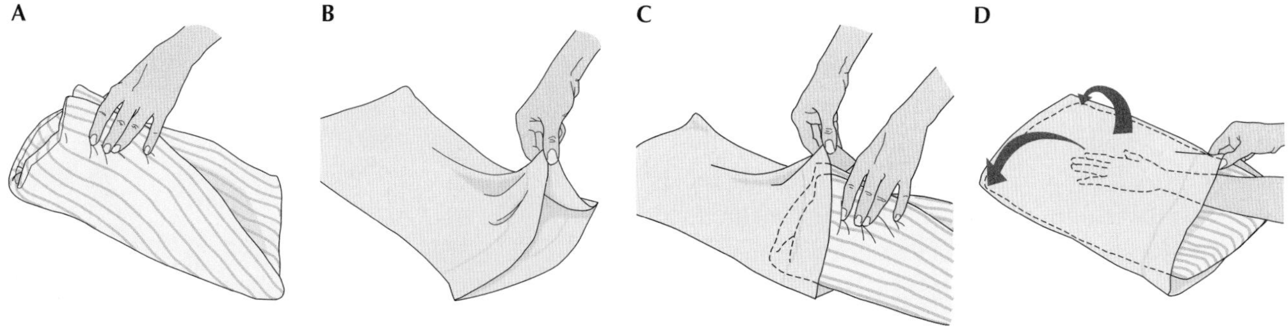

Figure 26–20 Putting a pillowcase on a pillow. **A,** Grasp the corners of the pillow at the seam end and form a "V" with the pillow. **B,** The pillowcase is flat on the bed; the pillowcase is opened with the free hand. **C,** The "V" end of the pillow is guided into the pillowcase. **D,** The "V" end of the pillow falls into the corners of the pillowcase.

The Open Bed

An *open* bed is made shortly before the bed is to be occupied. Top linens are folded back so that the client can easily get into bed (Figure 26–21). An open bed is made when the client is out of bed only for a short time, or it is made just before the client goes to bed.

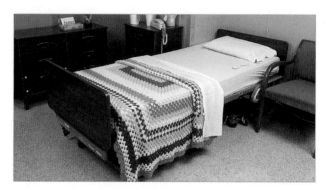

Figure 26–21 An open bed. **Source**: Sorrentino, S.A. & Gorek, B. (2003). *Mosby's textbook for long-term care assistants* (4th ed., p. 277). St Louis: Mosby.

1 2 3 MAKING AN OPEN BED

Remember to promote:

• Dignity • Independence • Preferences • Privacy • Safety

Procedure

1 Perform hand hygiene.
2 Collect linen for a closed bed.
3 Make a closed bed (see *Making a Closed Bed,* page 474).
4 Fanfold top linens to the foot of the bed (see Figure 26–21).
5 Attach the call bell to the bed.*
6 Lower the bed to its lowest position.*
7 Put towels, wash cloth, pyjamas, and bath blanket on the bedside stand.*
8 Remove the laundry bag from the room. Follow employer policy for dirty linen.
9 Perform hand hygiene.

*Steps marked with an asterisk may not apply in community settings.

The Occupied Bed

An *occupied bed* is made with the client in it (Figure 26–22) because the client cannot get out of bed for reasons of illness or injury. You must keep the client in good body alignment. If the client is too heavy or unable to turn independently, make sure to get help to move the client. Mechanical lifts may be used to lift the client out of the bed while it is being made. Before you start, you must know about restrictions or limits in the client's movement or positioning. Explain each step of the procedure to the client before it is done. Always explain what you are doing even if the client cannot respond to you or is in a coma. Remember to use good body mechanics.

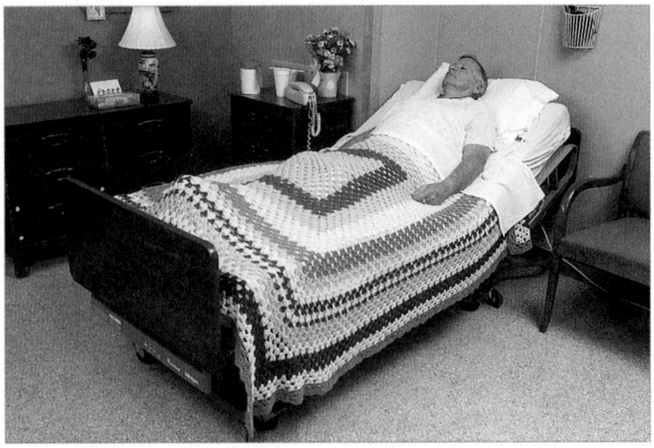

Figure 26–22 An occupied bed. **Source**: Sorrentino, S.A. & Gorek, B. (2003). *Mosby's textbook for long-term care assistants* (4th ed., p. 277). St Louis: Mosby.

1 2 3 MAKING AN OCCUPIED BED

Remember to promote:

• **D**ignity • **I**ndependence • **P**references • **P**rivacy • **S**afety

Pre-Procedure

1 Identify the client, according to employer policy.
2 Explain the procedure to the client.
3 Perform hand hygiene.
4 Collect the following:
- Laundry bag
- Clean linen (see *Making a Closed Bed,* page 474)

5 Place linen on a clean surface.
6 Provide for privacy.
7 Remove the call bell.*
8 Place the laundry bag near the bed.
9 Raise the bed to a comfortable working height. Follow the care plan for bed rail use.*
10 Lower the head of the bed. It should be as flat as possible. Lower the bed rail near you, if it is up.*

Procedure

11 Put on gloves if linens are soiled with blood, body fluids, secretions, or excretions.
12 Loosen top linens at the foot of the bed.
13 Remove the bedspread and blanket separately. Fold them as shown in Figure 26–23 if you will reuse them. Place each over a chair.
14 Cover the client with a bath blanket to provide warmth and privacy:
- **a** Unfold a bath blanket over the top sheet.
- **b** Ask the client to hold on to the bath blanket. If he or she is not able to, tuck the top part under the client's shoulders.
- **c** Grasp the top sheet under the bath blanket at the shoulders. Bring the sheet down to the foot of the bed. Remove the sheet from under the blanket (Figure 26–24).
- **d** If a bath blanket is not available, the existing top sheet can be used if it is not soiled or wet.

15 Move the mattress to the head of the bed.
16 Position the client on the side of the bed opposite to where you will begin changing the bed. Adjust the pillow for comfort.
17 Loosen bottom linens from the head of the bed to the foot of the bed.
18 Fanfold bottom linens one at a time toward the client. Start with the cotton drawsheet (Figure 26–25). If you will be reusing the mattress pad, do not fanfold it.
19 Place a clean mattress pad on the bed. Unfold it lengthwise, with the centre crease in the middle. Fanfold the top part toward the client. If you will be reusing the mattress pad, straighten and smooth any wrinkles.

(continued on page 479)

1 2 3 MAKING AN OCCUPIED BED

Procedure (cont'd)

20 Place the bottom sheet on the mattress pad, with the hem stitching away from the client. Unfold the sheet so that the crease is in the middle and the small hem even with the bottom of the mattress. Fanfold the top part toward the client. In the community and in some facilities, fitted bottom sheets are used. They should be placed and unfolded the same as an unfitted sheet.

21 Make a mitred corner at the head of the bed. Tuck the sheet under the mattress from the head to the foot.

22 Pull the plastic drawsheet toward you over the bottom sheet, and tuck excess material under the mattress. Do the following for a clean plastic drawsheet (Figure 26–26):

- **a** Place the plastic drawsheet on the bed about 35 cm (14 in.) from the mattress top.
- **b** Fanfold the top part toward the client.
- **c** Tuck in the extra fabric.

23 Place the cotton drawsheet over the plastic drawsheet. It must cover the entire plastic drawsheet. Fanfold the top part toward the client. Tuck in the extra fabric.

24 Raise the bed rail, if it was used. Go to the other side and lower the bed rail.

25 Explain to the client that he or she will roll over a bump. Assure the client that he or she will not fall.

26 Help the client turn to the other side. Adjust the pillow for the client's comfort.

27 Loosen the bottom linens. Remove one piece at a time, and place each piece in the laundry bag.

28 Remove and discard the gloves, if they were worn. Wash your hands.

29 Straighten and smooth the mattress pad.

30 Pull the clean bottom sheet toward you. Make a mitred corner at the top. Tuck the sheet under the mattress from the head to the foot of the bed.

31 Pull the drawsheets tightly toward you. Tuck both under together or separately.

32 Position the client supine in the centre of the bed. Adjust the pillow for comfort.

33 Put the top sheet on the bed. Unfold it lengthwise. The crease is in the middle, and the large hem is even with the top of the mattress. Hem stitching is on the outside.

34 Ask the client to hold on to the sheet so that you can remove the bath blanket. Or tuck the top sheet under the client's shoulders. Remove the bath blanket.

35 Place the blanket on the bed. Unfold it so that the crease is in the middle and it covers the client. The upper hem should be 15 to 20 cm (6 to 8 in.) from the top of the mattress.

36 Place the bedspread on the bed. Unfold it so that the centre crease is in the middle and it covers the client. The top hem is even with the mattress top.

37 Turn the top hem of the bedspread under the blanket to make a cuff.

38 Bring the top sheet down over the bedspread to form a cuff.

39 Go to the foot of the bed.

40 Make a toe pleat. Make a 5-cm (2-in.) pleat across the foot of the bed. The pleat is about 15 to 20 cm (6 to 8 in.) from the foot of the bed.

41 Lift the mattress corner with one arm. Tuck all top linens under the mattress together. Make a mitred corner.

42 Raise the bed rail, if it was used. Go to the other side and lower the bed rail.

43 Straighten and smooth top linens.

44 Tuck the top linens under the mattress. Make a mitred corner.

45 Change the pillowcase(s).

46 Raise the head of the bed to a level appropriate for the client, or use pillows to position the client.

Post-Procedure

47 Provide for safety and comfort.

48 Place the call bell within reach.*

49 Lower the bed to its lowest position. Follow the care plan for bed rail use.*

50 Put towels, wash cloth, pyjamas, and bath blanket in the bedside stand.*

51 Remove privacy measures, as needed.

52 Remove linen bag from the room. Follow employer policy for dirty linen.

53 Perform hand hygiene.

*Steps marked with an asterisk may not apply in community settings.

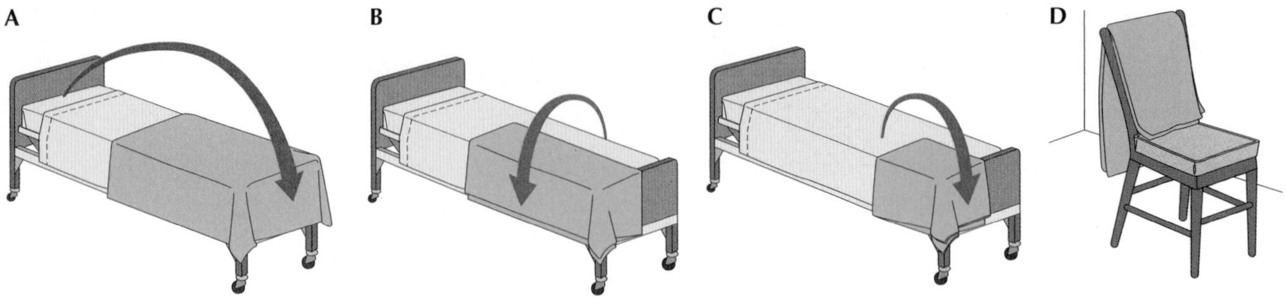

Figure 26–23 Folding linen for reuse. **A,** Fold the top edge of the blanket down to the bottom edge. **B,** Fold the blanket from the far side of the bed to the near side. **C,** Fold the top edge of the blanket down to the bottom edge again. **D,** Place the folded blanket over the back of a straight chair.

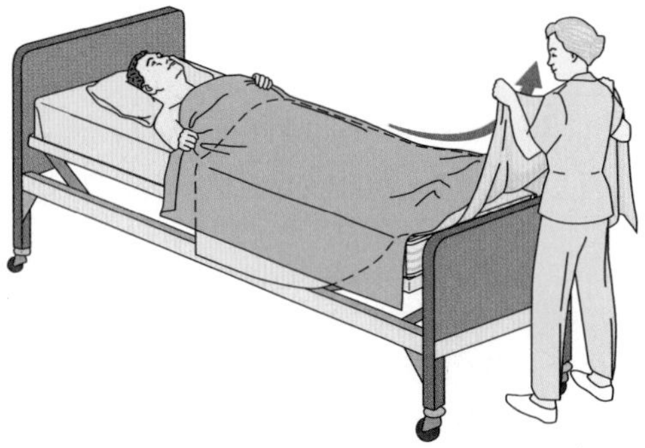

Figure 26–24 Ask the client to hold on to the bath blanket. Remove the top sheet from under the bath blanket.

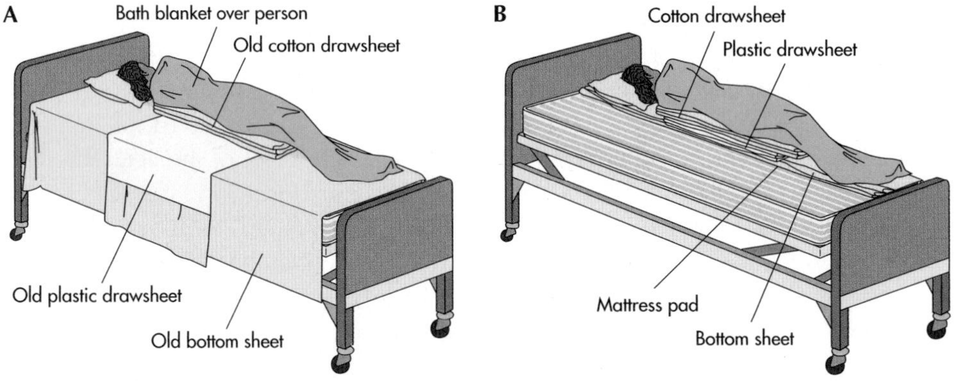

Figure 26–25 An occupied bed. **A,** The cotton drawsheet is fanfolded and tucked under the client. **B,** All bottom linens are tucked under the client.

Figure 26–26 A clean bottom sheet and plastic drawsheet are on the bed, with both fanfolded and tucked under the client.

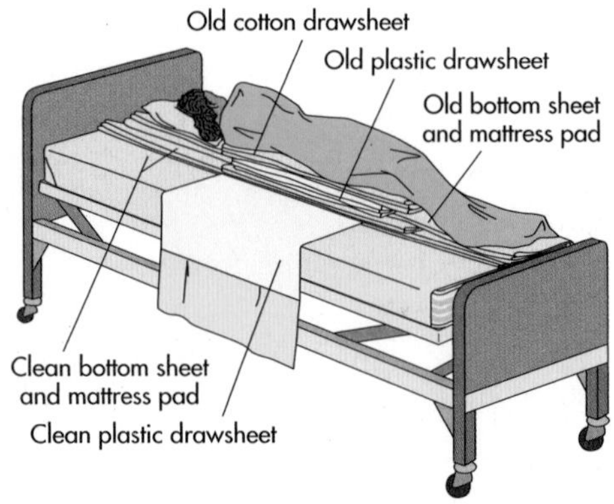

REVIEW

Answers to these questions are at the bottom of the page.

Circle the BEST answer.

1. **A hospital bed:**
   - A. Cannot be raised or lowered
   - B. Cannot be controlled by the client
   - C. Usually has bed rails
   - D. Is kept in the highest position at all times

2. **The Trendelenburg bed position is:**
   - A. A semi-sitting position
   - B. When the head of the bed is lowered, and the foot of the bed is raised
   - C. A flat position for sleeping
   - D. When the head of the bed is raised, and the foot of the bed is lowered

3. **Which of the following requires a linen change?**
   - A. Soiled linen
   - B. Loose linen
   - C. After the client has had an afternoon nap
   - D. Wrinkled linen

4. **When handling linens:**
   - A. Put dirty linens on the floor
   - B. Hold linens away from your body and uniform
   - C. Shake linens to remove crumbs
   - D. Take the extra linen to another client's room

5. **A cotton drawsheet is:**
   - A. Placed over the middle of the bottom sheet and over the plastic drawsheet
   - B. Waterproof
   - C. Placed under the bottom sheet
   - D. Placed under the plastic drawsheet

6. **You are using a plastic drawsheet. Which is *true*?**
   - A. A cotton drawsheet must completely cover the plastic drawsheet.
   - B. Disposable bed protectors are needed.
   - C. The client's consent is needed.
   - D. The plastic must be in contact with the client's skin.

7. **The following are crib safety rules. Which one is *true*?**
   - A. Bumper pads should remain in the crib until the baby moves to a bed.
   - B. The mattress must fit snugly in the crib frame.
   - C. Plastic garbage bags and dry-cleaning bags may be used to protect the mattress.
   - D. Pillows, fluffy comforters, and heavy blankets are safe to use in the crib with the baby in it.

8. **An open bed is made:**
   - A. When the bed will be unoccupied for a period of time
   - B. Shortly before the bed is to be occupied
   - C. With the client in it
   - D. So that a client can be moved to or from a stretcher

9. **When making an occupied bed you should:**
   - A. Cover the client with a bath blanket
   - B. Remove all pillows
   - C. Lower the bed rails if bed rails are used
   - D. Fanfold top linens to the foot of the bed

Answers: 1.C, 2.B, 3.A, 4.B, 5.A, 6.A, 7.B, 8.B, 9.A

CHAPTER 27

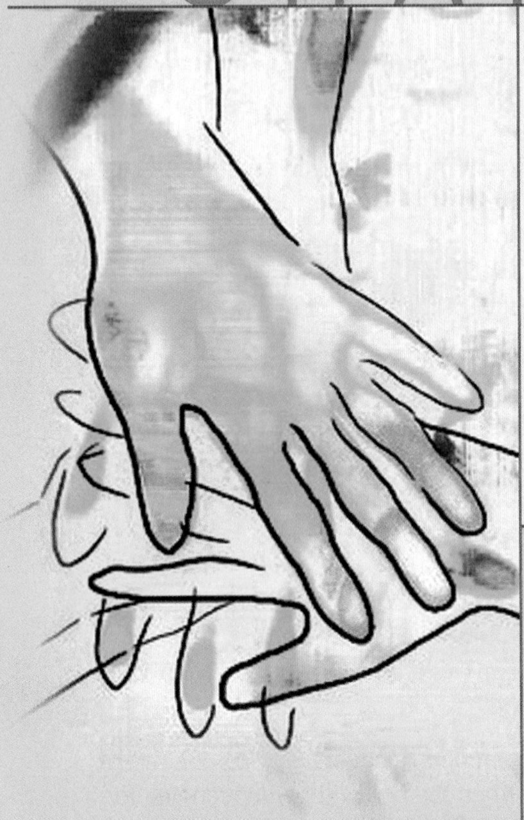

Basic Nutrition and Fluids

OBJECTIVES

- Define the key terms listed in this chapter.
- Describe the functions and major sources of protein, carbohydrates, fats, vitamins, minerals, and water.
- Explain the principles of *Canada's Food Guide to Healthy Eating*.
- Explain the purpose of food labels.
- Explain how nutrient requirements change throughout the life cycle.
- Explain factors that affect eating and nutrition.
- Explain your role in meal planning and preparation.
- Explain why food safety is important.
- Describe special diets.
- Explain your role in assisting clients to eat.
- Explain how to feed clients.
- Describe adult fluid requirements and the common causes of edema and dehydration.
- Describe three common special fluid orders.
- Explain the purpose of intake and output records.
- Perform the procedures described in this chapter.

key terms

allergy Sensitivity to a substance that causes the body to react with signs and symptoms.

aspiration Inhaling fluid or an object into the lungs.

calorie The amount of energy produced as the body burns food.

cross-contamination The spread of pathogens from one source to another.

Daily Value (DV) How a serving fits into the daily diet; expressed as a percentage based on recommended daily intake.

dehydration A decrease in the amount of water in body tissues.

dysphagia Difficulty (*dys*) swallowing (*phagia*).

edema Swelling of body tissues with water.

foodborne illness An illness transmitted by contaminated food products, which includes improperly cooked or stored foods.

intake The amount of fluids taken in by the body.

nutrients Substances that are ingested, digested, absorbed, and used by the body

nutrition The many processes involved in the ingestion, digestion, absorption, and use of foods and fluids by the body.

output The amount of fluid lost by the body.

pathogen Disease-causing microbe.

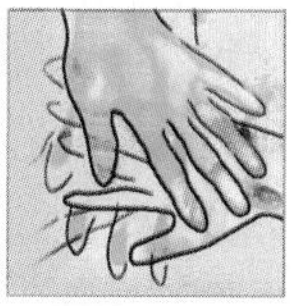

Food and water are necessary for life and health. The amount and quality of foods and fluids in the diet are important, as they affect a person's current as well as future health and well-being. A poor diet affects physical and mental function, increases the risk for disease, and slows healing. Poor physical and mental functioning increases the risk for accidents and injuries.

Food and drink contribute to social and emotional health also. Eating and drinking are part of social activity with family and friends (Figure 27–1).

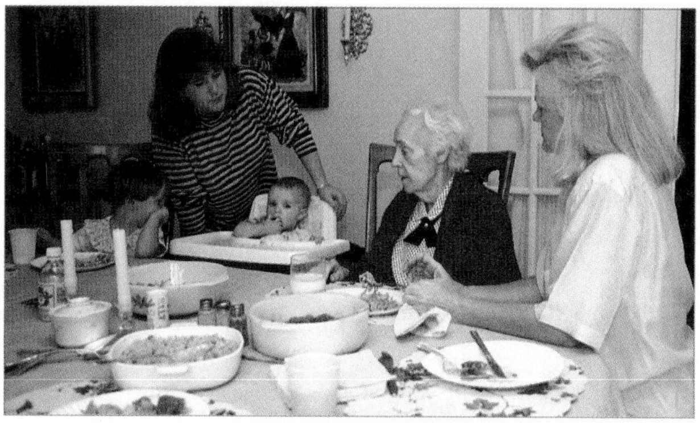

Figure 27–1 Meals are enjoyed when shared with family and friends. **Source**: Sorrentino, S.A. & Gorek, B. (2003). *Mosby's textbook for long-term care assistants* (4th ed., p. 414). St Louis: Mosby.

Many people need a friendly, social setting for meals; or they eat poorly.

As a support worker, you will serve food and fluids to clients and assist them with eating. In home care settings, you may also prepare meals for clients. This chapter introduces you to the basics of nutrition.

BASIC NUTRITION

Nutrition refers to the many processes involved in the ingestion, digestion, absorption, and use of foods and fluids by the body. *Ingestion* is the process of taking food and fluids into the body. *Digestion* is the process of physically and chemically breaking down food so that it can be absorbed for use by the cells. *Absorption* is the process by which substances pass through the intestinal wall into the blood. Review the description of the digestive system in Chapter 14.

Good nutrition is needed for growth, healing, and the maintenance of body functions. Selected foods must provide a well-balanced diet and the correct amounts of calories. A diet high in fat and calories causes weight gain and obesity; and weight loss occurs when a person consumes fewer calories than needed.

Nutrients

Foods and fluids contain **nutrients**—substances that are ingested, digested, absorbed, and used by the body. Nutrients are grouped into proteins, carbohydrates, fats, vitamins, minerals, and water.

Proteins, fats, and carbohydrates give the body fuel for energy. The amount of energy provided by a nutrient is measured in calories. A **calorie** is the amount of energy produced as the body burns food.

- 1 g of carbohydrate supplies the body with 4 calories
- 1 g of protein supplies the body with 4 calories
- 1 g of fat supplies the body with 9 calories

Protein. Protein is needed for tissue growth and repair. Protein sources include meat, fish, poultry, eggs, milk and milk products, cereals, beans, peas, and nuts. Animal products are the best sources of protein; so people who do not eat animal products must consume sufficient protein from plant sources, which are best eaten in combinations, for example, beans and rice. Protein deficiency can result in severe malnutrition. Children and older adults who do not eat properly are at higher risk.

Carbohydrates. Carbohydrates provide energy for the body and fibre for bowel elimination. Most carbohydrates come from plants. There are three main kinds of carbohydrates:

- ***Simple sugars*** are found in table sugar, fruit, and fruit juices.
- ***Starches*** are found in bread, pasta, rice, and potatoes.
- ***Fibre*** is found in bran, nuts, seeds, and raw fruits with skins. Fibre cannot be digested and passes through the intestines undigested.

During digestion, most carbohydrates (except fibre) are broken down into sugars, which are then absorbed into the bloodstream.

Fats. Fats provide energy, help the body to use certain vitamins, and add flavour to food, so some fat is necessary in the diet. Dietary fat not needed by the body is stored as body fat. There are three main types of dietary fat:

- ***Saturated fat*** is found in animal and dairy products (for example, meat, butter, milk, and cheeses).
- ***Unsaturated fat*** is found in fish and many vegetable oils (for example, canola oil and olive oil).
- ***Trans fat*** is found in margarine, shortening, store-bought cookies, cakes, pies, doughnuts, and fried foods. Trans fat is created when liquid oil is chemically altered to form a more solid substance. It is used to increase the flavour and shelf life of foods.

Unsaturated fat is healthier than saturated fat and trans fat.

Vitamins. Vitamins are needed daily for normal function and growth, but they do not provide calories. Each vitamin is needed for specific body functions (Table 27–1)—for example, vitamin A is necessary for vision. Vitamins are an essential part of a healthy diet, and the lack of a specific vitamin may result in illness. Older adults are at risk for developing vitamin deficiencies because the aging process affects the body's ability to absorb certain vitamins.

Minerals. Minerals are chemical substances found in both plant and animal foods. Each mineral is needed for specific body functions—for example, calcium and phosphorus are used to form strong bones and teeth. Table 27–2 lists the major functions and sources of minerals.

Water. Water is the most important nutrient necessary for life. The body needs water for maintaining cell function, regulating body temperature, delivering nutrients, and removing waste and for other body processes. Water enters the body through fluids and foods and is lost through urine and feces, through the skin as perspiration, and through the lungs with expiration. There must be a balance between the amount of fluid taken in and the amount lost. Death can result from inadequate water intake or from excessive fluid loss.

CANADA'S FOOD GUIDE TO HEALTHY EATING

Canada's Food Guide was developed by Health Canada to promote wise food choices. Healthy eating is needed to:

- Ensure a daily diet of the essential nutrients

Table 27–1 Vitamins: Major Functions and Sources

	Major Functions	Sources
Vitamin A	Growth; vision; healthy hair, skin, and mucous membranes; resistance to infection	Liver, spinach, leafy green and yellow vegetables, yellow fruits, fish liver oils, egg yolk, butter, cream, whole milk
Vitamin B_1 (thiamin)	Muscle tone, nerve function, digestion, appetite, normal elimination, carbohydrate metabolism	Pork, fish, poultry, eggs, liver, breads, pastas, cereals, oatmeal, potatoes, peas, beans, soybeans, peanuts
Vitamin B_2 (riboflavin)	Growth, vision, protein and carbohydrate metabolism, healthy skin and mucous membranes	Milk and milk products, liver, leafy green vegetables, eggs, breads, cereals
Vitamin B_3 (niacin)	Protein, fat, and carbohydrate metabolism; nervous system function; appetite; digestive system function	Meat, pork, liver, fish, peanuts, breads and cereals, green vegetables, dairy products
Vitamin B_{12}	Formation of red blood cells, protein metabolism, nervous system function	Liver, meats, poultry, fish, eggs, milk, cheese
Folic acid	Formation of red blood cells, intestinal function, protein metabolism	Liver, meats, fish, poultry, leafy green vegetables, whole grains
Vitamin C (ascorbic acid)	Formation of substances that hold tissues together; healthy blood vessels, skin, gums, bones, and teeth; wound healing; prevention of bleeding; resistance to infection	Citrus fruits, tomatoes, potatoes, cabbage, strawberries, green vegetables, melons
Vitamin D	Absorption and metabolism of calcium and phosphorous; healthy bones	Fish liver oils, milk, butter, liver, exposure to sunlight
Vitamin E	Normal reproduction, formation of red blood cells, muscle function	Vegetable oils, milk, eggs, meats, cereals, green leafy vegetables
Vitamin K	Blood clotting	Liver, green leafy vegetables, egg yolk, cheese

- Promote health and an overall sense of physical and mental well-being
- Reduce the risk of health problems related to nutritional deficiencies

The *Food Guide* divides foods into four groups, each containing different foods and nutrients.

- ***Vegetables and fruit***—fresh, canned, frozen, and dried vegetables and fruit; fruit juices
- ***Grain products***—cereals, pasta, rice, and other foods made with flour
- ***Milk products***—milk (fresh, powdered, or evaporated), cream, cheese, yogurt, and ice cream
- ***Meat and alternatives***—fresh and canned meat, poultry, fish, eggs, beans, lentils, dried peas, nuts, peanut butter, and tofu

A healthy diet contains foods from each food group. In the *Food Guide*, the four food groups are shown in a rainbow design (Figure 27–2 on page 487). Most food servings should come from the green band, representing fruits and vegetables. Unfortunately, most Canadians eat too much fat. Eating more carbohydrates (whole bread, cereal, grains, vegetables, fruit, peas, beans, and lentils) helps reduce fat intake. Foods high in carbohydrates are filling, allowing a person to feel satisfied with smaller quantities of food.

Table 27–2 Minerals: Major Functions and Sources

	Major functions	Sources
Calcium	Formation of teeth and bones, blood clotting, muscle contraction, heart function, nerve function	Milk and milk products, leafy green vegetables, whole grains, egg yolk, dried peas and beans, nuts
Phosphorus	Formation of bones and teeth; use of proteins, fats, and carbohydrates; nerve and muscle function	Meat, fish, poultry, milk and milk products, nuts, egg yolk, dried peas and beans
Iron	Enables red blood cells to carry oxygen	Liver, meat, eggs, leafy green vegetables, breads and cereals, dried peas and beans, nuts
Iodine	Thyroid gland function, growth, metabolism	Iodized salt, seafood, and shellfish
Sodium	Fluid balance, nerve function and muscle function	Almost all foods
Potassium	Nerve function, muscle contraction, heart function	Fruits, vegetables, cereals, meats, dried peas and beans
Zinc	Growth process, healing process, immune system	Meat, poultry, whole grains, dried peas and beans, eggs

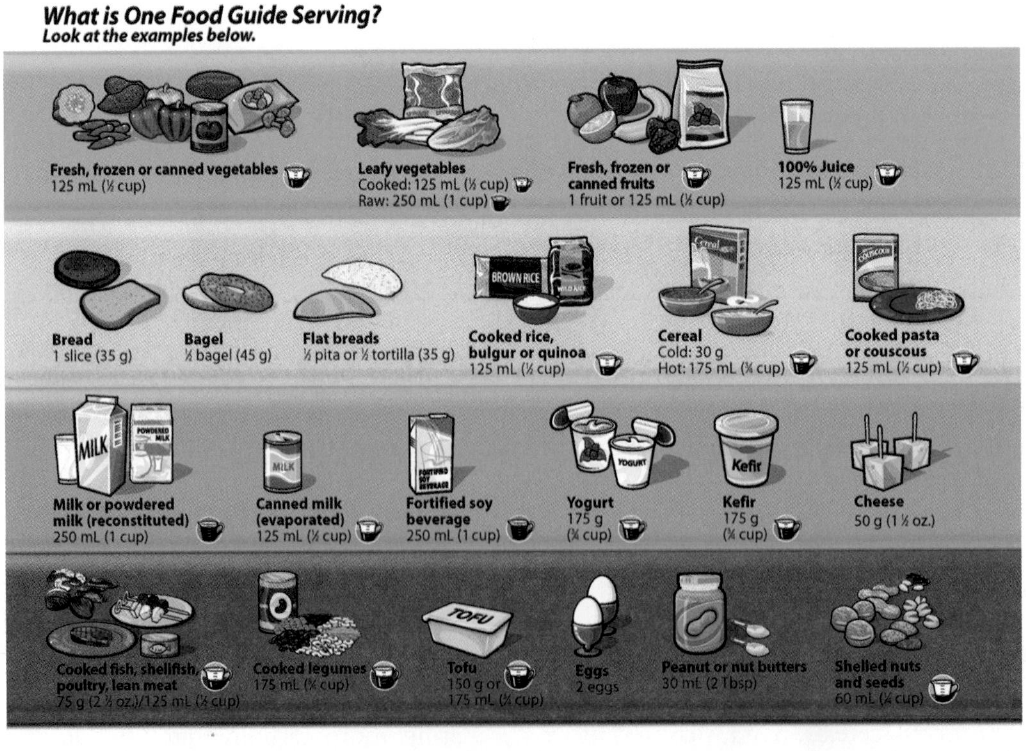

Figure 27–2 *Canada's Food Guide.* **Extracted from:** Health Canada. (2007). *Eating Well with Canada's food guide* (Cat. No. H164-38/I-2007E. Retrieved October 17, 2007, from http://www.hc-sc.gc.ca/fn-an/food-guide-aliment/order-commander/index_e.html. Reproduced with permission of the Minister of Public Works and Government Services Canada, 2007.

Box 27–1 Recommended Number of Food Guide Servings per Day

	Children			Teens		Adults			
Age in Years	**2–3**	**4–8**	**9–11**	**12–18**		**19–50**		**50+**	
Sex	**Girls and Boys**			**Females**	**Males**	**Females**	**Males**	**Females**	**Males**
Vegetables and Fruit	4	5	6	7	8	7–8	8–10	7	7
Grain Products	3	4	6	6	7	6–7	8	6	7
Milk and Alternatives	2	2	3–4	3–4	3–4	2	2	3	3
Meat and Alternatives	1	1	1–2	2	3	2	3	2	3

The chart above shows how many Food Guide Servings you need from each of the four food groups every day.

Having the amount and type of food recommended and following the tips in Canada's Food Guide will help:

- Meet your needs for vitamins, minerals and other nutrients.
- Reduce your risk of obesity, type 2 diabetes, heart disease, certain types of cancer and osteoporosis.
- Contribute to your overall health and vitality.

Extracted from: Health Canada. (2007). *Eating Well with Canada's food guide* (Cat. No. H164-38/1-2007E). Retrieved October 17, 2007, from http://www.hc-sc.gc.ca/fn-an/food-guide-aliment/order-commander/index_e.html. Reproduced with permission of the Minister of Public Works and Government Services Canada, 2007.

The *Food Guide* recommends a small amount of oils and fats be included in the diet—30–45 mL (2 to 3 tablespoons) of unsaturated fat per day. This would include oil used for cooking, salad dressings, margarine, and mayonnaise. Vegetable oils (such as canola, olive and soybean) and soft margarines that are low in saturated and trans fats are recommended. Butter, hard margarine, lard, and shortening should be used in limited amounts.

Many diseases—heart disease, high blood pressure, stroke, diabetes, osteoporosis, and certain cancers—are related to diet and the kinds of foods eaten. Therefore, the goal and benefits of healthy eating are better overall health, lower risk of disease, and a healthy body weight. A person who eats well will have more energy, feel and look better, and have stronger muscles and bones.

Servings From the Food Groups

The number of servings a person needs depends on age and gender (see Box 27–1 for the number of servings recommended by age). Young children have small appetites and need more calories than do adults for growth and development. Children have definite likes and dislikes, so they should be offered a variety of foods from the four food groups and small nutritious meals and snacks each day.

Women who are pregnant or breastfeeding need an extra two to three *Food Guide* servings each day. Women of childbearing age who plan to become pregnant or are breastfeeding need to take a multivitamin supplement containing folic acid every day. Adults over 50 need to increase their intake of vitamin D and should take a daily vitamin D supplement of 400 IU.

Vegetables and Fruit. Vegetables and fruits (including juices) provide carbohydrates, vitamins C and A, iron, and magnesium and are naturally low in fat. Eat a least one dark green vegetable (such as broccoli, romaine lettuce, or spinach) and one orange vegetable (such as carrots, sweet potatoes, or winter squash) each day. Try to prepare vegetables and fruits with little or no added fat, sugar, or salt. Fresh vegetables and fruits are more beneficial than juices. Frozen or canned fruit should be unsweetened, as sweetened and syrupy products are high in sugar and calories.

Vegetables provide the best value when steamed, baked, or stir-fried, and not deep fried, which can make vegetable preparations high in fat. For example, french fries are very high in fat compared with baked or boiled potatoes. Butter, oil, mayonnaise, salad dressing, sour cream, and sauces—toppings that are high in fat—are often added to vegetables. Small amounts of low-fat toppings help keep vegetable preparations low in fat.

Grain Products. It is recommended that at least half of the grain products consumed each day are those made from whole grain, such as whole grain bread, oatmeal, or whole wheat pasta. Eat a variety of whole grains such as barley, rice, oats, quinoa or wild rice. Carbohydrates (especially fibre), protein, iron, thiamin, niacin, riboflavin, folic acid, iron, and zinc are the main nutrients in this group. Choose grain products that are low in fat, sugar, and salt. Enriched products are also recommended because of their higher content of iron and B vitamins (see Box 27–2).

Milk Products. Milk and milk products are high in protein, calcium, carbohydrates, fat, riboflavin, and vitamins A and D. They are the richest source of calcium, which is needed to form and maintain strong bones. It is recommended that you drink 500 mL (2 cups) of milk every day for adequate vitamin D. Lower-fat milk products have less fat than whole-milk products and still provide the protein and calcium essential to a healthy diet. For example, one cup of skim milk has only a trace of fat (86 calories), whereas one cup of whole milk has about 150 calories—72 of the calories come from fat. Choose products low in milk fat and butter fat. Skim, 1%, and 2% milk are healthy choices. Other low-fat foods in this group include cheeses made with skim milk, low-fat or nonfat yogurt, and ice milk, rather than ice cream.

If you do not drink milk, drink fortified soy beverages instead.

Meat and Alternatives. Protein, fat, thiamin, vitamin B_{12}, and iron are the main nutrients in this group. The foods in this group vary in fat content. Wise food choices help lower the fat intake through foods in this group. Cold cuts and some luncheon meats are high in fat, so choose leaner meats, poultry, and fish. Chicken and turkey have less fat than do veal, beef, pork, and lamb, and skinless chicken and turkey are even lower in fat. Veal is lower in fat than beef. Egg yolks have more fat than do egg whites. Low-fat egg substitutes can be used for cooking and baking. Dried peas, lentils, and beans are recommended as meat alternatives, as they are low in fat and provide fibre and protein.

The type of cooking can help keep the fat in foods lower. Trim fat from meat and poultry. Baking, broiling, roasting, or microwaving is better than deep frying. Gravies and sauces also add fat.

Eat at least two servings of fish each week. Choose char, herring, mackerel, salmon, sardines, and trout.

Meat, poultry, and seafood are high in calories, so serving size is important. Restaurants frequently serve large portions of meat—for example, a 360-gram (12-ounce) steak would equal four to six servings from this group.

Box 27–2 Fortified and Enriched Foods

Food processing removes valuable nutrients from food. To replace losses or to enhance nutrient content, foods are *enriched* or *fortified.* In enriched foods—for example, wheat flour, cereal, and pasta—nutrients are replaced to their original level or higher. In fortified foods, nutrients are added, for example, milk fortified with vitamin D. Labels on products usually indicate whether a food has been fortified or enriched.

FOOD LABELS

Food labels are useful in planning a healthy diet and following special diets ordered by physicians, dietitians, or RNs. Nutrition labels are now mandatory on packaged food. Food labels have three components: a list of ingredients, nutrition facts, and nutrition claims.

List of Ingredients

Ingredients in products are usually listed starting with the major ingredient. Use the list to compare two or more products. For example, Brand A lists sodium first, followed by wheat flour, and Brand B lists wheat flour first and then sodium. So, Brand A has more sodium than Brand B. Use the lists on food products to also check for ingredients that cause allergies or food intolerance (see page 491).

Nutrition Facts

The *Nutrition Facts Table* (Figure 27–3) contains information on calories and 13 nutrients, including fat, carbohydrates, and protein. **Daily Value (DV)** shows how a serving fits into the daily diet of an adult and is expressed as a percentage based on recommended daily intake. Health Canada recommends the following daily intake of major nutrients:

- 60% of total calories per day should come from carbohydrate.
- 10% of total calories per day should come from protein.
- 30% (or less) of total calories per day should come from fat.
- 10% (or less) of total calories per day should come from saturated fat.

Nutrition Claims

Manufacturers' nutrition claims about foods (such as "low in fat," or "high in fibre") must meet government requirements. The following diet-related health claims are allowed:

Nutrition Facts Per 125 mL (87 g)	
Amount	**% DV***
Calories 80	
Fat 0.5 g	1 %
Saturated 0 g + Trans 0 g	0 %
Cholesterol 0 mg	
Sodium 0 mg	0 %
Carbohydrate 18 g	6 %
Fibre 2 g	8 %
Sugars 2 g	
Protein 3 g	
Vitamin A	2 %
Vitamin C	10 %
Calcium	0 %
Iron	2 %
* DV = Daily Value	

3.6 cm x 7.7 cm = 27.7 cm²

Valeur nutritive par 125 mL (87 g)	
Teneur	**% VQ***
Calories 80	
Lipides 0,5 g	1 %
saturés 0 g + trans 0 g	0 %
Cholestérol 0 mg	
Sodium 0 mg	0 %
Glucides 18 g	6 %
Fibres 2 g	8 %
Sucres 2 g	
Protéines 3 g	
Vitamine A	2 %
Vitamine C	10 %
Calcium	0 %
Fer	2 %
* VQ = valeur quotidienne	

3.6 cm x 7.7 cm = 27.7 cm²

Figure 27–3 The *Nutrition Facts Table.* **Source:** Health Canada. *The nutrition facts—to help you make informed choices.* Retrieved October 17, 2007, from http://www.hc-sc.gc.ca/fn-an/label-etiquet/nutrition/education/cons-res/cr_tearsheet-cr_fiche_e.html

- A healthy diet low in sodium and high in potassium may reduce the risk of high blood pressure.
- A healthy diet adequate in calcium and vitamin D may reduce the risk of osteoporosis.
- A healthy diet low in saturated fat and trans fat may reduce the risk of heart disease.
- A healthy diet rich in vegetables and fruit may reduce the risk of some types of cancer.

Some manufacturers will claim their products have "controlled fat" but this can be misleading as they have not indicated how much, if at all, the level of fat has been decreased. Be careful of products labelled "controlled sugar" or "added sugar."

CAFFEINE INTAKE

Health Canada has been conducting research into caffeine consumption levels that can be recommended for various age groups. Their research has shown that consumption of 400 mg/day is not associated with any adverse effects in adults. For the majority of the adult population, small amounts of caffeine can help increase alertness and concentration. For some people, small or larger amounts of caffeine can cause insomnia, headaches, irritability, and nervousness.

For women who are pregnant, planning to become pregnant, or breastfeeding, the recommended intake is 300 mg/day. If you asked your friends and family how much caffeine they consumed in a day, they would probably only count the number of cups of coffee or tea they had. For example, they may say they had three coffees, but they do not specify if each cup was 240 mL (135 mg of caffeine), 480 mL, or 600 mL (595 mg of caffeine), and they do not add the caffeine from colas, chocolates, energy drinks, and over-the-counter (OTC) medications.

Just one 600-mL cup of coffee contains more caffeine than the daily limit recommended for adults. How coffee is made also determines how much caffeine it contains. A 240-mL cup of instant decaffeinated coffee has 5 mg of caffeine, whereas a 240-mL cup of roasted, ground, filter-dripped coffee contains 179 mg of caffeine.

We know that caffeine has been identified in tea, coffee, chocolate, and some energy drinks. Certain herbs, such as guarana and yerba mate, that are added to energy drinks and bars also contain caffeine. Currently, these products are not required to identify the amount of caffeine added.

Recommended caffeine amounts for children are even less:

- 4–6 years 45 mg/day
- 7–9 years 62.5 mg/day
- 10–12 years 85 mg/day

As a support worker, be aware of the amounts of caffeine you are consuming and the amounts your client is consuming, as too much caffeine can cause significant side effects.

NUTRITION THROUGHOUT THE LIFE CYCLE

Nutritional requirements differ throughout the life cycle of a person.

Infancy and Childhood

Infancy is a period of rapid growth and development. Babies can be either breastfed or bottlefed. Breastmilk provides the best source of nutrients and antibodies during the baby's first 6 months. Formula milk can provide adequate nourishment but lacks antibodies. The pediatrician or the public health nurse usually provides guidance to parents on feed times for infants.

At 4 to 6 months, iron-fortified cereals are introduced, followed by puréed foods. Most babies are ready for finger foods and chopped foods at 10 months to 1 year. After the first year, the growth rate slows down.

Children usually have strong likes and dislikes for foods, which can make meal planning a challenge. Regular meals and physical activity are important for them. It must be remembered that children under 4 should not be given a low-fat diet, as fat is needed for brain development and energy.

When you care for infants and children, your supervisor will provide instructions about their dietary requirements. Follow the care plan.

Adolescence

In both boys and girls, the biggest growth spurt after infancy occurs during puberty, and increased nutrients are needed for this rapid growth. Many adolescents, however, have unhealthy eating habits—for example, they may skip meals, consume fast foods and soft drinks only, diet, and drink alcohol. Poor eating habits can lead to eating disorders, iron deficiency, and poor health.

Young and Middle Adulthood

Nutritional requirements in young and middle adulthood depend on age, gender, body size, and activity levels. Unless extremely active, most adults have lower energy needs than adolescents, and energy needs continue to decline into the 40s and 50s. If calorie intake exceeds energy needs, adults gain weight. A healthy diet containing essential nutrients is, therefore, extremely important.

Pregnancy. Pregnant women and their developing fetuses require nutrient-rich food, about 500 additional calories per day.

Pregnant women are advised not to smoke, drink alcohol, or take drugs. Pregnant women who do not usually consume meat and dairy products need to discuss their diets with their physician.

Health Canada suggests that pregnant and breastfeeding women increase folic acid, iron, and calcium intake. Low folic acid intake before and during pregnancy increases the risk of spinal cord and brain abnormalities in infants (see Chapter 39).

Late Adulthood

Older adults have wide variations in their health and nutritional status, as it is affected by emotional, social, and physical factors.

Many older adults are used to cooking for and eating with a family group. Preparing a meal for just one may hold no interest. Some older adults do not drive and may not be able to carry heavy grocery bags on public transit. Some may not have family or friends nearby who can help them with shopping and meal preparation. Those with low incomes may avoid buying high-protein foods, such as meat and cheese, which are usually expensive. Those living in long-term care facilities may not like the food that is served.

Loss of hearing, smell, and taste can affect appetite and social enjoyment of food, and poor vision may make shopping and meal preparation more challenging. Decreases in saliva may cause **dysphagia**—difficulty (*dys*) in swallowing (*phagia*). (See page 499.) Secretion of digestive juices also declines with age. As a result, fried and fatty foods are hard to digest and may cause indigestion, and nutrients are not absorbed as easily. Medications may have side effects, such as nausea, constipation, and loss of appetite. Loss of teeth and ill-fitting dentures can affect chewing. Decreased peristalsis, common among older adults, results in slower emptying of the stomach and colon, causing flatulence and constipation.

Energy levels are usually lower in older adults. Fewer calories are needed to sustain weight, but nutritional requirements remain high. High-protein foods are needed for tissue growth and repair. Foods high in calcium help keep bones strong; high-fibre foods, such as raw vegetables, help avoid constipation, but they can be hard to chew and can cause indigestion. Foods providing soft bulk, such as cooked fruits and vegetables, are often preferred for older clients with constipation or chewing problems. Drinking more fluids may also aid digestion, kidney function, chewing, and swallowing.

Good oral hygiene and well-fitted dentures can help prevent irritation of gums and mouth sores and improve the ability to eat and taste.

FACTORS THAT AFFECT EATING AND NUTRITION

Many factors affect nutrition and eating habits; some of them begin during infancy and continue throughout life, while others develop later:

- ***Personal choice.*** Likes and dislikes of certain foods is a matter of personal preferences that begin in childhood. They are influenced by the way foods taste, smell, and look and the way it is prepared.
- ***Allergies.*** An **allergy** is sensitivity to a substance that causes the body to react with signs and symptoms. Common allergic reactions are swelling of the lips, throat, tongue, or face; skin rash; coughing or difficulty breathing; abdominal cramps; nausea; or diarrhea. In severe cases, *anaphylactic shock*—a life-threatening sensitivity to a substance that can be fatal—can occur. For some people, food allergies are just an annoyance, while for others, avoiding certain foods is a matter of life and death. Nuts and shellfish cause the most severe reactions.
- ***Food intolerances.*** A food intolerance is a noticeable reaction to food, such as indigestion and diarrhea, but it does not involve the immune system and is not as serious as a food allergy. For example, lactose intolerance occurs in people who lack the enzyme lactase, which is needed to break down the sugar (lactose) in milk. Therefore, people who are lactose-intolerant cannot digest milk.
- ***Culture.*** Culture influences dietary practices, food choices, and food preparation (see the *Respecting Diversity: Food Practices* box). The way food is cooked—frying, baking, smoking, and roasting food—or eaten raw depends on cultural practices. The use of sauces and spices is also related to culture.
- ***Religion.*** Religious practices can often influence the selection, preparation, and eating of food. Members of a religious group may follow all, some, or none of the dietary practices of their faith. You need to be aware of and respect your clients' religious practices.

RESPECTING DIVERSITY

Food Practices

Food practices vary among cultures. For example, rice and beans are common protein sources in Mexico. Rice is also common in the Philippines, China, and Japan. A diet high in starch and fat is common in Poland. A low-fat, high-sodium diet is common in China. In some countries (such as India) beef is not eaten by most people.

Adapted from: D'Avanzo & Geissler, E.M. (2003). *Pocket guide to cultural assessment* (3rd ed.). St. Louis: Mosby.

- ***Finances.*** People with limited incomes often buy cheaper foods, so their diets may lack proteins and certain vitamins and minerals.
- ***Appetite.*** Appetite relates to the desire for food. When hungry, a person seeks food and eats until the appetite is satisfied. Aromas and thoughts of food can also stimulate the appetite. However, illness, medications, anxiety, pain, and depression, as well as unpleasant sights, thoughts, and smells, can cause lack of appetite.
- ***Illness.*** Appetite usually decreases during illness and during recovery from injuries, but nutritional needs increase. The body must fight infection, heal tissues, and replace blood cells and nutrients lost though vomiting and diarrhea. Some diseases and medications can cause a sore mouth, which makes eating painful. Loss of teeth affects chewing, especially protein foods. Illness makes it difficult to prepare and serve meals. Poor nutrition is common among long-term care residents, so they need good nutrition to correct or prevent health problems. (See the *Focus on Long-Term Care: Food and Quality of Life* box.)
- ***Age.*** Age affects nutrition (see pages 490–491).

focus on ›› LONG-TERM CARE

Food and Quality of Life

Food is important to a long-term care client's quality of life. Legislation ensures that:

- Each client's dietary and nutritional needs are met
- Nourishing, tasty, attractive, and well-balanced meals are served
- Hot food is served hot and cold food is served cold
- Special diets are provided, as needed
- Special eating utensils are provided (Figure 27–4), as needed. The client's hands, wrists, and arms may be affected by disease or injury; special eating utensils help the client to eat with minimum assistance

In some long-term care facilities, clients can dine with guests—for example, spouses, partners, family members, or friends. The dietary department may provide the meal or it may be brought by the visitor.

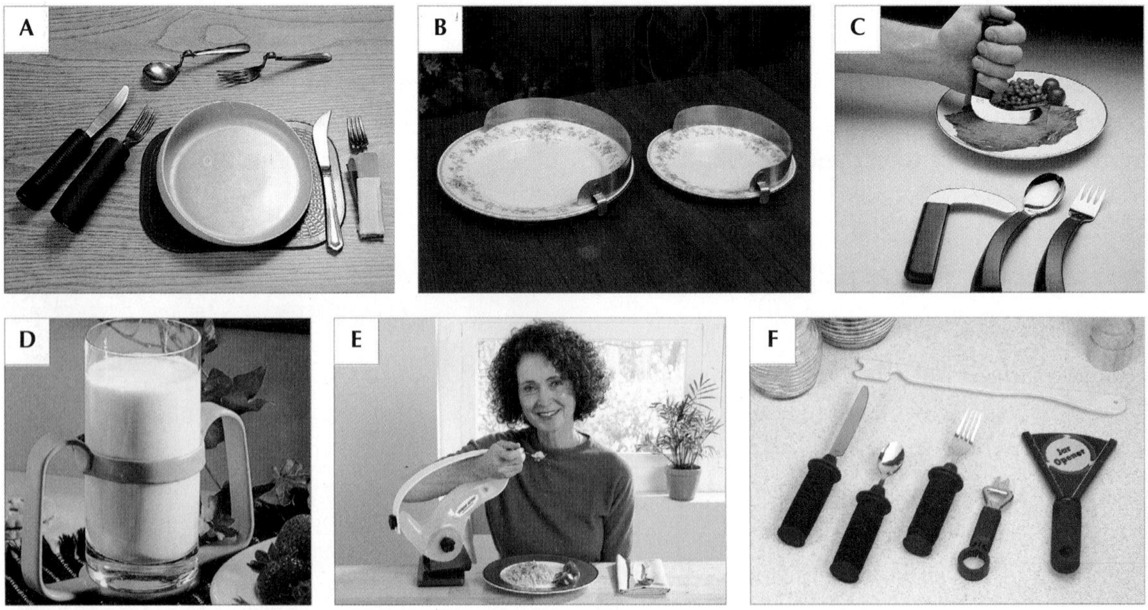

Figure 27–4 Eating utensils for clients with special needs. **A,** The curved fork fits over the hand. The rounded plate helps keep food on the plate. Special grips and swivel handles are helpful to some clients. **B,** Plate guards help keep food on the plate. **C,** Knives with rounded blades are rocked back and forth to cut food. The client does not need a fork in one hand and a knife in the other. **D,** Glass or cup holder. **E,** Arm Support. **F.** Arthritis Kitchen Kit. **Courtesy:** Sammons Preston; An AbilityOne Company, Bolingbrook, IL.

MEAL PLANNING AND PREPARATION

Your role in meal planning and preparation depends on the care plan and on your client's needs. Most home care agencies expect clients' families to provide groceries and main meals. The case manager arranges for Meals on Wheels, if desired by the family and client. Meals on Wheels provides clients with their main meal of the day. You may need to prepare a light meal for a client, for example, toast for breakfast or a sandwich for lunch. Sometimes, you may have to prepare several meals and freeze them for future use. Occasionally, you may be required to plan menus and shop for groceries.

When preparing meals for clients, consider their dietary requirements, food preferences, and eating habits.

- ***Dietary requirements.*** The care plan includes special diets, mealtime instructions, dietary practices, and food allergies and food intolerances. If there is no information in the care plan, ask your supervisor for guidance. A good cookbook is a helpful guide for planning and preparing meals.
- ***Food preferences.*** Many clients have strong food preferences and definite ideas about preparing meals. Follow the client's wishes. Never give clients food that they are not allowed. If you have concerns about a client's diet, speak with your supervisor.
- ***Eating habits.*** Clients may choose to have the main meal in the evening or at noon. Some clients eat several meals of the same size but never snack. Others snack between meals. Some clients eat the same things for breakfast and lunch every day.

Shopping for Groceries

You may be expected to shop for a client's food. Use shopping lists to remember needed items. If your client is on a special diet, read food labels carefully. The labels will tell you if the product is "diet," "low fat" and so on. Keep the list in one place, and encourage the client to add to it throughout the week. Add personal care items, as needed. On shopping day, check and finalize the list.

Checking Expiry Dates. By law, expiry or "best before" dates must appear on products that have a limited shelf life. If stored properly, the product can be safely used before the date listed. There are three commonly used dates:

- ***Sell by …:*** This is the last recommended date of sale. Most products will keep for at least 3 days beyond this date.
- ***Best before …:*** This is the last date at which the manufacturer will guarantee freshness.
- ***Expiry date …:*** This is the last date at which the product can be safely consumed.

Some products, for example, packaged meats and fish, contain only the date on which they were packaged. Select the products that were packaged most recently.

Handling Clients' Money. Some clients have running accounts at the grocer's, while some others may provide cash for groceries. Always handle someone else's money carefully. You must be honest, efficient, and organized. Keep a separate wallet or purse for the client's money, change, and receipts. Use the receipts to total the money spent, and return the right amount of change to the client. Most employers have strict policies about handling clients' money. Be sure to follow these policies.

Following Recipes

Use a recipe to prepare meals. If necessary, consult a basic cookbook that has key terms. You may have to substitute ingredients if your client does not have an ingredient required for the recipe. For example, canola oil and margarine can usually be substituted for olive oil. Never substitute an ingredient without getting the client's permission and checking the care plan. Do not use a substitute ingredient if the client is on a special diet or has a food allergy or intolerance. Consult your supervisor for guidance.

Canada uses the metric system, which has quantities such as millilitres (mL) and grams (g). However, household units of measurement, such as tablespoons or cups, are also commonly used in recipes. Table 27–3 provides some common equivalents for metric units.

Table 27–3 Approximate Equivalent Measurements

Liquids	
1 cup = 250 millilitres	
1 pint = 473 millilitres	
1 quart = 1 litre	
1/2 teaspoon = 2 millilitres	
1 teaspoon = 5 millilitres	
1 tablespoon = 15 millilitres	
Weights	
1 ounce = 30 grams	
1 pound = 454 grams	

Food Safety

Food safety is an important consideration for all, since foodborne illnesses can cause serious illness and death. A **foodborne illness** is an illness caused by improperly cooked or stored food. Diarrhea, nausea, and vomiting are common signs and symptoms of a foodborne illness. Some people are particularly at high risk—for example, infants, children, older adults, people with chronic illnesses, and clients with weakened immune systems.

Pathogens are disease-causing microbes (see Chapter 20) commonly called "germs." When pathogens are present in or on food, the food is said to be *contaminated.* Many foods naturally have pathogens in them in their raw state, for example, meat, fish, poultry, and eggs. When food is cooked properly, however, most pathogens are killed. However, raw food may spread pathogens to other, ready-to-eat foods—referred to as **cross-contamination**. For example, when fluids from raw chicken meat drip onto vegetables in the refrigerator, the vegetables become contaminated. If they are eaten before they are properly washed, they could cause illness.

It is usually hard to tell by sight, smell, or taste if something is contaminated. Safe food-handling practices and effective cooking can prevent cross-contamination and foodborne illnesses. Most pathogens thrive at room temperature, but they die at temperatures below 4°C (40°F) and above 60°C (140°F) (Table 27–4 on page 496). Therefore, it is important to cook foods well and preserve them in the refrigerator. Never leave foods sitting out at room temperature for more than a few minutes.

If you prepare and serve meals to clients, you must know safe food-handling practices. Observe safety practices when grocery shopping and when storing, cooking, reheating, and serving food (see Box 27–3).

SPECIAL DIETS

Physicians may order special diets for clients because of a nutritional deficiency or a disease, to eliminate or decrease certain substances in the diet, or for weight control (Table 27–5 on page 497). Special diets are common before and after surgery and for people with diabetes. People with diseases of the heart, kidneys, gallbladder, liver, stomach, or intestines may receive special diets. Allergies, food intolerances, obesity, and other disorders also require special diets.

When a special diet is ordered, the RN and dietitian work together to plan the client's nutritional needs. The plan takes into consideration the client's preferences, culture, religion, and food allergies and intolerances, as well as any eating problems, such as dysphagia (see page 499).

In facilities, the terms *regular diet, general diet,* and *house diet* mean that there are no dietary limits or restrictions. Two common special diets are the sodium-controlled diet and diabetes meal planning.

The Sodium-Controlled Diet

The average amount of sodium found in the daily diet of a person is 3000 to 5000 mg, twice the daily amount required by the body. Healthy people excrete the excess sodium in the urine. Heart and kidney diseases, as well as some drugs and some complications of pregnancy cause the body to retain the extra sodium.

Sodium causes the body to retain water. If there is too much sodium, the body retains more water. Tissues swell with water, and there are excess amounts of fluid in the blood vessels, which makes the heart work harder. The extra workload for the heart can cause serious complications and even

Box 27–3 Guidelines for Safe Food Practices

Shopping

- Packaging should be secure. Do not buy ripped packages, broken seals, and dented cans.
- Check the "best before" date. Do not buy expired items.
- Select refrigerated and frozen foods last. Do not buy items with ice crystals on the package.
- Put meats, poultry, and seafood in bags to avoid cross-contamination.

Food Storage

- Do not leave groceries in a warm car. Freeze or refrigerate items promptly.
- Store raw meat, poultry, and seafood in plastic bags on the bottom shelf of the refrigerator. This prevents their fluids from dripping onto other foods.
- Store leftovers in small, shallow containers in the refrigerator. This allows rapid cooling and prevents the growth of pathogens. Cover the containers with lids, foil, or plastic wrap. Write the date you store the leftovers on the containers.
- Do not refreeze food.

Food Preparation

- Wash your hands before and after preparing food. Wash your hands immediately before and after handling raw meat, poultry, seafood, or eggs to avoid cross-contamination of other foods.
- Do not cough or sneeze over food. Wear a hair net.
- Wear gloves if you have cuts on your hands or wrists.
- Defrost foods in the refrigerator, in the microwave, or under cold running water. Do not defrost food at room temperature.
- Prevent contact between raw and ready-to-eat food.
- Wash vegetables and fruits to remove pathogens and pesticides.
- Discard food with expired "best before" dates. Discard food if it has mould on it. If in doubt about freshness, discard the product.
- Do not keep leftovers longer than 2 to 3 days.
- Use clean utensils to take food items from containers that will be refrigerated.
- Rinse raw meats, poultry, and seafood before use. Wash the sink thoroughly (see Chapter 25).
- Avoid recipes that call for eggs not having to be cooked.
- Use different cutting boards for raw meats and poultry; seafood; cooked food; cheese; and washed fruits and vegetables. For added safety, cut raw meats, poultry, and seafood on disposable waxed paper placed on top of the board. Wash the cutting board thoroughly (see Chapter 25).
- Wash and dry the tops of cans to remove pathogens. Wash can openers to prevent pathogens from entering cans.
- Wash knives or scissors used to cut open food packages.
- Follow the guidelines for cleaning kitchens (see Chapter 25).

Cooking and Reheating Food

- Cook foods to at least their minimum safe temperature (Table 27–4). Cooking foods at the right temperature kills pathogens.
- Cook food thoroughly, especially meat, poultry, seafood, and eggs. Use a meat thermometer to determine if the meat is cooked. Eggs should be firm when eaten.
- Reheat sauces and gravy to a rolling boil.
- Stir and rotate food reheated in microwaves to prevent cold or hot spots.

Serving Food

- Serve food immediately after cooking it or removing it from the refrigerator. Remember, pathogens grow rapidly at room temperature.
- Serve food on a clean plate. Wash plates, platters, or containers used for raw meats, poultry, seafood, or eggs immediately after use.
- Use clean table linens, plastic mats, and eating surfaces.
- Do not use chipped or cracked dishes.

death. Restricting sodium in the diet helps the body retain less water, and less water in the tissues and blood vessels reduces the amount of work for the heart.

The physician may order sodium control (restriction) for the client. Many low-salt or salt-free foods are available in the market, and you can use food labels to determine salt content.

Table 27–4 Minimum Safe Temperatures	
Ground beef/pork	71°C (160°F)
Ground chicken/turkey	80°C (175°F)
Beef, lamb, and veal roasts/steaks	63°C (145°F) Medium-rare 71°C (160°F) Medium 77°C (170°F) Well
Pork chops/roasts/fresh cured ham	71°C (160°F) Medium
Ham, ready-to-eat, fully cooked	Cold or 60°C (140°F)
Whole turkey (stuffed) or chicken (stuffed or not)	82°C (180°F)
Whole turkey (without stuffing)	77°C (170°F)
Stuffing	77°C (170°F)
Chicken/turkey pieces	77°C (170°F)
Rolled stuffed beef roasts or steaks (e.g., London Broil)	71°C (160°F)
Mechanically tenderized/delicate meats	71°C (160°F)
Egg dishes/casseroles	71°C (160°F)
Leftovers, reheated	74°C (165°F)

Source: The Canadian Partnership for Consumer Food Safety Education. (2006). *Food safety at home: Your guide to safe food handling* (brochure), p. 6. Cambridge, ON. Retrieved on February 22, 2008, from http://www.canfightbac.org/en/_pdf/SafetyKraftEng.pdf

- ***2000–3000-mg sodium diet***—this is called the *low-salt diet* or *no-added-salt diet.* Sodium restriction is mild, and all high-sodium foods are omitted. A minimum amount of salt is used for cooking, and salt is not added to foods at the table.
- ***1000-mg sodium diet***—sodium restriction is moderate. Food is cooked without salt, and foods high in sodium are omitted. Vegetables high in sodium are restricted in amount. Salt-free products, such as salt-free bread, are used. Diet planning is necessary.
- ***500-mg sodium diet***—sodium restriction is severe. Restrictions for the mild and moderate sodium diets are followed. In addition, vegetables high in sodium are omitted. Other restrictions are: milk 1 cup per day; egg 1 per day; and meat 120 grams (4 ounces) per day. Diet planning is essential.

Diabetes Meal Planning

Diabetes meal planning is done for clients with diabetes. *Diabetes* is a chronic condition resulting from a lack of insulin (see Chapter 18). In healthy people, the pancreas produces and secretes insulin, which enables the body to use the sugar consumed. In people who lack insulin, sugar builds up in the bloodstream rather than being used by cells for energy. Diabetes is usually treated with insulin or medication, diet, and exercise.

The dietitian and the client develop a meal plan together. Consistency is the key. The plan involves:

- ***The client's food preferences.*** It may be necessary to limit amounts or change the way food is prepared.
- ***The calories needed.*** The same amount of carbohydrates, protein, and fat are eaten each day. The dietician teaches clients, families and other

Table 27–5 Special Diets

Diet	Use	Foods Allowed
Clear-liquid: foods that are liquid at body temperature and that leave small amounts of residue; nonirritating and non–gas-forming	Postoperatively; for acute illness; infection; nausea, and vomiting; and in preparation for gastro-intestinal exams	Water, tea, and coffee (without milk or cream); carbonated beverages; gelatin; clear fruit juices (apple, grape, and cranberry); fat-free clear broth; hard candy, sugar, and popsicles
Full-liquid: foods that are liquid at room temperature or that melt at body temperature	Advance from clear-liquid diet postoperatively; for stomach irritation; fever; nausea and vomiting; and for people unable to chew, swallow, or digest solid foods	Foods on the clear-liquid diet; custard; eggnog; strained soups; strained fruit and vegetable juices; milk and milkshakes; strained, cooked cereals; plain ice cream and sherbet; pudding; yogurt
Mechanical soft: semi-solid foods that are easily digested	Advance from full-liquid diet; for chewing problems; gastro-intestinal disorders; and infections	All liquids; eggs (not fried); broiled, baked, or roasted meat, fish, or poultry that is chopped or shredded; mild cheeses (American, Swiss, cheddar, cream, and cottage); strained fruit juices; refined bread (no crust) and crackers; cooked cereal; cooked or puréed vegetables; cooked or canned fruit without skin or seeds; pudding; plain cakes and soft cookies without fruit or nuts
Fibre and residue restricted: food that leaves a small amount of residue in the colon	Diseases of the colon; diarrhea	Coffee, tea, milk, carbonated beverages, strained fruit juices; refined bread and crackers; creamed and refined cereal; rice; cottage and cream cheese; eggs (not fried); plain puddings and cakes; gelatin; custard; sherbet and ice cream; strained vegetable juices; canned or cooked fruit without skin or seeds; potatoes (not fried); strained, cooked vegetables; plain pasta; *no raw fruits* and vegetables
High-fibre: foods that increase the amount of residue and fibre in the colon to stimulate peristalsis	Constipation and other gastro-intestinal disorders	All fruits and vegetables; whole wheat bread; whole grain cereals; fried foods; whole grain rice; milk, cream, butter, and cheese; meats
Bland: foods that are mechanically and chemically nonirritating and low in roughage; foods served at moderate temperatures; no strong spices or condiments	Ulcers; gallbladder disorders; some intestinal disorders; after abdominal surgery	Lean meats; white bread; creamed and refined cereals; cream or cottage cheese; gelatin, plain puddings, cakes, and cookies; eggs (not fried); butter and cream; canned fruits and vegetables without skin and seeds; strained fruit juices; potatoes (not fried); pastas and rice; strained or soft cooked carrots, peas, beets, spinach, squash, and asparagus tips; creamed soups from allowed vegetables; no fried foods

(continued on page 498)

Table 27–5 Special Diets (cont'd)

Diet	Use	Foods Allowed
High-calorie: calorie intake is increased to about 3000 to 4000; includes three full meals and between-meal snacks	For weight gain; some thyroid imbalances	Dietary increases in all foods; large portions of a regular diet with three between-meal snacks
Calorie-controlled: provides adequate nutrients while controlling calories to promote weight loss and reduction of body fat	For weight reduction	Foods low in fats and carbohydrates and lean meats; avoid butter, cream, rice, gravies, salad oils, noodles, cakes, pastries, carbonated and alcoholic beverages, candy, potato chips, and similar foods
High-iron: foods that are high in iron	Anemia; following blood loss; for women during the reproductive years	Liver and other organ meats; lean meats; egg yolks; shellfish; dried fruits; dried beans; leafy green vegetables; lima beans; peanut butter; enriched breads and cereals
Fat-controlled (low-cholesterol)**:** foods low in fat and foods prepared without adding fat	Heart disease; gallbladder disease; disorders of fat digestion; liver disease; diseases of the pancreas	Skim milk or buttermilk; cottage cheese (no other cheeses allowed); gelatin; sherbet; fruit; lean meat, poultry, and fish (baked, broiled, or roasted); fat-free broth; soups made with skim milk; margarine; rice, pasta, breads, and cereals; vegetables; potatoes
High-protein: aids and promotes tissue healing	Burns; high fever; infection; some liver diseases	Meat; milk, eggs, and cheese; fish and poultry; breads and cereals; green leafy vegetables
Sodium-controlled: a certain amount of sodium is allowed	Heart disease; fluid retention; liver disease; some kidney diseases	Fruits and vegetables and unsalted butter are allowed; adding salt at the table is not allowed; highly salted foods and foods high in sodium are not allowed; the use of salt in cooking may be restricted
Diabetes meal planning: the same amount of carbohydrates, protein, and fat are eaten at the same time each day	Diabetes	Determined by nutritional and energy requirements

team members about portion control, food group regulations and food substitutions.

- ***Eating meals and snacks at regular times.*** The client eats at the same time every day.

The same meal and snack times are maintained daily. You must serve the client's meal and snack on time, and the client must eat at regular times to maintain a certain blood sugar level. Some clients require a between-meal snack to maintain their sugar level. The nourishment makes up for what was not eaten at the regular meal. If all the food is not eaten during a meal, it is important to report it to your supervisor. For example, if your client did not eat the meat at lunch, at snack time a possible substitute for the meat serving would be a quarter cup of cottage cheese along with their regular snack. The amount of insulin given is also based on the client's daily food intake. Report to your supervisor any changes in the client's eating habits. Dieticians are an important member of the health care team of a diabetic client.

ASSISTING CLIENTS WITH EATING

A client's appetite and ability to eat can be affected by weakness and illness; odours; unpleasant equipment; an uncomfortable position; the need for oral hygiene; the need to eliminate; and pain. You can help control some of these factors by helping your clients prepare for meals.

- Assist with oral hygiene, elimination, and hand washing.
- Change clothing and provide clean linens for incontinent clients.
- Be sure dentures, eyeglasses, and hearing aids are in place.
- Help clients get to the dining room.
- Ensure a comfortable position for eating. Help clients transfer from beds to chairs or move to a sitting position in bed.

Making Meals Enjoyable

Some clients lose interest in eating because of illness or other factors. Small details can help a client enjoy a meal. Some of the following may not apply to clients on special diets. Check their individual care plans.

- ***Assist with menu choices.*** Help home care clients make choices from the Meals on Wheels menu. Help long-term care clients select a meal from the facility menu. If planning and preparing meals, involve the client in the decisions.
- ***Make the setting attractive.*** In the client's home, let the client choose table linens and utensils.
- ***Serve hot meals immediately.*** Lukewarm meals lack appeal.
- ***Serve moderate portions.*** Some clients lose their appetite at the sight of too much food. Ask the client how much food he or she wants. Place the desired amount on the plate.
- ***Make mealtimes social occasions.*** To avoid loneliness at mealtimes, encourage long-term care clients to dine with others. In home care settings, provide company to the client by staying by their side while you do quiet tasks, such as folding laundry.

Assisting Clients With Eating Problems

Changes resulting from aging, illness, and disabilities can cause eating problems. These include chewing and swallowing problems, weakness, and vision loss.

Chewing Problems. Foods that provide soft bulk are served (see soft diet, page 497) to clients with chewing problems. A food processor or blender is used to purée foods. Follow the care plan. To help overcome chewing problems:

- Offer plenty of fluids
- Offer small mouthfuls
- Give the client time to chew

Swallowing Problems (Dysphagia). Clients can have difficulty swallowing for many reasons. Certain medications (including chemotherapy) decrease saliva production, resulting in dry mouth. Clients with paralysis may have difficulty swallowing because their throat muscles are affected. A swallowing assessment is completed by an occupational therapist, a physiotherapist, or a nurse who has received training in this assessment tool. Clients who have difficulty swallowing thin liquids often must drink thickened liquids. There are three common consistencies of thickened liquids.

- ***Nectar thickened or easily pourable***—comparable to thicker cream soup, milkshake
- ***Honey thickened or slightly thicker***—comparable to honey, pours very slowly
- ***Pudding thickened***—will hold its shape when scooped; usually eaten with a spoon; comparable to the consistency of pudding

If your client requires thickeners, do not give them anything that melts, such as ice cream or ice cubes. Clients with dysphagia often do not get enough fluids. Thickened liquids are still considered part of their fluid intake.

Thick, soft, moist foods are served to clients. The care plan may include the following measures to help a client swallow:

- Help the client sit upright, leaning slightly forward.
- Ask the client to lower the chin while swallowing.
- Offer plenty of fluids.
- Give the client time to chew and swallow before offering more food.
- Ask the client to remain sitting for at least 30 minutes after the meal.

A recent recommendation is that when feeding clients with swallowing problems, you should give them one third of a teaspoon at a time. However, some feel that being fed such a small amount, which would involve many spoonfuls, could tire the client. Follow the care plan regarding the amount you should feed each time.

Clients with swallowing problems are at risk for choking and aspiration. **Aspiration** is inhaling fluid or an object into the lungs. If you find a client being unable to talk or cough, he or she may be choking, and you should call for help immediately. If no help is available, follow the emergency measures for choking (foreign-body airway obstruction) that you have been taught.

Weakness. Some clients are too weak to chew and swallow, and when they do not eat well, they become even weaker and have even less energy to eat. Never force a client to eat. If the client cannot eat, tell your supervisor. To encourage a client to eat, offer frequent, small, high-calorie meals, and serve nutritious drinks, including liquid dietary supplements. Soft foods that do not need much chewing are preferred. Follow the care plan, and do the following:

- Allow the client to rest before and after meals.
- Provide a straw to drink so the client does not need to lift the glass (if allowed).
- Provide cups, glasses, and utensils that are light and easy to handle.

Vision Loss. Clients with vision loss are often keenly aware of food aromas and often can identify foods served to them. Most of these clients can eat independently, with some guidance. To assist these clients to eat:

- Identify the location of foods and fluids on the tray or table.
- Use the numbers on a clock to identify the location of foods and fluids (Figure 27–5).
- Describe what you are offering, if you are feeding the client.

Serving Meal Trays

Most clients in hospitals eat their meals in their rooms. However, long-term care clients are encouraged to eat in the dining room (see the *Focus on Long-Term Care: Dining Programs* box), but those who are too ill to move about eat in their rooms.

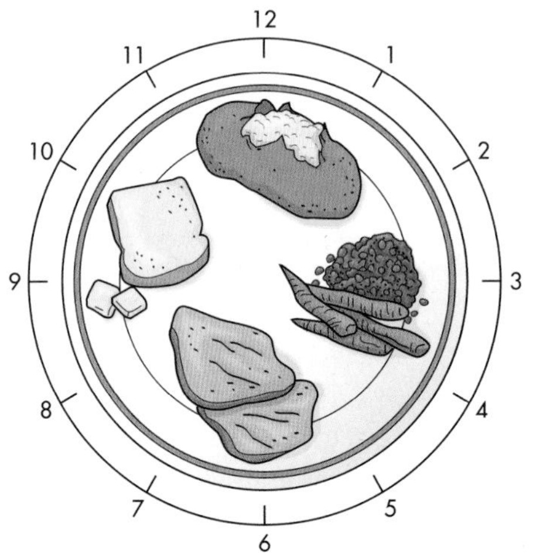

Figure 27–5 The numbers on a clock are used to help a client with vision loss locate food on a plate.

focus on »LONG-TERM CARE

Dining Programs

Many long-term care facilities have special dining programs:

- *Social dining*—clients eat in the dining room. Each table has four to six residents (Figure 27–6). Food is served as in a restaurant. Just as in many homes, clients usually prefer to sit in the same spot for each meal.
- *Family dining*—food is placed in bowls and on platters, and clients serve themselves as they would at home.
- *Assistive dining*—the dining room has circular or horseshoe-shaped tables. Clients who need assistance with eating are seated around the tables. In this arrangement, the support worker sits at the centre of the table and is able to feed as many as four clients (Figure 27–7).

1 2 3 SERVING MEAL TRAYS

Remember to promote:

• Dignity • Independence • Preferences • Privacy • Safety

Pre-Procedure

1 Identify the client, according to employer policy.
2 Perform hand hygiene.
3 Prepare the client for the meal. Assist with hand washing.
4 Provide for privacy only if requested by your client.
5 Make sure the tray contains everything needed. Make sure special utensils are included, if needed.

Procedure

6 Help client to a sitting position.
7 Place tray on the overbed table or other table. If the client is in bed and there is no overbed table, position the tray on the client's lap.
8 Remove lids from dishes. Open milk cartons and cereal boxes, cut the meat, and butter the bread, if indicated in the care plan (Figure 27–8).
9 Place the napkin, clothes protector (if needed), and utensils within reach.
10 Measure and record intake, if ordered (see page 507). Note the amount and type of foods eaten.
11 Check for and remove any food in the mouth (pocketing). Wear gloves.
12 Remove the tray.
13 Assist with hand washing. Offer oral hygiene.
14 Clean any spills, and change soiled linen.
15 Help the client to return to bed, if indicated.

Post-Procedure

16 Provide for safety and comfort.
17 Place the call bell within reach.*
18 Follow the care plan for bed rail use.*
19 Remove privacy measures.
20 Perform hand hygiene.
21 Report and record your actions and observations according to employer policy. Include the amount and kind of food eaten.

*Steps marked with an asterisk may not apply in community settings.

Some long-term clients may choose to eat in their rooms. Home care clients usually eat in the dining room or kitchen. If they are weak or ill, they may eat in bed or sitting in a chair in their bedroom. Meals served in beds and bedrooms are delivered on trays, with the food served in containers that keep hot and cold foods at the correct temperature. You should serve meal trays after helping clients prepare for eating. Serve meal trays promptly, as prompt service keeps food at the right temperature.

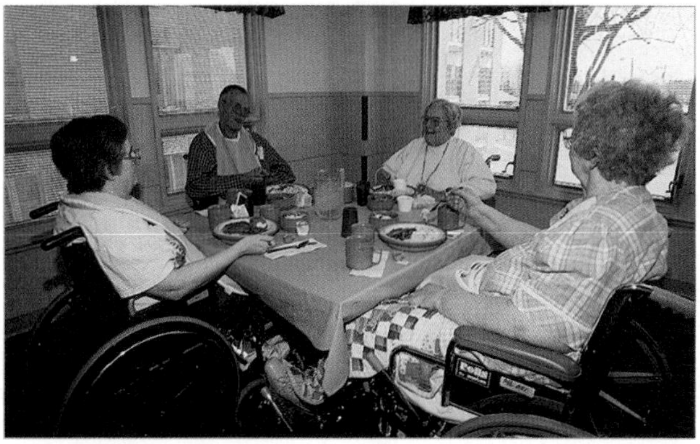

Figure 27–6 Clients enjoy a pleasant meal in the dining room.

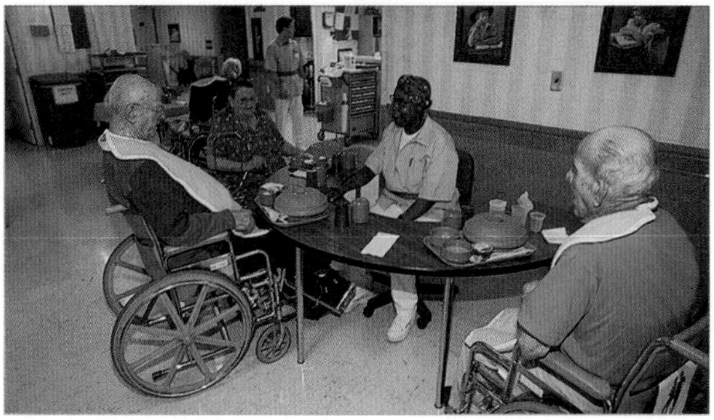

Figure 27–7 Special tables are used for assistive dining programs. A support worker feeds three clients at one time. Clients are in the company of others.

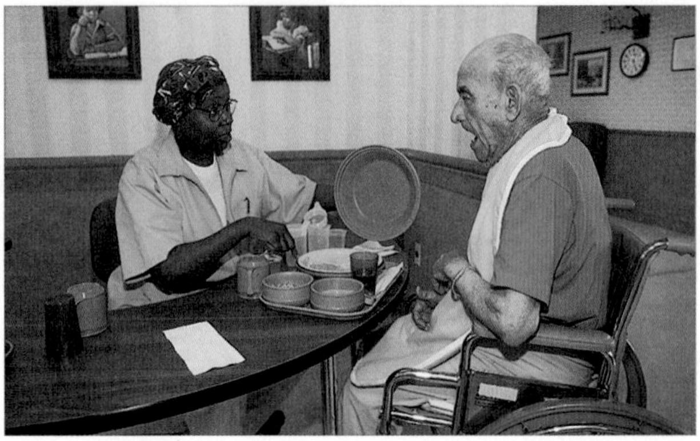

Figure 27–8 Open cartons and other containers for the client.

Feeding a Client

Some clients who cannot feed themselves due to weakness, paralysis, casts, and other physical limits need to be fed. This can be difficult for the client to accept, so you need to be kind and supportive when feeding clients (see the *Providing Compassionate Care: Feeding A Client* box below.)

Between-Meal Nourishments

Many special diets involve between-meal nourishments—such as crackers, milk, juice, milkshake, cake, wafers, sandwich, gelatin, and custard. Provide nourishments according to the care plan. There are many types of pre-packaged nutritional liquid food supplements, such as Ensure or Boost, which are only meant to be supplements and not intended to be meal replacements for an extended period of time, as they do not provide adequate nutritional balance. In home care settings, you may have to prepare the between-meal nourishments. In facilities, these are supplied to the unit. Provide eating utensils, a straw, and a napkin to the client. Follow the procedures for serving meals and feeding clients.

Calorie Counts

For some clients, it is important to keep a record of calorie intake. A flow sheet is provided for this purpose, and you must note what the client ate and how much. For example, a client is served a chicken breast, a baked potato, green beans, a roll, pudding, and two pats of butter. You note that the client finished all the chicken, half the potato, the roll, and one pat of butter but left the beans and the pudding, and you record this on the form. The care plan tells you which clients require calorie counts.

PROVIDING COMPASSIONATE CARE

Feeding a Client

- **Dignity.** Clients who cannot feed themselves may feel embarrassed, humiliated, or angry, and some clients can become depressed or resentful. Some of these clients may refuse to eat. Be gentle, patient, and encouraging, and ensure comfort. Sit facing the client, as it is more relaxing and shows that you have time for the client. Standing communicates that you are in a hurry, and clients should never be made to feel rushed. Clean up dribbles and spills in a tactful way to save the client from embarrassment.
- **Independence.** Encourage the client to participate in some part of the meal, and allow the client to set the pace. The client may be able to gesture or nod to show preferences.
- **Preferences.** If the client wants to pray before eating, provide time and privacy for it. Describe the food on the tray, and ask the client the order in which foods and fluids should be served. Ask questions and use paraphrasing (see Chapter 13) to make sure that you understand the client's feelings and wishes. Engage the client in pleasant conversation.

(continued on page 503)

PROVIDING COMPASSIONATE CARE (cont'd)

- **Privacy.** Some clients do not like others to see them being fed. Be sensitive to your client's needs and feelings. Provide for privacy if desired by the client.
- **Safety.** Follow the care plan. Use spoons, not forks, as they are less likely to cause injury. The spoon should be only one third full (Figure 27–9) each time, as this portion is easy to chew and swallow. Some clients need even smaller portions. Sit facing the client so that you can see immediately choking or any problems with eating, chewing, or swallowing. Give the client enough time to chew and swallow. Remember to offer fluids during the meal as they help with chewing and swallowing.

1 2 3 FEEDING THE CLIENT

Remember to promote:

• **D**ignity • **I**ndependence • **P**references • **P**rivacy • **S**afety

Pre-Procedure

1 Identify the client, according to employer policy.
2 Explain the procedure to the client.
3 Perform hand hygiene.
4 Prepare the client for mealtime. Assist with hand washing.
5 Provide for privacy only if requested by the client.
6 Help the client to a comfortable sitting position. Ensure the client is at a level which will not cause you risk of injury.
7 Place the tray on the overbed table, other table, or the client's lap.

Procedure

8 Drape a napkin across the client's chest and under the chin.
9 Prepare the food for eating.
10 Tell the client what foods are on the tray.
11 Serve foods in the order the client prefers. Alternate between solid and liquid foods. Use a spoon for safety (see Figure 27–9). Allow time for chewing. Do not rush the client.
12 Use straws if the client cannot drink out of a glass or cup. Use one straw for each liquid. Use a short straw if the client is weak.
13 Follow the care plan if the client has dysphagia. (Some clients with dysphagia do not use straws.) Give thickened liquids with a spoon.
14 Talk with the client.
15 Encourage the client to eat.
16 Wipe the client's mouth with a napkin as soon as a spill occurs.
17 Note how much was eaten and which foods were eaten.
18 Measure and record intake, if ordered.
19 Remove the tray.
20 Assist with oral hygiene (if in the care plan) and hand washing. Wear gloves for this step.

Post-Procedure

21 Provide for safety and comfort.
22 Place the call bell within reach.*
23 Follow the care plan for bed rail use.*
24 Remove privacy measures.
25 Perform hand hygiene.
26 Report and record your actions and observations according to employer policy. Include:
- The amount of food eaten and the kind of food eaten
- Complaints of nausea or dysphagia
- Signs of aspiration

*Steps marked with an asterisk may not apply in community settings.

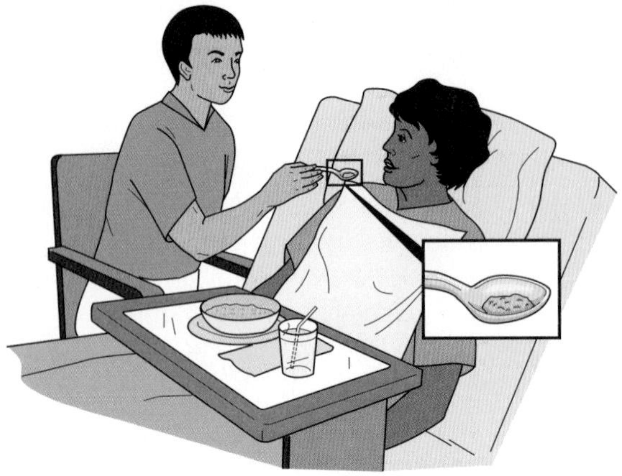

Figure 27–9 A spoon is used to feed a client. The spoon is no more than one third full.

FLUID BALANCE

Harm, even death can result from too much or too little water in the body, so fluid balance is essential for health. The amount of fluid taken in (**intake**) and the amount lost (**output**) must be equal. If fluid intake exceeds fluid output, tissues swell with water—this is called **edema.** Edema is common in clients with heart and kidney diseases. **Dehydration** is a decrease in the amount of water in body tissues, which occurs when fluid output exceeds intake. Common causes are low fluid intake, vomiting, diarrhea, bleeding, excess sweating, and increased urine production.

Normal Fluid Requirements

An adult needs 1500 mL of water daily to survive. About 2000 to 2500 mL of fluid per day is needed for normal fluid balance, but water requirements increase in certain conditions—such as hot weather, exercise, fever, illness, and excessive fluid loss. Minimum water requirements vary with age (see the *Focus on Children: Fluid Requirements* and *Focus on Older Adults: Fluid Requirements* boxes).

Special Orders

The physician may specify the amount of fluid that a client can have in a 24-hour period. This is done to maintain fluid balance. Common orders in the care plan are:

- ***Encourage fluids***—The client needs to drink more fluids. The order states the amount to ingest. A variety of allowed fluids are provided. Fluids are kept within the client's reach and are offered regularly to clients who cannot feed themselves. Intake records are kept.
- ***Restrict fluids***—Fluids are restricted to a certain amount. They are offered in small amounts and in small containers. The water pitcher is removed or kept out of sight. The client needs frequent oral hygiene, as it helps keep the mucous membranes of the mouth moist. Intake records are kept.
- ***Nothing by mouth***—The client cannot eat or drink anything—NPO stands for the Latin term *nil per os,* meaning nothing (*nil*) by (*per*) mouth (*os*). Clients are usually NPO before and after surgery, before certain laboratory tests and x-ray procedures, and in the treatment of certain ill-

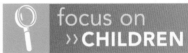

focus on
»CHILDREN

Fluid Requirements

Infants and young children have more body water than do adults and therefore need higher fluid intake. Excessive fluid loss can quickly cause death in infants and children.

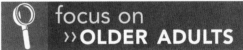

focus on
»OLDER ADULTS

Fluid Requirements

Older adults are at risk for diseases, such as heart disease, kidney disease, cancer, and diabetes, that affect fluid balance. Many older adults also take medications that cause the body to lose fluids or retain water. Older adults are thus at risk for edema and dehydration.

Older adults may have a decreased sense of thirst. Their bodies need water, but they may not feel thirsty. Offer water often to your older clients.

nesses. Clients who are tube fed may be NPO, and an NPO sign is posted above the bed. The water pitcher and glass are removed. Frequent oral hygiene is important, but you must ensure that the client does not swallow any fluid.

Intake and Output Records

The physician or nurse may want a client's fluid intake and output measured. This means keeping intake and output (I&O) records, which are used to evaluate fluid balance and kidney function and to plan medical treatment. They also are kept when the client has special fluid orders.

All fluids taken by mouth, as well as fluids given in IV therapy and tube feedings (see Chapter 28) are measured and recorded. The obvious fluids are measured—water, milk, coffee, tea, juices, soups, and soft drinks—as well as the fluid content in soft and semi-solid foods such as ice cream, sherbet, custard, pudding, gelatin, and popsicles. Output measure includes urine, vomitus, diarrhea, and wound drainage.

Measuring Intake and Output. Intake and output are measured in millilitres (mL) or in cubic centimetres (cc). These metric system measurements are equal in amount.

- 30 mL equals 1 ounce
- 500 mL is about 1 pint
- 1000 mL is about 1 quart

You need to know the serving size of bowls, cups, glasses, and other containers. The information may be on the I&O record.

A container called a *graduate* is used to measure fluids, including leftover fluids, urine, vomitus, and drainage from suction (see Chapter 42). Similar to a measuring cup, the graduate is marked in millilitres or cubic centimetres as well as in ounces (Figure 27–10). Plastic urinals and kidney basins are also marked with measurements.

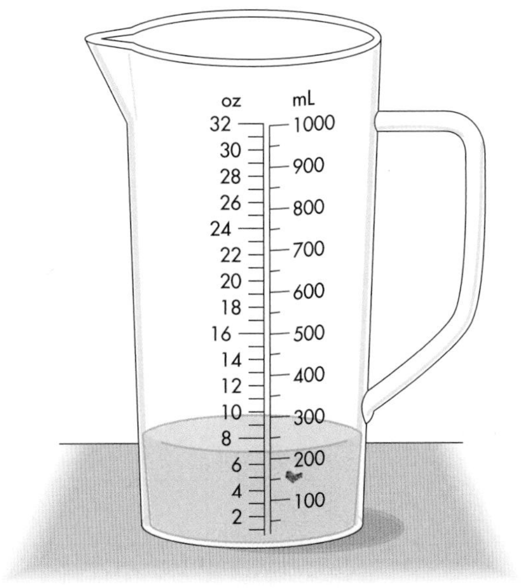

Figure 27–10 A graduate marked in millilitres and ounces.

When intake or output is measured, the amount is recorded in the correct column on the I&O record (Figure 27–11). Amounts are totalled at the end of the shift and recorded on the client's chart. In facilities, totals are shared among staff during end-of-shift report.

Recording intake and output is ordered for many different reasons. As mentioned on page 502, fluid balance is needed for health. Unequal intake and output amounts will alert the health care team to carry out interventions needed to correct the fluid balance.

The purpose of measuring I&O and how this can help are explained to the client. Some clients measure and record their intake themselves, and sometimes family members may help. For output measurement, the urinal, commode, bedpan, or specimen pan is used. Remind the client not to void in the toilet and not to put toilet tissue into the container that will be used for taking measurements.

Follow medical asepsis and Standard Practices when measuring intake and output.

CODE (Intake): O - Oral; IV - Intravenous; NG - Nasogastric; GT - Gastrostomy Tube

CODE (Output): U - Urine; E - Emesis

	INTAKE										OUTPUT									
DATE	NIGHT	CODE	INIT.	DAY	CODE	INIT.	EVE	CODE	INIT.	24 HR TOTAL	NIGHT	CODE	INIT.	DAY	CODE	INIT.	EVE	CODE	INIT.	24 HR TOTAL

Initials		NURSE'S SIGNATURE	Initials		NURSE'S SIGNATURE	Initials		NURSE'S SIGNATURE	Initials		NURSE'S SIGNATURE
1			3			5			7		
2			4			6			8		

Name ____________________ Birthdate ____________________

Admission Date ____________________ Medical Rec. # ____________________

Physician ____________________

GSS #242

INTAKE & OUTPUT RECORD

Rev. 2-12-82

Figure 27–11 An intake and output record. **Source**: Sorrentino, S.A. (2000). *Mosby's textbook for nursing assistants* (5th ed., p. 384). St. Louis: Mosby.

1 2 3 MEASURING INTAKE AND OUTPUT

Remember to promote:

• Dignity • Independence • Preferences • Privacy • Safety

Pre-Procedure

1 Identify the client, according to employer policy.
2 Explain the procedure to the client.
3 Perform hand hygiene.
4 Collect the following:
- Intake and output (I&O) record
- Graduates
- Gloves

5 Provide for privacy.

Procedure

6 Put on gloves.
7 Measure intake as follows:
- a Pour remaining liquid in the serving container into the graduate.
- b Measure the amount at eye level. Keep the graduate level.
- c Check the consumed amount as recorded on the I&O record.
- d Subtract the amount consumed from the full serving amount and record the amount of intake.
- e Repeat steps a through d above for each liquid.
- f Total the intake amounts of all liquids.
- g Record the time and amount on the I&O record.

8 Measure output as follows:
- a Pour the fluid into the graduate used to measure output.
- b Measure the amount at eye level. Keep the graduate level.

9 Dispose of fluid in the toilet, taking care to avoid splashes.
10 Clean and rinse the graduate. Dispose of rinse into the toilet. Return the graduate to its proper place.
11 Clean and rinse the bedpan, urinal, kidney basin, or other drainage container. Discard the rinse into the toilet. Return the item to its proper place.
12 Remove gloves. Perform hand hygiene.
13 Record the amount on the I&O record.
14 Remove privacy measures.

Post-Procedure

15 Report and record your actions and observations, according to employer policy.

*Steps marked with an asterisk may not apply in community settings.

REVIEW

Answers to these questions are at the bottom of the page.

Circle the BEST answer.

1. **Nutrition is:**
   - A. Fats, proteins, carbohydrates, vitamins, minerals, and water
   - B. The many processes involved in the ingestion, digestion, absorption, and use of foods and fluids by the body
   - C. The *Food Guide* rainbow
   - D. The balance between calories taken in and used by the body
2. **Protein is needed for:**
   - A. Tissue growth and repair
   - B. Energy and fibre
   - C. Body heat and the protection of organs from injury
   - D. Improving the taste of food
3. ***Canada's Food Guide to Healthy Eating* encourages:**
   - A. A low-carbohydrate diet
   - B. A high-fat diet
   - C. A low-fibre diet
   - D. A low-fat diet
4. **How many daily servings of grain product does the *Food Guide* recommend for women over 50 years of age?**
   - A. 5
   - B. 6
   - C. 4
   - D. 3
5. **Which food groups contain the most fat?**
   - A. Grain products and milk products
   - B. Grain products and meat and alternatives
   - C. Milk products and meat and alternatives
   - D. Grain products and vegetables and fruit
6. **The Daily Value (DV) is an amount that indicates:**
   - A. The number of calories an adult of average weight should consume daily
   - B. Intake and output measured in millilitres (mL) or in cubic centimetres (cc)
   - C. The nutrients in each meal served in hospitals and long-term care facilities
   - D. Whether there is a little or a lot of a nutrient in a serving of food
7. **Older adults:**
   - A. Have lower nutrient requirements than do younger adults
   - B. Should eat a high-fat diet
   - C. Should eat foods high in protein and calcium
   - D. Should consume at least 3000 calories per day
8. **Which of the following is an acceptable food safety practice?**
   - A. Washing your hands immediately after handling raw chicken
   - B. Defrosting frozen chicken on the kitchen counter
   - C. Cutting raw chicken and vegetables on the same cutting board
   - D. Serving chicken that is crisp on the outside and pink on the inside
9. **People with diabetes must:**
   - A. Restrict their intake of fluids
   - B. Eat a diet high in saturated fat and protein
   - C. Eat a high-fibre diet
   - D. Eat the same amount of carbohydrates, protein, and fat each day
10. **Which of the following is suggested for clients who are weak and fatigued?**
    - A. A straw for drinking liquids
    - B. Large portions
    - C. Foods that are high in calories
    - D. Hard to chew foods
11. **Adult fluid requirements for normal fluid balance are about:**
    - A. 1000 to 1500 mL daily
    - B. 1500 to 2000 mL daily
    - C. 2000 to 2500 mL daily
    - D. 2500 to 3000 mL daily
12. **A person is NPO. You should:**
    - A. Provide a variety of fluids
    - B. Offer fluids in small amounts and small containers
    - C. Remove the water pitcher and glass
    - D. Prevent the person from having oral hygiene

Answers: 1.B, 2.A, 3.D, 4.B, 5.C, 6.D, 7.C, 8.A, 9.D, 10.C, 11.C, 12.C

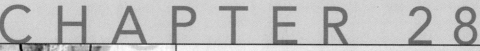

CHAPTER 28

Enteral Nutrition and IV Therapy

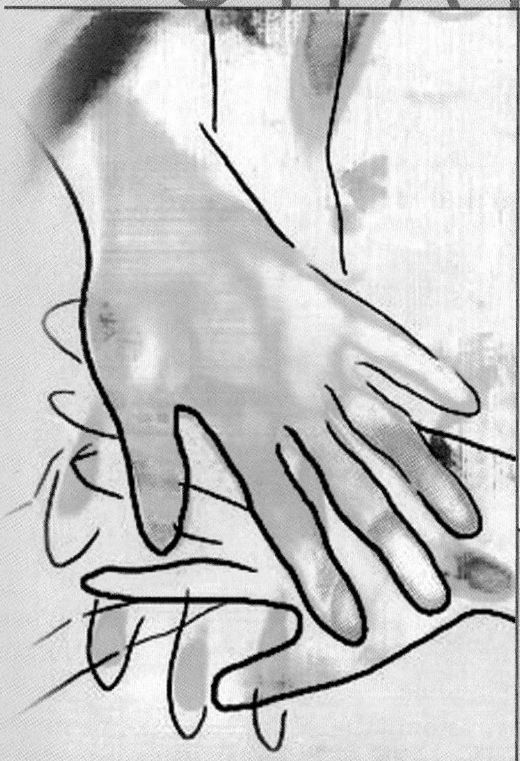

OBJECTIVES

- Define the key terms listed in this chapter.
- Explain the purpose of enteral nutrition and necessary comfort measures.
- Explain how to prevent aspiration and regurgitation.
- Identify the signs and symptoms of aspiration.
- Identify the solutions, equipment, and complications involved in intravenous (IV) therapy.
- Explain the safety measures necessary for IV therapy and your role in maintaining the flow rate.

key terms

aspiration Inhaling fluid or an object into the lungs.

enteral nutrition Giving nutrients by way of the intestine (*enteral*).

flow rate The volume of fluid over a prescribed period.

gastro-jejunostomy tube A tube that connects the stomach to the jejunum.

gastrostomy tube A tube inserted through an opening (*stomy*) into the stomach (*gastro*).

gavage Tube feeding.

intravenous (IV) therapy Fluids given through a needle or catheter inserted into a vein; also referred to as IV, IV therapy, and IV infusion.

jejunostomy tube A tube inserted into the intestines through an opening (*stomy*) into the middle part of the small intestine (*jejunum*).

nasogastric (NG) tube A tube inserted through the nose (*naso*) into the stomach (*gastro*).

nasointestinal tube A tube inserted through the nose (*naso*) into the small intestine (*intestinal*).

percutaneous endoscopic gastrostomy (PEG) tube A tube inserted into the stomach (*gastro*) through a puncture wound (*stomy*) made through (*per*) the skin (*cutaneous*); a lighted instrument (*scope*) allows the physician to see inside the body cavity or organ (*endo*).

regurgitation The backward flow of food from the stomach into the mouth.

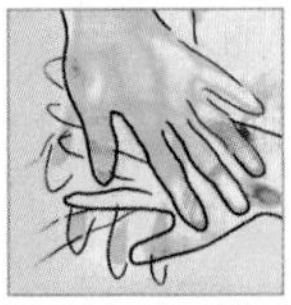

Some clients have special requirements with regard to nutrition and fluids. Because of illness, injury, or surgery, some clients have difficulty eating, drinking chewing, or swallowing. Using various methods, nutrition and fluids as well as medications are provided though tubes, as ordered by a physician. Only a qualified nurse or other professional administers the procedures. As a support worker, you care for clients who have had these procedures.

ENTERAL NUTRITION

People who cannot chew or swallow often require **enteral nutrition,** which involves giving nutrients through the gastro-intestinal tract (*enteral*). A nurse gives formula through a feeding tube. **Gavage** is another term for tube feeding.

- A **nasogastric (NG) tube** is inserted through the nose (*naso*) into the stomach (*gastro*) (Figure 28–1). A physician or an RN performs the procedure.
- A **nasointestinal tube** is inserted through the nose (*naso*) into the small intestine (*intestinal*) (Figure 28–2). A physician or an RN performs the procedure.
- A **gastrostomy tube** is inserted into the stomach. A surgically created opening (*stomy*) in the stomach (*gastro*) is needed for this procedure (Figure 28–3).
- **A gastro-jejunostomy tube** connects the stomach to the jejunum.
- A **jejunostomy tube** is inserted into the intestines. A surgically created opening (*stomy*) in the middle part of the small intestine (*jejunum*) is needed for this procedure (Figure 28–4).
- A **percutaneous endoscopic gastrostomy (PEG) tube** is inserted with an endoscope, which is a lighted instrument (*scope*) that allows the physician to see inside a body cavity or organ (*endo*), such as the stomach. The physician inserts the endoscope through the person's mouth and esophagus and into the stomach. A stab or puncture wound (*stomy*) is made through (*per*) the skin (*cutaneous*) and into the stomach (*gastro*). A tube is inserted into the stomach through the puncture wound (Figure 28–5).

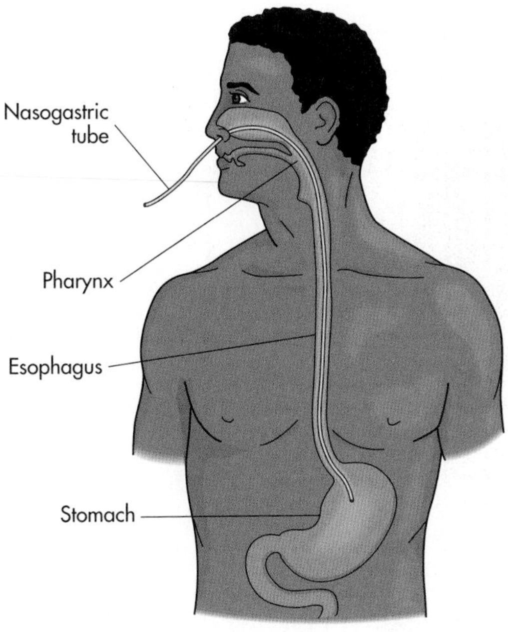

Figure 28–1 A nasogastric tube is inserted through the nose and esophagus into the stomach.

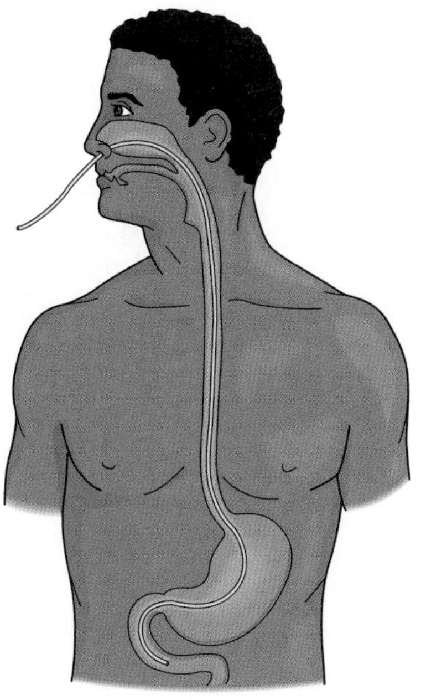

Figure 28–2 A nasointestinal tube is inserted through the nose into the duodenum or jejunum of the small intestine.

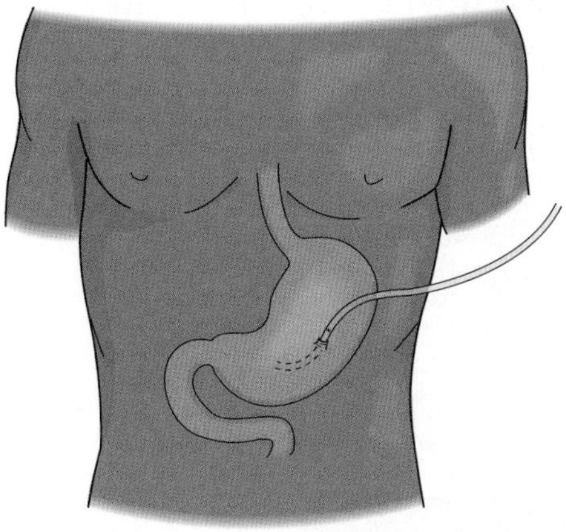

Figure 28–3 A gastrostomy tube.

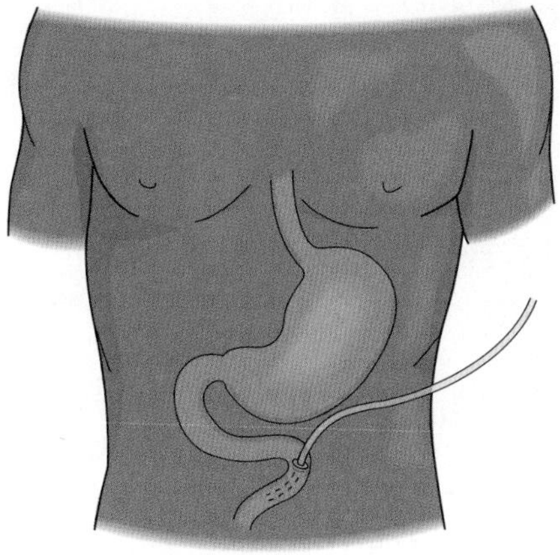

Figure 28–4 A jejunostomy tube.

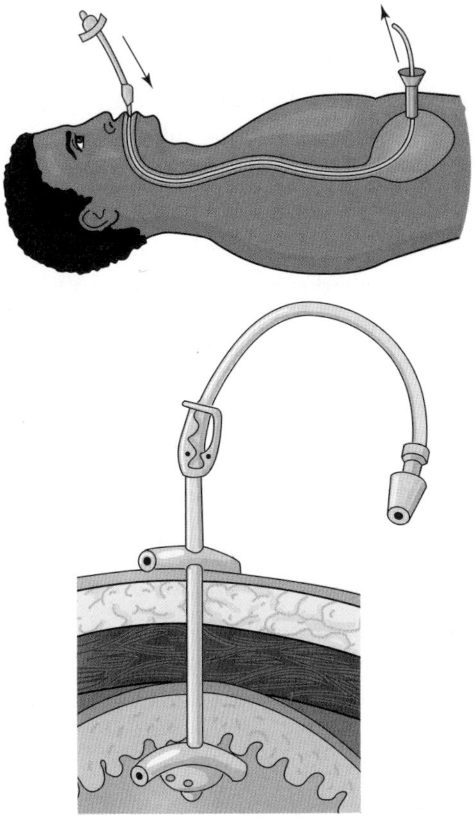

Figure 28–5 A percutaneous endoscopic gastrostomy.

Feeding tubes are used when food cannot pass normally from the mouth into the esophagus and then into the stomach. Causes include cancers of the head, neck, and esophagus; trauma or surgery to the face, mouth, head, or neck; and coma dysphagia caused by paralysis. Some people with dementia no longer know how to eat and may require tube feedings. Gastrostomy, jejunostomy, and PEG feedings are used for long-term enteral nutrition. The ostomy may be temporary or permanent.

Formulas

The physician orders the type of formula and the amount to be given to the client. Most formulas contain protein, carbohydrates, fat, vitamins, and minerals. Commercial formulas are commonly used, and sometimes formulas are prepared by the facility's dietary department.

Scheduled and Continuous Feedings

The physician orders scheduled or continuous feedings. Scheduled feedings usually are given four times a day using a syringe, a rigid plastic container, or feeding bag (Figure 28–6). Usually about 400 mL is given over 20 minutes during a scheduled feeding. The amount and rate are the same as regular meals. The physician will also specify how much water is to be given to the client each day, the usual recommended amount being 2000 mL/day.

Continuous feedings require electronic feeding pumps (Figure 28–7). Nasointestinal and jejunostomy tube feedings are always continuous.

Formula is given at room temperature, as cold fluids can cause stomach cramping. Sometimes (depending on regional differences) continuous feedings are kept cold with ice chips around the container to prevent the growth of microbes. The formula warms to room temperature as it drips from the bag and passes through the connecting tubing to the feeding tube. The nurse adds formula, as needed (see the *Focus on Home Care: Enteral Nutrition* box).

Preventing Aspiration

Aspiration, which is inhaling fluid or an object into the lungs, is a major complication of nasogastric and nasointestinal tube feedings. Nasogastric and

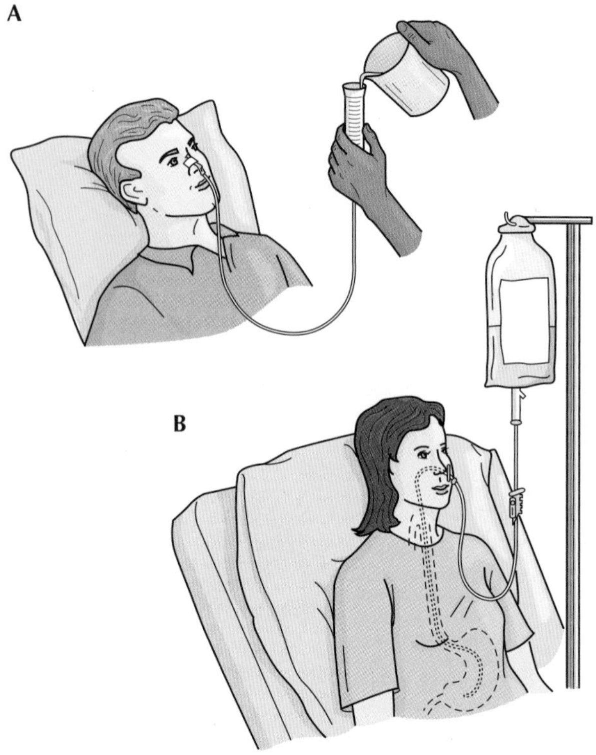

Figure 28–6 **A,** A tube feeding is given with a syringe. **B,** Formula drips from a feeding bag into the feeding tube.

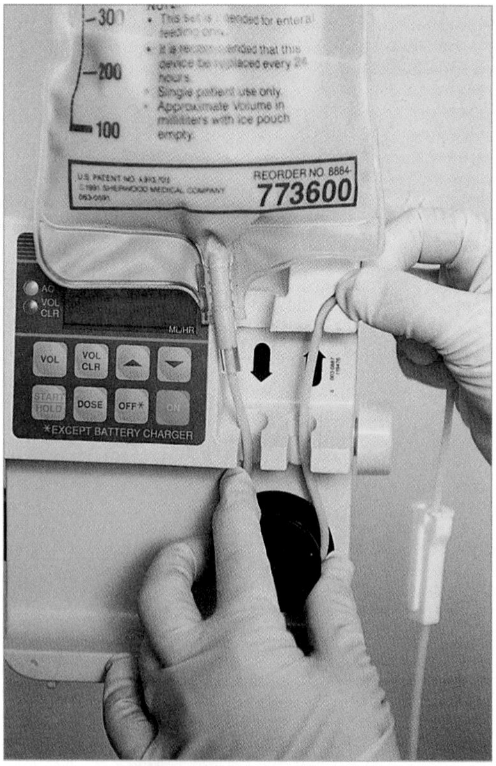

Figure 28–7 Feeding pump. **Source**: Potter, P.A. & Perry, A.G. (2005). *Fundamentals of nursing: Concepts, process, and practice* (6th ed.). St. Louis: Mosby.

focus on ›› HOME CARE

Enteral Nutrition

As a support worker you may provide home care to clients who are being fed by tubes, or in a facility, you may assist the nurse with a tube feeding. ***You should take care to never:***

- ***Insert feeding tubes***
- ***Test the position of the tube***
- ***Give the first dose of a tube feeding***

However, some home care agencies do permit support workers to start the feeding pumps and pour formula into feeding bags or containers. However, this is done only with gastrostomy tubes and jejunostomy tubes and only if the tube has been established. These tasks are *always* delegated by a nurse. A home care nurse may teach you the task; or the nurse may teach your supervisor the task, and your supervisor will, in turn, teach you. Another method of learning the procedure may be to attend a course given by a nurse in your agency. The agency supervises and monitors your performance closely. In most circumstances, you will need to be retrained to perform the task for each new client you work with. This process is needed to ensure competency in the delegated task. The person who teaches you the task has full responsibility for the tube feeding.

nasointestinal tubes are passed through the esophagus and then into the stomach or small intestine. During insertion, the tube could accidentally slip into the respiratory tract causing aspiration, which can cause pneumonia and even death. An X-ray taken after insertion is the best way to determine correct tube placement.

The tube can move out of place from coughing, sneezing, vomiting, suctioning, and poor positioning. A confused client can also move the feeding tube by pulling on it. The tube can move from the stomach or intestines into the esophagus and then into the airway. ***The nurse therefore checks tube placement before every scheduled tube feeding. In case of continuous tube feedings, the nurse checks tube placement every 4 to 8 hours.*** To do so, the nurse attaches a syringe to the tube and aspirates gastro-intestinal secretions. Then the nurse measures the pH of the secretions.

Aspiration can also occur from **regurgitation,** which is the backward flow of food from the stomach into the mouth. This can occur with nasogastric, gastrostomy, and PEG tubes. Delayed stomach emptying and overfeeding are common causes of regurgitation. To prevent regurgitation, the client is in the sitting or semi-Fowler's position for the feeding. The client remains in this position 1 to 2 hours after the feeding as well, as it promotes movement of the formula through the gastro-intestinal system and prevents aspiration. The left side-lying position has to be avoided, as it prevents emptying of the stomach.

The risk of regurgitation is less with nasointestinal and jejunostomy tubes. Formula is given at a slow rate and passes directly into the small intestine. Remember, during digestion, food passes slowly from the stomach to the small intestine and that the stomach can handle larger amounts of food at one time than can the small intestine.

Observations. Besides aspiration, which is the major risk, diarrhea, constipation, and delayed stomach emptying can also occur with tube feeding. Report the following immediately:

- Nausea
- Discomfort during the tube feeding
- Vomiting
- Diarrhea
- Distended (enlarged and swollen) abdomen
- Coughing
- Complaints of indigestion or heart burn
- Redness, swelling, drainage, odour, or pain at the ostomy site
- Elevated temperature
- Signs and symptoms of respiratory distress (see Chapter 44)
- Increased pulse rate
- Complaints of flatulence (see Chapter 32)

Comfort Measures

The client with a feeding tube is usually NPO (*NPO* stands for the Latin term *nil per os,* which means nothing by mouth). When dry mouth, dry lips, and sore throat cause discomfort, clients can suck on hard candy or chew gum. The client's needs include frequent oral hygiene, lubricant for the lips, and mouth rinses. The nose and nostrils also are cleaned every 4 to 8 hours. Give care as directed by your supervisor and the care plan.

Nasogastric and nasointestinal tubes can irritate and cause pressure on the nose. Sometimes they alter the shape of the nostrils or cause pressure ulcers. Securing the tube using tape or a tube holder helps prevent these problems (Figure 28–8). Tube holders have foam cushions that prevent pressure on the nose and eliminate the need for retaping; frequent taping can irritate the nose. The tube also is secured to the client's clothes with a tape or by looping a rubber band around the tube and pinning the rubber band to the client's clothes with a safety pin.

IV THERAPY

Intravenous (IV) therapy—also referred to as *IV* and *IV infusion*—involves giving fluids through a needle or catheter inserted into a vein. Physicians order IV therapy to:

- Provide needed fluids when a client cannot take fluids by mouth
- Replace minerals and vitamins lost because of illness or injury
- Provide sugar for energy
- Administer medications and blood
- Provide *hyperalimentation*—a solution highly concentrated with nutrients

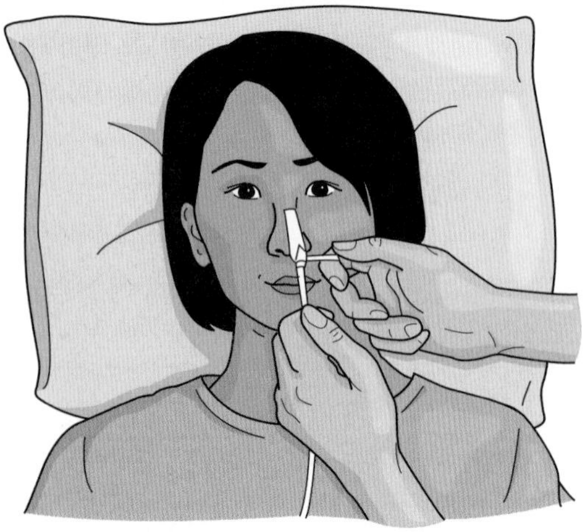

Figure 28–8 The feeding tube is taped to the nose.

IV therapy is given in hospital, outpatient, subacute care, long-term care, and home care settings. Nurses are responsible for IV therapy—they start and maintain the infusion according to the physician's orders and also give IV medications and administer blood.

Sites

Peripheral and central venous sites are used for IV therapy. Periphery means around (*peri*) a boundary (*phery*). The boundary is the centre of the body near the heart. *Peripheral IV sites* are away from the centre of the body. In adults, the back of the hand, forearm, and crease of the elbow are used as IV sites (Figure 28–9) (see the *Focus on Children: IV Sites* box.)

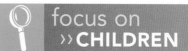

> **focus on ›› CHILDREN**
>
> **IV Sites**
>
> The hand, wrist, foot, crease of the elbow, and occasionally scalp veins are peripheral sites used for infants and children (Figure 28–10).

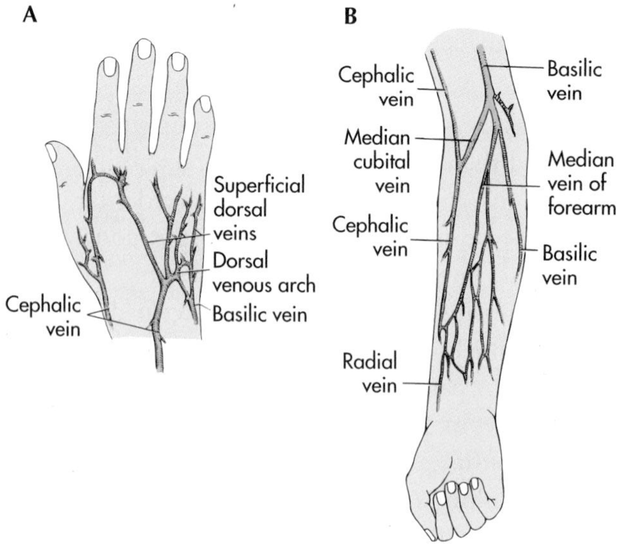

Figure 28–9 Peripheral IV sites for adults. **A,** Back of the hand. **B,** Forearm and crease of the elbow. **Source:** Potter, P.A., & Perry, A.G. (1997). *Fundamentals of nursing: Concepts, process, and practice* (4th ed.) St Louis: Mosby.

The subclavian vein and the internal jugular vein—located close to the heart—are *central venous sites.* A physician inserts a long catheter—called a *central venous catheter* or *central line*—into a central vein. The catheter tip is then threaded into the superior vena cava or right atrium (Figure 28–11, *A* and *B*). The cephalic and basilic veins in the arm also are used at times for IV therapy. Catheters inserted into these sites are called *peripherally inserted central catheters (PICC).* The catheter tip is threaded into the subclavian vein or the superior vena cava (Figure 28–11, *C*). Only physicians and specially trained nurses can insert PICCs.

Central venous sites are used to give large amounts of fluid and for long-term IV therapy. They also are used for IV medications that irritate the peripheral veins. Sometimes surgery is necessary to insert a central venous catheter (see the *Focus on Home Care: IV Therapy* box).

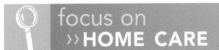

focus on ››HOME CARE

IV Therapy

Clients receiving IV therapy in their homes often have central venous catheters. The nurse teaches the client and family about administering IV medications and managing the catheter.

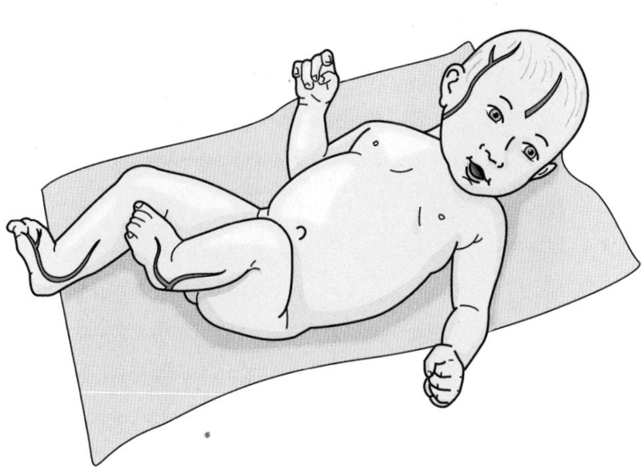

Figure 28–10 The scalp and foot provide peripheral IV sites in infants.

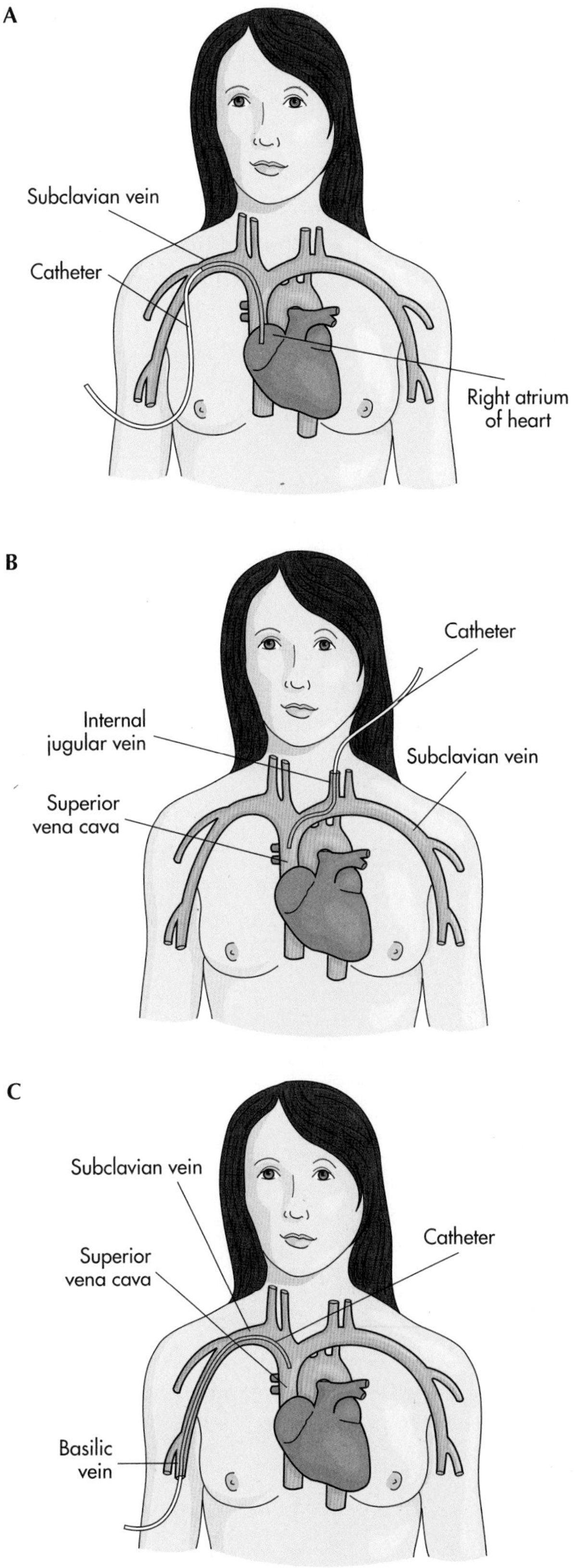

Figure 28–11 Central venous sites. **A,** Subclavian vein. The catheter tip is in the right atrium. **B,** Internal jugular vein. The catheter tip is in the superior vena cava. **C,** Basilic vein. This is a peripherally inserted central catheter (PICC).

Assisting With IV Therapy

You help meet the hygiene and activity needs of clients receiving IV therapy. You are *never* responsible for starting or maintaining IV therapy, but you may be expected to provide safe care. Follow the safety measures in Box 28–1. Complications can occur from IV therapy. Report at once if you see any of the signs and symptoms listed in Box 28–2.

Box 28–1 Safety Measures for IV Therapy

- Follow Standard Practices.
- The position of the IV needle or catheter must be maintained. Do not move the needle or catheter. If the needle or catheter is moved, it may come out of the vein and fluid will flow into the tissues (infiltration) or the flow will stop.
- Sometimes the nurse may apply splints or restrains to prevent movement of the extremity (Figure 28–12) and thus the movement of the needle or catheter.
- Protect the IV bag, tubing, and needle or catheter when ambulating the client. Portable IV stands are rolled along next to the client (Figure 28–13).
- Assist the client with turning and repositioning. Move the bag to the side of the bed where the client is lying. Always allow enough slack in the tubing, as otherwise the needle may dislodge due to pressure on the tube.
- Notify your supervisor immediately if bleeding occurs from the insertion site. Follow Standard Practices.
- Notify your supervisor immediately if there is any leaking of fluid from the IV site.
- Notify your supervisor immediately of any signs and symptoms listed in Box 28–2.

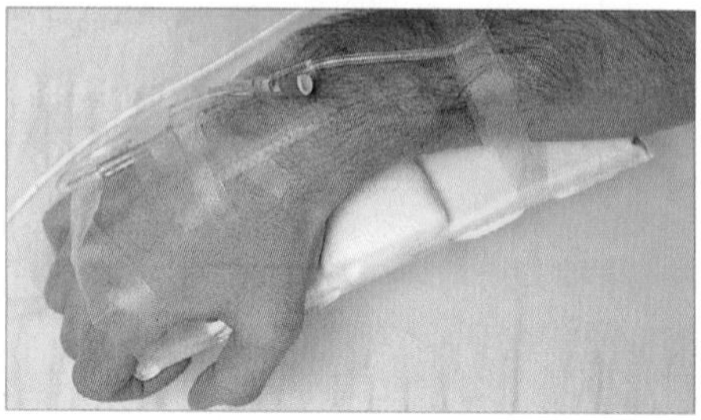

Figure 28–12 An armboard prevents movement at an IV site. **Source:** Elkin, M.K., Perry, A.G., & Potter, P.A. (2007). *Nursing interventions and clinical skills* (4th ed.). St Louis: Mosby.

Box 28–2 Signs and Symptoms of IV Therapy Complications

Local—At the IV Site

- Bleeding
- Puffiness or swelling
- Pale or reddened skin
- Complaints of pain at or above the IV site
- Hot or cold skin near the site
- Leaking of fluid from the site

Systemic—Involving the Whole Body

- Fever
- Itching
- Drop in blood pressure
- Tachycardia (pulse rate more than 100 beats per minute)
- Irregular pulse
- Cyanosis
- Changes in mental function
- Loss of consciousness
- Difficulty breathing (dyspnea)
- Shortness of breath
- Decreasing or no urine output
- Chest pain
- Nausea
- Confusion

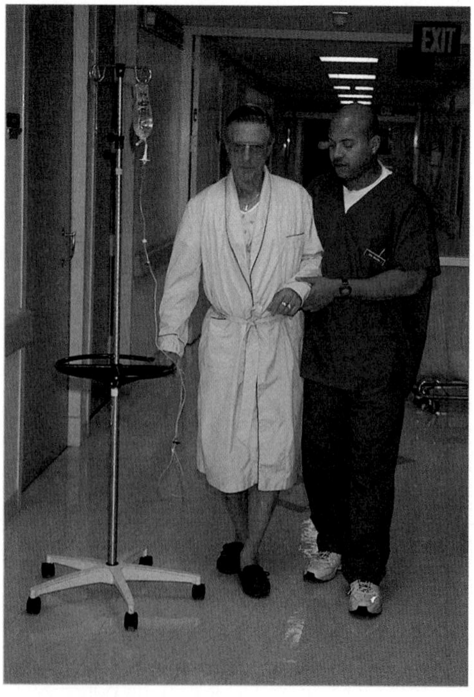

Figure 28–13 A client ambulating with an IV.

REVIEW

Answers to these questions are at the bottom of the page.

Circle the BEST answer.

1. **A gastrostomy tube is inserted into the:**
   A. Small intestine
   B. Stomach
   C. Colon
   D. Nose
2. **Which is a common reason for tube feedings?**
   A. Cancer of the lung
   B. Surgery to the mouth
   C. Chronic obstructive pulmonary disease (COPD)
   D. Pneumonia
3. **Continuous feedings require:**
   A. Electronic feeding pumps
   B. IV bags
   C. Catheters
   D. Syringes
4. **Aspiration is a major complication of:**
   A. Hyperalimentation
   B. IV therapy
   C. Nasogastric and nasointestinal tubes
   D. Central venous catheters
5. **A client with a feeding tube is usually:**
   A. NPO
   B. On bed rest
   C. Allowed a regular diet
   D. In a coma
6. **Care of a person who is NPO includes:**
   A. Frequent oral hygiene
   B. Frequent repositioning of the client
   C. Lubrication of nostrils
   D. Frequent drinks of water
7. **Which is a common IV site for adults?**
   A. Back of the hand
   B. Upper arm
   C. Scalp
   D. Foot
8. **A client is bleeding from an IV site. You should:**
   A. Remove the IV catheter or needle
   B. Apply direct pressure
   C. Call your supervisor at once
   D. Apply a dressing to the site
9. **Which is a sign of IV therapy complication?**
   A. Swelling at the IV site
   B. Changes in appetite
   C. Frequent urination
   D. Constipation

Answers: 1.B, 2.B, 3.A, 4.C, 5.A, 6.A, 7.A, 8.C, 9.A

CHAPTER 29

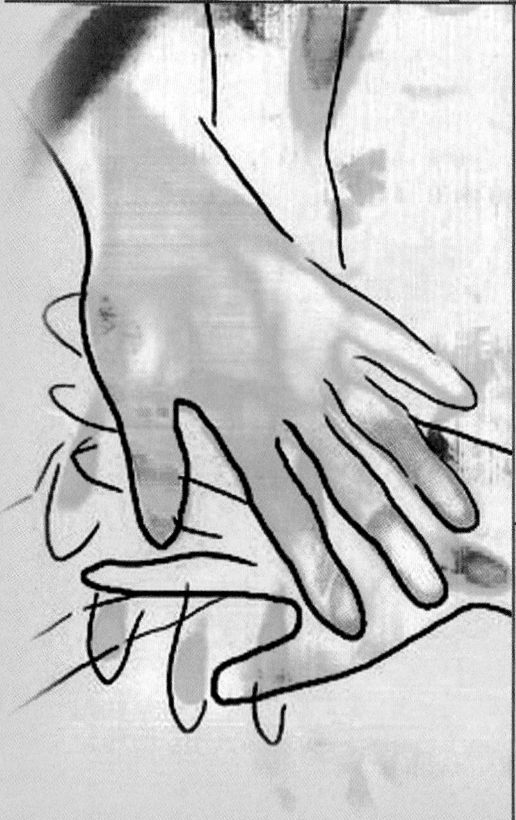

Personal Hygiene

OBJECTIVES

- Define the key terms listed in this chapter.
- Explain the importance of personal hygiene.
- Describe oral hygiene and the observations to report.
- Describe the guidelines for bathing and the observations to report.
- Identify the safety precautions for clients taking tub baths or showers.
- Explain the purposes of a back massage.
- Identify the purposes of perineal care.
- Describe menstrual care.
- Perform the procedures described in this chapter.

key terms

afternoon care Routine care given in a facility that occurs between lunch and the evening meal.

AM care Routine care given in a facility before lunch. AM care sometimes occurs before breakfast. Also known as **early morning care** and **morning care**.

aspiration Inhaling fluid or an object into the lungs.

biofilm A thin film that sticks to the teeth; it contains saliva, microbes, and other substances.

early morning care See **AM care**.

evening care See **HS care** or **PM care**.

HS care Routine care given in a facility in the evening at bedtime (HS means hour of sleep). Also known as **evening care** or **PM care.**

morning care See **AM care**.

oral hygiene Measures performed to keep the mouth and teeth clean; mouth care.

perineal care (pericare) Cleansing the genital and anal areas.

PM care See **HS care**.

tartar Hardened biofilm on teeth.

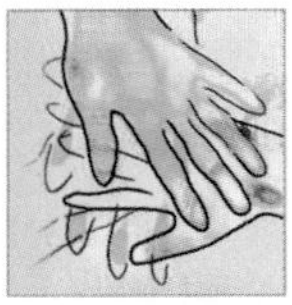

Personal hygiene—which involves activities to clean the skin, teeth, mouth, genital area, and anus—promotes comfort, safety, and health.

Good hygiene helps keep teeth, skin, and mucous membranes intact and healthy. When microbes enter the body through breaks in the skin or mucous membranes, infections can result. Therefore, intact skin and mucous membranes are the body's first line of defence against disease. As well as keeping the body clean and healthy, personal hygiene prevents body and breath odours, promotes relaxation, and increases circulation.

Support workers often help clients with personal hygiene. Some clients need only minimal help, while some others may need hygiene care done for them. Illness, disability, and changes associated with aging affect the ability to practise hygiene. Many factors affect hygiene and skin care—perspiration, elimination, vomiting, drainage from wounds or body openings, bed rest, and activity.

Culture and personal choice also affect hygiene practices (see the *Respecting Diversity: Personal Hygiene Practices of Hindus* box). Most clients have established hygiene routines and habits—for example, a bath at bedtime or in the morning; brushing teeth and washing face and hands on awakening, and so on. Usually these and other hygiene measures are done before and after meals and at bedtime. The care plan lists what personal hygiene measures are needed for a client and when to provide them. You are required to assist with personal hygiene whenever needed. If you have questions, check with your supervisor (see the *Focus on Long-Term Care: Daily Care* box on page 520).

Clients may feel frustrated, angry, or embarrassed because they need help with such personal care. Remember the priorities of support work when assisting with hygiene. Promote DIPPS—dignity, independence, preferences, privacy, and safety. This will help the client feel more at ease during hygiene procedures (see the *Providing Compassionate Care: Assisting With Personal Hygiene* box on page 521).

RESPECTING DIVERSITY

Personal Hygiene Practices of Hindus

Personal hygiene is very important to Hindus, as their religion requires at least one bath a day. However, some Hindus believe that bathing right after a meal can cause harm to the body. They also believe that eye injuries can occur from bath water that is too hot. When preparing a bath, hot water can be added to cold water. However, cold water is not added to hot water. After bathing, the body is carefully rubbed dry with a towel.

Remember, not all individuals in a group may follow every belief and practice of their culture and religion. Each client is unique.

Adapted from: Giger, J.N. & Davidhizar, R.E. (1999). *Transcultural nursing: Assessment and intervention* (3rd ed.). St. Louis: Mosby.

focus on ››LONG-TERM CARE

Daily Care

Facilities provide routine hygiene care at set times of the day. The amount of care given at each time and the terminology used vary from facility to facility.

- **AM care (early morning care** and **morning care)**—routine care provided before lunch. Most clients are toileted, given a partial bath that includes perineal care, dressed, groomed, and provided mouth care before they go to the dining room for breakfast. If there is enough time, clients requiring a tub bath or shower would have this completed before breakfast. If this is not possible, these clients might go to the dining room in their pyjamas or robe. GentleCare technique involves allowing clients to continue sleeping, if they so desire, and providing them with a late breakfast.

  In some facilities, tub baths or showers are done after breakfast. The client is also assisted with grooming—hair care, shaving, and dressing, mouth care, and perineal care.
- **Afternoon care**—routine care given after lunch and before the evening meal. Many clients like to have the afternoon care completed before naps, visiting time, or activity programs. Afternoon care usually includes assisting with oral hygiene, face and hand washing, and hair care.
- **HS care (evening care** or **PM care)**—care provided at bedtime. (*HS* means hour of sleep.) HS care, aimed at relaxing the client and increasing comfort, includes face and hand washing, oral hygiene, perineal care, and back massages. Bed linens and units are made neat and comfortable, and the client is helped into sleepwear.

ORAL HYGIENE

Oral hygiene (mouth care) keeps the mouth and teeth clean; prevents mouth odours, infections, and *cavities* (*dental caries*); increases comfort; and makes food taste better. It also prevents *periodontal disease* (*gum disease, pyorrhea*), which is an inflammation of the tissues around the teeth.

Poor oral hygiene allows the buildup of biofilm and tartar. **Biofilm**—which contains saliva, microbes, and other substances—is a thin film that sticks to teeth and leads to tooth decay, or cavities. When biofilm hardens, it is called **tartar.** Tartar builds up at the gum line near the neck of the tooth, which leads to periodontal disease. The gums become red and swollen and bleed easily. As the disease progresses, bone is destroyed and teeth become loosened, eventually resulting in tooth loss.

Illness and disease often cause a bad taste in the mouth. Some medications and diseases cause a whitish coating on the mouth and tongue, and some others cause redness and swelling of the mouth and tongue. Dry mouth is common from oxygen administration, smoking, decreased fluid intake, mouth breathing, and anxiety. Some medications cause dry mouth.

Your supervisor and the care plan will tell you the type of mouth care and assistance needed. Oral hygiene is given on awakening, after each meal, and at bedtime. Many clients also practise oral hygiene before meals.

Equipment

For oral hygiene, a toothbrush, toothpaste, dental floss, and mouthwash are needed. Ensure that the toothbrush has soft bristles, and replace tooth brushes every 3 months. Use toothpaste that contains fluoride. Clients with dentures need a denture cleaner, denture cup, and denture brush or toothbrush. Use only those products that are recommended for cleaning dentures, as otherwise you could damage the dentures.

You also need a kidney basin or small bowl, water glass, straw, tissue, towels, and gloves.

Sponge swabs are used for clients with sore, tender mouths and for unconscious clients. However, be careful when using sponge swabs. Always check the foam pad to make sure it is tight on the stick. The client could choke on the foam pad if it comes off the stick. Lip moisturizers are often used to relieve dry lips.

PROVIDING COMPASSIONATE CARE

Assisting With Personal Hygiene

- **Dignity.** Hygiene is a very personal and private matter. Most clients feel embarrassed that someone else needs to provide hygiene care for them, more so when the caregiver is of the opposite sex. Remember, personal hygiene is necessary for the client's health and well-being. Never show embarrassment or hesitation when assisting with hygiene procedures, as the client is likely to sense your discomfort. Talk to the client before and during the procedure. Let him or her know what you will be doing. Listen to what the client has to say about the procedure, and address any concerns or questions. If appropriate, chat with the client about anything he or she is interested in. Your calm, professional manner will help put the client at ease. Minimizing exposure of the body during bathing promotes dignity.
- **Independence.** Allow and encourage clients to do as much self-care as possible. Sometimes you only need to assist with a task. Give the client enough time to do what he or she can independently. Check with your supervisor and the care plan to determine the client's abilities and limitations.
- **Preferences.** Clients usually have hygiene preferences and routines. Routines provide a sense of order and control. Clients have a say about when and how a hygiene procedure is done. Personal choice is allowed in such matters as bath times and products used. The care plan should reflect the client's preferences and cultural practices. If there is a conflict between the care plan and the client's wishes, inform your supervisor.
- **Privacy.** Protecting the client's privacy is very important when assisting with hygiene. All procedures must be done in a private area with minimal exposure of the client's body. Close doors, privacy curtains, and drapes before giving care. Ask family members or visitors to leave the room. If a family member or friend wants to help, the client must consent to this. Do not unnecessarily expose the client's body when assisting with the bath. Provide appropriate covers to clients when taking them to and from tubs or shower rooms.
- **Safety.** Some clients have skin that can be easily damaged. Always be gentle; never scrub the skin or use rough sponges or cloths. Make sure your fingernails are trimmed, and remove rings before giving skin care. This prevents scratching or tearing the client's skin. Remember to wash your hands with soap and warm water before and after every procedure. Wear gloves when giving perineal care, oral care, and whenever you may have contact with blood, body fluids, secretions, or excretions. Gloves should be worn when you have cuts or rashes on your hands. Always check the water temperature before bathing the client.

When giving oral hygiene, you will come in contact with the client's mucous membranes. During oral hygiene procedures, the client's gums may bleed, which is a sign of inflammation and usually means more mouth care is needed, not less. The mouth contains many microbes, so wear gloves and follow Standard Practices when giving oral hygiene.

Observations

Report and record the following if observed when assisting with oral hygiene:

- Dry, cracked, swollen, or blistered lips
- Redness, swelling, irritation, sores, or white patches in the mouth or on the tongue
- Bleeding, swelling, or redness of the gums
- Loose teeth
- Rough, sharp, or chipped areas on dentures
- Complaints of pain or discomfort

Brushing Teeth

Many clients can perform oral hygiene procedures themselves, but the majority of long-term care clients cannot perform them adequately. Others may need help gathering and setting up equipment. Encourage the client to be as independent as possible according to his or her abilities and the care plan. The client may choose to brush his or her teeth in the bathroom, at the kitchen sink, or at the bedside.

You may have to brush the teeth of clients who are very weak or confused or who cannot use or move their arms. It can be difficult to provide mouth care to clients with dementia, but remember that even a small amount of mouth care is better than none. There is no consensus among dentists as to the proper brushing technique. Some recommend a circular motion, some the up-and-down motion, and others the side-to-side motion. All, however, agree that the brushing should start at the gum line (see the *Focus on Children: Brushing Teeth* box.)

focus on ›› CHILDREN

Brushing Teeth

Children learn to brush their teeth around 3 years of age. However, they may not be thorough, so they need help with brushing. Though older children can do a thorough job, it is often necessary to remind them to brush.

1 2 3 ASSISTING THE CLIENT TO BRUSH TEETH AT THE BEDSIDE

Remember to promote:

• Dignity • Independence • Preferences • Privacy • Safety

Pre-Procedure

1 Identify the client, according to employer policy.
2 Explain the procedure to the client.
3 Perform hand hygiene.
4 Collect the following:
- Toothbrush
- Toothpaste
- Mouthwash (or solution specified in the care plan)
- Dental floss (if used)
- Lip moisturizer (if used)
- Water glass with cool water
- Straw
- Kidney basin or small bowl
- Face towel
- Paper towels
- Gloves

5 Place paper towels on the overbed table (in facilities) or on a work area that the client can easily reach from the bedside. Arrange items on top of paper towels.
6 Provide for privacy.
7 Raise bed to a comfortable working height. Follow the care plan for bed rail use.*

Procedure

8 Lower the bed rail near you, if it is up.
9 Position the client so that he or she can brush with ease.
10 Place a towel over the client's chest. This protects garments and linens from spills.
11 Adjust the overbed table in front of the client.*
12 Let the client perform oral hygiene. This includes brushing teeth, rinsing the mouth, flossing, and using mouthwash or other solution. The client spits into the kidney basin or small bowl.
13 Remove the towel when the client is done.
14 Adjust the overbed table next to the bed.*

Post-Procedure

15 Provide for safety and comfort.
16 Place the call bell within reach.*
17 Return the bed to its lowest position. Follow the care plan for bed rail use.*
18 Clean and return equipment to its proper place. Wear gloves for this step.
19 Wipe off the overbed table or work area with the paper towels. Discard the paper towels.
20 Remove privacy measures.
21 Follow employer policy for dirty linen.
22 Perform hand hygiene.
23 Report and record your actions and observations, according to employer policy.

*Steps marked with an asterisk may not apply in community settings.

1 2 3 BRUSHING THE CLIENT'S TEETH

Remember to promote:

• Dignity • Independence • Preferences • Privacy • Safety

Pre-Procedure

1 Identify the client, according to employer policy.
2 Explain the procedure to the client.
3 Perform hand hygiene.
4 Collect gloves and items listed in *Assisting the Client to Brush Teeth at the Bedside* on page 522.
5 Place paper towels on the overbed table (in facilities) or on a work area within easy reach. Arrange items on top of paper towels.
6 Provide for privacy.
7 Raise the bed to a comfortable working height. Follow the care plan for bed rail use.*

Procedure

8 Lower the bed rail near you, if it is up.
9 Assist the client to a sitting or side-lying position facing you.
10 Place a towel over the client's chest.
11 Adjust the overbed table so that you can reach it with ease.*
12 Put on gloves.
13 Apply toothpaste to the toothbrush.
14 Hold the toothbrush over the kidney basin or bowl. Pour some water over the brush.
15 Brush the client's teeth gently (Figure 29–1).
16 Brush the client's tongue gently, if needed.
17 Allow the client to rinse the mouth with water. Hold the kidney basin or bowl under the client's chin (Figure 29–2). Repeat this step, as needed.
18 Floss the client's teeth (see *Flossing the Client's Teeth* on page 524).
19 Let the client use mouthwash or other solution. Hold the kidney basin or bowl under the client's chin.
20 Remove the towel.
21 Remove and discard gloves. Perform hand hygiene.
22 Adjust the overbed table next to the bed.*

Post-Procedure

23 Follow steps 15 through 23 for *Assisting the Client to Brush Teeth at the Bedside* on page 522.

*Steps marked with an asterisk may not apply in community settings.

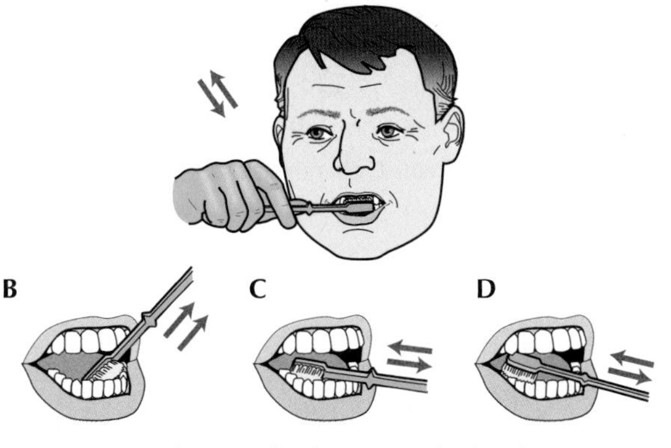

Figure 29–1 Brushing teeth. **A,** Position the brush at a 45-degree angle to the gums. Brush with short strokes. **B,** Position the brush at a 45-degree angle against the inside of the front teeth. Brush from the gum to the crown of the tooth with short strokes. **C,** Hold the brush horizontally against the inner surfaces of the teeth. Brush back and forth. **D,** Position the brush on the biting surfaces of the teeth. Brush back and forth.

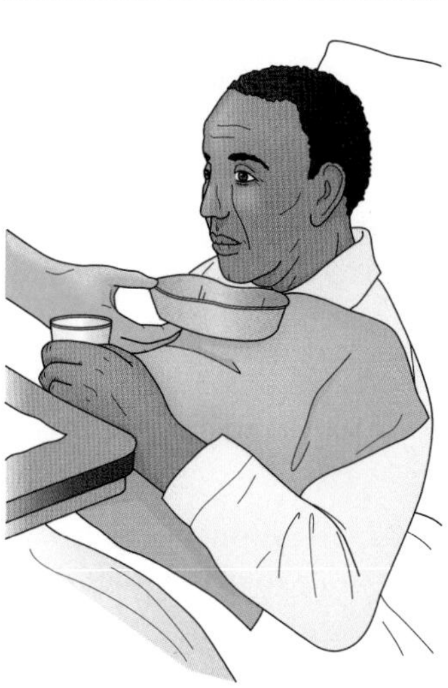

Figure 29–2 Hold a kidney basin under the client's chin. **Source**: Sorrentino, S.A. & Gorek, B. (2003). *Mosby's textbook for long-term care assistants* (4th ed., p. 297). St Louis: Mosby.

Flossing

Flossing is a preventive measure. It removes plaque and tartar, which cause serious gum disease that leads to loosening and loss of teeth. Flossing also removes food lodged between teeth. It is usually done after brushing but can be done at other times, for example, after meals. If flossing is done only once a day, bedtime is the best time to floss.

You will be required to floss for clients who cannot do it themselves. Follow the care plan (see the *Focus on Children: Flossing* and *Focus on Older Adults: Flossing* boxes).

1 2 3 FLOSSING THE CLIENT'S TEETH

Remember to promote:

• Dignity • Independence • Preferences • Privacy • Safety

Pre-Procedure

1 Identify the client, according to employer policy.
2 Explain the procedure to the client.
3 Perform hand hygiene.
4 Collect the following:
- Kidney basin or small bowl
- Water glass with cool water
- Dental floss
- Face towel
- Paper towels
- Gloves

5 Place paper towels on the overbed table (in facilities) or on a work area within easy reach. Arrange items on top of paper towels.
6 Provide for privacy.
7 Raise bed to a comfortable working height. Follow the care plan for bed rail use.*

Procedure

8 Lower the bed rail near you, if it is up.
9 Assist the client to a sitting or side-lying position facing you.
10 Place a towel over the client's chest.
11 Adjust the overbed table so that you can reach it with ease.*
12 Put on gloves.
13 Break off a 45-cm (18-in.) piece of floss from the dispenser.
14 Hold the floss between the middle fingers of each hand (Figure 29–3, *A*).
15 Stretch the floss with your thumbs.
16 Start at the upper back tooth on the right side. Work around to the left side.
17 Move the floss gently up and down between the teeth (Figure 29–3, *B*). Move the floss up and down from the top of the tooth to the gum line.
18 Use a new section of floss after every second tooth.
19 Floss the lower teeth. Hold the floss with your index fingers (Figure 29–3, *C*). Use up-and-down motions, and go under the gums as for the upper teeth. Start on the right side. Work round to the left side.
20 Allow the client to rinse his or her mouth. Hold the kidney basin or bowl under the the client's chin. Repeat rinsing, as necessary.
21 Remove the towel.
22 Remove and discard gloves. Perform hand hygiene.
23 Adjust the overbed table next to the bed.*

Post-Procedure

24 Follow steps 15 through 23 for *Assisting the Client to Brush Teeth at the Bedside* on page 522.

*Steps marked with an asterisk may not apply in community settings.

focus on ››CHILDREN

Flossing

Both preschoolers and older children need to floss. Older children can floss themselves, but you need to floss for preschoolers. Older children need reminding and some supervision.

focus on ››OLDER ADULTS

Flossing

Flossing was not a common oral hygiene practice in the past, so some older adults may have never flossed their teeth. A client may refuse to floss or to let you do it. Respect the client's wishes. Inform your supervisor so that the client's care plan may be changed, as needed.

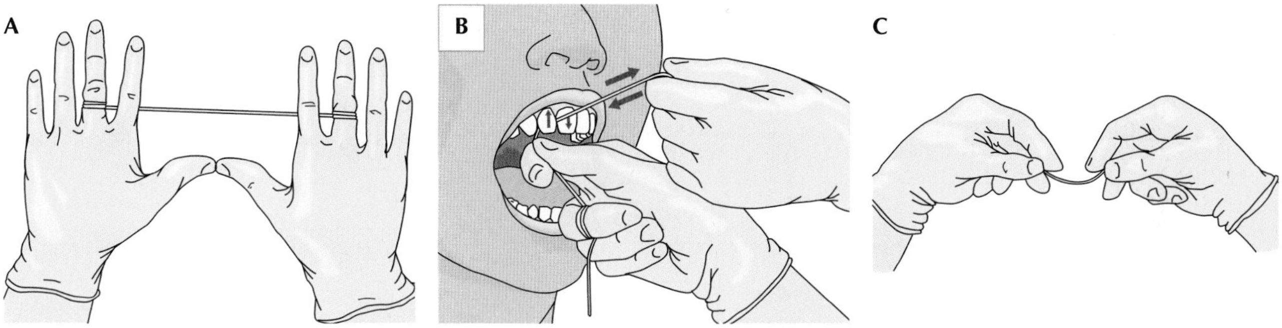

Figure 29–3 Flossing. **A,** Hold dental floss between the middle fingers to floss the upper teeth. **B,** Move floss in up-and-down motions between the teeth. Move floss up and down from the top of the tooth to the gum line. **C,** Hold floss with the index fingers to floss the lower teeth.

Mouth Care for an Unconscious Client

Unconscious clients need special mouth care procedures. They cannot eat or drink, they may breathe with their mouths open; and many receive oxygen therapy (see Chapter 44), all of which cause mouth dryness and crusting on the tongue and mucous membranes. Oral hygiene helps keep the mouth clean and moist and prevents infection.

The care plan tells you what cleaning agent to use. Use sponge swabs to apply the cleaning agent. To prevent cracking of lips, apply a lubricant (check the care plan) to the lips after cleaning.

Unconscious clients usually cannot swallow and need to be protected from choking and aspiration. **Aspiration** is the inhaling of fluid or an object into the lungs, which increases the risk of pneumonia and death. To prevent aspiration:

- Position the client on one side, with his or her head turned well to the side (Figure 29–4) so that excess fluid runs out of the mouth.
- Use only a small amount of fluid. Sometimes oral suctioning is needed (see Chapter 44).

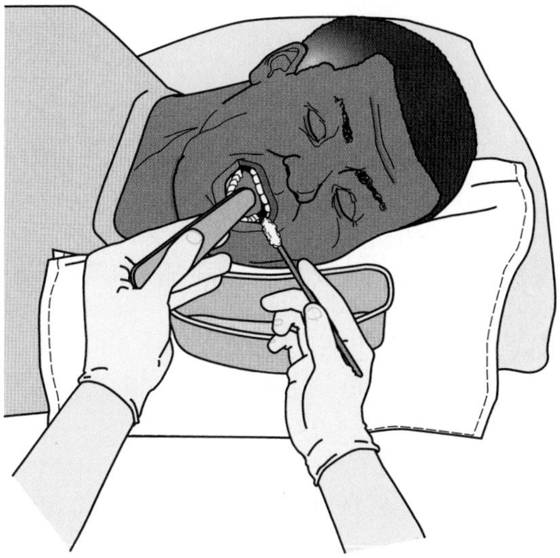

Figure 29–4 Turn the head of the unconscious client well to the side to prevent aspiration. Use a padded tongue blade to keep the mouth open while cleaning the mouth with swabs.

1 2 3 PROVIDING MOUTH CARE FOR AN UNCONSCIOUS CLIENT

Remember to promote:

• Dignity • Independence • Preferences • Privacy • Safety

Pre-Procedure

1 Identify the client, according to employer policy.
2 Explain the procedure to the client.
3 Perform hand hygiene.
4 Collect the following:
- Cleaning agent (check the care plan)
- Sponge swabs
- Padded tongue blade
- Water glass with cool water
- Face towel
- Kidney basin or small bowl
- Lubricant for lips
- Paper towels
- Gloves

5 Place paper towels on the overbed table (in facilities) or on a work area within easy reach. Arrange items on top of paper towels.
6 Provide for privacy.
7 Raise bed to a comfortable working height. Follow the care plan for bed rail use.*

Procedure

8 Lower the bed rail near you, if it is up.
9 Position the client in a side-lying position facing you. Turn his or her head well to the side.
10 Place a towel under the client's chin.
11 Place the kidney basin or bowl under the client's chin.
12 Adjust the overbed table so that you can reach it with ease.*
13 Put on gloves.
14 Separate the upper and lower teeth with the padded tongue blade. Be gentle. Do not use force.
15 Clean the mouth with sponge swabs moistened with the cleaning agent (see Figure 29–4 on page 525):
- **a** Clean the chewing and inner surfaces of the teeth.
- **b** Clean the outer surfaces of the teeth.
- **c** Swab the roof of the mouth, inside of the cheeks, and the lips.
- **d** Swab the tongue.
- **e** Moisten a clean swab with water, and swab the mouth to rinse.
- **f** Place used swabs in the kidney basin or bowl.

16 Dry the client's mouth with the towel.
17 Apply lubricant to the lips.
18 Remove the towel.
19 Remove gloves. Perform hand hygiene.

Post-Procedure

20 Explain to the client that you are going to reposition him or her.
21 Reposition the client, and provide for safety and comfort.
22 Place the call bell within reach.*
23 Return bed to its lowest position. Follow the care plan for bed rail use.*
24 Clean and return equipment to its proper place. Discard disposable items. Wear gloves for this step.
25 Wipe off the overbed table or work area with the paper towels. Discard the paper towels.
26 Remove privacy measures.
27 Tell the client that you are leaving the room.
28 Follow employer policy for dirty linen.
29 Perform hand hygiene.
30 Report and record your actions and observations, according to employer policy.

*Steps marked with an asterisk may not apply in community settings.

Keep the client's mouth open with a padded tongue blade. If one is not available, make a padded tongue blade as shown in Figure 29–5. Do not use your fingers to hold the client's mouth open, as he or she could bite down on them. Remember, breaks in the skin create a portal of entry for microbes and may cause an infection to develop.

Unconscious clients cannot say anything or respond to what is happening, but many can hear. Always assume that unconscious clients can hear, and explain what you are doing step by step. Also, tell the client when you are done and when you are leaving the room.

Mouth care is given at least every 2 hours. Check with your supervisor and the care plan. They tell you how often to do oral hygiene and what to use. Unconscious clients are also repositioned at least every 2 hours. Combining mouth care, skin care, and other comfort measures increases their comfort and safety.

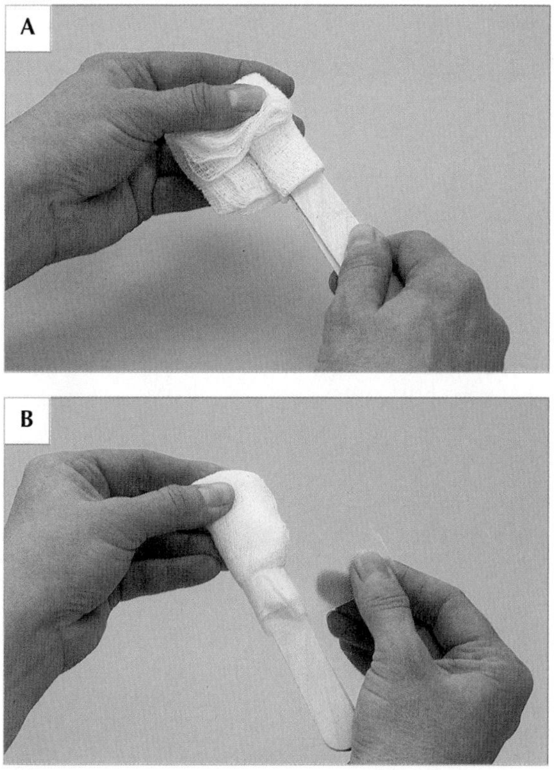

Figure 29–5 Making a padded tongue blade. **A,** Place two wooden tongue blades together and wrap gauze around the top half. **B,** Tape the gauze in place.

Denture Care

Dentures are artificial teeth. A client may have a complete set of dentures or a partial set. Mouth care is given and dentures are cleaned as often as are natural teeth. Dentures are very costly, so handle them carefully. They are slippery when wet and easily break or chip if dropped onto a hard surface (floors, sinks). During cleaning, firmly hold the dentures over a basin of water lined with a towel. Wear gloves and use gauze or a clean cloth to grasp the dentures.

The cleaning agent will have the manufacturer's instructions on how to use it and the water temperature required. Very hot water causes warping. If the dentures are not going to be worn after cleaning, store them in a container. Dentures are usually removed at bedtime. Some clients do not wear their dentures all the time; they may wear them for eating and remove them after meals. Remind them not to wrap dentures in tissues or napkins, as there is a risk of easily discarding them.

Many clients clean their own dentures and may need help to collect the cleaning items or to get to the bathroom. You are required to clean dentures only for those clients who cannot do it themselves.

Many clients do not like being seen without their dentures. After you have cleaned the dentures, return them to the client as quickly as possible. Provide privacy for clients who clean their own dentures.

1 2 3 PROVIDING DENTURE CARE

Remember to promote:

• Dignity • Independence • Preferences • Privacy • Safety

Pre-Procedure

1 Identify the client, according to employer policy.
2 Explain the procedure to the client
3 Perform hand hygiene.
4 Collect the following:
- Denture brush or toothbrush (soft bristle)
- Denture cup
- Denture cleaner agent
- Water glass with cool water
- Straw
- Mouthwash (or other specified solution)
- Kidney basin or small bowl
- Two face towels
- Paper towels
- Gauze squares
- Gloves

5 Provide for privacy.

Procedure

6 Lower the bed rail near you, if it is up.
7 Place a towel over the client's chest.
8 Put on gloves.
9 Ask the client to remove the dentures. Carefully place them in the kidney basin or bowl.
10 Remove the dentures using gauze if the client cannot do so. (The gauze lets you get a good grip on slippery dentures.)
  a Grasp the upper denture with your thumb and index finger (Figure 29–6). Move the denture up and down slightly to break the seal. Gently remove the denture once the seal is broken. Place the denture in the kidney basin or bowl.
  b Remove the lower denture by grasping it with your thumb and index finger. Turn it slightly, and lift it out of the client's mouth. Place it in the kidney basin or bowl.
11 Raise the bed rail if used.
12 Take the kidney basin, denture cup, brush, and cleaning agent to the sink.
13 Line the sink with a towel, and fill it with water.
14 Rinse the dentures under warm running water. Return them to the denture cup.
15 Apply the cleaning agent to the brush.
16 Brush the dentures as shown in Figure 29–7.
17 Rinse dentures under running water. Use warm or cool water, as directed by the cleaning agent manufacturer.
18 Place the dentures in the denture cup.
19 Clean the kidney basin or bowl.
20 Bring the denture cup and kidney basin to the client.
21 Lower the bed rail if it is up.
22 Position the client for oral hygiene.
23 Assist the client to rinse his or her mouth with mouthwash or specified solution. Hold the kidney basin under the client's chin.
24 Ask the client to insert the dentures. If the client cannot do this, insert them in the following manner:
  a Grasp the upper denture firmly with your thumb and index finger. Raise the upper lip with the other hand, and insert the denture. Use your index fingers to gently press on the denture to make sure it is securely in place.
  b Grasp the lower denture securely with your thumb and index finger. Pull down slightly on the lower lip, and insert the denture. Gently press down on it to make sure it is in place.
25 Store the dentures in a safe location if they are not going to be worn.
26 Remove the towel.
27 Remove gloves. Perform hand hygiene.

Post-Procedure

28 Provide for safety and comfort.
29 Place the call bell within reach.*
30 Follow the care plan for bed rail use.*
31 Clean and return equipment to its proper place. Discard disposable items. Wear gloves for this step.
32 Remove privacy measures.
33 Follow employer policy for dirty linen.
34 Perform hand hygiene.
35 Report and record your actions and observations, according to employer policy.

*Steps marked with an asterisk may not apply in community settings.

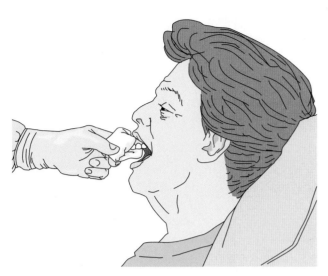

Figure 29–6 Remove the upper denture. Grasp it with the thumb and index finger of one hand. Use a piece of gauze to grasp slippery dentures.

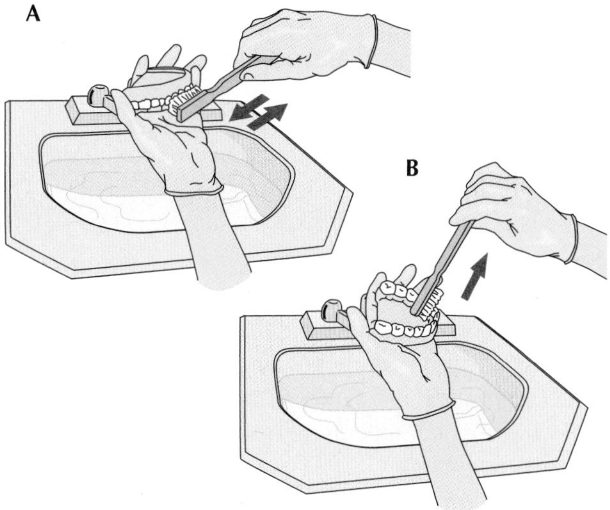

Figure 29–7 Cleaning dentures. A, Brush the outer surfaces of the upper denture with back-and-forth motions. Note that the denture is held over the sink, which is lined with a towel and filled halfway with water. B, Position the brush vertically to clean the inner surfaces of the denture. Use upward strokes.

BATHING

Bathing helps keep the skin as well as the genital and anal areas clean by removing microbes, dead skin, perspiration, and excess oils. A bath is refreshing and relaxing, stimulates circulation, and exercises body parts. During the bath, you are able to make important observations about the client and you have time to get to know him or her.

A client may require a complete bath or a partial bed bath, a tub bath, or a shower depending on the client's condition, self-care abilities, and personal choice. In facilities, bathing usually occurs after breakfast or the evening meal. The client's choice of bath time is respected, whenever possible.

Bathing frequency is a matter of personal choice. Some clients may bathe daily, while some others may choose to take a complete bath only once or twice a week. Besides personal choice, weather, physical activity, and illness also affect bathing frequency. Bathing may need to be more frequent because of increased perspiration caused by high environmental temperatures or a fever. Some illnesses and dry skin may limit bathing to once in 2 or 3 days. In some cultures, only a family member can bathe a person.

Guidelines to observe when assisting with bed baths, showers, and tub baths are listed in Box 29–1 on page 530. Table 29–1 on page 531describes common skin care products (see the *Focus on Older Adults: Bathing* box).

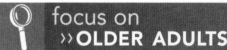

focus on ››OLDER ADULTS

Bathing

Aging and soap cause dry skin, which is easily damaged. Therefore, older adults usually need a complete bath or shower only two times a week, and partial baths on other days. Some older clients may bathe daily but do not always use soap. When using soap, thorough rinsing is needed. Lotions and oils help keep the skin soft. Special skin cleansing products are now available that do not require rinsing. Follow the manufacturers' guidelines for use.

Box 29–1 Guidelines for Bathing Clients

- Follow the care plan for bathing method and skin care products. Allow personal choices, whenever possible.
- Follow Standard Practices.
- Make sure the client fully understands the procedure before you begin. Talk with your supervisor if you are not sure the client fully understands and agrees to the procedure.
- Collect needed items before starting the procedure.
- Provide for privacy. Close doors, shades, drapes, or privacy curtains.
- Cover the client for warmth and privacy.
- Eliminate drafts. Close doors and windows.
- Protect the client from falling.
- Use good body mechanics at all times (see Chapter 23).
- Protect the client from burns and scalds. Make sure water is not too hot, particularly for older adults. Check water temperature with a bath thermometer, the inside of your wrist, or your elbow. Water temperature for a complete bed bath is usually 43.3°C to 46.1°C (110°F to 115°F) for adults. However, older adults may need lower temperatures. Follow the care plan.
- Keep bar soap in the soap dish between latherings to prevent soapy water. It reduces the chance of slips and falls in showers and tubs.
- Wash from the cleanest areas to the dirtiest areas.
- Encourage the client to help as much as is safely possible.
- Rinse the skin thoroughly to ensure that all soap is removed.
- Pat the skin dry to avoid irritating or breaking the skin. Never rub the skin.
- Dry under the breasts, between skinfolds, in the perineal area, and between the fingers and toes.
- Bathe the skin thoroughly to wash off stool or urine, if present. Follow Standard Practices.

Observations

Observe the client's skin during bathing procedures. Report and record the following:

- The colour of the skin, lips, nail beds, and sclera (whites of the eyes)
- The location and description of rashes
- Dry skin
- Bruises or open skin areas
- Pale or reddened areas, particularly over bony parts
- Drainage or bleeding from wounds or body openings
- Swelling of the feet and legs
- Corns or calluses on the feet
- Skin temperature
- Complaints of pain or discomfort

The Complete Bed Bath

The *complete bed bath* involves washing the entire body while the client is still in bed and is given to clients who cannot bathe themselves—clients who are unconscious, paralyzed, in casts or traction, or weak from illness or surgery.

Ask your supervisor about the client's ability to assist with the bath and about any activity or position limits. Remember to follow Standard Practices. Also, remember to allow the client to make choices during the bath.

A bed bath is a new experience for many clients. Some may be embarrassed that another person can see their bodies, and some fear exposure and loss of privacy. Explain to the client how a bed bath is given and that you will cover the body for privacy.

The bed bath procedure on page 532 applies to adults. Follow the adult procedure for bathing toddlers and older children. See Chapter 38 for bathing infants. Infants, young children, and older adults have fragile skin, so lower water temperatures must be used for them. Ask your supervisor about what water temperature to use. Always remember to test the bath water before bathing a client.

Towel Baths. With a *towel bath*, usually an oversized towel is used so that it covers the client's body from neck to feet. The bath towel is saturated with a cleaning solution, which contains water, a cleaning agent, and a skin-softening agent. It also has a drying agent so that the client's body dries quickly. The towel bath is quick, soothing, and relaxing. Clients with dementia often accept this type of bath well. Your supervisor and the care plan will tell you when to use the towel bath. Follow employer policies and procedures.

Table 29–1 Common Skin Care Products

Type	Purpose	Considerations
Soaps	Clean the skin Remove oil, dirt, dead skin, skin oil, some microbes, and perspiration	Tend to dry and irritate the skin Dry skin is easily injured and causes itching and discomfort Skin must be rinsed well to remove all soap Not needed for every bath; plain water can clean the skin Plain water is often used for older adults and clients with very dry skin
Bath oils	Keep the skin soft and prevent drying	Some soaps contain bath oil Liquid bath oil can be added to bath water Bath oils can cause showers and tubs to become slippery; safety precautions are necessary to prevent falls
Creams and lotions	Protect the skin from the drying effect of air and evaporation	Do not feel greasy but leave an oily film on the skin Should not contain alcohol because it will dry the skin Most are scented Lotion is used for back massage; applying lotion to bony points helps prevent skin breakdown Apply lotion to the back, elbows, knees, and heels after bathing Never apply to an area receiving radiation, as the aluminum in the lotion could cause skin burns
Powders	Absorb moisture and prevent friction when two skin surfaces rub together	Many agencies do not recommend the use of powder, as its use encourages the growth of microbes. If your employer allows the use of powder, follow procedures carefully. If used, powder is usually applied under the breasts, under the arms, in the groin area, and sometimes between the toes To apply powder, turn away from the client and sprinkle a small amount onto your hands or a cloth; apply in a thin, even layer Excessive amounts cause caking and crusts that can irritate the skin and allow microbes to grow Do not shake or sprinkle powder onto the client; inhaled powder can irritate the airway and lungs Should not be used near clients with respiratory diseases. Never use on an area that is receiving radiation, as the aluminum in the powder will cause skin burns Check the care plan before applying powder
Deodorants and antiperspirants	Deodorants mask and control body odours Antiperspirants reduce the amount of perspiration	Applied to the axillae (underarms) Should not be applied to irritated skin Are not a substitute for bathing

1 2 3 GIVING A COMPLETE BED BATH

Remember to promote:

• **D**ignity • **I**ndependence • **P**references • **P**rivacy • **S**afety

Pre-Procedure

1 Identify the client, according to employer policy.
2 Explain the procedure to the client.
3 Offer the bedpan or urinal (see Chapter 31). Provide for privacy.
4 Perform hand hygiene.
5 Collect the following:
- Wash basin
- Soap
- Bath thermometer
- Orange stick, nail file, or soft nail brush
- Wash cloth
- Two bath towels and two face towels
- Bath blanket
- Clean gown, pyjamas, or clothing of the client's choice
- Items for oral hygiene
- Lotion
- Powder
- Deodorant or antiperspirant
- Brush and comb
- Other grooming items, if requested by client
- Paper towels
- Gloves (Wear when contact with blood, body fluids, secretions, or excretions is likely. Gloves are not necessary for bathing a continent client with intact skin. However, wear gloves when bathing the genital and rectal [perineal] areas.)

6 Place paper towels on the overbed table (in facilities) or on a work area within easy reach. Arrange items on top of paper towels.
7 Close doors and windows to prevent drafts.
8 Provide for privacy.
9 Raise the bed to a comfortable working height. Follow the care plan for bed rail use.*

Procedure

10 Lower the bed rail near you, if it is up. Remove the call bell.*
11 Provide oral hygiene, if necessary (see *Brushing the Client's Teeth* on page 523.)
12 Cover the client with a bath blanket. Remove top linens (see *Making an Occupied Bed* on page 478).
13 Lower the head of the bed until flat.* Ensure the client has at least one pillow.
14 Raise the bed rail near you, if bed rails are used. Fill the wash basin two thirds full with water. Check the care plan for the right water temperature—usually 43.3°C to 46.1°C (110° to 115°F) for adults. Measure the water temperature using a bath thermometer, or test the bath water by dipping your elbow or inner wrist into the basin.
15 Place the basin on the overbed table or work area.
16 Lower the bed rail, if it is up.
17 Help the client move to the side of the bed near you.
18 Place a bath towel over the client's chest.
19 Make a mitt with the wash cloth (Figure 29–8) and use it for the entire bath.
20 Wash around the client's eyes with water. Do not use soap. Gently wipe from the inner part of the eye to the outer with a corner of the mitt (Figure 29–9). Clean around the far eye first. Repeat this step to clean around the near eye, using a clean part of the mitt.
21 Ask the client if you can use soap on the face.
22 Wash the face, ears, and neck. Rinse and pat dry with the towel on the chest.
23 Remove the client's garments, but take care to not expose the client. (Having waited until this time to remove garments helps the client feel less exposed and more comfortable with the bath.)
24 Place a bath towel lengthwise under the far arm.
25 Support the arm, with your palm under the client's elbow and the client's forearm resting on your forearm.
26 Wash the arm, shoulder, and underarm (axilla) using long, firm strokes (Figure 29–10). Rinse and pat dry.
27 Place the basin on the towel, and place the client's hand into the water (Figure 29–11). Wash it well, and clean under fingernails with an orange stick, nail file, or soft nail brush.
28 Have the client exercise the hand and fingers.
29 Remove the basin, and dry the hand well. Cover the arm with the bath blanket.
30 Repeat steps 24 to 29 for the near arm.
31 Place basin back on the bedside work area.

(continued on page 533)

1 2 3 GIVING A COMPLETE BED BATH

Procedure (cont'd)

32 Place a bath towel over the chest crosswise, and hold the towel in place. Pull the bath blanket from under the towel to the waist. While washing the chest and abdomen, observe the skin condition under the breasts, in the abdominal folds, and in the groin.
33 Lift the towel slightly, and wash the chest (Figure 29–12). Do not expose the client. Rinse and pat dry, especially under the breasts.
34 Move the towel lengthwise over the chest and abdomen. Do not expose the client. Pull the bath blanket down to the pubic area.
35 Lift the towel slightly, and wash the abdomen (Figure 29–13). Rinse and pat dry.
36 Pull the bath blanket up to the shoulders, covering both arms. Remove the towel.
37 Change soapy, soiled, or cooled water. Measure temperature as in step 14. If bed rails are used, raise the bed rail before leaving the bedside. Lower it when you return.
38 Uncover the far leg. Do not expose the genital area. Place a towel lengthwise under the foot and leg.
39 Bend the knee, and support the leg with your arm. Wash the leg with long, firm strokes. Rinse and pat dry.
40 Place the basin on the towel near the foot.
41 Lift the leg slightly. Slide the basin under the foot.
42 Place the foot in the basin (Figure 29–14). Use an orange stick, nail file, or soft nail brush to clean under toenails, if necessary. If the client cannot bend the knees:
- **a** Wash the foot. Carefully separate the toes. Rinse and pat dry.
- **b** Clean under toenails with an orange stick, nail file, or soft nail brush, if necessary.

43 Remove the basin. Dry the leg and foot. Cover the leg with the bath blanket. Remove the towel.
44 Repeat steps 38 to 43 for the near leg.
45 Change the water. Measure temperature as in step 14. If bed rails are used, raise the bed rail near you before leaving the bedside. Lower it when you return.
46 Turn the client onto his or her side facing away from you. Keep him or her covered with the bath blanket.
47 Uncover the back and buttocks. Do not expose the client. Place a towel lengthwise on the bed along the back.
48 Wash the back. Work from the back of the neck to the lower end of the buttocks. Use long, firm, continuous strokes (Figure 29–15). Rinse and dry well.
49 After the bath, give a back massage (see *Giving a Back Massage* on page 543), if the client wants one.
50 Turn the client onto his or her back.
51 Change the water to provide perineal care. Measure water temperature as in step 14. If bed rails are used, raise the bed rail near you before leaving the bedside. Lower it when you return.
52 Allow the client to wash the genital area. Place the wash basin, soap, and towels within easy reach. Place the call bell (in facilities) within reach. Ask the client to call you when finished. Make sure the client understands what to do. Answer calls for assistance promptly. If the client cannot do perineal self-care, put on gloves, and provide perineal care for the client (see *Perineal Care* on page 544).
53 Give a back massage if you have not already done so.
54 Apply deodorant or antiperspirant, lotion, and powder, as directed by the care plan or client.
55 Put clean garments on the client.
56 Comb and brush the hair (see Chapter 30).
57 Make the bed.

Post-Procedure

58 Provide for safety and comfort.
59 Return the bed to its lowest position. Attach the call bell. Follow the care plan for bed rail use.*
60 Empty and clean the wash basin. Return it and other supplies to their proper places.
61 Wipe off the overbed table or work area with the paper towels. Discard the paper towels.
62 Remove privacy measures.
63 Follow employer policy for dirty linen.
64 Perform hand hygiene.
65 Report and record your actions and observations, according to employer policy.

*Steps marked with an asterisk may not apply in community settings.

Bag Baths. *Bag baths* are prepared commercially or by the employer. Eight to ten wash cloths are provided in a plastic bag. The wash cloths are moistened with a cleaning agent that does not require rinsing. Before use, the wash cloths are warmed in the microwave. Check with your supervisor and manufacturer's instructions about the microwave setting. A new wash cloth is used for each body part, and the skin is air-dried, so towels are not needed.

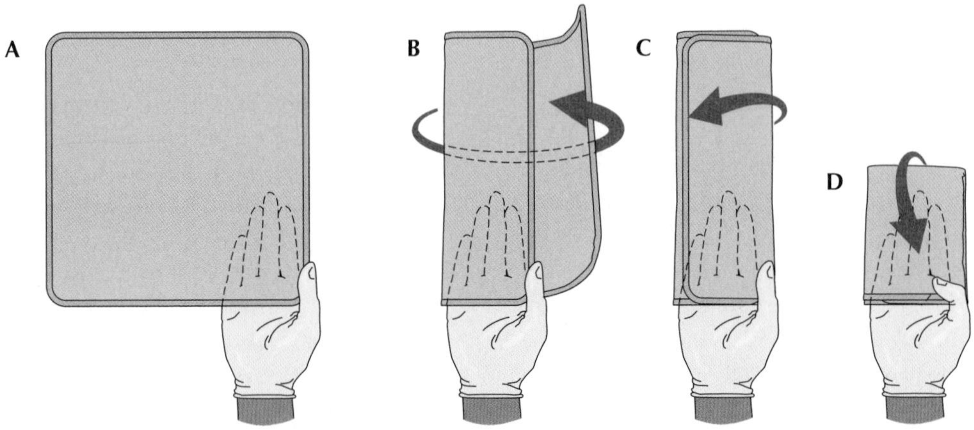

Figure 29–8 Making a mitted wash cloth. **A,** Grasp the near side of the wash cloth with your thumb. **B,** Bring the wash cloth around and behind your hand. **C,** Fold the side of the wash cloth over your palm as you grasp it with your thumb. **D,** Fold the top of the wash cloth down and tuck it under next to your palm.

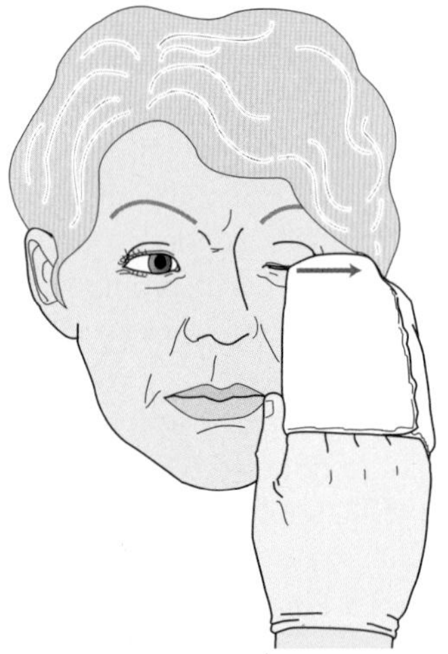

Figure 29–9 Wash around the client's eyes with a mitted wash cloth. Wipe from the inner area to the outer area of the eye.

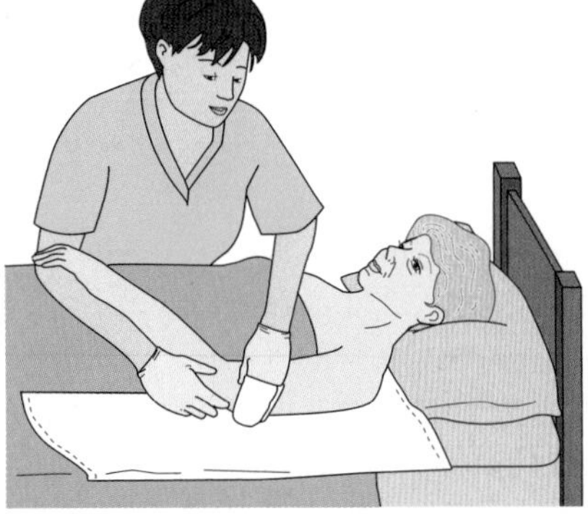

Figure 29–10 Wash the client's arm with firm, long strokes using a mitted wash cloth.

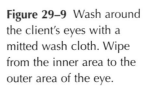

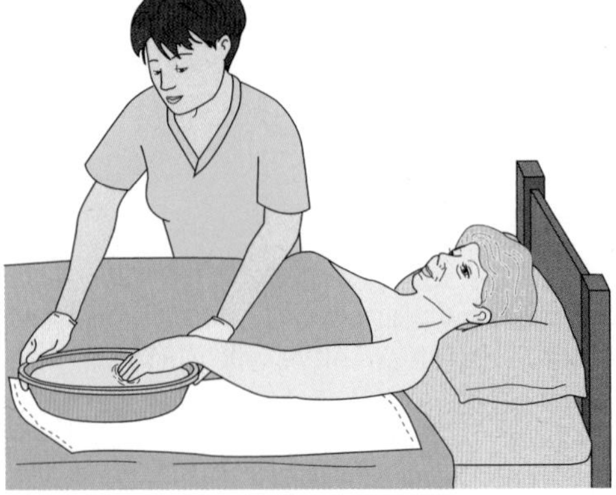

Figure 29–11 Place the wash basin on the bed. Wash the client's hands in the wash basin.

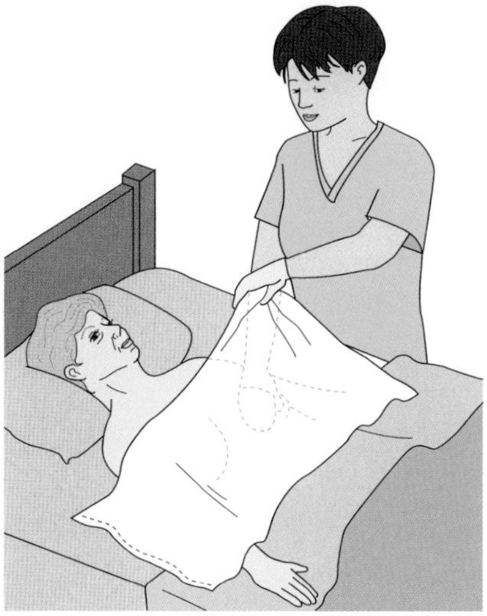

Figure 29–12 Do not expose the client's breasts during the bath. Place a bath towel horizontally over the chest area. Lift the towel slightly to reach under to wash the breasts and chest and to observe skin condition.

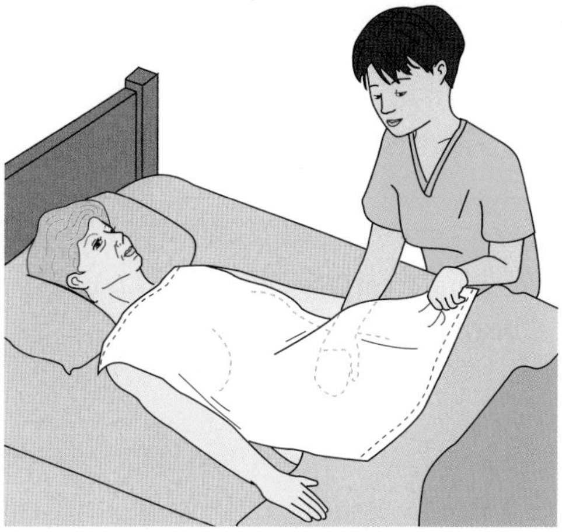

Figure 29–13 Turn the bath towel vertically to cover the breasts and abdomen. Lift the towel slightly to bathe the abdomen. The bath blanket covers the pubic area. Check the skin condition in abdominal folds.

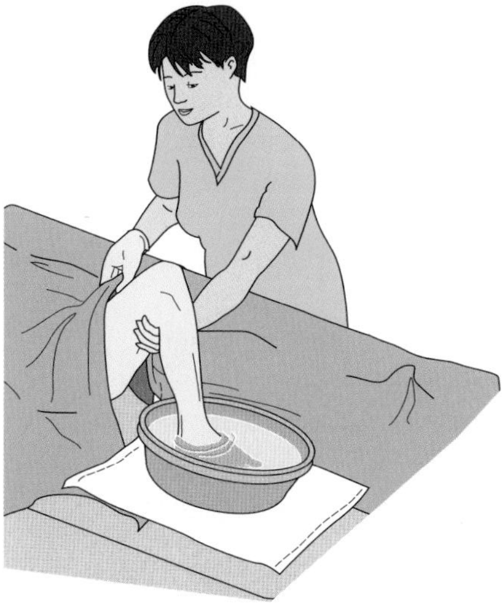

Figure 29–14 Wash the foot after placing it in the wash basin on the bed.

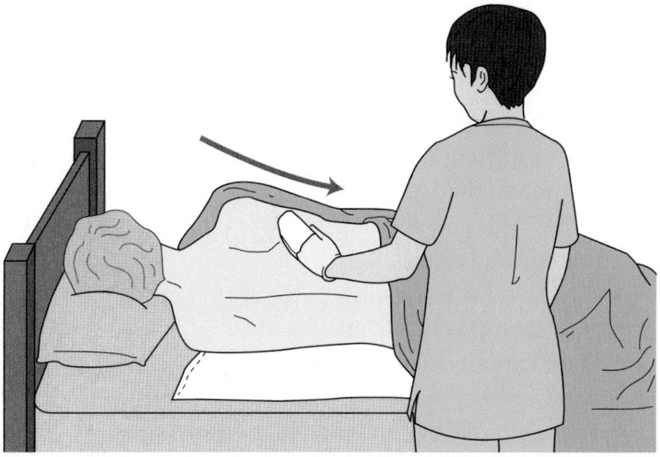

Figure 29–15 Wash the back with long, firm, continuous strokes. Note that the client is in a side-lying position. A towel is placed lengthwise on the bed to protect the linens from getting wet.

The Partial Bath

The *partial bath* involves bathing the face, hands, axillae (underarms), back, buttocks, and perineal area. These areas develop odours or cause discomfort if not clean. Partial bed baths are given to clients who cannot bathe themselves. Some clients may be able to bathe themselves in the bed or at the bathroom sink (Figure 29–16). You will be required to assist them, as needed, especially with washing the back.

The guidelines for bathing as well as the considerations involved (see Box 29–1 on page 530) also apply for partial bed baths.

1 2 3 GIVING A PARTIAL BATH

Remember to promote:

• **D**ignity • **I**ndependence • **P**references • **P**rivacy • **S**afety

Pre-Procedure

1 Follow steps 1 through 8 in *Giving a Complete Bed Bath* (see page 532). Put on gloves, if that is your employer's policy.

Procedure

2 Make sure the bed is in the lowest position.*

3 Assist with oral hygiene.

4 Remove top linen. Cover the client with a bath blanket.

5 Place paper towels on the overbed table (in facilities) or on a work area that the client can easily reach from the bedside.

6 Fill the wash basin with water. Water temperature should be 43.3°C to 46.1°C (110°F to 115°F) or as directed by your supervisor and the care plan. (Use a bath thermometer to measure water temperature, or test the bath water by dipping your elbow or inner wrist into the basin.)

7 Place the basin on the overbed table or work area.

8 Position the client in Fowler's position. Or assist him or her to sit at the bedside.

9 Adjust the overbed table so that the client can reach the basin and supplies.*

10 Help the client undress.

11 Ask the client to wash easy-to-reach body parts. Explain that you will wash the back and the areas the client cannot reach.

12 Place the call bell within reach. Ask the client to use it if help is needed or when he or she is done bathing.*

13 Perform hand hygiene. Leave the room if it is safe to do so. Stay within hearing distance.

14 Return when the client calls for assistance. Knock before entering.

15 Change the bath water. (Measure the bath water temperature as in step 6.)

16 Raise the bed to a comfortable working height. Adjust the overbed table as needed.*

17 Ask the client to specify which parts were washed by him or her. Wash and dry areas the client could not reach. The face, hands, underarms, back, buttocks, and genital and rectal areas (perineal area) are washed for the partial bath. Wear gloves for perineal care.

18 Give a back massage.

19 Apply deodorant or antiperspirant, as requested by the client.

20 Help the client put on clean garments.

21 Assist with hair care.

22 Assist the client to a chair (see *Transferring the Client to a Chair or Wheelchair* on page 416.) Otherwise, turn the client onto the side away from you.

23 Make the bed.

24 Return the bed to its lowest position.*

Post-Procedure

25 Provide for safety and comfort.

26 Place the call bell within reach.*

27 Follow the care plan for bed rail use.*

28 Empty and clean the basin. Return the basin and supplies to their proper places.

29 Wipe off the overbed table or work area with the paper towels. Discard the paper towels.

30 Remove privacy measures.

31 Follow employer policy for dirty linen.

32 Perform hand hygiene.

33 Report and record your actions and observations, according to employer policy.

*Steps marked with an asterisk may not apply in community settings.

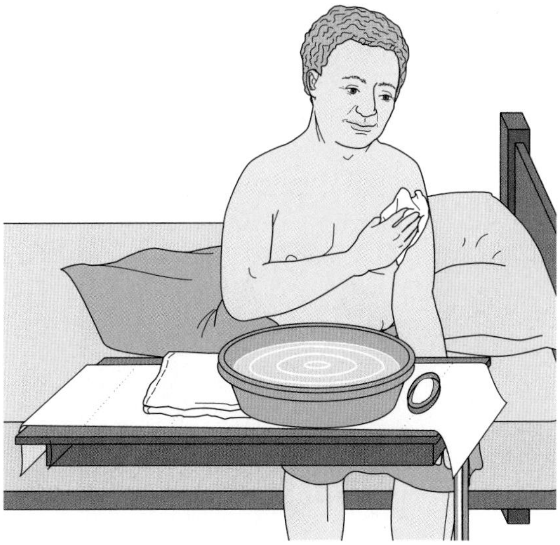

Figure 29–16 The client is bathing himself in bed. Necessary equipment is within his reach.

Tub Baths and Showers

Some clients prefer tub baths, while some others may prefer showers. In both cases, falls and burns from hot water are risks, so ensuring safety is important (see Box 29–2). You must prevent slipping, falls, chills, and burns. *Only give a tub bath or shower if it is specified in the care plan.* Check with your supervisor and the care plan for special instructions.

Tub Baths. Many clients find tub baths relaxing, but they can cause a client to feel faint, weak, or tired. The risks are greater for clients who are on bed rest, so a bath should last no longer than 20 minutes.

In a facility, you will need to reserve the tub room for the client. The tub is cleaned before and after use. This prevents the spread of microbes and infection.

Box 29–2 Safety Guidelines for Assisting Clients With Tub Baths and Showers

- Know the right water temperature. Check with your supervisor and the care plan. Usually the optimal temperature is 40.5°C (105°F).
- Clean the tub or shower before and after use. This prevents the spread of microbes and infection.
- Dry the bathroom or shower room floor.
- Check hand rails, grab bars, hydraulic lifts, and other safety aids. They must be in working order.
- Place a bath mat in the tub or on the shower floor. The mat is not needed if there are nonskid strips or a nonskid surface.
- Cover the client for warmth and privacy during transport to and from the shower room or tub.
- Place needed items within the client's reach.
- Place the call bell (in facilities) within the client's reach. Show the client how to use the call bell in the shower or tub room.
- Have the client use safety bars when getting in and out of the tub or shower. The client must not use towel bars for support.
- Use good body mechanics when transferring clients to and from tubs and showers (see Chapter 23). If necessary, ask for help before beginning the transfer.
- Turn cold water on first and then the hot water. Turn hot water off first and then the cold water.
- Adjust water temperature and pressure to prevent chilling or burns. Do this before the client gets into the shower. If a shower or bath chair is used, position the chair first.
- Direct water away from the client while adjusting water temperature and pressure.
- Fill the tub before the client gets into it.
- Measure the water temperature by using a bath thermometer. Or use the digital display for showers and tub baths in facilities (see Figure 29–23 on page 541).
- Keep the water spray directed toward the client during the shower. This helps keep him or her warm.
- Avoid using bath oils, as they make tub and shower surfaces slippery.
- Keep the bar soap in the soap dish to prevent soapy water. It also reduces the chance of slips and falls in the tub or shower.
- Do not leave weak or unsteady clients unattended in the tub or shower.
- Stay within hearing distance if the client can be left alone. Wait outside the door or shower curtain. You will be nearby if the client calls for you or has an accident.
- Drain the tub before the client gets out of the tub.

Some facilities have portable tubs. The sides are lowered to transfer the client from the bed to the tub (Figure 29–17) and raised after the transfer. The client is transported to the tub room in the portable tub. There the tub is filled and the client bathed in the usual manner. Remember to cover the client with a blanket for privacy and warmth during the transfers and transports.

Whirlpool tubs have hydraulic lifts (Figure 29–18). The client is transported to the tub room in a special wheelchair or stretcher. The client and the chair or stretcher are lifted into the tub (Figure 29–19). The whirlpool action cleans the client's lower body, and you will wash the upper body. Carefully wash under breasts, between skinfolds, and the perineal area. Dry the client after the bath.

In a client's home, the bathroom should be as safe as possible. Make sure there is a rubber bath mat or nonskid strips on the tub floor. Safety devices such as grab bars, transfer boards, and bath or shower chairs are helpful for some clients (Figure 29–20), so the case manager and other members of the health care team arrange for these devices. Make sure they are in place and used when necessary. Bring a straight chair into the bathroom so that the client can sit when the bath or shower is being prepared. Make sure the bathroom is warm and well lit and the floor is free of clutter and water spills.

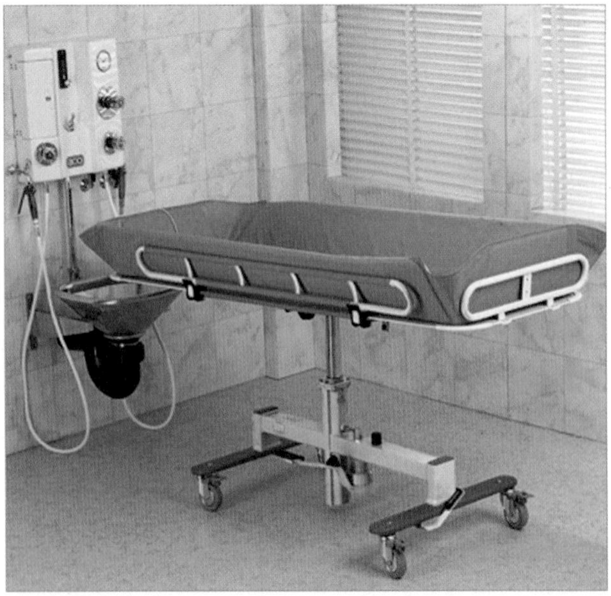

Figure 29–17 Portable tub. **Courtesy:** ARJO, Inc., Roselle, IL.

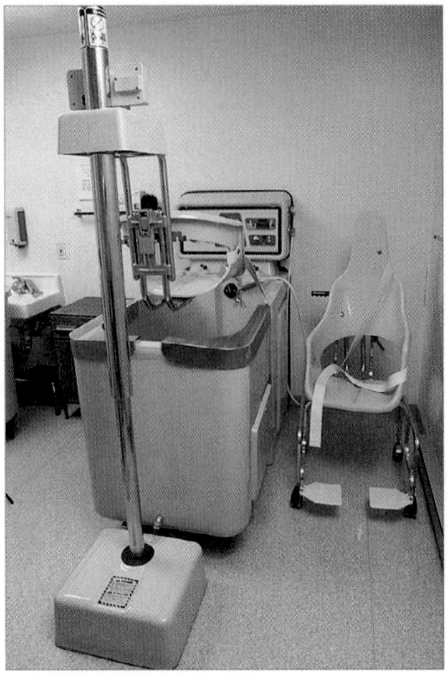

Figure 29–18 Whirlpool tub with a hydraulic lift.

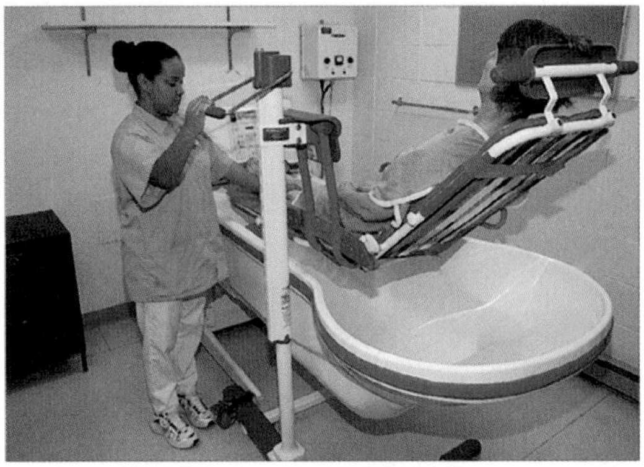

Figure 29–19 The stretcher and client are lowered into the tub.

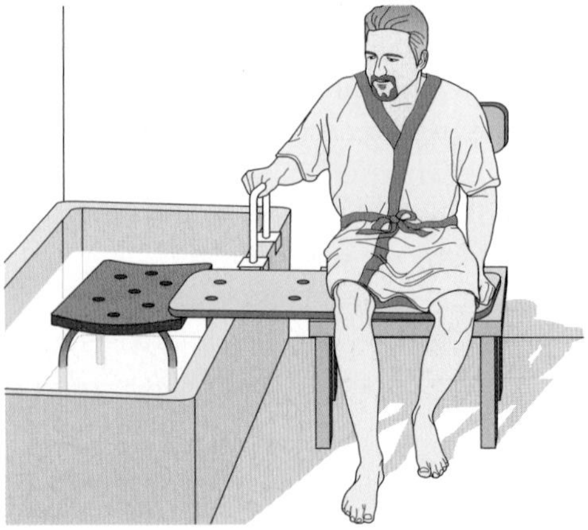

Figure 29–20 A client using a transfer board, bath chair, and grab bar when taking a bath at home.

Showers. Some facilities provide private baths or showers in the client's room. Other facilities have common baths or shower rooms that must be reserved before use. Shower rooms have shower stalls or shower cabinets (Figure 29–21). The client walks into the stall or cabinet or is wheeled in on a shower chair. An open part of the plastic seat lets water drain off the chair. The chair can be used to transport the client to and from the shower room. The wheels are locked during the shower to prevent the chair from moving.

The shower room may have more than one stall or cabinet. Protect the client's right to privacy. The client has the right to not have his or her body seen by others, so screen and cover the client properly, and close doors and the shower curtain.

Shower stalls and bathtub-shower units are common in most homes. If the client has to step into the bathtub to take a shower, make sure there are safety bars for the client's use. Assist the client with getting into and out of the shower, as needed.

Home care clients can buy or rent a shower chair for home use, or a sturdy chair, for example, a sturdy lawn chair, can be used. The case manager will assist the client or family in finding a safe chair for shower use. Before every use, make sure the chair is steady and will not slide.

Turn on the water, and test its temperature before the client enters the shower. If the client can stand in the shower, encourage him or her to use the grab bars, if available, for support during the shower. Like tubs, showers floors should have nonskid surfaces. If not, a rubber bath mat is used, but make sure the bath mat does not cover the drain. Never let weak or unsteady clients stand in the shower. They must use a shower chair. Contact your supervisor if you are concerned about the client's safety (see the *Focus on Children: Showers* box).

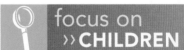

focus on
›› CHILDREN

Showers

Many older children enjoy showers. Your supervisor will tell you how much help and supervision to give the child. Remember, independence and privacy are important to older children.

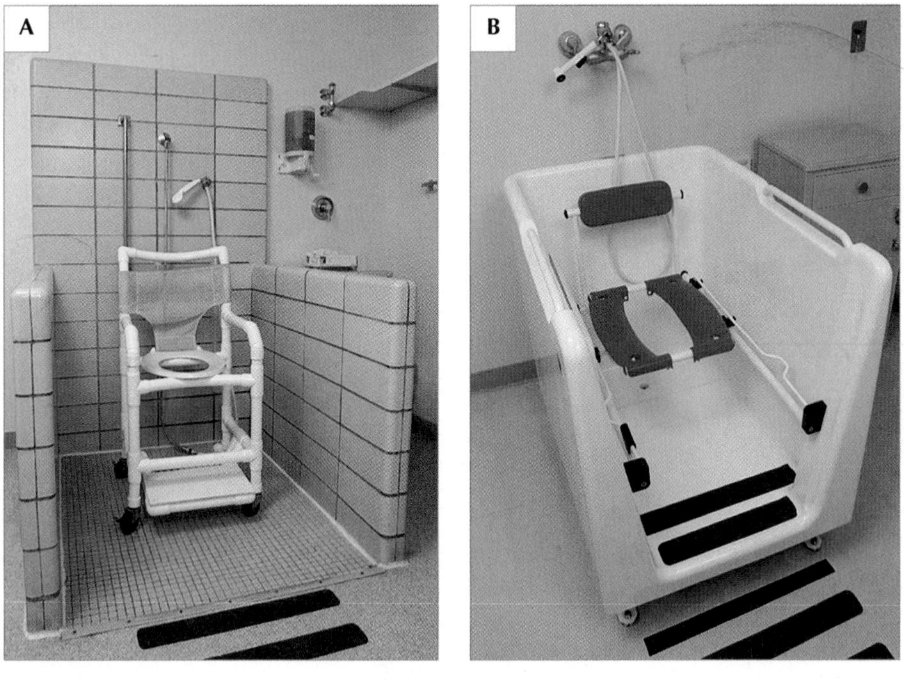

Figure 29–21 Common showers in facilities. **A,** Shower chair in a shower stall. **B,** Shower cabinet.

1 2 3 ASSISTING WITH A TUB BATH OR SHOWER

Remember to promote:

• Dignity • Independence • Preferences • Privacy • Safety

Pre-Procedure

1 Reserve the bathtub or shower.*
2 Identify the client, according to employer policy.
3 Explain the procedure to the client.
4 Perform hand hygiene.
5 Collect the following:
- Wash cloth and two bath towels
- Soap
- Bath thermometer (for a tub bath)
- Straight chair (optional)
- Bath or shower chair, as necessary
- Transfer board, if necessary
- Clean garments
- Grooming items, as requested by the client
- Robe and nonskid footwear
- Rubber bath mat, if needed
- Disposable floor mat, if needed
- Gloves

Procedure

6 Place items in the bathroom or shower room. Use the space provided or a chair.
7 Clean the tub or shower.*
8 Place a rubber bath mat in the tub or on the shower floor. Make sure it does not block the drain.
9 Place a bath mat on the floor in front of the tub or shower.
10 Place the bath or shower chair in position. Lock the wheels. Position the transfer board, if one is used.
11 Put the *Occupied* sign on the door.*
12 Return to the client's room after completion of the bath. Provide for privacy.
13 Help the client sit on the side of the bed.
14 Help the client put on a robe and nonskid footwear.
15 Assist the client to the bathroom or shower room. Use a wheelchair, if necessary.
16 *For a tub bath:*
  a Have the client sit on the chair by the tub.
  b Fill the tub halfway with warm water (40.5°C or 105°F). (See Figure 29–22.) Measure water temperature with the bath thermometer, or check the digital display (Figure 29–23).

  For a shower:
  a Turn on the shower.
  b Adjust water temperature and pressure.
17 Help the client undress and remove footwear.
18 Assist the client into the tub or shower (see Chapter 23). Have the client use grab bars for support.
19 Assist with washing if necessary (a bath should last no longer than 20 minutes).
20 Place a towel across the chair.
21 Turn off the shower, or drain the tub. Cover the client while the tub drains.
22 Help the client out of the tub or shower and onto the chair. Encourage the client to use the grab bars.
23 Help the client dry off by patting gently. Dry under breasts, between skinfolds, around the perineal area, and between toes.
24 Assist with applying lotion and other grooming items, as needed.
25 Help the client dress and put on footwear.
26 Help the client return to the room. Assist the client into the bed or to a chair.
27 Provide for privacy.
28 Give a back massage, if the client returns to bed.
29 Assist with hair care and other grooming needs.

Post-Procedure

30 Provide for safety and comfort.
31 Place the call bell within reach.*
32 Follow the care plan for bed rail use.*
33 Return to bathroom or shower room. Remove soiled linen. Discard disposable items. Wear gloves for this step.
34 Put the *Unoccupied* sign on the door.*
35 Return supplies to their proper places.
36 Follow employer policy for dirty linen.
37 Perform hand hygiene.
38 Report and record your actions and observations, according to employer policy.

*Steps marked with an asterisk may not apply in community settings.

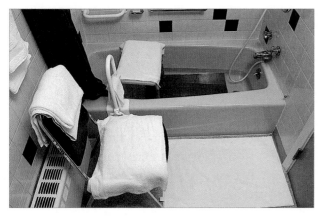

Figure 29–22 A bath mat is in the tub; the tub is filled halfway with water; a floor mat is in front of the tub; and a straight chair is next to the tub.

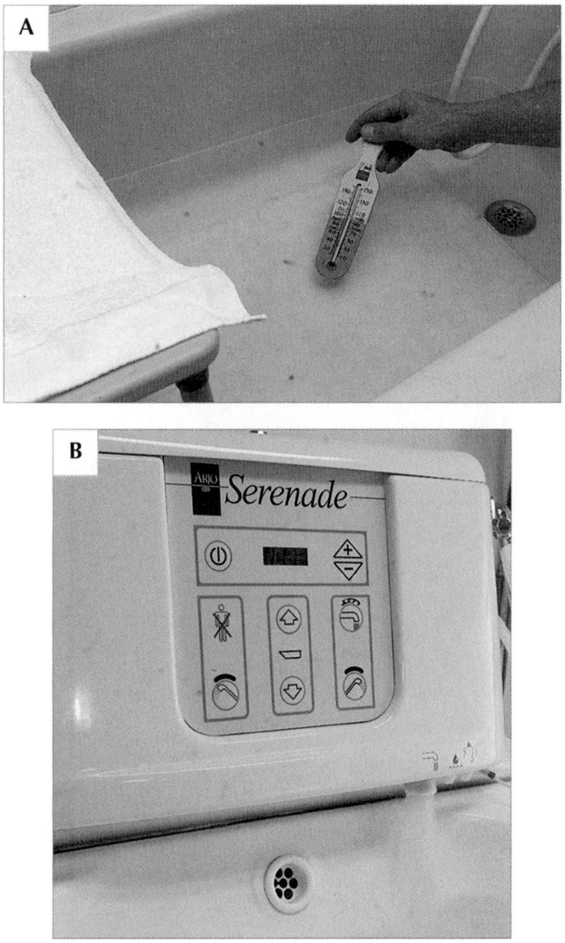

Figure 29–23 Measuring bath water temperature. **A,** A bath thermometer is used to measure water temperature. **B,** The digital display shows water temperature.

Dealing With Bathing Problems

Problems can arise when bathing a client. The client may refuse the bath. Bathing procedures can frighten clients with dementia. The client may urinate or defecate during the procedure. You need to be prepared for these and other problems.

The Client Refuses the Bath. As with all procedures, the client has the right to refuse a bath. You cannot perform a bathing procedure without the client's informed consent. Sometimes people feel too ill or weak to bathe. Some are afraid of falling or getting chilled, and some may be just embarrassed. Listen carefully to the client to learn how you can provide reassurance. Did the client get cold during the last bath? If so, offer to raise the room temperature before you start. If the bathing area has a heat lamp, use it to provide extra warmth during bathing. Does the client think a bath is not needed? If so, remind the client that bathing promotes hygiene, comfort, and relaxation. If the client continues to refuse the bath, talk to your supervisor. Do not bathe the client against his or her wishes.

The Client Has Dementia. Clients with dementia are often frightened by bathing procedures. They do not understand what is happening or why and may fear harm or danger. So they may resist care and become agitated and combative. They may shout at you and cry for help.

The guidelines in Box 29–1 on page 530 apply when you are bathing clients with dementia. The client's care plan lists measures to help him or her through the bathing procedure. Such measures include:

- Not rushing the client
- Using a calm, pleasant voice
- Diverting the client's attention (see Chapter 35)
- Calming the client and trying the bath again later

The Client Cannot Tolerate the Bathing Position. Some clients cannot sit or lie on their backs or sides for long periods of time due to disease, injury, surgery, or shortness of breath. You must adapt the procedure to meet the client's needs. Follow your supervisor's directions and the care plan. You may need to scale down to a partial bath, or you may need to ask for help so that the client can be bathed quickly.

You may have to adapt your technique to whatever position the client finds more comfortable.

The Client Urinates or Defecates. Some clients may have urinary or fecal incontinence (see Chapters 31 and 32). If they urinate or defecate during a bed bath, put on gloves if you are not wearing them already. Turn the client away from you, and clean the client with toilet tissue and discard it in a bedpan. Change the soiled linens, and clean the bedpan. Remove your gloves, wash your hands, and put on clean gloves. Change the bath water and wash cloths to prevent contamination of other body areas.

If the client is taking a tub bath, drain the bath. Cover the client with a towel to prevent chilling. Help the client out of the tub. Remove stool with toilet tissue, and dispose of it in the toilet. Clean and refill the tub. Then help the client back into the tub. Use a clean wash cloth for the bath. Remember to control your verbal as well as nonverbal reactions, taking care to not embarrass the client.

Hardened Secretions or Stool on the Client's Body. To remove hardened secretions or stool, use unscented lotion or petroleum jelly. Place some on a clean, damp wash cloth. Gently clean the area. Repeat this step, as needed. Use a clean wash cloth and more lotion or petroleum jelly. Do not rub or scratch. You can irritate the skin and cause skin breakdown.

A Client Has an Erection. Privacy is important when a male client has an erection during the bath. In a professional and calm manner, tell him that you will give him some time alone. Provide for safety, leave the room, and close the door. When you return, knock on the door before entering the room. Identify yourself, and ask if you can enter the room. Continue with the bath.

An erection is a normal reaction to physical contact, especially to the genital area. Try not to show any embarrassment. Remember, the client is probably embarrassed, too. A professional manner will help both of you.

THE BACK MASSAGE

The back massage (back rub) relaxes muscles and stimulates circulation. A massage is normally given after the bath and before bedtime. It should last 3 to 5 minutes. Observe the skin before giving the massage. Look for breaks in the skin, bruises, reddened areas, and other signs of skin breakdown.

Application of lotion reduces friction during the massage. Before applying the lotion, warm it by placing the bottle in the bath water, holding it under warm water, or rubbing some lotion between your hands.

The prone position is best for a massage. Older or disabled people may find the side-lying position more comfortable. Use firm strokes, and always keep your hands in contact with the client's skin. After the massage, apply some lotion to the client's elbows, knees, and heels to keep the skin in those areas soft. These bony areas are at risk for skin breakdown. Report any reddened areas or signs of skin breakdown at once.

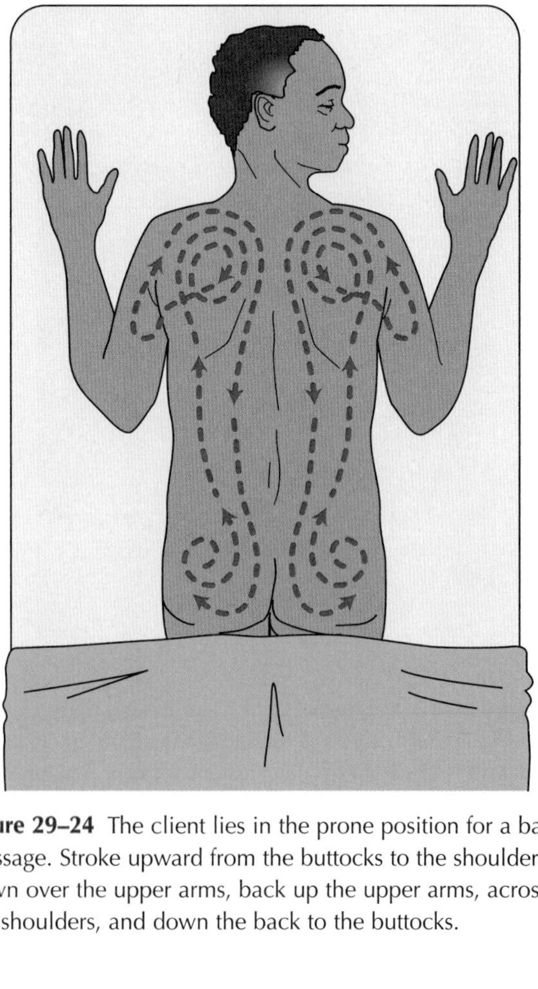

Figure 29–24 The client lies in the prone position for a back massage. Stroke upward from the buttocks to the shoulders, down over the upper arms, back up the upper arms, across the shoulders, and down the back to the buttocks.

1 2 3 GIVING A BACK MASSAGE

Remember to promote:

• Dignity • Independence • Preferences • Privacy • Safety

Pre-Procedure

1 Identify the client, according to employer policy.
2 Explain the procedure to the client.
3 Perform hand hygiene.
4 Collect the following:
- Bath blanket
- Bath towel
- Lotion

5 Provide for privacy.
6 Raise the bed to a comfortable working height. Follow the care plan for bed rail use.*

Procedure

7 Lower the bed rail near you, if it is up.
8 Position the client in the prone or side-lying position. The back is toward you.
9 Expose the back, shoulders, upper arms, and buttocks. Cover the rest of the body with the bath blanket.
10 Lay a towel on the bed along the back.
11 Warm the lotion.
12 Explain that the lotion may feel cool and wet.
13 Apply lotion to the lower back area.
14 Stroke up from the buttocks to the shoulders. Then stroke down over the upper arms. Stroke up the upper arms, across the shoulders, and down the back to the buttocks (Figure 29–24). Use firm strokes. Keep your hands in contact with the client's skin.
15 Repeat step 14 for at least 3 minutes, unless the client asks you to stop sooner.
16 Knead by grasping skin between your thumb and fingers (Figure 29–25). Knead half of the back, starting at the buttocks and moving up to the shoulder. Then knead down from the shoulder to the buttocks. Repeat on the other half of the back.
17 Apply lotion to bony areas. Use circular motions with the tips of your index and middle fingers. Do not massage bony areas that are reddened (see Chapter 42).
18 Use fast movements to stimulate and slow movements to relax the client.
19 Stroke with long, firm movements to end the massage. Tell the client that you are about to finish.
20 Cover the client. Remove the towel and bath blanket.

Post-Procedure

21 Provide for safety and comfort.
22 Place the call bell within reach.*
23 Return the bed to its lowest position. Follow the care plan for bed rail use.*
24 Return the lotion to its proper place.
25 Remove privacy measures.
26 Follow employer policy for dirty linen.
27 Perform hand hygiene.
28 Report and record your actions and observations, according to employer policy.

*Steps marked with an asterisk may not apply in community settings.

Back massages as described in this procedure can be dangerous to some clients, for example, those with certain heart diseases, back injuries, back surgeries, skin diseases, and some lung disorders. Check with the care plan and your supervisor before giving back massages.

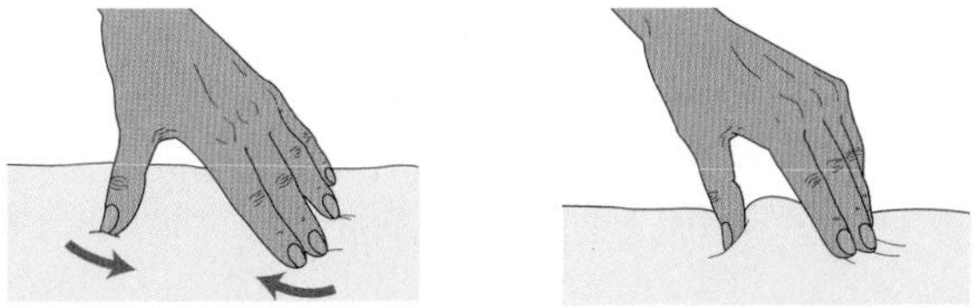

Figure 29–25 Kneading is done by grasping skin between the thumb and fingers.

PERINEAL CARE

Perineal care (pericare) involves cleaning the genital and anal areas, which provide a warm, moist, and dark place suitable for microbes to grow. Cleaning prevents infection, odours, and skin breakdown and promotes comfort.

Perineal care is done at least once every day during the bath. The procedure is also done whenever the area is soiled with urine or stool. Clients with certain disorders need perineal care more often. Your supervisor and the care plan tell you when the client needs perineal care.

Clients do their own perineal care if they can. Some may need assistance with perineal care. Clients may not know the terms *perineum* and *perineal.* Most understand terms such as *privates, private parts, crotch, genitals,* or the *area between the legs.* Use terms the client understands. The term must also be in good taste professionally.

Follow Standard Practices and medical asepsis when providing perineal care. Wear gloves. Work from the cleanest area to the dirtiest. The urethral area is the cleanest and the anal area the dirtiest, so clean from the urethra to the anal area. Clean around the perineum. When cleaning the perineum, use three strokes. Clean down each side and then down the centre. The perineal area is very delicate and easily injured. Use warm water, not hot water. Test the water temperature, according to employer policy. Use wash cloths, towelettes, cotton balls, or swabs, according to employer policy. Rinse the area thoroughly. Pat dry after rinsing to reduce moisture and to promote comfort.

1 2 3 GIVING PERINEAL CARE TO A FEMALE CLIENT

Remember to promote:

• **D**ignity • **I**ndependence • **P**references • **P**rivacy • **S**afety

Pre-Procedure

1. Identify the client, according to employer policy.
2. Explain the procedure to the client.
3. Perform hand hygiene.
4. Collect the following:
   - Wash basin
   - Soap
   - At least four wash cloths
   - Bath towel
   - Bath blanket
   - Bath thermometer
   - Waterproof pad
   - Gloves
   - Paper towels
5. Place paper towels on an overbed table (in a facility) or on a work area within easy reach from the bedside. Arrange items on top of the paper towels.
6. Provide for privacy.
7. Raise the bed to a comfortable working height. Follow the care plan for bed rail use.*

Procedure

8. Lower the bed rail near you, if it is up.
9. Cover the client with a bath blanket. Move top linens to the foot of the bed.
10. Position the client on her back. Remove garments from the waist down.
11. Position waterproof pad under the client's buttocks.
12. Drape the client as in Figure 29–26.
13. Raise the bed rail, if used.
14. Fill the wash basin. Water temperature must be 40.5°C to 42.7°C (105°F to 109°F). Measure water temperature, according to employer policy.
15. Place the basin on the overbed table or work area.
16. Lower the bed rail, if up.
17. Help the client flex her knees and spread her legs. If she cannot flex her knees, help her spread her legs as much as possible with her knees straight.
18. Put on gloves.
19. Fold the corner of the bath blanket between the client's legs onto her abdomen.
20. Wet the wash cloths. Squeeze out excess water from wash cloths before using them.
21. Apply soap to a wash cloth.
22. Separate the labia. Clean downward from front to back with one stroke (Figure 29–27).

(continued on page 545)

1 2 3 GIVING PERINEAL CARE TO A FEMALE CLIENT

Procedure (cont'd)

23 Repeat steps 21 and 22 until the area is clean. Use a clean part of the wash cloth for each stroke. Use more than one wash cloth, if needed.
24 Rinse the perineum with a clean wash cloth. Separate the labia. Stroke downward from front to back. Go down each side and then down the centre. Repeat as necessary. Use a clean part of the wash cloth for each stroke. Use more than one wash cloth, if needed.
25 Pat the area dry with the towel.
26 Fold the blanket back between the client's legs.
27 Help the client lower her legs and turn onto her side away from you.
28 Apply soap to a wash cloth.
29 Clean the rectal area. Separate buttocks and clean from the vagina to the anus with one stroke (Figure 29–28).
30 Repeat steps 28 and 29 until the area is clean. Use a clean part of the wash cloth for each stroke. Use more than one wash cloth, if needed.
31 Rinse the rectal area with a wash cloth. Stroke from the vagina to the anus. Repeat as necessary using a clean part of the wash cloth for each stroke. Use more than one wash cloth, if needed.
32 Pat the area dry with the towel.
33 Remove the waterproof pad.
34 Remove gloves. Wash your hands.

Post-Procedure

35 Provide for safety and comfort.
36 Cover the client.
37 Remove the bath blanket.
38 Place the call bell within reach.*
39 Return the bed to its lowest position. Follow the care plan for bed rail use.*
40 Empty and clean the wash basin.
41 Return the basin and supplies to their proper places.
42 Wipe off the overbed table or work area with the paper towels, and discard the paper towels.
43 Remove privacy measures.
44 Follow employer policy for dirty linen.
45 Perform hand hygiene.
46 Report and record your actions and observations, according to employer policy.

*Steps marked with an asterisk may not apply in community settings.

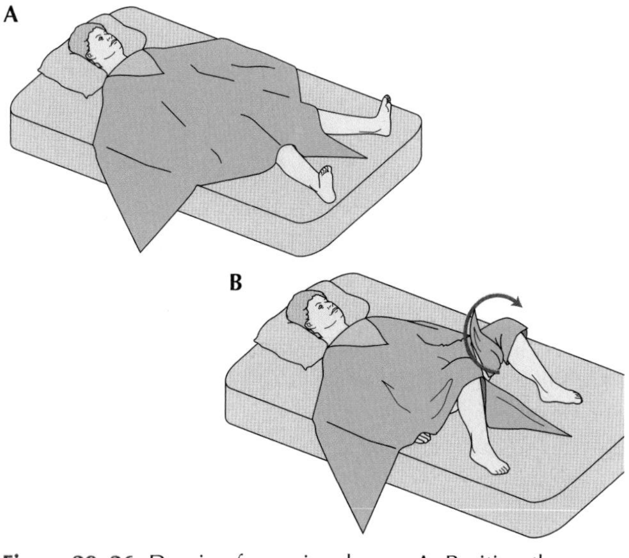

Figure 29–26 Draping for perineal care. **A,** Position the bath blanket like a diamond: one corner is at the neck, one corner is at each side, and one corner is between the client's legs. **B,** Wrap the blanket around the leg by bringing the corner around under the leg and over the top. Tuck the corner under the hip.

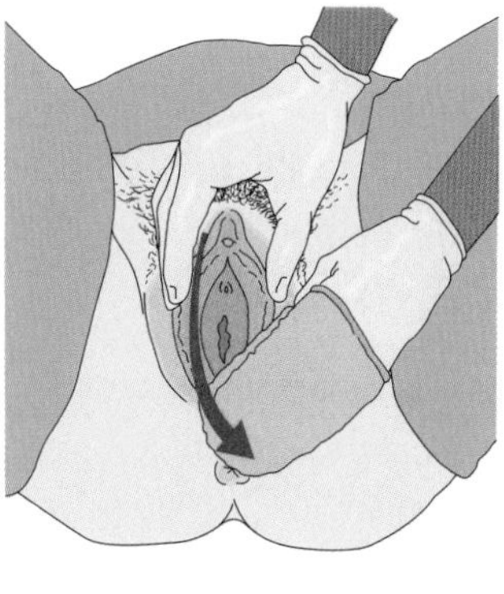

Figure 29–27 Female perineal care. Separate the labia with one hand. Use a mitted wash cloth to cleanse between the labia with downward strokes.

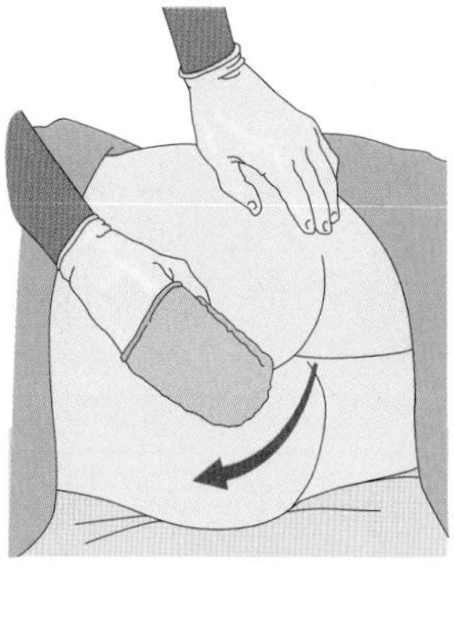

Figure 29–28 Cleaning the rectal area. Wipe from the vagina to the anus. The side-lying position allows thorough cleaning of the anal area.

When washing a client who has soiled himself or herself, wash the buttocks area and then the anal area. Some clients with dementia may put their hands into their briefs or put their hands in the area you are cleaning. Wash their hands first and give them something, for example, a wash cloth or a towel, to hang on to while you clean the area (see the *Focus on Children: Perineal Care* box.)

Report and record the following if observed when providing perineal care:

- Odours
- Redness, swelling, discharge, or irritation
- Complaints of pain, burning, or other discomfort
- Signs of urinary or fecal incontinence (see Chapters 31 and 32)
- Presence of hemorrhoids
- A male client's foreskin not retracting

focus on »CHILDREN

Perineal Care

Children of all ages need perineal care. In children who wear diapers, the perineal area is often exposed to urine and stool. Inadequate wiping after urinating and defecating is a common problem in younger children. Older children may hesitate to clean the genital and anal areas.

1 2 3 GIVING PERINEAL CARE TO A MALE CLIENT

Remember to promote:

• Dignity • Independence • Preferences • Privacy • Safety

Pre-Procedure

1 Follow steps 1 through 21 in *Giving Perineal Care to a Female Client* on page 544.

Procedure

2 Retract the foreskin, if the client is uncircumcised (Figure 29–29).
3 Grasp the penis.
4 Clean the tip using a circular motion. Start at the urethral opening, and work outward (Figure 29–30). Repeat this step as necessary. Use a clean part of the wash cloth each time.
5 Rinse the area with another wash cloth.
6 Return the foreskin to its natural position.
7 Clean the shaft of the penis with firm downward strokes. Rinse the area.
8 Help the client flex his knees and spread his legs. If he cannot flex his knees, help him spread his legs as much as possible with his knees straight.
9 Clean the scrotum and rinse well. Observe for redness and irritation in the skinfolds.
10 Pat dry the penis and scrotum.
11 Fold the bath blanket back between his legs.
12 Help him lower his legs and turn onto his side away from you.
13 Clean the rectal area (see steps 28 to 32 of *Giving Perineal Care to a Female Client*). Rinse and dry well.
14 Remove the waterproof pad.
15 Remove and discard the gloves. Perform hand hygiene.

Post-Procedure

16 Follow steps 35 through 46 in *Giving Perineal Care to a Female Client.*

*Steps marked with an asterisk may not apply in community settings.

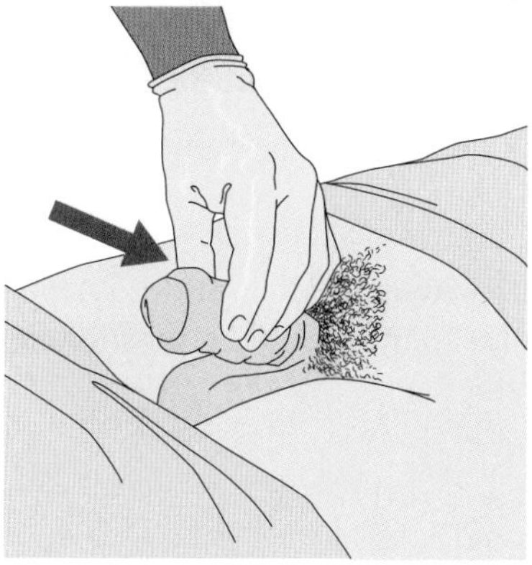

Figure 29–29 Male perineal care. Pull back the foreskin of the uncircumcised male. Return the foreskin to its normal position immediately after cleaning.

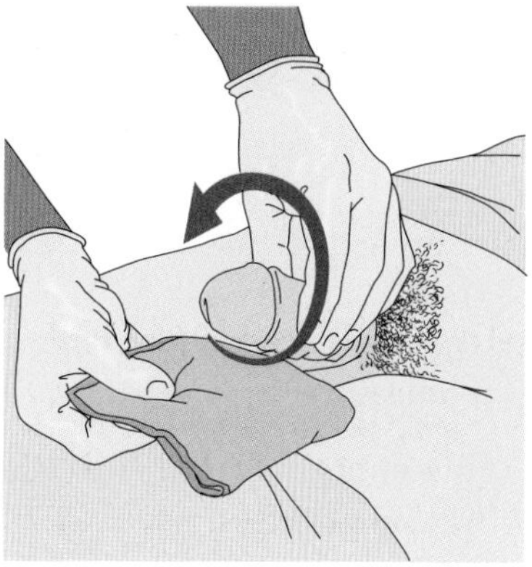

Figure 29–30 Clean the penis with circular motions starting at the urethra.

MENSTRUAL CARE

Menstruation is a woman's monthly bleeding, when blood flows from the uterus through the vaginal opening (see Chapter 15). Sanitary pads absorb menstrual blood. Most menstrual periods last 3 to 5 days. Some clients need assistance with menstrual care, as they may be too ill or weak to change their sanitary pads.

Usually women use disposable sanitary pads, which have an adhesive strip to hold them in place in the woman's panties. Sanitary pads containing perfumes can irritate the skin and should be avoided. In some hospitals, female clients may use disposable sanitary pads that are held in place with sanitary belts or reusable mesh panties.

Sanitary pads should be changed often. This promotes good hygiene and comfort and prevents odours and infection. Follow the care plan for when to change the woman's sanitary pad. Frequency depends on the amount of menstrual flow. Usually the pads need to be changed at least every 3 to 5 hours. However, they should be changed before they become soaked with blood.

Contact with the client's blood and mucous membranes is likely, so always wear gloves when removing or applying sanitary pads. Wash your hands, and help the client wash her hands after menstrual care. Dispose of sanitary pads, according to employer policy. Also, follow employer policy for disposing of soiled sanitary belts and mesh panties.

Record and report the following if observed while providing menstrual care:

- Odours
- Fever
- Redness, swelling, or irritation in the perineum
- Complaints of pain, burning, difficulty urinating, or other discomforts
- Heavy bleeding; for example, the sanitary pad becomes soaked within one hour of application (report this at once)
- Large number of blood clots on the pad (report this at once)

REVIEW

Answers to these questions are at the bottom of the page.

Circle **T** if the answer is true or circle **F** if the answer is false.

1. T F **Hygiene is needed for comfort, safety, and health.**
2. T F **Culture and personal choice affect hygiene practices.**
3. T F **Mrs. Lam's toothbrush has hard bristles. They are good for oral hygiene.**
4. T F **Unconscious clients are kept in the supine position for mouth care.**
5. T F **You use your fingers to keep an unconscious client's mouth open for oral hygiene.**
6. T F **Mrs. Lam has a lower denture. It is placed on a hard surface and washed in warm water.**
7. T F **Bath oils cleanse and soften the skin.**
8. T F **Powders absorb moisture and prevent friction.**
9. T F **Deodorants reduce the amount of perspiration.**
10. T F **The care plan says that Mrs. Lam can have a tub bath. You can allow her to take a 30-minute bath.**
11. T F **Weak clients can be left alone in the shower if they are sitting.**
12. T F **A back massage relaxes muscles and stimulates circulation.**
13. T F **Perineal care helps prevent infection.**
14. T F **The foreskin is returned to its normal position after cleaning.**
15. T F **Sanitary pads should be changed at least every 3 to 5 hours.**

Circle the **BEST** answer.

16. **When providing mouth care to an unconscious client, the client should be positioned:**
    - A. On the back
    - B. On the side
    - C. Sitting up
    - D. On the stomach
17. **What is the purpose of bathing?**
    - A. Increasing circulation
    - B. Preventing odours and cleansing skin
    - C. Refreshing and relaxing the person
    - D. All of the above
18. **Soaps do the following:**
    - A. Remove dirt and dead skin
    - B. Remove pigment
    - C. Remove hair
    - D. Moisten the skin
19. **Which action is correct when bathing Mrs. Smith?**
    - A. Removing all of the covers
    - B. Rinsing the skin thoroughly to remove all soaps
    - C. Washing from the dirtiest to the cleanest area
    - D. Rubbing the skin dry
20. **Water for Mrs. Lam's complete bed bath should be approximately**
    - A. 37.8°C (100°F)
    - B. 40.5°C (105°F)
    - C. 43.4°C (110°F)
    - D. 48.9°C (120°F)
21. **You are going to give Mrs. Lam a back massage. How long should it last?**
    - A. 3 to 5 minutes
    - B. 1 to 2 minutes
    - C. 10 minutes
    - D. 6 to 7 minutes

Answers: 1.T, 2.T, 3.F, 4.F, 5.F, 6.F, 7.F, 8.T, 9.F, 10.F, 11.F, 12.T, 13.T, 14.T, 15.T, 16.B, 17.D, 18.A, 19.B, 20.C, 21.A

CHAPTER 30

Grooming and Dressing

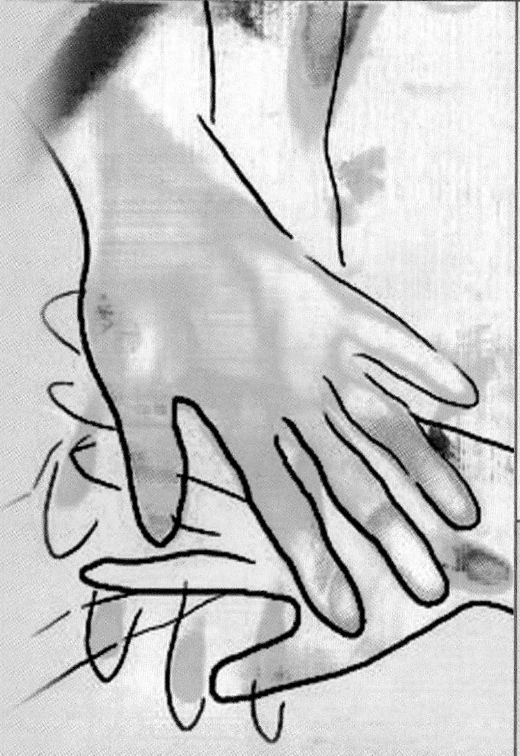

OBJECTIVES

- Define the key terms listed in this chapter.
- Explain the importance of hair care and shaving.
- Identify the factors that affect hair care.
- Explain how to care for matted and tangled hair.
- Describe how to shampoo hair.
- List the steps taken to shave a client.
- Explain why nail and foot care is important.
- Describe how to dress and undress clients.
- Explain the purpose of elastic stockings and bandages and when you assist with them.
- Apply the procedures described in this chapter to your clinical practice by providing culturally sensitive grooming.

key terms

alopecia Hair loss.

dandruff Excessive amount of dry, white flakes on the scalp.

hirsutism Excessive and increased hair growth in women in locations where the occurrence of visible, coarse hair is normally minimal or absent (such as on the face or neck). Men who are described as being *hirsute* have an abundant (or above average) amount of body hair or have coarse, visible body hair in areas of the body where men usually do not, such as on the forehead, nose, or back.

ingrown hair A hair that curls into the side wall of the hair follicle or into the skin surface, which causes the skin to become inflamed. Also known as **razor bumps**.

ingrown nails Toenails that grow in at the side of the nailbed.

lice Small, insect-like parasites that live on the human body, most commonly on the skin, hair, and genital area. They feed on human blood and lay their eggs on body hair and in clothing. The word "lice" is plural for the word "louse."

mites Small, often microscopic, invertebrates that can infest stored food and are parasitic to animals and plants.

parasite Animals that live off other animals.

pediculosis Infestation with lice.

pediculosis capitis Infestation of the scalp (*capitis*) with lice.

pediculosis corporis Infestation of the body (*corporis*) with lice.

pediculosis pubis Infestation of the pubic (*pubis*) hair with lice.

podiatrist A physician who specializes in the evaluation and treatment of diseases of the foot.

razor bumps See **ingrown hair**.

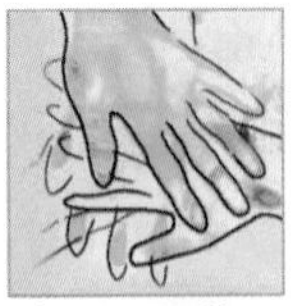

As you already know, personal grooming—which involves clean hair, nails, and clothes—is not only important to health care workers but also to all people, whatever their nationality or culture. Good grooming not only helps with emotional well-being and self-confidence, it also helps prevent infection and promote comfort.

Clients' degree of attention varies with regard to their own grooming. Some are satisfied if their hair is just clean, while some others are very particular about the way it is washed and styled. While some clients are content to have their hands just cleaned, others may want their nails to be cleaned, manicured, and polished as well. With regard to body hair, shaving and beard grooming are important to many men, and many women would like to shave their legs and underarms. Most women who have facial hair would prefer to have this unwanted hair removed.

When you provide grooming care, keep in mind that it should be done in a considerate manner, which respects the client's dignity and right to privacy. Most workers understand that certain acts of grooming (such as shaving legs or underarms) in women need to be done in private but forget to provide the same privacy when shaving a man's face!

HAIR CARE

How the hair looks and feels can affect a person's emotional well-being. People generally feel better about themselves when they are well groomed. Unfortunately, illness and disability can interfere with hair care, especially when clients are too ill to care for their hair themselves. It is the support worker's responsibility to assist with hair care (or any grooming for that matter) whenever needed, as stated on the client's care plan.

The care plan should address the individual client's hair care needs. Culture, personal choice, skin and scalp condition, physical and mental health, and self-care abilities should always be taken into consideration for providing hair care, and this should be indicated on the client's care plan. Some common terms related to hair that may be used in care plans include:

- ***Alopecia*** (hair loss)—may be complete or partial. Male pattern baldness occurs due to aging or heredity. In women, hair thins with aging. Cancer treatments (radiation therapy to the head, and chemotherapy) often cause alopecia in both men and women. Other causes include skin disease, stress, poor nutrition, pregnancy, some medications, and hormone changes. In many cases (but not all), the hair grows back once these issues have been resolved.
- ***Hirsutism*** (from Latin *hirsutus* = shaggy, hairy)—excessive and increased hair growth in women in locations where the occurrence of visible, coarse hair is normally minimal or absent (such as on the face or neck). It refers to a male pattern of body hair and is therefore usually a cosmetic and psychological concern. However, hirsutism may be a sign of a more serious medical indication, especially if it develops well after puberty.
- ***Dandruff***—excessive amount of dry, white flakes on the scalp. It often causes itching of the scalp, sometimes involving the eyebrows and ear canals as well. Medicated shampoos usually can solve the problem.
- ***Pediculosis (lice)***—infestation with lice, which are small, insect-like parasites that live on the human body, most commonly on the skin, hair, and genital area. Lice (singular, louse) feed on human blood and lay their eggs on body hair and in clothing (Figure 30–1).

  Lice do not cause dangerous infections but may carry pathogens that cause more serious diseases, such as trench fever and typhus. Lice tend to be a problem primarily found in overcrowded areas or places that have inadequate bathing and laundry facilities, such as among the homeless or in military or refugee camps. All humans are equally at risk to infestation by lice, but elderly people are more prone to develop complications from it.

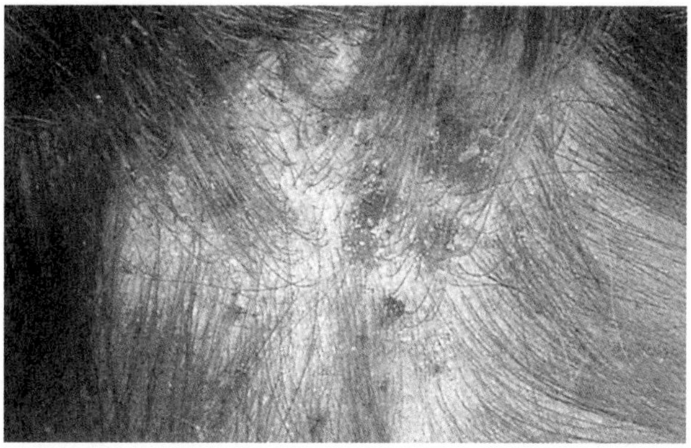

Figure 30–1 Pediculosis capitis. **Source:** Habif, T.P. (1996). *Clinical dermatology: A guide to diagnosis and therapy* (3rd ed.). St. Louis: Mosby.

Lice are **parasites**, and their bites cause severe itching in the affected body area. **Pediculosis capitis** is the infestation of the scalp (*capitis*) with lice, and **Pediculosis pubis** is the infestation of the pubic (*pubis*) hair with lice. Both head lice and pubic lice attach their eggs to hair shafts. **Pediculosis corporis** is the infestation of the body (*corporis*) surfaces with lice.

Lice eggs (nits) (Figure 30–2) attach to clothing and furniture and can easily spread to other people through clothing, furniture, bed linen, and physical contact, as well as by sharing of combs and brushes. They can be difficult to remove but all lice and their eggs must be destroyed with due diligence.

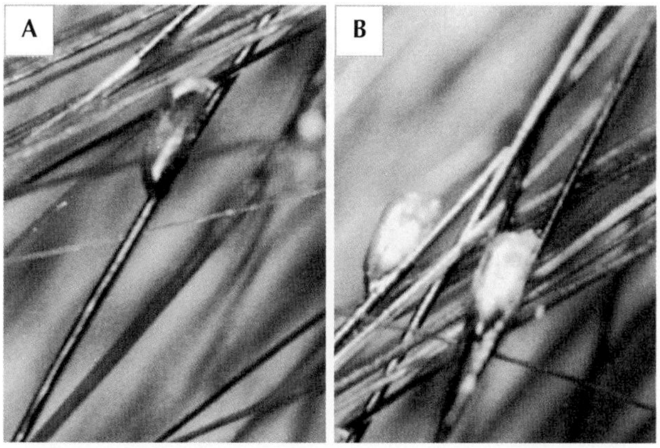

Figure 30–2 **A,** Empty nit case. **B,** Viable nits. **Source:** *The contemporary approach to the control of head lice in schools and communities.* (1991). Pittsburgh: SmithKline Beecham.

Lice can be eradicated by using medicated shampoos, lotions, and creams (following manufacturers' directions carefully). Several applications of these products as well as manual removal of the nits are usually necessary. In addition, clients (and anyone they have shared items with) will need a thorough tub bath and must have their clothing and linens washed in hot water. Items that cannot be washed should be thoroughly vacuumed and placed in a sealed, airtight bag and stored for several weeks till the lice are destroyed. Report any signs of lice to your supervisor immediately, and follow your agency's policies.

Brushing and Combing Hair

Brushing and combing hair are part of the client's daily routine, and usually the client's hair is groomed in the morning (after the bath or shower) and at bedtime. However, assist with brushing and combing, as needed, during the day—for example, some clients may want their hair styled before visitors arrive.

Encourage clients to do their own hair care, but you may assist, as needed. It is your responsibility to perform hair care for clients who cannot do it by themselves. Clients should be allowed to decide how to brush, comb, and style their hair (see *Focus on Children: Grooming Preferences* box).

You should never cut a client's hair; only a professional barber or hairstylist should cut hair. Some facilities have barber shops or beauty shops, where residents or patients can have their hair shampooed, cut, and styled. Some hairstylists make visits to homes or long-term care (complex care) facilities to provide their services.

focus on ›› CHILDREN

Grooming Preferences

Hairstyles are important to adolescents as well as other school-age children. Do not make judgements about any child's hairstyle. Style hair in a manner that pleases both the child and his or her parents. Take care not to impose your hairstyle preferences on your client.

Remember that people who have had chemical permanent treatments to their hair may have drier and more brittle hair that is more prone to tangling. Remember to brush hair that has been chemically treated gently, starting at the ends, and working up toward the roots. Chemically treated hair may get flattened during sleep, so it may need to be recombed or "fluffed up" after the client wakes up.

How to Brush or Comb Hair. Before giving hair care, you should place a towel over the client's shoulders to protect his or her garments. If the client is confined in bed, give hair care *before* changing the pillowcase. If it has to be done after a linen change, place a towel over the pillow to collect falling hair, as hair on the client's pillowcase is unsightly and, in some situations, poses the risk of being inhaled or swallowed.

When brushing/combing hair, start at the scalp, and brush/comb to the hair ends. Handle hair gently to avoid hurting the client or damaging the hair. Always brush slowly, never pulling or tugging at the client's hair. If you find the client has matted or tangled hair, discuss with your supervisor about what can be done. You may be directed to comb/brush through the matting and tangling. To do this, take a small section of hair near the ends, and gently comb/brush through to the ends. Work up to the scalp in small sections. and eventually you will be able to brush/comb from the scalp to the hair ends. ***Never cut hair to remove tangles.***

Cultural Differences With Respect to Hair. Hair of African-Canadian (also known as Black) people is extremely fragile, so you should be very gentle and careful in order to avoid unnecessary breakage and hair loss. Always use a wide-tooth comb/pick when combing the hair, and avoid fine-tooth combs because they tend to snag and pull out curly/kinky hair. If possible, use a good-quality, natural boar brush. Curly/kinky hair needs a lot of moisture, so you need to avoid drying products, such as hair spray, mousse, or holding gels.[1]

Black textured hair tends to produce less sebum (oily secretion created by the sebaceous gland) than does Caucasian hair. Black hair therefore requires more oil, so use products that contain moisturizers, leave-in conditioners, and styling lotions.[1] Remember that just because a product claims to be created for "curly hair" it does not guarantee that it will be suitable for Black curly hair as well.

Special measures are needed for curly, coarse, and dry hair. Using a wide-toothed comb, start at the neckline, comb the hair, and work upward, lifting and fluffing hair outward. Continue until you reach the forehead. Wetting the hair or applying a conditioner or petroleum jelly may make combing easier.[1]

The client may have certain practices or use special hair care products, and these should become part of the client's care plan. The client can guide you about these when giving hair care (see the *Respecting Diversity: Corn Braids* and *Respecting Diversity: Dreadlocks* boxes).

Cutting Hair. You should never cut a client's hair unless you have been specifically instructed to do so. In many long-term care facilities, the client (or his or her substitute decision maker) is required to sign a consent form giving permission for a hair cut. Some facilities provide the option of a salon where clients may pay to have their hair cut, washed, and groomed.

If you *must* cut a client's hair (for example, to remove a section of hair that is matted), ensure that proper consent has been obtained and details have been specified in the client's care plan.

These steps should then be followed:

- Cut the smallest amount of hair possible to help the client get rid of the matted hair.
- Make every attempt to ensure the client's hair appears attractive. For instance, the haircut should not be lopsided and uneven, drawing attention to the client's hair.
- Cut the hair using the correct type of hair shears (scissors). Never cut hair with scissors meant for other purposes, as they can tear the hair, causing discomfort to the client.

Observations to Make. Report and record the following if observed when brushing or combing:

- Scalp sores
- Flaking
- The presence of lice (check for tiny, white, oval-shaped specks in the hair; these are the nits, or egg cases)
- Patches of hair loss
- Very dry or very oily hair

RESPECTING DIVERSITY

Corn Braids

Styling hair in corn braids is a common practice in some cultural groups. The braids are left intact even while shampooing. Remember that you should never do or undo braids without the client's consent, and it may also be required by your supervisor. Some agencies have permission forms that the client has to sign, so know your agency's policy regarding this.

Caring for corn braids differs from caring for hair that is braided into a single large braid. If the client has a single braid, the braid should be undone each night, as the braid would cause discomfort if the client were to lie on it.

RESPECTING DIVERSITY

Dreadlocks

Dreadlocks are coils of hair that are twisted, rubbed or backcombed together in a specific way. They should not be combed out. Dreadlocks should be washed with a residue-free product, with the frequency depending on the client. If the client perspires considerably, frequent washing will reduce the salt build-up that sweat can produce on the client's scalp. For clients who do not perspire a lot, hair should be washed about once a week. The client's care plan will specify the specifics of his or her hair care.

Gently massaging the client's scalp for a few minutes each day will help to release natural oils from the client's scalp sebaceous glands. The client's care plan will specify the frequency and specific care that they require.

Source: *Dreadlock maintenance turns drab dreads into luscious locks in 5 easy steps.* (2007). Retrieved September 4, 2007, from http://www.mydreadlocks.com/dreadlock-maintenance.html

1 2 3 BRUSHING AND COMBING HAIR

Remember to promote:

• **D**ignity • **I**ndependence • **P**references • **P**rivacy • **S**afety

Pre-Procedure

1 Identify the client, according to employer policy.
2 Explain the procedure to the client. Ask the client how he or she would like you to style the hair.
3 Practise proper hand hygiene.
4 Collect the following:
- Comb and brush
- Bath towel
- Other grooming items, as requested by the client

5 Arrange items on a work area within easy reach.
6 Provide for privacy.

Procedure

7 Position the client:
  a If the client can get out of bed, provide a comfortable chair. Help the client to the chair (see *Transferring the Client to a Chair or Wheelchair*, page 416). The client should put on a robe and footwear when out of bed.
  b If the client remains in bed, raise the bed to a comfortable working height. Follow the care plan for bed rail use. Lower the bed rail near you, if it is up. Assist the client to semi-Fowler's position, if allowed by the care plan.

8 Place the towel over the client's shoulders or the pillow.
9 Ask the client to remove the eyeglasses and put them in their case. Place the case in a safe location.
10 Part the hair into two sections (Figure 30–3, *A*). Divide one side into two sections (Figure 30–3, *B*).
11 Brush the hair. Start at the scalp, and brush toward the hair ends (Figure 30–4).
12 Style the hair as the client prefers.
13 Remove the towel.
14 Help the client put on eyeglasses.

Post-Procedure

15 Provide for safety and comfort.
16 Place the call bell within reach.*
17 Return the bed to its lowest position. Follow the care plan for bed rail use.*
18 Remove privacy measures.
19 Clean and return equipment to its proper place.
20 Follow employer policy for dirty linen.
21 Practise proper hand hygiene.
22 Report and record your actions and observations, according to employer policy.

*Steps marked with an asterisk may not apply in community settings.

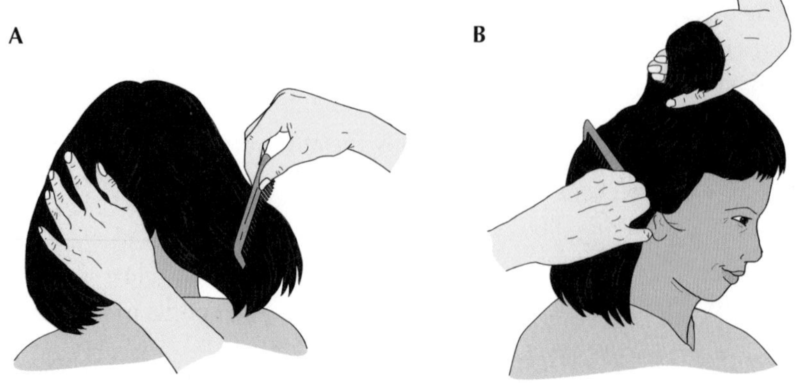

Figure 30–3 Parting hair. **A,** Part hair down the middle. Divide it into two sections. **B,** Then part each section into two smaller sections.

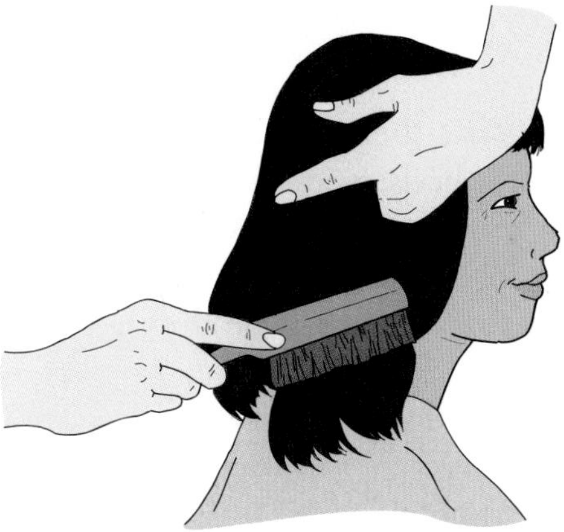

Figure 30–4 Brush hair by starting at the scalp. Then brush down to the hair ends.

Shampooing

The frequency of shampooing —once a week, two or three times a week, or every day—varies among clients based on such factors as the condition of the hair and scalp, hairstyle, and personal choice. Shampoo and hair conditioner products also involve personal choice (see the *Focus on Children: Shampooing* box.)

Many clients need help with shampooing, and if you are asked to assist a client, you should always keep in mind their personal preferences and need for privacy and safety. Whenever your client requests a shampoo, you should be sure to check your client's care plan for instructions regarding special care that is needed for each specific client's hair.

The shampooing method depends on the client's condition, safety factors, and personal choice (if permitted). Follow the care plan. Dry and style hair as quickly as possible after shampooing. If female clients want their hair curled or placed in hair rollers (rolling up) before it is dried, consult with your supervisor before doing it (see the *Focus on Long-Term Care: Shampooing* box.)

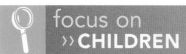

focus on »CHILDREN

Shampooing

Oil gland secretion increases during puberty, so adolescents tend to have oily hair. Frequent shampooing is therefore necessary for them.

focus on »LONG-TERM CARE

Shampooing

Shampooing is usually done once or twice weekly on a resident's bath/shower day. If a female client has had her hair done in the beauty shop, do not shampoo her hair. Protect her hair with a shower cap during the tub bath or shower.

Guidelines for shampooing are listed in Box 30–1. Report and record the following observations after shampooing:

- Scalp sores
- Hair falling out in clumps
- How the client tolerated the procedure
- The presence of lice

Box 30–1 Guidelines for Shampooing a Client's Hair

- Shampoo hair only if instructed to do so by your supervisor.
- Ask your supervisor and check the care plan about what method to use (shampooing during the shower or tub bath, at the sink, or in bed).
- Check if the client has position restrictions or limits.
- Return medicated shampoos to their proper storage place or give them to your supervisor. Do not leave them at the client's bedside, unless instructed to do so.
- Wear gloves, and follow Standard Practices if the client has scalp lesions or head lice or if you have to use certain medicated shampoos. The client's care plan will specify if gloves are required.
- Check what water temperature to use. Usually water temperature should be 40.5°C (105°F). Measure the water temperature, according to employer policy. ***Re-test the water temperature frequently as in some facilities it can cool down quickly.***
- Prevent shampoo getting into the client's eyes by having the client hold a face towel or wash cloth over the eyes.
- Cup your hand against the client's forehead when rinsing the hair, to keep soapy water from running down the client's forehead and into the eyes.

Shampooing During the Shower or Tub Bath. Clients who shower or bathe in a tub can usually be shampooed using a hand-held shower nozzle. The client should tip the head back to keep shampoo and water out of the eyes. Support the back of the client's head with one hand, and shampoo with your other hand. Those who are not be able to tip their head back should be assisted to lean forward and hold a folded wash cloth over the eyes. Support the forehead with one hand as you shampoo with the other. Be sure that the client can breathe easily.

Shampooing a Client's Hair at the Sink. Clients who can sit up may have their hair washed at a sink. However, they must be able to tilt their head forward or backward. Many older or disabled people have limited range of motion in their necks and upper backs, so they may not be able to use this method. It is your responsibility to follow the client's care plan.

For shampooing at a sink, the client can sit facing away from the sink or facing the sink. If the client uses a wheelchair, make sure the wheels are securely locked.

Facing the Sink. If the client chooses to sit facing the sink and the sink is low enough:

- Have the client lean forward over the sink.
- Place a towel over the shoulders.
- Give the client a folded wash cloth to hold over the eyes.
- Wet and rinse the hair using a water pitcher or hand-held nozzle.

Leaning Back. If the client prefers to lean back over the sink:

- Place the chair or wheelchair so it faces away from the sink.
- Place a folded towel over the sink edge to protect the neck.
- Help the client tilt the head back over the edge of the sink.
- Give the client a folded wash cloth to hold over the eyes.
- Wet and rinse the hair using a water pitcher or hand-held nozzle.

Lying Down. If the client has to lie on a stretcher while the hair is shampooed at the sink:

- Place the stretcher in front of the sink; lock the stretcher wheels; and apply the safety straps. Follow the care plan for side rail use.
- Place a folded towel over the edge of the sink.
- Help the client tilt the head over the edge of the sink.
- Place a folded wash cloth over the client's eyes.
- Wet and rinse the hair using a water pitcher or hand-held nozzle.

Assistive Devices. Assistive devices may make shampooing a client's hair easier. For example, you could use a plastic cape to drape over the client's shoulders and into the sink, or you may use a wheelchair shampoo rinse tray, which is made of plastic and clamps onto the back of the wheelchair, extending over the sink. The client's head rests directly on it. The water runs down the tray and into the sink (Figure 30–5), and its sides keep the water from spilling over the edges.

Shampooing in Bed. Clients who cannot tolerate sitting long enough to have their hair washed at the sink may have their hair shampooed while in bed. To begin, the client should be moved as close to the edge of the bed as possible. This will ensure that the client is in proper body alignment and will reduce the amount of stretching that you will have to do. A shampoo tray is placed under the client's head to protect the linens and mattress from

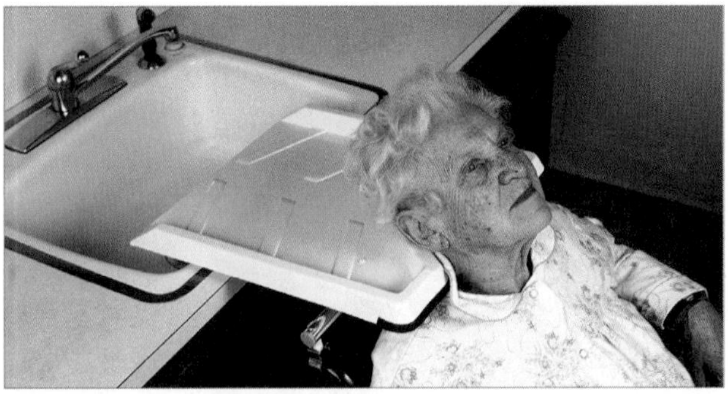

Figure 30–5 Shampooing at the sink. The wheelchair is in front of the sink, with its wheels locked in place. A wheelchair shampoo rinse tray may be useful. **Courtesy**: DeRoyal. http://www.deroyal.com/Catalog/Catalogs/CatalogMain.aspx?CatalogCode=COMPCAT&CatalogGroup=ADL49.

1 2 3 SHAMPOOING A CLIENT'S HAIR IN BED

Remember to promote:

• Dignity • Independence • Preferences • Privacy • Safety

Pre-Procedure

1 Identify the client, according to employer policy.
2 Explain the procedure to the client.
3 Practise proper hand hygiene.
4 Collect the following:
- Two bath towels
- Face towel or wash cloth
- Shampoo
- Hair conditioner (if requested by client)
- Bath thermometer
- Pitcher or nozzle (if needed)
- Shampoo tray (if needed)
- Basin or pail (if needed)
- Waterproof pad (if needed)
- Gloves (if needed)
- Comb and brush
- Hair dryer

5 Arrange the items close at hand.
6 Provide for privacy.

Procedure

7 Position the client as close to the edge of the bed as possible for the method you will use. Place the waterproof pad and shampoo tray under the head and shoulders, if needed.
8 Place a bath towel over the shoulders or over the pillow.
9 Brush and comb hair to remove snarls and tangles.
10 Raise the bed rail, if used.
11 Obtain water. Water temperature should be about 40.5°C (105°F). Test temperature using a bath thermometer, according to employer's policy. Allow the client to test the water temperature with his or her hand.
12 Lower the bed rail, if used.
13 Put on gloves, if needed.
14 Ask the client to hold a dampened face towel or wash cloth over the eyes, making sure that it does not cover nose or mouth. (A wet cloth will not slip off as easily as a dry cloth.)
15 Use the pitcher or nozzle to wet the hair.
16 Use a small amount of shampoo.
17 Work up a lather with both hands. Start at the hairline. Work toward the back of the head. If the client is leaning forward, start at the back of the head and work toward the hairline.
18 Massage the scalp with your fingertips. Take care not to scratch the scalp with your fingernails.
19 Rinse the hair.
20 Repeat steps 15 through 18.
21 Rinse the hair completely.
22 Apply conditioner following directions on the container.
23 Squeeze water from the client's hair.
24 Cover hair with a bath towel.
25 Dry the client's face with the towel.
26 Help the client raise the head, if appropriate.
27 Rub the hair and scalp with the towel. Use the second towel if the first becomes wet.
28 Comb hair to remove snarls and tangles.
29 Dry and style the hair as quickly as possible.
30 Remove gloves, if used. Practise proper hand hygiene.

Post-Procedure

31 Provide for safety and comfort.
32 Place the call bell within reach.*
33 Follow the care plan for bed rail use.*
34 Remove privacy measures.
35 Clean and return equipment to its proper place. Discard disposable items.
36 Follow employer policy for dirty linen.
37 Practise proper hand hygiene.
38 Report and record your actions and observations, according to employer policy.

*Steps marked with an asterisk may not apply in community settings.

getting wet. The tray also drains the water into a basin placed on a chair next to the bed (see Figure 30–6). Use a water pitcher to wet and rinse the hair (see the *Focus on Home Care: Shampoo Trays* box.)

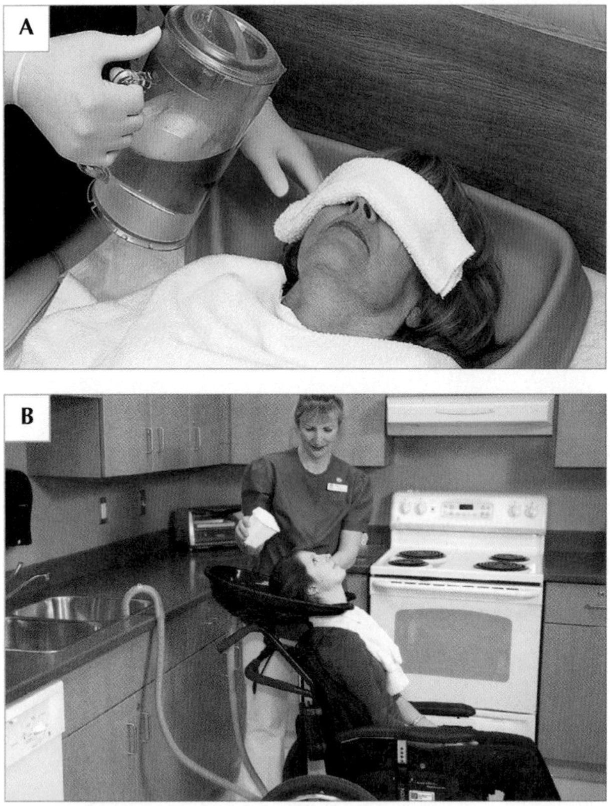

Figure 30–6 A, A shampooing tray is used when shampooing a client in bed. The tray is directed to the side of the bed so that water drains into a collecting basin. **B,** A wash basin for use in the home. Note the drain that is designed to empty rinse water into the sink or a bucket on the floor. **Courtesy (for B):** Brian Hillier.

focus on ››HOME CARE

Shampoo Trays

You can make a shampoo tray with a plastic shower curtain, a tablecloth, or even a plastic drop cloth used for painting. However, avoid using plastic garbage bags, as they slip and slide too easily and are not sturdy. To make a shampoo tray, first place the plastic under the client's head. To prevent water from spilling over the sides, make a raised edge by rolling up the plastic sheet round the edges. Place the ends of the plastic into the basin to direct the water into the basin. Check the care plan, and consult with your supervisor before starting the procedure.

SHAVING

Men shave for comfort and a sense of well-being. Younger women usually shave their legs and underarms, while some older women have coarse facial hair that they would like removed. You may be asked to remove unwanted hair in female clients by shaving, depilation, electrolysis, or waxing. You must be aware of what your client's care plan has specified, and consult with your supervisor if you have any questions about the technique you should use.

Depending on the their conditions, clients may prefer to shave themselves or may require your assistance. Shaving may be done at the sink, bedside, or in bed. You may need to use electric or manual shavers, depending on the client's condition, preference, and what is specified in the care plan. Shaving guidelines and precautions are listed in Box 30–2.

Electric Shaver Maintenance

Simple cleaning routines performed on a regular basis help prolong the life of the electric shaver and can reduce skin irritation or injury in the client.[2]

- Many problems with electric shavers can be avoided very easily by simply removing the cutting head and tapping the hair particles into a tissue after each use. Discard the tissue into the garbage.
- Most electric shavers come with a cleaning brush, which also should be used after each shave to remove hair particles that cannot be removed by blowing on them.
- Some manufacturers advise spraying the shaver every week or so with a special lubricating spray to both lubricate and de-grease the cutting blades.
- In addition, aging cutters and the foil surface should be replaced periodically (according to the manufacturer's directions).

Caring for Mustaches and Beards

Beards and mustaches need daily care to prevent food as well as mouth and nose drainage from collecting in the hair. Daily washing and combing usually are enough to keep beards and moustaches clean. Ask the client how he would like his beard or mustache groomed. ***Never trim or shave a beard or mustache without the client's consent.***

Shaving Legs and Underarms for Female Clients

Many women shave their legs and underarms, although this practice varies among cultures. Some women shave only the lower legs, while others shave to mid-thigh or even shave the entire leg.

Female clients' legs and underarms should be shaved after the bath when the skin is soft. Collect the client's shaving items along with the bath items to save time. When shaving, use soap and water or a shaving cream to work up a lather. Rinse the razor in a kidney basin and not in the bathwater. The guidelines in Box 30–2 (see page 559) also apply when shaving the underarms and legs.

Box 30–2 Guidelines for Shaving Clients

- While shaving a client, always follow Standard Practices, such as practising proper hand hygiene and wearing gloves.
- Because of the risk of transmitting pathogens (see Chapter 20) from one client to another, the same razors or shavers should not be used between clients. Each client should have his or her own.
- Follow the care plan for the type of shaver used for each client.
- Protect bed linens by placing a towel under the part that is being shaved. If you are shaving the client's face, you might want to place a towel over the client's shoulders to protect the clothing.
- Soften the client's facial hair before shaving by applying a warm, moist cloth onto the skin. If using a manual razor, use shaving cream (after applying the warm, moist cloth) to soften the skin and hair, making it easier to shave.
- Encourage the client to do as much as is safely possible.
- Stretch the skin taut, as needed.
- Shave in the direction of hair growth when shaving the face and underarms.
- When shaving the leg, shave up from the ankles, against the direction of hair growth.
- Rinse the shaved area completely.
- Shaving can potentially cut, nick, or irritate the skin. Ensure that you shave carefully and only after properly preparing the client's skin and hair.
- Razor blades can cause nicks or cuts. Follow Standard Practices to prevent contact with blood. Handle razor blades and disposable shavers extremely carefully to protect yourself from cuts; discard them in the sharps container (see Chapter 19).
- Apply direct pressure to nicks or cuts on the client (wear gloves).
- Report nicks, cuts, or skin irritation to your supervisor at once.
- Discard disposable razors and blades in the sharps container. Handle them carefully.
- Follow employer policy for disposing of sharps.
- If using an electric razor, make sure the shaver is in good working order before each use. Follow the safety rules for electrical equipment (see Chapter 19).

You may be given the following shaving instructions for certain clients:

- ***Manual shavers with open blades should never be used on clients receiving medications that slow down blood clotting (anticoagulants). In these clients, a nick or cut could cause serious bleeding problems. Electric shavers are preferable for clients taking these types of medications.***
- ***Electric shavers are not used on clients receiving oxygen.*** A spark from the electric shaver could cause a fire.
- ***Manual shavers are also not used on clients with dementia.*** Clients with dementia may not understand what you are doing so they may resist care and make sudden movements. As this increases the risk for serious nicks and cuts, only electric shavers should be used for these clients.
- ***If an electric razor scratches the client's face, have the shaver repaired at once.*** Report and record the scratches; most agencies require that an incident report be completed.
- ***Never rinse out an electric razor under a running tap***, unless the manufacturer specifies that this is allowed. ***Electric razors should also never be immersed in water.***

1 2 3 SHAVING A CLIENT

Remember to promote:

• Dignity • Independence • Preferences • Privacy • Safety

Pre-Procedure

1 Identify the client, according to employer policy.
2 Explain the procedure to the client.
3 Practise proper hand hygiene.
4 Collect the following:
- Wash basin
- Bath towel
- Face towel
- Wash cloth
- Blade razor or electric shaver, according to the client's care plan
- Mirror
- Shaving cream, soap, or lotion
- Shaving brush (optional)
- Aftershave lotion (men only)
- Tissues
- Paper towels
- Gloves

5 Arrange paper towels and supplies on the overbed table (in facilities) or on a work area within easy reach.
6 Provide for privacy.
7 Raise the bed to a comfortable working height. Follow the care plan for bed rail use.*

Procedure

8 Fill the basin with warm water.
9 Place the basin on the overbed table or work area.
10 Lower the bed rail near you, if it is up.
11 Assist the client to semi-Fowler's position, if allowed. If this is impossible, assist the client to the supine position.
12 Adjust lighting to see the client's face clearly.
13 Place the bath towel over the chest. Allow the client to use a mirror, if he or she would like to.
14 Adjust the overbed table for easy reach.*
15 If using a manual shaver:
- **a** Fix the razor blade to the shaver tightly.
- **b** Wash the client's face. Do not dry.
- **c** Wet a wash cloth or face towel. Wring it out.
- **d** Apply the wash cloth or towel to the client's face for a few minutes.
- **e** Put on gloves.
- **f** Apply shaving cream with your hands or using a shaving brush.
- **g** Hold the client's skin taut with one hand.
- **h** Shave in the direction of hair growth. Use shorter strokes around the chin and lips (Figure 30–7).
- **i** Rinse the razor frequently. Shake off excess water and lather.
- **j** Apply direct pressure to any bleeding area.
- **k** Wash off remaining shaving cream or soap from the client's face. Dry with a towel.

16 If using an electric shaver:
- **a** Put on gloves.
- **b** Make sure the client's face is dry. Do not apply shaving cream or a warm cloth to the face.
- **c** Hold skin taut with one hand.
- **d** Turn the razor on.
- **e** Place the razor over the hair growth. Move the razor back and forth or in a circular pattern.
- **f** Apply direct pressure to any bleeding area.

17 Apply aftershave lotion, if requested by client.
18 Remove the towel and gloves. Practise proper hand hygiene.
19 Move the overbed table to the side of the bed.*

Post-Procedure

20 Provide for safety and comfort.
21 Place the call bell within reach.*
22 Return the bed to its lowest position. Follow the care plan for bed rail use.*
23 Clean and return equipment and supplies to their proper place. Discard disposable items. Wear gloves for this step.
24 Wipe off the overbed table or work area with paper towels. Discard paper towels.
25 Remove privacy measures.
26 Follow employer policy for dirty linen.
27 Practise proper hand hygiene.
28 Report nicks or bleeding to your supervisor.

*Steps marked with an asterisk may not apply in community settings.

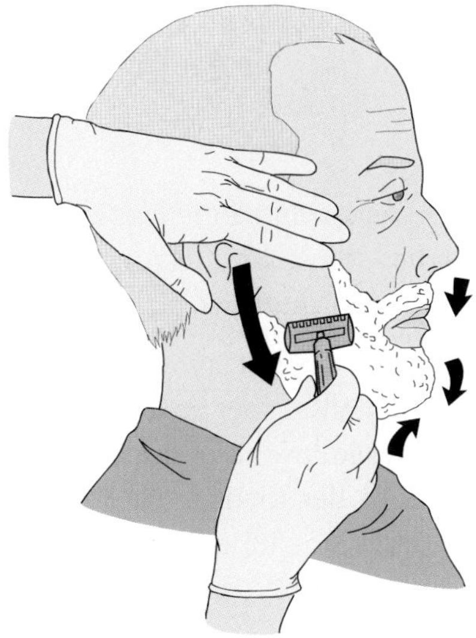

Figure 30–7 Shave in the direction of hair growth. Use longer strokes on the larger areas of the face. Use short strokes around the chin and lips.

Pubic Hair

Pubic hair is found in the frontal genital area, in the crotch, and the top inside of the legs. In most cases, pubic hair begins to appear within 3 years following puberty. As a person ages, he or she will have less body hair, and the body hair may grey or turn white, much like the hair on the head. Many consider the care of pubic hair to be an important part of grooming, so they may chose to remove it. Some cultures, such as the Islamic cultures, have rules that insist on women trimming or removing their pubic hair.

Hair removal of any kind, including that of pubic hair, can result in **ingrown hairs** (also known as **razor bumps**), which may be painful and red. An ingrown hair (Figure 30–8) does not grow straight out of the follicle opening. Instead, it curls into the side wall of the hair follicle or into the skin surface causing the skin to become inflamed. This inflammation can result in the development of a pimple (such as a papule or a pustule) or a cyst (nodule), both of which are usually tender. The hair tip may continue to grow into the adjacent skin outside the follicle and may produce a larger and more inflamed area, which can produce permanent scarring or changes in the colour of the skin. If you observe any ingrown hairs, you should report and record them, according to your agency's policies.

As a support worker, you would rarely be asked to remove pubic hair. The pubic area is a very delicate one and can easily be nicked by razors or cut by sharp scissors. However, if you are required to, you should do it in a tactful, professional manner, ensuring that the client's rights to privacy and dignity are preserved at all times. The client's care plan would specify the steps involved in removing or trimming pubic hair.

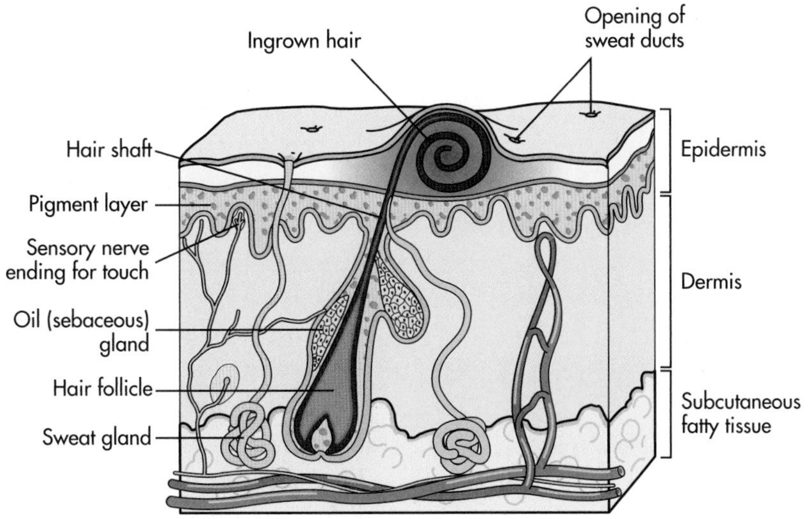

Figure 30–8 Ingrown hair.

CARE OF NAILS AND FEET

Foot and nail care is a very important part of daily personal care to prevent infection, injury, and odours. Long or broken nails can scratch skin or snag clothing. Hangnails, **ingrown nails** (nails that grow in at the side), and nails torn away from the skin cause skin breaks, which can easily provide portals of entry for microbes and pathogens.

Feet are easily infected and injured. Dirty or moist feet, socks, and stockings harbour microbes and cause odours, and shoes and socks provide a warm, moist environment for the growth of microbes. Injuries occur from stubbing of toes, stepping on sharp objects, or being stepped on. Shoes that fit poorly can cause bunions, calluses, corns, blisters, or ingrown nails, all of which can be considerably painful!

Infections or foot injuries are particularly serious in older adults and people with circulatory disorders. Poor circulation in the feet prolongs healing because it prevents white blood cells (WBCs) and oxygenated blood entering that area. WBCs engulf and eat infected material, and oxygen provides the necessary energy for cells to function well. Diabetes and vascular disease are common causes of poor circulation, and gangrene and amputations are serious complications (see Chapter 18).

Important Things to Watch for. It is your responsibility to check the client's feet every day. This is especially important if the client has a circulatory disorder or diabetes, or takes medications that affect blood clotting. Notify your supervisor if you observe any of the following:

- Very dry skin
- Foot odours
- Cracks or breaks in the skin, especially between the toes
- Ingrown nails
- Loose nails
- Reddened, irritated, or calloused areas on the feet, heels, or ankles
- Drainage or bleeding
- Change in colour or texture of nails, especially black, thick, or brittle nails
- Corns, bunions, or blisters

When Not to Trim Toenails. Trimming and clipping toenails can easily cause injuries, and if the client has a disease or illness that makes them more likely to develop an infection, you should be aware of this. Support workers do not cut or trim toenails if the client:

- Has diabetes
- Has poor circulation to the legs and feet
- Takes medications that affect blood clotting
- Has very thick or ingrown nails

Some employers do not allow support workers to cut or trim toenails under any circumstances, so you should always follow your employer policy. If a client needs his or her toenails trimmed, tell your supervisor, and never assume that you can go ahead and trim them yourself. Also, support workers do not treat corns, bunions, or blisters, as these are foot problems that may require a podiatrist. A **podiatrist** is a physician who specializes in the evaluation and treatment of diseases of the foot.

Soak the Nails First. Fingernail and foot soaks may be part of the client's care plan, and you may be responsible for providing them. Generally, nails are easier to trim and clean when they have been softened, ***but you should not cut a client's toenails immediately after soaking, as the tissue around the nail will be puffy from water absorption and more prone to nicks and cuts.*** Follow your agency's policies and the client's care plan about the right method to soften the client's nails. Some agencies advise the use of specific lotions for this purpose.

Tub baths are a good time for soaking feet and fingernails. If soaking is done at other times, the client can sit on the side of the tub and soak the feet. Make sure the client can step into and out of the tub. Otherwise, soak the feet in a basin. If the client is comfortable doing it, he or she can soak the fingers in the sink or in a small basin or bowl. Usually fingernail or foot soaks should last 15 to 20 minutes. Feet are easily burned, so you should check with your supervisor about the correct water temperature for foot soaks. ***You must be very careful when preparing soaks for people with decreased sensation or circulatory problems. They may not feel hot temperatures and are at risk for scalding or burning of their feet.***

Nail clippers should be used to cut fingernails. ***Never use scissors.*** Use extreme caution to prevent damage to nearby tissue. Cut fingernails only if instructed to do so by your supervisor and the care plan.

1 2 3 PROVIDING NAIL AND FOOT CARE

Remember to promote:

• Dignity • Independence • Preferences • Privacy • Safety

Pre-Procedure

1 Identify the client, according to employer policy.
2 Explain the procedure to the client.
3 Practise proper hand hygiene.
4 Collect the following:
- Wash basin
- Soap
- Bath thermometer
- Bath towel
- Face towel
- Wash cloth
- Kidney basin
- Nail clippers
- Orange stick
- Emery board or nail file
- Lotion or petroleum jelly
- Paper towels
- Disposable bath mat
- Gloves

5 Arrange paper towels and other items on the overbed table (in facilities) or on a work area within easy reach.
6 Provide for privacy.
7 Help the client to a bedside chair. Place the call bell (in facilities) within reach.

Procedure

8 Place the bath mat under the client's feet.
9 Fill the wash basin. The care plan tells you what temperature to use. Measure the water temperature, according to employer policy.
10 Place the basin on the bath mat.
11 Help the client remove his or her shoes and socks.
12 Help the client put his or her feet into the basin (Figure 30–9).
13 Adjust the overbed table or work area in front of the client. It should be low and close to the client.
14 Fill the kidney basin. Measure the water temperature, according to employer policy.
15 Place the kidney basin on the overbed table or work area.
16 Put the client's fingers into the basin. Position the arms for comfort.
17 Allow the feet and fingernails to soak for 15 to 20 minutes. Warm the water again, as needed.
18 Remove the kidney basin. Thoroughly dry the client's hands, especially between the fingers.
19 Put on your gloves.
20 Clean under fingernails with the orange stick. Use a towel to wipe the orange stick after each nail.
21 Clip fingernails straight across with nail clippers (Figure 30–10).
22 Shape nails with an emery board or nail file.
23 Push the cuticles back with a wash cloth or orange stick (Figure 30–11).
24 Move the overbed table to the side.*
25 Wash the client's feet with soap and a wash cloth. Wash between the toes.
26 Rinse the feet and between the toes.
27 Remove the feet from the basin. Dry thoroughly, especially between the toes.
28 Clean under the toenails with an orange stick.
29 Apply lotion or petroleum jelly to the tops and soles of the feet, but not between the toes. Warm the lotion before applying it by pouring a small amount into your hand and rubbing your palms together.
30 Remove your gloves. Practise proper hand hygiene.
31 Help the client put socks and shoes on.

Post-Procedure

32 Provide for safety and comfort.
33 Place the call bell within reach.*
34 Follow the care plan for bed rail use.*
35 Clean and return equipment and supplies to their proper places. Discard disposable items. Wear gloves for this step.
36 Remove privacy measures.
37 Follow employer policy for soiled linen.
38 Practise proper hand hygiene.
39 Report and record your actions and observations, according to employer policy.

*Steps marked with an asterisk may not apply in community settings.

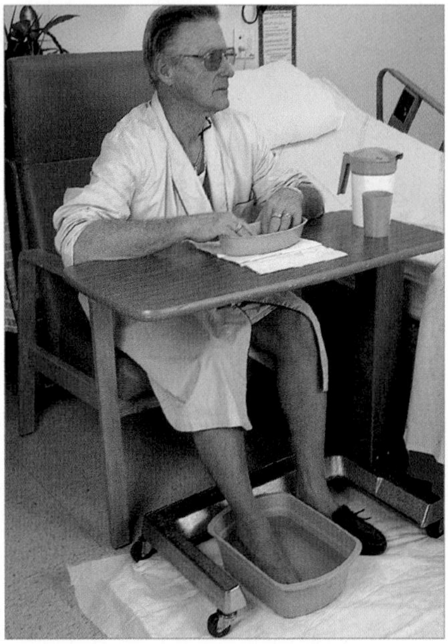

Figure 30–9 Nail and foot care. The feet soak in a foot basin, and the fingers soak in a kidney basin.

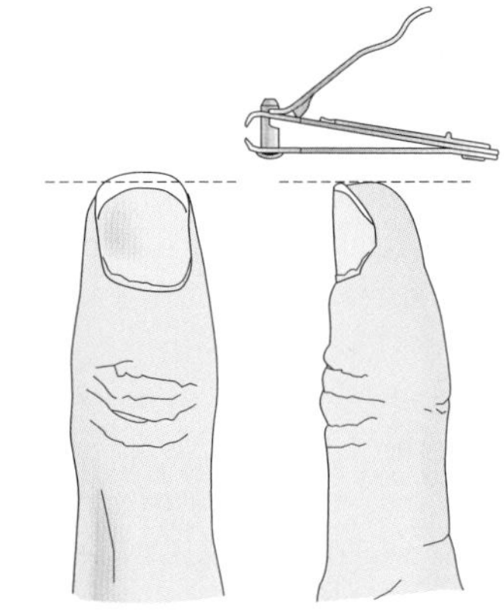

Figure 30–10 Clip fingernails straight across. Use a nail clipper.

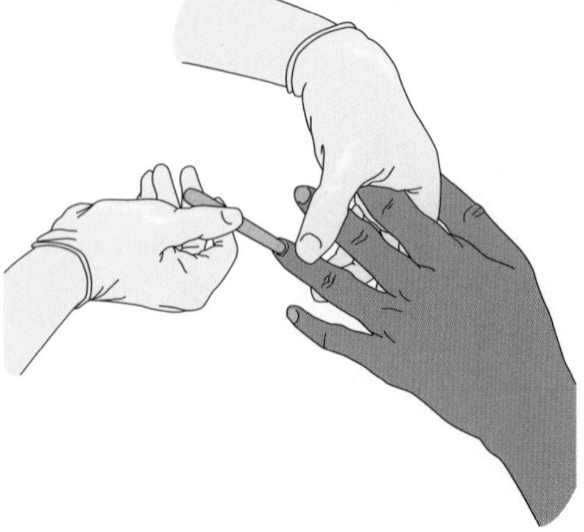

Figure 30–11 Push the cuticle back with an orange stick.

CHANGING CLOTHING AND HOSPITAL GOWNS

Like everyone else, clients who live in the community or in long-term care (complex care) facilities also dress and undress at least once a day. They usually wear more formal clothes during the day and change to sleepwear at bedtime. Incontinent clients may require more frequent changes of clothing. Some clients who are ill or confined to bed choose to wear sleepwear and robes through the day. Clients who are hospitalized wear hospital gowns, especially if they are receiving IV therapy. Hospital gowns are put on and removed in a certain way when the client is receiving IV therapy (see page 570).

Among clients who need help dressing and undressing, changing is easier when they can move their arms and legs. In clients with arm or leg injuries or paralysis, special techniques are required to dress and undress them safely, comfortably, and quickly. Follow the guidelines in Box 30–3 when dressing and undressing clients.

Pay particular attention to the client's comfort when you are dressing them. Moving the joints can sometimes be very uncomfortable for the client, so you should always be organized, efficient, and as quick as possible. Never jerk or pull the client, which can be very uncomfortable and distressing.

Box 30–3 Guidelines for Changing Clients' Clothing or Hospital Gowns

- Provide for privacy. Do not expose the client.
- Encourage the client to do as much as possible.
- Allow the client to choose what to wear. Make sure the right undergarments are chosen.
- Support the arm or leg when removing or putting on a garment.
- Put clothing on the *affected side* (the weak side affected by disease or disability) first. Never call the affected side the "bad" side. When dressing a client, remember the acronym **DAF**—**D**ress **A**ffected side **F**irst.
- Remove clothing from the *unaffected side* (the strong side not affected by disease or disability) first. When undressing a client, remember the acronym **RUF**—**R**emove from **U**naffected side **F**irst.

When assisting a client with putting socks and pants on, put the client's socks on first before putting their pants on. By dressing the client in this order, loose threads or the hem of the pants will not catch on the client's toes. Ensure that the client's socks go on smoothly and are not binding or bunched at the top.

Report and record the following observations after helping a client dress or undress:

- How much help was given
- How the client tolerated the procedure
- Any complaints from the client

1 2 3 UNDRESSING A CLIENT

Remember to promote:

• Dignity • Independence • Preferences • Privacy • Safety

Pre-Procedure

1 Identify the client, according to employer policy.
2 Explain the procedure to the client.
3 Practise proper hand hygiene.
4 Collect a bath blanket.
5 Provide for privacy.
6 Raise the bed to a comfortable working height. Follow the care plan for bed rail use.*
7 Lower the bed rail (if it is up) on the client's affected side.
8 Place the client in the supine position.
9 Cover the client with the bath blanket. Fanfold linens to the foot of the bed. Do not expose the client during the procedure.

Procedure

10 Paying particular attention to the client's comfort, remove the back-opening garments:
- **a** Raise the client's head and shoulders (see *Raising the Client's Head and Shoulders,* page XXX), or turn him or her onto the side away from you.
- **b** Undo buttons, zippers, ties, or snaps.
- **c** Bring the sides of the garment to the client's sides (Figure 30–12). If he or she is in the side-lying position, tuck the far side under the client. Fold the near side onto the chest (Figure 30–13).
- **d** Place the client in the supine position.
- **e** Slide the garment off the shoulder on the unaffected side. Remove the garment from the arm (Figure 30–14).
- **f** Repeat the above step for the affected side also.

11 Paying particular attention to the client's comfort, remove front-opening garments.
- **a** Undo buttons, zippers, snaps, or ties.
- **b** Slide the garment off the shoulder and arm on the unaffected side.
- **c** Raise the client's head and shoulders. Bring the garment over to the affected side (Figure 30–15). Lower the client's head and shoulders.
- **d** Remove the garment from the affected side.
- **e** If you cannot raise the client's head and shoulders:
  - i. Turn the client toward you. Tuck the removed part of the garment under the client.
  - ii. Turn him or her onto the side away from you.
  - iii. Pull the side of the garment out from under the client. Make sure he or she will not lie on it when supine.
  - iv. Return the client to the supine position.
  - v. Remove the garment from the affected side.

12 Paying particular attention to the client's comfort, remove pullover garments.
- **a** Undo any buttons, zippers, ties, or snaps.
- **b** Remove the garment from the client's unaffected side.
- **c** Raise the client's head and shoulders, or turn him or her onto the side away from you. Bring the garment up to the client's neck (Figure 30–16).
- **d** Remove the garment from the affected side.
- **e** Bring the garment over the client's head.
- **f** Place the client in the supine position.

(continued on page 566)

1 2 3 UNDRESSING A CLIENT

Procedure (cont'd)

13 Paying particular attention to the client's comfort, remove pants or slacks.
- **a** Remove footwear.
- **b** Place the client in the supine position.
- **c** Undo buttons, zippers, ties, snaps, or buckles.
- **d** Remove the belt, if one is worn.
- **e** Ask the client to lift the buttocks off the bed. Slide the pants down over the hips and buttocks (Figure 30–17). Have the client lower the hips and buttocks.
- **f** If the client cannot lift his or her hips off the bed:
  - i. Turn the client toward you.
  - ii. Slide the pants off the hip and buttock on the unaffected side (Figure 30–18).
  - iii. Turn the client away from you.
  - iv. Slide the pants off the hip and buttock on the affected side (Figure 30–19).
- **g** Slide the pants down the legs and over the feet.

14 Paying particular attention to the client's comfort, dress the client (see *Dressing a Client*, page 568).

15 Help the client get out of bed if he or she has to be up. If the client will stay in bed:
- **a** Cover the client and remove the bath blanket.
- **b** Provide for safety and comfort.
- **c** Return the bed to its lowest position. Follow the care plan for bed rail use.*

Post-Procedure

16 Place the call bell within reach.*

17 Remove privacy measures.

18 Follow employer policy for dirty linen.

19 Practise proper hand hygiene.

20 Report and record your actions and observations, according to employer policy.

*Steps marked with an asterisk may not apply in community settings.

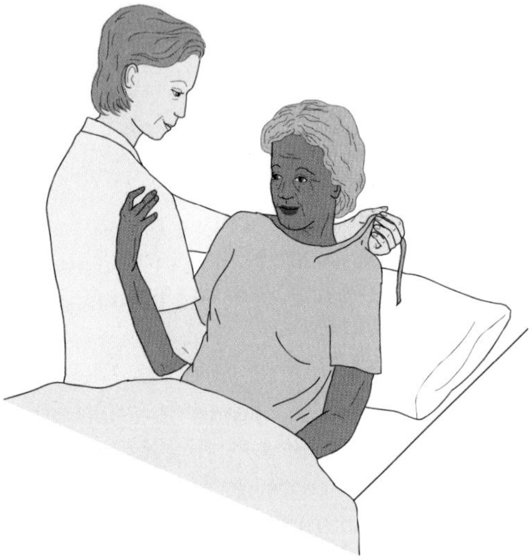

Figure 30–12 Bring the sides of the garment from the back to the sides of the client.

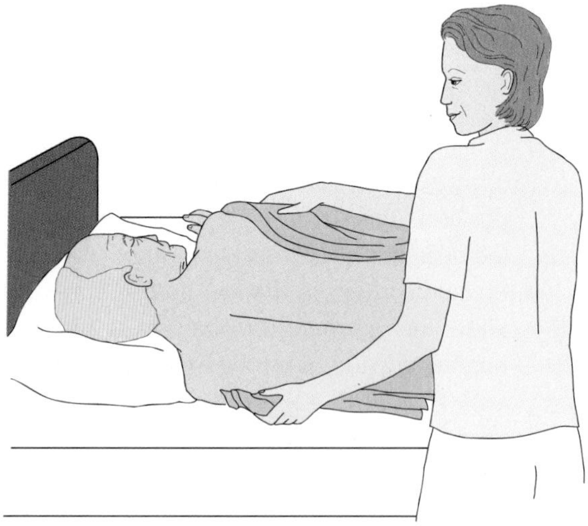

Figure 30–13 Assist the client to the side-lying position to remove a back-opening garment. Tuck the far side of the garment under the client. Fold the near side onto the client's chest.

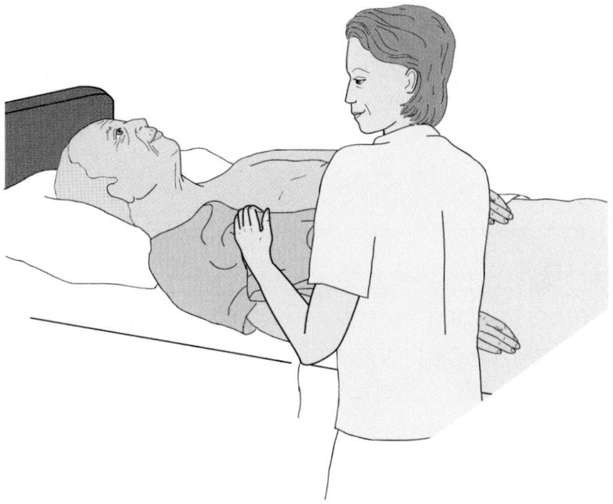

Figure 30–14 Remove the garment from the unaffected side first.

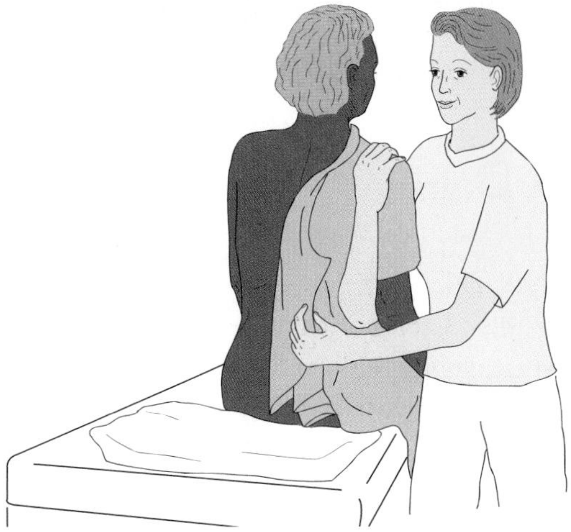

Figure 30–15 Raise the client's head and shoulders to remove the front-opening garment. Remove the garment from the unaffected side first. Then bring it around the back to the affected side.

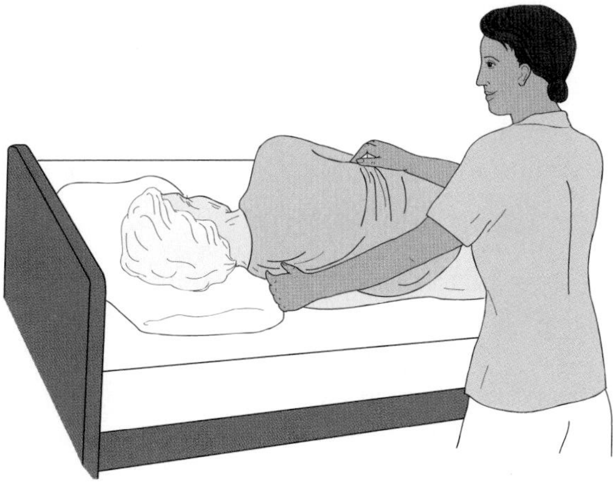

Figure 30–16 Remove a pullover garment from the unaffected side first. Then bring the garment up the client's neck to remove it from the affected side.

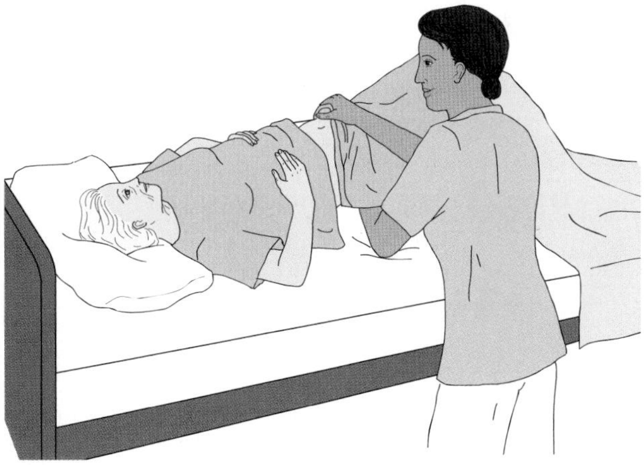

Figure 30–17 The client lifts the hips and buttocks for removing the pants. Slide the pants down over the hips and buttocks.

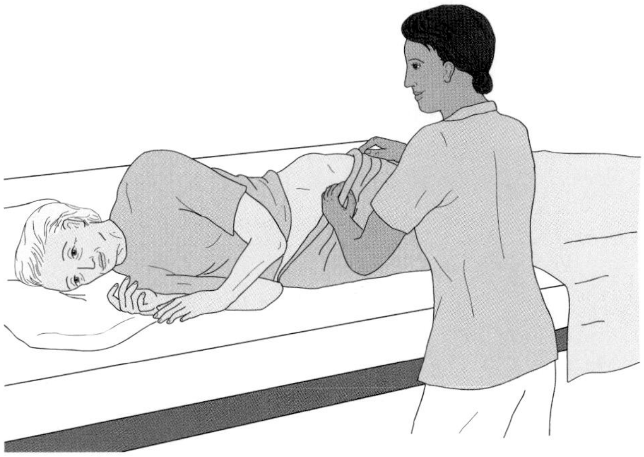

Figure 30–18 Pants are removed with the client in the side-lying position. Remove them from the unaffected side first. Slide them over the hips and buttocks.

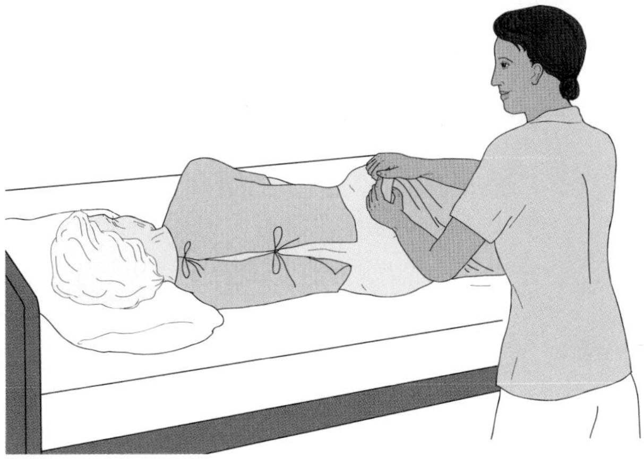

Figure 30–19 Turn the client onto the other side. Remove the pants from the affected side.

1 2 3 DRESSING A CLIENT

Remember to promote:

• Dignity • Independence • Preferences • Privacy • Safety

Pre-Procedure

1 Identify the client, according to employer policy.
2 Explain the procedure to the client.
3 Practise proper hand hygiene.
4 Collect a bath blanket and clothing requested by the client.
5 Provide for privacy.
6 Raise the bed to a comfortable working height. Follow the care plan for bed rail use.*
7 Undress the client (see *Undressing a Client,* page 565).
8 Lower the bed rail (if it is up) on the client's unaffected side.
9 Place the client in the supine position.

Procedure

10 Cover the client with the bath blanket. Fanfold linens to the foot of the bed. Do not expose the client during the procedure.
11 Paying particular attention to the client's comfort, put on back-opening garments:
- **a** Slide the garment onto the arm and shoulder of the affected side.
- **b** Slide the garment onto the arm and shoulder of the unaffected side.
- **c** Raise the client's head and shoulders.
- **d** Bring the sides of the garment to the back.
- **e** If the client is in the side-lying position:
  - i. Turn the client toward you.
  - ii. Bring one side of the garment to the client's back (Figure 30–20, *A*).
  - iii. Turn the client away from you.
  - iv. Bring the other side of the garment to the client's back (Figure 30–20, *B*).
- **f** Fasten buttons, snaps, ties, or zippers.
- **g** Place the client in the supine position.

12 Put on the front-opening garments:
- **a** Slide the garment onto the arm and shoulder on the affected side.
- **b** Raise the client's head and shoulders. Bring the side of the garment around to the back. Help the client lie down. Slide the garment onto the arm and shoulder of the unaffected arm.
- **c** If the client is not able to raise the head and shoulders:
  - i. Turn the client toward you.
  - ii. Tuck the garment under the client.
  - iii. Turn the client away from you.
  - iv. Pull the garment out from under the client.
  - v. Turn the client back to the supine position.
  - vi. Slide the garment over the arm and shoulder of the unaffected side.
- **d** Fasten buttons, snaps, ties, or zippers.

13 Paying particular attention to the client's comfort, put on pullover garments:
- **a** Place the client in the supine position.
- **b** Bring the neck of the garment over the head.
- **c** Slide the arm and shoulder of the garment onto the client's affected side.
- **d** Raise the client's head and shoulders.
- **e** Bring the garment down.
- **f** Slide the arm and shoulder of the garment onto the unaffected side.
- **g** If the client is not able to assume the semi-sitting position:
  - i. Turn the client toward you.
  - ii. Tuck the garment under the client.
  - iii. Turn the client away from you.
  - iv. Pull the garment out from under the client.
  - v. Place the client in the supine position.
  - vi. Slide the arm and shoulder of the garment onto the unaffected side.
- **h** Fasten buttons, snaps, ties, or zippers.

(continued on page 569)

1 2 3 DRESSING A CLIENT

Procedure (cont'd)

14 Paying particular attention to the client's comfort, put socks and footwear on the client.

15 Paying particular attention to the client's comfort, put pants or slacks on the client:

- **a** Slide the pants over the feet and up the legs.
- **b** Ask the client to raise the hips and buttocks off the bed.
- **c** Bring the pants up over the buttocks and hips.
- **d** Ask the client to lower the hips and buttocks.
- **e** If the client is not able to raise the hips and buttocks:
  - i. Turn the client onto the unaffected side.
  - ii. Pull the pants over the buttock and hip on the affected side.
  - iii. Turn the client onto the affected side.
  - iv. Pull the pants over the buttock and hip on the unaffected side.
  - v. Place the client in the supine position.
- **f** Fasten buttons, ties, snaps, zipper, and belt buckle.

16 Help the client get out of bed. If the client will stay in bed:

- **a** Cover the client. Remove the bath blanket.
- **b** Provide for safety and comfort.
- **c** Return the bed to its lowest position. Follow the care plan for bed rail use.*

Post-Procedure

17 Place the call bell within reach.*

18 Remove privacy measures.

19 Follow employer policy for dirty linen.

20 Practise proper hand hygiene.

21 Report and record your actions and observations, according to employer policy.

*Steps marked with an asterisk may not apply in community settings.

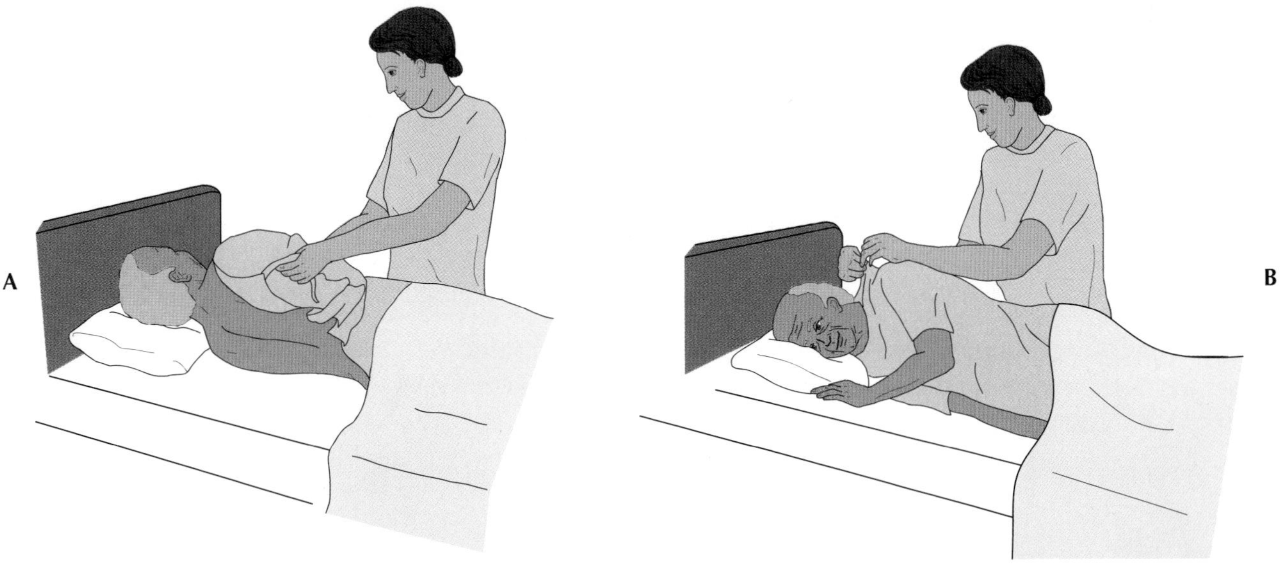

Figure 30–20 Putting on back-opening garments. **A,** The side-lying position can be used to put on back-opening garments. Turn the client toward you after the garment is put on the arms. Bring the side of the garment to the client's back. **B,** Then turn the client away from you. Bring the other side of the garment to the back. Fasten the garment.

1 2 3 CHANGING THE GOWN OF A CLIENT WITH AN IV

Remember to promote:

• Dignity • Independence • Preferences • Privacy • Safety

Pre-Procedure

1 Identify the client, according to employer policy.
2 Explain the procedure to the client.
3 Practise proper hand hygiene.
4 Collect a clean gown and a bath blanket.
5 Provide for privacy.
6 Raise the bed to a comfortable working height. Follow the care plan for bed rail use.*

Procedure

7 Lower the bed rail near you, if it is up.
8 Cover the client with a bath blanket. Fanfold linens to the foot of the bed.
9 Untie the gown. Free the parts that the client is lying on.
10 Remove the gown from the arm with no IV.
11 Gather up the sleeve of the arm with the IV. Slide it over the IV site and tubing. Remove the arm and hand from the sleeve (Figure 30–21, *A*).
12 Keep the sleeve gathered. Slide your arm along the tubing to the bag (Figure 30–21, *B*).
13 Remove the IV bag from the pole. Slide the bag and tubing through the sleeve (Figure 30–21, *C*). Do not pull on the tubing. Keep the bag above the client.
14 Hang the IV bag on the pole.
15 Gather the sleeve of the clean gown that will go on the arm with the IV infusion.
16 Remove the bag from the pole. Slip the sleeve over the bag at the shoulder part of the gown (Figure 30–21, *D*). Hang the bag.
17 Slide the gathered sleeve over the tubing, hand, arm, and IV site. Then slide it onto the shoulder.
18 Put the other side of the gown on. Fasten the back.
19 Cover the client. Remove the bath blanket.

Post-Procedure

20 Provide for safety and comfort.
21 Place the call bell within reach.*
22 Return the bed to its lowest position. Follow the care plan for bed rail use.*
23 Remove privacy measures.
24 Follow employer policy for dirty linen.
25 Practise proper hand hygiene.
26 Report and record your actions and observations according to employer policy. (In facilities, ask your supervisor to check the flow rate.)

*Steps marked with an asterisk may not apply in community settings.

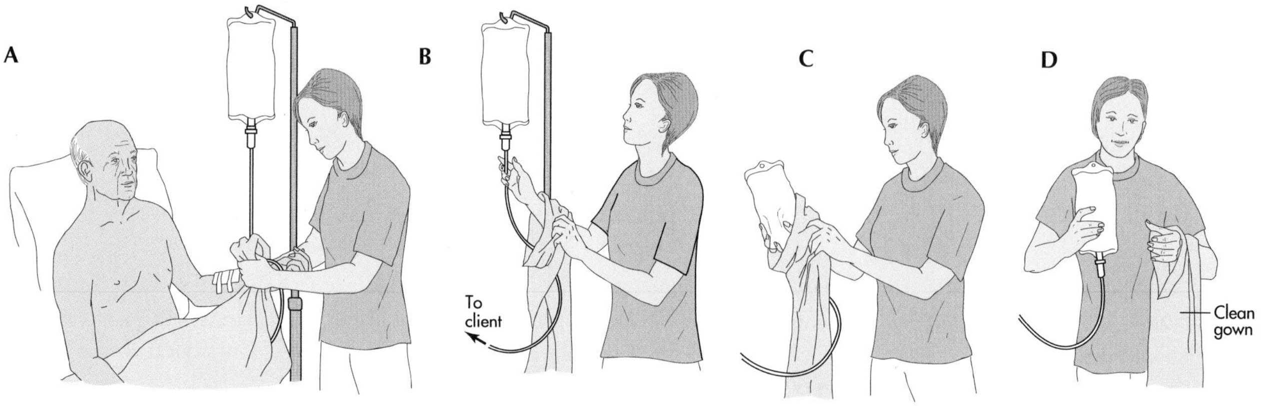

Figure 30–21 Changing a hospital gown. **A,** Remove the gown from the arm with no IV. Gather up the sleeve on the arm with the IV, slide it over the IV site and tubing, and remove it from the arm and hand. **B,** Slip the gathered sleeve along the IV tubing to the bag. **C,** Remove the IV bag from the pole and pass it through the sleeve. **D,** Slip the gathered sleeve of the clean gown over the IV bag at the shoulder part of the gown.

Changing Hospital Gowns

Hospitalized clients wear hospital gowns, such as when they are receiving IV therapy. Some facilities and agencies have special gowns for IV therapy, where the gowns open along the sleeve and close with ties, snaps, or Velcro, but many facilities and agencies still use standard hospital gowns. If this is the case at your agency, you should use the procedure described in Figure 30–21. You should not, however, when clients have IV pumps that control their infusions. If the client has an IV pump and a standard hospital gown, do not use this procedure. To avoid pulling on the IV, the client is usually dressed without his or her arm placed in the sleeve. The article of clothing is simply draped over the client's arm with the IV in, and the shirt is buttoned up.

APPLYING ELASTIC STOCKINGS AND BANDAGES

Some clients need to wear elastic stockings or bandages on their legs as ordered by their physicians. These must be applied as part of their daily dressing routine and are used to help prevent blood clots (thrombi). A blood clot (thrombus) can form in deep leg veins (see Figure 46–3 on page 883), break loose, travel through the bloodstream, and lodge in a distant vessel. If the clot lodges in the lungs, severe respiratory problems and death can result. Clients with circulatory disorders and heart disease and those on bed rest are at risk for blood clots.

Elastic stockings and bandages help to prevent thrombi. The elastic exerts pressure on the veins, which promotes venous blood flow to the heart. They also provide support and reduce swelling from injuries. However, elastic stockings and bandages can harm the client if applied incorrectly. Therefore, most hospitals do not allow support workers to apply them to acute care patients. Some employers do not allow support workers to apply them at all. You may be asked to apply them on clients in stable condition. It is your responsibility to know and follow your employer's policy.

Applying Elastic Stockings

Elastic stockings come in a variety of sizes and lengths (thigh-high or knee-high). The care plan lists the correct size to use. Stockings are applied in the morning before the client gets out of bed, as otherwise, the client's legs can swell from sitting or standing, making the stockings very difficult to put on. They are removed every 8 hours for 30 minutes or according to the care plan. The client lies in bed whenever they are off in order to prevent the legs from swelling. Most stockings have an opening near the toes. Others have an opening at the top or bottom of the foot. The opening is used to check circulation as well as skin colour and temperature.

The client usually has two pairs of stockings. One pair is washed while the client wears the other pair. Wash the stockings by hand with a mild soap, and then hang them to dry.

Make sure that the stockings are smooth and not bunched up or binding, without twists, creases, or wrinkles after you apply them. Bunching, binding, or twisting stockings can affect circulation, and creases and wrinkles can cause skin breakdown. Report and record the following observations after applying elastic stockings:

- Skin colour and skin temperature
- Leg and foot swelling
- Signs of skin breakdown
- Complaints of pain, tingling, or numbness

Applying Elastic Bandages

Elastic bandages are applied to the upper or lower extremities and have the same purposes as elastic stockings; they also hold dressings in place.

The bandage is applied from the lower (distal) part of the extremity to the top (proximal) part. Your supervisor and the care plan will tell you which area to bandage and the proper width of the bandage to use for that client. If the roll of bandage is not long enough to cover the part, another roll of bandage may be added.

1 2 3 APPLYING ELASTIC STOCKINGS

Remember to promote:

• Dignity • Independence • Preferences • Privacy • Safety

Pre-Procedure

1 Identify the client, according to employer policy.
2 Explain the procedure to the client.
3 Practise proper hand hygiene.
4 Collect elastic stockings in the correct size and length.
5 Provide for privacy.
6 Raise the bed to a comfortable working height. Follow the care plan for bed rail use.*

Procedure

7 Lower the bed rail near you, if it is up.
8 Place the client in the supine position.
9 Expose the legs. Fanfold top linens toward the client's thighs.
10 Turn the stocking inside out down to the heel (Figure 30–22, *A*).
11 Slip the foot of the stocking over the toes, foot, and heel (Figure 30–22, *B*).
12 Grasp the stocking top. Slip it over the foot and heel. Pull it up the leg. It turns right side out as it is pulled up. The stocking must be even and snug (Figure 30–22, *C*).
13 Remove twists, creases, or wrinkles.
14 Repeat steps 10 through 13 for the other leg.

Post-Procedure

15 Cover the client.
16 Provide for safety and comfort.
17 Place the call bell within reach.*
18 Return the bed to its lowest position. Follow the care plan for bed rail use.*
19 Remove privacy measures.
20 Practise proper hand hygiene.
21 Report and record your actions and observations, according to employer policy.

*Steps marked with an asterisk may not apply in community settings.

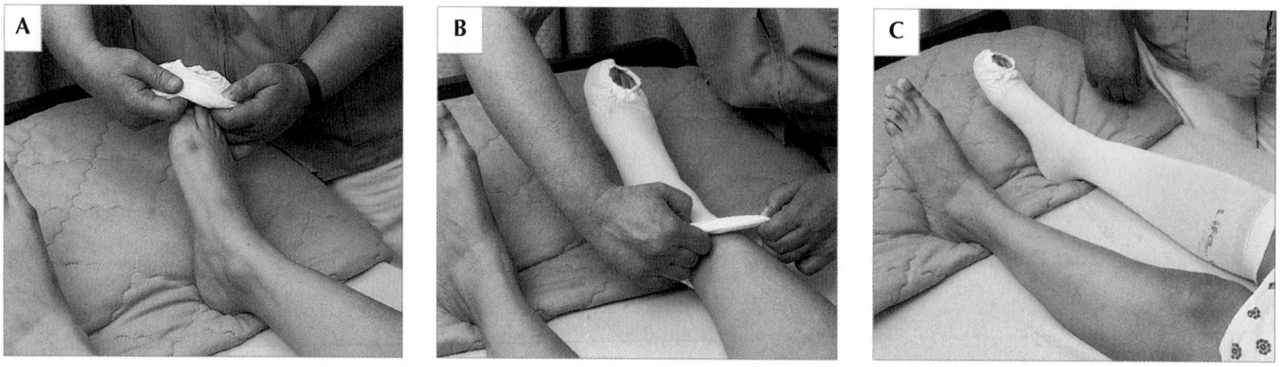

Figure 30–22 Applying elastic stockings. **A,** Turn the stocking inside out down to the heel. **B,** Slip the stocking over the toes, foot, and heel. **C,** The stocking turns right side out as it is pulled up over the leg.

Elastic bandages are removed every 8 hours for 30 minutes. If specified in the client's care plan, bandages may be washed in mild soap and water, rinsed well, patted dry, and then hung up to dry overnight. This is especially important if the client perspires on the bandage or has soiled the bandage in any way.

Follow these guidelines when applying elastic bandages:

- Use the correct length and width.
- Position the body part in good alignment.
- Face the client during the procedure.
- Expose fingers or toes, if possible. This allows circulation checks.
- Apply the bandage with firm, even pressure.
- Make sure the bandage is firm and snug. It must not be tight, as a tight bandage can affect circulation.
- Check the colour and temperature of the extremity every hour.
- Re-apply a loose, wrinkled, moist, or soiled bandage.

Report and record the following observations after applying elastic bandages:

- Skin colour and skin temperature
- Swelling in the leg and foot
- Signs of skin breakdown
- Complaints of pain, tingling, or numbness

1 2 3 APPLYING ELASTIC BANDAGES

Remember to promote:

• **D**ignity • **I**ndependence • **P**references • **P**rivacy • **S**afety

Pre-Procedure

1 Identify the client, according to employer policy.
2 Explain the procedure to the client.
3 Practise proper hand hygiene.
4 Collect the following:
- Elastic bandage, as directed by the care plan
- Tape or metal clips (unless the bandage has Velcro)

5 Provide for privacy.
6 Raise the bed to a comfortable working height. Follow the care plan for bed rail use.*

Procedure

7 Lower the bed rail near you, if it is up.
8 Help the client to a comfortable position. Expose the part you will bandage.
9 Make sure the area is clean and dry.
10 Hold the bandage so that the roll is up. The loose end must be on the bottom (Figure 30–23, *A*).
11 Apply the bandage to the smallest part of the wrist, foot, ankle, or knee.
12 Make two circular turns around the part (Figure 30–23, *B*).
13 Make overlapping spiral turns in an upward direction. Each turn overlaps about two thirds of the previous turn (Figure 30–23, *C*).
14 Apply the bandage smoothly with firm, even pressure. It must not be tight.
15 Secure the bandage in place with Velcro, tape, or a clip. Ensure that the bandaged area does not put pressure on the clip, as this could injure underlying tissues.
16 Check the fingers or toes for coldness or cyanosis (bluish colour). Ask about pain, itching, numbness, or tingling. Report and record any unusual or abnormal observations. Remove the bandage if you note any, and report it to your supervisor.

Post-Procedure

17 Follow steps 16 through 21 of *Applying Elastic Stockings.*

*Steps marked with an asterisk may not apply in community settings.

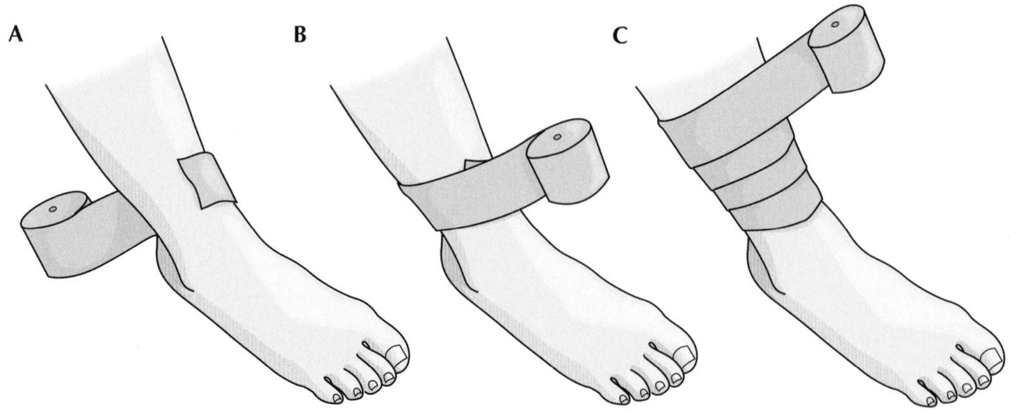

Figure 30–23 Applying an elastic bandage. **A,** The roll of the bandage is up, and the loose end is at the bottom. **B,** Apply the bandage to the smallest part with two circular turns. **C,** Apply the bandage with spiral turns in an upward direction.

COMPASSIONATE CARE

When helping with grooming and dressing, remember to focus on the whole client rather than only on the task. Promote the client's dignity, independence, preferences, privacy, and safety (see the *Providing Compassionate Care: Assisting Clients with Grooming and Dressing* box).

Care of Wigs

Wigs are worn for a variety of reasons. Some Orthodox Jewish married women remove all the hair and wear only a head covering, while others wear a wig to cover their hair. Some clients may have lost their hair due to natural aging or as a result of chemotherapy for cancer. Some clients may be bald from birth, while some others may have become bald after an illness or an injury to their scalp.

Whatever the reason, many people—both men and women—wear wigs for warmth, modesty, or their own body image. Wigs can be very expensive, so it is important to care for them properly so that they are kept fresh, attractive, and comfortable. When caring for a client's wig, you should follow the maintenance steps that are in client's care plan. Here are some tips on maintenance.[3]

Storage. After removing the wig, keep it on a wig stand (or "head form") to maintain the shape. Smooth out straight hair or fluff curls with a wire brush or pick. Cover the wig with a hair net that maintains the style without matting. Avoid leaving the wig near heat (radiators, vents), humidity (showers), or dusty areas.

Washing. Shampooing frequency depends on wearing frequency. Generally, a wig should be washed after every 6 to 8 uses in warm climates or after every 12 to 15 uses in cooler ones. However, if the client is especially active, uses heavy hairspray, or lives in an especially humid climate or in one with poor air quality, the wig should be washed about once a week to remove excess perspiration and dirt.

Before washing, smooth out a straight-hair wig or fluff a curly-hair wig gently and completely with a wire brush or pick. Add a cap of wig shampoo or baby shampoo to a basin of cool (never hot) water. Immerse the wig gently and soak for 2 minutes. Rinse well by swishing in clean, cool water. Gently squeeze out excess water without twisting the wig. For extra shine and softness, apply wig conditioner and leave it on for 5 minutes. Rinse again in clean, cool water. Gently squeeze out excess water without twisting the wig.

PROVIDING COMPASSIONATE CARE

Assisting Clients With Grooming and Dressing

- **Dignity.** Being clean and well-groomed helps the client maintain dignity. People often feel good about themselves when they have a neat appearance and clean clothing. When assisting with grooming, handle the client's hygiene products, shaver, hair dryer, brush and comb, perfumes, and other personal care items carefully. When handling clothing, take care not to break zippers, tear clothing, lose buttons, or cause other damage. Treat the client's property with care and respect. If damage occurs, notify your supervisor.
- **Independence.** Encourage the client to be as independent as possible. Provide assistance only when needed. Like other activities of daily living (ADLs), dressing and undressing stimulate circulation and increase muscle strength and flexibility. They also increase the client's confidence and self-esteem. Sometimes allowing clients to do what they can for themselves requires patience and understanding. Give the client extra time to dress and undress independently.

  If the client has self-care devices, encourage him or her to use them. Many self-care devices that promote independence with dressing and undressing include:
  - Button hooks (see Figure 33–2, *A* on page 633)
  - Sock pullers (see Figure 33—2, *B*)
  - Shoe removers (see Figure 33–2, *C*)
  - Pantyhose aids
  - Trouser pulls
  - Pant clips
- **Preferences.** Encourage personal choices, whenever possible. Each client will have his or her own grooming practices. Do not impose your standards on the client. Ask clients how they want their hair styled, what hair or shaving products they use, and what clothing they want to wear.
- **Privacy.** Providing for privacy is important when dressing and undressing the client. Do not expose the client when you are performing the procedures described in this chapter. Also, provide privacy when assisting with grooming.
- **Safety.** Remember to dress the affected side first (DAF) and remove clothing from the unaffected side first (RUF). Also, remember to frequently check clients with elastic stockings and bandages. Check for signs of reduced circulation, swelling, or skin breakdown. Report your observations to your supervisor. This information is needed to provide complete care to the client.

Drying. After washing the wig, tightly finger-squeeze each curl. Gently towel-blot both straight-hair and curly-hair wigs to remove excess water. Let the wig air-dry on a clean, dry towel or on a wire head form that allows air circulation. Do not set the wig stand near heat sources or in direct sunlight. Never use blow dryers or other heat appliances on synthetic wigs. Also, be sure not to comb, brush, or pick a wet wig unless you are completely re-styling it. As the wig dries, shake it out periodically for fast drying. Once the wig is fully dry, style it in the normal manner.

Wearing. Once the client has become accustomed to the wig, he or she can wear it for daily activities. Advise the client to avoid blasts of heat—for example, when quickly opening an oven door—on synthetic wigs.

REVIEW

Answers to these questions are at the bottom of page 577.

Circle the **BEST** answer.

1. **Mr. Lee has alopecia. This is:**
   A. Excessive body hair
   B. Dry, white flakes on the scalp
   C. An infestation of lice
   D. Hair loss
2. **When brushing hair that is not matted or tangled, start at:**
   A. The forehead, and brush backward
   B. The hair ends
   C. The scalp, and brush toward the hair tips
   D. The back of the neck, and brush forward
3. **Brushing is important to keep the hair:**
   A. Soft and shiny
   B. Clean
   C. Free from lice
   D. Long
4. **Mr. Lee wants his hair washed. You should:**
   A. Wash his hair during his shower
   B. Wash his hair at the sink
   C. Shampoo him in bed
   D. Follow the care plan
5. **When shaving Mr. Lee with a blade razor, you need to do the following:**
   A. Remove any beard or mustache that he has
   B. Moisten the beard before shaving to soften it
   C. Shave perpendicular to the direction of hair growth
   D. Shave when the skin is dry
6. **Mr. Lee is nicked during shaving. Your first action should be to:**
   A. Practise proper hand hygiene
   B. Apply direct pressure
   C. Tell your supervisor
   D. Apply a bandage
7. **When shaving a man's face, you should shave in the __________ direction from his neck to his chin.**
   A. Left to right, from one side to another
   B. Right to left, from one side to another
   C. Up to down from chin to neck
   D. Down to up from neck to chin
8. **Fingernails are cut with:**
   A. Toenail clippers
   B. Scissors
   C. A nail file
   D. Nail clippers
9. **You should never attempt to trim nails on clients who are:**
   A. Alert and oriented
   B. Diabetic
   C. Paralyzed
   D. Awake
10. **Elastic stockings are used to:**
   A. Reduce swelling in the legs
   B. Improve the appearance of the legs
   C. Exert pressure on the veins
   D. Reduce circulation
11. **Elastic stockings are applied:**
   A. Before the client gets out of bed
   B. When the client is standing
   C. After the client's shower or tub bath
   D. Before the client goes to sleep
12. **When applying an elastic bandage:**
   A. The body needs to be in good alignment
   B. The fingers or toes are covered
   C. It is applied from the largest to the smallest part of an extremity
   D. It is applied from the upper to the lower part of the extremity

REVIEW

Answers to these questions are at the bottom of the page.

13. **When dressing a client who has hemiplegia (paralysis) on her right side, you should place her right arm in her sleeve:**
    - A. First
    - B. Last
    - C. Not place her arm in a sleeve
    - D. You should not be dressing clients with hemiplegia.

Circle T if the answer is true or circle F if the answer is false.

14. T F **You can shave a client's beard and mustache if you think he would be more comfortable without facial hair.**
15. T F **You can cut and trim toenails for a client who has diabetes.**
16. T F **Clothing is removed from the unaffected side first.**
17. T F **The client chooses what to wear.**
18. T F **Wigs should never be washed. They should only be dry-cleaned.**

Answers: 1.D, 2.C, 3.A, 4.D, 5.B, 6.B, 7.D, 8.D, 9.B, 10.C, 11.A, 12.A, 13.A, 14.F, 15.F, 16.T, 17.T, 18.F

CHAPTER 31

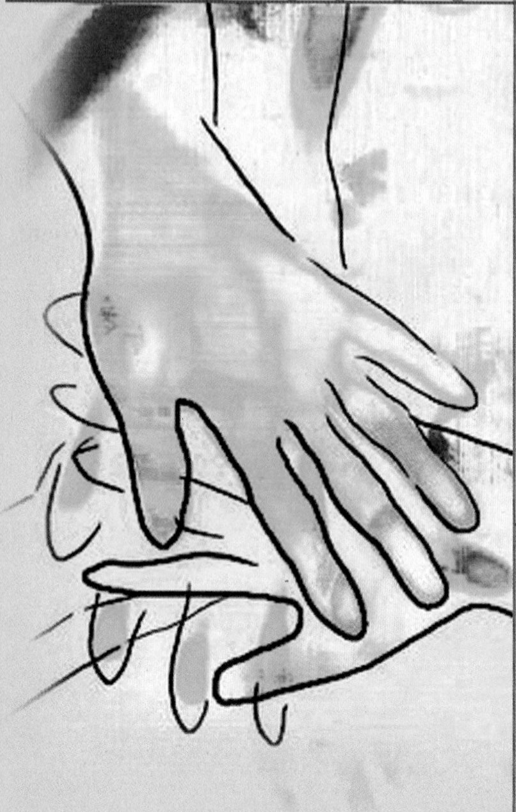

Urinary Elimination

OBJECTIVES

- Define the key terms listed in this chapter.
- Identify the characteristics of normal urine.
- Describe the guidelines for maintaining normal urinary elimination.
- List the observations to make about urine.
- Describe urinary incontinence and the care required.
- Explain why catheters are used.
- Explain the differences between straight, indwelling, suprapubic, and condom catheters.
- Describe the guidelines for caring for clients with indwelling catheters.
- Describe two methods of bladder training.
- Describe the guidelines for collecting urine specimens.
- Explain how to care for a client with a ureterostomy.
- Apply the procedures described in this chapter to your clinical practice properly.

key terms

acetone A compound that appears in the urine from the rapid breakdown of fat for energy.

catheter A tube used to drain or inject fluid through a body opening.

catheterization The process of inserting a catheter.

condom catheter A sheath that slides over the penis; tubing connects the catheter and drainage bag.

dysuria Painful or difficult (*dys*) urination (*uria*).

Foley catheter See **indwelling catheter**.

fracture pan A small thin rimmed bedpan that is about 1 cm deep at one end. It is often given to clients who cannot manoeuvre themselves onto a larger bedpan, for example, someone who has had a hip fracture. Also called a **slipper pan**.

functional incontinence Urinary incontinence caused by physical conditions or environmental barriers that prevent the client from reaching the toilet on time.

glucosuria Sugar (*glucos*) in the urine (*uria*).

hematuria Blood (*hemat*) in the urine (*uria*).

ileal conduit An artificial bladder fashioned out of a section of the ileum. Urine drains from the ureters into this newly created artificial bladder and then through the client's stoma.

indwelling catheter A catheter that is inserted into the bladder, through the urinary meatus and urethra, so urine drains constantly into a drainage bag. Also known as **Foley** or **retention catheter**.

ketone body A byproduct of the metabolism of protein.

micturition See **urination**.

nocturia Frequent urination (*uria*) at night (*noct*).

oliguria Scant amount (*olig*) of urine (*uria*); usually less than 500 mL in 24 hours.

ostomy Surgical creation of an artificial opening.

overflow incontinence The leaking of urine when the bladder is too full.

polyuria The production of abnormally large amounts (*poly*) of urine (*uria*).

reflex incontinence The loss of urine at predictable intervals.

retention catheter A **Foley** or **indwelling catheter**.

slipper pan See **fracture pan**.

stoma A surgically created opening from a portion of the body cavity to the outside environment.

straight catheter A catheter that is inserted to drain the bladder and is then removed.

stress incontinence The leaking of urine during exercise and certain movements.

suprapubic catheter A catheter that is surgically inserted into the bladder through the abdomen.

ureterostomy An artificial opening (*stomy*) between the ureter (*uretero*) and the abdomen.

urge incontinence The loss of urine in response to a sudden, urgent need to void.

urinary frequency The need to urinate at frequent intervals.

urinary incontinence The inability to control the passage of urine from the bladder; the loss of bladder control.

urinary urgency The need to void immediately.

urination The process of emptying urine from the bladder. Also known as **micturition** or **voiding**.

voiding See **urination**.

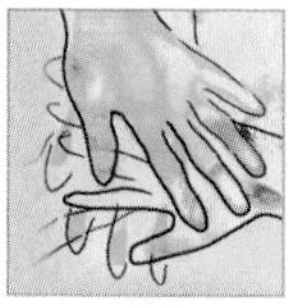

Eliminating waste is one of the important functions of the body. The body's waste products are removed through various body systems—digestive, respiratory, integumentary, and urinary. The digestive system rids the body of solid wastes; the lungs rid the body of carbon dioxide; the skin sweats, getting rid of water and other substances; and the urinary system removes waste products from the blood (from body cells burning food for energy) and maintains the body's water balance (see Chapter 14 to review the urinary system).

When assisting a client with elimination, you may be exposed to urine or stool (feces) directly, as well as indirectly on linens and clothing that are soiled with these bodily fluids. Protect yourself and your client by following the rules of medical asepsis and Standard Practices (see Chapter 20). Follow the infection control precautions in Box 31–1 when assisting with elimination.

NORMAL URINATION

The healthy adult excretes about 1500 mL (millilitres) of urine a day. Many factors such as age, disease, the amount and kinds of fluid ingested, dietary salt, and medications affect urine production. Some substances such as coffee, tea, alcohol, and some medications increase urine production. A diet high in salt causes the body to retain water; when water is retained, less urine is produced.

Urination, micturition, and **voiding** all mean the process of emptying urine from the bladder. The amount of fluid intake, personal habits, and available toilet facilities, as well as activity, work, and illness, affect frequency. People usually void at bed time, after getting up, and before meals. Some people void every 2 to 3 hours, while others void less frequently. The need to void at night often causes sleep disturbance in many people. You should be aware that while many of the clients that you may see in various facilities may be incontinent of urine, ***it is not a normal part of aging.***

Clients may need help with urinary elimination. You should be aware of the transmission control precautions with regard to assisting a client with toileting (see Box 31–1). Some clients may need help getting to the bathroom, and others may use bedpans, urinals, or commodes. Follow the guidelines listed in Box 31–2 to help maintain normal elimination. Remember that it is your responsibility to follow the client's care plan when assisting with urinary elimination.

Box 31–1 Transmission Control Precautions When Assisting With Elimination

- Perform hand hygiene before and after wearing gloves.
- Wear gloves whenever there is a risk of contact with urine, feces, secretions, or mucous membranes. Examples include:
  - Assisting clients who have diarrhea, urinary incontinence (page 587), or fecal incontinence (see Chapter 32)
  - Handling or cleaning bedpans, urinals, commodes, toilets, or bathroom floors
  - Handling soiled clothing or linens
  - Changing incontinence products
  - Measuring client's output
  - Collecting specimens
- Change gloves between procedures on the same client, as the gloves may be contaminated. For example, change gloves after perineal care and before cleaning an indwelling catheter.
- Remove contaminated gloves before touching a clean surface. For example, remove soiled gloves before raising the bed rails.
- Remember that soiled incontinence briefs should never be placed on the floor. This is both unhygienic practice (see Chapter 20) and a source of offensive odour. If client safety is at risk while changing incontinence briefs, you should place them at the foot of the bed, ensure safety and privacy, and then discard the briefs into the proper container. Ensure that the lid is placed on the container for odour control.
- Wear a protective apron or gown if there is a chance that you might be sprayed or splashed with blood, body fluids, secretions, or excretions. This could occur when you are emptying bedpans or commodes.
- Cover bedpans and tightly cap urinals when carrying them. Avoid splashing when disposing of bedpan, urinal, or commode contents. If splashing occurs, clean the area immediately. Dispose of body wastes immediately and carefully. Clean and disinfect bedpans, urinals, and commodes immediately after use.
- Place soiled disposable materials in leak-proof plastic bags. Seal them tightly. Immediately discard the bags according to employer policy.
- Place soiled linen and clothing in a leak-proof plastic bag. Launder it as soon as possible, according to employer policy. In a client's home, wash soiled linen separately from other laundry.

Adapted from: Birchenall J., & Streight, E. (1997). *Mosby's textbook for the home care aide* (p. 262). St. Louis: Mosby.

1 2 3 GIVING THE BEDPAN

Remember to promote:

• **D**ignity • **I**ndependence • **P**references • **P**rivacy • **S**afety

Pre-Procedure

1 Identify the client, according to employer policy.
2 Explain the procedure to the client.
3 Provide for privacy.
4 Practise proper hand hygiene. Put on gloves.
5 Collect the following:
- Bedpan
- Bedpan cover (or paper towels)
- Toilet tissue
- Talcum powder (optional)
- Extra gloves

6 Arrange equipment on the chair or bed.

Procedure

7 Warm and dry the bedpan, if necessary. Lightly dust the rim of the bedpan with talcum powder (optional).
8 Lower the bed rail near you, if it is up.
9 Place the client in the supine position, keeping the bed as flat as possible. You may use pillows to raise the client's head and shoulders.
10 Fold the top linens and the client's gown out of the way. Keep the lower body covered.
11 Ask the client to flex the knees and raise the buttocks by pushing against the mattress with the feet.
12 Slide your hand under the lower back, and help raise the buttocks.
13 Slide the bedpan under the client (Figure 31–4).
14 If the client cannot assist in getting on the bedpan:
  a Turn the client onto the side away from you.
  b Place the bedpan firmly against the buttocks (Figure 31–5, *A*).
  c Push the bedpan down and toward the client (Figure 31–5, *B*).
  d Hold the bedpan securely. Turn the client onto the back.
  e Make sure the bedpan is centred and under the client.
15 Cover the client.
16 Raise the head of the bed so that the client is in the sitting position. If the bed is not adjustable, assist the client into the sitting position, using pillows for support.
17 Make sure the client is correctly positioned on the bedpan (Figure 31–6).
18 Raise the bed rail, if used.
19 Place the toilet tissue and call bell (in facilities) within reach.
20 Ask the client to call when done or when help is needed.
21 Practise proper hand hygiene.
22 Leave the room, and close the door.
23 Return when the client calls. Knock before entering.
24 Practise proper hand hygiene. Put on gloves.
25 Raise the bed to a comfortable working height. Lower the bed rail (if used) and the head of the bed.* Or remove the pillows, and place the client in the supine position.
26 Ask the client to raise the buttocks, and remove the bedpan. If the client cannot raise the buttocks, hold the bedpan securely, and turn the client onto the side away from you.
27 Clean the genital area, if the client cannot do so. Clean from the front (urethra) to the back (anus) with toilet tissue, using a fresh tissue for each wipe. Provide perineal care.
28 Cover the bedpan and take it to the bathroom. Remember to lower the bed and raise the bed rail (if used) before leaving the bedside.
29 Note the colour, amount, and character of urine or stool.
30 Empty and rinse the bedpan with cold water. Clean it with a disinfectant.
31 Remove soiled gloves. Practise proper hand hygiene.
32 Put bedpan and lid away.
33 Help the client practise proper hand hygiene.
34 Remove gloves. Practise proper hand hygiene.

Post-Procedure

35 Provide for safety and comfort.
36 Place the call bell within reach.*
37 Follow the care plan for bed rail use.*
38 Remove privacy measures.
39 Follow employer policy for soiled linen.
40 Practise proper hand hygiene.
41 Report and record your actions and observations, according to employer policy.

*Steps marked with an asterisk may not apply in community settings.

hooks to the bed rail, the back of a chair, or any place within the client's reach that is sturdy enough to support a filled urinal. The urinal should ***never*** be placed on the client's overbed table, bedside table, or stand, as these surfaces are used as work areas, for eating, or for keeping the client's items. Follow employer policy on where to place urinals.

If possible, while using the urinal, the male client should stand, sit on the side of the bed, or lie in bed. For some clients who cannot stand without the support of one or two people, you may have to place and hold the urinal for them.

Remind clients to cap the urinal after voiding to prevent urine spilling. You should also remind clients

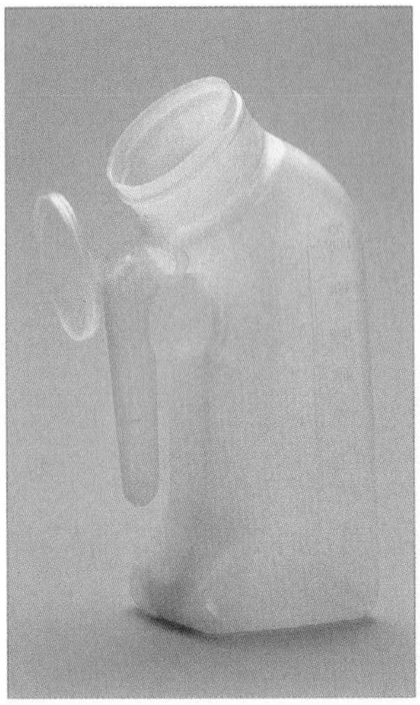

Figure 31–3 A urinal.

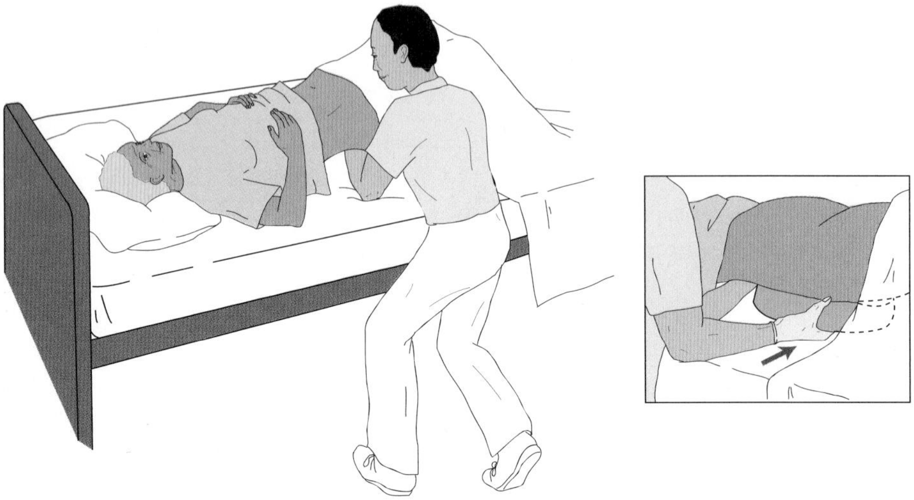

Figure 31–4 The client raises the buttocks off the bed with help. Slide the bedpan under the client.

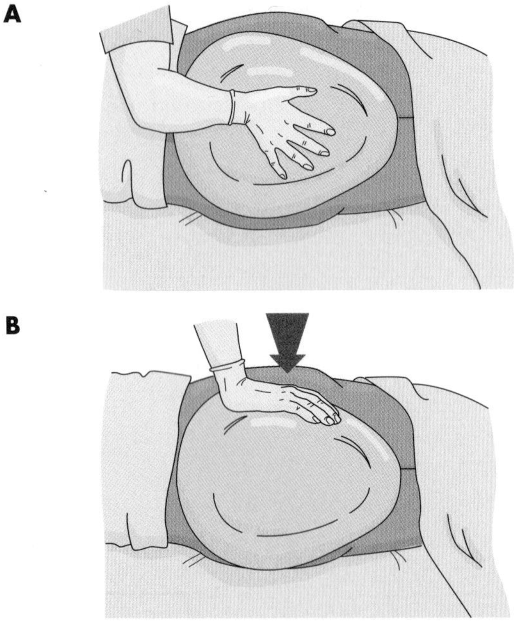

Figure 31–5 Giving a bedpan. **A,** Position the client on one side, and place the bedpan firmly against the buttocks. **B,** Push downward on the bedpan and toward the client.

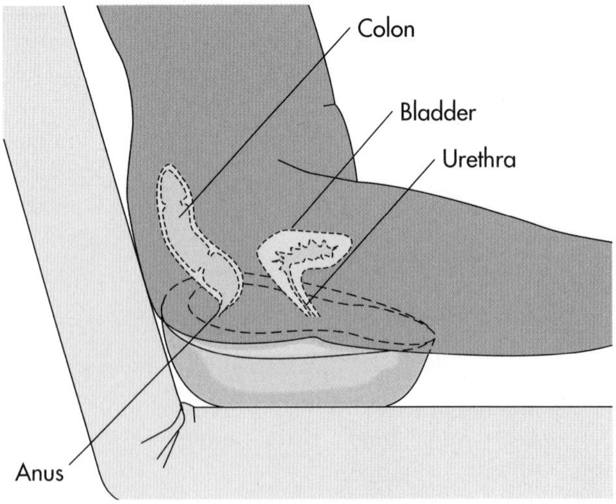

Figure 31–6 Position the client on the bedpan so that the urethra and anus are directly over the opening.

to hang used urinals on bed rails or the backs of chairs, and to call you when their urinals need emptying. Follow medical asepsis and Standard Practices when handling urinals and their contents. A filled urinal spills easily, causing safety hazards. Also, it may be embarrassing for the client to have the filled urinal around. You should always empty urinals promptly and thoroughly rinse and clean them (in the same manner as bedpans) after each use to prevent odours and the buildup and spread of microbes.

Commodes

A commode is a portable chair or wheelchair with an opening for a bedpan or container, which allows a normal position for elimination (Figure 31–7 on page 587). Some chairs have wheels so that they can be moved, while others do not. Clients who are unable to walk to the bathroom often use commodes. The commode arms and back provide support and help prevent falls while allowing for a more natural and comfortable position for elimination.

1 2 3 PROVIDING A URINAL TO A MALE CLIENT

Remember to promote:

• Dignity • Independence • Preferences • Privacy • Safety

Pre-Procedure

1 Provide for privacy.
2 Determine if the client will stand, sit, or stay in bed.
3 Practise proper hand hygiene. Put on gloves.

Procedure

4 Give the client the urinal if he is in bed. Remind him to tilt the bottom down to prevent spills.
5 If the client is going to stand:
  a Help him sit on the side of the bed.
  b Help him put on nonskid footwear.
  c Help him stand. Provide support if he is unsteady.
  d Give him the urinal.
6 Position the urinal, if necessary. Position his penis in the urinal if he cannot do so.
7 Provide for privacy.
8 Place the call bell within reach.*
9 Ask the client to call when done or when he needs help.
10 Remove gloves. Practise proper hand hygiene.
11 Leave the room, and close the door.
12 Return when he calls for you. Knock before entering.
13 Practise proper hand hygiene. Put on gloves.
14 Close the cap on the urinal. Take it to the bathroom.
15 Note the colour, amount, and character of the urine.
16 Empty the urinal, rinse it with cold water, and clean it with disinfectant.
17 Return the urinal to its proper place.
18 Remove gloves. Practise proper hand hygiene. Put on clean gloves.
19 Help the client wash his hands.
20 Remove gloves. Practise proper hand hygiene.

Post-Procedure

21 Provide for safety and comfort.
22 Place the call bell within reach.*
23 Follow the care plan for bed rail use.*
24 Remove privacy measures.
25 Follow employer policy for soiled linen.
26 Practise proper hand hygiene.
27 Report and record your actions and observations, according to employer policy.

*Steps marked with an asterisk may not apply in community settings.

The bedpan or container should be cleaned after each use, as in the case of the regular bedpan, following Standard Practices. If a specimen is not required, placing a small amount of water in the commode container will allow for easier cleaning after use.

For clients who cannot sit unsupported on the toilet, some commodes are wheeled into the bathroom and positioned over the toilet, after the bedpan or container have been removed. This helps clients unable to walk to the bathroom have privacy and safety during elimination. It is your responsibility to ensure that the commode wheels are locked and that the commode is positioned correctly over the toilet. ***Note that clients should never be tied or***

1 2 3 HELPING THE CLIENT TO THE COMMODE

Remember to promote:

• Dignity • Independence • Preferences • Privacy • Safety

Pre-Procedure

1 Explain the procedure to the client.
2 Provide for privacy.
3 Practise proper hand hygiene. Put on gloves.
4 Collect the following:
- Commode
- Toilet tissue
- Bath blanket
- Extra gloves
- Transfer belt (optional)

Procedure

5 Bring the commode next to the bed. Remove the cushion and lift the container lid.
6 Help the client sit on the side of the bed.
7 Help the client put on a robe and nonskid footwear.
8 Assist the client to the commode. Use a transfer belt, if necessary.
9 Cover the client with a bath blanket for warmth.
10 Place the call bell (in facilities) and toilet tissue within reach.
11 Ask the client to call when done or when help is needed. (Stay with the client if necessary. Be respectful. Provide as much privacy as possible.)
12 Remove gloves. Practise proper hand hygiene.
13 Leave the room, and close the door.
14 Return when the client calls. Knock before entering.
15 Practise proper hand hygiene. Put on gloves.
16 Help the client clean the genital area, as needed. Remove gloves. Practise proper hand hygiene.
17 Help the client back to the bed. Remove the robe and footwear. Follow the care plan for bed rail use.
18 Put on clean gloves. Remove and cover the commode container. Clean the commode.
19 Take the container to the bathroom.
20 Check urine and stool for colour, amount, and character.
21 Empty, clean, and disinfect the container.
22 Return the container to the commode. Return other supplies to their proper places.
23 Return the commode to its proper place.
24 Remove soiled gloves. Practise proper hand hygiene. Put on clean gloves.
25 Help the client with hand washing.
26 Remove gloves. Practise proper hand hygiene.

Post-Procedure

27 Provide for safety and comfort.
28 Place the call bell within reach.*
29 Follow the care plan for bed rail use.*
30 Remove privacy measures.
31 Follow employer policy for soiled linen.
32 Practise proper hand hygiene.
33 Report and record your actions and observations, according to employer policy.

*Steps marked with an asterisk may not apply in community settings.

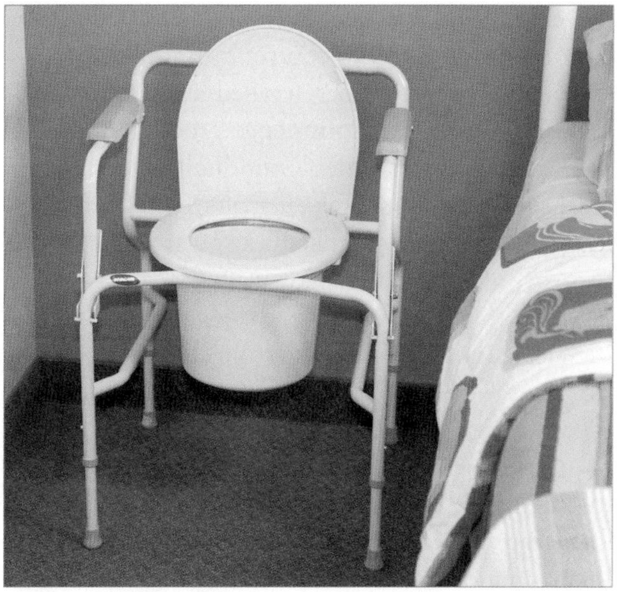

Figure 31–7 The bedside commode has a toilet seat with a container beneath it. The container slides out from under the toilet seat for emptying. This commode is extra-wide to accommodate large clients. **Source:** Brian Hillier.

restrained to a commode. While commodes are very useful, they can tip easily. Clients who cannot sit up on their own should not be placed on a commode chair. The longest time a client should be on a commode chair is 20 to 30 minutes.

The client may be lowered onto a commode chair, which is then wheeled and positioned over a toilet. To prevent injury to the client, it is your responsibility to ensure that the client's buttocks do not rub against the toilet while positioning the commode chair over it. In addition, you must ensure that the commode chair's wheels are locked and secured so that they do not roll. This helps stabilize the client and prevent falls.

URINARY INCONTINENCE

Urinary incontinence—the loss of bladder control—may be temporary or permanent. The different types of incontinence are:

- ***Stress incontinence***—the leaking of urine during exercise and certain movements. Urine loss is small (less than 50 mL). Often called *dribbling*, it occurs with laughing, sneezing, coughing, lifting, or other activities. Late pregnancy and obesity are other causes. The problem is common in women, as pelvic muscles weaken from pregnancies and with aging.
- ***Urge incontinence***—the loss of urine in response to a sudden, urgent need to void. The client cannot get to a toilet in time. Urinary frequency, urinary urgency, and night-time voidings are common. Causes include urinary tract infections, nervous system disorders, bladder cancer, and an enlarged prostate.
- ***Overflow incontinence***—the leaking of urine when the bladder is too full. The client feels as though the bladder is never completely empty and experiences only dribbling or a weak urine stream. Diabetes, enlarged prostate, and some medications are causes.
- ***Functional incontinence***—the loss of urine that occurs when the client has bladder control but cannot get to the toilet in time. Immobility, restraints, unanswered calls for help, lack of a call bell within reach, confusion, disorientation, difficulty removing clothing, and not knowing where to find the bathroom are all causes of functional incontinence.
- ***Reflex incontinence***—the loss of urine at predictable intervals. Urine is lost whenever the bladder becomes full, even when the client does not feel the need to void. Nervous system disorders and injuries are common causes.

Sometimes incontinence results from surgeries to the intestinal, rectal, and reproductive systems. When more than one type of incontinence can be present, it is called *mixed incontinence.*

Problems Related to Urinary Incontinence. Incontinence is embarrassing for the client. Clothing and linens get wet, odours develop, and the client is usually cold and uncomfortable. The client can develop skin irritation, skin breakdown, and infection. The urge to urinate can be so strong that some clients may rush to the washroom and sustain injury by slipping or falling on the way.

You can minimize incontinence by ensuring the client toilets regularly, for example, before and after each meal, before and after activities, and before going to sleep and upon wakening. Incontinence can affect clients' pride, dignity, and self-esteem and cause them to avoid participating in activities, going out, or visiting with others out of fear of being incontinent in public. These clients need your support, understanding, and compassion.

Check with your supervisor and consult the care plan for the best ways to meet the client's needs. Care measures depend on the type of incontinence. The client's care plan may include some of the measures listed in Box 31–3. ***It is essential that you provide frequent, proper skin care and change the client into clean, dry garments after each episode. Promptly changing wet bed linens is also essential, and failure to do so is considered a form of neglect.*** Following the guidelines for maintaining normal urination will prevent urinary incontinence in some clients. Other clients may need bladder training (page 598), and occasionally, some clients require the use of catheterization to control incontinence.

For clients with uncontrolled urinary incontinence, a variety of incontinence products are available, and the most suitable product for each client is selected by a nurse, the client, or the client's family. In addition, some clients use garment protectors or incontinence pads (Figure 31–8). It is essential that you keep the client's skin and clothing clean and dry, even when the client uses incontinence products. You need to frequently check the incontinence products for wetness, and change them, as needed, following the manufacturer's instructions. The client should receive proper perineal care and be thoroughly dried each time the incontinence product is checked or changed. Observe the skin frequently (at least every 2 to 4 hours), checking for signs of redness or rash.

Box 31–3 Care Measures for Clients With Urinary Incontinence

- Record the client's voidings. This includes episodes of incontinence as well as successful use of the toilet, commode, bedpan, or urinal.
- Answer all calls for assistance promptly. The client may have an urgent need to void.
- Promote normal urinary elimination (see Box 31–2 on page 581).
- Promote normal bowel elimination (see Chapter 32).
- Encourage urination at scheduled intervals.
- Monitor the client's bladder training program.
- Encourage the client to wear clothing that is easy to remove. Incontinence can occur as the client is trying to deal with buttons, zippers, and undergarments.
- Encourage the client to do pelvic muscle exercises, as directed by the care plan.
- Help prevent urinary tract infections:
  - Encourage adequate fluid intake, as directed by the care plan.
  - Encourage the client to wear cotton undergarments.
  - Provide perineal care, as needed (see Chapter 29). Keep the perineal area clean and dry.
- Decrease fluid intake before bedtime (the client's *daily* fluid intake is usually not restricted, however).
- Provide proper skin care (see Chapter 29).
- Provide dry garments and linens.
- Observe for signs of skin breakdown (see Chapter 42).
- Use incontinence products, as directed by the care plan. Follow manufacturer's instructions. Remove when they become wet and discard or wash them (depending on the type of product and the manufacturer's instructions).
- If a catheter is used on a client, many agencies use an adhesive strip that secures the catheter tubing to the client's leg to prevent the tubing from being pulled and the injury that could result from this (see Figure 31–11 on page 592).
- Catheters are not very effective in managing incontinence and are usually avoided because they can cause urinary infections, which can make a client very ill.
- Many agencies no longer use condom catheters as a means to manage urinary incontinence in men. If applied incorrectly or not observed often enough, they can cause painful sores on the client's penis and can be very irritating to the client's skin.

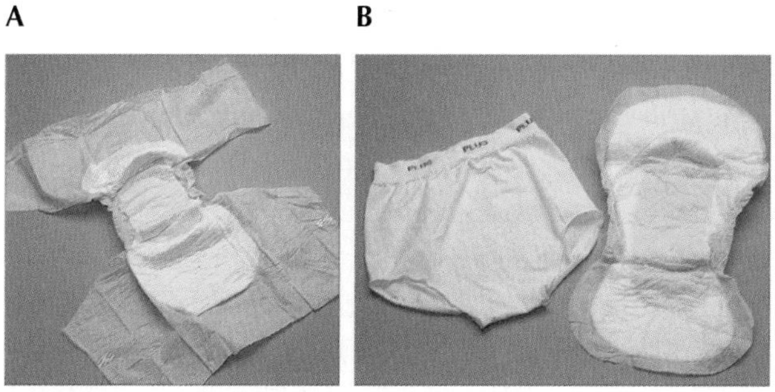

Figure 31–8 Garment protectors. **A,** Complete incontinence brief. **B,** Pant liner and undergarment.

Stress for the Caregiver. Caring for people with incontinence can be stressful. Some family members who are caregivers cannot cope with problems associated with incontinence and often seek long-term care for the client. As a professional caregiver, even you may find caring for these clients stressful, as they may need frequent care with changing wet garments and linens and skin care within very short intervals. Do not lose patience. The client's needs are great, and your role is to meet these needs. If you find yourself becoming short-tempered and impatient, discuss it with your supervisor immediately. Remember, the client has the right to be free from abuse, mistreatment, and neglect. The incontinence is beyond the client's control and is not something he or she chooses to let happen. Kindness, empathy, understanding, and patience are very important.

Drawsheets and Incontinence Pads. Incontinence drawsheets help keep bed linens dry. Placed over the bottom sheet, the drawsheet has two layers and a waterproof back. Fluid passes through the first layer and is absorbed by the lower layer. When the drawsheet becomes wet or soiled, change it and any damp bed linens. Do not place a dry drawsheet over wet bed linen to save time, as this could be considered neglect.

CATHETERS

A **catheter** is a tube used to drain or inject fluid through a body opening. A *urinary catheter* is a tube which is inserted into the bladder to drain urine. Catheter insertion (**catheterization**) is done by a nurse or physician, or even by the client himself or herself, if the client can learn how to do it.

Occasionally, a physician might order a client to be catheterized after he or she has voided to determine how much urine is left in the bladder. If a client was catheterized for 300 mL but voided only 200 mL, this would indicate inadequate emptying of the bladder and the need for medical treatment.

- A **straight catheter** drains the bladder and is removed after use. It is inserted through the urethra into the bladder.
- An **indwelling catheter** (**retention** or **Foley catheter**) is left in the bladder. Most indwelling catheters are inserted through the urethra into the bladder. Urine drains constantly into a drainage bag. A balloon near the tip is inflated after the catheter is inserted. The balloon prevents the catheter from slipping out of the bladder (Figure 31–9). Tubing connects the catheter to the drainage bag.

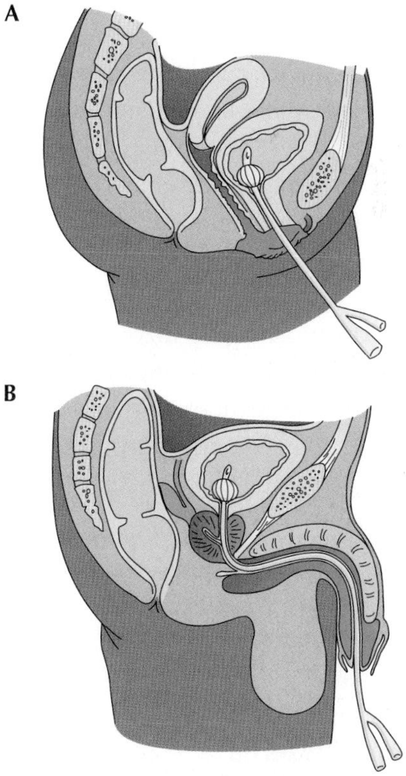

Figure 31–9 **A,** Indwelling catheter in the female bladder. The inflated balloon at the top prevents the catheter from slipping out through the urethra. **B,** Indwelling catheter with the balloon inflated in the male bladder.

- A **suprapubic catheter** is a catheter that is surgically inserted through the abdomen, above the pubic bone, into the bladder. It is a type of indwelling catheter; that is, it is left in the bladder and is attached to a drainage bag with tubing. Suprapubic catheters may be used in clients needing long-term catheterization or after certain types of surgeries. The insertion site (the opening on the abdomen) and the tubing must be cleaned daily with soap and water and covered with dry gauze. Follow the care plan and your assignment sheet.

Purposes of Catheters.

- Catheters often are used before, during, and after surgery to keep the bladder empty. This reduces the risk of accidental bladder injury during surgery, and after surgery, it prevents pressure on nearby organs that could be caused by a full bladder.
- Catheters also allow hourly urinary output measurements in critically ill people.
- Catheters are the last resort for managing incontinence, since they do not treat the cause of incontinence, and the risk of infection is high. However, some clients have wounds and pressure ulcers that must be protected from contamination by urine.
- Some clients are too weak or disabled to use the bedpan, commode, or toilet, for example, those who are dying. In them, catheters can promote comfort by managing incontinence.
- Catheters also have diagnostic uses, such as collecting sterile urine specimens and measuring *residual urine.* For such purposes, the catheter is inserted after the client voids.

As a support worker, you will be required to care for clients with indwelling catheters. Follow the guidelines listed in Box 31–4 to promote comfort and safety.

Drainage Systems

A closed drainage system is used for indwelling catheters (including suprapubic catheters) so that nothing enters the system from the catheter to the drainage bag. The urinary system must remain sterile, otherwise infection can occur when microbes enter the drainage system and travel up the tubing or catheter into the bladder and kidneys. A urinary tract infection can threaten the client's health and even life.

The drainage system consists of tubing and a drainage bag. Tubing attaches to the catheter at one end and the drainage bag at the other end. The bag hangs from the bed frame, chair, or wheelchair but must not touch the floor. The bag must always be lower than the client's bladder (see Figure 31–11 on page 592). Clients may feel embarrassed if the drainage bag can be seen by visitors. Carefully drape a bed sheet or robe over the drainage bag when visitors are present. Some clients wear leg bags when up and about. The bag is attached to the thigh or calf (see page 596), and the pant leg or the robe can cover it.

As stated earlier, ***it is important to never hang the drainage bag on a bed rail because when the bed rail is raised, the bag is at a higher level than the bladder.*** When the client walks, the bag must be held at a lower level than the bladder.

Measuring Urine Drainage. The urine drainage bag is emptied at routine times, according to your agency's policy. If you are responsible for this task, follow the guidelines to empty and measure the urine from a drainage bag:

- Always follow Standard Practices when handling any bodily fluids.
- Never use the measurements marked on the drainage bag to measure the amount of urine collected. These measurements are often inaccurate and unreliable.
- Unclip the drainage latch at the bottom of the bag, and pour the urine in the drainage bag into a measuring cup or a see-through graduated cup.
- Ensure that the drainage bag is clipped securely, and replace the drainage plug of the drainage bag.
- Place the see-through graduated cup or measuring cup on a flat surface to read the urine measurement. Try to read the measurement by looking at it as close to eye level as possible. Holding the measuring cup in the air will result in inaccurate measurements.
- After you have obtained your urine measurement, discard the urine down the toilet or bedpan flusher. Do not pour the urine down a

sink, as it would contaminate the sink and produce an unpleasant odour.

- Rinse and wash out the measuring cup, according to your agency's policy.

Accidental Disconnection. Sometimes drainage systems are disconnected accidentally. If that happens, re-attach the catheter and inform your supervisor immediately. Do not touch the ends of the catheter or tubing. Do the following:

- Wash your hands, and put on gloves.
- Wipe the end of the tube and the end of the catheter with antiseptic wipes. Use a separate wipe for the tube end and catheter end (Figure 30–10).
- Do not put the ends down. Do not touch the ends after you clean them.
- Connect the tubing to the catheter.
- Discard the wipes into a biohazard plastic bag.
- Remove the gloves, and practise proper hand hygiene.

Box 31–4 Guidelines for Caring for Clients With Indwelling Catheters

- Follow the rules of medical asepsis and Standard Practices.
- Make sure urine flows freely through the catheter or tubing. Tubing should not have kinks, and the client should not lie on the tubing.
- When the client is being moved, the catheter tube must remain slack, never taut or pulled.
- Make sure the catheter is connected to the drainage tubing. If the catheter and drainage tube become disconnected, follow the measures described above.
- Urine provides the ideal environment for the growth of microbes. If the drainage bag is higher than the bladder, urine can flow back into the bladder, and an infection can develop. ***Keep the drainage bag below the bladder*** to prevent urine from flowing backward into the bladder.
- Attach the drainage bag to the bed frame, to the back of a chair, or to the lower part of an IV pole. ***Never attach the drainage bag to the bed rail, otherwise the drainage bag is higher than the bladder when the bed rail is raised.***
- Move the drainage bag to the side of the bed to which the client will be turned. You must remember to move the drainage bag *before* turning the client.
- Do not let the drainage bag rest on the floor because this can contaminate the system.
- Coil the drainage tubing on the bed. Secure it to the bottom linen (Figure 31–11). Use a clip, tape, or a safety pin and rubber band, according to your employer policy. Tubing must not loop below the drainage bag.
- In women, secure the catheter to the inner thigh as in Figure 31–11, *A*, and in men, secure it to the thigh (Figure 31–11, *B*). This prevents excessive movement of the catheter and reduces friction at the insertion site. Secure the catheter with tape or other devices as ordered by the care plan. ***Many agencies no longer tape the catheters to the client. Always check your client's care plan and your agency's policy on this.***
- Check for leaks at the site where the catheter connects to the drainage bag. Report any leaks immediately.
- Provide catheter care, if ordered, once or twice a day. It includes cleaning the part of the tube that extends outside of the body. This helps prevent bladder or urethra infections (see *Giving Catheter Care* on page 593). Some employers consider perineal care sufficient. Catheter care is sometimes needed after bowel movements and when there is vaginal drainage. Follow the care plan.
- Provide perineal care daily, after bowel movements, and when vaginal drainage is present. Follow the care plan.
- Empty the drainage bag at the end of the shift or at intervals specified in the care plan. Measure and record the amount of urine (see *Emptying a Urinary Drainage Bag* on page 595). Report increases or decreases in the amount of urine.
- Use a separate measuring container for each client. This prevents the spread of microbes from one client to another.
- Do not let the drain or the drainage bag touch any surface.
- Immediately report any complaints of pain, burning, urge to urinate, or irritation. Also report the colour, clarity, and odour of urine and the presence of particles.
- Encourage fluid intake, as instructed by the care plan.

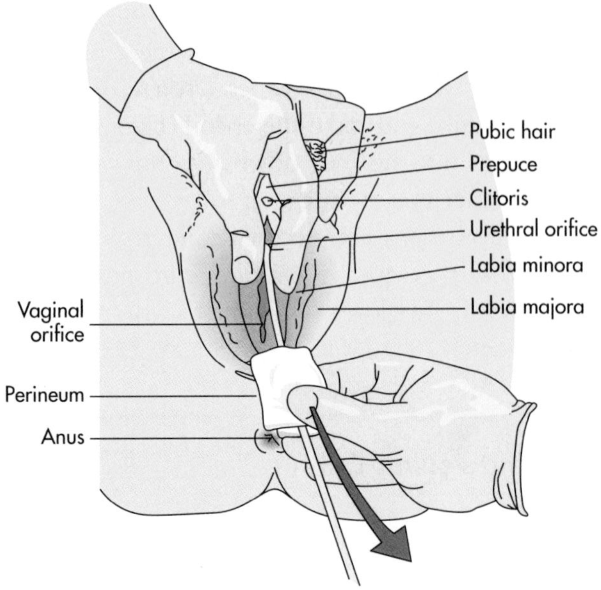

Figure 31–10 Hold the catheter near the meatus (insertion point). Clean the catheter starting at the meatus and moving down about 10 cm (4 in.).

Leg bags are replaced by drainage bags when the client is in bed. You will have to open the drainage system that was previously closed, while taking care to prevent microbes from entering the system. Review the principles of surgical asepsis in Chapter 20.

Some employers do not allow support workers to replace leg bags with drainage bags, as the risk of infection is high. If you are delegated to replace a leg bag with a drainage bag, make sure this procedure is part of your job description. You must be formally trained, supervised, and monitored. Follow employer policy and procedures.

Drainage bags are emptied, according to the care plan. Usually this task is completed:

- At the end of each shift
- When replacing a leg bag with a drainage bag
- When replacing a drainage bag with a leg bag
- When a leg bag is becoming full

In many instances, you will be required to measure the amount of urine that is in the drainage bag prior to emptying it. This is called ***measuring output*** (see page 507 for a description of how to measure intake and output [I&O]).

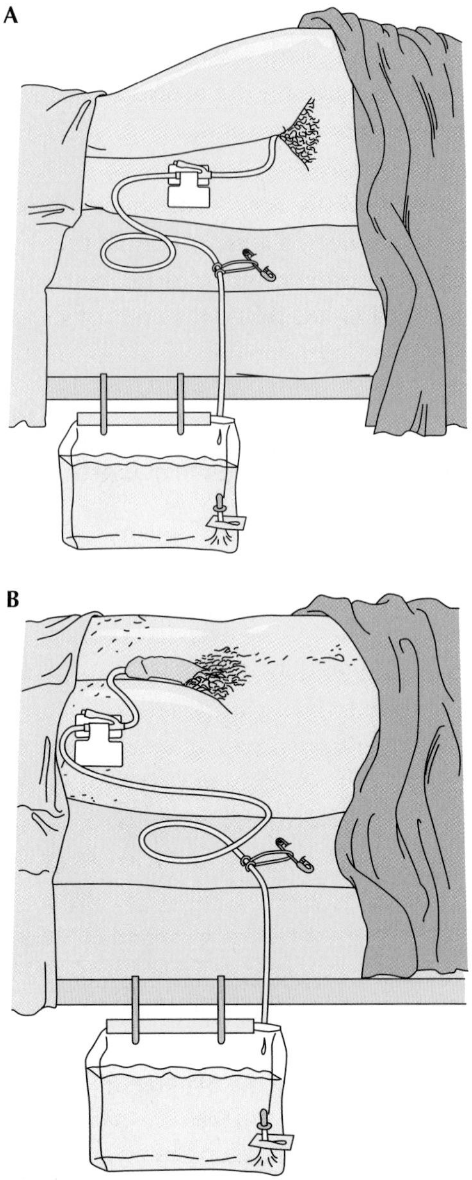

Figure 31–11 Securing catheters. **A,** The drainage tubing is secured to the female client's thigh to prevent it from being pulled. Enough slack is left on the catheter to prevent friction at the urethra. **B,** The catheter is secured to the male client's upper thigh leaving enough slack so that the client's penis is not being pulled.

Report and record the following:

- The amount of urine measured
- The colour, clarity, and odour of urine
- Particles in the urine
- Complaints of pain, burning, irritation, or the need to urinate
- Drainage system leaks

1 2 3 GIVING CATHETER CARE

Remember to promote:

• Dignity • Independence • Preferences • Privacy • Safety

Pre-Procedure

1 Identify the client, according to employer policy.
2 Explain the procedure to the client.
3 Practise proper hand hygiene.
4 Collect the following:
- Items for perineal care (page 544)
- Gloves
- Bed protector
- Bath blanket

5 Provide for privacy.
6 Raise bed to a comfortable working height. Follow the care plan for bed rail use.

Procedure

7 Lower the bed rail near you, if it is up.
8 Put on gloves.
9 Cover the client with a bath blanket. Fanfold top linens to the foot of the bed.
10 Drape the client for perineal care (see Figure 29–26 on page 545).
11 Fold back the bath blanket to expose the genital area.
12 Place the bed protector under the buttocks. Ask the client to flex the knees and raise the buttocks off the bed.
13 Give perineal care (see *Giving Female Care* to a Female Client on page 544 or *Giving Perineal Care to a Male Client* on page 546).
14 Apply soap to a clean, wet wash cloth.
15 Separate the labia (female) as in Figure 29–27 on page 546. Or retract the foreskin (uncircumcised male) as in Figure 29–29 on page 547. Check for presence of crusts, abnormal drainage, or secretions.
16 Hold the catheter near the meatus (insertion point).
17 Clean the catheter from the meatus down the catheter about 10 cm (4 in.) (see Figure 31–10). Clean downward, away from the meatus with one stroke. Do not tug or pull on the catheter. Repeat, as needed, with a clean area of the wash cloth. Use a clean wash cloth, if needed.
18 Rinse the catheter. Clean from the meatus down the catheter about 10 cm (4 in.). Clean downward, away from the meatus with one stroke. Do not tug or pull on the catheter. Repeat, as needed, with a clean area of the wash cloth. Use a clean wash cloth, if needed.
19 Secure the catheter. Coil and secure tubing (see Figure 31–11).
20 Remove the bed protector.
21 Cover the client. Remove the bath blanket.
22 Remove gloves. Practise proper hand hygiene.

Post-Procedure

23 Provide for safety and comfort.
24 Place the call bell within reach.*
25 Return the bed to its lowest position. Follow the care plan for bed rail use.*
26 Clean and return equipment to its proper place. Discard disposable items. (Wear gloves for this step.)
27 Remove privacy measures.
28 Follow employer policy for soiled linen.
29 Practise proper hand hygiene.
30 Report and record your actions and observations, according to employer policy.

*Steps marked with an asterisk may not apply in community settings.

1 2 3 CHANGING A DRAINAGE BAG TO A LEG BAG

Remember to promote:

• Dignity • Independence • Preferences • Privacy • Safety

Pre-Procedure

1 Identify the client, according to employer policy.
2 Explain the procedure to the client.
3 Practise proper hand hygiene.
4 Collect the following:
- Gloves
- Drainage bag and tubing
- Antiseptic wipes
- Bed protector
- Sterile cap and plug
- Catheter clamp
- Paper towels
- Bedpan
- Bath blanket

5 Arrange paper towels and equipment on the work area.
6 Provide for privacy.

Procedure

7 Have the client sit on the side of the bed.
8 Put on gloves.
9 Help the client lie down. Raise the bed to a comfortable working height.*
10 Cover the client with a bath blanket. Expose the catheter and drainage tubing. Place the bed protector under the leg.
11 Clamp the catheter (Figure 31–12) to prevent urine from draining from the catheter into the drainage tubing.
12 Let urine drain from below the clamp site into the drainage tubing. This empties the lower end of the catheter.
13 Open the antiseptic wipes. Set them on the paper towels.
14 Open the package with the sterile cap and plug. Set the package on the paper towels. Do not let anything touch the sterile cap or plug (Figure 31–13).
15 Open the package with the leg bag drainage tubing, and attach the drainage bag to the bed frame.
16 Disconnect the catheter from the drainage tubing. Do not let anything touch the ends.
17 Remove the cap from the leg bag drainage tubing. Do not let anything touch the ends.
18 Insert the end of the catheter into the leg bag drainage tubing.
19 Place the sterile cap on the end of the drainage bag tubing (Figure 31–14). (If you contaminate the tubing end, wipe it with an antiseptic wipe. Do so before you put the sterile cap on.)
20 Remove the clamp from the catheter.
21 Loop the tubing, and secure it to the client's leg.
22 Remove the drainage tubing from the bed. Place it in the bedpan.
23 Remove and discard the bed protector.
24 Cover the client. Remove the bath blanket.
25 Take the bedpan to the bathroom.
26 Drain the drainage bag into a measuring cup, make a note of the measurement, and empty the measuring cup into the toilet (see *Emptying a Urinary Drainage Bag* on page 595) and rinse it out.

Post-Procedure

27 Remove gloves. Practise proper hand hygiene.
28 Provide for safety and comfort.
29 Place the call bell within reach.*
30 Return the bed to its lowest position. Follow the care plan for bed rail use.*
31 Remove privacy measures.
32 Discard the drainage tubing and bag or clean the bag, according to employer policy.
33 Return the bedpan and other supplies to their proper place.
34 Report and record your actions and observations, according to employer policy.
35 Reverse the procedure to attach a drainage bag to the catheter.

*Steps marked with an asterisk may not apply in community settings.

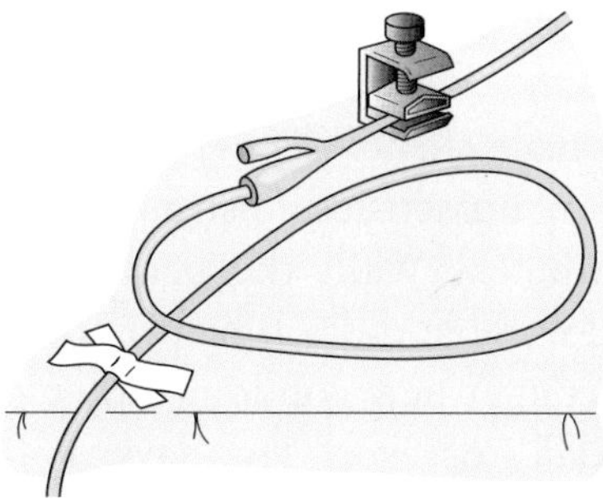

Figure 31–12 The catheter is clamped. The clamped catheter prevents urine from draining out of the bladder. The clamp is applied to the catheter, not to the drainage tubing.

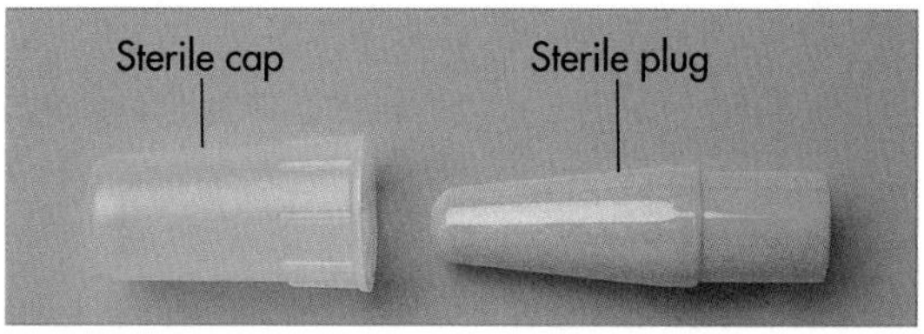

Figure 31–13 Sterile cap and catheter plug. The inside of the cap is sterile. It is inserted into the catheter. Touch only the end of the plug.

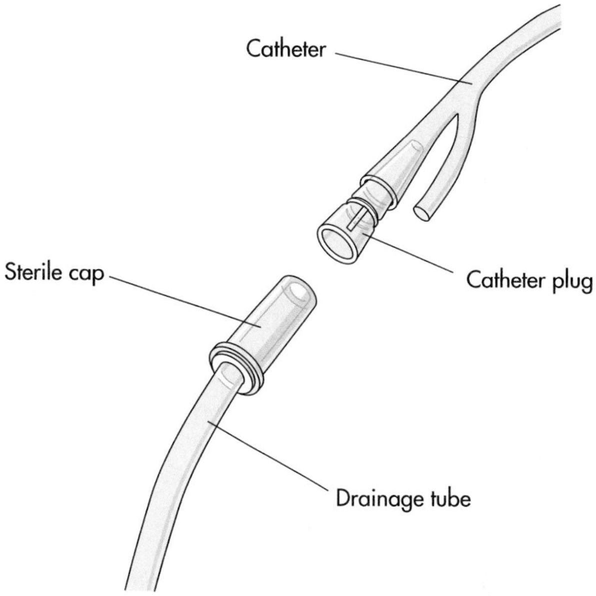

Figure 31–14 Sterile plug inserted into the end of the catheter. A sterile cap is on the end of the drainage tube.

1 2 3 EMPTYING A URINARY DRAINAGE BAG

Remember to promote:

• **D**ignity • **I**ndependence • **P**references • **P**rivacy • **S**afety

Pre-Procedure

1 Identify the client, according to employer policy.
2 Explain the procedure to the client.
3 Practise proper hand hygiene.
4 Collect the following:
- Graduate (measuring container)
- Gloves
- Paper towels

5 Provide for privacy.

Procedure

6 Put on gloves.
7 Place the paper towel on the floor. Place the graduate on top of the paper towel.
8 Position the graduate under the drainage bag drain.
9 Open the clamp on the drainage bag.
10 Allow all the urine to drain into the graduate. Do not let the drain touch the graduate (Figure 31–15).
11 Close and position the clamp (see Figure 31–11 on page 592).
12 Measure the urine.
13 Remove and discard the paper towel.
14 Dispose of the urine in the toilet.
15 Rinse the graduate, and dispose of the rinse water in the toilet.
16 Return the graduate to its proper place.
17 Remove gloves. Practise proper hand hygiene.
18 Record the time and amount on the intake and output (I&O) record (see Chapter 27).

Post-Procedure

19 Remove privacy measures.
20 Report and record the amount and other observations (Figure 31–16). Follow employer policy.

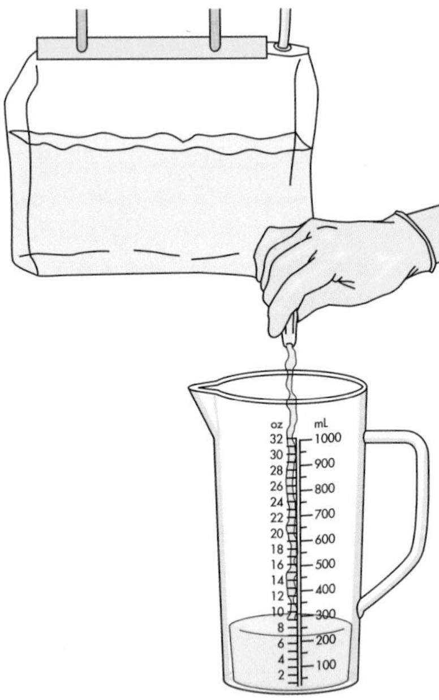

Figure 31–15 Open the clamp on the drainage bag, and direct the drain into the measuring container. The drain must not touch the inside of the container.

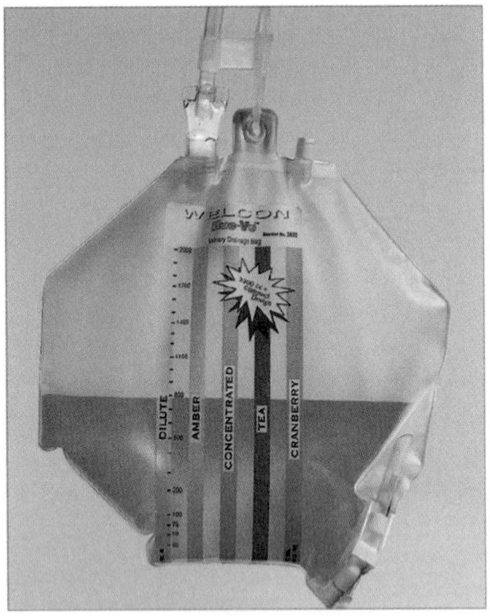

Figure 31–16 This urinary drainage bag has a comparison chart for the urine colour. **Courtesy:** Welcon, Inc., Fort Worth, TX.

The Condom Catheter

Condom catheters—also called *external catheters* and *urinary sheaths*—are often used in incontinent male clients. A **condom catheter** is a soft sheath that slides over the penis. Tubing connects the condom catheter and the drainage bag; leg bags are used in many male clients (Figure 31–17).

Follow the manufacturer's instructions to apply a condom catheter.. Wash the penis thoroughly with soap and water and dry it before applying the condom catheter. A new condom catheter is usually applied daily or every few days. Follow the care plan.

Elastic tape secures the catheter in place. Use the elastic tape packaged with the condom catheter. Some condom catheters come with the elastic tape already lining the catheter. The elastic tape expands according to changes in penis size, which allows blood flow to the penis. ***Never use adhesive tape to secure condom catheters. As adhesive tape does not expand, blood flow to the penis would be cut off, harming the penis.*** Follow medical asepsis and Standard Practices when removing and applying condom catheters.

Report and record the following:

- Reddened or open areas on the penis
- Swelling of the penis
- Colour, clarity, and odour of urine
- Particles in the urine

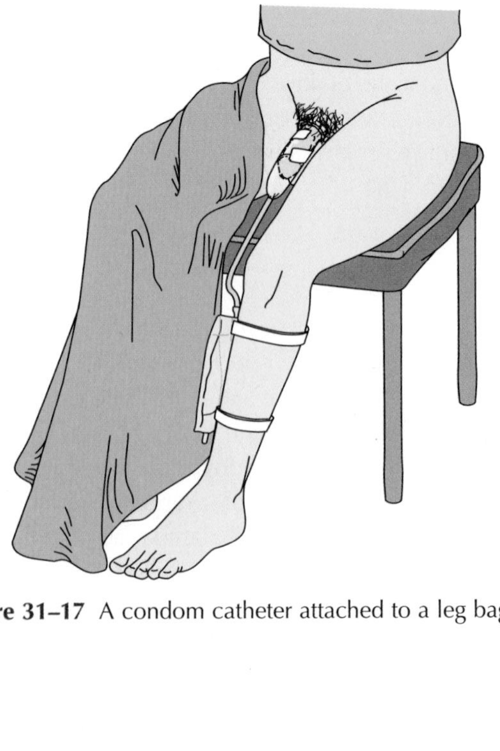

Figure 31–17 A condom catheter attached to a leg bag.

1 2 3 REMOVING AND APPLYING A CONDOM CATHETER

Remember to promote:

• Dignity • Independence • Preferences • Privacy • Safety

Pre-Procedure

1 Identify the client, according to employer policy.
2 Explain the procedure to the client.
3 Practise proper hand hygiene.
4 Collect the following:
- Condom catheter
- Elastic tape
- Drainage bag/leg bag
- Cap for the drainage bag
- Basin of warm water
- Soap
- Towel and wash cloths
- Bath blanket
- Gloves
- Bed protector
- Paper towels

5 Place paper towels on the work area. Arrange equipment on top of the paper towels.
6 Provide for privacy.
7 Raise the bed to a comfortable working height. Follow the care plan for bed rail use.*

Procedure

8 Lower the bed rail near you, if it is up.
9 Cover the client with a bath blanket. Lower top linens to the knees.
10 Ask the client to raise his buttocks off the bed, or turn him onto his side away from you.
11 Slide the bed protector under his buttocks.
12 Have the client lower his buttocks, or turn him onto his back.
13 Secure the drainage bag to the bed frame (not the bed rails), or have a leg bag ready. Close the drain.
14 Expose the genital area.
15 Put on gloves.
16 Remove the condom catheter:
   a Remove the tape. Roll the sheath off the penis.
   b Disconnect the drainage tubing from the condom. Cap the drainage tube.
   c Discard the tape and condom.
17 Provide perineal care (see *Giving Perineal Care to a Male Client* on page 546). Observe the penis for skin breakdown or irritation.
18 Remove the protective backing from the condom. This exposes the adhesive strip.
19 Hold the penis firmly. Roll the condom onto the penis. Leave a 2.5-cm (1-in.) space between the penis and the catheter end (Figure 31–18).
20 Secure the condom with elastic tape. Apply tape in a spiral (see Figure 31–18). Do not apply tape completely around the penis.
21 Connect the condom to the drainage tubing. Coil excess tubing on the bed (see Figure 31–11 on page 592), or attach a leg bag.
22 Remove the bed protector.
23 Remove gloves. Practise proper hand hygiene.
24 Cover the client. Remove the bath blanket.

Post-Procedure

25 Provide for safety and comfort.
26 Place the call bell within reach.*
27 Return the bed to its lowest position. Follow the care plan for bed rail use.*
28 Remove privacy measures.
29 Practise proper hand hygiene. Put on clean gloves.
30 Measure and record the amount of urine in the bag. Clean or discard the drainage bag, according to employer policy.
31 Discard disposable items.
32 Clean and return the wash basin and other equipment. Return items to their proper places.
33 Remove gloves. Practise proper hand hygiene.
34 Report and record your actions and observations, according to employer policy.

*Steps marked with an asterisk may not apply in community settings.

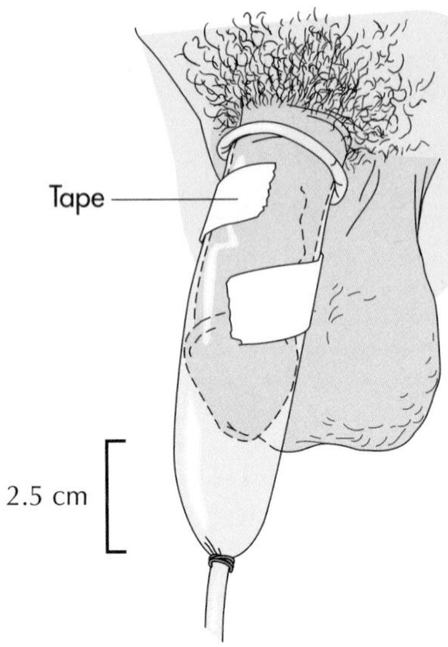

Figure 31–18 A condom catheter applied to the penis. There is a 2.5 cm (1 in.) space between the penis and the end of the catheter. Apply tape in a spiral fashion to secure the condom catheter to the penis.

BLADDER TRAINING

Bladder training programs have been developed for clients with urinary incontinence. Some clients need bladder training after indwelling catheter removal. After having an indwelling catheter for some time, they may have lost muscle tone in their bladder and their bladder may no longer be able to stretch sufficiently to hold urine. These clients may have urinary incontinence until their bladder tone is restored. Voluntary control of urination is the goal of the bladder training program, which is part of the care plan. You are required to assist with bladder training, as directed by your supervisor and the care plan.

There are two basic methods for bladder training:

- The client uses the toilet, commode, bedpan, or urinal at scheduled times. The client is given 15 or 20 minutes to initiate voiding. The guidelines for maintaining normal urination are followed. The normal position for voiding is assumed if possible. Privacy is important. Help the client relax, and provide encouragement. This can help the client succeed.
- The client has a catheter. The catheter is clamped to prevent urine from draining out of the bladder (see Figure 31–12 on page 595). Usually the catheter is clamped for 1 hour at first, and eventually it is clamped for 3 to 4 hours at a time. Urine drains from the bladder when the catheter is unclamped. When the catheter is removed, you will encourage the client to void every 3 to 4 hours or as directed by your supervisor and the care plan.

COLLECTING URINE SPECIMENS

Urine specimens (samples) are collected for urine tests. Physicians use test results to make a diagnosis or evaluate treatment. Follow the guidelines in Box 31–5 when collecting specimens.

Box 31–5 Guidelines for Collecting Urine Specimens

- Explain the procedure to the client thoroughly and ensure their cooperation.
- Follow the rules of medical asepsis and Standard Practices. Wear gloves when collecting specimens.
- Use a clean container for each specimen.
- Use a container appropriate for the specimen.
- Label the container accurately. Write the client's full name, address or room and bed number, date, and time the specimen was collected. If preprinted labels are used, place a label on the container.
- Do not touch the inside of the container or lid.
- Collect the specimen at the time specified.
- Ask the client not to defecate during specimen collection. The specimen must not contain feces.
- Ask the client to dispose of used toilet tissue in the toilet and to ensure that the specimen does not contain tissue.
- Put the lid on the specimen container.
- Place the specimen container in a plastic bag for transportation. In a facility, take the specimen and requisition slip to the laboratory or storage area. In community settings, follow your supervisor's instructions for storing the specimen. Tell the client or family members where the specimen is stored. Follow your supervisor's instructions for sending the specimen to the laboratory.
- Report and record the following observations:
  - Difficulty in obtaining the specimen
  - Colour, clarity, and odour of urine
  - Particles in the urine
  - Complaints of pain, burning, urgency, dysuria, or other problems

The Random Urine Specimen

The random urine specimen is collected for a urinalysis. No special measures are needed, and the specimen is collected at any time. Often clients can collect the specimen themselves, but weak and very ill clients will need assistance.

It is difficult to collect any type of urine specimen from the elderly and the young, and especially from people who are unable to follow instructions, for example, clients who have dementia or a severe mental disorder. Your supervisor will have suggestions on how you may successfully obtain specimens from these clients, while ensuring that their right to dignity and privacy are respected.

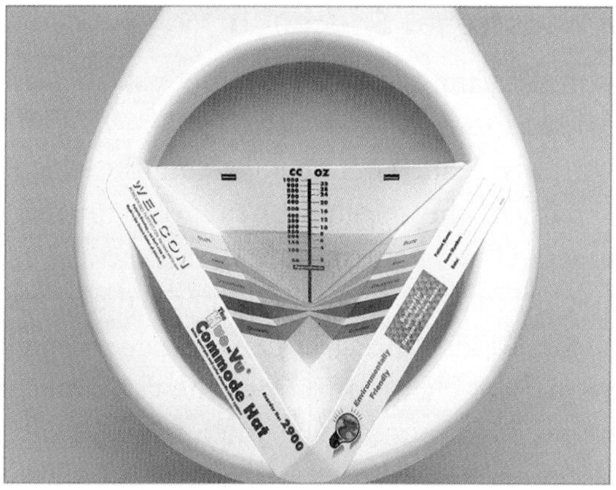

Figure 31–19 The specimen pan is placed on the rim of the toilet. It has a colour chart for urine. **Courtesy:** Welcon, Inc., Fort Worth, TX.

1 2 3 COLLECTING A RANDOM URINE SPECIMEN

Remember to promote:

• Dignity • Independence • Preferences • Privacy • Safety

Pre-Procedure

1 Identify the client, according to employer policy.
2 Explain the procedure to the client.
3 Practise proper hand hygiene.
4 Collect the following:
- Bedpan and cover, urinal, or specimen pan (Figure 31–19)
- Specimen container and lid
- Label
- Gloves
- Plastic bag

Procedure

5 Label the container.
6 Put the container and lid in the bathroom.
7 Provide for privacy.
8 Put on gloves.
9 Ask the client to urinate in the receptacle (the bedpan, urinal, or specimen pan). Remind him or her to put toilet tissue into the wastebasket or toilet, not in the bedpan or specimen pan.
10 Take the receptacle to the bathroom.
11 Measure urine if intake and output (I&O) is ordered.
12 Pour about 120 mL (4 oz) of urine into the specimen container. Dispose of excess urine.
13 Place the lid on the specimen container. Put the container in the plastic bag.
14 Clean and return the receptacle to its proper place.
15 Help the client with hand washing.
16 Remove gloves. Practise proper hand hygiene.

Post-Procedure

17 Provide for safety and comfort.
18 Place the call bell within reach.*
19 Follow the care plan for bed rail use.*
20 Remove privacy measures.
21 Practise proper hand hygiene.
22 Report and record your actions and observations, according to employer policy.
23 Follow your supervisor's instructions for storage and transportation of the specimen.

*Steps marked with an asterisk may not apply in community settings.

The Midstream Specimen

The midstream specimen is also called a *clean-voided specimen* or a *clean-catch specimen*. The perineal area is cleaned before collecting the specimen. This reduces the number of microbes in the urethral area. The client starts to void into the toilet, bedpan, urinal, or commode. Then the stream is stopped and a sterile specimen container is held in position. The client voids into the container until the required amount of specimen is obtained.

Stopping the stream of urine midway is hard for many people. You may need to hold the container in place and collect the specimen after the client starts to void.

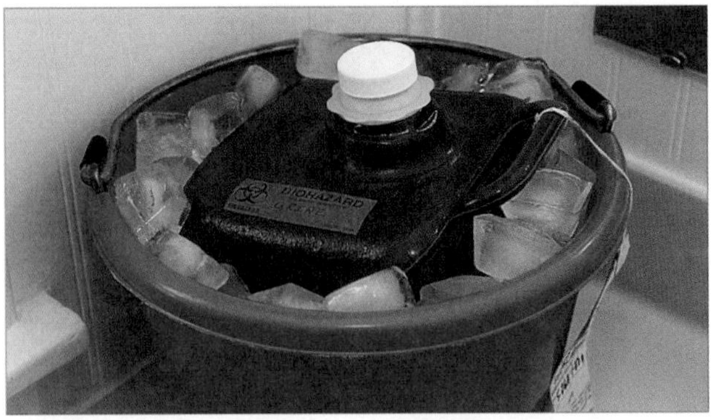

Figure 31–20 To preserve the 24-hour urine specimen, the urine container may be stored in a bucket of ice. **Source:** Birchenall J., and Streight, E. (1997). *Mosby's textbook for the home care aide* (p. 315). St. Louis: Mosby.

The 24-Hour Urine Specimen

All urine voided during a 24-hour period is collected for a 24-hour urine specimen. The collected urine is kept chilled on ice or refrigerated during the collection period (Figure 31–20) to prevent the growth of microbes. A preservative is added to the collection container for some tests.

To start the collection, the client voids, and this first voiding is discarded. *All* voidings during the next 24 hours are then collected. The client and staff must have a clear understanding of the procedure and the test period. In home care settings, the client and primary caregiver need to collect some of the specimen on their own. Make sure they understand what needs to be done. Contact your supervisor if they are unsure. Follow the guidelines for collecting urine specimens.

Collecting Specimen from an Infant or Child

Sometimes specimens are needed from infants and children who are not toilet trained. A collection bag is applied over the urethra. A parent or another staff member assists you if the child is agitated. This procedure may also be adapted for clients who are in wheelchairs or who are incontinent.

1 2 3 COLLECTING A MIDSTREAM SPECIMEN

Remember to promote:

• **D**ignity • **I**ndependence • **P**references • **P**rivacy • **S**afety

Pre-Procedure

1 Identify the client, according to employer policy.
2 Explain the procedure to the client.
3 Practise proper hand hygiene.
4 Collect the following:
- Clean-voided specimen kit (with antiseptic solution)
- Label
- Disposable gloves
- Sterile gloves (if not in the kit)
- Bedpan, urinal, or commode, if needed
- Plastic bag
- Supplies for perineal care

5 Provide for privacy.
6 Label the container.
7 Wear gloves, and provide perineal care. Remove gloves. Practise proper hand hygiene.
8 Open the sterile kit. Use sterile technique (see Chapter 20).
9 Put on the sterile gloves.
10 Pour the antiseptic solution over the cloth intended for perineal care.

(continued on page 601)

1 2 3 COLLECTING A MIDSTREAM SPECIMEN (cont'd)

Procedure

11 Open the sterile specimen container. Do not touch the inside of the container or lid. Set the lid down so that the inside is up.

12 *For a female: Clean the perineum with the cloth intended for perineal care:*

- **a** Spread the labia with your thumb and index finger. Use your nondominant hand. (This hand is now contaminated. It must not touch anything sterile.)
- **b** Clean down the urethral area from front to back. Use a clean corner of the cloth intended for perineal care for each stroke.
- **c** Keep the labia separated to collect the urine specimen (steps 14 to 17).

13 *For a male: Clean the penis with the cloth intended for perineal care:*

- **a** Hold the penis with your nondominant hand. (This hand is now contaminated. It must not touch anything sterile.)
- **b** Clean the penis starting at the urethral opening. Use the cloth intended for perineal care and clean in a circular motion.
- **c** Keep holding the penis until the specimen is collected (steps 14 to 17).

14 Ask the client to void into the toilet, bedpan, commode, or urinal (as well as into a sterile bedpan, commode container, or urinal).

15 Hold the specimen container to collect the stream of urine. Keep the labia separated, if possible.

16 Collect about 30 to 60 mL of urine (1 to 2 oz).

17 Remove the specimen container before the client stops voiding.

18 Let go of the labia or penis.

19 Allow the client to finish voiding into the toilet, bedpan, commode, or urinal.

20 Put the lid on the specimen container. Touch only the outside of the container or lid.

21 Wipe the outside of the container.

22 Place the container in a plastic bag.

23 Provide toilet tissue after the client finishes voiding.

24 Remove and empty the bedpan, commode container, or urinal.

25 Clean the bedpan, urinal, or commode container and other items. Return the equipment to its proper place.

26 Remove gloves. Practise proper hand hygiene.

27 Put on clean gloves.

28 Help the client with hand washing.

29 Remove gloves. Practise proper hand hygiene.

Post-Procedure

30 Follow steps 17 through 23 in *Collecting a Random Urine Specimen* on page 599.

1 2 3 COLLECTING A URINE SPECIMEN FROM AN INFANT OR CHILD

Remember to promote:

- **D**ignity • **I**ndependence • **P**references • **P**rivacy • **S**afety

Pre-Procedure

1 Identify the child, according to employer policy.

2 Explain the procedure to the child and parents.

3 Practise proper hand hygiene.

4 Collect the following:

- Collection bag
- Wash basin
- Cloth intended for perineal care
- Bath towel
- Two diapers, one with a 2.5-cm (1 in.) hole cut into the bottom (over the area of the child's urethra)
- Specimen container
- Gloves
- Plastic bag
- Scissors

5 Provide for privacy.

(continued on page 602)

COLLECTING A URINE SPECIMEN FROM AN INFANT OR CHILD (cont'd)

Procedure

6 Remove and dispose of the diaper.
7 Clean the perineal area with the cloth intended for perineal care. Use a new corner for each stroke. Rinse and dry the area.
8 Practise proper hand hygiene.
9 Position the child on the back. Flex the child's knees, and separate the legs.
10 Remove the adhesive backing from the collection bag.
11 Apply the bag to the perineum. Do not cover the anus (Figure 31–21).
12 Put a new diaper on the child.
13 Pull the collection bag through a 2.5 cm (1 in.) hole in the bottom of the diaper.
14 Practise proper hand hygiene.
15 Raise the head of the crib, if allowed. This helps urine to collect in the bottom of the bag.
16 Raise the crib rail.
17 Check the bag periodically to see if the child has voided. (Wear gloves, and provide for privacy.)
18 Provide for privacy if the child has urinated.
19 Put on gloves.
20 Lower the crib rail.
21 Remove the diaper.
22 Remove the collection bag gently.
23 Press the adhesive surfaces of the bag together, or transfer the urine to the specimen container through the drainage tab.
24 Clean the perineal area, rinse, and dry well.
25 Put a new diaper on the child.
26 Remove gloves. Practise proper hand hygiene.

Post-Procedure

27 Provide for safety and comfort. Raise the crib rail.
28 Remove privacy measures.
29 Write the requested information on the specimen container. Place the container in the plastic bag.
30 Clean and return the equipment to its proper place. Discard disposable items. (Wear gloves for this step.)
31 Practise proper hand hygiene.
32 Report and record your actions and observations, according to employer policy.
33 Follow your supervisor's instructions for storage and transportation of the specimen.

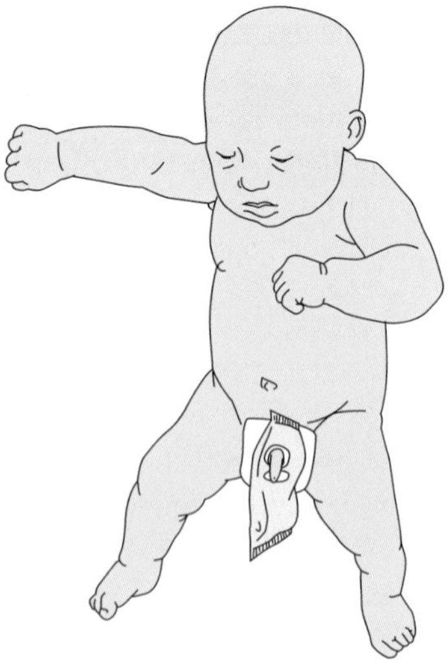

Figure 31–21 A disposable collection bag is applied to the perineal area of the infant. Urine collects in the bag for a specimen.

TESTING URINE

You may be asked to perform simple urine tests—for example, for measuring pH, glucose, ketones, and blood—using reagent strips. Straining urine for stones is another simple test. A physician orders the type and frequency of urine tests, and you must ensure accuracy when performing the tests. Ensure that the reagent strips are not outdated by checking the expiry date on the container. Promptly report the results, according to employer policy.

- ***Testing pH***—Urine pH measures indicate whether urine is acidic or alkaline. Changes in normal pH (4.6 to 8.0) occur due to illness, foods, and medications. A routine urine specimen is needed.

- ***Testing for glucose and ketones***—In diabetes, the pancreas does not secrete enough insulin (see Chapter 18), which is needed by the body to use sugar for energy. If not used by the body, sugar builds up in the blood, and some of it will appear in the urine. **Glucosuria** means sugar (*glucos, glycos*) in the urine (*uria*). The diabetic client may also have **acetone (ketone bodies)** in the urine. These appear in urine because of the rapid breakdown of fat for energy, which happens when the body cannot use sugar. Urine is also tested for ketones. These tests are usually done four times a day: 30 minutes before each meal (ac) and at bed-time (hs). The physician uses the test results to regulate the client's medication and diet.

  You should follow the instructions that are printed on the side of the reagent bottle to test for glucose and ketones. You should first dip the reagent strip into the urine and wait for the specified length of time. The reagent strip may turn certain colours, and you need to compare the colour that is on the reagent strip with that on the reagent strip bottle (see Using Reagent Strips below).
- ***Testing for blood***—Normal urine is free of blood. Injury and disease can cause blood (*hemat*) to appear in the urine (*uria*). This is called **hematuria.** Sometimes blood can be seen in the urine, and at other times it is not visible (*occult*), So a routine urine specimen is needed.

Using Reagent Strips

Reagent strips are chemically treated "dipsticks." They have different sections that change colour when they react with urine. To use a reagent strip, dip the strip into the urine specimen, and compare the colour on the strip with the colour chart on the bottle (Figure 31–22). You will probably need a watch or a clock to keep track of the time, according to the instructions. Instructions vary depending on the test. Your supervisor will tell you how to perform the urine test that has been ordered by the physician.

1 2 3 TESTING URINE WITH REAGENT STRIPS

Remember to promote:

• Dignity • Independence • Preferences • Privacy • Safety

Pre-Procedure

1 Identify the client, according to employer policy.
2 Explain the procedure to the client.
3 Practise proper hand hygiene.
4 Put on gloves.
5 Collect the following:
- Urine specimen (check with your supervisor for method to obtain)
- Reagent strip, as ordered
- Gloves

Procedure

6 Remove a strip from the bottle. Recap the bottle immediately. The cap must be on tight.
7 Dip the reagent strip into the specimen.
8 Remove the strip after the correct amount of time (follow manufacturer's instructions).
9 Tap the strip gently against the container to remove excess urine.
10 Wait the required amount of time (follow manufacturer's instructions).
11 Compare the colour on the strip with the colour chart on the bottle. Read the results.
12 Discard disposable items and the specimen.

Post-Procedure

13 Clean and return equipment to its proper place.
14 Remove gloves. Practise proper hand hygiene.
15 Report and record the results and other observations, according to employer policy.

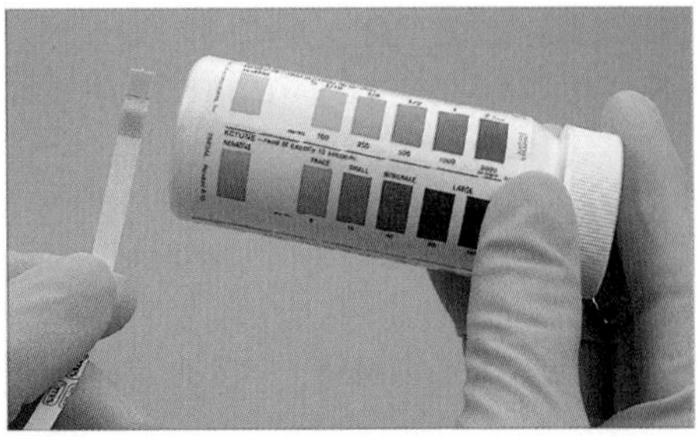

Figure 31–22 Reagent strip for sugar and ketones.

You must read the manufacturer's instructions before you begin. Always check the date on the container. Do not use the product past its expiry date.

Straining Urine

Stones (*calculi*) can develop in the kidneys, ureters, or bladder. Stones vary in size—some are the size of

1 2 3 STRAINING URINE

Remember to promote:

• **D**ignity • **I**ndependence • **P**references • **P**rivacy • **S**afety

Pre-Procedure

1 Identify the client, according to employer policy.
2 Explain the procedure to the client. Also, explain that the urinal, bedpan, commode, or specimen pan is used for voiding.
3 Practise proper hand hygiene.
4 Collect the following:
- Strainer, and 10 x 10 cm. (4 x 4 in) gauze
- Specimen container
- Urinal, bedpan, commode, or specimen pan
- Two labels stating that all urine has been strained
- Gloves
- Plastic bag

Procedure

5 Arrange items in the client's bathroom. Place the specimen pan in the toilet.
6 Place one label in the bathroom. Place the other near the bed.
7 Put on gloves.
8 Offer the bedpan or urinal, or assist the client to the bedside commode or bathroom.
9 Provide for privacy.
10 Tell the client to call you after voiding.
11 Remove gloves. Practise proper hand hygiene.
12 Return when the client calls you. Knock before entering the room.
13 Practise proper hand hygiene. Put on gloves.
14 Place the strainer or gauze over the specimen container.
15 Pour urine into the specimen container. Urine passes through the strainer or gauze (Figure 31–23).
16 Discard the urine.
17 Place the strainer or gauze in the container if any crystals, stones, or particles appear.
18 Provide perineal care, if needed.
19 Clean and return equipment to its proper place.
20 Remove soiled gloves. Practise proper hand hygiene. Put on clean gloves.
21 Help the client with hand washing.
22 Remove gloves. Practise proper hand hygiene.

Post-Procedure

23 Provide for safety and comfort.
24 Place the call bell within reach.*
25 Follow the care plan for bed rail use.*
26 Remove privacy measures.
27 Label the specimen container with the requested information. Put the container in the plastic bag. (Wear gloves for this step.)
28 Practise proper hand hygiene.
29 Report and record your actions and observations, according to employer policy.
30 Follow your supervisor's instructions for storage and transportation of the specimen.

*Steps marked with an asterisk may not apply in community settings.

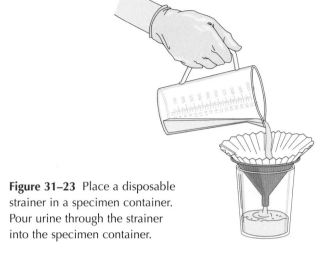

Figure 31–23 Place a disposable strainer in a specimen container. Pour urine through the strainer into the specimen container.

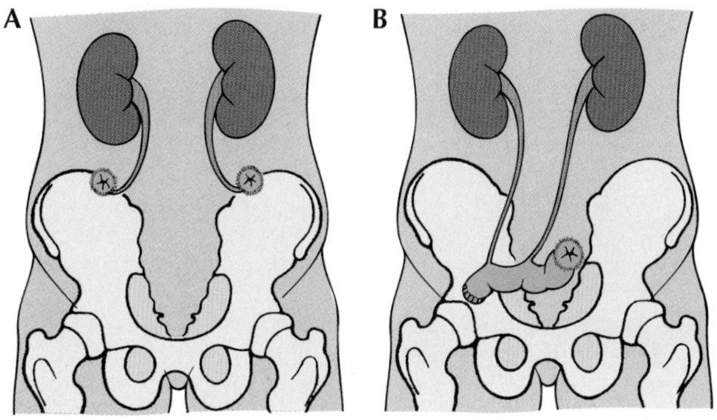

Figure 31–24 Ureterostomies. **A,** Both ureters are brought through the skin onto the abdomen. The client has two stomas, one for each ureter. **B,** The ileal conduit. A small section of the small intestine is removed and one end sutured closed to form an artificial bladder. The other end is brought through the skin onto the abdomen to form a stoma. The ureters are attached to this part of the small intestine, and urine collects in the newly created artificial bladder, and drains through the stoma. **Source:** Beare, P.A., & Myers, J.L. (1998). *Principles and practices of adult health nursing* (3rd ed.). St. Louis: Mosby.

a pinhead; others are the size of an orange. Stones that cause severe pain and damage to the urinary system may require surgical removal. Some stones exit the body through urine. When the care plan calls for the client's urine to be strained, all the urine is poured through a disposable strainer. If any stones are found, they are sent to the laboratory for examination.

THE CLIENT WITH A URETEROSTOMY OR ILEAL CONDUIT

Sometimes the bladder is surgically removed to treat cancer and bladder injuries. Since provision must be made for urine to leave the body, a new pathway—called a *urinary diversion*—is created.

There are many types of urinary diversions, the most common one being an **ostomy,** which is the surgical creation of an artificial opening. A **ureterostomy** is an artificial opening (*stomy*) between the ureter (*uretero*) and the abdomen. The artificial opening is called a **stoma** (Figure 31–24). Stomas do not have nerve endings, so they are not painful. In the case of an **ileal conduit**, an artificial bladder is fashioned out of a section of the ileum, and urine drains from the ureters into the newly created artificial bladder and then through the stoma.

An ostomy appliance (which some call a "pouch") is applied over the stoma (Figure 31–25). The ostomy appliance is a disposable plastic bag that is adhered to the skin around the stoma, and urine drains into it. The ostomy appliance is replaced anytime it leaks, as leaking urine can cause skin irritation, skin breakdown, and infection. Leaks often cause clients to worry about odours and embarrassing wetness. Immediately after this type of surgery, the client will receive care from a nurse, but you may be required to care for clients with longstanding ureterostomies, and the client assists with care as much as he or she is able to.

It is your responsibility to provide good skin care to the client with an ureterostomy. Skin breakdown, which can occur around the stoma, is caused by the draining urine as well as by the adhesive side of the ostomy appliance and must be prevented. You need to report and record changes in the client's skin around the stoma.

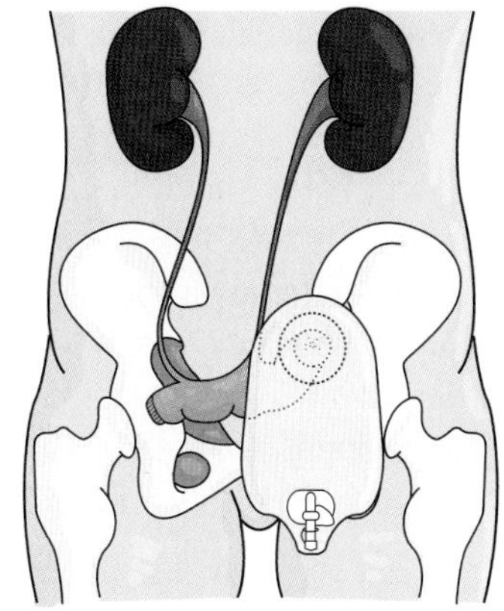

Figure 31–25 Ureterostomy pouch.

1 2 3 CHANGING A URETEROSTOMY POUCH

Remember to promote:

• **D**ignity • **I**ndependence • **P**references • **P**rivacy • **S**afety

Pre-Procedure

1 Identify the client, according to employer policy.
2 Explain the procedure to the client.
3 Practise proper hand hygiene.
4 Collect the following:
- Clean pouch with skin barrier
- Skin barrier (if not part of pouch)
- Pouch clamp, clip, or wire closure
- Clean ostomy belt (if used)
- Four to eight 5 x 5 cm. (2 × 2 in.) gauze squares
- Adhesive remover
- Cloth for applying adhesive remover
- Bedpan with cover
- Waterproof pad
- Bath blanket
- Toilet tissue
- Wash basin
- Bath thermometer
- Soap or cleansing agent, according to the care plan
- Pouch deodorant
- Paper towels
- Gloves
- Disposable bag

5 Arrange the paper towels on the work area. Place items on top of paper towels.
6 Provide for privacy.
7 Raise bed to a comfortable working height. Follow the care plan for bed rail use.*

Procedure

8 Lower the bed rail near you if up. (*Note*: This procedure can be performed while the client is sitting on the toilet, provided the client is able to sit for any length of time without assistance, and it is preferred by the client and the support worker).
9 Cover the client with a bath blanket. Fanfold linens to the foot of the bed.
10 Place the waterproof pad under the client's buttocks.
11 Put on gloves.
12 Disconnect the pouch from the belt. Remove the belt.
13 Remove the pouch gently. Gently push the skin down and away from the skin barrier. Place the pouch in the bedpan.
14 Place one or two gauze squares over the stoma to absorb the urine.
15 Wipe around the stoma with toilet tissue or a gauze square. Place soiled tissue in the bedpan. Discard gauze squares into the disposable bag.
16 Apply adhesive remover on a piece of cloth. Clean around the stoma to remove any remaining skin barrier. Clean from the stoma outward.
17 Cover the bedpan, and take it to the bathroom. (If bed rails are used, raise them before leaving the bedside.)
18 Measure the urine. Report any abnormality in the urine. Empty the pouch and bedpan into the toilet. Note the colour, clarity, and odour of the urine. Put the pouch in the disposable bag.
19 Remove gloves. Practise proper hand hygiene. Put on clean gloves.
20 Fill the wash basin with warm water. (Measure the temperature of the water with a bath thermometer. Check the care plan for the correct temperature to use.) Place the basin on the work area on top of paper towels. Lower the bed rail near you, if it is up.
21 Clean the skin around the stoma with water. Rinse and pat dry. Use soap or other cleansing agent.
22 Observe the stoma and skin around the stoma. Report any irritation or skin breakdown.
23 Apply the skin barrier, if it is a separate device.
24 Put a clean ostomy belt on the client (if a belt is worn).
25 Add deodorant to the new pouch.
26 Remove adhesive backing on the pouch.
27 Remove the gauze square that was used to absorb the urine from the stoma.
28 Centre the pouch over the stoma. The drain points downward.

(continued on page 607)

1 2 3 CHANGING A URETEROSTOMY POUCH

Procedure (cont'd)

29 Press around the skin barrier so that the pouch seals to the skin. Apply gentle pressure from the stoma outward.
30 Maintain pressure for 1 to 2 minutes.
31 Connect the belt to the pouch (if a belt is worn).
32 Remove the waterproof pad.
33 Remove gloves. Practise proper hand hygiene. (If the client uses bed rails, raise the bed rails before leaving the bedside.)
34 Cover the client. Remove the bath blanket.

Post-Procedure

35 Provide for safety and comfort.
36 Place the call bell within reach.*
37 Return the bed to its lowest position. Follow the care plan for bed rail use.*
38 Remove privacy measures.
39 Clean the bedpan, wash basin, and other equipment. Put on gloves for this step.
40 Return equipment to its proper place.
41 Discard the disposable bag, according to employer policy. Follow employer policy for soiled linen.
42 Remove gloves. Practise proper hand hygiene.
43 Report and record your actions and observations, according to employer policy.

*Steps marked with an asterisk may not apply in community settings.

COMPASSIONATE CARE

Elimination is a very personal and private act. Be sensitive to the client's feelings of embarrassment or discomfort. You should try to make the client feel better about accepting your help. Tell your supervisor if the client refuses care. It is your responsibility to promote the client's dignity, independence, preferences, privacy, and safety (see the *Providing Compassionate Care: Assisting Clients with Elimination* box.)

PROVIDING COMPASSIONATE CARE

Assisting Clients With Elimination

- **Dignity.** Never do anything to increase the client's embarrassment. Always be encouraging and positive when providing care. Do not show disgust at the sights or odours associated with elimination and ostomy care. Remember that your nonverbal behaviours and expressions reveal your feelings. For example, do not wrinkle your nose or grimace while you are assisting the client.
- **Independence.** Respond promptly to all requests for help with elimination, as the need may be urgent. Believe clients when they ask for help, even if they just used the toilet, bedpan, urinal, or commode. Your prompt response gives the client some sense of control.
- **Preferences.** Respect the client's preferences, whenever possible. For example, some male clients may want to use the urinal sitting up, while some others may prefer to do it lying down.
- **Privacy.** Provide as much privacy as possible. Lack of privacy may inhibit the client and interfere with elimination. Pull privacy curtains, and close doors, shades, and drapes. Ask visitors or family members to step out of the room. If allowed by the care plan, leave the room after assisting the client to the bathroom or providing a bedpan, urinal, or commode. Or, to be immediately available, stand just outside the door, stand on the other side of the privacy curtain, or stay by the client's side but look away, if safe to do so. Ask your supervisor for advice on ways to protect the client's privacy.
- **Safety.** Do not leave clients who are weak or dizzy. If you can leave the client and a call bell is available, make sure it is always within reach. Stay close enough so that you can hear the client's call for help. Remember to follow Standard Practices.

REVIEW

Answers to these questions are at the bottom of the page.

Circle the BEST answer.

1. **Which of the following statements is true?**
   - A. Urine normally has a foul odour.
   - B. A client normally voids about 1500 mL a day.
   - C. Urine is normally cloudy and amber or brown in colour.
   - D. Micturition usually occurs after going to bed and before rising.

2. **Which will help normal elimination?**
   - A. Helping the client assume a supine position for urination
   - B. Talking to the client while they are trying to void
   - C. Helping the client to the bathroom or commode or providing the bedpan or urinal as soon as requested
   - D. Always staying with the client who is using a bedpan

3. **The best position for using a bedpan is:**
   - A. Fowler's position
   - B. The supine position
   - C. The prone position
   - D. The side-lying position

4. **After using the urinal, the male client should:**
   - A. Put the urinal on the bedside stand
   - B. Hook the urinal from his bedrail
   - C. Put the urinal on the overbed table
   - D. Empty the urinal

5. **Urinary incontinence:**
   - A. Is permanent
   - B. Requires urine tests
   - C. Requires good skin care
   - D. Is always treated with an indwelling catheter

6. **Which of the following is your responsibility when supporting Mrs. Jones, who has an indwelling catheter?**
   - A. Hook the drainage bag from the bedrails
   - B. Keep the drainage bag below the level of her bladder
   - C. Hide the tubing by placing it underneath the client who is sitting
   - D. Insist that the client's urge to void is all in her head

7. **Mr. Powers has a condom catheter. You should apply elastic tape:**
   - A. Completely around the penis
   - B. To the inner thigh
   - C. To the abdomen
   - D. In a spiral fashion

8. **The goal of bladder training is to:**
   - A. Remove the catheter
   - B. Allow the client to walk to the bathroom
   - C. Gain voluntary control of urination
   - D. Heal the stoma

9. **When collecting a random urine specimen into a bedpan, you should do the following:**
   - A. Label the bedpan with the requested information
   - B. Wash the client's perineum first with antiseptic soap
   - C. Collect the specimen at the time specified
   - D. Allow the client to use toilet tissue and then place it in the bedpan

10. **The perineum is cleaned immediately before collecting:**
    - A. Random specimens
    - B. Midstream specimens
    - C. 24-hour urine specimens
    - D. Random and 24-hour urine specimens

11. **A 24-hour urine specimen involves:**
    - A. Collecting all urine voided by a client during a 24-hour period
    - B. Collecting a random specimen every hour for 24 hours
    - C. Not allowing the client to urinate for 24 hours
    - D. Testing the urine for sugar and blood

12. **Straining of urine is done to find:**
    - A. Hematuria
    - B. Stones
    - C. Nocturia
    - D. Urgency

13. **Which of the following should you do for the client who has a ureterostomy?**
    - A. Pull off the adhesive ostomy appliance every hour
    - B. Tape the ostomy appliance down whenever it leaks
    - C. Report any changes in the skin around the stoma
    - D. Provide incontinence briefs

Answers: 1.B, 2.C, 3.A, 4.B, 5.C, 6.B, 7.D, 8.C, 9.C, 10.B, 11.A, 12.B, 13.C

CHAPTER 32

Fecal Elimination

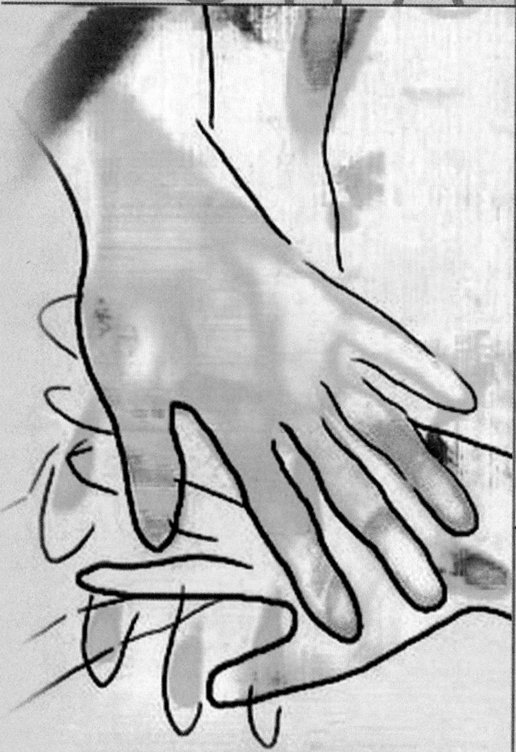

OBJECTIVES

- Define the key terms listed in this chapter.
- Describe normal stools and the normal pattern and frequency of bowel movements.
- List the observations to make about bowel movements.
- Identify the factors that affect fecal elimination.
- Describe common fecal elimination problems.
- Describe the measures that promote comfort and safety during defecation.
- Describe bowel training.
- Explain why enemas are given.
- Know the common enema solutions.
- Describe the comfort and safety measures for giving enemas.
- Explain the purpose of rectal tubes.
- Describe how to care for a client with an ostomy pouch.
- Explain why stool specimens are collected.
- Perform the procedures described in this chapter.

key terms

colostomy An artificial opening (*stomy*) between the colon (*colo*) and the abdominal wall.

constipation A condition in which bowel movements are less frequent than usual; the stool is hard, dry, and difficult to pass.

defecation The process of excreting feces from the rectum through the anus; bowel movement.

dehydration The excessive loss of water from tissues.

diarrhea The frequent passage of liquid stools.

enema The introduction of fluid into the rectum and lower colon.

fecal impaction The prolonged retention and accumulation of feces in the rectum.

fecal incontinence The inability to control the passage of feces and gas through the anus. Also known as *anal incontinence.*

feces The semisolid mass of waste products in the colon.

flatulence The excessive formation of gas in the stomach and intestines.

flatus Gas or air from the stomach or intestines passed through the anus.

ileostomy An artificial opening (*stomy*) between the ileum (small intestine; *ileo*) and the abdominal wall.

melena Dark, tarry stools containing decomposing blood that is usually an indication of bleeding in the upper part of the alimentary canal and especially in the esophagus, stomach, and duodenum.

ostomy The surgical creation of an artificial opening.

peristalsis The alternating contraction and relaxation of intestinal muscles.

stoma A surgically created opening through which a portion of the body cavity is brought to the outside environment.

stool Excreted feces.

suppository A cone-shaped, solid medication that is inserted into a body opening; it melts at body temperature.

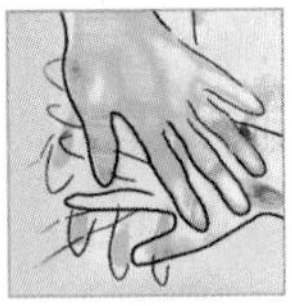

Like urinary elimination, fecal elimination—the excretion of wastes from the digestive system—is a basic physical need (see Chapter 14). Many factors affect bowel elimination—for example, privacy, personal habits, age, diet, exercise and activity, fluids, and medications. Promoting normal bowel elimination is important, as problems related to any of these factors may occur easily. As a support worker, you are required to assist clients in meeting their elimination needs.

Bowel elimination problems and treatments for them may be uncomfortable, frustrating, embarrassing, and humiliating for the client. Be sensitive and offer emotional support (see the *Providing Compassionate Care: Assisting Clients with Elimination* box). Follow Standard Practices and the infection control guidelines listed in Box 31–1 on page 580.

NORMAL BOWEL MOVEMENTS

Foods and fluids that are partially digested in the stomach are called *chyme,* and these pass from the stomach into the small intestine and enter the large intestine (large bowel or colon), where the fluids are absorbed. Chyme thus becomes more solid in consistency. **Feces** are the semi-solid mass of waste products in the colon.

Feces move through the intestine by **peristalsis**—the alternating contraction and relaxation of intestinal muscles. Feces move through the colon to the rectum, where they are stored until they are excreted from the body. **Defecation** (bowel movement [BM]) is the process of excreting feces from the rectum through the anus. **Stool** is the term for excreted feces.

Normally, people have a bowel movement every day or every 2 to 3 days. Some people have even two or three bowel movements a day. People defecate at different times—for example, after breakfast or in the evening. Many older adults expect to have a bowel movement every day, and the slightest irregularity causes them concern. Reassurance from the nurse can help relieve their anxiety about this.

Stools are normally brown in colour. However, bleeding in the stomach and small intestine will cause the stools to appear black or tarry, and bleeding in the lower colon and rectum or eating beets will make the stools appear red. A diet that contains a lot of green vegetables can cause green stools. Some diseases and infections can cause clay-coloured, white, pale, orange-coloured, or green-coloured stools.

Stools are normally soft, formed, moist, and shaped like the rectum and have a characteristic odour, which is caused by bacterial action in the intestines. Certain foods and medications also cause odours in the stools.

Observations

Your careful observations about the client's stools are important for the care planning process. When you observe abnormal stools, ask the nurse (in a facility setting) and your supervisor (in a community setting) to also observe them. You need to report any abnormalities in the following: colour, amount, consistency, odour, shape, size, frequency, and any complaints of pain.

FACTORS AFFECTING BOWEL MOVEMENT

Normal, regular defecation, including frequency, consistency, colour, and odour of stools, can be affected by many factors:

- ***Privacy***—Like urination, defecation is a private act. Lack of privacy deters many people from defecating despite having the urge. Odours associated with defecation are embarrassing. Some clients ignore the urge to defecate when others are present, which can lead to constipation.
- ***Personal habits***—Many clients routinely have a bowel movement after breakfast. Some do relaxing activities—for example, drinking a hot beverage, reading a book or newspaper, or taking a walk—which make defecation easier.
- ***Diet***—A well-balanced diet and bulk are needed to promote regular bowel movement. High-fibre foods, such as fruits, vegetables, and whole grain cereals and breads, leave a residue that provides needed bulk. However, many older adults do not eat enough fruits and vegetables, as some do not have teeth or have poorly fitting dentures, which makes chewing difficult. Some clients think they will not be able to digest fruits and vegetables, so they refuse to eat them. Bran, prunes, and juices help prevent constipation. Certain foods can cause diarrhea or constipation—for example, milk causes constipation in some people and diarrhea in others. Other foods and chocolate can cause similar reactions. Spicy foods can irritate the intestines, resulting in frequent stools or diarrhea. Gas-forming foods, such as onions, beans, cabbage, cauliflower, radish, and cucumber, stimulate peristalsis, and increased peristalsis results in defecation. But many people avoid gas-forming foods because they cause stomachache or bloating.
- ***Fluids***—Stool consistency depends on the amount of water absorbed in the colon. The amount of fluid ingested, urine output, and vomiting can affect stool consistency. Feces become hard and dry when large amounts of water are absorbed by the colon and when fluid intake is poor. Hard, dry feces move through the intestines at a slower rate, resulting in constipation. Drinking 6 to 8 glasses of water every day promotes normal bowel movement. Warm fluids—coffee, tea, hot cider, and warm water—increase peristalsis.
- ***Activity***—Exercise and activity maintain muscle tone and stimulate peristalsis. Irregular elimination and constipation often occur due to inactivity and bed rest resulting from disease, surgery, injury, and aging.

- ***Medications***—On the one hand, medications can prevent constipation or control diarrhea; on the other hand, some medications can cause diarrhea or constipation as side effects. Medications for pain relief often cause constipation, and antibiotics to fight or prevent infection often cause diarrhea. Diarrhea occurs when the antibiotics kill normal flora (bacteria which are always present) in the large intestine. Normal bacteria are necessary for stools to form.
- ***Aging***—As people age, feces tend to pass through their intestines at a slower rate, resulting in constipation. Some clients may lose bowel control but incontinence is *not* a normal consequence of aging. Some older adults may not completely empty the rectum. They often need to defecate again 30 to 45 minutes after the first bowel movement.
- ***Disability***—Some clients with disabilities are not able to control their bowel movements and defecate whenever feces enter the rectum. Such clients need a bowel training program (page 614), with the goal of having a bowel movement at the same time each day.

COMFORT AND SAFETY

The care plan lists comfort and safety measures to meet the client's elimination needs. These measures may involve diet, fluids, and exercise. The actions in Box 32–1 are routinely practised to promote comfort and safety during defecation.

COMMON PROBLEMS

Common problems that affect normal bowel movement include constipation, fecal impaction, diarrhea, fecal incontinence, and flatulence.

Constipation

Constipation is a condition in which bowel movements are less frequent than usual, and the stool is hard, dry, and difficult to pass, causing the client to strain to have a bowel movement. Clients may complain of abdominal discomfort, a feeling of fullness, or increased gas (flatus). Stools could be large in size or marble-sized. Large-sized stools cause pain as they pass through the anus. Constipation occurs when feces move through the intestine slowly, allowing more time for water absorption in the colon. Common causes include a low-fibre diet, ignoring

Box 32–1 Comfort and Safety During Defecation

- Assist the client to the toilet or commode, or provide the bedpan, as soon as the client requests it.
- To promote privacy, wheel the client into the bathroom on the commode, if possible. Position the commode over the toilet. Support workers must, however, be cautious transporting clients on commodes, as these normally have small wheels that make them difficult to manoeuvre over uneven surfaces. They also do not have adequate, if any, safety belts to prevent the client from tipping forward. Smaller clients and male clients who have a pendulous scrotum are at risk of having their bottoms rubbed or pinched between the commode seat and the toilet bowl.
- Provide for privacy. Ask visitors or family members to leave the room. Close doors, pull privacy curtains, and close window curtains, blinds, or shades.
- Make sure the bedpan is warm.
- Position the client in the normal sitting position.
- Cover the client for warmth and privacy.
- Allow enough time for defecation. Do not rush the client.
- Place the call bell (in facilities) and toilet tissue within the client's reach.
- Stay with the client if he or she is weak or unsteady.
- Leave the room if the client can be left alone. Stay within hearing distance.
- Provide perineal care.
- Dispose of stools promptly. This reduces odours and prevents the spread of microbes.
- Assist the client with hand washing after elimination.
- If the client has fecal incontinence, follow the care plan, which will tell you when to assist with elimination.
- Follow Standard Practices.

the urge to defecate, decreased fluid intake, inactivity, medications, aging, and certain diseases.

A client may be too embarrassed to tell you that he or she is constipated. If you note that the client is having fewer bowel movements than normal, inform your supervisor. If a client is prone to constipation, it can be helpful to keep a record of how often this happens. Common measures used to prevent or relieve constipation include changing the diet (increasing fibre, increasing fluids) and encouraging physical activity. The physician may order medications or enemas for prolonged constipation.

As a support worker, you play a very important role in preventing constipation in your clients by ensuring adequate activity, fluids, privacy, and so on. Prevention of constipation is much better than treatment.

It is essential to accurately chart your client's bowel movements during your shift to enable team members to recognize and treat constipation in a timely manner.

Fecal Impaction

Fecal impaction is the prolonged retention and accumulation of feces in the rectum. Feces are hard or puttylike in consistency. Fecal impaction results if constipation is not relieved. The person with fecal impaction is unable to defecate. More water gets absorbed from the already hard feces. If left untreated, a fecal impaction can lead to complete bowel obstruction, which will require surgery.

The client may try many times to defecate. If a client shows any of the following signs or symptoms of a fecal impaction, report it at once:

- Abdominal discomfort and swelling
- Cramping
- A feeling of fullness or pain in the rectum
- Nausea or vomiting
- Fever
- Increased urge or decreased ability to urinate
- Liquid feces seeping from the anus. Seepage may look like diarrhea but is, in fact, liquid feces passing around the hardened fecal mass.

A physician or nurse performs a digital (finger) exam to check for impaction. In Alberta, support workers' competencies include rectal touch, which is done by inserting a gloved finger into the rectum and feeling for a hard mass. The client may feel uncomfortable after the procedure. The physician may order medications and enemas to remove the impaction, and on occasion, the physician or nurse may remove the fecal mass manually with a gloved finger. This is called *digital removal of an impaction.*

Diarrhea

Diarrhea is the frequent passage of liquid stools. Feces move through the intestines rapidly, which reduces the time for fluid absorption in the colon. The need to defecate is urgent, and some clients may not be able to get to a bathroom in time. Abdominal cramping, nausea, and vomiting may also occur.

Causes of diarrhea include infections, certain medications, foods that irritate the stomach, and pathogens in food and water. Diet and medications reduce peristalsis and stop the diarrhea. You need to:

- Assist with the client's elimination needs promptly.
- Dispose of stools promptly. This prevents odours and the spread of microbes.
- Provide good skin care, as liquid feces and frequent wiping with toilet tissue can irritate the skin, which may lead to skin breakdown and pressure ulcers.

Fluid lost through diarrhea must be replaced, as otherwise **dehydration**—the excessive loss of water from tissues—will result. Signs and symptoms of dehydration include oliguria (scant amount of urine), dark urine, pale or flushed skin, dry skin, coated tongue, cracked lips, sunken eyes, thirst, weakness, dizziness, and confusion. Falling blood pressure and increased pulse and respirations are serious signs, which may precede death. The care plan tells you how to meet the client's fluid needs. The physician orders intravenous fluids in severe cases (see *Focus on Children: Dehydration* and *Focus on Older Adults: Dehydration* boxes).

Pathogens often cause diarrhea, so preventing the spread of infection is important. Always follow Standard Practices when you come in contact with stools.

focus on ›› CHILDREN

Dehydration

The bodies of infants and young children contain large amounts of water. Infants and children are at risk for dehydration, and death from dehydration can occur quickly in them. Report any liquid or watery stool immediately. Note the number of wet diapers in 24 hours. Infants wet less when dehydrated. Fewer than six wet diapers in 24 hours may indicate that an infant is dehydrated. Report any concerns immediately.

focus on ›› OLDER ADULTS

Dehydration

Older adults also are at risk for dehydration, as the amount of body water decreases with aging. Diarrhea is therefore very serious in older adults and any signs of diarrhea should be reported immediately, as death can result from unrecognized and untreated dehydration.

Fecal Incontinence

Fecal incontinence (or **anal incontinence**) is the inability to control the passage of feces and gas through the anus due to intestinal and nervous system diseases, injuries, fecal impaction, diarrhea, and some medications. Fecal incontinence can also occur because of delayed requests for help to use the bathroom, commode, or bedpan.

Clients with mental health problems, dementia, or cognitive disorders (see Chapters 34 and 35) may not recognize the urge to defecate, and as a result, some may soil themselves, the furniture, and the walls. In such situations, a common problem encountered by support workers is resistance to care from clients, so it may be difficult to get the client cleaned up. Follow the client's care plan. Also, talk to your supervisor if you have problems getting the client cleaned up.

Flatulence

Gas and air are normally found in the stomach and intestines and are expelled through the mouth (belching, eructating) and the anus. Gas and air passed through the anus is called **flatus**. **Flatulence** is the excessive formation of gas or air in the stomach and intestines. Common causes are:

- Swallowing air while eating and drinking, especially when chewing gum, eating quickly, drinking through a straw, and drinking carbonated beverages. Tense or anxious people tend to swallow large amounts of air when drinking.
- Bacterial action in the intestines
- Gas-forming foods (onion, beans, cabbage, cauliflower, radish, cucumber)
- Constipation
- Bowel and abdominal surgeries
- Medications that decrease peristalsis

If flatus is not expelled, the intestines distend, that is, they swell or enlarge due to the pressure of the gases. Abdominal cramping or pain (sometimes severe), shortness of breath, a swollen abdomen, belching, burping, and eructating can occur. "Bloating" is a common complaint. Exercise, walking, and the left side-lying position often produce flatus. Physicians may order enemas, medications, or rectal tubes to relieve flatulence.

BOWEL TRAINING

Bowel training has two goals:

- To gain control of bowel movement
- To develop a regular pattern of elimination, which will prevent fecal impaction, constipation, and fecal incontinence.

The urge to defecate is usually felt after a meal, usually after breakfast. The client's usual time of day for a bowel movement is noted on the care plan, and the use of the toilet, commode, or bedpan should be offered at this time. Factors that promote elimination are part of the care plan and bowel training program. These include a high-fibre diet, increased fluids, warm fluids, activity, and privacy. Your supervisor will tell you about a client's bowel training program.

The physician may order a suppository to stimulate defecation. A **suppository** is a cone-shaped, solid medication that is inserted into a body opening. It eventually dissolves at body temperature. A nurse inserts a rectal suppository into the rectum, or the client applies it himself or herself, and you may assist, as needed (see Chapter 40). A bowel movement occurs after about 30 minutes. It takes time for the suppository to dissolve and work in the body.

ENEMAS

An **enema**—the introduction of fluid into the rectum and lower colon—is ordered by physicians to remove feces and to relieve constipation or fecal impaction. Clients with severely limited mobility or who are paralyzed are at risk for these problems. Enemas also are ordered to clean the bowel of feces before certain surgeries or radiographic procedures. Sometimes enemas are ordered to relieve excessive flatulence and intestinal distension.

Enemas are usually safe procedures, and often clients can give themselves enemas at home. However, enemas can be dangerous for older adults and those with certain heart and kidney diseases. Enemas are invasive and involve inserting a tube into a body opening. Therefore, giving an enema is a delegated task (see Chapter 5). You may or may not be allowed to give enemas. If you are delegated to give one, make sure of the following:

- Provincial or territorial laws and your employer's policies allow you to perform the procedure. Policies vary among different regions of the country.
- The procedure is in your job description.
- You have the necessary education and training.
- You have reviewed the procedure with a nurse.
- A nurse is available to answer questions and to supervise you.

Comfort and safety measures should be practised when giving an enema. Follow the guidelines in Box 32–2.

Box 32–2 Comfort and Safety Measures for Giving Large-Volume Enemas

- Measure the temperature of the solution with a bath thermometer—usually 40.5°C (105°F) for adults. Your supervisor and the care plan tell you what temperature to use.
- Give the amount of solution ordered by the physician and specified in the care plan—usually 500 to 1000 mL.
- Position the client, as directed by your supervisor and the care plan. Sims' position on the client's left side is preferred. Some clients cannot be placed in Sims' position, so it is acceptable to place the client on the left side with the right leg as close to 90 degrees at the knee and hip as possible.
- Ask your supervisor and check your employer's policies about the depth of insertion of the enema tubing. In adults, the tube is usually inserted 7.5 to 10 cm (3 to 4 in.). Stop if you feel resistance, the client complains of pain, or bleeding occurs.
- Lubricate the enema tip before inserting it.
- Ask your supervisor about how high the enema bag should be raised. For adults, it is usually held 30 cm (12 in.) above the level of the anus.
- Force air out of the enema tubing before inserting it into the anus. Do this by dribbling a small amount of water from the tubing into a bedpan before insertion.
- Administer the enema solution slowly. Usually it takes 10 to 15 minutes to give 750 to 1000 mL.
- Hold the enema tube in place while administering the solution.
- Ask your supervisor how long the client should retain the enema solution. The length of time depends on the amount and type of solution.
- Make sure the bathroom is available when the client needs to defecate.
- A nurse should observe the enema results.
- Make sure you report the lack of returns from the enema.
- Follow Standard Precautions.

Enema Solutions

A physician orders the enema solution. The kind of solution ordered depends on the purpose for the enema:

- ***Tap water enema***—water obtained from a faucet.
- ***Soap suds enema*** *(SSE)*—3 to 5 mL (½ to 1 teaspoon) of castile soap added to 500 to 1000 mL of tap water.
- ***Saline enema***—5 to 10 mL (1 to 2 teaspoons) of table salt added to 500 to 1000 mL of tap water.
- ***Oil retention enema***—mineral oil or commercial oil is used.
- ***Microlax enema***—about 120 mL (4 oz) of solution.
- ***Mayo enema*** (baking soda, granulated sugar, and water)—still used in some care facilities; only given by a nurse.

Other enema solutions may be ordered, for example, a fleet enema (there are two types of fleet enemas—sodium phosphates (most common) and mineral oil). Consult your supervisor and your employer's procedure manual to safely prepare and administer enemas. Do not administer enemas that contain medications, as only nurses are allowed to give these enemas.

The Cleansing Enema

Cleansing enemas clean the bowel of feces and flatus and relieve constipation and fecal impaction. They are also needed before certain surgeries and diagnostic procedures.

The physician may order a soap suds, tap water, or saline enema and may order *enemas until clear*. This means that enemas are given until the return solution is clear and free of feces. Ask your supervisor about the required number of enemas. Employer policy may allow repeating cleansing enemas only two or three times.

Tap water enemas can be dangerous. The large intestine may absorb some of the water into the bloodstream, which may create fluid imbalance in the body. A tap water enema should be given only once and not repeated, since that can increase the risk of excessive fluid absorption. The tap water enema takes effect in 15 to 20 minutes.

Soap suds enemas may irritate the bowel's mucous lining. Repeated enemas can damage the bowel, as can using more than 3 to 5 mL (1 teaspoon) of castile soap or stronger soap. The soap suds enema takes effect in about 10 to 15 minutes.

The saline enema solution is similar to body fluid. However, some of the salt solution may be absorbed, which can also cause fluid imbalance. When there is excess salt in the body, the body retains water. The saline enema takes effect in about 15 to 20 minutes (see the *Focus on Children: Saline Enemas* box).

The Commercial Enema

Commercial enemas stimulate and distend the rectum and cause defecation. They are often ordered to relieve constipation or when complete cleansing of the bowel is not needed.

Manufacturers prepare and package the commercial enema that is ready to administer. The solution is usually administered at room temperature. To give the enema, squeeze and roll up the plastic bottle from the bottom. Do not release pressure on the bottle, as that would cause the solution to be drawn from the rectum back into the bottle.

Encourage the client to retain the solution until he or she feels the urge to defecate. The enema usually takes 5 to 10 minutes to take effect. Remaining in Sims' on the left side helps the client retain the enema longer.

focus on
›› CHILDREN

Saline Enemas

Only saline enemas are used in children. The amount of enema solution varies for infants and children. If you are delegated to give an enema to a child, your supervisor will give you the necessary instructions.

1 2 3 GIVING A CLEANSING ENEMA TO AN ADULT

Remember to promote:

• **D**ignity • **I**ndependence • **P**references • **P**rivacy • **S**afety

Pre-Procedure

1 Identify the client, according to employer policy.
2 Explain the procedure to the client.
3 Perform hand hygiene.
4 Collect the following:
- Disposable enema kit as directed by your supervisor (enema bag, tube, clamp, and waterproof pad)
- Bath thermometer
- Waterproof pad
- Water-soluble lubricant
- Gloves
- Material for enema solution: 3 to 5 mL (1 teaspoon) castile soap or 5 to 10 mL (1 to 2 teaspoons) salt
- Toilet tissue
- Bath blanket
- IV pole
- Robe and nonskid footwear
- Bedpan or commode
- Paper towels

5 Provide for privacy.
6 Raise the bed to a comfortable working height. Follow the care plan for bed rail use.*

Procedure

7 Lower the bed rail near you, if it is up.
8 Cover the client with a bath blanket. Fanfold top linens to the foot of the bed.
9 Position the IV pole so that the enema bag is 30 cm (12 in.) above the anus or is at a height specified in the care plan.
10 Raise the bed rail, if used.
11 Prepare the enema:
a Close the clamp on the tube.
b Adjust water flow until it is lukewarm.
c Fill the enema bag for the amount ordered.
d Measure water temperature. For adults it is usually 40.5°C (105°F).
e Prepare the enema solution as directed in the care plan.
i. Saline enema: add 5 to 10 mL (1 to 2 teaspoons) of salt
ii. Soapsuds enema: add 3 to 5 mL (1 teaspoon) of castile soap
iii. Tap-water enema: add nothing to the water
f Stir the solution with the bath thermometer. Scoop off any suds in SSEs.
g Seal the bag.
h Hang the bag on the IV pole.
12 Lower the bed rail near you, if it is up.
13 Position the client on the left side.
14 Put on gloves.
15 Place waterproof pad under the buttock.
16 Expose the anal area.
17 Place the bedpan behind the client.
18 Position the enema tube in the bedpan.
19 Remove the cap from the enema tubing.
20 Open the clamp. Let the solution flow through the tube to remove air. Clamp the tube.
21 Lubricate the tube 7.5 to 10 cm (3 to 4 in.) from the tip.
22 Separate the buttocks to see the anus.
23 Ask the client to take a deep breath through the mouth.
24 Insert the tube gently 7.5 to 10 cm (3 to 4 in.) into the rectum when the client is exhaling (Figure 32–1). Stop if the client complains of pain, if you feel resistance, or if bleeding occurs.
25 Check the amount of solution in the bag.
26 Unclamp the tube. Administer the solution slowly (Figure 32–2).
27 Ask the client to take slow, deep breaths. This helps the client relax.
28 Clamp the tube if the client needs to defecate, has cramping, or starts to expel solution. Unclamp when symptoms subside.
29 Administer the amount of solution ordered. Stop if the client cannot tolerate the procedure.
30 Clamp the tube before it is empty. This prevents air from entering the bowel.

(continued on page 618)

1 2 3 GIVING A CLEANSING ENEMA TO AN ADULT

Procedure (cont'd)

31 Hold toilet tissue around the tube and against the anus. Remove the tube.
32 Discard the toilet tissue into the bedpan.
33 Wrap the tubing tip with paper towels. Place it inside the enema bag.
34 Help the client onto the bedpan. Raise the head of the bed, or help the client into a sitting position. Raise the bed rail, if used, or assist the client to the bathroom or commode. The client should wear a robe and nonskid footwear when up. The bed should be in the lowest position.
35 Place the call bell (in facilities) and toilet tissue within reach. Remind the client not to flush the toilet.
36 Discard disposable items.
37 Remove gloves. Perform hand hygiene.
38 Leave the room if the client can be left alone. Stay within hearing distance.
39 Return when the client calls. Knock before entering.
40 Perform hand hygiene. Put on gloves. Lower the bed rail, if it is up.
41 Provide perineal care, as needed.
42 Observe results of the enema for amount, colour, consistency, and odour. Call your supervisor to observe the results (in a facility).
43 Remove the bed protector.
44 Empty, clean, and disinfect the bedpan or commode. Flush the toilet. Return items to their proper place.
45 Remove gloves. Perform hand hygiene.
46 Help the client with hand washing. Wear gloves, if needed.
47 Return top linens, and remove the bath blanket.

Post-Procedure

48 Provide for safety and comfort.
49 Place the call bell within reach.*
50 Return the bed to its lowest position. Follow the care plan for bed rail use.*
51 Remove privacy measures.
52 Follow employer policy for soiled linen and used supplies. Wear gloves for this step.
53 Perform hand hygiene.
54 Report and record your actions and observations, according to employer policy.

*Steps marked with an asterisk may not apply in community settings.

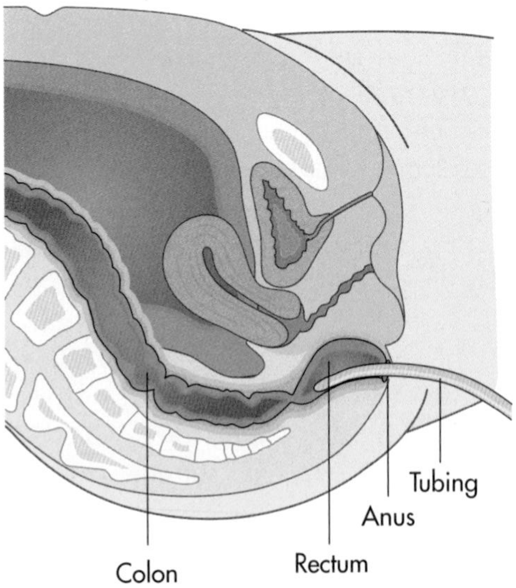

Figure 32–1 Enema tubing inserted into the adult rectum.

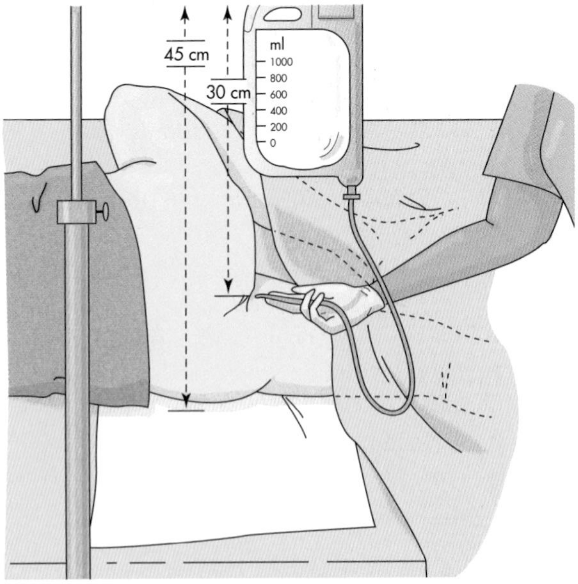

Figure 32–2 Administering an enema. The client is in Sims' position. The enema bag hangs from an IV pole. The enema bag is 30 cm (12 in.) above the level of the anus and 45 cm (18 in.) above the mattress.

1 2 3 GIVING A COMMERCIAL ENEMA TO AN ADULT

Remember to promote:

• Dignity • Independence • Preferences • Privacy • Safety

Pre-Procedure

1 Identify the client, according to employer policy.
2 Explain the procedure to the client.
3 Perform hand hygiene.
4 Collect the following:
- Commercial enema
- Bedpan or commode
- Waterproof pad
- Toilet tissue
- Gloves
- Robe and nonskid footwear
- Bath blanket

5 Provide for privacy.
6 Raise the bed to a comfortable working height. Follow the care plan for bed rail use.*

Procedure

7 Lower the bed rail near you, if it is up.
8 Cover the client with a bath blanket. Fanfold top linens to the foot of the bed.
9 Position the client in Sims' position on the left side.
10 Put on gloves.
11 Place the waterproof pad under the buttocks.
12 Expose the anal area.
13 Position the bedpan near the client.
14 Remove the cap from the enema tip.
15 Add lubricating jelly to coat the tip.
16 Separate the buttocks to see the anus.
17 Ask the client to take a deep breath through the mouth.
18 Insert the enema tip 5 cm (2 in.) into the rectum when the client is exhaling (Figure 32–3). Stop if the client complains of pain, you feel resistance, or bleeding occurs.
19 Squeeze and roll the bottle gently. Release pressure on the bottle *after* removing the tip from the rectum.
20 Put the bottle into the box, tip first.
21 Help the client onto the bedpan; raise the head of the bed, or help the client into a sitting position. Raise the bed rail, if used, or assist the client to the bathroom or commode. The client should wear a robe and nonskid footwear when up. The bed should be in the lowest position.
22 Place the call bell (in facilities) and toilet tissue within reach. Remind the client not to flush the toilet.
23 Discard disposable items.
24 Remove gloves. Wash your hands.
25 Leave the room if the client can be left alone. Stay within hearing distance.
26 Return when the client calls. Knock before entering.
27 Perform hand hygiene. Put on gloves.
28 Lower the bed rail, if it is up.
29 Observe results of the enema for amount, colour, consistency, and odour. Call your supervisor to observe the results (in a facility).
30 Help the client clean the perineal area.
31 Remove the bed protector.
32 Empty, clean, and disinfect the bedpan or commode. Flush the toilet.
33 Return equipment to its proper place.
34 Remove gloves. Perform hand hygiene.
35 Help the client with hand washing. Wear gloves, if necessary.
36 Return top linens, and remove the bath blanket.

Post-Procedure

37 Follow steps 48 through 54 in *Giving a Cleansing Enema to an Adult* on page 617.

*Steps marked with an asterisk may not apply in community settings.

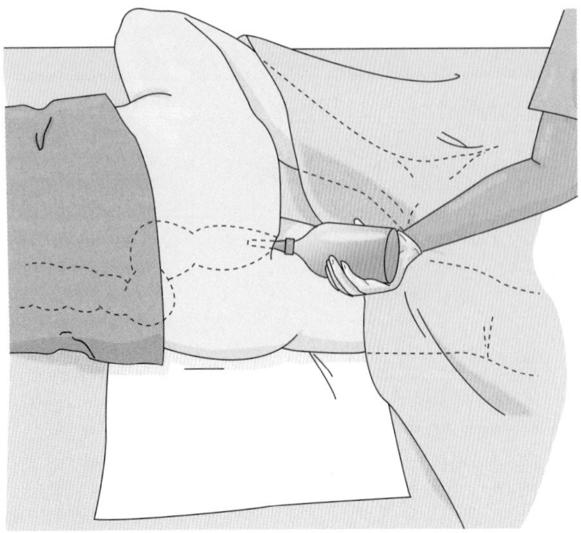

Figure 32–3 Insert the commercial enema tip 5 cm (2 in.) into the rectum.

RECTAL TUBES

A nurse inserts a rectal tube into the rectum to relieve flatulence and intestinal distention. Flatus is passed without effort or straining.

The rectal tube is usually inserted 10 cm (4 in.) into the adult rectum. It is left in place for 20 to 30 minutes, which helps prevent rectal irritation. It can be reinserted every 2 to 3 hours.

Often the tube is connected to a flatus bag or to a water container (Figure 32–4). The bag inflates as gas passes into it. If the tube is connected to a container with water, the water bubbles as gas passes through the tube into the water. For this system, the rectal tube is attached to connecting tubing, which is placed in the water container.

Feces may be expelled along with flatus. If a flatus bag is not used, the open end of the tube is placed in a folded, waterproof pad.

THE CLIENT WITH AN OSTOMY

Sometimes surgical removal of part of the intestines is necessary as part of the treatment for cancer, diseases of the bowel, or trauma (such as stab or bullet wounds). Following the surgery, an **ostomy**—the surgical creation of an artificial opening (**stoma**)—is sometimes needed. The client wears a pouch over the stoma to collect feces and flatus.

Colostomy

A **colostomy** is the surgically created opening (*stomy*) between the colon (*colo*) and abdominal wall. Part of the colon is brought out onto the abdominal wall, and a stoma is created. Feces and flatus pass through the stoma, not through the anus. Colostomies may be permanent or temporary. The colostomy is permanent if the diseased part of the colon has been removed. A temporary colostomy gives the diseased or injured bowel time to heal, and eventually another surgery reconnects the bowel.

Stomas will usually appear pink, but occasionally some can appear red and "angry." Both are, in fact, healthy stomas. Some support workers may be needlessly concerned that the red stomas would be painful to touch or cleanse.

The location of the colostomy depends on the site of colon disease or injury (Figure 32–5). Stool consistency ranges from liquid to formed. The more colon that is left remaining to absorb water, the more solid and formed the stools will be. If the colostomy is near the beginning of the colon, stools will be liquid, whereas the colostomy near the end of the large intestine results in formed stools.

Feces can irritate the skin, so skin care is essential to prevent skin breakdown around the stoma. Skin is washed and dried whenever the pouch is removed and a skin barrier applied around the

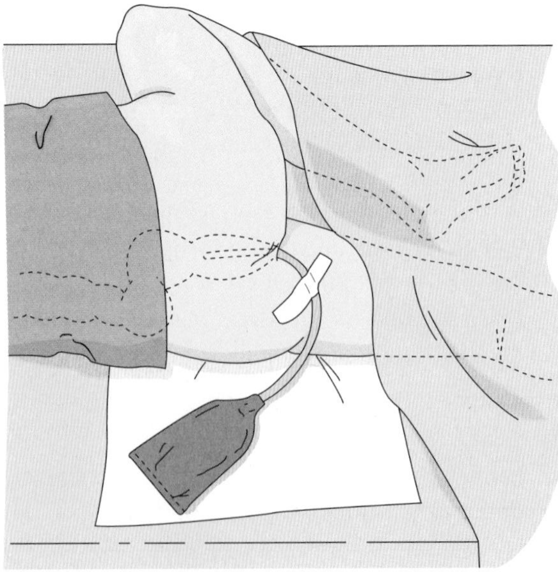

Figure 32–4 A rectal tube. A nurse inserts the rectal tube 10 cm (4 in.) into the adult rectum. The rectal tube is taped to the buttocks. The flatus bag rests on the bed.

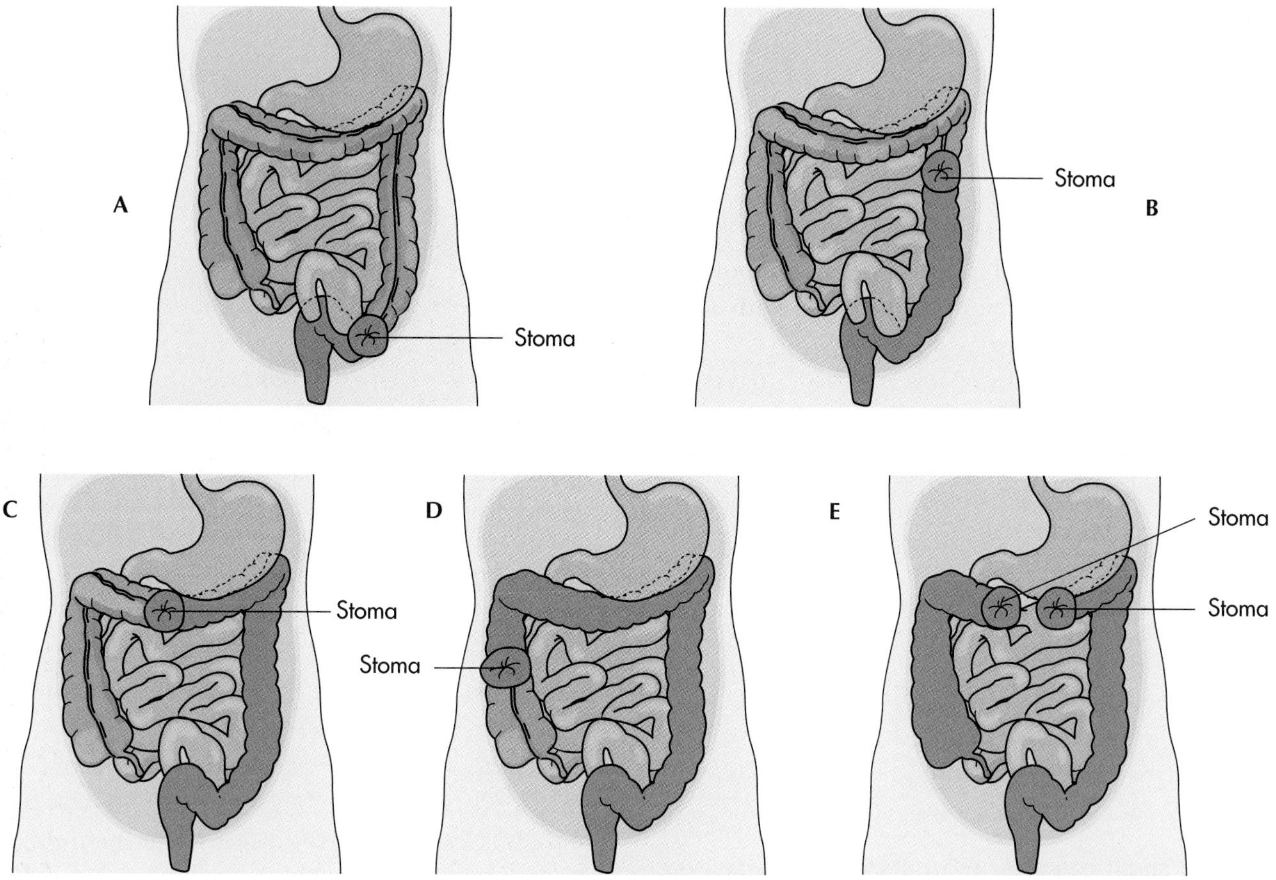

Figure 32–5 Colostomy sites. *Shading* shows the part of the bowel that was surgically removed. **A,** Sigmoid colostomy. **B,** Descending colostomy. **C,** Transverse colostomy. **D,** Ascending colostomy. **E,** Double-barrel colostomy—two stomas are created: one for the excretion of feces and the other for the administration of medicine into the bowel to help it to heal. This type of colostomy is usually temporary.

stoma. The skin barrier prevents feces from coming in contact with the skin. The skin barrier may be part of the pouch or a separate device.

Ileostomy

An **ileostomy** is the surgically created opening (*stomy*) between the ileum (small intestine [*ileo*]) and the abdominal wall. Part of the ileum is brought out onto the abdominal wall, and a stoma is created. The entire colon is removed (Figure 32–6), and liquid feces drain constantly from an ileostomy. Water is not absorbed because the colon has been removed. Feces in the small intestine contain digestive juices that are extremely irritating to the skin. The ileostomy pouch must fit well so that feces do not touch the skin to avoid excoriation and breakdown. Good skin care is essential.

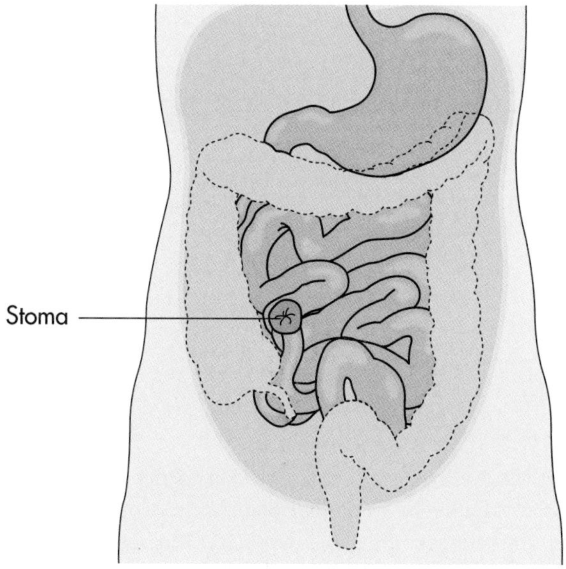

Figure 32–6 An ileostomy. The entire colon has been surgically removed.

Ostomy Pouches. The pouch has an adhesive backing that is applied to the skin (Figures 32–7 through 32–9). Some clients who have had a colostomy for many years may have the pouch attached to a belt. Many pouches have a drain at the bottom that is closed with clips, clamps, or wire closures. The drain is opened to empty the pouch of feces. It is opened when the bag balloons or bulges with flatus. The drain is wiped with toilet tissue before it is closed.

The pouch is changed every 3 to 7 days and when it leaks. Some clients want the pouch changed daily or whenever it becomes soiled. However, frequent pouch changes can damage the skin. Many clients manage their ostomy pouches without help.

Odours are prevented by the following:

- Good hygiene
- Emptying the pouch regularly
- Avoiding gas-forming foods
- Placing deodorants into the pouch. The care plan tells you which products to use.

The client can wear normal clothes when using an ostomy pouch. However, tight undergarments can prevent feces from entering the pouch. Also, bulging from feces and flatus can be seen through tight clothes.

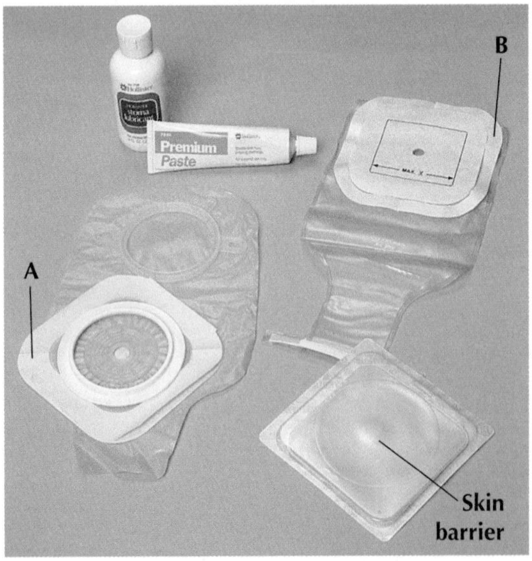

Figure 32–7 Ostomy pouches and skin barriers. **A,** Two piece detachable system (*Note:* Skin barrier would need to be custom cut according to stoma size.) The pouch opening is already precut by the manufacturer to fit the size of the flange on the skin barrier. **B,** One-piece pouch with skin barrier attached. **Source:** Potter, P.A., Griffin A., Perry, Ross-Kerr, J.C., & Wood, M.J. (2001). *Canadian fundamentals of nursing* (3rd ed., p. 1424). Toronto: Harcourt Canada.

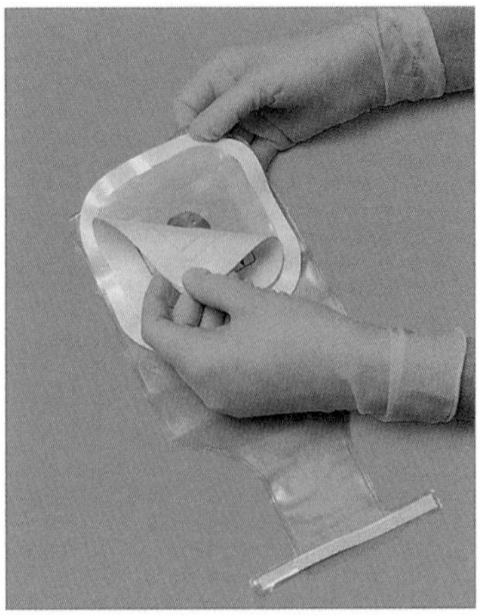

Figure 32–8 Preparing an ostomy pouch. **Source:** Potter, P.A., Griffin A., Perry, Ross-Kerr, J.C., & Wood, M.J. (2001). *Canadian fundamentals of nursing* (3rd ed., p. 1426). Toronto: Harcourt Canada.

Peristalsis increases after eating, so stomas are usually inactive before breakfast; that is, expulsion of feces is less likely at this time. If the client prefers to shower or bathe with the pouch off, it is best done before breakfast. Showers and baths are delayed 1 or 2 hours after applying a new pouch. This gives the adhesive backing on the pouch time to stick to the skin.

Do not flush pouches down the toilet. Follow employer policy for disposing of used pouches (see the *Focus on Children: Ostomy Pouches* box on page 624).

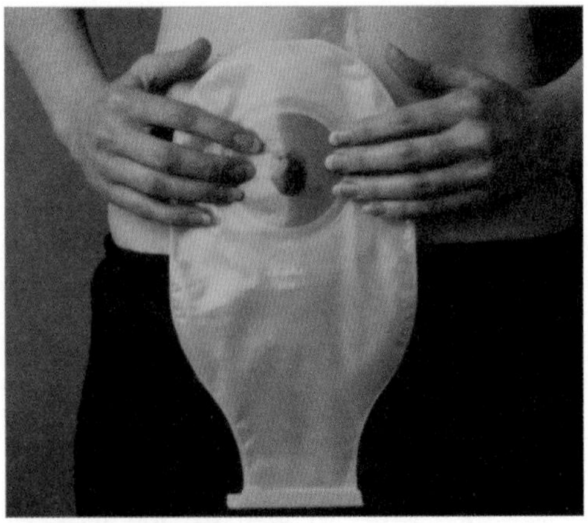

Figure 32–9 Applying a one-piece pouch. **Source:** Potter, P.A., Griffin A., Perry, Ross-Kerr, J.C., & Wood, M.J. (2001). *Canadian fundamentals of nursing* (3rd ed., p. 1427). Toronto: Harcourt Canada.

1 2 3 CHANGING AN OSTOMY POUCH

Remember to promote:

• Dignity • Independence • Preferences • Privacy • Safety

Pre-Procedure

1 Identify the client, according to employer policy.
2 Explain the procedure to the client.
3 Perform hand hygiene.
4 Collect the following:
- Clean pouch with skin barrier
- Skin barrier as ordered (if not part of pouch)
- Pouch clamp, clip, or wire closure
- Clean ostomy belt (if used)
- 4 to 8 gauze squares
- Adhesive remover
- Cotton balls
- Bedpan with cover
- Waterproof pad
- Bath blanket
- Toilet tissue
- Wash basin
- Bath thermometer
- Soap or cleansing agent, according to the care plan
- Pouch deodorant
- Paper towels
- Gloves
- Disposable bag

5 Arrange paper towels on a work area. Place items on top of paper towels.
6 Provide for privacy.
7 Raise bed to a comfortable working height. Follow the care plan for bed rail use.*

Procedure

8 Lower the bed rail near you, if it is up.
9 Cover the client with a bath blanket. Fanfold linens to the foot of the bed.
10 Place the waterproof pad under the client's buttocks.
11 Put on gloves.
12 Disconnect the pouch from the belt if one is worn. Remove the belt.
13 Remove the pouch gently. Gently push the skin down and away from the skin barrier. Place the pouch in the bedpan.
14 Wipe around the stoma with toilet tissue or a gauze square. This removes mucus and feces. Place soiled tissue in the bedpan.
15 Moisten a gauze square with adhesive remover. Clean around the stoma to remove any remaining skin barrier. Clean from the stoma outward.
16 Cover the bedpan, and take it to the bathroom. (If bed rails are used, raise them before leaving the bedside.)
17 Measure the feces, as directed by the care plan.
18 Note the colour, amount, consistency, and odour of feces. Report any abnormal feces. Then empty the pouch and bedpan into the toilet. Put the pouch in the disposable bag.
19 Remove gloves. Perform hand hygiene. Put on clean gloves.
20 Fill the wash basin with warm water. (Measure the temperature of water with a bath thermometer. Check the care plan for correct temperature.) Place the basin on the work area on top of paper towels. Lower the bed rail near you, if it is up.
21 Using soap or other cleansing agent, clean the skin around the stoma with water. Rinse and pat dry.
22 Observe the stoma and skin around the stoma. Report any irritation or skin breakdown.
23 Apply the skin barrier, if it is a separate device.
24 Put a clean ostomy belt on the client (if a belt is worn).
25 Add deodorant to the new pouch.
26 Remove adhesive backing on the pouch.
27 Centre the pouch over the stoma. The drain points downward.
28 Press around the skin barrier so the pouch seals to the skin. Apply gentle pressure from the stoma outward.
29 Maintain pressure for 1 to 2 minutes.
30 Connect the belt to the pouch (if a belt is worn).
31 Remove the waterproof pad.
32 Remove gloves. Perform hand hygiene. (If bed rails are used, raise them before leaving the bedside.)
33 Cover the client. Remove the bath blanket.

(continued on page 624)

1 2 3 CHANGING AN OSTOMY POUCH

Post-Procedure

34 Provide for safety and comfort.
35 Place the call bell within reach.*
36 Return the bed to its lowest position. Follow the care plan for bed rail use.*
37 Remove privacy measures.
38 Clean the bedpan, wash basin, and other equipment. Put on gloves for this step.
39 Return equipment to its proper place.
40 Discard the disposable bag, according to employer policy. Follow employer policy for soiled linen.
41 Remove gloves. Perform hand hygiene.
42 Report and record your actions and observations, according to employer policy.

*Steps marked with an asterisk may not apply in community settings.

focus on ››CHILDREN

Ostomy Pouches

Child clients of different ages, even premature infants, can have ostomies. If changing a child's ostomy pouch is assigned to you, your supervisor will give you the necessary instructions.

STOOL SPECIMENS

When internal bleeding is suspected, feces are checked for blood. Stools are also analyzed to identify fat, microbes, worms, and other abnormal contents. The guidelines for collecting urine specimens (see Chapter 31) apply when collecting stool specimens. Follow Standard Practices.

The stool specimen must not be contaminated with urine. Some tests require warm (fresh) stools. The specimen is taken to the laboratory immediately in that case.

Testing Stools for Blood

Blood can appear in stools for many reasons, including ulcers, colon cancer, and hemorrhoids. Often blood in stools is clearly visible. Bright red blood could be from hemorrhoids or cuts/abrasions in the anal area and can usually be seen if bleeding is low in the gastrointestinal (GI) tract. Stools are black and tarry (**melena**) if there is bleeding in the stomach or upper GI tract. When reporting blood in the stool, it is important to describe the colour as it may be an important clue when investigating the source.

Sometimes bleeding may occur in very small amounts, which will be difficult to detect by just observing the stools. So stools are tested for the presence of *occult (hidden* or *unseen) blood,* often done to screen for colon cancer.

There are many types of tests. Follow the manufacturer's instructions for the test ordered, and follow Standard Practices. The care plan and your assignment sheet will tell you when to collect the specimen. Many factors can affect the test results—for example, eating red meat. Therefore the client cannot eat red meat for 3 days before the test. Bleeding from hemorrhoids and menstrual periods also affects test results.

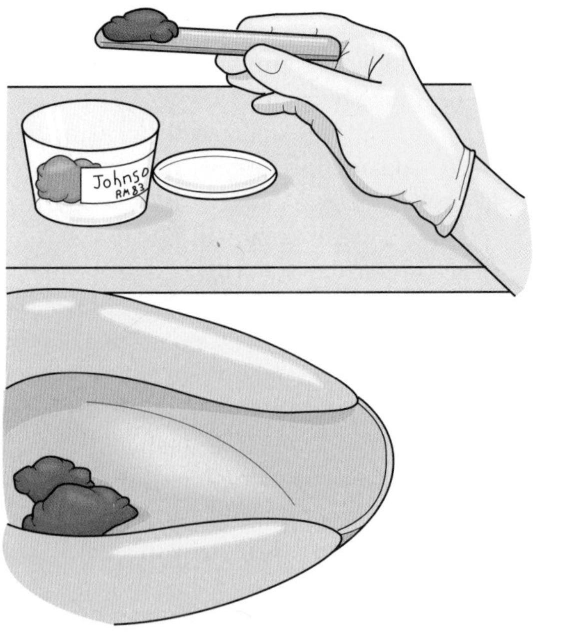

Figure 32–10 A tongue blade is used to transfer a small amount of stool from the bedpan to the specimen container.

1 2 3 COLLECTING A STOOL SPECIMEN

Remember to promote:

• Dignity • Independence • Preferences • Privacy • Safety

Pre-Procedure

1 Identify the client, according to employer policy.
2 Explain the procedure to the client.
3 Perform hand hygiene.
4 Collect the following:
- Bedpan and cover or bedside commode
- Urinal (or bedpan with cover) for voiding
- Specimen pan for the toilet or commode
- Specimen container and lid
- Tongue blade
- Disposable bag
- Gloves
- Toilet tissue
- Laboratory requisition slip
- Plastic bag

5 Label the container.
6 Provide for privacy.

Procedure

7 Ask the client to void. Provide the bedpan, commode, or urinal if the client does not use the bathroom. Empty and clean the device. Wear gloves.
8 Place the specimen pan under the toilet seat if the client uses the bathroom.
9 Assist the client onto the bedpan or to the toilet or commode. The client should wear a robe and nonskid footwear when up.
10 Ask the client not to put toilet tissue in the bedpan, commode, or specimen pan. Provide a disposable bag for toilet tissue.
11 Place the call bell (in facilities) and toilet tissue within reach. Raise or lower bed rails, according to the care plan.
12 Perform hand hygiene, and leave the room, if safe to do so. Stay within hearing distance.
13 Return when the client calls. Knock before entering. Perform hand hygiene.
14 Lower the bed rail near you, if it is up.
15 Put on gloves. Provide perineal care, if needed.
16 Use a tongue blade to take about 30 mL (2 tablespoons) of feces from the bedpan, commode, or specimen pan to the specimen container (Figure 32–10). Take the sample from the middle of a formed stool. If required by employer policy, take stool from two different areas on the specimen.
17 Put the lid on the specimen container. Do not touch the inside of the lid or container. Place the container in the plastic bag.
18 Wrap the tongue blade in toilet tissue and dispose of it, according to your employer's policy.
19 Empty, clean, and disinfect the equipment.
20 Remove gloves. Perform hand hygiene.
21 Return equipment to its proper place.
22 Assist the client with hand washing. Wear gloves, if needed.

Post-Procedure

23 Provide for safety and comfort.
24 Place the call bell within reach.*
25 Return the bed to its lowest position. Follow the care plan for bed rail use.*
26 Remove privacy measures.
27 Follow your supervisor's instructions for specimen storage and transportation.
28 Perform hand hygiene.
29 Report and record your actions and observations, according to employer policy.

*Steps marked with an asterisk may not apply in community settings.

1 2 3 TESTING A STOOL SPECIMEN FOR BLOOD

Remember to promote:

• **D**ignity • **I**ndependence • **P**references • **P**rivacy • **S**afety

Pre-Procedure

1 Explain the procedure to the client.
2 Perform hand hygiene.
3 Collect a stool specimen (see *Collecting a Stool Specimen* on page 625).
4 Collect the following:
- Paper towel
- Hemoccult test kit (includes developer)
- Tongue blades
- Gloves

5 Put on gloves.

Procedure

6 Open the test kit.
7 Use a tongue blade to obtain a small amount of stool.
8 Apply a thin smear of stool on box A on the test paper (Figure 32–11, *A*).
9 Use another tongue blade to obtain some stool from another area of the specimen.
10 Apply a thin smear of stool on box B on the test paper (Figure 32–11, *B*).
11 Close the test packet.
12 Turn the test packet to the other side. Open the flap. Apply developer to boxes A and B. Follow the manufacturer's instructions (Figure 32–11, *C*).
13 Wait for the specified amount of time, as in the manufacturer's instructions—from 10 to 60 seconds.
14 Note and record the colour changes (Figure 32–11, *D*). Follow the manufacturer's instructions.
15 Dispose of the test packet.
16 Wrap the tongue blades in toilet tissue, then discard them, according to your employer's policy.
17 Dispose of the rest of the stool.
18 Remove gloves. Perform hand hygiene.
19 Report and record your actions and observations, according to employer policy.

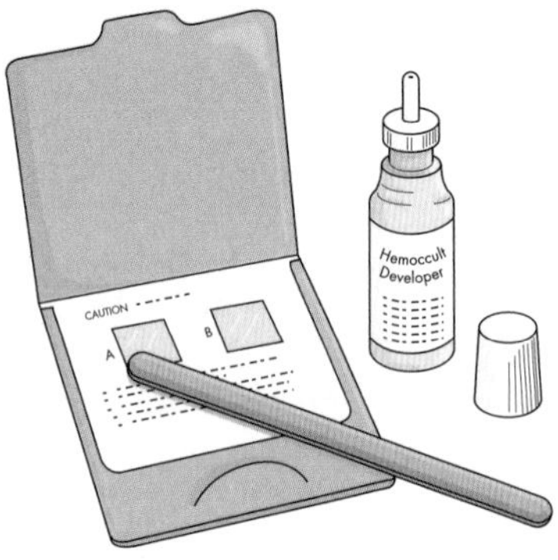

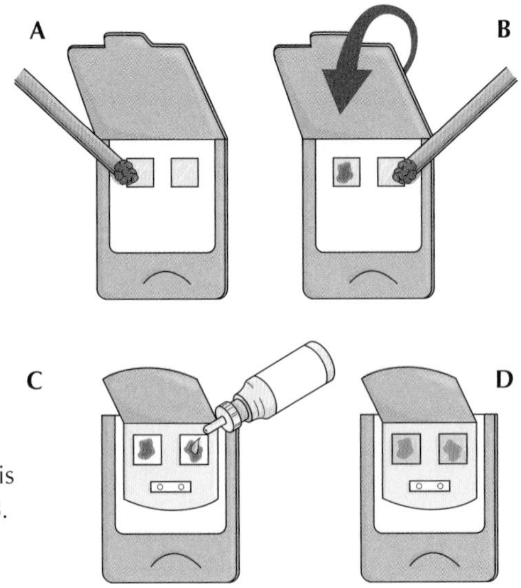

Figure 32–11 Testing for occult blood. **A,** Stool is smeared on box A. **B,** Stool is smeared on box B. **C,** Developer is applied to boxes A and B. **D,** Colour changes are noted.

REVIEW

Answers to these questions are at the bottom of the page.

Circle the **BEST** answer.

1. **Which is *true?***
   A. Most people have a bowel movement every day.
   B. Stools are normally black and runny.
   C. Diarrhea occurs when feces move slowly through the intestines.
   D. Constipation results when feces move through the large intestine rapidly.

2. **The prolonged retention and accumulation of feces in the rectum is called:**
   A. Constipation
   B. Fecal impaction
   C. Diarrhea
   D. Anal incontinence

3. **Which will promote comfort and safety in bowel movement?**
   A. Not asking visitors to leave the room
   B. Helping the client assume a sitting position
   C. Offering the bedpan only when asked.
   D. Telling the client to hurry

4. **Bowel training is aimed at:**
   A. Gaining control of bowel movements and developing a regular elimination pattern
   B. Ostomy control
   C. Preventing fecal impaction, constipation, and anal incontinence
   D. Preventing bleeding

5. **Which is used for a cleansing enema?**
   A. Vegetable oil
   B. An enema containing medication
   C. Mineral oil
   D. Tap water

6. **Which is *true?***
   A. Enema solutions should have a temperature of 42.5°C.
   B. Sims' position or left side with leg raised to as close to 90 degrees as is comfortable for the client, is used for administering an enema.
   C. The enema bag is held 50 cm (12 in.) above the anus.
   D. The enema solution is administered rapidly.

7. **In adults, the enema tube is inserted:**
   A. 5 cm (2 in.)
   B. 7.5 to 10 cm (3 to 4 in.)
   C. 13 to 15 cm (5 to 6 in.)
   D. 20 cm (8 in.)

8. **The commercial enema:**
   A. Must be prepared before it is administered
   B. Is ordered when complete cleansing of the bowel is needed
   C. Is retained until the person feels the urge to defecate
   D. Is retained for 60 to 90 minutes

9. **Rectal tubes are left in place no longer than:**
   A. 60 minutes
   B. 30 minutes
   C. 20 minutes
   D. 10 minutes

10. **Which statement about ostomies is *true?***
    A. Good skin care around the stoma is essential.
    B. Deodorants cannot control odours.
    C. The client does not wear a pouch.
    D. Feces are always liquid.

11. **A client wears an ostomy pouch. It is usually emptied:**
    A. Every 4 to 6 hours
    B. Every morning
    C. Every 3 to 7 days
    D. When feces are present

12. **Black, tarry stool is called:**
    A. Melena
    B. Feces
    C. Hemostool
    D. Occult blood

Answers: 1.A, 2.B, 3.B, 4.A, 5.D, 6.B, 7.B, 8.C, 9.B, 10.A, 11.D, 12.A

CHAPTER 33

Rehabilitation Care

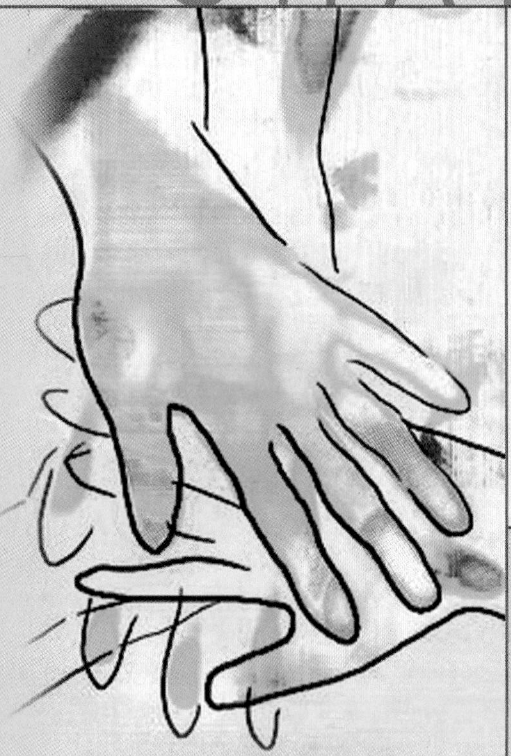

OBJECTIVES

- Define the key terms listed in this chapter.
- Describe the goals of rehabilitation.
- Explain how rehabilitation involves the whole client.
- Explain the family's role in the rehabilitation process.
- Explain the role of therapy and training in rehabilitation.
- Describe the four rehabilitation settings.
- Explain the role of the rehabilitation team in the rehabilitation process.

key terms

orthosis The process of straightening or correcting a deformity.

orthotic Apparatus worn for support or alignment of parts of the musculo-skeletal system and to prevent or correct problems associated with it.

prostheses (singular, prosthesis) Artificial replacements for missing body parts.

rehabilitation The process of restoring a client to the highest level of functioning possible through the use of therapy, exercise, or other methods.

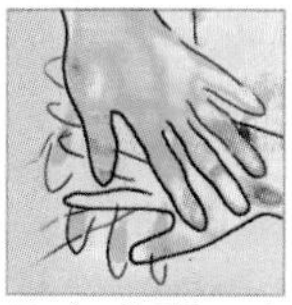

Rehabilitation is the process of restoring a client to the highest level of functioning possible through the use of therapy, exercise, or other methods. Rehabilitation may follow an acute injury or illness, or it may be part of the treatment for a chronic illness or disability. Rehabilitation helps the client function at his or her highest level of independence.

Among clients who are too weak to perform activities of daily living (ADLs), rehabilitation may involve measures that promote:

- Self-care
- Elimination
- Positioning
- Mobility
- Communication
- Cognitive function

The term "restorative care" is used in some agencies, and it is difficult to distinguish the definition of this term from that for "rehabilitation." The focus of rehabilitation and restorative care is to:

- Help maintain the highest level of functioning
- Prevent unnecessary decline in function

GOALS OF REHABILITATION

Goals depend on the client's condition and circumstances. For some clients, the goal is to return to work, and some others only want to be able to meet self-care needs and perform ADLs. Most clients want to reduce their reliance on others and to become more independent. The following goals are common:

- ***To restore function to former levels.*** A full restoration of function is the goal for most clients with acute or temporary conditions. For example, a healthy client with a simple leg fracture aims at full recovery.
- ***To improve functional abilities.*** A return to former levels of functioning is not possible for some clients. They aim to improve their abilities to the best extent possible. For example, they may want to work on mobility skills or carrying out ADLs independently.
- ***To learn new skills.*** Some clients need to learn new skills in order to adjust to their disability or limitations. For example, Mr. Liptak's larynx was surgically removed because of cancer, and he is not able to speak any more. His goal is to learn to communicate using, for example, sign language.
- ***To prevent further disability and illness.*** Complications that cause further disability and illness must be prevented. For example, immobility can lead to pressure ulcers or contractures, so proper skin care, exercise and activity, good alignment, and frequent repositioning are essential.

Consider the rehabilitation goals of the following clients:

- Chantal, 17, was in a car accident, which left her a hemiplegic. She needs to maintain her current range of motion, adapt to a wheelchair, and perform self-care.
- Mr. Cunningham, 27, is addicted to cocaine. His goals include restoring healthy physical and psychological functions and preventing a relapse

into addiction. He will learn how to avoid situations where drugs are present, and he will be encouraged to join NA (Narcotics Anonymous).

- Mr. Khan, 49, had a heart attack. His goal is to prevent another heart attack. His rehabilitation program includes exercise, nutrition counselling, and stress management techniques.
- Mr. Egri, 68, suffered hemiplegia and severe speech impairment as a result of a stroke. He needs to learn communication methods and to restore function. Prevention of another stroke through medication, exercises, and diet is a goal as well. His family needs to learn how to help with his care.
- Mrs. Boucher, 82, fractured her hip in a fall. Her goal is to remain in her own home. She needs to restore her ability to function at former levels. She also needs to take measures to prevent another fall (see the *Focus on Older Adults: Rehabilitation* box).

THE REHABILITATION PROCESS

Rehabilitation can be a short process—for example, a healthy person with a shoulder injury may need to do only a few simple exercises. However, rehabilitation is often a long, difficult process. The *Case Study* box on the next page shows the rehabilitation process experienced by a client who suffered a serious brain injury.

The Rehabilitation Team

Rehabilitation is a multidisciplinary team effort. Members of the team vary depending on the client's needs. The team usually includes the client, family members, physicians, nurses, occupational therapists, physiotherapists (physical therapists), support workers, and others—all can help the client regain function and independence. The team meets often to discuss the client's progress, and changes are made in the rehabilitation plan, as needed. The client and family attend the meetings, whenever possible. Family members are key to the team.

Restorative care usually involves the client and family, nurses, and support workers. Therapists and other professionals may be consulted, as needed, but the care is usually provided by nurses and support workers.

> **focus on »OLDER ADULTS**
>
> **Rehabilitation**
>
> Rehabilitation often takes longer for older clients than for others. Age-related changes affect healing, mobility, vision, hearing, and other functions (see Chapter 17). Older clients often have chronic health problems that slow down their recovery. They are also at risk for injuries. Because older clients do not tolerate long or fast-paced programs, their rehabilitation is usually slow.

Emphasis on the Whole Person

Illness and disability can affect a client's physical, emotional, social, intellectual, and spiritual health, so rehabilitation is aimed at the whole person. It addresses all dimensions of health, not only the physical:

- ***Physical health.*** The client's physical condition and ability to perform ADLs are assessed. Complications are prevented. Range-of-motion (ROM) exercises are done. The client learns or re-learns self-care and mobility skills.
- ***Emotional and social health.*** Emotional and social health as well as work skills are assessed. Family counselling and assistance for re-entering the community and workplace are provided, as needed.
- ***Intellectual health.*** Thinking, speech, memory, and organization are assessed. Measures to improve cognitive functioning are planned.
- ***Spiritual health.*** Counselling from spiritual advisers is provided, as needed.

All aspects of rehabilitation are interconnected—for example, following a stroke, Mr. Silva learns how to care for himself (physical health) and how to follow instructions (intellectual health), which increases his self-esteem (emotional health); family and friends visit often (social health), and his spiritual adviser visits every week (spiritual health).

CASE STUDY
REHABILITATION FOLLOWING A BRAIN INJURY

High school teacher Jeffery Butler, 34, was cycling to school when he was hit by a van. He sustained a severe blow to the head and broke several bones. After emergency care and surgery, he was placed in the intensive care unit (ICU). Because he had acquired a serious brain injury, he could not speak or recognize his family. After 10 days in the ICU, he was moved to the acute care unit, where he stayed for 2 months.

Eventually Mr. Butler was transferred to the hospital's rehabilitation unit, and 3 months later, he was discharged home. He received rehabilitation services at home and in the community for the next 6 months. During his long rehabilitation, Mr. Butler's rehabilitation team worked with him and his family (see the chart below). The team's main goals were helping Mr. Butler regain lost function and helping the family learn new skills for his care.

Rehabilitation Team	Role
Mr. Butler and his family	Made decisions regarding rehabilitation goals Were involved in every aspect of care Learned new skills and re-learned old skills
Neurosurgeon	Led surgical team and aspects of rehabilitation after surgery
Orthopedic surgeon	Led surgical team and aspects of rehabilitation after surgery
Nurses	Coordinated and provided care at every stage
Specialist in rehabilitation medicine	Led and coordinated rehabilitation
Neuropsychologists	Evaluated thinking, memory, emotions, behaviour, and personality Planned behaviour management treatment Headed adult day program
Case manager	Coordinated home care Arranged for adult day programs
Social workers	Provided counselling Headed adult day program
Occupational therapists	Assessed performance of activities of daily living Conducted home assessment prior to discharge Provided treatment, equipment, and devices to help client attain independence
Physiotherapists (Physical therapists)	Evaluated strength, flexibility, and balance Taught mobility exercises and equipment use
Speech-language pathologist	Tested speech Taught family communication strategies
Family physician	Provided medical care after discharge
Support workers	Assisted with personal care and range-of-motion exercises Assisted with household management Assisted with eating Helped with physical therapy exercises
Volunteers	Provided company to Mr. Butler when the family was not around Assisted with household tasks

The *Case Study* box on page 631 shows a rehabilitation team addressing all five dimensions of a client's health. The client's quality of life is central to care and treatment. The rehabilitation team encourages the client to control as many aspects of his or her care as possible. Being a key member of the rehabilitation team gives the client some control.

Role of the Family

Rehabilitation of clients also involves their family members, who need to learn about the illness, injury, or disability and how to care for their loved ones. Care often involves helping the client practise new skills. The family also learns new skills—for example, how to communicate with a spouse who has lost the ability to speak, how to cope with the behaviour of a mentally ill teenager, or how to dress a child with physical disabilities. Counselling is provided, as needed, to help cope with changes affecting the family. Families dealing with the rehabilitation of a client with a chronic health problem will need constant support from team members, as the challenges to a normal family life can be overwhelming, and family members need to know that the team is listening to their concerns.

Therapy and Training

The professionals on the rehabilitation team choose the therapy and training needed to meet the client's goals. The client is taught how to improve a skill or how to perform a task and practises what was learned either independently or with a caregiver or a family member. You may be required to help clients practise skills or tasks (see Chapter 14).

The client's therapy and training may involve learning to use self-help devices. Specific equipment to meet the client's needs is obtained and the client is taught how to use the equipment:

- ***Prostheses.*** **Prostheses** are artificial replacements for missing body parts—for example, feet, knees, lower limbs, upper limbs, hands, breasts, and eyes. The goal for a prosthesis is to be like the missing body part in function and appearance. Artificial limbs are made from a variety of materials—such as wood, aluminum, and plastic. Most artificial limbs are powered by the client's muscles, either by muscles in the stump or by other nearby muscles, so a physiotherapist works with the client to strengthen the muscles. The client learns how to use and care for the prosthesis. As a support worker, you might help a client get used to wearing and using a prosthesis. You might also assist the client with care of the skin at the prosthesis site (see Chapter 18).
- ***Orthotics.*** **Orthosis** is the process of straightening or correcting a deformity. An **orthotic** is an apparatus worn to support and align parts of the musculo-skeletal system and prevent or correct problems associated with it. Examples are splints, foot supports, and knee and back braces (see Chapter 24). The client learns how to put on, use, and care for the orthotic. You might help a client to put on an orthotic and practise moving or walking.
- ***Eating and drinking devices.*** These include glass holders, plate guards, and utensils with curved handles or cuffs (see Chapter 27).
- ***Self-care devices.*** These include electronic toothbrushes, combs, brushes, and sponges with long handles (Figure 33–1), as well as devices that help with dressing, cooking, writing, making phone calls, and other tasks (Figure 33–2).
- ***Devices to aid mobility.*** These include crutches, canes, walkers, and braces, as well as wheelchairs for some clients. If possible, the client learns how to transfer himself or herself to and from the wheelchair using a transfer board, which helps one move from one seat to another (Figure 33–3). The client also learns to transfer to and from the bed, toilet, bathtub, sofas and chairs, and cars.
- ***Other equipment.*** Some clients need feeding tubes (see Chapter 28) or mechanical ventilation (see Chapter 44). Some of them are eventually weaned from the ventilator, while others must adapt themselves to lifelong ventilation.

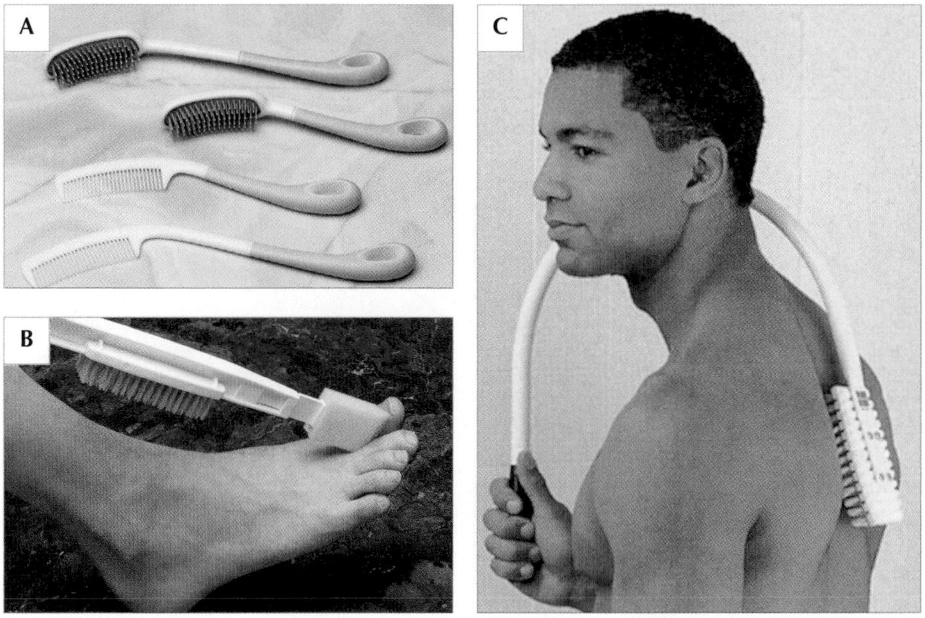

Figure 33–1 **A,** Long-handled combs and brushes for hair care. **B,** Long-handled brushes for bathing. **C,** Brush with a curved handle. **Courtesy:** Northcoast Medical, Inc., Morgan Hill, CA (A and B); Sammons Preston: An AbilityOne Company, Bolingbrook, IL. (C).

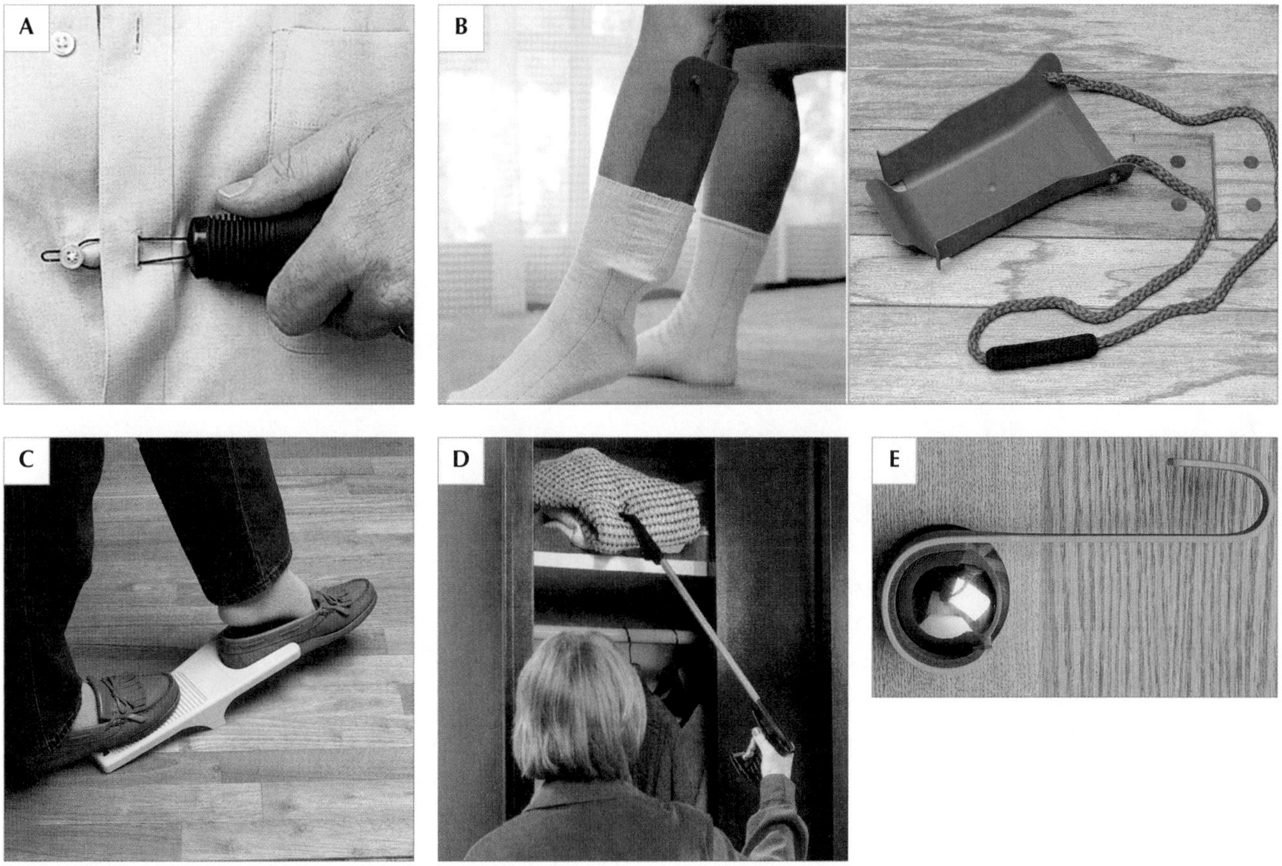

Figure 33–2 **A,** A button hook is used to button and zip clothing. **B,** A sock assist is used to pull on socks and stockings. **C,** A shoe remover is used to take off shoes. **D,** Reachers help remove items from high shelves. **E,** A doorknob turner increases leverage to help turn the knob. **Courtesy:** Northcoast Medical Inc., Morgan Hill, CA. (A, B, C, E); AbilityOne Corporation, Germantown, WI. (D).

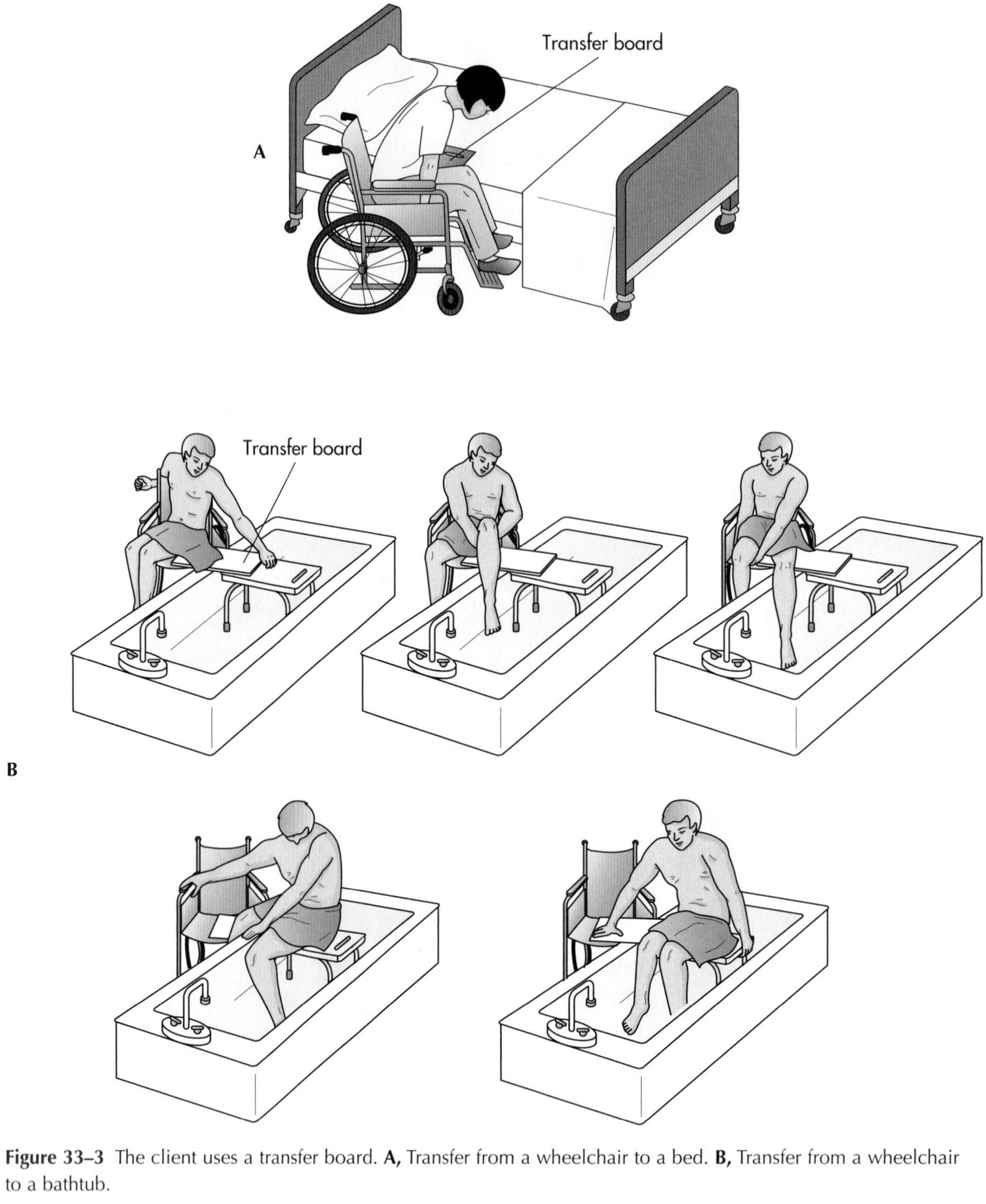

Figure 33–3 The client uses a transfer board. **A,** Transfer from a wheelchair to a bed. **B,** Transfer from a wheelchair to a bathtub.

REHABILITATION SETTINGS

Many common health problems require rehabilitation services (Box 33–1), which are offered in most health care facilities and in the community.

- ***Hospitals.*** Most hospitals have rehabilitation units for inpatients and outpatients. Many programs in these units focus on brain injury and tumours, spinal cord injury, and stroke. Some hospitals offer cardiac and respiratory rehabilitation, and some have programs for complex medical and surgical conditions, such as wound care and unstable diabetes.
- ***Specialized facilities.*** Some health care facilities focus on specific problems, for example, mental illness and substance abuse/addiction.
- ***Long-term care facilities.*** Most provide rehabilitation services similar to those found in hospitals.
- ***Community care.*** Home care services (see the *Focus on Home Care: Home Assessment* box) and adult day programs are offered as part of community care. A program for clients with brain injuries may teach life skills, social behaviour, and work techniques.

ASSISTING WITH REHABILITATION AND RESTORATIVE CARE

As a support worker, you will encounter a number of clients undergoing some form of rehabilitation or restorative care, some of whom will be adjusting to overwhelming change. Rehabilitation is often slow and frustrating, as improvement may not be seen for weeks or months. Some clients improve quickly at first, but the pace of improvement may slow down, causing great frustration and hardship to clients, so you must be patient, supportive, and empathetic (see the *Providing Compassionate Care: Assisting With Rehabilitation* box).

Box 33–1 Common Health Problems Requiring Rehabilitation

- Acquired brain injury
- Alcoholism
- Amputation
- Brain tumour
- Burns
- Cerebral palsy
- Chronic obstructive pulmonary disease
- Mental illness
- Myocardial infarction (heart attack)
- Parkinson's disease
- Spinal cord injury
- Spinal cord tumour
- Stroke
- Substance abuse

focus on ›› HOME CARE

Home Assessment

After the rehabilitation team assesses the client's home (Box 33–2), the case manager or occupational therapist discusses with the client and the family any safety risks and health hazards that have been identified. You may be asked to assist a member of the rehabilitation team to complete the assessment. If necessary, changes are made to make the home environment more appropriate for the client. The support worker should continue to be on the lookout for any safety risks during future contacts with the client and then gently suggest changes to the client/family to ensure a safe environment. If there are any problems, you must report them to your supervisor.

Box 33–2 Home Assessment

Outdoors

- Where is the parking area located? What is the distance from the parking area to the door?
- Where is the mailbox?
- Where is the motor vehicle parked?
- What is the width of car doors?
- Can the client turn the key?
- Can the client open and close doors?
- Are ramps needed?
- Are handrails needed?
- Are entrances well-lit?
- Does the client have access to private or public transportation?
- Can the client operate a motor vehicle?
- What are the width and height of ramps and sidewalks, if any?

Indoors

- Are there any obstructions on floors?
- Are there steps in the house? Where are they located?
- How is furniture arranged?
- Can the client use the furniture?
- Where are telephones located?
- Can the client raise and lower windows?
- How are floors covered (wall-to-wall carpeting, tile, hardwood, throw rugs)?
- Can the client use a wheelchair throughout the house?
- Where is the fuse or circuit-breaker box located?
- Can the client control the heat?
- Are walkways, doors, and halls wide enough for the client's wheelchair?
- Is there an elevator, if the client lives in an apartment or condominium building?

Kitchen

- Does the client have access to the stove, sink, cupboards, storage areas, workspace, refrigerator, and other appliances?
- What is the height of the sink and countertops?
- Is there an open space under the sink to bring the wheelchair close to the sink?
- Can the client turn faucets on and off?
- Can the client use the microwave oven?
- Can the client reach stove knobs?
- Are appliances arranged for the client's convenience?

Bathroom

- What are the heights of the sink, toilet, shower, and tub?
- Can the client reach the faucets?
- Can the client turn the faucets on and off?
- Is there space for using a wheelchair and other mobility devices?
- Can the client get into and out of the tub or shower?
- Are there grab bars by the toilet, shower, and tub?

Bedroom

- What is the height of the client's bed?
- Can the client access the closet? Can the client reach rods and shelves?
- Can the client transfer himself or herself in and out of bed safely? Is there enough space around the bed for the client to move about?
- How is furniture arranged?
- Does the furniture arrangement allow for the use of a wheelchair or mobility devices?
- Where is the nearest bathroom?

Safety

- Is the house number clearly visible and readable during an emergency?
- Do deadbolts and locks provide complete security? Can the client use the locks?
- Can the client see and talk to a visitor at the door without being seen?
- Are steps, porch, and front door well-lit?
- Are the steps, porch, and front door protected from rain, sleet, and snow?
- Is there a nonslip doormat?
- Can the client use the telephone?
- Are emergency telephone numbers kept close at hand?
- Can the client control water temperature?
- Do electrical outlets have childproof covers?
- Where are the smoke detectors? Are they working?
- Are rooms and hallways well-lit?
- Can the client control indoor and outdoor lighting?
- Can the client exit the home quickly in an emergency?
- Is oxygen used in the home? Are safety measures in place?

(continued on page 637)

Box 33–2 Home Assessment (cont'd)

- Does the client have access to the telephone, television, radio, and lights while in bed?
- Are space heaters used in the house? Are safety measures in place?
- Does the client have good judgement with regard to cooking and stove use?
- Is there a safe play area for children?
- Can the client safely dispose of blood, body fluids, secretions, and excretions?
- Is there a pest-free method of trash storage?

Adapted from: Hoeman, S.P. (1996). *Rehabilitation nursing: Process and application* (2nd ed.). St. Louis: Mosby.

PROVIDING COMPASSIONATE CARE

Assisting With Rehabilitation

- **Dignity.** Treat your clients with respect, and protect their right to dignity. Clients do not need your pity, but they do need encouragement and support. Focus on the positive by reminding them of their progress and highlighting their abilities and strengths. Provide emotional support and reassurance; when clients need someone to talk to, be a good listener.

  The process of regaining independence is often very slow, and you may grow impatient with your client when repeated explanations seem to have little or no result. Never show your impatience. Put yourself in the client's shoes and try to understand that having little control over one's own body movements or functions can be extremely frustrating. For many clients, having to learn new tasks is a reminder of their disability. Give praise when even a little progress is made. Remember that illness, disability, and fatigue can affect a client's ability to learn. Clients with brain injuries may have a particularly hard time learning new activities.
- **Independence.** Independence is a key rehabilitation goal. Encourage the client to perform activities of daily living (ADLs) as independently as possible. Do not rush the client, and allow time for him or her to complete each task. Familiarize yourself with the client's self-help devices, and encourage the client to use them whenever necessary. When assisting the client, apply the methods developed by the rehabilitation team and practise with the client the tasks that he or she must perform. This helps you guide and direct the client.
- **Preferences.** Ask clients about their preferences, and allow for personal choice, whenever possible. Freedom of choice helps clients feel in control. Follow the client's daily routine and care plan.
- **Privacy.** Some clients may feel embarrassed to practise skills (such as eating and walking) in front of others. Provide privacy for practising skills, as well as for care procedures and elimination. Keep information about clients confidential.
- **Safety.** Illness, disability, and fatigue increase the risk for accidents and injuries, so take the necessary measures to ensure safety (see Chapter 19). Never force clients to do more than they are able, and allow time for rest. Follow the care plan for safety measures needed for each client. Keep the client in good body alignment. Use safe transfer methods (see Chapter 23). Perform range-of-motion exercises, and turn and reposition the client, as directed. Report signs and symptoms of complications, such as pressure ulcers, contractures, elimination problems, and depression. In facility settings, make sure that the call bell and overbed table are placed on the client's unaffected side.

REVIEW

Answers to these questions are at the bottom of the page.

Circle the **BEST** answer.

1. **Which of the following is a common goal for rehabilitation?**
   A. To restore function to former levels
   B. To prepare for surgery
   C. To prepare for relocation to a long-term care facility
   D. To prepare for chemotherapy

2. **Rehabilitation is often slower for:**
   A. Toddlers
   B. Adolescents
   C. Middle-aged adults
   D. Older adults

3. **Which member of the rehabilitation team evaluates a client's strength and balance?**
   A. The physical therapist
   B. The occupational therapist
   C. The primary caregiver
   D. The speech therapist

4. **The rehabilitation process addresses:**
   A. What the client cannot do
   B. Only physical health
   C. The whole person
   D. Only emotional health

5. **Rehabilitation takes place:**
   A. Only in long-term care facilities
   B. Only in hospitals
   C. Only in specialized facilities
   D. In a variety of facility and community settings

Questions 6 to 9 relate to the following situation: Mr. Graziano, 72, has had a stroke and needs rehabilitation, since his right side is paralyzed.

6. **Mr. Graziano's personal care is:**
   A. Done by him to the extent possible
   B. Done by you
   C. Postponed until he can use his right side
   D. Supervised by his physician

7. **Mr. Graziano asks for some music to be played. You should:**
   A. Tell him music is not allowed
   B. Choose some music for him
   C. Ask him to choose some music
   D. Ask a therapist to choose some music

8. **The call bell is on Mr. Graziano's right side. Since his right side is weak, you move it to the left side of the bed. You have provided compassionate care to Mr. Graziano by:**
   A. Protecting him from abuse
   B. Providing for his safety
   C. Allowing personal choice
   D. Promoting his privacy

9. **Mr. Graziano puts on his shirt using one arm. His progress is slow. You:**
   A. Focus his attention on learning a new task
   B. Encourage him as he completes the task
   C. Ask him to sit down and rest
   D. Tell him he will learn the next task more quickly

Answers: 1.A, 2.D, 3.A, 4.C, 5.D, 6.A, 7.C, 8.B, 9.B

CHAPTER 34

Mental Health Disorders

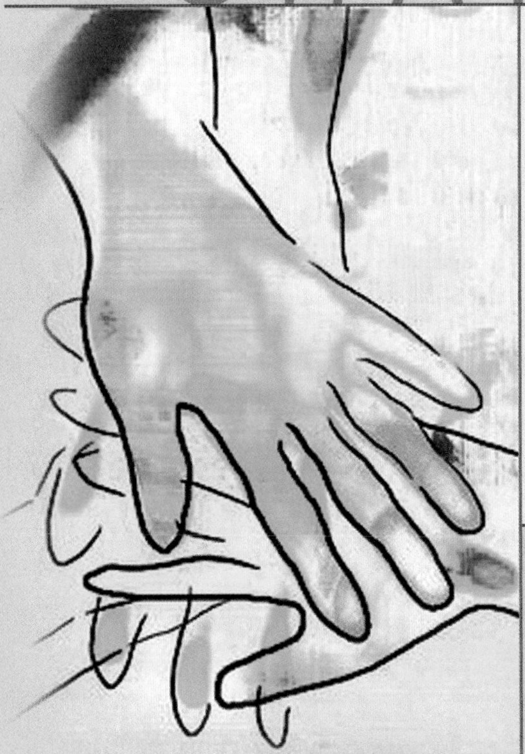

OBJECTIVES

- Define the key terms listed in this chapter.
- Describe the effects of mental health disorders on everyday life.
- List factors that may contribute to mental health disorders.
- Describe the major mental health disorders.
- Describe the stigma experienced by people with mental health disorders.
- Describe the effect of mental health disorders on families.
- Explain how to support clients with mental health disorders.
- Differentiate between reactive depression and major depression.
- List signs and symptoms of depression.
- List ways to reduce the number of episodes of depression in a person.
- Define body dysmorphic disorder.
- Differentiate between anorexia nervosa and anorexia bulimia.
- List the warning signs for suicide intent.
- Describe various ways to support clients with substance dependence disorder.
- List and describe various personality disorders.
- Describe various ways to support clients with personality disorders.
- Apply the information provided in this chapter in your practice by providing culturally sensitive care to clients with mental health disorders and to their families.

key terms

affect A word that describes a person's feelings, emotions and moods, and the way the person demonstrates them.

affective disorders A group of mental disorders involving feelings, emotions, and moods.

amenorrhea Absence of at least three consecutive menstrual periods as normally expected to occur.

anxiety disorders A group of mental disorders in which anxiety is the main symptom.

binge eating A compulsive disorder, in which an individual has periods of uncontrolled, impulsive, or continuous eating.

binge An episode where an individual eats a much larger amount of food than most people would in a similar situation. Binge eating is not a response to intense hunger but is usually a response to depression, stress, or low self-esteem.

bipolar affective disorder An illness characterized by periods of serious depression, followed by episodes of mania (mental hyperactivity or "highs," irritable moods, and disorganized behaviour).

body dysmorphic disorders Altered body image perceptions, which lead to disturbances in eating behaviours and an abnormal concern with body weight and shape. Also known as **eating disorders.**

clinical depression See **major depression.**

delusion A fixed, false belief that is not based on reality.

delusions of grandeur False and exaggerated beliefs about one's importance, talent, or wealth. For example, a woman believes that she is a goddess or the prime minister.

delusions of persecution False beliefs that one is being mistreated, abused, or harassed. For example, a man believes that his neighbour wants to kill him.

detoxification A process that involves allowing abused substances to exit the body naturally or medically removing the substance from the body. The person being detoxified may go into **drug withdrawal**.

drug tolerance A state in which a person abusing a substance needs larger and larger amounts of it to experience the same effect.

drug withdrawal A physical reaction that occurs when a person abusing a substance stops taking it. Signs and symptoms of withdrawal may include depression, agitation, abdominal cramps, nausea, diarrhea, and painful muscle spasms, and the symptoms can be severe.

DSM-IV (Diagnostic and Statistical Manual of Mental Disorders, Fourth Edition) A manual published by the American Psychiatric Association, used throughout North America to classify mental illnesses.

eating disorders See **body dysmorphic disorders**.

electroconvulsive therapy (ECT) A procedure in which an electric current is briefly applied to the brain to produce a seizure for quick relief of severe symptoms of depression or when there is no response to other forms of treatment. It is not known exactly how ECT works, but it is believed that ECT works by altering brain chemicals, serotonin, endorphins, and adrenalin.

emotional illness See **mental illness**.

hallucination Seeing, smelling, hearing, or feeling something that is not real.

Major depression A state of mind in which a person has severe feelings of worthlessness, self-blame, sadness, disappointment, and emptiness that last for weeks and interfere with the person's ability to perform activities of daily living. Also known as **clinical depression**.

mental disorder See **mental illness**.

mental health disorder See **mental illness**.

mental health A state of mind in which a person copes with and adjusts to the stresses of everyday living in socially acceptable ways. It is influenced by three factors: inherited characteristics, childhood nurturing, and life circumstances.

mental illness A disturbance in a person's ability to cope with or adjust to stress; thinking, mood, or behaviours are affected, and functioning is impaired;. Also known as **mental health disorder, emotional illness**, or **psychiatric disorder.**

panic An intense and sudden feeling of fear, anxiety, terror, or dread for no obvious reason.

paranoia Extreme suspicion about a person or a situation.

personality disorder A group of disorders involving rigid and socially unacceptable behaviours.

key terms

phototherapy A treatment for **seasonal affective disorder (SAD);** involves exposure to light directed from a box containing white fluorescent light tubes.

psychiatric disorder See **mental illness.**

psychosis A mental state in which perception of reality is impaired.

psychotherapy A form of therapy in which a client explores his or her thoughts, feelings, and behaviours with help and guidance from a mental health specialist.

reactive depression A term that some health care professionals use to describe normal reactions, such as feelings of loss and sadness, to what a person has just experienced.

remission Periods when the signs and symptoms of a disease lessen or disappear.

repression Keeping (or "burying") unpleasant or painful thoughts from the conscious mind.

schizophrenia An extremely complex mental health disorder characterized by delusions, hallucinations, disturbances in thinking, and withdrawal from social activity. The exact causes are still a mystery, but it is believed to be caused by a biochemical imbalance.

seasonal affective disorder (SAD) A type of depression that occurs each year at the same time, usually starting in fall or winter and ending in spring or early summer. It is common in colder regions, where people tend to spend a majority of their winter months indoors. Signs and symptoms may range from mild to severe, and the condition is often mistaken for major depression.

stigma A characteristic that marks a person as different or flawed.

substance-dependence disorder (substance-abuse disorder) The deliberate misuse of medications, illegal drugs, alcohol, or other substances.

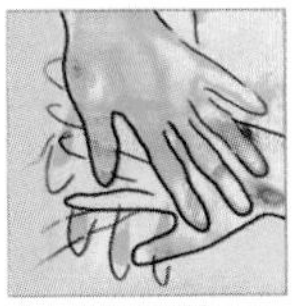

Mental disorders can affect all dimensions of a person's life—physical, emotional, spiritual, social, and intellectual. As a support worker, you will care for and support clients and family members with physical health problems, mental health problems, or both. The physical and mental health problems may not be related in some clients, but in others, physical problems can result from mental health problems, or the reverse.

In order for you to provide care to your clients and their families ensuring dignity, respect, and compassionate care, you need to understand what they are experiencing and be aware of your own attitude toward mental health and mental illness. Be sensitive to the feelings of your clients and their families (see *Providing Compassionate Care: Supporting Clients With Mental Health Disorders* box).

MENTAL HEALTH AND MENTAL ILLNESS

Mental illness, which can be caused by a combination of genetic, biological, personality, and environmental factors, is a disturbance in a person's ability to cope with or adjust to stress; the person's thinking, mood, and behaviours are affected, and functioning is impaired. Twenty percent of Canadians (one in five) will personally experience a mental illness during their lifetime.[1] Mental illnesses affect people of all ages, cultures, and educational and income levels. The onset of most mental illnesses occurs during adolescence and young adulthood. The terms **mental disorder, mental health disorder**, **emotional illness**, and **psychiatric disorder** all refer to mental illness.

Mental health is a state of mind in which a person copes with and adjusts to the stressors of

PROVIDING COMPASSIONATE CARE

Supporting Clients With Mental Health Disorders

- **Dignity.** Treat clients with mental health disorders as you would any other client. Show respect, and promote dignity. Do not label them—for example, it is not acceptable to say that a client *is* a schizophrenic or a drug addict. It is acceptable to say the client *has* schizophrenia or a substance dependence disorder.

  Be patient and understanding. Do not patronize (talk down to) the client. Do not feel offended or hurt by the client's remarks or actions. Remember, the client may have difficulty relating to others. Help the client feel good about himself or herself; accept the client for who he or she is. Treat the client as a valued, worthy individual.
- **Independence.** Clients with mental health disorders have the right to autonomy. They should be encouraged to be as independent as is safely possible. Those with mental health disorders are impaired in *some* areas but are rarely impaired in *all* areas. For example, a client with schizophrenia usually has no problems with ambulation.
- **Preferences.** Allow clients to make choices in their care, according to the care plan. This gives them a greater sense of control. Feelings of loss of control can cause some people with mental health disorders to become withdrawn, so encourage clients to express their wishes, likes, and dislikes.
- **Privacy.** Discuss the client only with the health care team. Respect the client's and the family's need for confidentiality and privacy.
- **Safety.** Stress, fatigue, and physical illness make mental health disorders worse and may trigger episodes. Observe the client carefully for any signs of stress or illness, and report them at once. Provide a calm, stress-free, and safe environment. The client's care plan lists activities and situations that should be avoided. Follow the safety guidelines in Chapter 19. For guidance on handling abusive situations, see Chapter 21.

everyday living in socially acceptable ways. It is influenced by three factors: inherited characteristics, childhood nurturing, and life circumstances. If a person has good mental health, he or she can cope with life's problems and challenges and can "bounce back" or recover from difficult situations.

People who are mentally healthy may feel anxiety, sadness, grief, and loneliness from time to time, but they can handle normal amounts of stress and are able to express and control their emotions appropriately. They feel capable and competent, know their own needs, can form stable and satisfying relationships, and lead an independent life.

The Impact of Mental Health Disorders

It is estimated that one in five Canadians will experience a mental illness in his or her lifetime and that over one million Canadians currently live with a severe or persistent mental illness. Most Canadians are affected by mental illnesses at some time or another because of the mental health disorders, ailments or addictions that may involve a family member, friend, a co-worker, or even themselves.

Mental illnesses are costly to the individual, the family, the community, and the health care system. The economic cost of mental illnesses in Canada was estimated to be at least $7.331 billion in 1993. In 1999, 3.8% of all admissions in general hospitals (1.5 million hospital days) were for anxiety disorders, bipolar disorders, schizophrenia, major depression, personality disorders, eating disorders, and suicidal behaviour.[2]

Today, 86% of hospitalizations for mental illness in Canada occur in general hospitals. In Canada, diagnosed mental illness is responsible for one third of the total number of hospital days each year, and the estimated cost of mental illness and addictions to the Canadian economy is about $18 billion each year. It is estimated that by 2020, depressive illnesses will become the second leading cause of disease burden worldwide and the leading cause in developed countries such as Canada, representing a global cost of hundreds of billions of dollars.[2]

How Do I Know if I Have a Mental Health Disorder?

Most people, at one time or another, have asked themselves this question. If you ask yourself: "Are my problems or symptoms getting in the way of my life?" and if you think the answer is "yes," then you may have a mental health disorder.

The **DSM-IV** (**Diagnostic and Statistical Manual of Mental Disorders, Fourth Edition**) published by the American Psychiatric Association is used throughout North America to classify mental illnesses. The manual states that you may have a mental health disorder if what you feel is severe enough to cause "clinically significant distress or impairment in [your] social, occupational, or other important areas of functioning."

People with a *mental disorder* or *mental illness* experience a disturbance in their ability to cope with or adjust to stress. They may have an alteration in their thinking, mood, or behaviour or some combination of alterations in these aspects. They may feel high levels of distress and fear and often have trouble coping with everyday life. They may have difficulties keeping a job, staying in school, forming strong family and social relationships, and performing daily routines. People with mental health disorders often behave differently from what is considered "normal," and their thinking, mood, or behaviours may be affected or impaired, with symptoms ranging from mild to severe.

If you think that you may have a mental health disorder, you should have yourself thoroughly evaluated by your doctor as soon as possible. When you see your doctor, you should describe how you are feeling as completely as you can. Your doctor may then take a complete medical history and examine you for any physical conditions that might have contributed to your condition. He or she may also advise you to refrain from drinking alcohol; to avoid taking any nonprescribed medications or drugs; to eat properly, reducing sugar and caffeine intake; to get plenty of exercise; and to get at least 8 hours of sleep.

If you still feel that you have a mental health disorder after making these changes to your lifestyle, your doctor may then prescribe medications, propose another course of treatment, or refer you to a mental health professional. Remember that it is always best to seek treatment as early as possible!

The **stigma** (a characteristic that marks a person as different or flawed) attached to mental illnesses presents a serious barrier not only to diagnosis and treatment but also to acceptance of the affected person in the community.

The Causes of Mental Health Disorders

The causes of mental health disorders are complex, as there are many contributing factors, including:

- ***Biological factors.*** Chemical imbalances in the body can cause mental health disorders. Some disorders run in families, which suggests that they can be inherited (passed from parent to child).
- ***Childhood experiences.*** Childhood traumas or conflicts, particularly when memories of them are repressed, can cause mental health disorders. **Repression** means to keep (or "bury") unpleasant or painful thoughts from the conscious mind. For example, a female client says she cannot remember being sexually abused during childhood.
- ***Social and cultural factors.*** These include poverty, discrimination, and social isolation.
- ***Stressful life events.*** Family situations and workplace pressures can be stressful. Change is also stressful (see Chapter 9), especially when associated with loss (such as the death of a loved one or divorce), and can be a source of extreme stress, which can lead to physical and mental health problems.
- ***Poor physical health or disability.*** People who are seriously ill, injured, or disabled are at risk for certain mental health disorders.

Supporting Clients and Their Families

It is now known that mental illnesses can be treated successfully in the vast majority of circumstances. Until the 1960s, many people with chronic or severe mental health disorders lived in psychiatric facilities. Today, only those who are severely ill live in facilities. Unfortunately, a few people with mental health disorders end up living on the streets, as they are too ill to hold a job or apply for financial assistance, may fear receiving treatment, or are not aware of their own illness.

Most people with mental health disorders are able to live in the community, where they may be offered treatment and assistance with life skills and employment. People with chronic or moderately severe mental health disorders are able to live in their homes, in group homes, or in assisted-living facilities, depending on their needs. Support workers provide valuable care and support to clients with mental health disorders and to their families in a wide variety of settings.

Remember DIPPS. While you are caring for and providing support to a person with a mental health disorder, your actions should always focus on respect and acceptance of the client and the family. Remember the principles of DIPPS *(see the Providing Compassionate Care: Supporting Clients with Mental Health Disorders* box on page 642*).* Box 34–1 lists the principles that govern health care workers' care and support for clients with mental health disorders and for their families.

Mental health disorders affect people in different ways, and often, people with mild disorders may have fewer problems than those with more pronounced mental health issues. Severe mental illness, however, almost always causes distress not only to the affected individuals but to their families as well. The ill person may be unable to function, and his or her behaviour may become disruptive at times. The support worker often provides the needed reassurance and support to these clients and also to their families.

Because they might have been exposed to negative attitudes in the past, your clients and their families may be particularly sensitive to your verbal or nonverbal signs that may indicate that you disapprove of them or that you *stigmatize* people with mental illness. You need to pay particular attention to your body language and verbal language and should make every attempt to convey to them that you are

Box 34–1 Principles of Mental Health Care

1. ***Follow the care plan.*** Tell your supervisor if support measures are not working.
2. ***Do no harm.*** Provide a safe, comfortable setting for the client. You need to provide both safe care and protection from harm at all times. A safe, quiet, and neat setting can calm the client. You should remember to act as the client's advocate, whenever necessary.
3. ***Accept each client as a whole person.*** You should accept the client as he or she is and refrain from making any judgements.
4. ***Be patient and supportive.*** Speak calmly, and avoid speaking in loud or sharp tones.
5. ***Develop mutual trust.*** Remember to ***do what you say you will do.*** Being on time, providing the care as promised, and explaining all procedures will all promote trust and reduce your client's anxiety.
6. ***Explore behaviours and emotions.*** Many clients will share with you what they are feeling and thinking when they trust you and if you take the time to listen to them.
7. ***Observe the client carefully.*** Observe for any changes in the client's behaviour, mood, and thinking, such as signs and symptoms of fatigue, stress, anxiety, fear, and frustration, as well as signs and symptoms of illness. Report and record all of your observations, according to employer policy.
8. ***Encourage responsibility.*** Taking responsibility for his or her own actions helps the client build self-worth, dignity and confidence.
9. ***Encourage effective adaptation.*** Clients who are mentally stressed may behave in socially unacceptable ways or may be harmful to themselves or others. It is often your responsibility to intervene when this happens and to help the client find better ways of coping.
10. ***Provide consistency.*** Maintaining a routine promotes a sense of control. Consistency and reliability of your care will also provide security and stability to the client. This will, in turn, help reduce the client's stresses and anxieties.

respectful, nonjudgemental, and accepting of their behaviours (see Chapter 13 for a discussion on ways to communicate with acceptance and respect).

Team approach. The care planning process aims at addressing the needs of clients with mental health disorders, including physical, safety, and emotional needs, and usually requires input from various members of the health care team. The physician may order medications, depending on the client's illness, signs, and symptoms, as a number of mental health disorders can be controlled effectively with medication.

The health care team may include a family physician, nurse, social worker, occupational therapist (who helps the person learn or relearn skills for the performance of life tasks), social workers (who can also provide assistance, such as helping a client resolve problems with employment), support workers, and one or more of the following mental health specialists:

- ***Psychiatrists***—physicians who specialize in mental health disorders, who can prescribe medications for treatment.
- ***Psychologists and psychotherapists***—health care professionals educated in treatments for mental health disorders that do not involve prescribing medications.

Treatment of mental health disorders often involves **psychotherapy**, which is a form of therapy in which a client explores his or her thoughts, feelings, and behaviours with help and guidance from a mental health specialist. The various forms of psychotherapy include:

- ***Psychoanalysis***—explores unconscious conflicts and the reasons behind the problems.
- ***Behaviour therapy***—attempts to change behaviour by using various techniques. The focus is on the behaviour, not on the underlying reasons for the behaviour.
- ***Group therapy***—a group of people who meet regularly to discuss their problems under the guidance of a mental health specialist.
- ***Family therapy***—family members meet regularly with a mental health specialist to discuss their problems.

The Stigma of Mental Health Disorders

In Chapter 4, we discussed that some people feel uncomfortable or fearful when they are with ill or disabled people. They may stare or avoid eye contact and may treat ill and disabled people differently from those who are well and able-bodied. This is certainly true for people with mental health disorders, who are often discriminated against due to lack of understanding of mental health disorders. Some fear being with a mentally ill person, as they do not know what to expect and may believe a mentally ill person is dangerous. Some people may blame the mentally ill person for his or her problems. Such attitudes lead people to avoid and exclude those with mental health disorders causing them to often feel ashamed, rejected, and isolated.

As mentioned earlier, a stigma is a characteristic that marks a person as different or flawed. A report from Health Canada (2002) states that stigma against individuals with mood disorders is a major cause for the affected person not seeking treatment, taking prescribed medication, or attending counselling.[3] It also states that stigma affects men more than it does women and also influences the person's successful reintegration into his or her family or into society in general. The stigma extends to the workplace, when employers are concerned about the person's ability to function at the level of other employees. Although it is against current human right legislation to openly discriminate against people with mental illnesses, many employers still do.

The Canadian Alliance for Mental Illness and Mental Health (CAMIMH) is an organization that represents mental health professionals and individuals concerned with mental health. The main goal of the CAMIMH is to prevent stigma and discrimination against people with mental health disorders. Through educational programs, the organization promotes greater understanding and acceptance of people with mental health disorders.[3]

As a support worker, it is imperative that you remember that all clients (and their families) have the right to caring, nonjudgemental support and the right to be treated with dignity and respect, as stressed throughout this textbook.

Effect on the Family. Family members of clients with mental health disorders must make difficult decisions about care, treatment, and housing. They may feel anxious about an uncertain future, and the financial burden of caring for a loved one who is ill may be a significant one. Some family members may feel guilty and blame themselves for the illness, and some others may be at risk for depression.

Family members are also affected by the stigma of mental health disorders. If friends and acquaintances feel uncomfortable, they may not offer their time or social support. One woman described how people reacted differently to her husband's physical illness and her son's mental illness: "When my husband had cancer, neighbours and friends were very kind. The phone rang constantly with offers to help. People brought over meals and sent flowers and cards. When my son was diagnosed with schizophrenia, everything was different. Nobody called. Nobody asked how we were doing. They pretended everything was fine. We felt very much alone."

Culture and Its Influence on Mental Health Disorders and Treatment

The need for understanding cultural differences among clients receiving support care has been stressed repeatedly in this book and was discussed at length in Chapter 12. Culture has a profound influence on understanding mental illness and its treatment. Clients in one culture may not find it hard to seek medical attention for their mental illness, while clients in some other culture may prefer to consult their local healer for herbal treatments or other remedies. People in certain cultures even refuse to acknowledge that they may have a mental illness, while some others may readily seek help and be open about their illness.

Interpretations of the signs and symptoms of what some call mental illness varies greatly from culture to culture, and even from person to person. What may be appropriate behaviour in one culture may be considered insanity in another. For example, someone who has lived through severe poverty might be afraid or hesitant to throw anything away, even items like rubber bands or paper clips, which some may consider odd behaviour. Understanding your clients' cultural background before caring for them will help you consider their cultural differences and preferences as you provide care. Make sure that you follow the DIPPS principles.

Refugees. It is important to understand the unique status of refugees. A *refugee* is someone who had to escape from his or her former home or country to seek safe shelter elsewhere. Many refugees have seen or experienced imprisonment, torture, murder of loved ones, extreme hunger, and poverty. They must learn to cope with life in a new country, learn new customs and language, and adjust to the new country's laws. Because of their particularly difficult circumstances, many refugees have a higher incidence of depression, anxiety, and stress disorders and may be distrustful of the support care that they are receiving. Some of your clients may exhibit some of these behaviours because may have had terrible experiences in another country or as soldiers in wars. As a support worker, you should know when to report your observations to your supervisor (see *Supporting Mr. Awondo* for an example of the changes that occurred when a support worker reported his client's behaviours to his supervisor).

Providing Care and Support for Clients With Mental Health Disorders

There are many different types of mental health disorders, and this book briefly addresses the most common of these, paying particular attention to the role of the support worker caring for clients with these disorders and for their families. Common mental health disorders include anxiety disorders; mood disorders (such as major depression and bipolar disorder); body dysmorphic disorders; sleeping disorders; schizophrenia; impulse control disorders (both outward- and inward-focused); substance-related disorders; and personality disorders.

Confusion, delirium, and dementia, which are conditions and mental health disorders of particular significance in the elderly, are discussed in Chapter 35.

supporting MR. AWONDO

Jesus Awondo, 44, single, fled to Canada 20 years ago from a South American country. Last week, at work, he fell from a scaffold and broke numerous bones in his body. After being discharged from hospital, he was cared for at home by Bob, a support worker. Bob came to Mr. Awondo's house every day to assist him with his activities of daily living (ADLs).

While caring for him, Bob noticed that Mr. Awondo usually fell asleep after his bed bath but never had a quiet sleep. Yesterday, while he was sleeping, Mr. Awondo started to scream, mumble loudly, and tried to swing his cast-covered arms around in the air. When Mr. Awondo woke up, Bob told him about what he had observed.

Mr. Awondo said that in his home country, he had watched his wife and child being killed with machetes by the local drug gangs. He had been bound, gagged, and placed in a cage, where rats were allowed to crawl on him. He told Bob that he had frequent nightmares of this, and since his injury at work, his nightmares had increased in their length and frequency. Bob reported this to his supervisor, who arranged for Mr. Awondo's doctor to see him at his home. Mr. Awondo's medical treatment was then changed, which resulted in Mr. Awondo sleeping more peacefully at night, in spite of an occasional nightmare.

ANXIETY DISORDERS

Anxiety disorders are a group of mental health disorders in which anxiety is the main symptom. Anxiety is a vague, uneasy feeling in response to stress. An anxious person has a sense of dread, danger, or harm. Some amount of anxiety is normal, but clients with anxiety disorders experience extreme anxiety. Their fears and worries are disproportionate for the situation, so their normal functioning is affected. Many anxiety disorders can be treated with medication, and clients will generally notice a reduction of symptoms as long as they take their medications continuously and regularly. The main types of anxiety disorders are discussed in this chapter.

Supporting Clients With Anxiety Disorders.

- ***Avoid situations that are known to cause anxiety.*** For example, if a client is afraid of small, closed spaces, keep him or her away from these.
- ***Avoid discussing subjects that cause anxiety.*** Keep the conversation on other subjects.
- ***Provide comfort during periods of anxiety.*** Stay with the client if he or she is extremely anxious or is having a panic attack. Use touch to reassure the client, if appropriate. Report the situation to your supervisor.

Panic Disorder

Panic is an intense and sudden feeling of fear, anxiety, terror, or dread for no obvious reason. A client who has panic disorder experiences panic attacks, during which the client is unable to function normally. He or she may experience a rapid heart rate, shortness of breath, chest pain, or dizziness. Panic attacks can last for a few minutes or hours and can occur several times a week. As a support worker, when you witness a panic episode, you should report and record in the client's chart the following information to your supervisor:

- Signs and symptoms
- How long the episode lasted
- What caused it to happen (triggering events)
- What you did to help the client

Obsessive-Compulsive Disorder (OCD)

An *obsession* is a persistent thought or desire, and a *compulsion* is the uncontrollable urge to perform an act. The obsession may be violent in nature and is usually disturbing to the person; he or she may try to ignore the obsessive thought or deal with it by repeating an act over and over again.

Examples of common obsessions include:

- Fearing that your thoughts will cause someone harm
- Ruminating (being preoccupied) about hurting someone

As the support worker caring for a client with OCD, you should observe the repeated behaviours, and report them to your supervisor. You should be aware that the client performs these behaviours to help relieve his or her stress, and he or she may not be able to stop without feeling extremely stressed and anxious.

Example of common compulsions include:

- Repeatedly washing hands, bathing, or cleaning household items
- Checking things several times a day, such as checking if the stove is off, windows locked, etc.
- Repeating a name, phrase, or tune
- Preoccupations with throwing things away that have little value

Post-traumatic Stress Disorder (PTSD)

Any traumatic event, such as war, fires, accidents, burns, torture, kidnapping, concentration camps, incest, or violent crimes can overwhelm the normal psychological coping mechanisms of the person witnessing these events. PSTD can occur in people of all ages, races, cultures, or genders.

Signs and symptoms include:

- Feelings of helplessness
- Terror
- Rage
- Feelings of loss of control

Survivors with PTSD are more likely to experience substance abuse, phobias, chronic pain, poor concentration, sleep disturbances, and extreme anxiety. Some survivors with PTSD might become easily angered, while others may feel overwhelming guilt because others have died and they have survived. The client in the box *Supporting Mr. Awondo* fits the description of someone living with PTSD.

PTSD in Children. Children who have experienced traumatic events may develop fear of the dark, fear of being alone, separation anxiety, nightmares, stomachaches, or headaches. They are often afraid to talk about the events to their parents for fear of upsetting them.[4]

PTSD in Older Adults. The signs and symptoms of PTSD in older adults are often the same as in children. Many older adults may have been traumatized when they were much younger, and extreme changes in their lives may trigger PTSD symptoms—for example, deaths of friends and family members or sudden loss of daily social contact. In long-term care facilities, rough treatment or a feeling of a loss of control when receiving care may trigger symptoms of PTSD in residents.[4]

As a support worker, you should be aware of the following:

- The client with PTSD should be treated according to all the DIPPS principles.
- Personal care should be provided in a gentle manner, respectful of the client's right to privacy.
- Clients should be given the opportunity to verbalize or reminisce about their experiences.
- Clients may have witnessed traumatic events in their past and PTSD may be triggered at anytime.
- Change in a client's willingness to be toileted, dressed, undressed, bathed, or fed may be a clue that the client has PTSD, and this should be reported to the supervisor immediately and always be documented.

Phobic Disorder

Phobia means fear, panic, or dread. A person with a phobic disorder has intense fear of a particular thing or situation. Often phobias occur after an event—for example, a fear of flying may develop after a person hears reports of a recent plane crash. Clients who struggle with phobias often feel embarrassed and stupid because they know their fear is exaggerated. Common phobias include *agoraphobia* (fear of open, crowded, public places) and *claustrophobia* (fear of small, enclosed places).

Panic Disorder

Panic attacks are part of panic disorder and are characterized by intense physical symptoms and sudden overpowering feelings of terror. The physical symptoms of fear (shortness of breath, racing heart, sweat) escalate very quickly. Many clients have symptoms that are similar to a heart attack.

Clients who wonder if they have panic disorder should ask themselves the following questions:

- Do I have sudden bursts of fear for no reason?
- Do I feel awful when they happen?

- Are there times when, for no reason, I experience chest pains, a racing heart, dizziness, sweating, stomach problems, nausea, and a feeling of loss of control?
- Am I afraid that I am dying or going crazy?

Panic attacks can happen anytime, anywhere, and without warning. The client who has panic attacks may live in fear of having another attack and may avoid places where they had an attack in the past. In the case of some clients, fear takes over their lives, and they are not able to leave their homes.

Panic disorder is more common in women than in men. It usually starts when the client is a young adult often during times of excessive stress. Panic disorder can last for months or years.

The treatment for panic disorder includes teaching the client to recognize and change thinking patterns before they lead to a panic attack, as well as medications prescribed by a doctor.

MOOD DISORDERS

Mood disorders are a group of mental health disorders that involve feelings, emotions, and mood that become troubling and difficult to manage on their own. They usually occur in three phases: (1) the acute phase (when the symptoms are escalating), (2) the continuation phase (when the symptoms are still visible and the client is usually being treated), and (3) the maintenance phase (when the client's acute symptoms have subsided). There are several major mood disorders, but this chapter focuses on the two main ones: *major depression* and *bipolar affective disorder*. It also includes seasonal affective disorder (SAD), which is common in northern regions with long cold winters.

Most people feel depressed at one time or another—for example, after the loss of a loved one, after a job loss, or any other major event in life. Grief is a normal and natural feeling that all people experience during their lives (see Chapter 47 for a discussion on the normal stages of grief and loss). Feelings of loss and sadness are normal reactions to recent experiences, and are sometimes referred to as **reactive depression**. This is different from **major depression** (also called **clinical depression),** which comprises severe feelings of worthlessness, self-blame, sadness, disappointment, and emptiness that last weeks and interfere with the person's ability to perform the activities of daily living. See Table 34–1 for a description of phases of treatment of mood disorders and the role of the support worker.

Table 34–1 Phases of Treatment of Mood Disorders and the Role of the Support Worker

Phase	Time Period	Goal of Treatment	Your Role
Acute treatment: Symptoms are beginning to escalate	6–12 months	To reduce symptoms and inappropriate behaviours	Observe for changes in the client's behaviour Report these changes to your supervisor Provide a safe, secure, consistent environment for the client
Continuation: Symptoms are still evident, but they are beginning to decrease with treatment	4–9 months	To prevent relapses into distressing emotional states	Observe the client for any sign or symptoms of depression (see Box 34–2) Report these to your supervisor
Maintenance: The client does not have acute symptoms	Indefinite	To prevent recurrences, as some clients think they are "cured," and stop taking their medication	Same as above

Major Depression

Major depression involves intense and prolonged feelings of sadness, hopelessness, and worthlessness and has physical and emotional effects. Sleep, eating, work, study, and other activities are affected. A person with depression may think about or attempt suicide. Major depression may occur only once, caused by a stressful event such as the death of a loved one, divorce, or job loss. Episodes of Major depression can occur throughout some clients' lives and at any age. It is, however, common among older adults (see the *Focus on Older Adults: Depression* box). For signs and symptoms of depression, see Box 34–2.

Major depression is usually treated by any of the following:

- ***Psychotherapy***—a form of therapy in which a person explores his or her thoughts, feelings, and behaviours with help and guidance from a mental health specialist
- ***Drug therapy***—various medications may be prescribed by a doctor with health benefits as the goal. Drugs and alcohol, which normally interfere with the helping action of medicines, will usually be discouraged
- ***ECT*** **(electroconvulsive therapy)**—a short-term treatment for severe depression. Before

Box 34–2 Signs and Symptoms of Depression

- Depressed mood—for example, feeling sad, "blue," "empty," pessimistic, or hopeless
- Irritability (especially in children and adolescents)
- Reduced interest in almost all activities
- Significant weight gain, or weight loss without dieting
- Insomnia or too much sleep
- Too much or too little motor activity
- Fatigue or loss of energy
- Feelings of worthlessness or guilt
- Reduced ability to concentrate or think
- Difficulties making decisions
- Loss of interest or pleasure in activities once enjoyed, including sex
- Chronic pain or other persistent bodily symptoms that are not caused by physical illness or injury
- Recurrent thoughts of death or suicide, or suicide attempts

Source: American Psychological Association. (1994). *Diagnostic and statistical manual of mental disorders (DSM-IV)* (4th ed. Text Revision.) Washington, DC: American Psychiatric Association.

focus on ››OLDER ADULTS

Depression

Depression is common in older adults, as they usually experience many losses—death of family members and friends, loss of health, loss of body functions, and loss of independence. Other factors that may trigger depression in older adults include:

- Loneliness
- The loss of a beloved pet
- Poor nutrition
- Overuse or underuse of prescribed medications
- Taking medications incorrectly
- Side effects of some medications
- Loss of control over finances
- Loss of memory

Depression in older adults is often overlooked or misdiagnosed. Sometimes the client is thought to have dementia (see Chapter 34), so the depression goes untreated. Ways to reduce the likelihood of depression in older adults include:

- Ensuring adequate nourishing food and water
- Ensuring regular bowel movements
- Having regular medical checkups by a family physician or nurse practitioner
- Taking medications correctly
- Avoiding excessive use of over-the-counter medications or alcohol
- Providing support and encouraging involvement with others
- Providing opportunities for physical activity
- Providing opportunities to be outside in the fresh air and sunlight
- Providing opportunities to interact with pets that they can see and pet
- Providing opportunities for stimulation of the senses
- Providing opportunities to interact with reminiscence groups
- Providing situations that allow the client to feel wanted and needed

ECT, clients are administered anaesthesia to put them in a dream-like state and medications to relax their muscles. An electrical current is then briefly sent to the brain through electrodes placed on the client's temples, which causes a seizure. It is not known exactly how ECT works, but it is believed that ECT works by altering brain chemicals, serotonin, endorphins, and adrenalin.

Supporting Clients With Major Depression.

- ***Show that you enjoy being with the client.*** Listen to your client. Show an interest in the client's life.
- ***Know that most clients do not know that they are depressed if they have never been diagnosed with depression.*** Many clients will not say they are depressed because they do not know they are.
- ***Do not minimize the client's problems.*** Do not say, "Cheer up," or "Snap out of it." Such statements suggest that the client is exaggerating the problem.
- ***Be positive.*** One positive experience may encourage further positive experiences.
- ***Encourage rest.*** It can refresh the client.
- ***Encourage activity and social interactions.*** It can improve the client's outlook and sense of well-being. However, do not tire the client with activities.
- ***Be alert for warning signals of suicidal intent*** (see Box 34–2 on page 659). Report any signals to your supervisor at once.
- ***Provide a safe, secure, stable environment.***
- ***Follow the care plan.*** The care plan may state that the client may not have access to his or her medication bottles but that he or she may take medications *from a* ***dosette*** *or* ***blister-packaged*** *container only* (see Chapter 40).
- ***Ensure safety.*** Sharp items, belts, cords, or items similar to these may be locked away if the client is voicing intentions of suicide.
- ***Encourage normal activities.*** The client should be encouraged and assisted with bathing, meals, and taking adequate fluids, as these measures can maintain the body's homeostasis and avoid other health issues.

Seasonal Affective Disorder (SAD)

SAD is a type of depression that occurs each year at the same time, usually starting in fall or winter and ending in spring or early summer. It is common in colder regions, where people tend to spend the majority of their winter months indoors. Signs and symptoms may be mild to severe, and the condition is often mistaken for major depression. The signs and symptoms of major depression can be the same as with any other type of depression (see Box 34–2), but the treatment may be different. It is usually treated with **phototherapy**, which involves exposure to light from a box containing white fluorescent light tubes.

Bipolar Affective Disorder

Bipolar disorder, also known as manic-depressive illness, is a brain disorder that causes unusual shifts in a person's mood, energy, and ability to function. Different from the normal ups and downs that everyone goes through, the symptoms of bipolar affective disorder involve extreme swings in mood, energy, and ability to function. A client with bipolar affective disorder has emotional lows (depression) and emotional highs (mania) and thoughts, moods, and behaviours that swing from normal to grandiose and then to depressed. This can result in damaged relationships, poor job or school performance, and even suicide. Bipolar affective disorder is, however, treatable, and with proper treatment, those with this illness can lead full and productive lives.

Bipolar affective disorder tends to run in families. Signs and symptoms can range from mild to severe and typically develop in late adolescence or early adulthood. However, some exhibit the first symptoms during childhood and some late in life. It is often not recognized as an illness, and some of the affected may suffer for years before it is properly diagnosed and treated. Like diabetes or heart disease, bipolar affective disorder is a long-term illness that must be carefully managed throughout a person's life.

Signs and Symptoms of Mania (or a Manic Episode).

- Increased energy, activity, and restlessness
- Excessive "high"; overly good, euphoric mood
- Extreme irritability

- Racing thoughts and talking very fast, jumping from one idea to another
- Distractibility, inability to concentrate
- Little need for sleep
- Unrealistic beliefs in one's abilities and powers
- Poor judgement
- Spending sprees
- A prolonged period of behaviour that is different from usual
- Increased libido (sex drive)
- Abuse of drugs, particularly cocaine, alcohol, and sleep medications
- Provocative, intrusive, or aggressive behaviour
- Denying that anything is wrong

Diagnosis. A manic episode is diagnosed if elevated mood occurs with three or more of the other symptoms most of the day, nearly every day, for 1 week or longer. If irritable mood is seen, four additional symptoms must be present for the diagnosis.

Children and adolescents can also develop bipolar affective disorder and it is more likely to occur in children of parents who have the illness themselves. Unlike many adults with bipolar affective disorder, whose episodes tend to be more clearly defined, children and young adolescents with the illness often experience very fast mood swings between depression and mania many times within a day. Children with mania are more likely to be irritable and prone to destructive tantrums than to be overly happy and elated. Mixed symptoms also are common in youths with bipolar disorder. Older adolescents who develop the illness may have the more classic, adult-type episodes and symptoms.

Bipolar affective disorder in children and adolescents can be hard to distinguish from other problems, such as drug abuse, that may occur in these age groups and have similar symptoms.

As with any illness, effective treatment depends on accurate diagnosis. Children or adolescents with emotional and behavioural symptoms should be carefully evaluated by a mental health professional.

Treatment. Most people with bipolar affective disorder—even those with the most severe forms—can achieve substantial stabilization of their mood swings and related symptoms with proper treatment. Because bipolar affective disorder is a recurrent illness, those affected need long-term preventive treatment. In most cases, the disorder is much better controlled if treatment is continuous than if it is periodical. However, even when there are no breaks in treatment, mood changes can occur and should be reported immediately to the doctor, who may be able to prevent a full-blown episode by making timely adjustments to the treatment plan. Working closely with the doctor and communicating openly about treatment concerns and options can contribute significantly to treatment effectiveness. The support worker can assist in keeping a chart of daily mood symptoms, treatments, sleep patterns, and life events to help the client and his or her family to better understand and cope with the illness.

Supporting Clients With Bipolar Affective Disorder.

- ***During depression:***
  - Follow the guidelines for major depression.
- ***During manic periods:***
  - Provide a calm environment, with few distractions.
  - Encourage periods of rest.
  - Encourage self-care; assist, as required.
  - Do not argue. This could irritate the client.
  - Offer limited, clear choices to make decision making easier.

BODY DYSMORPHIC DISORDERS

Body dysmorphic disorders, also known as **eating disorders**, arise from altered body image perceptions that lead to disturbances in eating behaviours and an abnormal concern about body weight and shape. These occur mainly in teenage girls and young women and can be life-threatening. Some affected individuals recover, but some do not. The two most common eating disorders are anorexia nervosa and anorexia bulimia.

Body dysmorphic disorders are not the same as the anorexia seen in a client in an extended (long-term) care facility. Body dysmorphic disorders usually occur in the young and may signal a much deeper, more complex psychological problem. An older adult who refuses to eat may be afraid of choking, may feel unwell, may be depressed, or may not like the texture or taste of the food.

Supporting Clients With Body Dysmorphic Disorders.

- Fortunately, most of the complications experienced by clients with anorexia nervosa are reversible when their normal weight is restored.
- Clients with anorexia bulimia may have permanently damaged their bodies, especially wearing out the enamel on the teeth. With these clients, proper dental care should be emphasized.
- Clients with eating disorders should be diagnosed and treated as early as possible for a successful outcome of treatment.
- Some clients can be treated as outpatients, but some may need hospitalization to correct their dangerously low weight and food bingeing behaviours.
- Weight gain of 2.2 to 6.6 Kg. (1 to 3 lb) per week is considered safe and desirable.
- The most effective strategies for treating a client have been weight restoration within 10% of normal and individual, family, and group therapies.

Anorexia Nervosa

Anorexia nervosa is a serious, often chronic, life-threatening eating disorder defined by a refusal to maintain minimal body weight within 15% of an individual's normal weight.

Some people have an intense fear of gaining weight, a distorted body image, and **amenorrhea** (absence of at least three consecutive menstrual periods as normally expected to occur). In addition to this, some will also engage in recurrent binge eating and purging episodes. Starvation, weight loss, and related medical complications can result in death.

People who have an ongoing preoccupation with food and weight, even when they are thin, would benefit from exploring their thoughts and relationships with help and guidance from a therapist. People with anorexia nervosa ignore hunger and thus control their desire to eat, and this desire is frequently masked by cooking for others or hiding food in personal spaces. Obsessive exercising may accompany the starving behaviour, which may mislead others to think that the person is healthy.

Like all eating disorders, anorexia nervosa tends to occur around puberty but can develop during any major life change. Anorexia nervosa predominately affects adolescent girls and young adult women, although it also occurs in men and older women. One reason younger women are particularly vulnerable to eating disorders is their tendency to go on strict diets to achieve an "ideal" figure. This obsessive dieting behaviour is a result of today's societal pressure to be thin, as seen in advertising and the media. Others especially at risk for eating disorders include athletes, actors, dancers, models, and TV personalities for whom thinness has become one of the professional requirements.

For the person with anorexia nervosa, the satisfaction of achieving control over weight and food becomes very important even though the rest of her or his life is chaotic and emotionally painful. Generally, if a person fears he or she has anorexia nervosa, a doctor who specializes in eating disorders should make the diagnosis and rule out other physical disorders. Other psychiatric disorders, such as *depression* and *obsessive-compulsive disorder*, can occur along with anorexia nervosa. Anorexia nervosa has the highest mortality rate (6%) among all other psychiatric conditions.

Signs and Symptoms.

- Obsession with food and weight
- Refusal to maintain minimally normal body weight
- Thoughts of looking fat in spite of being bone-thin
- Brittle nails and hair
- Dry and yellow skin
- Cessation (stoppage) of menstruation
- Depression
- Frequent complaints of feeling cold (because body temperature drops)
- Lanugo (a term for the fine hair on a newborn) on the body
- Strange eating habits, such as cutting food into tiny pieces
- Refusal to eat in front of others
- Fixing elaborate meals for others and not eating the meals
- Abuse of laxatives and enema to rid the body of food

- Abuse of diuretics (drugs that cause the kidneys to produce large amounts of urine, through which extra fluid in the body is lost, causing weight loss).

Causes. Certain personality traits common in persons with anorexia nervosa are low self-esteem, social isolation (which usually occurs after behaviours associated with anorexia nervosa begin), and perfectionism. These clients tend to be good students and excellent athletes. It does seem clear (although not to the client) that focusing on weight loss and food allows the client to ignore other problems that are too painful or seem impossible to resolve.

Eating disorders also tend to run in families, with female relatives most often affected—for example, a girl has a 10 to 20 times higher risk of developing anorexia nervosa if she has a sibling who has the disease. Behavioural and environmental influences, as well as stressful events, are likely to increase the risk of eating disorders.

Medical Complications.

- Damage to vital organs such as the heart and brain
- Irregular heart rhythms or heart failure
- Calcium loss from bones, which can become brittle and prone to breakage

The worst outcome is that people with anorexia can starve themselves to death.

Anorexia Bulimia

Anorexia bulimia is a psychological eating disorder that is characterized by episodes of binge eating followed by inappropriate methods of weight control (purging). **Binge eating** is a compulsive disorder, in which an individual resorts to uncontrolled, impulsive, or even continuous eating.

Signs and Symptoms.

- Eating uncontrollably
- Purging
- Strict dieting
- Fasting
- Vigorous exercising
- Vomiting, or abusing laxatives or diuretics in an attempt to lose weight
- Vomiting blood
- Using the bathroom frequently after meals
- Preoccupation with body weight
- Depression or mood swings, feeling "out of control"
- Swollen glands in neck and face
- Heart burn
- Bloating
- Indigestion
- Constipation
- Irregular menstrual periods
- Dental problems
- Sore throat
- Weakness and exhaustion
- Bloodshot eyes
- Compulsive exercising
- Excessive concern about shape and weight

A **binge** is an episode that occurs when an individual eats a much larger amount of food than most people would in a similar situation; it is not a response to intense hunger but usually to depression, stress, or self-esteem issues. During the binge eating episode, the individual experiences a loss of control, which is followed by a short-lived calmness and later self-loathing. The cycle of overeating and purging usually becomes an obsession and is repeated often.

People with anorexia bulimia can look perfectly normal. Most of them are of normal weight, but some may be overweight. Women with bulimia tend to be high achievers. It is often difficult to recognize bulimia because bingeing and purging are done in secret and those with the condition often deny having it.

Sufferers consume huge quantities of food, sometimes up to 20,000 calories at a time. The foods they binge on are usually considered "comfort foods"—sweet foods that are high in calories, or smooth and soft foods such as ice cream, cake, and pastry. An individual may binge eat anywhere from twice a day to several times daily.

Causes. Currently, the causes of bulimia are not definitely known but are generally thought to be similar to those that trigger anorexia nervosa.

Medical Complications.

- Erosion of tooth enamel because of repeated exposure to acidic gastric contents through vomiting
- Dental cavities, sensitivity to hot or cold food
- Swelling and soreness in the salivary glands (from repeated vomiting)
- Stomach ulcers
- Rupture of the stomach and esophagus
- Disruption in the normal bowel release function
- Electrolyte imbalance
- Dehydration
- Irregular heartbeat
- A greater risk for suicidal behaviour
- Decreased libido (sex drive)

SLEEP DISORDERS

Sleep is absolutely essential for normal, healthy function. Scientists and medical professionals do not fully understand this complex physiological phenomenon. It is not clear exactly why the body requires sleep, although inadequate sleep can have severe detrimental effects on health.

Studies have shown that sleep is essential for normal immune system function to maintain the ability to fight disease and sickness, for normal nervous system function, and for the ability to function both physically and mentally. In addition, sleep is necessary for learning and for normal, healthy cell growth. The more than 70 sleep disorders recognized so far are generally classified into one of three categories:

1. Lack of sleep (e.g., *insomnia*)
2. Disturbed sleep (e.g., *obstructive sleep apnea*, a medical condition)
3. Excessive sleep (e.g., *narcolepsy*, a medical condition)

In most cases, sleep disorders can be easily managed once they are properly diagnosed. Insomnia is the most common sleep disorder, which occurs more often in women and older adults.

The amount of sleep that a person needs to function normally depends on several factors (e.g., age). Infants sleep most of the day (about 16 hours); teenagers usually need about 9 hours of sleep a day; and adults need an average of 7 to 8 hours of sleep a day. Although older adults require about as much sleep as do younger adults, they usually sleep for shorter periods and spend less time in the deep stages of sleep. About 50% of adults over the age of 65 have some type of sleep disorder, although it is not clear whether this is a normal part of aging or a result of medications that older adults commonly use.

Both REM (rapid eye movement) and deep sleep are essential parts of the normal sleep cycle. Sleepwalking and bedwetting occur during deep sleep, and dreams occur during REM sleep when the muscles of the body stiffen, the eyes move, the heart rate increases, breathing becomes more rapid and irregular, and the blood pressure rises.

Supporting Clients With Sleep Disorders.

- Instruct the client to avoid foods and medicines that alter the balance of chemicals that affect how well we sleep. Caffeine, for example, can cause insomnia (lack of sleep). Antidepressant medications can cause loss of REM sleep. Smoking and alcohol can cause loss of REM sleep as well as deep sleep.
- If the client appears to have periods where he or she does not breathe, or if the client wakes up with a headache every morning, sleep apnea should be suspected. Encourage the client to seek medical attention, as this is a medical disorder that must be treated. The client might also benefit from sleeping on the side, with a pillow between the knees.
- Clients with problems of sleeping too much should see the doctor for a physical checkup to rule out narcolepsy, which is a medical condition.
- You should observe, report, and record how long the client is sleeping during each stage of sleep. Make a note of the client's use of prescription or nonprescription drugs or alcohol, which might be causing the sleep problems.

SCHIZOPHRENIA

Schizophrenia, which affects 1% of Canadians,[5] is an extremely complex mental health disorder characterized by delusions, hallucinations, disturbances in thinking, and withdrawal from social activity.

The exact causes are still a mystery, but schizophrenia is believed to be caused by a biochemical imbalance.[5] This disorder affects a person's ability to function in all aspects of life, including work, school, social life, family relationships, and self-care.

The term "schizophrenia" means split (*schizo*) mind (*phrenia*), but it does not mean split personality, as was once commonly believed. "Split mind" refers to the person's feelings of being "split off" from reality and not knowing what is real and what is not. The following are common with schizophrenia:

- ***Psychosis***—a mental state in which perception of reality is impaired. The person cannot view or interpret reality correctly.
- ***Delusions***—false beliefs. The person may believe he or she is a robot or some other person.
- ***Delusions of grandeur***—false and exaggerated beliefs about one's importance, talent, or wealth. For example, a woman believes she is a goddess or the prime minister.
- ***Delusions of persecution*** are false beliefs that one is being mistreated, abused, or harassed. For example, a man believes that his neighbour wants to kill him.
- ***Hallucinations***—seeing, hearing, tasting, smelling, or feeling things that are not real. For example, the person may see faces and hear voices that are not really there.
- ***Paranoia***—extreme suspicion about a person or situation. For example, a person may feel that he or she is being watched, followed, or controlled by someone else and may have delusions of persecution.

Without treatment, a person with schizophrenia suffers severe mental impairment. He or she has problems relating to others; responses are inappropriate; and communication is disturbed. The person may ramble in their speech or repeat what others say. Sometimes the person's speech cannot be understood.

Some people with schizophrenia may have one severe psychotic episode. Most suffer signs and symptoms throughout their lives but may have periods of **remission** when the signs and symptoms of the disease lessen or disappear.

Some people with schizophrenia have frightening hallucinations and hear voices ordering them to harm themselves or others, and some may have friendly, peaceful hallucinations. Some people with severe schizophrenia withdraw from others (stay away from others) and the world and may sit alone for hours without moving, speaking, or responding.

Supporting Clients With Schizophrenia.

- ***Focus on one task or activity at a time.*** This helps the client focus.
- ***Be aware of your nonverbal communication.*** Avoid body language and facial expressions that could be considered threatening.
- ***Do not argue.*** Never argue with the client about a delusion or hallucination not being real: it is real to the client. You can suggest gently to the client that the delusion is not real, but do not pretend that the delusion or hallucination is real. Comfort the client, and show empathy. Tell your supervisor if your client is having a delusion or hallucination.
- ***Use distractions.*** Distract the client to avoid disturbing subjects. For example, play music, or take the client for a walk.

IMPULSE-CONTROL DISORDERS: OUTWARD-FOCUSED EMOTIONS —ANGER AND AGGRESSION

This section deals with anger in clients (or someone you may know!) who is cognitively alert and has control over their reactions to life's events.[6] Clients with dementia who may display aggressive behaviours will be discussed in Chapter 35.

Anger is caused by the inability to mentally cope with some situation. If your clients (or others you know) have persistent problems with anger, there may be important underlying issues that they have not yet resolved—for example, loss of control perceived in their important values not being met. They also may be using ineffective emotional coping methods. Many of the internal and external methods that help in dealing with negative emotion can help in dealing with anger as well.

Identifying important values of life and understanding the lack confidence in one's ability to be happy may be helpful to overcome anger in your client (or someone you know). Clients need to real-

Dealing With Your Own Anger

- ***Understand the hurt and fear underlying the anger.*** Remember that anger stems from fear and a sense of helplessness, such as feeling that you are losing control of the situation. The real threat may not be the surface issue (being late to the movie) as may be the underlying issue (not being important to someone you love or being mistreated). Identifying emotions of fear and hurt will open the door to recognizing and dealing with these underlying issues.
- ***Develop empathetic understanding.*** If you choose to decrease your anger at someone, the first step is to make every effort to see the situation from the other person's point of view. You might begin by asking that person to explain his or her point of view and then try to understand that person's situation, point of view, and the reasons for his or her beliefs and behaviour. Not having empathetic understanding is usually the major hurdle to getting control of anger. "Forgiving is not forgetting, it is remembering and letting go."[6]
- ***Assume the best intentions (whenever possible).*** Try to assume the best intentions in others until there are repeated indications for other motives.
- ***Understand that sometimes "life is not fair."*** There is nothing "fair" about some people being born into happy, prosperous families and living prosperous, long, happy lives while other people are born into miserable situations and die young after leading a life filled with suffering. This is reality, and it is pointless to get angry about it. Make the most out of what *you* have.
- ***Do not hold on to anger for motivation.*** Do you want do something just to punish the person you are angry with or to "get even"? Holding on to anger or hurt can only hurt you! Wait until you have calmed down, and then talk to the person, stating reasons for your actions calmly. This is much more effective than giving punishment out of anger!
- ***Examine underlying expectations in other people.*** Unfulfilled expectations can lead to anger. What are your expectations of yourself and of others for a situation? Are you expecting more than is realistic from this person in this particular situation? People are who they are, and one of the root causes of anger is not accepting people (or events) as they are.
- ***Choose happiness instead of anger.*** People who habitually choose anger over happiness lead frustrated, angry lives—not happy lives. Remind yourself of this fact to get more control of your anger. Say to yourself, "Self, why choose anger when you can choose thoughts that produce happiness?"

ize that anger is a choice they have made. Blaming others (or themselves) and remaining angry can be the easiest way out. Finding new ways to think about the situation and to make oneself happy requires skillful effort and mental control.

Supporting Clients With an Anger Disorder.

- Remember that as a support worker, you must accept clients in a caring, nonjudgemental way. They may lack insight into their feelings to be able to deal with them at the present time.
- Avoid doing anything that might escalate the situation. Do not touch the client, as this can cause his or her actions to escalate.
- If clients are verbally aggressive but not physically aggressive, try to determine the cause of their anger. Determine if they are cold, hungry, in pain, or frightened about something.
- Try to understand the client's anger in his or her cultural context. Some men, for example, would rather yell and scream than admit that they are frightened or in pain.
- You do have the right to ask the client to speak to you politely as to a professional. Do not yell back, but remain calm and professional yourself.
- Most employers or agencies that provide support services to clients with anger management issues will offer (or encourage you to take on your own) courses such as "Managing Disruptive Behaviours" so that you can learn to deal with aggressive clients in a nonconfrontational manner.
- If the client is verbally aggressive, your main concern is your safety as well as the safety of others. You should leave the situation, and immediately call your supervisor. If the client is threatening to harm you physically, you should get to a safe

place and call the police immediately. Refer to the section in Chapter 35 "Managing Disruptive Behaviours" on page 684.

IMPULSE-CONTROL DISORDERS: INWARD-FOCUSED EMOTIONS —SUICIDE

Suicide—to kill (*caedere*) oneself (*sui*)—is a common cause of death in both males and females from adolescence through middle age, although it has also been found to be the cause of death among some school-age children as well as older adults.[7] People with mental health disorders are at high risk for suicide. People who attempt suicide view life as unbearable and may believe that their families and friends are better off without them. Suicide is more common among men than among women, although statistically, women attempt suicide more often than do men. Men tend to use violent means to kill themselves (hanging, firearms), so their attempts are often fatal. Women usually choose less violent means (taking an overdose of pills), so they often tend to survive their attempts.

Attempted suicide is a sign of a serious mental health problem, and the person attempting suicide needs professional care and to be put on a suicide prevention program. Any child or adolescent who has suicidal feelings, talks about suicide, or attempts suicide should be taken seriously and should receive immediate help from a mental health specialist (see the *Focus on Older Adults: Suicide* box).

Risk Factors.

- Mental illness, especially depression, bipolar disorder, or schizophrenia
- A history of abuse
- A family history of suicide
- The suicide of a friend
- A prior suicide attempt
- A major crisis such as the loss of a relationship, family problems, loss of position in society, and work, money, or legal problems
- Pressure to succeed
- Isolation
- Early losses in life
- Sexual identity issues
- Feelings of deep hopelessness and helplessness

> **focus on ››OLDER ADULTS**
>
> **Suicide**
>
> Older adults are at risk for suicide because they experience many losses: death of family members and friends, loss of physical health, and loss of cognitive (mental) abilities. Depression is common in older adults (see *Focus on Older Adults: Depression*, page 650). Some older adults choose suicide to avoid loneliness. For some who are facing death because of serious illness, suicide may seem better than prolonged suffering or causing hardship for their families. As with any person who speaks of committing suicide, the older adult who speaks of suicidal intentions should be carefully monitored and should be given medical treatment as soon as possible.

- Recent diagnosis of a life-threatening illness
- Substance abuse

The common warning signals of suicide are listed in Box 34–3.

Supporting Clients Who Have Suicidal Intent.

- If a client talks about suicide, take him or her seriously.
- Tell your supervisor at once.
- Do not leave the client alone.
- Encourage the client to talk. This gives your supervisor time to get help. It also shows the client that you care. Be a good listener.
- Do not minimize the client's concerns. Do not make comments such as: "You shouldn't have such thoughts," "Things will work out," or "Look on the bright side."
- In a home care setting, stay with the client until help arrives. Your supervisor may send a nurse, case manager, or emergency personnel to help the client.

SUBSTANCE DEPENDENCE DISORDERS

A **substance dependence disorder** or **substance-abuse disorder** is the deliberate misuse of prescription medications, illegal drugs, alcohol, or other substances. People with this disorder often develop relationship and work problems but are unable to stop the substance abuse.

Box 34–3 Warning Signs of Suicidal Intent

It is important to understand that suicidal feelings and actions are symptoms of an illness that can be treated. While some suicide attempts are carefully planned over time, others are impulsive acts that have not been thought through.

Warnings signs of suicidal intent include:

- Signs and symptoms of depression (see Box 34–2 on page 650).
- Repeated expressions of hopelessness, helplessness, or desperation
- Expressions of interest in committing suicide
- Having a plan for suicide, such as taking pills or hanging oneself at a specific place and time
- Loss of interest in friends, hobbies, or previously enjoyed activities
- Giving away prized possessions or putting personal affairs in order
- Telling someone else about final wishes
- A change in personality or mood—for example, sudden and unusually happy behaviour after a period of depression
- A change in appearance—for example, a person who is usually well groomed is untidy and unwashed
- Failure to recover from a loss or crisis
- A sudden tendency to take big risks
- Refusing to eat, drink, or take medications

If you are feeling suicidal or know someone who is:

- Call a doctor, emergency room, or 9-1-1 right away to get immediate help
- Make sure you, or the suicidal person, are not left alone
- Make sure that access is prevented to large amounts of medication, weapons, or other items that could be used for self-harm

With proper treatment, suicidal feelings can be overcome.

Sources: Health Canada. (2002). *A report on mental illness in Canada* (p. 90, Cat. No. 0-662-32817-5). Retrieved March 6, 2008, from http://www.hc-sc.gc.ca; The Canadian Mental Health Association. (1993). *Preventing suicide.* Toronto: National Office. Retrieved March 6, 2008, from http://www.cmha.ca/english/info_centre/mh_pamphlets/mh_pamphlet_12.htm

Abused substances affect the central nervous system—some have a calming or depressing effect, while others have a stimulating effect on the mind and thinking. Many are also mood altering—that is, after taking the substance, users may feel happy, self-confident, and relaxed, but some drugs cause hallucinations, an exaggerated sense of one's own abilities, or an emotional or aggressive state.

People with this disorder may show evidence of tolerance and withdrawal. **Drug tolerance** occurs when the person needs larger and larger amounts of the substance to experience the same effect. **Drug withdrawal** is a physical reaction that occurs when the person stops taking the substance. Signs and symptoms of withdrawal, which can be severe, may include depression, agitation, abdominal cramps, nausea, diarrhea, and painful muscle spasms. Some people turn to criminal acts to support their habit. Without treatment, death is a risk. Common causes of death are overdoses, suicide, and diseases contracted from using contaminated needles. Treatment depends on the substance being abused.

If a person has abused any type of drugs, alcohol, or a combination of these, they will need **detoxification**—a process that involves allowing abused substances to exit the body naturally or medically removing the abused substance from the body. The person being detoxified usually goes into drug withdrawal. Hospital care is usually required. Almost all treatment programs involve psychotherapy involving mental health professionals who help clients manage their problems.

Alcohol Abuse

Alcohol is abused more than any other substance. Signs and symptoms of alcohol abuse include intoxication (drunkenness), memory problems, difficulty concentrating, tremors, and loss of interest in family and friends. Liver, pancreas, and heart problems may develop. Fetal alcohol syndrome can result in a baby when a woman drinks during pregnancy (see Chapter 38). Many people with alcohol problems have poor nutrition, and many also are addicted to nicotine (cigarettes), so they are at risk for lung disease and certain cancers.

For most people, even exceeding two drinks a day can do significant harm. Women who have more than 9 drinks a week have higher rates of cancer and other problems than women who drink less.[8] Men who have more than 14 drinks a week also have higher rates of alcohol-related problems.[8] Some people drink every day, and some go for days or weeks without drinking and then drink a great deal in a short period. People who are mentally ill, under stress, or lonely may turn to alcohol to feel better. Older adults who live alone are at risk for alcohol abuse.

People with alcohol problems may be emotional, aggressive, and abusive, and their families are at risk for abuse and other problems. Some people who are "happy drunks" or the "life of the party" may not be violent with others, but they certainly put their own health at risk, and if they drink and drive, they risk killing themselves and others on the road.

The main treatment is to avoid drinking. Groups such as Alcoholics Anonymous (AA) help people with drinking cessation. Individual and family counselling is often needed as part of the treatment.[8]

Supporting Clients With Substance-Dependence Disorders.

- ***Report suspicions of substance abuse.*** You may smell alcohol on a client's breath, or you may observe that a client's medication is running out more quickly than it should.
- ***Report suspected substance abuse to your supervisor at once.*** This information is confidential. Do not discuss the matter with anyone else.
- ***Avoid confrontation.*** If you think a client is abusing a substance, do not argue. Tell your supervisor immediately. Do not discuss the matter with anyone.
- ***Never buy alcohol, drugs, or other substances for clients.*** Purchasing alcohol, drugs, or other substances for clients is unethical. Report any such requests from clients to your supervisor.

PERSONALITY DISORDERS

Personality disorders are a group of disorders involving rigid and socially unacceptable behaviours that are not expected from a person's culture. A personality disorder is identified by a pervasive pattern of experience and behaviour that is abnormal with respect to any two of the following: thinking, mood, personal relations, and the control of impulses. Individuals with personality disorders have problems relating to others. They may be demanding, hostile, and manipulative. Because of their behaviours, people with personality disorders are not able to function well in society.

When the behaviour of a person is inflexible, maladaptive, and antisocial, that individual is diagnosed with a personality disorder. Most personality disorders that begin as problems in personal development and character peak during adolescence.

Personality disorders are not illnesses in a strict sense, as they do not disrupt emotional, intellectual, or perceptual functioning. However, those with personality disorders suffer a life that is not positive, proactive, or fulfilling. Not surprisingly, personality disorders are also associated with failures to reach one's potential.

According to the DSM-IV (*Diagnostic and Statistical Manual of Mental Disorders*, Fourth Edition), published by the American Psychiatric Association, some of the main types of personality disorders include the following:

- ***Antisocial Personality Disorder***—a lack of regard for the moral or legal standards in the local culture, marked inability to get along with others or abide by societal rules. People with this disorder are sometimes called "psychopaths" or "sociopaths."
- ***Avoidant Personality Disorder***—marked social inhibition, feelings of inadequacy, and extreme sensitivity to criticism.
- ***Borderline Personality Disorder***—lack of identity, rapid changes in mood, intense unstable interpersonal relationships, impulsiveness, and lack of stability in the way one reacts to things and in self-image.
- ***Dependent Personality Disorder***—an extreme need of other people, to a point where the person is unable to make any decisions or take an independent stand on his or her own. People with this disorder also have a fear of separation,

behave in a submissive manner, and lack decisiveness and self-confidence.

- ***Histrionic Personality Disorder***—exaggerated, almost theatrical, and often inappropriate displays of emotional reactions in everyday behaviour. People with this disorder shift their emotional expressions suddenly and rapidly.
- ***Narcissistic Personality Disorder***—general lack of empathy for others, a need to be admired by others, an inability to see the viewpoints of others, and hypersensitivity to the opinions of others.
- ***Obsessive-Compulsive Personality Disorder***—perfectionism and inflexibility. People with this disorder are preoccupied with uncontrollable patterns of thought and action.
- ***Paranoid Personality Disorder***—a marked distrust of others, including the belief, without reason, that others are exploiting, harming, or trying to deceive. People with this disorder have an overall lack of trust and believe that others are betraying them and that there are hidden meanings in messages.
- ***Schizoid Personality Disorder***—a very limited range of emotion, both in expression of and experiencing emotions. People with this disorder are indifferent to social relationships.

Common Signs and Symptoms.

- Self-centredness that manifests itself through a "me-first," self-preoccupied attitude
- Lack of individual accountability that results in a victim mentality and blame of others, society, and the universe for one's problems
- Lack of perspective-taking and empathy
- Manipulative and exploitative behaviour
- Unhappiness, depression, and other mood and anxiety disorders
- Vulnerability to other mental disorders such as obsessive-compulsive tendencies and panic attacks
- Distorted or superficial understanding of self and others' perceptions, being unable to see his or her objectionable, unacceptable, disagreeable, or self-destructive behaviours or the issues that may have contributed to the personality disorder.
- Socially maladaptive, changing the rules of the game, introducing new variables, or otherwise influencing the external world to conform to one's own needs.

Treatment.

- Healing is possible when individuals choose to be in control of their lives and are committed to changing their lives.
- Therapy and medications can help, but it is the individual's decision to take accountability for his or her own life that makes the difference.
- Individuals need to want to gain insight into and face their inner experience and behaviour. To heal, they must first have the desire to change in order to break through the enduring pattern of a personality disorder. (These issues may concern severe or repeated trauma during childhood, such as abuse.)
- Support systems (e.g., therapy, self-help groups, friends, family, medication), are usually necessary for full treatment of the person with the personality disorder.

Supporting Clients With Personality Disorders.

- Remember that as a support worker, you must accept clients in a caring, nonjudgemental way. They may lack insight into their feelings to be able to deal with them at the present time.
- Speak to your client in a factual, professional manner.
- Provide care and support as specified in the client's care plan, in a respectful, efficient manner.
- Just as you would with any client, you should refrain from giving your home phone number, e-mail address, or information about your private life to the client, to avoid any misunderstanding that it constitutes an invitation to private correspondence.
- As with any client, do not accept gifts, money, or other items from your client. This might be misinterpreted by your client as a sign of affection or special treatment.
- Consult with the client's significant other for ways to successfully deal with him or her.

REVIEW

Answers to these questions are at the bottom of page 664.

Circle the BEST answer.

1. **Which of the following is *true*?**
   A. People with mental health disorders usually create their own problems.
   B. Chemical imbalances in the body can cause mental health disorders.
   C. Treatment for mental health disorders might include physiotherapy and medication.
   D. Most people with mental health disorders should be hospitalized.

2. **Mr. Mueller sees a psychologist. They explore the unconscious conflicts and underlying reasons for Mr. Mueller's problems. This kind of psychotherapy is:**
   A. Psychoanalysis
   B. Occupational therapy
   C. Behaviour therapy
   D. Group therapy

3. **Mrs. Paré is afraid of catching a disease and washes her hands hundreds of times a day. Mrs. Paré likely has:**
   A. Panic disorder
   B. Phobic disorder
   C. Anorexia nervosa
   D. Obsessive-compulsive disorder

4. **Mr. Lau has bipolar disorder. This means he:**
   A. Has delusions
   B. Is hostile
   C. Is very suspicious
   D. Has severe mood swings

5. **Which BEST describes how culture can impact mental health? Culture:**
   A. Can dictate the way that the brain reacts to traumatic events
   B. Can influence the way a person's behaviours are interpreted
   C. Can predict the presence of mental health disorders in people
   D. Has no effect on mental health disorders

6. **Which of the following might have the biggest impact on whether or not Mike develops a mental health illness in the future? Mike:**
   A. Has been abused as a child
   B. Eats a balanced diet and gets 8 hours of sleep a night
   C. Has a parent who suffers from *major* depression
   D. Answers A & C

7. **Shira, 15, has lost 30 pounds. She is terrified of becoming fat, even though she is extremely thin. She avoids food. Shira likely has:**
   A. Anorexia bulimia
   B. Repression
   C. Anorexia nervosa
   D. Claustrophobia

8. **Mrs. Alam has major depression. You should avoid:**
   A. Showing her that you care
   B. Telling her how lucky she is
   C. Encouraging periods of rest
   D. Encouraging activity and social interactions

9. **A client with major depression suddenly seems happy. She asks you to leave early because she is expecting friends. You should:**
   A. Leave as requested
   B. Leave as soon as the friends arrive
   C. Call your supervisor to report the situation
   D. Stay until you are scheduled to leave

10. **You are supporting a client with bipolar disorder, who is in the manic phase of the illness. You should:**
    A. Offer limited choices
    B. Direct her to clean her house
    C. Provide a stimulating environment
    D. Allow her to get tired so that she will fall asleep

11. **Your client, who you meet with at a day-program for older adults, complains that she has not been able to sleep for weeks. Before reporting this, you should:**
    A. Ask her more about her lifestyle
    B. Advise her to get a new mattress
    C. Ask her if she is depressed
    D. Tell her that *you* never get enough sleep

REVIEW

Answers to these questions are at the bottom of page 664.

12. **Mrs. Smith, an older woman who has just been admitted to a long-term care facility, tells you that she hopes that she "will die soon." Before notifying your supervisor, you should:**
    A. Tell her that she will get used to her new environment soon
    B. Introduce her to the other residents on her ward
    C. Not respond, but observe her for signs of depression
    D. Ask questions that will allow her to elaborate on why she feels this way

13. **Jimmie, 16, who used to be a soccer star in his high school, failed to make the soccer team last week. He tells his sister that she can have all of his electronic equipment. What should his sister do?**
    A. Watch what he does next
    B. Talk to his friends about this
    C. Offer him money for the equipment
    D. Notify an adult immediately and stay with him till help arrives

14. **Mr. Wilder is a World War II veteran. How might going to his local branch of the Legion help him deal with the new feelings of depression he has?**
    A. It will give him a chance to talk openly about the horrors of war that he never talked about before.
    B. It will give him an opportunity to talk to other people his age.
    C. It will provide a stimulating environment and give him somewhere to go.
    D. All of the above.

15. **Kathy, 19, has schizophrenia. She usually insists on having her MP3 player and headphones on all day because she says she likes to listen to music. Today, you realize that the headphones are not attached to her player. Before notifying your supervisor, you should:**
    A. Take her headphones away from her
    B. Point out this fact and reattach them
    C. Ask her to remove her headphones
    D. Talk to her to try to find out if she is having hallucinations

16. **Kathy says giant insects are climbing up the wall. She is terrified. You see nothing on the wall. You should:**
    A. Insist that Kathy is seeing things
    B. Pretend you also see the insects
    C. Offer Kathy comfort and report the hallucination
    D. Leave Kathy alone and call for help

17. **You are supporting a client in the home, and you discover several half-empty bottles of gin in her bathroom cupboard. You should:**
    A. Replace the gin with water
    B. Notify your supervisor
    C. Point them out to your client
    D. Ask her to breathe on you to smell her breath

18. **Which of the following is true? People with substance dependence disorder:**
    A. Can overcome their addictions
    B. Have only themselves to blame
    C. Can only be addicted to street drugs
    D. Will not experience withdrawal symptoms from prescription medications

19. **The client that you are supporting in the community asks for your home phone number. You should:**
    A. Only give her your cell phone number
    B. Give her your friend's phone number
    C. Give a false number so that she cannot call you
    D. Explain that you do not give out your phone number to clients

20. **You are supporting a client in his own home, who is recovering from neurosurgery. On his care plan, it says that he has an addiction to drugs and alcohol. You should:**
    A. Go through his cupboards looking for alcohol
    B. Refuse to care for him because you don't drink
    C. Provide respectful care that is stated in his care plan
    D. Tell him about the time you got "wasted" last week to make him feel comfortable with you

REVIEW

Answers to these questions are at the bottom of the page.

Discuss the following situation:

21. **You are newly employed as a support worker at a group home for adult male clients who are recovering from addictions. One day, while you are observing some of the clients make pancakes in the kitchen, a fight breaks out in another room between two of the newly admitted clients over the television remote. You enter the room just as "Bob" punches "Joe" in the nose. Being the first worker at the scene, what should you do first?**
   - A. Get your supervisor to deal with this.
   - B. Separate the two clients and talk to them separately.
   - C. Grab both by their arms and shout at them: "Quit this, now!"
   - D. Instruct them to clean the mess they made, and observe them while they do this.

Answers: 1.B, 2.A, 3.D, 4.D, 5.B, 6.D, 7.C, 8.B, 9.C, 10.A, 11.A, 12.D, 13.D, 14.D, 15.D, 16.C, 17.B, 18.A, 19.D, 20.C, 21. You should separate the two clients and talk to them separately. Begin with Bob, the aggressor. You should speak in a firm but soft voice that is both professional and friendly. Never grab an aggressive client, as this might cause their anger to increase. Distance yourself just beyond arm's length to be prepared if the client tries to hit you. By separating the two, away from each other and from the other clients, you can help diffuse this situation. Try to discuss ways that they can deal with their issues in a nonconfrontational manner. After they calm down, you can try role playing with them, to reinforce what you have discussed.

CHAPTER 35

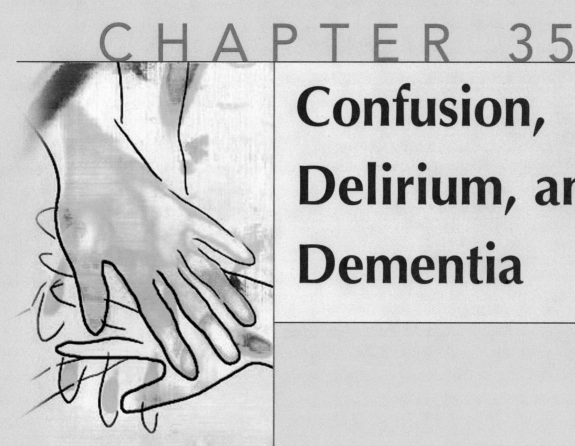

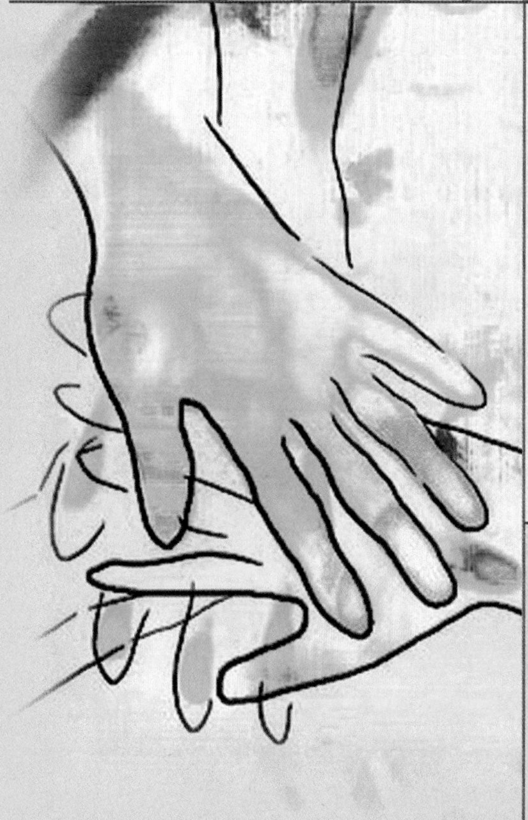

Confusion, Delirium, and Dementia

OBJECTIVES

- Define the key terms listed in this chapter.
- Describe confusion and delirium and their causes.
- List normal changes that happen with aging.
- Differentiate between normal and abnormal mental changes related to aging.
- List measures that help clients who are confused.
- Differentiate among confusion, delirium, and dementia.
- Summarize the role of the support worker when finding someone who is delirious.
- Describe dementia and its signs and symptoms.
- List different forms and causes of dementia.
- Describe the common stages of dementia.
- Describe the care needed for a client with dementia.
- Describe how caring for family members with dementia can affect primary caregivers.
- Apply the principles learned in this chapter to the care and support of a client with confusion, delirium, or dementia.
- List examples of challenging behaviours and possible causes.
- Apply the principles learned in this chapter to the care and support of clients with challenging behaviours.

key terms

Alzheimer's disease (AD) A progressive, degenerative disease that gradually destroys nerve cells (neurons) in most areas of the brain and causes thinking and memory to become seriously impaired; the most common form of dementia.

apathy An absence or lack of emotional feeling, which appears to be indifference.

apraxia Impairment of the skilled motor system, resulting in problems with feeding or dressing oneself.

atrophy Marked shrinkage or wastage of a specific body part or tissue.

cognitive function Brain function involving memory, thinking, reasoning, understanding, judgement, and behaviour functions of the brain.

cognitive impairment The loss of a person's ability to remember, think, reason, understand, or live independently.

confusion A mental state in which the person's memory and judgement are usually impaired and the person is disoriented to person, time, or place.

delirium A state of temporary mental confusion that can occur suddenly.

delusion A false belief.

dementia A general term that describes the progressive loss of brain functions, which include cognitive and social functions. It is not a single disease but a group of illnesses that involve memory, behaviour, learning, and communication.

disorientation Another name for **confusion**.

euphoria An exaggerated or abnormal sense of physical or emotional well-being that is not based on reality or truth.

hallucination Seeing, hearing, smelling, tasting, or feeling something that is not real.

hoarding Collecting things and putting them away in a guarded manner.

pseudo-dementia A word that means false (*pseudo*) dementia. Pseudo-dementia often occurs when severe depression causes cognitive changes that mimic dementia.

sundowning The name given for the condition in which the signs, symptoms, and behaviours of dementia increase at bedtime or during hours of darkness.

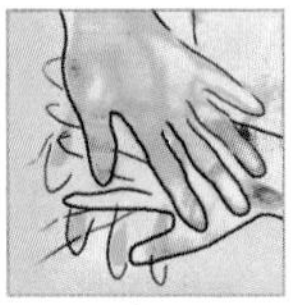

In Chapter 34, we discussed mental health disorders, most of which are changes in the brain's behaviour—which usually occur when the person is a teenager or a young adult—due to chemical imbalances or lifestyle choices. This chapter addresses the changes in behaviour that take place over time as the brain is affected by aging, illness, or, again, lifestyle. Although some changes in the brain and nervous system occur normally with aging (see Box 35–1), some other changes are caused by certain diseases. This chapter addresses confusion, delirium (which is sudden onset and sometimes reversible confusion), and dementia. You should be aware that ***confu-***

Box 35–1 Normal Changes in the Nervous System Associated With Aging

- Brain cells are lost.
- Nerve conduction slows.
- Response and reaction times are slower.
- Reflexes are slower.
- Vision and hearing decrease.
- Taste and smell decrease.
- Touch and sensitivity to pain decrease.
- Blood flow to the brain is reduced.
- Changes in sleep patterns occur.
- Mild word-finding problems occur.

sion, delirium, and dementia are NOT a normal part of aging. The reasons why a person may develop confusion, delirium, or dementia are discussed in this chapter.

The section on "Managing Disruptive Behaviours" at the end of this chapter describes some of the behaviours exhibited by people with dementia, which can be both disruptive and challenging. Diseases that affect the brain can affect **cognitive function** (the term *cognitive* relates to knowledge). Cognitive functioning involves the following functions of the brain:

- Memory
- Thinking
- Reasoning
- Ability to understand
- Judgement
- Behaviour

Loss of cognitive functioning affects all dimensions of a person's life. The state when a person has lost the ability to remember, think, reason, understand, or live independently is referred to as **cognitive impairment**.

CONFUSION

Confusion, also called **disorientation**, is the inability of a person to think with his or her usual speed or clarity. Confused people may have difficulty focusing attention and may feel disoriented to person, time, or place; the condition can be temporary or permanent or can occur suddenly or over a long period of time. Permanent confusion is caused by physical changes to the structure of the brain. Sudden confusion is called delirium, which is discussed later in this chapter. Confusion is more common in older adults and often occurs during hospitalization.

People with confusion often have behaviour changes and may be angry, restless, depressed, or irritable. Some confused people may behave aggressively. Other signs and symptoms of confusion include:

- Anxiety
- Tremors
- Hallucinations (page 685)
- Delusions (page 685)
- Decline in level of consciousness
- Disorganized thinking and speech
- Attention problems

Causes of Confusion.

- Urinary tract infection (main reason)
- Alcohol intoxication
- Low blood sugar
- Head trauma or head injury
- Concussion
- Fluid and electrolyte imbalance
- Nutritional deficiencies, particularly niacin, thiamine, vitamin C, or vitamin B_{12}
- Fever
- Sudden drop in body temperature (hypothermia)
- Low levels of oxygen (for example, from chronic lung disorders)
- Medications
- Infections
- Brain tumour
- Certain illnesses, especially in older adults
- Sleep deprivation
- Seizures

Diagnosing Confusion. People with ongoing confusion that has come on gradually (over weeks, months, or years) need to see a doctor to have the problem evaluated. The doctor will perform a physical examination and ask questions to determine if the client has any of the following signs or symptoms of confusion:

- Getting days and nights mixed up.
- Being awake during usual sleep time.
- Not recognizing people.
- Not knowing where they are.
- Not knowing the date and time.
- Not answering simple questions appropriately.
- Feelings of confusion that persist, or repeated episodes of confusion.
- Having confusion that is rapidly getting worse.
- Having confusion which comes and goes.

In addition, the doctor will ask about other conditions which may trigger confusion, such as:

- Having a recent illness, such as the flu.
- Having problems urinating.
- Having a recent head injury.

- Being diabetic.
- Having a lung disorder.
- Taking medications in the wrong combination or not as directed by the doctor or pharmacist.
- Having any exposure to other drugs or alcohol.

The physical examination will include a thorough evaluation of brain and nervous system functions. The doctor may also perform neurological cognitive tests, magnetic resonance imaging (MRI) of the head, blood and urine tests, and an electroencephalogram (EEG), depending upon signs and symptoms.

Ways to Prevent Confusion. While there are some types of confusion that cannot be prevented, other types of confusion can be prevented through good health practices and lifestyle choices, such as:

- Obtaining a regular amount of sleep
- Eating a balanced diet with plenty of vitamins and minerals
- Not drinking alcohol in excess

supporting MRS. THOMAS: PART I

Eileen Thomas is a 68-year-old woman, who lives with her husband in her own home. She used to be a chronic smoker for 40 years but quit 2 years ago when she was diagnosed with chronic obstructive pulmonary disease (COPD). Mrs. Thomas' husband reports to their family doctor that she has recently been leaving the stove on and forgetting to turn off the tap in the kitchen sink.

Mrs. Thomas' doctor tells the family that because of her long-term smoking (and other health issues), she has "hardening of the arteries" (atherosclerosis), which prevents oxygen from going to her brain in the normal manner. She is put on medication, but her family is told that her condition cannot be cured. As a support worker, it is your responsibility to assist Mrs. Thomas with bathing and cooking meals, while her husband buys the groceries for the family. You need to monitor her for unsafe behaviours and report your observations to your supervisor.

- Keeping careful control of blood sugar if diabetes is present
- Quitting smoking, which puts one at greater risk for lung diseases

Supporting Clients With Confusion.

- A good way to test for confusion is to ask the client to tell his or her name and age and the date. If the client is unsure or answers incorrectly, confusion can be diagnosed.
- Confusion interferes with a person's ability to make decisions and to remember, so it is *your* responsibility to meet a confused client's physical and safety needs.
- Confused clients should not be left alone.
- To ensure a confused client's safety, try to keep the surroundings calm, quiet, and peaceful.
- When visiting a client who has confusion (or dementia, which is discussed later in this chapter), you should always introduce yourself every time you see them, no matter how well he or she once knew you.
- Placing a calendar and clock near the client can help keep him or her oriented.
- When taking care of a client who is confused, frequently remind him or her of the location.
- Talk about current events and plans for the day.

DELIRIUM

Confusion which occurs suddenly is called **delirium**—a condition of severe confusion and rapid changes in brain function. It is usually caused by a treatable physical or mental illness; it is often temporary, as it disappears once the illness has been treated. It can occur due to a reaction to medications, infection or other illness, poor nutrition, food poisoning, dehydration, or emotional trauma. Major life changes—such as the death of a loved one or moving to a facility—can also cause delirium.

Delirium should always be treated as an emergency. It often is the first or only sign of physical illness in older adults and in people with dementia. If you observe any sudden occurrence of signs and symptoms of confusion, tell your supervisor at once. The cause must be found and treated immediately.

Signs and Symptoms of Delirium. Delirium involves a rapid alternation between mental states. For example, someone with delirium may become drowsy, then agitated, and then drowsy again. Other signs and symptoms include:

- Attention disturbance, such as an inability to maintain goal-directed, purposeful thinking or behaviour, or problems concentrating
- Incoherent speech and inability to stop the speech patterns or behaviours
- Disorientation to time or place
- Changes in sensation and perception (which increases the disorientation)
- Sign of illusions or hallucinations
- Altered level of consciousness or awareness
- Altered sleep patterns; drowsiness
- Varying levels of alertness may vary—usually more alert in the morning, less alert at night (drowsiness)
- Decrease in short-term memory and recall
- Changes in motor activities, movement
- Emotional or personality changes, such as anxiety, anger, **apathy**, depression, **euphoria**, or irritability

Diagnosis and Treatment of Delirium. The client with delirium should be seen as soon as possible by a physician, who will most likely order blood work (including blood and alcohol levels), EEG, computed tomography (CT), or MRI of the clients' head, chest X-ray, or a lumbar puncture (spinal tap) to determine the cause of the delirium. The client is usually admitted to a hospital and treated as an inpatient. Acute disorders that cause delirium may coexist with chronic disorders that cause dementia.

The goal of treatment is to control or reverse the cause of the symptoms, and treatment depends on the specific condition causing delirium. Sometimes, this means stopping the medications (or alcohol consumption). Disorders that contributed to confusion, such as heart failure, decreased oxygen, or psychiatric conditions (such as depression), will be treated. Correction of coexisting medical and psychiatric disorders often greatly improves mental functioning.

Some clients may require medications to control their aggressive, agitated behaviours or behaviours that are dangerous to themselves or to others. Medications are usually given in very low doses, with adjustments made as needed. For some clients, admission to a psychiatric facility may be necessary, especially if the dangerous behaviours continue. See *Supporting Mrs. Thomas: Part II.*

DEMENTIA

Dementia is a general term that describes the progressive loss of brain functions, including cognitive and social functions. It is not a single disease but a group of illnesses that involve memory, behaviour, learning, and communication. Usually dementia starts slowly and progresses gradually, that is, it gets worse. Dementia affects the ability to perform complex as well as simple tasks. Problems with complex tasks—such as driving, managing money, planning meals, and working—appear first. Over time, problems occur with simple tasks, such as

supporting MRS. THOMAS: PART II

Mrs. Thomas had been your client for several months now, and although she had occasionally displayed unsafe behaviours—such as leaving the stove on—her condition had remained unchanged. Today, Mrs. Thomas was acting completely differently. When you arrived, you found that she was very drowsy; then she woke up, became very tearful and agitated, threw some dishes on the floor, and finally fell asleep on the sofa.

As her support worker, you were understandably concerned, so you immediately notified your supervisor. Your supervisor advised you to call the paramedics and to accompany Mrs. Thomas to the hospital. In the hospital, it was found that the cause of this sudden, erratic behaviour was viral meningitis. The doctors expected that Mrs. Thomas would recover completely.

bathing, dressing, eating, using the toilet, and walking, and everyday skills are eventually lost.

Dementia is ***not*** a normal part of aging. The majority of older adults do not have dementia, and dementia can affect people in their 40s and 50s. However, dementia is more common after 65 years of age (see Box 35–2).

Supporting Clients With Confusion or Dementia.

Environment:

- Maintain the day–night cycle. Open curtains, shades, and drapes during the day. Close them at night. Use a night-light at night. The client wears regular clothes during the day—not sleepwear.
- Provide a calm, relaxed, and peaceful setting. Prevent loud noises, rushing, and congested hallways and rooms.
- Follow the client's established routine. Having a schedule for meals, bathing, exercise, TV, and other activities promotes a sense of order and what to expect.
- Break tasks into small steps when assisting the client.
- Do not rearrange furniture or the client's personal belongings.

Box 35–2 Signs and Symptoms of Dementia

Early Warning Signs of Dementia

- Memory loss that affects daily activities (e.g., misplacing items or putting them in odd places)
- Confusion (e.g., getting lost in familiar places or forgetting how to use simple, everyday items such as a microwave)
- Problems finding the right words or following conversations
- Poor judgement (e.g., going outdoors in the snow without shoes)
- Problems with common tasks (e.g., dressing, cooking, driving)
- Changes in mood, behaviour, or personality (e.g., unfounded jealousy, suspiciousness, or poor social behaviour)
- Loss of interest in activities or hobbies (e.g., an avid gardener now letting weeds overrun the garden)

Signs of Progression of Dementia

- Forgetting recent events
- Forgetting simple directions
- Forgetting conversations
- Forgetting appointments
- Forgetting names (including those of family members)
- Forgetting the names of everyday things (e.g., clock, radio, TV, and so on)
- Forgetting words
- Substituting unusual words and names for forgotten ones
- Loss of train of thought
- Forgetting English and speaking in the native language
- Cursing or swearing
- Misplacing items
- Putting things in odd places
- Having problems writing cheques or balancing cheque books
- Giving away large amounts of money
- Not recognizing or understanding numbers
- Having problems following conversations
- Having problems reading
- Having problems writing
- Becoming lost in familiar settings
- Forgetting where he or she is
- Wandering from home
- Not knowing how to get back home
- Not being able to tell or understand time
- Not being able to tell or understand dates
- Not being able to handle everyday tasks (e.g., leaving the iron or stove burners on, leaving the food burning on the stove, and so on)
- Not being able to perform activities of daily living (bathing, brushing teeth, and so on); this skilled motor system impairment is called apraxia.
- Distrusting others
- Being stubborn
- Withdrawal from society
- Being restless
- Becoming suspicious
- Becoming fearful
- Not wanting to do things
- Sleeping more than usual

- Encourage self-care.
- Be consistent.
- Place picture signs in rooms, bathrooms, dining rooms, and other areas (Figure 35–1). Follow your supervisor's directions.
- Keep personal items where the client can see them.
- Stay within sight to the extent possible.
- Place memory aids (large clocks and calendars) where the client can see them.
- Keep noise levels low.
- Play music and show movies from the client's past.
- Select tasks and activities specific to the client's cognitive abilities and interests.

Communication:

- Approach the client in a calm, quiet manner.
- Approach the client from the front. Do not approach from the side or back, as this can startle the client.
- Call the client by name every time you are in contact with him or her.
- State your name. Show your nametag.
- Give the date and time each morning. Repeat, as needed, during the day or evening.
- Explain what you are going to do and why.
- Give clear, simple directions and answers to questions.
- Ask clear and simple questions. Give the client time to respond.
- Keep calendars and clocks with large numbers in the client's room and in other areas (Figure 35–2). Remind the client of holidays, birthdays, and special events.
- Have the client wear his or her glasses and a hearing aid, if needed.
- Use touch to communicate (see Chapter 13).
- Place familiar objects and pictures within the client's view.
- Provide newspapers, magazines, TV, and radio. Read to the client, if appropriate.
- Discuss current events with the client.
- Identify other people by their names. Avoid using pronouns (he, she, them, and so on).
- Practise measures to promote communication (see Chapter 13).
- Use gestures and cues. Pointing to objects may improve the client's understanding.
- Speak in a calm, gentle voice.
- Speak slowly. Use simple words and sentences.
- Allow the client to speak by not interrupting or rushing him or her.
- Give the client time to respond.
- Do not criticize, correct, or argue with the client.
- Present one idea, question, or instruction at a time.
- Ask simple questions that require only simple answers. Do not ask complex questions.
- Do not present the client with many choices.
- Provide simple explanations of all procedures and activities.
- Give consistent responses.
- Provide frequent toileting at regular intervals.
- Repeat information frequently. Usually, the client cannot remember new information.

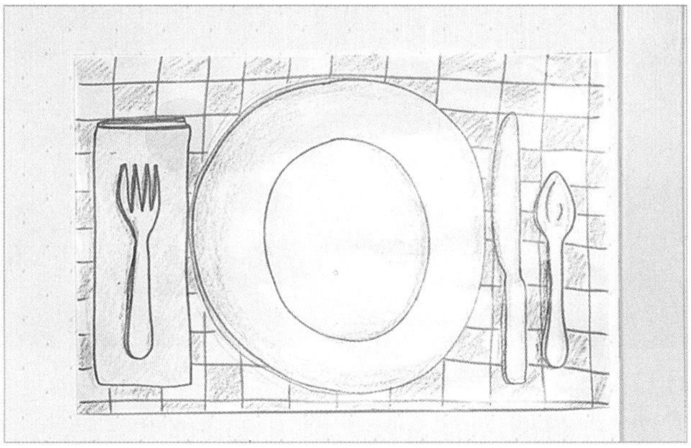

Figure 35–1 Signs provide cues to clients with dementia. **Source**: Sorrentino, S.A. & Gorek, B. (2003). *Mosby's textbook for long-term care assistants* (4th ed., p. 670). St Louis: Mosby.

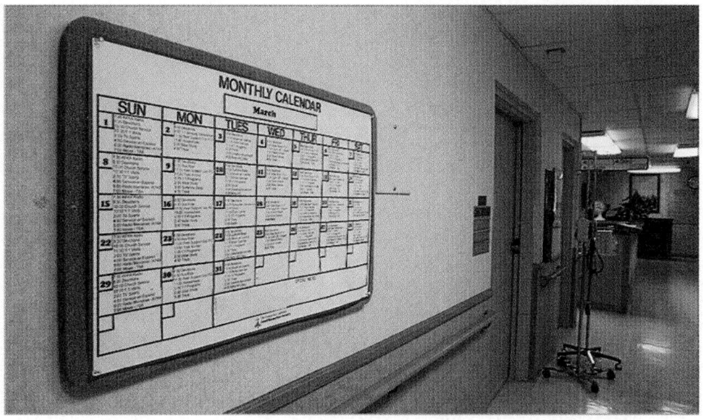

Figure 35–2 A large calendar can be helpful to clients with confusion or dementia. **Source**: Sorrentino, S.A. (2000). *Mosby's textbook for nursing assistants* (5th ed., p. 733). St. Louis: Mosby.

Safety:

- Remove harmful, sharp, and breakable objects—such as knives, scissors, glass, dishes, razors, and tools—from the area.
- Provide plastic eating and drinking utensils. This helps prevent breakage and cuts.
- Place safety plugs in electrical outlets.
- Keep cords and electrical equipment out of reach.
- Remove electrical appliances—for example, hair dryers, curling irons, make-up mirrors, and electric shavers—from the bathroom.
- Store personal care items—shampoo, deodorant, lotion, and so on—in a safe place.
- Store household cleaners and medications in locked storage areas.
- Store dangerous equipment and tools in a safe place.
- Supervise the client when he or she smokes.
- Store cigarettes, cigars, pipes, matches, and other smoking materials in a safe place.
- Practise safety measures to prevent falls, burns, choking, poisoning, and fires (see Chapter 19).
- Keep all doors to kitchens, utility rooms, and housekeeping closets locked.

Wandering:

- Follow facility policy for locking doors and windows. In community settings, locks are often placed at the tops and bottoms of doors (Figure 35–3), as the client is not likely to look for a lock in these places.
- Keep door alarms and electronic doors turned on. The alarm should be set to go off whenever the door is opened.
- Follow facility policy for fire exits. Everyone must be able to leave the building if a fire occurs.
- Make sure the client wears a facility ID bracelet or Alzheimer's Safe Home™ Registry ID at all times.
- Agencies may camouflage exits or hazardous equipment that cannot be put away (such as oxygen tanks) to reduce the risk of clients leaving the facilites or injuring themselves.
- Exercise the client, as ordered, as adequate exercise often reduces wandering.

Figure 35–3 A slide lock is placed at the top of the door.

- Involve the client in simple activities—folding napkins, dusting a table, sorting socks, rolling yarn, sweeping, sanding blocks of wood, or watering plants.
- Do not use restraints, as they tend to increase confusion and disorientation. Restraints require a physician's order.
- Do not argue with the client who wants to leave. He or she does not understand what you are saying.
- Go with the client who insists on going outside. Make sure he or she is properly dressed. Guide the client inside after a few minutes (Figure 35–4).
- Allow the client to wander in enclosed areas. Many long-term care facilities have enclosed areas that provide a safe place for clients to walk about.

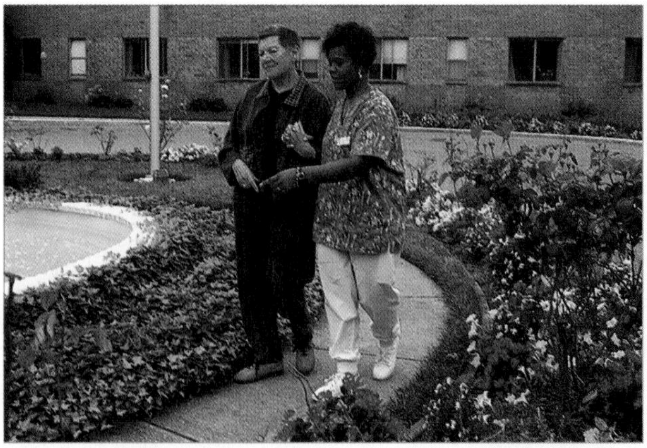

Figure 35–4 Walk with the client who wants to go outside. Then guide him or her back inside after a few minutes.
Source: Sorrentino, S.A. & Gorek, B. (2003). *Mosby's textbook for long-term care assistants* (4th ed., p. 670). St Louis: Mosby.

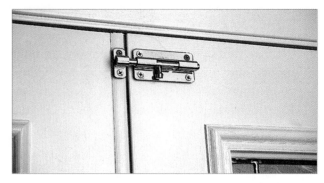

Sundowning:

- Complete treatments and activities early in the day.
- Provide a calm, quiet setting late in the day.
- Play soft music.
- Do not restrain the client.
- Encourage exercise and activity early in the day.
- Meet nutrition needs. Hunger can increase restlessness.
- Promote regular elimination. The need to eliminate can increase restlessness.
- Do not try to reason with the client, as communication is impaired and he or she cannot think or speak clearly.

Hallucinations and Delusions:

- Make sure the client wears eyeglasses or hearing aids, as needed. Follow the care plan.
- Do not argue with the client.
- Reassure the client. Say that you will protect him or her from harm.
- Distract the client with some item or activity. Taking the client for a walk may be helpful to him or her.
- Use touch to calm and reassure the client (Figure 35–5).
- Eliminate noises that the client could misinterpret and that could upset him or her, for example, noises created by TV, radio, stereos, furnaces, air conditioners, appliances, and other things.

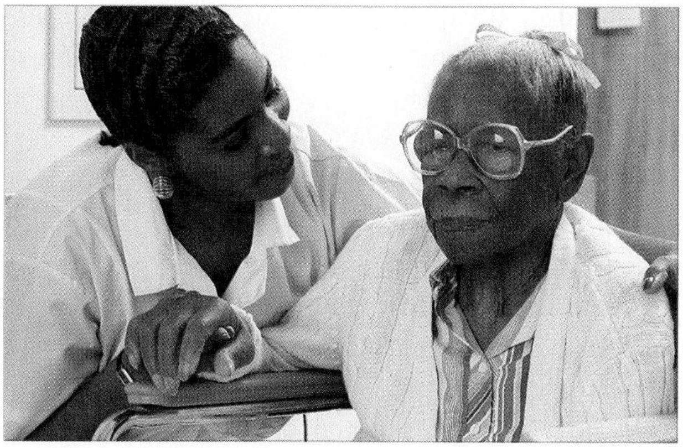

Figure 35–5 Use touch to calm the client with dementia.
Source: Sorrentino, S.A. & Gorek, B. (2003). *Mosby's textbook for long-term care assistants* (4th ed., p. 670). St Louis: Mosby.

- Check lighting. Make sure there are no glares, shadows, or reflections.
- Cover or remove mirrors. The client could misinterpret his or her reflection.

Sleep:

- Follow bedtime rituals.
- Use night-lights, which will help prevent accidents and disorientation.
- Limit caffeine intake during the day.
- Discourage naps during the day.
- Encourage exercise during the day.
- Reduce noises.

Basic Needs:

- Meet food and fluid needs (see Chapter 28). Provide finger foods. Cut food to small bits and pour out liquids, as needed.
- Provide good skin care (see Chapters 30 and 42). Keep skin free of urine and stool.
- Promote urinary and fecal elimination (see Chapters 32 and 33).
- Provide incontinence care, as needed (see Chapters 32 and 33).
- Provide frequent toileting at regular intervals throughout the day and night.
- Promote exercise and activity during the day (see Chapter 24). This helps reduce wandering and sundowning behaviours. The client may also sleep better.
- Reduce intake of coffee, tea, and cola drinks, which contain caffeine. Caffeine is a stimulant that can increase restlessness, confusion, and agitation.
- Provide a quiet, restful setting (see Chapter 22). Soft music is better than loud TV programs.
- Play soft music during care activities such as bathing and during meals.
- Promote personal hygiene (see Chapter 30), but do not force the client into a shower or tub, as clients with dementia are often afraid of bathing. Try bathing the client when he or she is calm, using his or her preferred bathing method—tub bath, shower, bed bath, towel bath. Follow the care plan. Provide privacy, and keep the client warm. Do not rush the client.

- Provide oral hygiene (see Chapter 30).
- Choose clothing that is comfortable and easy to put on, for example, front-opening garments. Pullover tops are harder to put on, and the client may become frightened when the head is inside the pullover top.
- Clothing that closes with Velcro is easy to put on and take off. Buttons, zippers, snaps, and other closures that are hard to handle can frustrate the client.
- Offer simple clothing choices. Let the client choose between two shirts or blouses, two pants or slacks, and so on.
- Lay out clothing in the order it will be put on. Hand the client one clothing item at a time. Describe or show what to do, and do not rush him or her.
- Have equipment ready for any procedure. This reduces the amount of time the client is involved in care measures.
- Observe for signs and symptoms of health problems (see Chapter 18).
- Prevent infection. Assist with hand washing, when necessary (see Chapter 20).

There are many different forms and causes of dementia. Sometimes dementia is caused by conditions that are treatable and the dementia is usually reversed (cured) or slowed.

Treatable Forms of Dementia. Dementias that may be treated, and hopefully reversed, are caused by the following:

- ***Brain injury.*** Some brain injuries result in internal bleeding in the skull, which can cause symptoms of dementia. Surgery to correct the bleeding can correct the dementia.
- ***Brain tumour.*** Delirium or dementia may result depending on the location, size, and type of the brain tumour. Surgery or chemotherapy may be used to treat the tumour.
- ***Alcohol.*** Long-term alcohol abuse can lead to dementia, which may or may not be reversible.
- ***Thyroid deficiency.*** When the thyroid gland is underactive, it can lead to dementia as well as delirium, which can be reversed when the thyroid condition is corrected.

Untreatable Forms of Dementia. Most forms of dementia cannot be reversed and have no prevention or cure. As a result, the client's brain function will decline over time. Irreversible dementia eventually interferes with all daily activities and will, unfortunately, lead to the client's death.

The most common forms of irreversible dementia are described below.

Alzheimer's Disease (AD)

Being the most common form of dementia, AD accounts for over 64% of all dementias in Canadians.[1] Alzheimer's disease was first identified by Dr. Alois Alzheimer in 1906. He described the two hallmarks of the disease: "plaques"—numerous tiny dense deposits scattered throughout the brain, which become toxic to brain cells at excessive levels, and "tangles" which interfere with vital processes, eventually "choking" off the living cells.[2] When these brain cells degenerate and die, the brain markedly shrinks in some regions. This shrinkage will continue over time, affecting how the brain functions.[2]

Alzheimer's disease is gradual in onset but is progressive and irreversible, gradually destroying nerve cells (neurons) in most areas of the brain and resulting in impaired cognitive function and behaviour changes. The progression of AD varies from client to client and can span 3 to 20 years (the average length of the disease is between 8 and 12 years). The progression can be described as a series of stages; this provides a guide to the pattern of the disease and helps make care decisions.

One system explains the three stages of the disease: (1) early, (2) middle, and (3) late. Most dementias are explained in these three stages (see the section on "Stages of Dementia" later in this chapter). Another staging system, used by medical professionals, is called the Global Deterioration Scale (also called the Reisberg Scale), which divides the disease into seven stages. More information about this scale is available on the Internet or from your local Alzheimer Society.

Whichever staging system is used, it is important to remember that the disease affects each client differently. ***The order in which the symptoms appear, as well as the length of each stage, will***

vary from client to client. There is no clear line between the end of one stage and the beginning of another. In many clients, stages will overlap; some may experience many of the symptoms in each stage, and others may experience only a few. There may be fluctuations in a client from day to day when he or she may appear more confused one day and less so on the next day.

Symptoms of AD will worsen over time, the rate of decline varying from client to client. AD usually occurs after 65 and is often diagnosed after 80. However, it can also affect people in their 40s and 50s. Currently, AD has no cure, but there are some medications that can slow its progress. The cause of AD is unknown, but a family history of AD is a known risk factor.[2]

Vascular Dementia (multi-infarct)

This type of dementia is caused by a series of small strokes, resulting in death of brain tissue. These strokes do not necessarily cause hemiplegia but might, instead, cause changes in memory or personality, depending on which part of the brain has been affected. These strokes can occur at any time and lead to progressive cognitive impairment.

Lewy Body Dementia

Dementia with Lewy bodies (DLB) is one of the most common types of progressive dementia. The central feature of DLB is progressive cognitive decline, combined with three additional defining features: (1) severe fluctuations in alertness and attention, such as frequent drowsiness, lethargy, lengthy periods of time spent staring into space, or disorganized speech; (2) recurrent visual hallucinations, and (3) Parkinson-like motor symptoms, such as rigidity and the loss of spontaneous movement. People with DLB may also suffer from depression. The symptoms of DLB are caused by the buildup of Lewy bodies—accumulated bits of protein—inside the nuclei of neurons in areas of the brain that regulate particular aspects of memory and motor control.

The similarity of symptoms between DLB and Parkinson's disease and between DLB and Alzheimer's disease can often make it difficult for the physician to make a definitive diagnosis. Lewy bodies are often found in the brains of people with Parkinson's disease and AD as well, which suggests that either DLB is related to these other causes of dementia or that an individual can have both diseases at the same time. DLB usually occurs sporadically, in people with no known family history of the disease. However, rare familial cases have occasionally been reported.

Pick's Disease

Pick's disease is a rare form of dementia, which accounts for about 5% of all dementia types. The clinical picture is fairly similar to AD but differences can be detected at autopsy. In Pick's disease, the brain tissue changes, affecting focal areas, unlike the generalized damage seen in AD. Pick's disease affects the frontal and temporal lobes of the brain. Marked shrinkage, or **atrophy**, of the frontal lobes of the brain occurs that can be seen on brain scans.[3]

Pick's disease is marked by the presence of abnormalities in brain cells, called Pick's bodies, which are found in the affected areas as well as elsewhere in the brain.

Many of the early symptoms of Pick's disease are frontal lobe symptoms, which tend to mark out the differences between Pick's dementia and the other types, such as AD. In AD, the initial symptoms tend to be memory impairment, but in Pick's disease, since the frontal lobes of the brain are affected, the first symptoms occur in emotional and social functioning. The mood changes, often leaning toward euphoria, lack of inhibitions, and deterioration in social skills, are clearly noticeable.

A client with Pick's disease may become excessively extroverted, or withdrawn, rude, impatient, and aggressive and make inappropriate remarks in public. He or she may exhibit altered sexual behaviour, with a markedly increased interest in sex, which can be linked to loss of inhibition; it can be very disturbing and can get the client involved with law enforcement agencies.[3]

Behavioural changes can sometimes be very subtle at first; when behaviour becomes more bizarre, dementia is recognized. Because of the type of brain damage, the disease also causes gluttony (gross overeating) and increased alcohol intake. Clients with Pick's disease may have the compulsion to put objects in their mouth.[3]

Problems with language can occur in the early stages but are not as striking as those in the early stages of AD. Difficulty finding words and naming objects occurs initially, and as the disease progresses, memory and **apraxia** become more marked.[4] Someone suffering from Pick's disease will have difficulty maintaining a line of thought, be easily distracted, and have difficulty maintaining conversation for any length of time.[5]

Pick's disease generally occurs between 40 and 60 years, and women are affected slightly more than are men.[5]

Creutzfeldt-Jakob Disease

First identified in the 1920s, Creutzfeldt-Jakob disease (CJD)[6] is a very rare disease that causes dementia. It is believed to be caused by something called *proteinaceous prions* that can live in the body for years before any signs of the disease become obvious. CJD occurs in people between the ages of 50 and 70 years and is a rapid, progressive neurological disease that can affect people as well as animals. In animals, prion diseases are also known as *scrapie* in sheep and *bovine spongiform encephalopathy (BSE)*—also known as "mad cow disease"—in cattle. A similar disease is also found in deer.

CJD appears to have a genetic link or susceptibility in 5% to 15% of cases and can be passed on through infected brain tissue. BSE is found to occur in people who have been treated with growth hormone and in those who are exposed to poorly sterilized instruments. A tribe in New Guinea that practises cannibalism and eats dead relatives' brains also suffers a prion dementia called Kuru.

Early signs and symptoms of CJD include fatigue, difficulty sleeping and insomnia, excessive sleepiness, changes in personality, anorexia, progressive deterioration of memory, behaviour disturbances, and spasms of the body. Depression and psychosis are seen in 10% of cases, along with delusions and hallucinations.

In later stages, the client will have poor balance and pain, which will cause increasing problems with stability and walking. Dementia becomes obvious and leads to a mute, rigid state. Once the signs of CJD become apparent, the progress of the disease is very rapid. There is no known cure for CJD; symptoms are treated to help alleviate distress and pain and to make the client as comfortable as possible. About 90% of patients with CJD die within 1 year of the first symptoms.

Many other health conditions that can also cause dementia include the following (see Chapter 18):

- Acquired immune deficiency syndrome (AIDS)
- Huntington's disease
- Multiple sclerosis

supporting
MRS. THOMAS: PART III

Mrs. Thomas has fully recovered and returned to her pre-meningitis state, but she is becoming increasingly more forgetful. Last week, you noticed that she needed help with buttoning up her clothing while she was getting dressed. Mrs. Thomas herself mentioned to you that she "forgot" to undo her pants when she had to go to the washroom and soiled herself. On your last two visits, she had not been able to recognize you but could read your nametag. Earlier this week, her husband told you that she did not recognize him when he was helping her undress for bedtime and started punching him, accusing him of trying to molest her. She also started to yell at her reflection in the mirror because she did not recognize herself.

Her husband took her to her doctor, and after numerous tests, the doctor told Mr. and Mrs. Thomas that she had dementia and that it was probably due to Alzheimer's disease. The doctor said that Mrs. Thomas' symptoms had progressed at a very rapid rate and her cognition would probably decline quickly over time. Mrs. Thomas' husband is very upset about the diagnosis; the couple had made plans to drive across Canada to visit their grown children and their grandchildren. Mr. Thomas tells you that he is very grateful for your support in his wife's care.

- Parkinson's disease
- Syphilis

Delirium and depression (see Chapter 34) can easily be mistaken for dementia, as they share many of the same signs and symptoms. For this reason, depression is sometimes called **pseudo-dementia**, meaning false (*pseudo*) dementia. However, with delirium and depression, there are no permanent changes in the brain. Sometimes delirium and depression may accompany dementia, so accurate diagnosis by a physician is very important.

Stages of Dementia

The three stages of dementia generally apply to AD and most other forms of dementia. In the early stages, different dementias can present quite differently but tend to become similar as they progress. Signs and symptoms become more severe with each stage. Eventually, the client is confined to bed and becomes totally dependent on others for care. Death occurs when the brain shuts down all body systems.[7]

Stage 1: Mild (Early Stage). A client with dementia is usually cared for at home until symptoms become severe (see table below). Some clients live with family members, but some live alone in their own homes, where they receive support from family, friends, volunteers, and home care workers. The primary caregiver may be the client's spouse, adult child, another family member, or friend. Other caregivers may periodically provide relief to the primary caregiver. Respite care through adult day care and home care may also provide temporary help.

Clients with dementia often need help getting organized, solving simple problems, and remembering appointments, occasions, and medications. They need support and supervision—for example, if a client wants to bake cookies, you will need to make sure that the setting is safe for the activity and that the oven is turned off when the client is finished. Safety is an ongoing concern for the client with dementia, since he or she may wander away, swallow a poisonous substance, or leave an appli-

Abilities Affected	Typical Symptoms of Early Stage of Dementia
Mental Abilities	Mild forgetfulness; forgetting recent events Difficulty learning new things and following conversations Difficulty concentrating, or limited attention span Problems with orientation, such as getting lost or not following directions Communication difficulties, such as finding the right word Problems finding words, finishing thoughts, following directions, and remembering names Poor judgement; bad decisions (including when driving) Occasional confusion occurs—disorientation to person, time, and place Lack of spontaneity—less outgoing or less interested in things Problems performing everyday tasks
Moods and Emotions	Blaming others for mistakes, forgetfulness, and other problems Mood shifts Symptoms of depression, irritability, or defensiveness; depression
Behaviours	Passive Withdrawn from usual activities Restless
Physical Abilities	Mild coordination problems

Source: Alzheimer Society. (1997–2008). *Alzheimer's disease: The progression of Alzheimer's disease.* Toronto, ON. Retrieved March 6, 2008, from http://www.alzheimer.ca/english/disease/progression-3stages.htm

ance on. Ensure a safe setting, and supervise the client at all times. It is your responsibility to follow the client's care plan.

You may need to help a client start an activity or task, and then provide only support and encouragement. Some clients with dementia will, however, have problems completing tasks, and they will need frequent cues, reminders, and restatements of facts and conversations. For example, a client wants to mail a letter but cannot remember the word for "stamps" or where they are kept. You help her to remember the word and then help her to find the stamps. Follow the care plan, which may specify that you should focus on the client's enjoyment of the activity rather than on achievement.

A client in this stage will usually be aware of the diagnosis and will be able to participate in decisions affecting future care. Symptoms can include mild forgetfulness and communication difficulties, such as finding the right word and following a conversation. Some clients are able to stay involved in activities. Some others may become passive or withdrawn, or become depressed or anxious because they may be frustrated by changing abilities. It is important to monitor the emotional well-being of the client.

Stage 2: Moderate (Middle Stage). Further decline occurs in the client's mental and physical abilities at this stage (see table on page 679). Memory will continue to deteriorate as the client forgets personal history and no longer recognizes family and friends. Some clients become restless and pace constantly or may wander off. Registering the client with the Safely Home™ Alzheimer Wandering Registry program will provide peace of mind to the client's family, as the client can be easily located should he or she become lost.

A client may react in a number of ways in response to the loss of abilities. For example, he or she may become less involved in activities or may repeat the same action or word over and over again. The local Alzheimer Society can provide education about the disease, resources, and support for clients and their families and can assist them to develop strategies to deal with difficult situations.

As the client's dementia progresses, the need for assistance increases. Usually there comes a time when family and friends can no longer deal with the situation or meet all of the client's needs. The client may be unable to tolerate wearing his or her dentures or eyeglasses, which can increase the client's risk of injury, so it should be detailed in the client's care plan and noted by caregivers. Increased confusion and disorientation to time and place will also necessitate assistance in many activities of daily living (ADLs), such as dressing, bathing, and using the toilet.

Adult day care, respite care, home care, and help from family members, friends, and volunteers are no longer enough at this stage. Long-term care is needed when at least one of the following occurs:

- Family members and friends are not able to meet the client's needs
- Family members themselves have health problems
- The client's behaviours present a danger to self or others
- The client no longer knows the caregiver

Many long-term care facilities have special care units for clients with dementia. The health care team ensures that their needs are met. Many facilities provide hospice care for those in the final stages of dementia.

When a client with dementia moves to a facility, the family or close friends usually continue to be involved in the care, as they are an important part of the health care team and help plan the client's care, whenever possible. Some of the family members and friends may take part in facility activities, and, for many clients with dementia, they can provide comfort and support.

Abilities Affected	Typical Symptoms of Middle Stage of Dementia
Mental Abilities	Memory loss increases—failure to recognize family and friends Forgetting personal history Disorientation to time and place Increasing restlessness during the evening hours (sundowning) Increased episodes of confusion Development of sleep problems Dulled senses—inability to tell the difference between hot and cold and to recognize dangers Movement and gait problems—walking slowly; having a shuffling gait Communication problems—inability to follow directions; problems with reading, writing, and math; speaking in short sentences or single words; statements not making sense
Moods and Emotions	Loss of impulse control—foul language, poor table manners, sexual aggression, rudeness Personality change Confusion Anxiety or apprehension Suspiciousness Mood shifts Anger, hostile behaviours; violent behaviour Sadness or depression
Behaviours	Declining ability to concentrate Restlessness (pacing, wandering) Repetition of movements and statements—moving things back and forth constantly Saying the same thing over and over again Delusions Aggression Uninhibited behaviours Passive behaviour
Physical Abilities	Bowel and bladder incontinence Need for help with activities of daily living (ADL)—bathing, feeding, and dressing self Fear of bathing; refusal to change clothes Disrupted sleep patterns Appetite fluctuations Language difficulties Visual spatial problems

Source: Alzheimer Society. (1997–2008). *Alzheimer's disease: The progression of Alzheimer's disease.* Toronto, ON. Retrieved March 6, 2008, from http://www.alzheimer.ca/english/disease/progression-3stages.htm

Stage 3: Severe (Late Stage). In this last stage, the client is incapable of remembering, communicating or self-care (see table below). Care is required 24 hours a day. Eventually, the client will become bed-ridden, have difficulty eating or swallowing, and lose control of bodily functions. This stage eventually ends with the client's death, often from secondary complications such as pneumonia.

Supporting Clients With Dementia. Each client with dementia has unique care needs, depending on the form of dementia, the stage of the dementia, and the care setting. Box 35–3 on page 684 lists general guidelines for caring for clients with dementia. The care plan and your supervisor will give you specific instructions for each client.

Meeting Basic Client Needs: Over time, clients with dementia become dependent on others for all care—safety, hygiene, grooming, dressing, and elimination, as well as nutrition and fluids, exercise, health, comfort, and therapy. Follow the care plan.

Safety: Clients need a safe, quiet setting. They do not recognize safety hazards and are at risk for falls. If a client with dementia falls, he or she may not understand why it is unsafe to move after the fall. You may need to allow the client move about. Talk to the client in a quiet and soothing voice until someone can assist you. Never use force or hold a client down.

Clients may feel fearful even in a safe, quiet setting. They do not understand what is happening to them, so always explain calmly what you are going to do. Be prepared to repeat information, since clients with dementia are not able to retain information.

Clients may be at increased risk for injury if they are combative or aggressive. Family members or caregivers (who are tired and weary) may be more likely to restrain or confine the client to be able to manage them.

Abilities Affected	Typical Symptoms of Late Stage of Dementia
Mental Abilities	Loss of ability to remember, communicate, or function Inability to process information Severe speaking difficulties Severe disorientation to time, place, and people Seizures (see Chapter 18) Constant state of confusion—inability to recognize self, family members, or others Total dependence on others for all activities of daily living Total urinary and fecal incontinence Inability to swallow—increased risk of choking and aspiration Increased sleep problems Confinement to bed—inability to sit or walk Coma, death
Moods and Emotions	Withdrawal from conversations
Behaviours	Nonverbal communication (eye contact, crying, groaning) Inability to speak (groaning, grunting, or screaming)
Physical Abilities	Sleeping longer and more often Immobility (being bed-ridden) Loss of ability to speak Loss of control of bladder and bowels Difficulty eating and swallowing Inability to dress or bathe Loss of weight

Source: Alzheimer Society. (1997–2008). *Alzheimer's disease: The progression of Alzheimer's disease.* Toronto, ON. Retrieved March 6, 2008, from http://www.alzheimer.ca/english/disease/progression-3stages.htm

Hygiene, Grooming, and Dressing: Clients with moderate and severe dementia do not understand the need for personal hygiene and aseptic practices. They have to rely on the health care team to prevent the spread of infection. You assist them with hand washing:

- After they have urinated or defecated
- After they have coughed, sneezed, or blown the nose
- Before or after they have handled or eaten food
- Anytime their hands are soiled

Good skin care is very important for clients with dementia, as it can help prevent skin breakdown. Skin care and other personal care can seem threatening to clients with moderate and severe dementia. During personal care, look for signs or symptoms of conditions that may cause pain (for example, skin lesions, rough pieces of clothing, or dental problems). Clients may resist efforts to keep them clean and dry, as they do not understand what is happening or why. They may fear harm or danger when you get too close or touch them, so they may resist care and become agitated and combative. They may shout and cry out for help, and some clients may pull away during care, while others may hit or kick. Sudden movements can cause skin tears. Refer to the section "Managing Challenging Behaviours" later in this chapter.

Elimination Needs: Clients with moderate and severe dementia may urinate in the wrong places, for example, garbage cans, planters, and heating vents. Some may remove incontinence products and throw them down on the floor or in the toilet. Some may soil themselves, the furniture, or the walls. Offer to assist with elimination needs frequently at regular times during both day and night. Provide perineal care after urinary and fecal elimination. Ask your supervisor for help if a client resists you. Never restrict fluid intake in an effort to control elimination.

Nutrition: Clients with dementia may become distracted during meals, or it may be hard for some to sit long enough to eat a meal. Some with later stage dementia forget how to use eating utensils, so finger foods can be offered to them. Some clients have problems swallowing (see Chapter 25), and some have to be fed. Some clients will resist efforts to assist them with eating, and confused clients may throw or spit food. A quiet and calm environment in the dining area and special mealtimes are often helpful. Clients may be able to eat small amounts more frequently, rather than three times per day.

Fluids: Clients with moderate and severe dementia are at risk for dehydration, as they do not recognize thirst. Encourage them to drink. Keep water and other fluids nearby, and offer fluids whenever you are around them. Remember that adequate fluids can reduce risks of serious problems such as urinary infections or constipation.

Exercise: Inactivity and immobility are risk factors for pneumonia and pressure ulcers. Exercise is therefore important for clients with dementia, but they may resist it because they do not understand what is happening and may fear harm. They may become agitated and combative or cry out for help. Do not force a client to exercise or take part in activities. Stay calm. Ask your supervisor for help, if needed. Follow the care plan.

Health Problems: Many clients with dementia have other health problems or injuries. However, they may not notice or recognize pain, fever, constipation, incontinence, or other signs and symptoms. Changes in usual behaviour may signal pain or discomfort. A client who normally moans and groans all the time may become quiet and withdrawn; a client who is usually friendly and outgoing may become agitated and aggressive; a client who is nonverbal and quiet may become restless and cry easily. Loss of appetite may also signal pain. Report any changes in a client's usual behaviour to your supervisor.

Comfort: Comfort is important in the care of a client with dementia, so make sure that the client is physically comfortable. A quiet environment, talking in a calm voice, massage, soothing touch, music, and aromatherapy are all comforting and relaxing. Make sure that the client's clothing is also comfortable.

Therapy and Activities: Clients with dementia need to feel worthy and useful and to remain active, as this will promote emotional and physical health. Clients should be encouraged to do what they can do and enjoy. For example, a man who used to be a good dancer can take part in dancing activities. A woman who likes to draw can be encouraged to join a painting group. The social contact may be as important as the activity itself.

Adult day programs and long-term care facilities provide therapy and activities—such as music programs, art programs, fitness programs, and support groups—to meet the client's needs and cognitive abilities. Therapists may work with one client, a small group, or a large group.

PROVIDING COMPASSIONATE CARE

The Client With Dementia

- **Dignity.** Clients with dementia do not choose to be forgetful, incontinent, agitated, angry, or rude. Nor do they choose to display other behaviours, signs, and symptoms of the disease. They cannot control what is happening to them; it is the disease that causes the behaviours. ***The dementia is responsible, not the client.***

  Treat all clients with dementia with dignity and respect. They have rights under human rights codes and long-term care legislation. In the advanced stages of dementia, they may not know or be able to exercise their rights, but they are still entitled to their rights. Be patient and calm when caring for clients with dementia. Do not assume that the client cannot understand you. Always explain what you are going to do.

  Take care to never to make the client feel foolish about forgetting or misplacing something. Even in the later stages of dementia, clients can still feel embarrassment and shame. Protect the client's dignity when you are providing care. Only those involved in the client's care should be present for care procedures.

- **Independence.** The client has the right to autonomy. Clients with dementia should be encouraged to be independent for as long as safely possible. Encourage clients to do what they can for themselves.

- **Preferences.** Personal choice is important. Clients with early stage dementia can voice their preferences. Encourage clients with moderate stage dementia to make simple choices—for example, choosing one of two sweaters, or watching or not watching TV. The family or substitute decision maker usually makes choices regarding bath times, menus, clothing, activities, and other care, if the client cannot.

  A client may choose to use a special pillow or blanket. He or she may insist on wearing a particular sweater or cardigan because the item may have special meaning, or it may provide comfort and security. Eventually, the client may not know why the item is important or may not even recognize it. However, do not remove the item, as it is still important to the person.

  With Alzheimer's disease and most other dementias, clients continue to experience all forms of emotions well into the final stages. When a client can no longer use language, being able to recognize his or her emotional state can help you determine wishes, preferences, fears, likes, and dislikes.

- **Privacy.** The client has the right to privacy and confidentiality. Provide space and privacy for the client to visit with others. Protect confidentiality. Do not share information about the client with others. Do not relate stories about the client's behaviour to others.

- **Safety.** A safe, quiet, and calm setting promotes quality of life. Follow the safety measures in Chapter 19. All clients have the right to be free from restraints, which require a physician's order in any case and are used only if it is the best way to protect the client, not for the convenience of the health care team. Restraints can worsen confused and agitated behaviours. Your supervisor will tell you when to use restraints.

  The client must be kept free from abuse and neglect. Caring for clients with dementia is often very frustrating because some behaviours can be hard to deal with. Family caregivers and health care providers can become short-tempered and angry. Protect clients with dementia from abuse. Report any signs of abuse to your supervisor at once. If you are becoming frustrated with a client, talk to your supervisor. An assignment change may be needed.

In adult community settings, you often work with clients with early stage dementia. Many of these clients have care requirements but may be able to make some decisions for themselves. Your support enables these clients to remain in their homes.

MANAGING CHALLENGING BEHAVIOURS

Clients with dementia often display challenging behaviours, many of which may be disruptive to other clients or residents around them and may even challenge the abilities of the caregivers to provide compassionate care. It is important to know that clients' challenging behaviours result from their dementia. The client with dementia cannot control his or her actions, so you should never take the client's behaviours personally, become upset or angry with the client, or blame yourself for the client's behaviour.

Challenging behaviours can sometimes be a response to an illness, infection, or physical discomfort. It is important for you to remember that ***all behaviour has meaning.*** A client with dementia may be unable to understand that he or she is cold or hungry because the brain may (a) no longer be able to sort out the vast number of messages that it receives; (b) no longer send out the correct message to other parts of the brain; or (C) not be able to understand the meaning behind certain actions. As a result, the client with dementia may act out, become very resistant to staff, or even become very vocal or physically combative. You should try to determine what the client is trying to tell you. You should also report unusual or increased instances of challenging behaviours. Your observations are very important in determining the causes of the person's behaviour (see Box 35–3).

Wandering

Clients with dementia are not oriented to person, time, and place, so they may wander away and not be able to find their way back. They may wander off very quickly by foot, car, bicycle, or other means—they may be with you one moment and gone the next.

Judgement in these clients is poor. They cannot tell what is safe or dangerous, so they are at high risk of life-threatening accidents. They can walk into traffic or into a nearby lake, river, or forest. If not properly dressed, they are at risk for heat or cold exposure.

Wandering may have no cause or may have a legitimate cause that the client cannot articulate (tell you). For example, the client may be looking for something or someone—the bathroom, the bedroom, a child, or a partner. The client may also be experiencing pain, side effects of medications, stress, restlessness, or anxiety.

For clients living at home or in facilities, for a small fee, the Alzheimer Society of Canada provides a nationwide service called the Alzheimer's Wandering Registry, which serves to identify and safely return people who wander off or become lost. A family member completes a form and provides a recent picture of the client. This information is entered into a national database, and the client is given an ID card and bracelet. Anyone finding a lost client can call the police, who then will call the family member or caregiver.

Sundowning

Sundowning occurs when signs, symptoms, and behaviours of dementia increase during the hours of darkness—in the late afternoon and evening hours. As daylight ends and darkness sets in, confusion and restlessness, anxiety, agitation, and other symptoms increase in the client. Behaviour worsens after the sun goes down and may deteriorate throughout the night.

The client who is experiencing sundowning may be tired or hungry, have to go to the washroom, or may forget where he or she is. The client may be afraid of the dark or may see things that are not there because of poor lighting or shadows.

If the client tells you, for example, that there is a "strange person" in his or her room, you should never ignore the client's statement. Turn the light on, and reassure the client. Remove things that may be casting a shadow or disturbing the client. Ensure that the client is clean, dry, and in no danger of falling, and provide the client with verbal reassurance. See *Supporting Reverend Green* on page 687.

Box 35–3 The ABCDs of Managing Challenging Behaviours

A = Activating Event

Remember that all behaviours have meaning.
Ask yourself:

- When and where did the behaviour occur?
- What was the client doing immediately before the behaviour occurred?
- What was happening around the client at the time?

Assess environmental factors *(Consult with your supervisor or nurse.)*

- Noise (e.g., loud TV, loud music, staff change of shift, meal time clatter)
- Clutter (e.g., furniture, people)
- Bright lights or glare on the floor
- Mirrors
- Room temperature (e.g., too hot or too cold)
- Recent changes in environment (e.g., renovations, staff or resident changes)
- Does the environment provide a safe area for residents to wander around?
- Does the environment encourage independence, dignity, and mobility?
- Does the environment accept the client's cultural and lifestyle habits?
- Has there been a recent change in medication?

Does the client have any of the following? *(Consult with your supervisor or nurse.)*

- Impaired vision or hearing
- Acute illness (e.g., urinary tract infection [UTI], pneumonia)
- Chronic illness (e.g., angina, diabetes)
- Chronic pain (e.g., arthritis, ulcers, headaches)
- Dehydration
- Constipation
- Fatigue or physical discomfort

Observe for psychological factors *(Consult with your supervisor or nurse.)*

- Does the client have a history of psychiatric illness?
- Has the client experienced a recent loss or an accumulation of losses?
- Does the client appear sad (e.g., tearful or withdrawn)?
- Are past events influencing present behaviours (e.g., post-traumatic stress disorder [PTSD], abuse)?
- Does the client appear to be responding to hallucinations?

B = Behaviour

Does the client have the following behavioural symptoms?

- Physical aggression
- Screaming
- Restlessness
- Agitation
- Wandering
- Culturally inappropriate behaviours
- Lack of sexual inhibitions
- Hoarding
- Constant questioning
- Cursing
- Shadowing (following someone, often imitating their actions)

Psychological symptoms
Other clients and relatives may describe the client as having symptoms indicating the following: (*Consult with your supervisor or nurse.*)

- Anxiety
- Depression
- Paranoia
- Hallucinations
- Delusions

C = Consequences

Ask yourself the following questions:

- What was the consequence of the behaviour for the client, for staff, and for other residents?
- Was the client told off, ignored, restrained, sedated, or guided back to where he or she was? The consequence of the behaviour is very much dependent on the staff's interpretation and reaction to the behaviour. At this stage, communication is the main factor to influence the behaviour and its consequence.
- Remember the three parts of communication:
  - i. body language (55%)
  - ii. tone and pitch of voice (38%)
  - iii. words used (7%)

The attitude and manner of the care staff are extremely important. Clients with cognitive impairment are extremely sensitive to nonverbal cues and mirror the affective behaviour of those around them. A patient, calm, and gentle manner is contagious and has a

(continued on page 685)

Box 35–3 The ABCDs of Managing Challenging Behaviours (cont'd)

positive effect. It is important to be aware that if your body language indicates that you feel tense, frustrated, or angry, it may contradict the words you are using.

D = DECIDE How to Support Clients; Help DECREASE Their Challenging Behaviours; and DEBRIEF Others.

- STOP before you approach the client and think about what you are about to do, and consider the best way to do it. Plan your actions and explain who you are, what you want to do, and why you want to do it. Never assume the client will not understand you!
- SMILE! Clients will take their cue from you and will mirror your relaxed and positive body language and tone of voice.
- GO SLOWLY! You may have a lot to do and be in a hurry but the client is not. How would you feel if someone came into your bedroom, pulled back your blankets, and started pulling you out of bed without giving you time to wake up properly?
- GO AWAY when it is necessary! If the client is resistive or aggressive but is not causing harm to self or others, leave them alone. Give them time to settle down and approach them again later.
- GIVE THEM SPACE! Any activity that involves invasion of personal space increases the risk of assault and aggression. Every time you provide care to a client, you are invading their space!
- STAND ASIDE! Always provide care from the side, not from the front, of the client where you are an easy target to hit, kick, and so on.
- DISTRACT THEM! Talk to the client about things he or she enjoyed in the past and give a face towel or something to hold on to while you are providing care.
- KEEP IT QUIET! Excess noise can confuse and agitate the client. Check the noise level, and if it is high, reduce it. Turn off the radio and TV if they are upsetting the client!
- DO NOT ARGUE! This will only confuse, irritate, and further agitate the client.
- BRAINSTORM AND DEBRIEF! Discuss with the rest of the team how all of you can best meet the physical, environmental, and psychological needs of the clients in your care.
- FOLLOW THE CARE PLAN.
- REPORT AND RECORD what caused the behaviours, all behaviours observed, and what you did to support the client.

(See Figure 35–6, A and B.)

Source: Regional Dementia Management Strategy Document Library. (2001, Bendigo Health Care Group). Bendigo, Australia. Retrieved March 6, 2008, from http://www.bendigohealth.org.au/Regional-Dementia-Management/Library.html. Reprinted by permission of the Centre for Rural Rehabilitation & Aged Care.

Hallucinations

A **hallucination** is seeing, hearing, or feeling something that is not real. Senses are dulled in the affected people, who see animals, insects, or people who are not present. Some may hear voices, may feel that bugs are crawling on them, or feel that they are being touched by someone.

Sometimes the problem is made worse by impaired vision or hearing, so the client needs to wear eyeglasses and hearing aids as prescribed.

Delusions

Delusions are false beliefs. Some clients with dementia may believe that a doll is a baby or that their spouse has been unfaithful. Some may believe that they are being held captive, killed, or attacked. A client may believe that the caregiver is someone else. Many other false beliefs that can cause intense fear or other emotions in the client can occur.

Catastrophic Reactions

These are extreme responses to what the client perceives as extreme danger, disaster, or tragedy. The client may scream, cry, or be agitated or combative. These reactions are commonly from too much stimulation that can overwhelm the client, for example, being in a noisy dining room, hearing radio or TV noises, and being asked questions all at the same time.

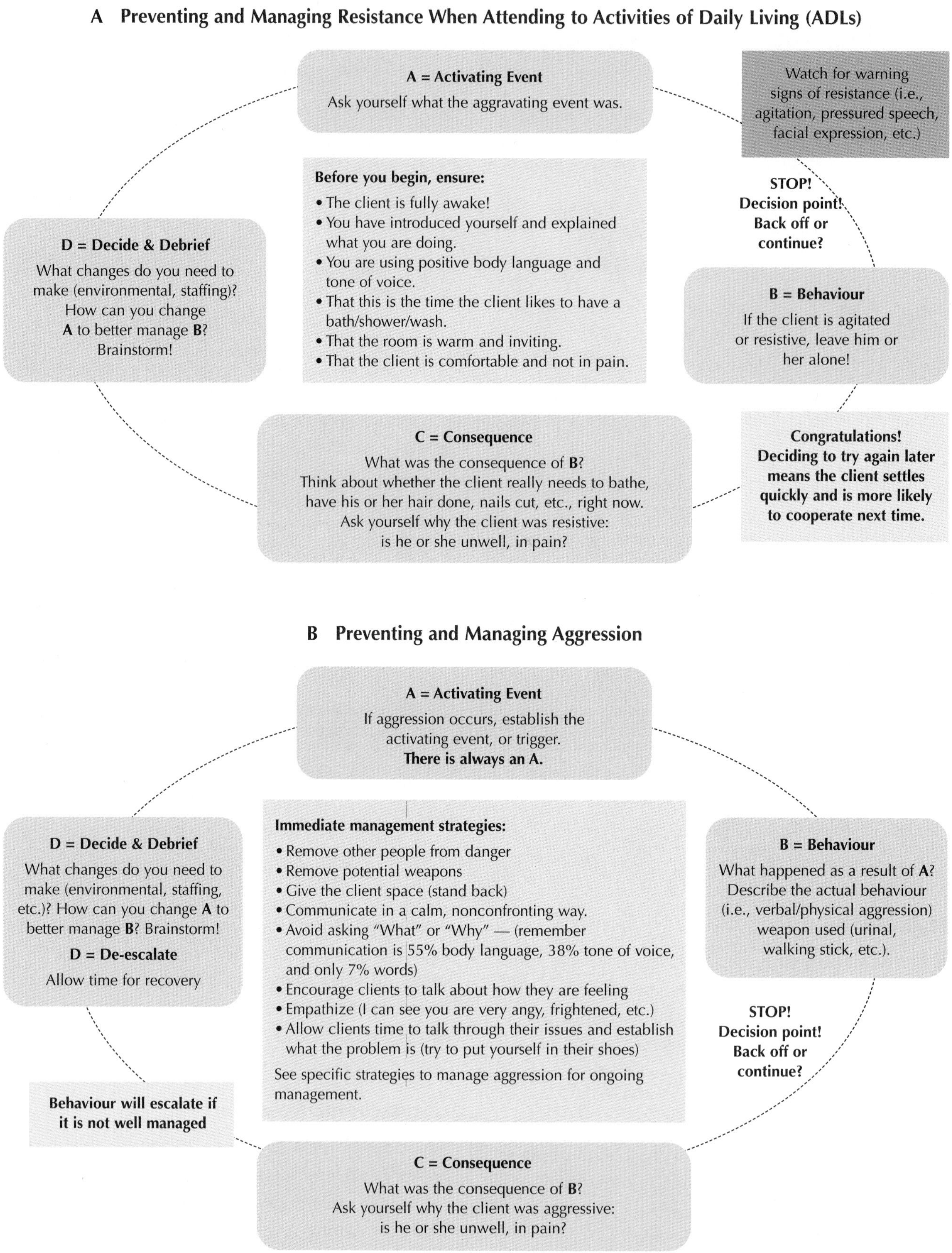

A Preventing and Managing Resistance When Attending to Activities of Daily Living (ADLs)
A = Activating Event
Ask yourself what the aggravating event was.
Watch for warning signs of resistance (i.e., agitation, pressured speech, facial expression, etc.)
STOP! Decision point! Back off or continue?
B = Behaviour
If the client is agitated or resistive, leave him or her alone!
Congratulations! Deciding to try again later means the client settles quickly and is more likely to cooperate next time.
C = Consequence
What was the consequence of B?
Think about whether the client really needs to bathe, have his or her hair done, nails cut, etc., right now.
Ask yourself why the client was resistive: is he or she unwell, in pain?
D = Decide & Debrief
What changes do you need to make (environmental, staffing)? How can you change A to better manage B? Brainstorm!
Before you begin, ensure:
• The client is fully awake!
• You have introduced yourself and explained what you are doing.
• You are using positive body language and tone of voice.
• That this is the time the client likes to have a bath/shower/wash.
• That the room is warm and inviting.
• That the client is comfortable and not in pain.
B Preventing and Managing Aggression
A = Activating Event
If aggression occurs, establish the activating event, or trigger.
There is always an A.
B = Behaviour
What happened as a result of A? Describe the actual behaviour (i.e., verbal/physical aggression) weapon used (urinal, walking stick, etc.).
STOP! Decision point! Back off or continue?
C = Consequence
What was the consequence of B?
Ask yourself why the client was aggressive: is he or she unwell, in pain?
Behaviour will escalate if it is not well managed
D = Decide & Debrief
What changes do you need to make (environmental, staffing, etc.)? How can you change A to better manage B? Brainstorm!
D = De-escalate
Allow time for recovery
Immediate management strategies:
• Remove other people from danger
• Remove potential weapons
• Give the client space (stand back)
• Communicate in a calm, nonconfronting way.
• Avoid asking "What" or "Why" — (remember communication is 55% body language, 38% tone of voice, and only 7% words)
• Encourage clients to talk about how they are feeling
• Empathize (I can see you are very angy, frightened, etc.)
• Allow clients time to talk through their issues and establish what the problem is (try to put yourself in their shoes)
See specific strategies to manage aggression for ongoing management.

Figure 35–6 The Cycle of Challenging Behaviours **A**, Preventing and Managing Resistance when Attending to Activities of Daily Living (ADLs), **B**, Preventing and Managing Aggression. **Source:** Regional Dementia Management Strategy Document Library. (2001, Bendigo Health Care Group). Bendigo, Australia. Retrieved March 6, 2008, from http://www.bendigohealth.org.au/Regional-Dementia-Management/Library.html. Reprinted by permission of the Centre for Rural Rehabilitation & Aged Care.

supporting REVEREND GREEN

Reverend Green, 72, a retired clergyman, lived at home with his wife until several months ago. He was admitted to an extended care facility due to dementia. Rev. Green was usually a quiet, soft spoken man, but the staff at this facility had begun to notice that Reverend Green was becoming increasingly more agitated in the evenings. One night, he took his pants down and started pulling on his penis while his wife and daughter were visiting him in the lounge area. They were horrified and embarrassed and could not understand why he was behaving this way.

The support staff took him to his room to provide him with privacy, assisted him to the bathroom, and then to bed. They then reported this behaviour to the nurse in charge, who conveyed the information to his doctor. It was later found that Rev. Green had a urinary infection, and because he was unable to state that something was wrong, he acted out to show his discomfort.

His wife and daughter were very relieved when this information was relayed to them. They decided to visit him earlier in the evenings when he was more "like himself." This helped make Mrs. Green's visits with her husband less distressing.

Sometimes clients have extreme reactions whenever anything out of the ordinary or unexpected happens. For example, a flickering light may be perceived as a fire, resulting in the client running away screaming. The client may even be frightened if someone approaches too quickly or stands too close to him or her.

Clients with dementia should never be "sneaked up on." Approach them from the side, in full view of them. Calmly address the client to get his or her attention, taking care not to startle the client.

Agitation and Restlessness

The client may fidget, pace, hit, or yell and may resist care. Common causes of such behaviour are pain or discomfort, anxiety, lack of sleep, and too much or too little stimulation, as well as hunger, thirst, and the need to eliminate. A calm, quiet setting and meeting basic needs help calm the client.

Do not overstimulate the client. Use a calm, gentle voice when talking to him or her. Do not overwhelm the client with instructions or choices. Do not rush the client or be impatient.

Aggression and Combativeness

These behaviours include hitting, pinching, grabbing, biting, or swearing. They may result from agitation and restlessness, which can frighten others.

Sometimes these behaviours may be caused by pain, fatigue, too much stimulation, caregiver stress, and feeling lost or abandoned. The behaviours can occur during care procedures (bathing, dressing) that upset or frighten the client. See Chapter 13 for ways to deal with an angry client. It is your responsibility to always follow the client's care plan regarding these procedures.

Screaming

Clients with dementia have communication problems. At first, it is hard to find the right word. As the dementia progresses, the client speaks in short sentences or in words, and often his or her speech is not understandable.

Sometimes clients in later stages of dementia may scream to communicate, which is common in those who are very confused and have poor communication skills. Clients may scream a word or a name or just make screaming sounds.

Possible reasons for screaming include hearing and vision problems, pain or discomfort, fear, and fatigue. Clients may have been overstimulated or understimulated. A confused client may react to a caregiver or family member by screaming.

Sometimes the following measures are helpful:

- Providing a calm, quiet setting
- Playing soft music
- Having the client wear their hearing aids and eyeglasses
- Having a family member or favourite caregiver comfort and calm the client
- Using therapeutic touch to calm the client

Abnormal Sexual Behaviours

Sexual behaviours can be labelled "abnormal" based on how and when they occur. Clients with dementia are not oriented to person, place, or time.

Abnormal sexual behaviours may involve the wrong person, the wrong place, and the wrong time. Sometimes clients with dementia are not able to control their behaviours.

Some clients may touch and fondle their genitals for pleasure. Masturbation in public is viewed as sexually aggressive behaviour, but some clients may not understand that their behaviour is socially offensive. Some clients with dementia may mistake someone else for a sexual partner and may try to kiss, hug, or touch that person.

Sometimes abnormal behaviours are not sexual in nature. Touching, scratching, and rubbing the genitals can signal infection, pain, or discomfort in the genito-urinary system, or some other underlying health problem that can cause soreness and itching. Other causes can be poor hygiene or being wet or soiled from urine or stool. Clean the client quickly and thoroughly after elimination to ensure that the client is not wet or soiled.

Sexually aggressive behaviours have many causes, including:

- Confusion or disorientation
- Nervous system disorders
- Side effects from medications
- Fever
- Dementia
- Acquired brain injury

Report when a client repeatedly touches his or her genitals. Try to determine the cause of the client's behaviour. Provide for privacy and safety. Tell your supervisor about the situation. A health care professional may assess the client for health problems and may encourage the client's sexual partner to show affection. Remember that normal practices such as hand holding, hugging, kissing, and touching are encouraged, and this may reduce the client's inappropriate behaviour. If you observe a client masturbating in public, lead the client to his or her room, and provide for privacy and safety.

Repetitive Behaviours

"Repetitive" means repeated over and over again. Clients with dementia sometimes repeat the same motions over and over. For example, a client may fold a napkin, may say the same words, or ask the same question over and over. Such behaviours are not hurtful to the client but can be annoying to caregivers and family members.

Harmless acts should be permitted, or the client can be distracted away from the act with music, picture books, exercise, movies, or a walk.

Hoarding

Hoarding means to collect things and put them away in a guarded manner. Clients who hoard items may hide them in drawers or under the beds. Some clients will hoard any and all items that they can find, while some will seek out specific items and hoard them. You should try to find out from the family why these items are significant to the client.

Secured Units. Some long-term care residents tend to wander throughout the facility or try to leave the building, which may put them at risk for injury. These residents may be moved to a secured unit—an area in the facility where entrances and exits are locked—which provides a safe setting for residents to move about but not wander away.

Secured units are considered a form of environmental restraint, so the facility must take care to use the least restrictive approach. A dementia diagnosis and a physician's order are needed to place a resident in a secured unit, and the health care team should regularly review the client's need to be placed in a secured unit, always taking care to protect the resident's rights.

As the dementia progresses to the advanced stage, a secured unit is no longer needed, as the client cannot sit or walk and is confined in bed. As wandering is not a risk any more, the client is transferred to another unit.

Legislation has standards of care for special care units. Staff must have special training in the care of people with dementia. The unit must have programs that promote dignity, personal freedom, and safety.

CAREGIVER NEEDS

Being a primary caregiver to a person with dementia can be extremely stressful physically, emotionally, socially, and financially. Many adult children in the "sandwich generation" have their energies divided between taking care of their children and their parents who both need attention. They not only care for two families but also have full-time jobs outside their homes, which can add to their stress.

Caregivers can therefore suffer from anger, anxiety, sleeplessness, and depression. Some find it difficult to concentrate on anything and are always irritable. Abuse may occur in very stressful caregiving situations.

Because they are constantly under stress, caregivers are susceptible to health problems, so they need to take care of their own health by ensuring healthy diet, exercise, and plenty of rest. The caregiver must ask family and friends for help when their responsibilities become overwhelming.

Caregivers need much support and encouragement, so many of them join support groups sponsored by hospitals, long-term facilities, and the Alzheimer Society of Canada, which has chapters in cities and towns across the country. People in similar situations voice their feelings, anger, frustration, guilt, and other emotions and share coping and caregiving strategies.

Caregivers, family members, and friends of a person with dementia often feel helpless. No matter what they do, the person only gets worse. Much time, money, energy, and emotion are needed to care for the person. Guilty feelings are common in these caregivers as well. Family and friends know that the person does not choose to have dementia. They know that the person does not choose to have its signs, symptoms, and behaviours. Nevertheless, sometimes behaviours are frustrating, embarrassing, or threatening. Family and friends may be upset and angry that their loved one cannot show love or affection.

As a support worker, you play a key role in caregiver relief. You may assist the primary caregiver or other caregivers, or you may care for the client to give the caregiver some time off from his or her responsibilities. Follow the care plan, and perform your tasks competently. The caregiver should have confidence in your skill and ability so that she or he is able to relax and let go of control for a time. The care plan may ask you to encourage the caregiver to take care of his or her own needs and to leave the home to have a break while you are there. You may observe signs and symptoms of caregiver stress and of depression and abuse. Report these observations immediately to your supervisor (see the *Support Workers Solving Problems: Supporting Caregivers of Clients with Dementia* box).

Support Workers Solving Problems

Supporting Caregivers of Clients With Dementia

<< Scenario >>

Mrs. Munroe, 70, has Alzheimer's disease. She has stage 2 (moderate) dementia. She lives at home with her husband, who is her primary caregiver. Leila is assigned to provide morning respite care. This is her fourth visit. Mrs. Munroe is incontinent; she also needs assistance with feeding, bathing, and dressing. She is frequently rude and aggressive. She becomes angry if someone stands too near her or tries to make her do something. Quick, sudden movements and loud noises also upset her. The care plan calls for Mr. Munroe to take a break—preferably away from the house—while Leila takes care of Mrs. Munroe's needs. Mr. Munroe is reluctant to leave, since he is anxious about his wife.

<< Discussion >>

Leila's visit is scheduled for 3 hours. She knows that Mr. Munroe will not leave until he is satisfied that his wife is in competent hands. Leila starts her visit by sitting down with Mrs. Munroe at the kitchen table and talking quietly and gently. She explains that she is going to make breakfast and gives Mrs. Munroe two food choices. Leila makes breakfast, while she continues talking with Mrs. Munroe in a quiet, reassuring voice. Mr. Munroe is anxiously watching everything from the living room. When Mrs. Munroe is settled, Leila suggests to Mr. Munroe that he go out for a coffee and he reluctantly agrees to go. When he comes back 1 hour later, Mrs. Munroe has been bathed and dressed, and she is sitting quietly watching TV. Mr. Munroe feels better for having had a break, and now he feels confident in Leila's ability to care for his wife.

REVIEW

Answers to these questions are at the bottom of page 691.

Circle the BEST answer.

1. **Cognitive function relates to:**
   A. Memory loss and personality
   B. Thinking and reasoning
   C. Ability to toilet oneself
   D. How emotional a person can get

2. **If a client is confused after moving to a long-term care facility, this confusion is likely to be:**
   A. Temporary due to medications he or she has been on
   B. Due to emotional stress caused by the move
   C. Due to an infection
   D. Due to brain injury

3. **Which of the following statements about delirium is true? It:**
   A. Is a permanent state of confusion
   B. Is unavoidable and happens to most clients
   C. Is an emergency and can be a reaction to medications
   D. Should be ignored so as to not embarrass the client

4. **Which of the following statements about dementia is true? Dementia:**
   A. Can affect people in their 40s
   B. Is a normal part of aging
   C. Is less common in people over 65 years of age
   D. Can result in colour-blindness

5. **Which of the following statements about Alzheimer disease (AD) is true?**
   A. It occurs only in older people
   B. Diet and medications can cure the disease
   C. AD and confusion are the same
   D. It is the most common form of dementia

6. **A common sign or symptom of dementia is:**
   A. Headache
   B. Paralysis
   C. Dyspnea
   D. Poor judgement

7. **People with early stage dementia:**
   A. Usually remain in their homes with support
   B. Are totally dependent on others for care
   C. Are confined to bed
   D. Are usually placed in secured units

8. **Joe Dunn has Alzheimer's disease (AD). Which statement is true?**
   A. AD only occurs in older people
   B. Diet and drugs can control the disease
   C. AD and delirium are the same thing
   D. There is no known cure for AD

9. **Mr. Dunn is screaming. You know that this is:**
   A. An agitated reaction
   B. His style of singing
   C. Caused by a delusion
   D. A repetitive behaviour

10. **Mr. Dunn is offered simple choices. This is because:**
    A. He is not really a choosy person
    B. He is not very smart
    C. His wife makes all of his decisions
    D. More choices would only confuse and agitate him

11. **Secured units:**
    A. Prevent the confused client from wandering and getting lost
    B. Are rarely used because they are restrictive and inhumane
    C. Are only necessary when a client is in the severe or late stage of dementia
    D. Prevent a client's family from visiting

12. **Mr. Dunn has moderate dementia and tends to wander. You should do the following:**
    A. Tell him which areas are safe for wandering
    B. Keep him in his pyjamas so he will not want to wander far
    C. Keep him on bedrest and give him comfort care
    D. Make sure door alarms are turned on

REVIEW

Answers to these questions are at the bottom of the page.

13. **Sundowning means that:**
    - A. The person becomes sleepy when the sun sets
    - B. Behaviours become worse in the late afternoon and evening hours
    - C. Behaviour improves at night
    - D. The person is in the third stage of dementia

14. **Which of the following safety points should you follow for Mr. Dunn?**
    - A. All safety hazards should be painted red
    - B. Mr. Dunn should wear a large sign that says he is a safety risk
    - C. Sharp and breakable objects should be removed from his environment
    - D. He can keep his smoking materials but should only smoke in designated areas

15. **Besides a quiet, calm environment, what else should you keep in mind when caring for Mr. Dunn in a facility?**
    - A. Introduce yourself every time you see him
    - B. Mr. Dunn no longer has rights, as he is too confused
    - C. Never touch any of the clients as it could scare them
    - D. Clients should be encouraged to bathe each other, as it gives them a sense of purpose

16. **Support workers usually have much contact with family members in the following ways:**
    - A. Offering advice to the family
    - B. Telling the family that they are not helping out enough
    - C. Providing support and relief to the family
    - D. Telling the family about other clients

17. **A type of dementia that is caused by a series of small strokes resulting in brain tissue death is called:**
    - A. Lewy body dementia
    - B. Creutzfeldt-Jakob disease
    - C. Pick's disease
    - D. Vascular dementia

Match each definition with the letter beside each correct key term on the list below.

- A. Agitation
- B. Catastrophic reactions
- C. Delusions
- D. Depression
- E. Hallucinations
- F. Hoarding
- G. Pacing
- H. Sundowning
- I. Wandering

18. __H__ **Becoming restless and agitated in the late afternoon or night**

19. __C__ **Believing things that are not true**

20. __E__ **Seeing things that are not there**

21. __G__ **Walking back and forth in the same area**

22. __D__ **Becoming withdrawn and having no energy or interest in doing things**

23. __A__ **Being excited, restless, or troubled**

24. __F__ **Collecting and putting things away in a guarded manner**

25. __I__ **Moving from one area to another aimlessly**

Answers: 1.B, 2.B, 3.C, 4.A, 5.D, 6.D, 7.A, 8.D, 9.A, 10.D, 11.A, 12.D, 13.B, 14.C, 15.A, 16.C, 17.D, 18.H, 19.C, 20.E, 21.G, 22.D, 23.A, 24.F, 25.I

CHAPTER 36

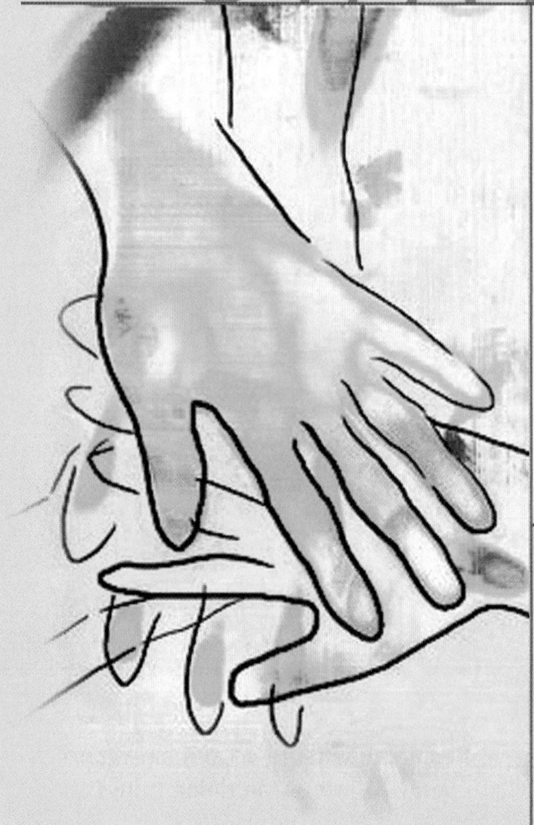

Speech and Language Disorders

OBJECTIVES

- Define the key terms listed in this chapter.
- Describe three types of aphasia.
- Describe apraxia of speech.
- Describe dysarthria.
- Describe how speech and language disorders are treated.
- Identify what communication aids are and how they assist the client.
- Describe how computers can assist clients with speech disorders.
- Describe the emotional effects of a language disorder.
- Describe how to communicate with clients with language disorders.
- Apply the procedures described in this chapter to your clinical practice properly.

key terms

aphasia Partial or complete loss (*a*) of speech and language skills (*phasia*), caused by brain injury.

apraxia of speech Inability (*a*) to move *(praxia)* the muscles used to speak. Apraxia is usually caused by a brain injury.

dementia A general term that describes the progressive loss of brain functioning, which includes cognitive and social functions. It is not a single disease but a group of illnesses that involve memory, behaviour, learning, and communication.

dysarthria Difficulty (*dys*) in speaking clearly (*arthria*), caused by weakness or paralysis in the muscles used for speech.

expressive aphasia Difficulty in speaking or writing.

expressive-receptive aphasia Difficulty in speaking and understanding language.

receptive aphasia Difficulty understanding language.

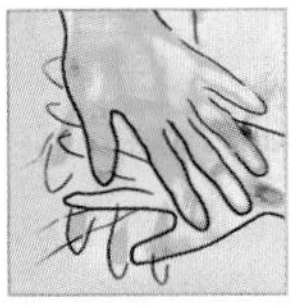

Imagine what it would be like if you were unable to speak or communicate! For those with speech and language disorders, this is a daily reality. Speech and language disorders are an inability to speak, understand, read, or write, and, unfortunately, they can occur at any age. There are many causes, including:

- Genetic problems or conditions present at birth
- Brain injury (may be caused by accident, infection, drug abuse, stroke, and so on)
- Disease
- Hearing loss
- Brain tumours
- Problems involving the structures used for speech

In Chapter 13, we discussed effective communication between people who have no physical communication challenges. This chapter builds on the information presented in Chapter 13, to apply it to the process of communicating effectively with clients with speech and language disorders. It should be noted that speech and language disorders are a result of injuries or decline in the brain's communication centre. They should not be confused with inability to understand English (by people who speak another language)!

APHASIA

Aphasia is the partial or complete loss (*a*) of speech and language skills (*phasia*) caused by brain injury. Stroke (*cerebral vascular accident*, or *CVA*), head trauma, and brain tumours are the most common causes for aphasia. Some people with aphasia regain some or all of their language skills, but in some, aphasia is permanent. Many people with **dementia** also have aphasia (see Chapter 35).

For communication to occur, a message must be sent, received, and interpreted. Some people with aphasia are unable to send messages, understand the message received, or both send and receive messages.

Types of Aphasia. There are three basic types of aphasia:

1. **Receptive aphasia**—difficulty understanding language, including both spoken and written words. People with receptive aphasia have difficulty understanding what is said or read. They cannot understand their own words, so their speech is mixed up or "muddled." They may make up words or use the wrong words but may not be aware of their mistakes. For example, they may use the word "orange" when they mean "apple." They also mix up sounds within words. A client trying to say "hospital" may

actually say "posital." A client trying to say, "Please give me a glass of water" may actually say "Ples put dat cat over tad counter."

2. **Expressive aphasia**—difficulty speaking and writing. People with expressive aphasia can understand spoken and written words, but their speech is jumbled or slurred and difficult to understand. They think one thing but say another. For example, a client may want food but ask for a newspaper. People with expressive aphasia cannot think of the right words or put the right sounds together to form words and sentences. They may leave out connecting words. For example, instead of saying "I want to go to the bathroom," a client may say "me ... uh ... room ... uh ... bathroom." Some people can only produce meaningless sounds. People with expressive aphasia are very aware of their mistakes because *they* can understand what they are saying, so this may lead to frustration or depression in them. They may also cry or swear for no apparent reason. They may be doing this out of frustration or for other reasons unknown to you.
3. **Expressive-receptive aphasia**—difficulty speaking and understanding language. Some people with expressive-receptive aphasia can only say "yes," "no," and make sounds such as "da da." Some others have lost all speech and language skills.

APRAXIA OF SPEECH

Apraxia of speech (*verbal apraxia*) is the inability (*a*) to move (*praxia*) the muscles used to speak. People with this disorder are not able to control their lip, jaw, or tongue movements. As a result, they are not able to say the desired sounds and words. Apraxia of speech is caused by brain injury resulting from stroke, accidents, brain tumour, or infection. Some children are born with this disorder. Apraxia of speech can occur alone or with aphasia.

It is difficult to understand the speech of people with apraxia of speech, as it is usually slow. They may use a word that sounds like the word they are trying to say. For example, a client may say "me" instead of "see." The order of sounds within words is mixed up. For example, a client may say "thootshub" instead of "toothbrush." Some people have problems putting words in the right order or finding the right words. Inconsistent speech is common—that is, a client may say something correctly one time and incorrectly another time.

DYSARTHRIA

Dysarthria is difficulty (*dys*) speaking clearly (*arthria*). It is caused by weakness or paralysis in the muscles used for speech. Some common causes of dysarthria include cerebral palsy, multiple sclerosis, head injury, tumour, and infection.

People who have dysarthria usually have slurred, slow, and soft speech and speak in flat, harsh, or nasal tones. They often have problems forming words, spacing their words, and breathing while speaking. Speech errors are usually consistent and predictable, so you may become familiar with a client's speech.

EMOTIONAL EFFECTS OF SPEECH AND LANGUAGE DISORDERS

Imagine what it would be like to have a speech and language disorder. How would you feel if you were not able to express your thoughts and feelings? How would you feel if you were not able to understand what others are saying? People with speech and language disorders experience many emotions, such as frustration, depression, and anger, as well as low-self esteem, shame, and guilt. Box 36–1 contains comments from people who have had aphasia.

Communication is important for functioning and for maintaining relationships with others. Being unable to communicate may cause a client to avoid social situations, or family and friends may avoid the client instead. Speech and language disorders can be very stressful for families, as the relations between all family members are usually affected.

For many of us, sharing our thoughts and feelings with others is often difficult. It is even more

Box 36–1 Comments From People Who Have Had Aphasia

"I wanted to speak, but no sounds came out of my mouth."

"I felt ... imprisoned in a tomb."

"I noticed a change in me. I was another person, someone who was unable to express the little I knew. I was ashamed."

"If you don't know words, you keep quiet ... When it's noisy, you can't talk ... People talk for us ... Anyway, when we talk, it's not the way it used to be ... you keep quiet."

"Once I had to answer the intercom. I said 'Hello? 'I heard the person speaking on the other end, but I couldn't understand him. So, to prove that it wasn't me who had the problem, I repeated 'Hello! Hello! Hello!' as if to signal the line was bad. That's how I got out of that situation."

"I feel useless ... slightly distanced from the family because I can only understand things after some time. My world has shrunk."

"I want to say something ... just before I start saying it, she helps. Sometimes if she would stay back and let me finish, I would be all right."

Source: Joanette, Y., Lafond, D., & Lecours, A.R. (1993). *The client with aphasia: Living with aphasia: Psychosocial issues* (pp. 19–36). San Diego: Singular Publishing Group.

difficult for someone who has a speech or language disorder or challenge, when even everyday conversations require great effort. In addition, the person with a speech and language disorder may not be able to work, so there may be the added stress of financial concerns. For some people, routine tasks like shopping, cooking, paying bills, and doing household repairs may also be impossible, and they are forced to depend on others to do what they used to be able to do themselves.

Emotional reactions vary from client to client and from family to family. Observe and listen to your clients and their families. Put yourself in their place. How would you feel and want to be treated in their position? Accept and understand displays of emotion.

TREATMENT FOR SPEECH AND LANGUAGE DISORDERS

A speech therapist (also called a speech-language pathologist) helps the client with a speech disorder learn to communicate and also helps family members learn new communication techniques. Methods used depend on the disorder, its cause, and severity. Practice and exercises may help the client relearn speech and language skills. For dysarthria, the client practises muscle-strengthening exercises and learns how to breathe while speaking.

People with speech and language disorders also learn how to improve existing skills. For example, a client learns to use body language and facial expressions to make communication more effective. Some people learn new skills such as sign language.

Those with severe speech and language problems may never regain their speech or ability to understand language. These clients may be helped by the following aids:

- ***Communication boards.*** These are boards with pictures or words that show functions or tasks (Figure 36–1). There are pictures or words related to activities of daily living, such as sleep, food, drink, medicine, and glasses. The client points to the things he or she needs. The type of communication board depends on the client's needs. For those who can read, words rather than pictures are often used. For those with quadriplegia who are not able to speak, eye-gaze boards are used. The client indicates his or her needs by gazing at the picture or word on the board and either blinking or using another signal to accept it.

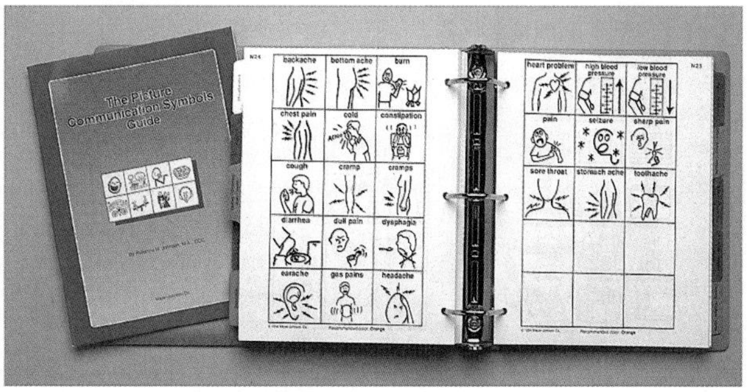

Figure 36–1 Communication board.

- ***Mechanical and electronic devices.*** These range in complexity and cost—from large computers that cannot be moved easily from place to place to hand-held devices such as electronic talking aids (Figures 36–2 and 36–3). The client touches a picture displayed on the screen, and the message is then voiced by the device. For example, the client touches a picture of a sad face. A recorded message says: "I am sad." The message may also be printed on a screen, and some devices convert words into pictures.

The Use of Computers That Assist Clients With Speech and Language Challenges

With the introduction of the personal computer, technology is now assisting many clients who have speech and language challenges to communicate more easily.[1] For example, people with verbal-expression communication disorders (such as dyslexia or expressive apraxia) often have difficulty reading or writing. Electronic devices that use a combination of screen reading, magnification systems, and alternate input provide computing access to persons with such impairments.

Systems that speak for the user can help individuals with speech impairments if they are able to type in the correct words or identify symbols that represent the words. Most of the software packages used for these applications can operate with a speech synthesizer. The speech that comes from the machine is electronically generated but can be adapted for a male or female voice.

These computer-assisted electronic aids are expensive and difficult for some to carry around, but they have proven to be invaluable in improving the quality of life for those with speech and language challenges.

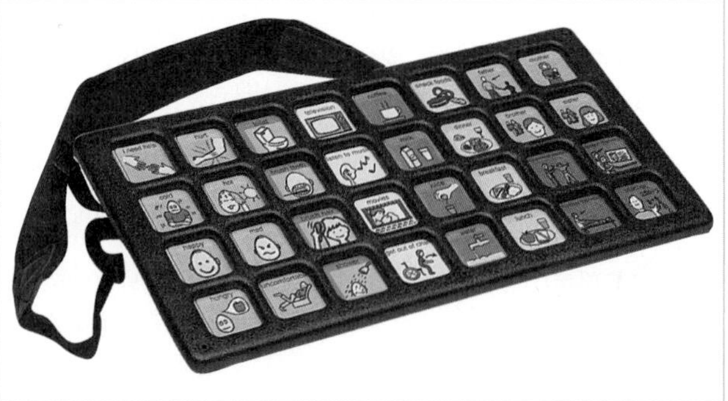

Figure 36–2 Electronic talking aid using symbols. **Courtesy:** Mayer-Johnson Co., Solana Beach, CA.

Figure 36–3 A computer that provides a speaking voice to its user. **Courtesy:** Special Needs Computer Solutions, St. Catharines, ON.

COMMUNICATING WITH CLIENTS

As a support worker, in order to effectively communicate with your clients who have speech and language disorders, you must know how you communicate effectively. Do you speak clearly, or do you mumble? Do you use gestures when you speak? You may have to change the way you speak. Follow the care plan and your supervisor's instructions. Use the communication methods that are best for your client. While you are speaking, you should remember to be mindful of your facial expressions, as they can reflect your impatience or frustration with the client.

The effort of understanding others and making oneself understood can be exhausting, especially to clients with speech and language disorders, so they often tire easily. Their other health problems may also cause fatigue. Be alert for signs of fatigue, such as drooping shoulders, irritability, lack of interest, and a decline in understanding.

Some clients with speech and language disorders will appear withdrawn and uninterested. Spend extra time with these clients. Social interaction can promote self-esteem and recovery. Always include them in conversations, even if they cannot understand you.

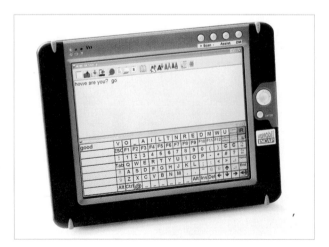

Clients with speech and language disorders should be treated with respect and empathy. Remember DIPPS—the five principles of support work (see the *Providing Compassionate Care: Communicating with Clients with Speech and Language Disorders* box). Follow the guidelines in Box 36–2.

PROVIDING COMPASSIONATE CARE

Communicating With Clients With Speech and Language Disorders

- **Dignity.** Showing respect, warmth, and compassion are important ways to promote dignity. Never talk about a client as if he or she were not present. Address questions and comments to the client, not to others who are present. Some people with language disorders are embarrassed to speak in front of others, especially strangers, so do not force a client to talk in front of others.
- **Independence.** People with speech and language disorders must gain, regain, or maintain independence and control. Support, encouragement, and patience are important. Never show impatience, frustration, or worry when a client is having problems speaking or understanding. Do not talk down to the client. (The *Support Workers Solving Problems* box describes a support worker patiently using body language and symbols to learn about a client's needs.) The care plan may list ways to encourage communication.
- **Preferences.** Limit the number of choices to help the client express preferences without difficulty. Be encouraging and supportive. A useful tip is to write down the available choices beforehand so that the client can pick one easily.
- **Privacy.** Keep information about your client confidential. Remember your role and relationship with the client at all times. Be professional in your communication. Learn to be comfortable with silence. Do not feel that you need to talk when the client is silent.
- **Safety.** Take extra time to explain procedures. Do not explain all the steps at once. Explain the step just before you do it. Avoid medical terms. Speak clearly and slowly. Be alert for signs the client has not understood you.

supporting MR. HAMILTON

Joshua Hamilton, 57, survived a cerebral vascular accident (CVA, or stroke) several months ago. In addition to a few other health challenges, he also has expressive aphasia. Marta, his support worker, has been assigned to Mr. Hamilton to assist him with his basic care at home.

Mr. Hamilton frequently asks Marta questions that she does not understand. Here is an example of a recent conversation:

Mr. Hamilton: Wuld ples git bassen eaten.
Marta: Could you please repeat that Mr. Hamilton?
Mr. Hamilton: (raises his voice) Plasin get eatin puck.
Marta: Would you like something to eat?
Mr. Hamilton: (looks puzzled and upset) Dat stan woo.
Marta: (pretends to eat) Would you like a snack?
Mr. Hamilton: (shakes his head, but says nothing)
Marta: (pretends to drink) Something to drink?
Mr. Hamilton: (nods his head and looks relieved)
Marta: (gets a glass and cup)
Mr. Hamilton: (gestures toward the cup)
Marta: (gets a tea bag): Would you like a cup of tea?
Mr. Hamilton: (nods)

In this situation, Marta was not sure what exactly Mr. Hamilton wanted. She thought the words "eaten" and "eatin" suggested that Mr. Hamilton wanted something to eat. He was, in fact, trying to say "tea." Marta did not know this, but she knew from reading his care plan and speaking to his family that Mr. Hamilton liked tea. Using body language and symbols, Marta discovered what Mr. Hamilton wanted; and by being patient and persistent, she was able to meet Mr. Hamilton's needs.

Box 36–2 Guidelines for Communicating With Clients With Speech and Language Disorders

- ***Minimize distractions.*** Distractions make concentration difficult and can also upset the client. Reduce background noise and activity. Close doors and windows. Turn off the television and radio (if the client agrees). Make sure there is nothing in your hands or on your lap.
- ***Adjust the lighting.*** Make sure the client can see your face clearly and that you can see the client's. Turn down lights and adjust window coverings to reduce glare. Do not position yourself between the client and a window. The client may not be able to see you in the glare.
- ***Give the client your full attention.*** Sit close by and face the client. Look directly into the client's eyes so that he or she can look at your face. Get the client's attention before you speak. Show that you are listening by using gestures and facial expressions. Do not perform other tasks while you are talking to the client.
- ***In the beginning of your work relationship with the client, you can start by asking questions to which you know the answer.*** This helps you become familiar with his or her speech.
- ***Determine the subject being discussed.*** This helps you understand the main points. Look for nonverbal clues. Do the client's gestures, eyes, and body language tell you anything? Does the client use words or partial words that might describe an item or concept?
- ***Follow the client's lead.*** Alter your communication method, as needed. For example, Mrs. Schmidt becomes frustrated when you ask her questions. You learn that she responds better when you use gestures to demonstrate your question. If Mrs. Schmidt seems tired or has lost interest, allow her to rest. Bring up the subject at a later time.
- ***Speak slowly, clearly, and in a normal tone of voice.*** Adjust your speech to suit the client's needs. Talk to adults in an mature, professional manner. Do not use slang or figures of speech. Some clients may not understand them.
- ***Give the client time to respond.*** Do not rush the client. Pause between sentences to allow the client time to think and respond. Do not answer questions, including your own questions and those from others, when they are addressed to the client.
- ***Use simple words and short sentences.*** Avoid long, complex sentences. Focus on key words—mostly action words and words for people, places, or things. For example, say "Let's go for lunch" instead of "It's time for me to transfer you to the dining room for lunch."
- ***Be patient.*** Repeat your words, as needed. Rephrase your sentences if the client does not understand you.
- ***Use positive statements.*** These are easier to understand than negative statements. For example, say: "Bend your arm" instead of "Don't straighten your arm."
- ***Use appropriate questioning and paraphrasing techniques.*** Ask questions that require only a short answer or a shake of the head. Paraphrase (summarize in your own words) what the client has said. Ask the client if you have understood him or her correctly (see Chapter 13).
- ***Provide cues, as needed.*** Help clients express themselves by giving them cues about a word they cannot recall. If it is an object, ask: "What does it look like?" "What is it used for?" and "Where is it found?" Encourage the use of gestures and pointing. If you think you understand what the client says, verify your assumption by asking the client to use gestures, pointing, or symbols. For example, Mrs. Lin points to her sweater. You get it for her and she puts it on. You have understood her need.
- ***Try other communication methods.*** Some people may write better than they speak. Follow the care plan. Use writing and communication boards, as needed.
- ***Pay attention to your own facial expressions and nonverbal cues.*** Your facial expressions can reveal if you are frustrated or impatient, and your client could easily detect this.

REVIEW

Answers to these questions are at the bottom of the page.

Circle the **BEST** answer.

1. **People with receptive aphasia have problems with:**
   A. Speaking and writing
   B. Pronouncing vowels
   C. Understanding language
   D. Moving the mouth, tongue, and lips

2. **People with expressive-receptive aphasia have problems with:**
   A. Speaking and writing
   B. Understanding language
   C. Moving the mouth, tongue, and lips
   D. Speaking and understanding language

3. **Apraxia of speech is caused by:**
   A. Brain injury
   B. Laziness of the client
   C. Increased tone in the muscles used to speak
   D. Lack of coordination in the muscles used to walk

4. **People with dysarthria:**
   A. Cannot read or write
   B. Understand what is said
   C. Make unpredictable speech errors
   D. Can control the muscles used to speak

5. **People with speech and language disorders:**
   A. Are not affected emotionally
   B. Cannot improve their communication
   C. Often have problems relating to family and friends
   D. Are consistent in the way they react emotionally to their disorders

6. **When communicating with clients who have speech and language disorders, you should:**
   A. Speak in a very loud voice
   B. Leave them out of conversations
   C. Ask others what they are trying to say
   D. Provide cues about words they cannot recall

7. **If you do not understand what a client has said, you should:**
   A. Use body language and symbols
   B. Ask to be assigned to another client
   C. Pretend that you did understand
   D. Ignore the client, hoping that he or she will stop asking

8. **Why should instructions be stated using positive phrases (Bend your leg) rather than negative phrases (Do not straighten your leg)?**
   A. Using negative terms may be confusing for the client
   B. Positive terms are usually more direct
   C. Negative terms usually focus on what the client has already done
   D. All of the above

Answers: 1.C, 2.D, 3.A, 4.B, 5.C, 6.D, 7.A, 8.D

CHAPTER 37

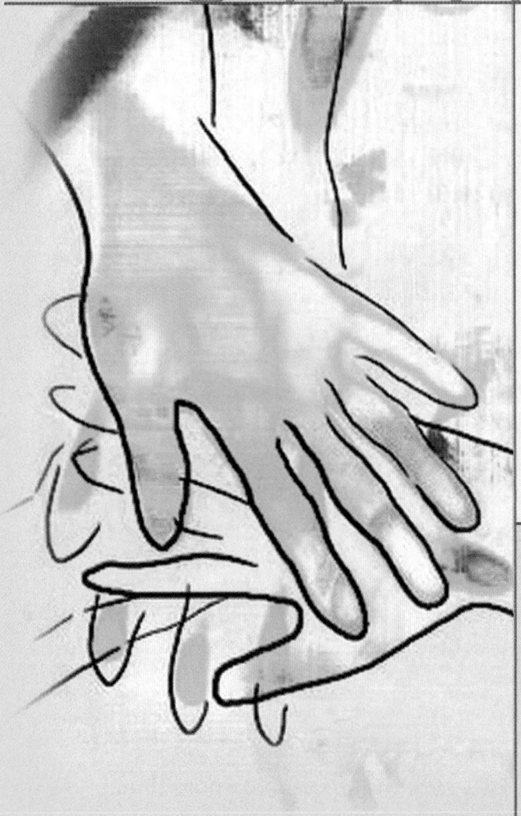

Hearing and Vision Problems

OBJECTIVES

- Define the key terms listed in this chapter.
- Describe the major ear disorders.
- Describe the effects of hearing problems.
- Describe aids for clients with hearing problems.
- Explain how to care for clients with hearing loss.
- Describe the major eye disorders.
- Describe aids for clients with vision problems.
- Explain how to care for clients with vision loss.
- Perform the procedures described in this chapter.

key terms

age-related macular degeneration (AMD; ARMD) The breakdown (degeneration) of the macula (the light-sensitive part of the retina).

Braille A writing system for the blind that uses raised dots for each letter of the alphabet.

cataract Clouding of the eye's lens.

diabetic retinopathy A disorder (*pathy*) caused by diabetes, in which the blood vessels in the retina are damaged.

dominant progressive hearing loss The impairment of nerves used to hear.

glaucoma An eye disease that causes pressure within the eye and vision loss.

Ménière's disease An increase of fluid in the inner ear causing pressure in the middle ear; vertigo, tinnitus, and hearing loss.

otitis media Infection (*itis*) of the middle (*media*) ear (*ot*).

otosclerosis a condition (*osis*) in which there is hardening (*sclero*) of the ossicles in the middle ear (*oto*).

presbycusis The gradual hearing (*cusis*) loss associated with aging (*presby*).

presbyopia The gradual inability to focus (*opia*) on close objects; a condition associated with aging (*presby*).

retinal detachment The separation of the retina from its supporting tissue.

tinnitus Ringing in the ear.

vertigo Dizziness.

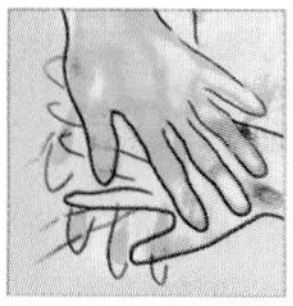

The senses of sight and hearing are important for communicating, learning, moving about, and performing activities of daily living (ADLs). They also help keep us safe by alerting us to danger.

Hearing and vision problems are common among all age groups, and common causes include conditions present at birth, diseases, and accidents. Some hearing and vision loss (and loss of other senses) is a natural part of aging.

As a support worker, you will care for many clients with hearing and vision problems. Some clients may have minor problems that can be corrected with hearing aids and glasses, while some others may have severe losses (see the *Providing Compassionate Care: Clients With Severe Hearing Loss and Vision Loss* box).

EAR DISORDERS AND HEARING PROBLEMS

The ear is needed for hearing and balance. Hearing problems range from slight hearing impairments to complete deafness. Hearing problems may occur suddenly, but usually they are gradual in onset. One or both ears may be affected. Ear structures are shown in Figure 37–1. See Chapter 14 for a review of the structure and function of the ear.

Common causes of hearing problems include:

- ***Otitis media***—infection (*itis*) of the middle (*media*) ear (*ot*). It is common in infants and children and may be acute or chronic. Chronic otitis media can damage the eardrum as well as the bones of the middle ear that conduct sound to the inner ear (the *ossicles*), which are essential for hearing. Permanent hearing loss can result from chronic otitis media.
- ***Otosclerosis***—a condition (*osis*) in which there is hardening (*sclero*) of the ossicles in the middle ear (*oto*). It is a hereditary condition that is a common cause of hearing loss in adults. The person experiences gradual and progressive hearing loss and **tinnitus** (ringing in the ear). Surgery can often restore some hearing.
- ***Ménière's disease***—an increase of fluid in the inner ear causing pressure in the middle ear. Usually only one ear is affected, resulting in

PROVIDING COMPASSIONATE CARE

Clients With Severe Hearing Loss and Vision Loss

- **Dignity.** Clients with hearing loss and vision loss need patience and respect, not pity. Speak clearly in a normal tone of voice. Do not shout, and do not mumble or use slang terms. Do not talk to the client as you would to a child. Include him or her in conversations with others. Never ask another person (such as a family member) to speak for the client. When speaking of a client, always state his or her name before the disability. For example, Mrs. Kabir has hearing loss. She is not "the deaf client." If a client uses sign language and has an interpreter, speak to the client, not to the interpreter.
- **Independence.** Remember, clients who are impaired in one area are not impaired in all areas. Do not make assumptions about their abilities or limitations. Clients with hearing loss and vision loss should be allowed to do as much for themselves as possible. Tell the client what you are doing step by step. Indicate when the procedure is over. When clients use self-care (assistive) devices to maintain independence, make sure they have access to these needed devices.
- **Preferences.** Follow your clients' choices and directions. Ask how you can help. Assist only if the client wants you to.
- **Privacy.** Respect your client's privacy. Always let the client know when you are in the room. If the client cannot hear you knock, make sure the client can see you entering the room. If the client cannot see you, announce your arrival clearly. Also, tell the client if others join you in the room.

  Always tell your client when you are leaving the room. Remember your role and relationship with your clients at all times. Keep information about clients confidential. Communicate in a professional manner.
- **Safety.** A safe setting is critical to clients with hearing loss and vision loss. Clients with hearing loss cannot hear sounds that signal danger, and those with vision loss cannot see obstacles in their path, so they are at great risk for falls. Follow the safety measures described in Chapter 19. Follow the care plan for safety measures specific for each client. In facilities, keep the call bell within easy reach.

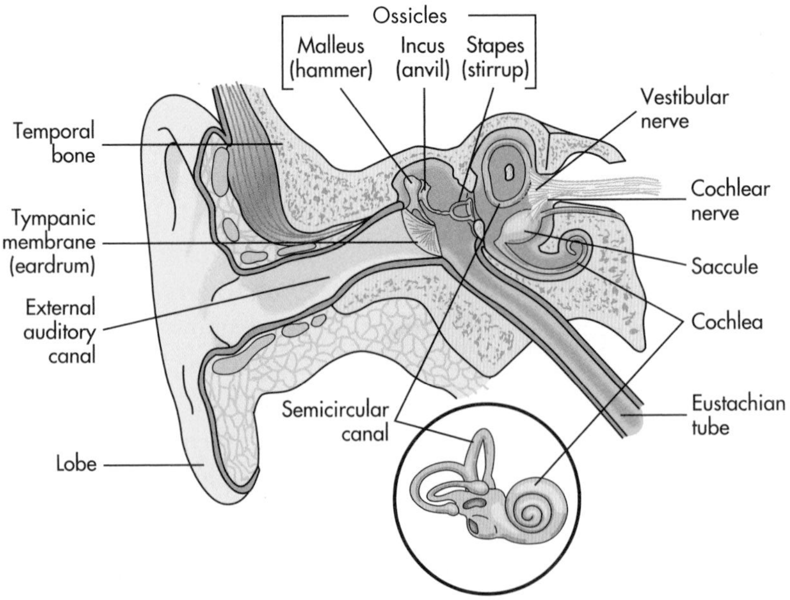

Figure 37–1 The ear.

vertigo (dizziness), tinnitus, and hearing loss. If the client feels dizzy, he or she must lie down to prevent a fall. Severe dizziness can cause nausea and vomiting.

- ***Dominant progressive hearing loss***—the impairment of nerves used to hear. Hearing loss is progressive. Sometimes the disease starts in early childhood, but usually it starts in early or middle adulthood.
- ***Presbycusis***—the gradual hearing (*cusis*) loss associated with aging (*presby*). It usually occurs after age 50. There is no cure, but hearing aids and speech reading are helpful to those affected.
- ***Temporary hearing loss***—The blockage of the ear canal with earwax. This is common in older adults. Hearing improves when the earwax is removed by a physician or a nurse.

The Effects of Hearing Problems

Signs and symptoms of hearing problems vary and are not always obvious. A person's behaviour or attitude may change because of hearing problems. For example, a person may not respond when others talk or ask questions, and he or she may become angry that others are not speaking loudly enough. Family and friends may not be aware of the hearing problems, and they may become frustrated when communicating with the affected person and may avoid talking with him or her.

Some people deny that they have hearing problems, as they may not want to believe that they are different from others or to admit to a sign of aging. Some people refuse to get or use a hearing aid.

The obvious signs of hearing problems in adults and children include:

- Speaking too loudly
- Leaning forward to hear
- Turning and cupping the unaffected ear toward the speaker
- Responding inappropriately
- Asking for words to be repeated

Hearing problems can affect all aspects of a person's health—physical, emotional, social, intellectual, and spiritual. For example, Mrs. Lopez has hearing loss and avoids social situations because she feels left out of conversations. She is afraid of embarrassing herself by giving the wrong response. Straining to hear a conversation makes her tired. She no longer listens to the radio or watches TV. She has stopped going to church because she cannot hear the sermon. She is alone so much that she feels isolated and bored.

Hearing loss may cause speech problems. A person can hear himself or herself talk, which has an influence on pronunciation and the volume of voice. Hearing loss may result in slurred speech and poor pronunciation. Some people with severe hearing loss speak in a flat tone and drop word endings, and some cannot speak at all.

The Canadian Hearing Society is an excellent resource for clients, families, and support workers for information on hearing problems as well as educational material and aids for the hearing impaired.

Aids for People With Hearing Loss

A number of aids help people with hearing problems to communicate. These include hearing aids, special telephone systems, and signalling devices.

Hearing Aids. A *hearing aid* is a device that fits inside the ear, behind the ear, or in the ear canal and makes sounds louder (Figure 37–2). It does not cure the hearing problem, but it improves a client's hearing. Both background noise and speech are made louder, so you should help minimize background noise to enable your client to adjust to the hearing aid. Remember that the hearing aid makes speech louder—not clearer.

Care of hearing aids: Hearing aids are expensive, so handle and care for clients' devices properly. Every day you should:

- Look for visual signs of damage, such as cracks, broken parts, clogged openings, or moisture droplets
- Place the battery in the hearing aid and turn it on (to "M" or microphone position). Make sure the '+' on the battery matches the '+' in the battery door.
- Check to make sure the battery is working by turning the hearing aid on, cupping it in your hand, and listening for a whistle.

- The type of hearing aid your client is using will determine the daily care you need to provide. The care plan will tell you what needs to be done. For example, some hearing aids must not be washed, but some need to be washed every time they are removed from the ear.
- Keep the hearing aid in a dry, temperate place, away from hairsprays and X-rays.
- Avoid getting the device wet.
- Turn the hearing aid off, remove the batteries, and keep the battery door open when the device is not in use.
- Avoid dropping the hearing aid.
- Report a missing or damaged hearing aid to your supervisor.

Technology Devices. Technology is advancing rapidly to provide assistance to hearing-impaired clients and clients with complete hearing loss.

- ***Special Telephone Systems***: *TTYs* (once called *telephone teletypes*) allow people with hearing loss to communicate through the telephone system. Users type messages back and forth to one another. *Amplified telephone handsets* make the caller's voice louder. *Extension bells* make the telephone ring more loudly.

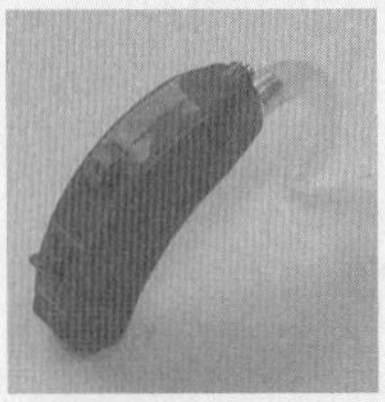

Behind-the-ear (BTE) hearing aids: As the name implies, the BTE hearing aid sits behind the pinna of the outer ear. It houses the microphone, amplifier, and receiver. The body of the BTE hearing aid is attached to an ear hook that sits on top of the pinna. The hook is attached to an earmould that directs the sound from the hearing aid down the earmould tubing into the canal of the hearing aid.

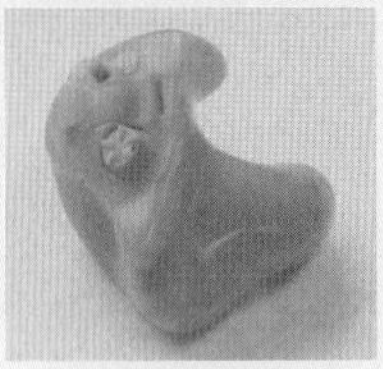

In-the-ear (ITE) hearing aids: The ITE hearing aid fits directly into the bowl of the ear and extends into the ear canal. All the parts are housed in the casing that is moulded to fit into the ear. ITE hearing aids fill most of the concha (bowl) of the ear.

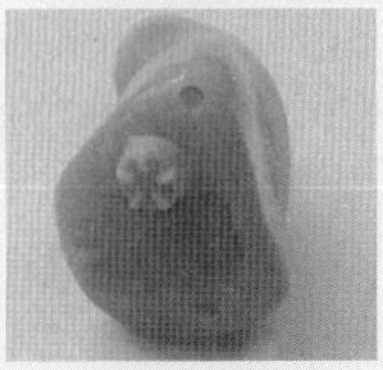

In-the-canal (ITC) hearing aids: The ITC hearing aid is a smaller version of an ITE hearing aid but operates in much the same manner.

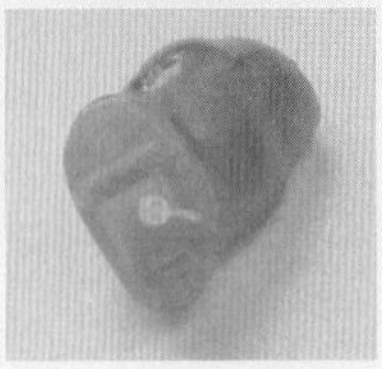

Completely-in-the-canal (CIC) hearing aids: As the name suggests, this is a very small hearing aid and fits right into the ear canal. Once in the person's ear it is very hard to see. It operates in much the same manner as the ITE, ITC, and MIC hearing aids.

Mini-Canal (MIC) hearing aids (look very much like ITC): The MIC hearing aid is smaller than the ITC hearing aid but operates in much the same manner.

Disposable hearing aids: Disposable hearing aids are available in a one-size-fits-all concept and they may not be covered by financial assistive programs. They perform much like in-the-ear hearing aids and are most beneficial to people with moderate hearing loss. The unit can last up to one month and then it needs to be replaced.

Figure 37–2 Types of hearing aids. **Source:** The Canadian Hearing Society. (2002). *Get connected: Facts on hearing aids. Fact sheet #4: Hearing aids.* Toronto, ON. Retrieved November 14, 2007, from http://www.chs.ca/info/ha/4.html. Reprinted with permission.

Box 37–1 Troubleshooting Common Hearing Aid Problems

Symptom	Cause	Possible Remedy
Dead	Not turned on	Turn the MTO switch to "M"
	Battery weak/dead	Replace with fresh battery
	Battery polarity reversed	Make sure the battery is properly inserted
	Blocked ear mould	Clean ear mould
	Aid clogged with wax	Clean receiver opening
	Volume too low	Turn up the volume
Aid whistles	Improper seating in the ear	Insert correctly
	Volume up too high	Reduce volume
	Excessive wax in the ears	Have wax removed by a doctor or by a nurse on a doctor's order
	Ear mould loose	Get new ear mould—need appointment with hearing aid dispenser
	Internal feedback	Factory repair
Intermittent	Battery weak	Replace battery
	Poor battery contacts	Clean contacts
	"ON" switch intermittent	Clean switch
	Moisture	Blow out moisture from the ear mould
	Damaged internal components	Factory repair
Not loud enough/ sound distorted	Volume too low	Turn up the volume
	Battery weak	Replace battery
	Ear mould loose	Get new ear mould—need appointment with hearing aid dispenser
	Blocked ear mould	Clean ear mould
	Excessive wax in the ears	Have wax removed by doctor or by a nurse on a doctor's order
	Change in hearing	Appointment for hearing test

Source: The Canadian Hearing Society. (2002). *Get connected: Facts on hearing aids. Fact sheet #7: Care of the hearing aids.* Toronto, ON. Retrieved November 14, 2007, from http://www.chs.ca/info/ha/7.html. Reprinted with permission.

- ***Signalling Devices:*** These attach to such items as telephones, doorbells, and smoke alarms. When the device makes a sound, a light flashes to alert the person. Some devices include a vibrating option that can be felt.
- ***E-mails:*** Text messaging through computers and personal digital assistants (PDAs) has improved the ability of hearing-impaired clients to communicate with those who can hear. There are now speaking computer software programs available as well.
- ***Dogs:*** Dogs are now being trained to alert a hearing-impaired person to different sounds by alerting him or her to the ringing phone, to someone at the door, to ringing alarms, to baby's crying, and so on.
- ***Closed Captioning:*** Since 1993, all TVs with screens over 13 inches have built-in decoder circuitry that allows hearing-impaired clients to enjoy the same programs as everyone else.

Caring for Clients With Hearing Problems

Some clients with hearing problems wear hearing aids, or they speech read (lip read) by watching facial expressions, gestures, and body language. Some learn sign language (Figure 37–3), and some have *hearing dogs* that alert them to such sounds as ringing phones, doorbells, sirens, and oncoming cars.

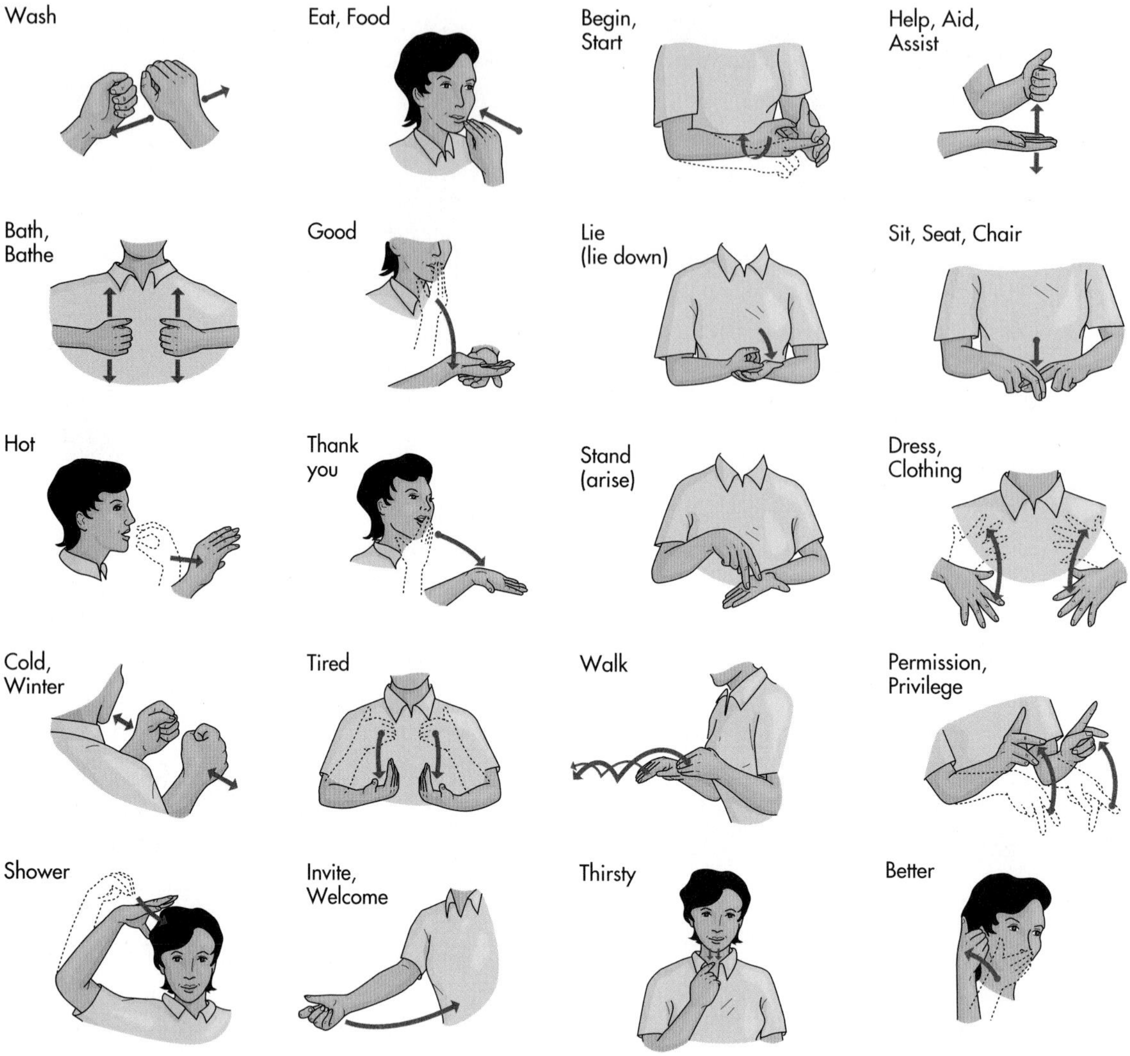

Figure 37–3 Sign language examples.

Follow the guidelines listed in Box 37–2 when caring for clients with severe hearing loss. Remember, some clients with hearing loss also have speech problems. Follow the guidelines listed in Chapter 36 for communicating with clients with speech problems.

EYE DISORDERS AND VISION PROBLEMS

Eye disorders and vision problems, ranging from very mild vision loss to complete blindness, can occur at all ages. Health conditions, accidents, and eye diseases are among the causes of blindness. The level of blindness varies—some people cannot sense light at all and have no vision; others can sense some light but cannot see details; and still others have some vision but cannot see well. The legally blind person is able to see objects at 6 m (20 ft), whereas a person with normal vision can see objects at 60 m (200 ft). Eye structures are shown in Figure 37–4. See Chapter 14 for a review of the structure and function of the eye.

Vision problems may occur suddenly or gradually, necessitating surgery, eyeglasses, or contact lenses. Common causes of vision problems include:

- ***Age-related macular degeneration (AMD; ARMD)***— the breakdown (*degeneration*) of the macula, the central part of the retina. The *retina* is the inner layer of the eye that senses light and colour. AMD is the most common cause of blindness in people over 50. More

Box 37–2 Guidelines for Caring for Clients With Hearing Loss

- ***Alert the client to your presence.*** Get the client's attention. Raise an arm or hand, or lightly touch the client's arm. Do not startle or approach the client from behind.
- ***Adjust the lighting.*** Stand or sit in good light. Clients with hearing loss may need to see your face for speech reading (lip reading). Shadows and glares affect their ability to see your face.
- ***Reduce background noise.*** Turn radios, televisions, air conditioners, and fans down or off, if possible.
- ***Focus your attention on the client.*** Face the client. Stand or sit on the side of the unaffected ear. Do not turn or walk away, and do not do other tasks while talking to the client.
- ***Speak in a normal tone.*** Speak slowly and clearly. Do not shout. Do not cover your mouth when talking.
- ***Check communication aids.*** Make sure the client is wearing his or her hearing aids, eyeglasses, or contact lenses. The client needs to see your face for speech reading. Help the client to put them on, if necessary.
- ***Adjust your language.*** State the topic of conversation clearly. Use simple words and short sentences. Focus on key words. Learn what works for the client. Try saying things in a different way if the client does not understand you.
- ***Use other communication methods.*** You may be unable to communicate using speech. Use nonverbal communication, including body language, to communicate messages (see Chapter 12), or write the key words on paper.
- ***Watch for signs of fatigue.*** Drooping shoulders and a decline in understanding are examples. Avoid tiring the client.

than 25% of people over 70 are affected.[1] The condition starts with slow or sudden partial loss of vision. The central vision becomes fuzzy or shadowy, and over time vision gets worse. AMD varies in severity—some people become completely blind; others may have some sight; and some may lose central vision but still have some *peripheral* vision (the sides, top, and bottom areas of vision). There is no cure for AMD. Macular degeneration can also affect younger adults and children.

- ***Retinal detachment***—the separation of the retina from its supporting tissue. The retina cannot function when detached, and permanent blindness can result. Vision may be saved by reattaching the retina surgically.
- ***Diabetic retinopathy***—a disorder (*pathy*) caused by diabetes, in which the blood vessels in the retina are damaged. Blood can leak from the blood vessels. New blood vessels grow over the retina creating scar tissue that pulls the retina away from the back of the eye. Retinal detachment and blindness may result.
- ***Glaucoma***—an eye disease that causes pressure within the eye, which damages the optic nerve. Vision loss and blindness eventually result. Glaucoma is usually an age-related disease that may be gradual or sudden in onset. Signs and symptoms include *tunnel vision* (the field of vision is reduced so the person can only see straight ahead), blurred vision, and blue-green halos around lights. Treatment involves medications and possibly surgery. The goal is to prevent further damage to the optic nerve. Damage that has already occurred cannot be reversed.
- ***Cataract***—the clouding of the eye's lens, which prevents light from entering the eye. The term

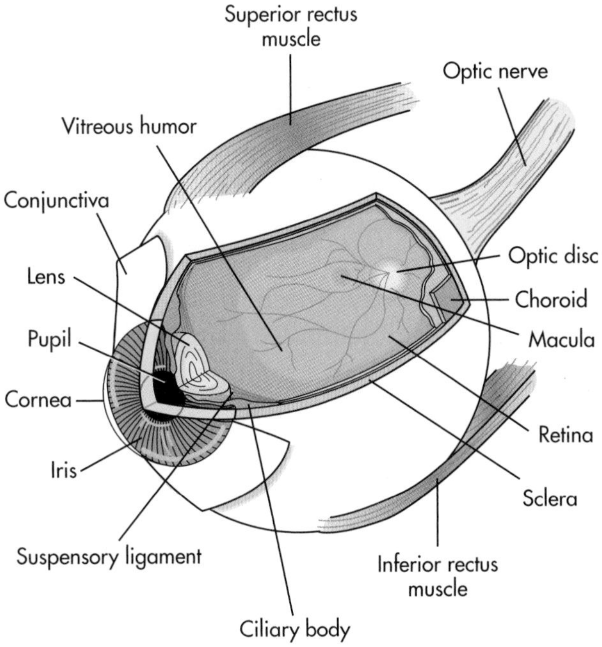

Figure 37–4 The eye.

"cataract" comes from the Greek word that means *waterfall.* It is most common in older adults. Gradual blurring and dimming of vision occur. A person with a cataract remains sensitive to light and glares, and vision is eventually lost. A cataract can occur in one or both eyes. Surgery is the only treatment. A tiny incision is made into the eye, the cloudy lens is removed, and a plastic lens is implanted into the eye. Following cataract surgery, vision returns to near normal.

- ***Presbyopia***—the gradual inability to focus (*opia*) on close objects. This condition is associated with aging (*presby*). Most people experience this normal decline in vision, usually after age 40. Corrective and contact lenses, as well as good lighting, can be helpful.

The Effects of Vision Problems

Severe vision loss affects a client's physical, emotional, social, intellectual, and spiritual health. For example, Mr. Barak, 78, has AMD. He feels the loss of his independence and self-esteem, as even simple tasks, such as dressing, take much longer, and he is not able to read the newspaper. He no longer goes out alone because he is afraid of falling or getting lost, so he no longer attends his mosque.

Although the process is long and hard, many people with severe vision loss learn to lead independent lives. They learn how to move about, complete activities of daily living, and learn new reading methods.

Some people learn how to move about independently using a guide dog or a special white cane with a red tip. Both are recognized worldwide as signs that the person using them is blind. The guide dog serves as the eyes of the blind person and recognizes danger and guides the person through traffic.

The Canadian National Institute for the Blind (CNIB) has excellent resources available to the blind—for example, talking books, many different types of aids, and support to clients and families.

Aids for People With Vision Problems

A number of aids are available to correct vision problems and help those affected. Examples include eyeglasses and contact lenses, reading aids, communication aids, devices for entertainment, and medical devices.

Eyeglasses. Eyeglasses correct vision problems and are worn for reading or seeing objects at a distance. Some people wear them all the time while awake. Some people initially feel upset when they first realize they need glasses, but adjustment is usually rapid. Most accept the fact that glasses will be needed as they grow older.

Glasses are costly, so protect the client's glasses from damage. When not worn, they should be kept in their case. Lenses are made of hardened glass or plastic to avoid breakage. Remove eye glasses carefully (Figure 37–5).

Glass lenses are washed with warm water and dried with soft tissue. Plastic lenses are easily scratched, so special cleaning solutions, tissues, and cloths are used to clean and dry them.

Contact Lenses. Contact lenses—hard or soft—fit directly on the eye. Many people prefer contacts

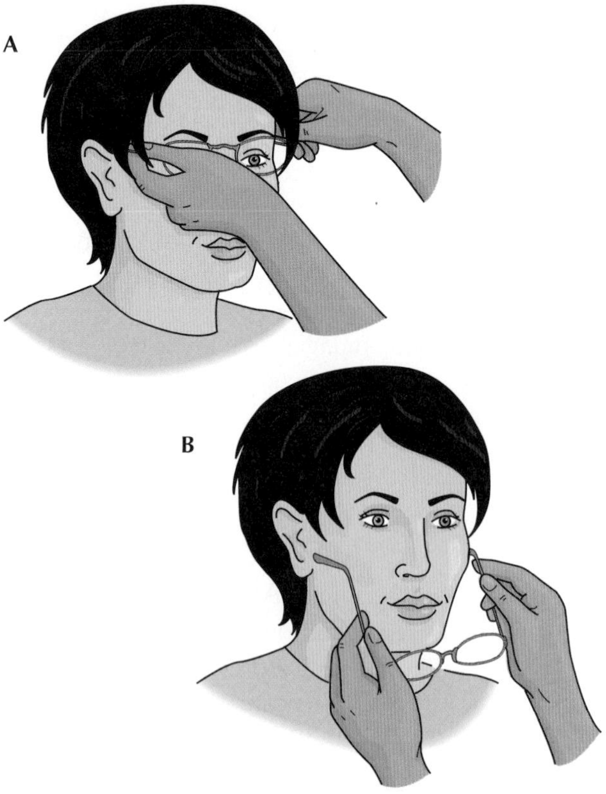

Figure 37–5 **A,** Remove eyeglasses by holding the part of the frames sitting on both ears. **B,** Lift the frames off the ears, and bring the glasses down and away from the face.

because they cannot be seen, they do not break easily and can be worn even while playing sports. The disadvantage is that contacts can be easily lost. Depending on the type of lens, contacts can be worn continuously for 12 to 24 hours or even for 1 week. Contacts are usually removed for swimming and sleeping.

Remove and clean clients' contact lenses, according to the manufacturer's instructions and employer policy. Report any eye redness or drainage to your supervisor. Also, report complaints of eye pain or blurred vision.

Aids for Reading. Many people learn to read **Braille**—a writing system for the blind that uses raised dots in a certain pattern for each letter of the alphabet. The first 10 letters also represent numbers 0 to 9 (Figure 37–6). The person feels the pattern of dots with his or her fingers (Figure 37–7) and makes out the letter.[2] Many books, magazines, newspapers, and computer keyboards are available in Braille. Braille is hard to learn, especially for older adults. Some blind people never learn to read Braille.

Other reading aids include books with large print, books on audiotape or compact discs (CDs), and magnifiers (some with reading lamps attached to them).

Communication Aids. Examples are calendars in Braille, large-print clocks that voice the time in hours or minutes, telephones with Braille keypads and extra large numerals, and cheque and envelope writing guides.

Devices for Entertainment. Examples are playing cards and bingo cards with large letters or in Braille.

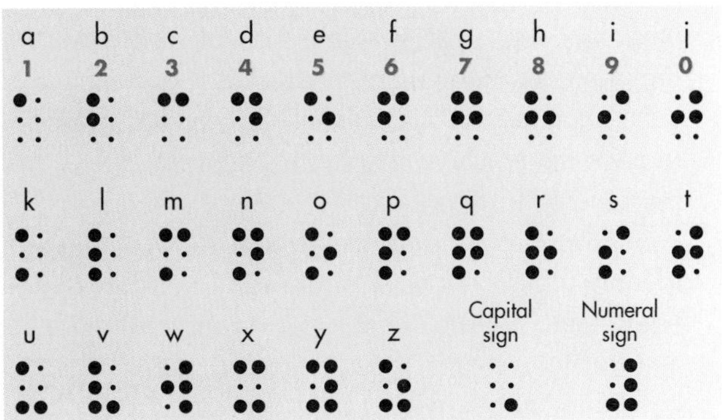

Figure 37–6 Braille.

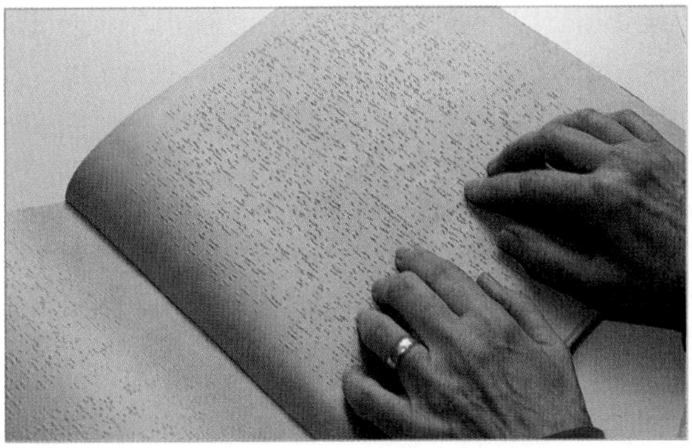

Figure 37–7 Braille is "read" with the fingers.

Medical Devices. Examples include pillboxes that let the person feel if the pill has been taken and "talking prescription devices" that have voice messages describing how to take the medication.

Artificial Eyes

Removal of an eye is sometimes necessary because of injury or disease. The person is then fitted with an *ocular prosthesis,* an artificial eye made of glass or plastic that matches the other eye in colour and shape (Figure 37–8). Prostheses may be permanent implants or removable. If the prosthesis is removable, the person is taught to remove, clean, and reinsert it and also to perform routine prosthesis care.

As a support worker, you may care for clients with artificial eyes, which are the client's property. As you would protect hearing aids, eyeglasses, and

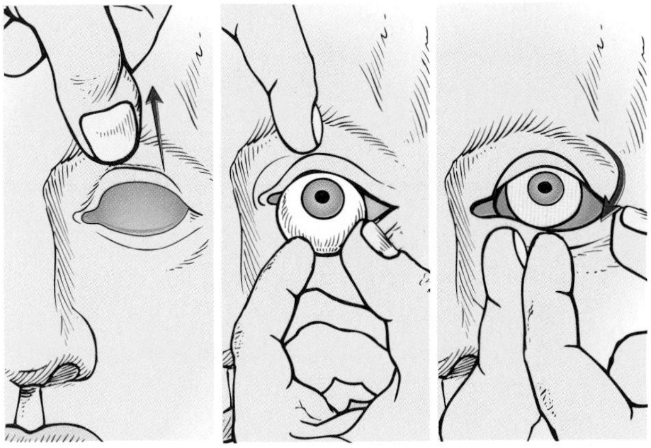

Figure 37–8 Inserting an artificial eye. **Source:** Lewis, S.M., Heitkemper, M.M., & Dirkson, S.R. (2000). *Medical-surgical nursing: Assessment and management of clinical problems* (5th ed.). St. Louis: Mosby.

other valuable devices, protect the artificial eye from loss and damage. Care for the artificial eye in a safe place. Do not hold it over a sink because it can easily roll down the drain if dropped. You may assist your client in caring for the artificial eye and the eye socket where it is placed. Follow these measures when the artificial eye is removed and will not be re-inserted:

- Wash the artificial eye with mild soap and warm water. Rinse it well.
- Line a container with a soft cloth or 4 × 4 gauze to prevent damage.
- Fill the container with water or a saline (salt) solution.
- Place the artificial eye in the container. Close the container.
- Label the container with the client's name (if in a facility, include the room number).
- Place the container in the drawer in the bedside stand or in another safe place, as directed by the client.
- Wash the eye socket with warm water or saline. Use a wash cloth or gauze square. Use a gauze square to remove excess moisture.
- Wash the eyelid with mild soap and warm water. Clean from the inner to the outer part of the eye (see Chapter 29). Dry the eyelid.

The client is blind on the side of the artificial eye, but vision in the other eye may be normal or only impaired.

Caring for Clients With Vision Problems

People with vision loss often have highly developed senses of hearing, touch, smell, and taste. They are sensitive to the tone of a person's voice. When talking with clients with vision loss, pay attention to your voice, which needs to convey nonverbal cues you usually give with body language. Your voice should communicate warmth and respect. Box 37–3 contains guidelines for caring for clients with vision loss.

Box 37–3 Guidelines for Caring for Clients With Vision Loss

- ***Adjust the lighting.*** Ask the client what type of lighting he or she prefers. Adjust blinds and shades to avoid glare (usually worse on bright, snowy days). Stand or sit in good light.
- ***Alert the client to your presence.*** Identify yourself when you enter the room. Give your name, title, and your reason for being there. Do not touch the client before indicating your presence. Address the client by name. Tell the client when you are leaving the room.
- ***Assist with walking.*** Walk slightly ahead of the client at a normal pace (Figure 37–9). Offer your right or left arm. Tell the client which arm you are offering, and the client can then take that arm. Never push, pull, or guide the client in front of you. Tell the client when approaching a curb or steps. Say if you will step up or down. Inform the client of doors, turns, furniture, and other obstructions. Give specific directions. For example, say "right behind you," "on your left," or "in front of you." Avoid phrases like "over here" or "over there."
- ***Assist with eating.*** Read menus to the client. Avoid table linens and china with patterns and designs. These items should be solid colours and provide contrast. For example, a white plate should be placed on a dark place mat. Explain the location of food and beverages on the tray. Use the face of a clock to describe their location (see Chapter 27), or guide the client's hand to each item on the tray. Cut meat into small bits, open containers, butter the bread, and perform other activities, as needed.
- ***Provide a safe setting.*** Outdoor walks and stairs must be clear of ice and snow. Tell your supervisor if they are not. Hallways and rooms must be free of clutter. Keep doors open or closed, never partially open, as otherwise the client could walk into the door. Remember that furniture and other items are arranged to suit the client's needs. Always replace items where you found them. Avoid rearranging furniture and other items. Orient the client to a new setting. Describe the layout, and identify the location and purpose of furniture or equipment. Let the client move about and touch and locate furniture, if he or she can. In facilities, keep the call bell within the client's reach.

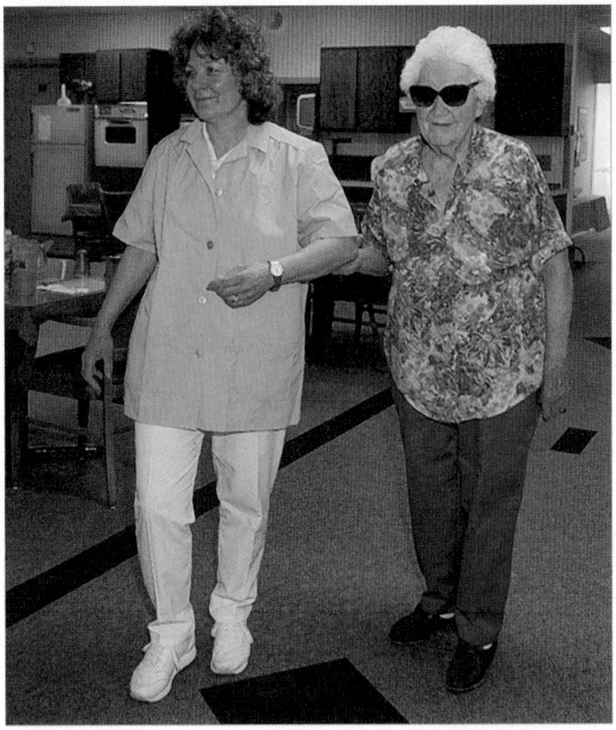

Figure 37–9 This client, who is blind, walks slightly behind the support worker, keeping her arm resting lightly on the support worker.

REVIEW

Answers to these questions are at the bottom of the page.

Circle the BEST answer.

1. **Mr. Poulin has Ménière's disease. Which of the following is likely *true*?**
   A. He has a middle ear infection
   B. Vertigo is a major symptom
   C. Hearing aids will correct the problem
   D. He has vision problems because of it

2. **Which effect of hearing problems is often not obvious to others?**
   A. Loneliness and social isolation
   B. Speaking too loudly
   C. Asking to repeat things
   D. Answering questions inappropriately

3. **You are talking to Mr. Poulin. You should do the following:**
   A. Speak clearly, distinctly, and slowly
   B. Sit out of direct light
   C. Shout
   D. Sit on the side of his affected ear

4. **Mr. Poulin's hearing aid is not working. First, you should:**
   A. See if it is turned on
   B. Wash the hearing aid with soap and water
   C. Have it repaired
   D. Change the batteries

5. **Which is true of age-related macular degeneration?**
   A. Surgery usually corrects the problem
   B. There is no cure
   C. Eyeglasses will improve vision
   D. It is most common in young adults

6. **Glaucoma is:**
   A. An ear disorder common among children
   B. Sign language for people with hearing loss
   C. A disease that damages the optic nerve
   D. A symptom of cataracts

7. **When not worn, glasses should be:**
   A. Left on the bed or chair within easy reach
   B. Left out of the case on the bedside table
   C. Kept in a cleaning solution
   D. Kept in their case

8. **Braille involves:**
   A. A white cane with a red tip for walking
   B. Raised dots arranged to represent letters of the alphabet
   C. An artificial eye
   D. Books on CD or audiotape

9. **Mrs. Ho is blind. You should do the following:**
   A. Offer her your arm and walk slightly behind her
   B. Speak loudly to her
   C. Announce your presence when entering her room and let her know when you leave the room
   D. Leave the room quickly

10. **Which of the following is unsafe for Mrs. Ho?**
   A. Keeping doors open or closed
   B. Informing her of steps and curbs
   C. Turning lights on
   D. Rearranging furniture

Answers: 1.B, 2.A, 3.A, 4.A, 5.B, 6.C, 7.D, 8.B, 9.C, 10.D

CHAPTER 38

Caring for Mothers and Infants

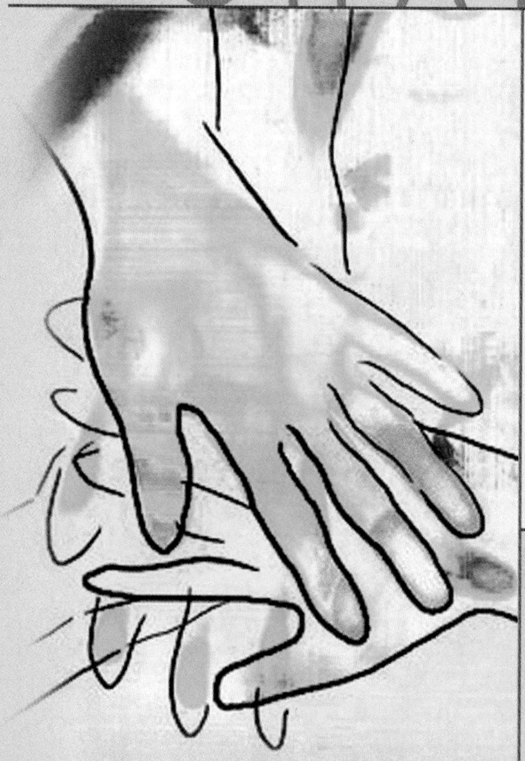

OBJECTIVES

- Define the key terms listed in this chapter.
- List physical and emotional changes a new mother may experience.
- Identify the signs and symptoms of postpartum complications.
- Identify some common problems in infants.
- Identify the signs and symptoms of serious illness in infants.
- Describe how to hold and comfort infants.
- List precautions that reduce the risk of sudden infant death syndrome (SIDS).
- Describe how to help mothers with breastfeeding and bottlefeeding.
- Describe how to burp and diaper an infant.
- Describe how to provide cord care and circumcision care.
- Describe how to bathe infants.
- State why infants are weighed.
- Describe your role in providing childcare.
- Apply the procedures described in this chapter to your clinical practice properly.

key terms

cervical mucus A viscous discharge secreted by the glands in the cervix.

Cesarean section A surgical incision into the abdominal and uterine walls; the baby is delivered through the incision.

circumcision The surgical removal of foreskin from the penis.

congenital Present at birth.

engorged breasts Breasts that are overfilled with milk, which makes them swollen, hard, and painful. Engorgement usually decreases once breastfeeding is established or within 1 to 2 days after breast milk dries up.

episiotomy An incision made in the perineum to increase the size of the vaginal opening for the delivery of the baby.

jaundice A yellowing of the skin and the white part (conjunctiva) of the eyes.

lactation The process of producing and secreting milk from the breast.

leukocytes White blood cells that are part of the blood; the cells are part of the immune system that fight infection.

lochia Postpartum vaginal discharge that begins as a bloody discharge and changes in colour and amount.

mastitis An infection of the breast.

postpartum After (*post*) childbirth (*partum*).

postpartum blues Feelings of sadness or mild depression in the mother during the first 2 weeks after childbirth; baby blues.

postpartum depression Major depression at any point during the first year after childbirth.

postpartum psychosis The most severe form of postpartum depression; the mother may experience delusions, hallucinations, and suicidal thoughts.

sudden infant death syndrome (SIDS) The sudden, unexplained death of an apparently healthy infant under 1 year of age.

toxic shock syndrome (TSS) A rare, often life-threatening, illness that develops suddenly after an infection. TSS can quickly affect several different organ systems including the liver, lungs, and kidneys. It has been linked to the use of tampons in postpartum women.

umbilical cord The structure that carries blood, oxygen, and nutrients from the mother to the fetus.

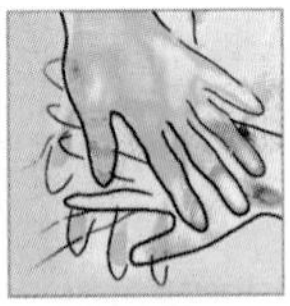

Support workers are sometimes required to care for new mothers and infants, usually in a home care setting. Caring for an infant provides a valuable service to the mother because it enables her to have more time and energy for herself and her family. It is important that you, as the support worker, respect the family's routines, schedules, and ways of doing things. Remember to follow the mother's standards and preferences, whenever possible. As with all of the duties that you perform, it is your responsibility to follow your clients' care plan and to know the limits of your scope of practice (see *Supporting Leslie and Milton*).

CARING FOR NEW MOTHERS

A new mother may require home care services if she:

- Experienced complications before or after the birth.
- Needs help caring for her other young children at home.
- Had a multiple birth (twins, triplets, or more).
- Has an infant with special needs who requires extra time and attention.
- Has a physical or mental disability.
- Has problems adjusting to her new responsibilities.

supporting LESLIE AND MILTON

Leslie X., 17, mother of 2-week old Milton, is a single mother who is new to your community. Milton's father left Leslie during her pregnancy while they were both in drug rehab, and she does not have any contact with her family. You are the support worker assigned to Leslie to find out if she has any difficulties with her new role as a mother. She is currently breastfeeding Milton. Milton weighed 17.6 kg (8 pounds) at birth and, according to his pediatrician, has grown and gained weight well. Leslie seems to have no trouble changing him, bathing him, or bringing him to his doctor for his weekly visits.

On your visit today, Leslie greets you at the door, carrying Milton in one arm and holding a cigarette in her other hand. She looks as if she has been crying. Milton is crying, wet, and obviously needs a diaper change. Leslie says that she thinks that her decision to keep Milton was a wrong one and that she wants to spend some time with her friends. While you watch Leslie change Milton's diaper, you notice her hands are shaking. Leslie then says that she has been feeling very lonely and sad lately and asks if smoking a "joint" (i.e., marijuana cigarette) to help her relax will be harmful to Milton.

You are unsure how to answer Leslie's question. What should you do? What can you say to her? Who can she turn to for help in your community?

When assisting a new mother, you usually do one or more of the following:

- Provide physical care for the mother.
- Provide care for the newborn.
- Help with child care when other young children are in the home.
- Help with home management tasks, such as meal preparation and housekeeping.

The **postpartum**—after (*post*) childbirth (*partum*)—period starts with the birth of the baby and ends 6 weeks later. During this time, the mother begins to adjust physically and emotionally to the effects of childbirth, and her body begins to return to its normal (pre-pregnant) state. Because of the many changes experienced during the postpartum period, the mother needs to rest and recover. Encourage her to rest or nap when the baby is sleeping and to take time for herself and her partner. During this time, she also has important nutritional needs (see Chapter 27).

Lochia. In the first few weeks to months after giving birth, the mother's hormone levels will change dramatically, and her uterus will begin to contract to its pre-pregnant size. Blood and other substances will be expelled from the uterus; this vaginal discharge, called **lochia** (from the Greek word *lochos*, which means *childbirth*), is made up of blood, mucus, and placental tissue.

Lochia will typically increase with breastfeeding (*nursing*) and activity, but the amount of flow should return to normal after the mother rests. The mother wears clean sanitary pads to absorb the discharge, which eventually decreases in amount. Lochia generally has an odour similar to that of normal menstrual discharge.

Any offensive odour indicates a possible infection and should be reported to a health care provider. The mother should shower daily, change her sanitary pad frequently (at least every 4 hours, or after each time she urinates), practise hand hygiene before and after changing her sanitary pad (see Chapter 20), and check her lochia for signs of infection (such as an offensive odour and greenish colour). You should check for fever and pelvic pain, which are also signs of infection (see Box 38–1).

Lochia typically continues for 4 to 6 weeks after childbirth and progresses through three stages. These stages describe the changes in the colour of the postpartum flow:

1. ***Lochia rubra***—the first discharge, red in colour because of the large amount of blood it contains. It typically lasts no longer than 3 to 5 days after birth.
2. ***Lochia serosa***—thinned discharge that has turned brownish or pink in colour. It contains blood, water, red blood cells, white blood cells,

Box 38–1 Signs and Symptoms of Postpartum Complications

- Fever of 38°C (100.4°F) or higher
- Chills, poor appetite, fatigue, nausea, or vomiting
- Lochia that soaks a sanitary pad within 1 hour of application
- Foul-smelling lochia
- Large number of clots in the lochia
- Painful, burning, or difficult urination
- Severe abdominal or perineal pain
- Bleeding, redness, swelling, or drainage from a Cesarean-section incision (see below)
- Leg pain, tenderness, or swelling
- Breast pain, tenderness, or swelling (see Box 38–2)
- Feelings of depression (see Box 38-3, on page 718, and Chapter 34)

and **cervical mucus**. This stage continues until around the tenth day after delivery.

3. ***Lochia alba***—discharge that has turned whitish or yellowish-white in colour. It typically lasts from the second through the third to sixth week after delivery. It contains fewer red blood cells and is mainly made up of **leukocytes**, epithelial cells, cholesterol, fat, and mucus.

It is important to note that the mother should not use tampons during the postpartum period, as the risk of toxic shock syndrome is very great, especially if the mother had an episiotomy. **Toxic shock syndrome (TSS)** is a rare, often life-threatening, illness that develops suddenly after an infection. TSS can quickly affect several different organ systems, including the liver, lungs, and kidneys.

It is important that you observe these changes, as postpartum hemorrhage, infection of the uterine lining, and other complications are possible. Tell your supervisor immediately if you notice any of the signs or symptoms listed in Box 38–1.

Perineal Care

Episiotomies. An **episiotomy** is an incision (*otomy*) in the perineum to increase the size of the vaginal opening for delivery of the baby. The physician or midwife performs this procedure, and the incision is sutured after the delivery. After the episiotomy, the perineal area may become swollen, sore, and tender. The episiotomy prevents perineal tearing, which will cause severe pain, swelling, or more severe problems in the mother's perineal area.

Some women do not require an episiotomy, especially if the woman (a) has had previous vaginal deliveries; (b) has a very long labour, allowing her perineum to have an opportunity to stretch sufficiently; or (c) if her doctor or birthing midwife think it is unnecessary. However, many women require episiotomies in order to prevent perineal tearing.

Complications can develop after an episiotomy, so it is very important that the mother practises good perineal care and proper hand hygiene (see Chapter 20) for as long as she has lochia. She should be instructed to clean her perineum with a clean, wet cloth (a baby wipe will do), change her sanitary pad, and practise good hand hygiene each time she urinates. Complications of an episiotomy include infection and wound separation (dehiscence). Tell your supervisor if the client complains of pain in the perineum.

The physician may order pain relief medications and cold packs to the perineum for the client's comfort. Physicians may also order sitz baths to promote comfort and hygiene (see Chapter 43). A warm bath also may relieve perineal pain and soreness. Make sure the tub is disinfected before each use, and have clean wash cloths and towels available for the client.

The client will be advised by her doctor, nurse practitioner, or midwife about when it is safe for her to resume sexual relations, which is usually 6 weeks after delivery.

Care of Abdominal Incisions

Some clients may have had Cesarean sections. A **Cesarean section** (C-section) is a surgical incision into the abdomen and uterine wall through which the baby is delivered. A Cesarean section is done when:

- The baby must be delivered quickly to save the baby's or the mother's life
- The baby is too large to pass through the birth canal

- The mother has a vaginal infection that could be transmitted to the baby
- A normal vaginal delivery would be difficult for the baby or the mother

The mother requires recovery time because she has not only just given birth, she has also had a major surgery (Cesarean section). In the first few weeks after surgery, she may feel weak and tired. The physician may order her to avoid any lifting or housework during at least the first week. You may be required to help with housekeeping tasks and child care, or you may bring the baby to her for feedings.

The Cesarean section incision also needs to heal (see Chapter 42). Tell your supervisor if the client complains of pain around the incision site. Also, tell your supervisor if you observe bleeding, redness, swelling, or drainage from the incision.

Breast Care

Lactation—the process of producing and secreting milk from the breasts—usually begins around the third day after childbirth. Occasionally, the new mother's breasts may become overfilled with milk. **Engorged breasts** are swollen, hard, and painful, but once breastfeeding is established or the milk dries up (if the mother chooses not to breastfeed), engorgement decreases within 1 or 2 days. Cold packs applied to the breasts or warm showers promote comfort. A good nursing bra worn day and night supports the breasts and increases comfort during engorgement. Follow the care plan to promote the client's comfort.

Sometimes clients feel a tender lump in a breast, which usually is a symptom of a *plugged duct*. Milk drains into ducts that open onto the nipple (see Figure 14–29). When the milk does not drain properly through the duct, it builds up within the breast. An untreated plugged duct can cause a breast infection. Tell your supervisor if you suspect the mother has a plugged duct. Treatment usually involves:

- Encouraging frequent nursing
- Keeping pressure off the clogged duct by ensuring that the clothes and bra are not too tight
- Applying warm wash cloths to the affected area or having warm showers to promote drainage

Mastitis—infection (*itis*) of the breast (*mast*)—occurs when bacteria enter a milk duct through a cracked nipple. One way the client can prevent mastitis is to practise proper hand hygiene each time she touches her nipples. Mastitis is usually very painful, so early treatment is essential. Tell your supervisor as soon as signs or symptoms appear (see Box 38–2). Medications and rest may be ordered by the client's doctor or nurse practitioner. Breastfeeding during treatment for mastitis is usually encouraged. The client should breastfeed as much as possible from the affected breast, even if it is painful at first. This keeps the milk flowing and speeds recovery.

When the client is started on antibiotics, she may be allowed to continue breastfeeding, but she must check with her doctor or nurse practitioner about this.

Postpartum Blues, Depression, and Psychosis

The postpartum period is also a time of emotional changes. Lack of sleep, more responsibilities, and her new role may affect the new mother's moods. These and other issues such as isolation, disappointment, anxiety, poor body image, or lack of support from a partner or spouse as well as the changes in hormone levels may contribute to **postpartum blues** ("baby blues"), which are feelings of sadness or mild depression during the first 2 weeks after childbirth.

Common symptoms of postpartum blues include:

- Insomnia
- Mood changes

Box 38–2 Signs and Symptoms of Mastitis

- Pain, heat, tenderness, red streaks, or swelling in a breast
- Tender lump or hardened area in the breast
- Fever: 38°C (100.4°F) or higher
- Chills
- Fatigue
- General body ache
- Cracked nipples or cracked skin around the nipples

- Weepiness
- Fatigue
- Headaches
- Poor concentration
- Feelings of sadness, anger, or anxiety

Health Canada estimates that up to 80% of Canadian women who give birth experience postpartum blues.[1] Symptoms usually begin in the first days after delivery and disappear, even without treatment, after 1 to 2 weeks. Your encouragement and emotional support during this time may be very helpful to the mother.

About 10 to 15% of Canadian women suffer postpartum depression after childbirth.[2] **Postpartum depression** is Major depression that begins any time within the first year after childbirth (see Chapter 34 for a discussion on major depression). Usually it begins within 2 weeks to 6 months after childbirth. Professional care is needed as soon as possible, as postpartum depression can worsen over time.

Postpartum psychosis is a severe form of postpartum depression. It is relatively rare, affecting about 1 woman per 1000.[3] The mother with postpartum psychosis loses touch with reality and has delusions, hallucinations, or suicidal thoughts (see Chapter 34). She could harm or neglect her child, so she must not be left alone with the infant or other children. ***Tell your supervisor immediately if the mother shows any of the signs or symptoms listed in Box 38–3.***

A client diagnosed with postpartum depression may be ordered medications and may need help with home management or child care so that she has time to rest. Your understanding and emotional support are essential at this time.

Box 38–3 Signs and Symptoms of Postpartum Depression

- Crying
- Feelings of sadness, hopelessness, or guilt
- Difficulties sleeping
- Inability to cope with everyday problems
- Avoiding visiting with others
- Feelings of anger toward the baby
- Fatigue
- Extreme anxiety
- Delusions or hallucinations
- Thoughts of harming the baby or self

CARING FOR INFANTS

Since infants are helpless and cannot care for or protect themselves and must depend on others for their basic needs, as a support worker, you must ensure their safety (see Chapter 19) as well as their physical and emotional needs while they are under your care. Because infants have a delicate immune system, it is important for everyone to remember to practise proper hand hygiene (see Chapter 20) each time infants are touched or picked up.

Newborns and infants change and grow quickly, and their physical and emotional needs will also change as they grow. Review the normal growth and development patterns of newborns and infants (see Chapter 15). Follow the care plan to meet the infant's needs.

Holding the Infant

Pay particular attention to hygienic measures when handling infants. You should always practise proper hand hygiene before and after handling the infant. You should wear a clean top (or gown) for each baby that you hold. If you are caring for a client and her baby in a home care setting, you should either change into your clean uniform when you arrive at the client's house, or if this is not feasible, you should protect your clean uniform by wearing a covering garment over it until you are in the client's home and are about to pick up the infant.

Most infants are comforted when they are held and cuddled, and it helps them feel loved and secure. Always handle a baby with gentle, smooth movements; avoid sudden or jerking movements, as these may startle or upset the baby.

Use both hands to lift a newborn. Always support the entire body, especially the head and the neck (because a baby's neck is very weak for about the first 3 months), when lifting and holding the infant. Do not let the baby's arms or legs dangle. Hold the baby securely and close to your body. Figure 38–1 shows how to hold a baby. Do not forget to practise proper hand hygiene before touching the infant.

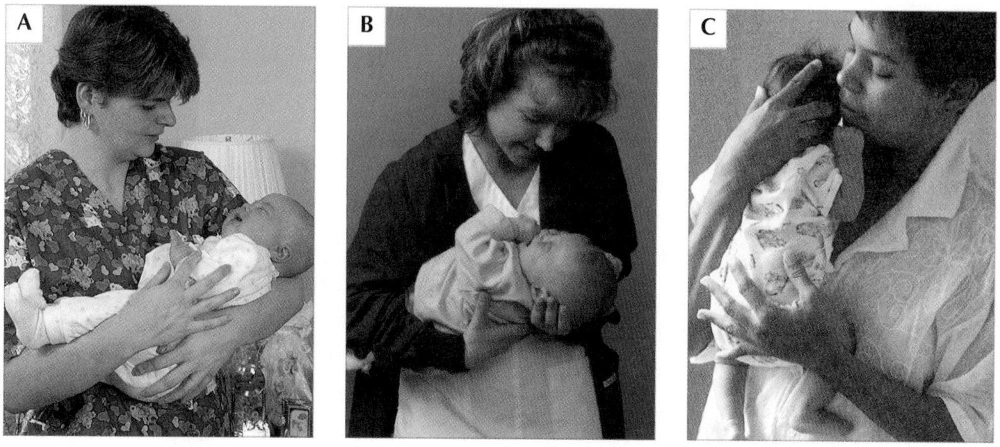

Figure 38–1 Support the head and neck with one hand and the legs and back with the other. Hold the baby close to your body. **A,** The cradle hold. **B,** The football hold. **C,** The shoulder hold. Note how each support worker is looking at the baby she is holding.

Swaddling the Infant

Swaddling an infant, a technique that is practised throughout the world in many cultures, provides warmth, comfort, and security to an infant. Many parents also report that their infants sleep better when they are swaddled. Swaddling holds infants securely so that they do not flail their limbs and startle themselves. Many infants sleep better on their backs (the proper way for babies to sleep) while they are swaddled. Some babies like being swaddled, but some dislike it, so you should always first check with the parents.

To swaddle an infant, begin by performing hand hygiene; when your hands are completely dry, lay a receiving blanket on a flat surface and fold a top corner down. Place the baby supine with his or her head on the folded corner (see Figure 38–2 A). Pull the corner of the blanket near the baby's right arm across the body, and tuck it under the baby's left arm (see Figure 38–2 B). Pull the bottom corner up over the baby's body and to the chest. Bring the last free corner of the blanket over the baby's left arm and across the chest, and tuck it under the back on the baby's right side (see Figure 38–2 C).

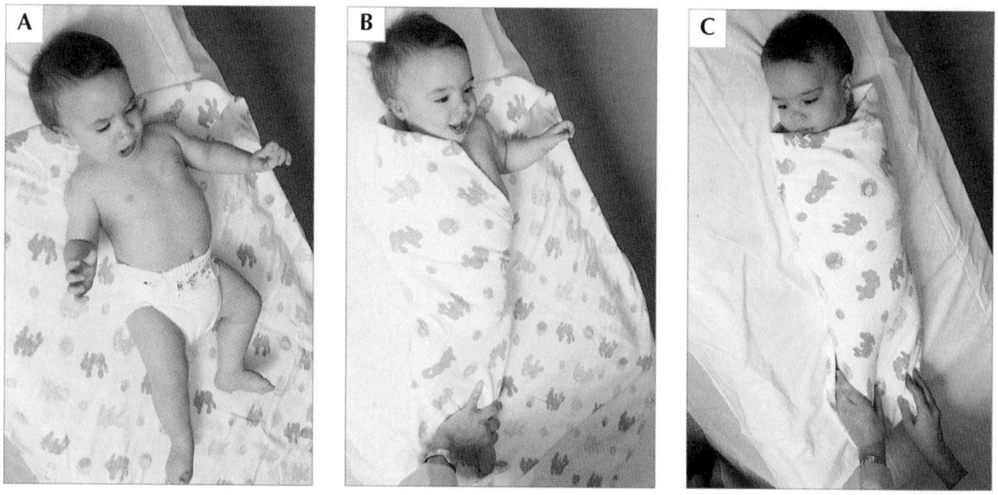

Figure 38–2 Swaddling an infant. Lay out the receiving blanket in a diamond shape, and bring the top corner of the blanket down. **A,** Place the baby's shoulders in line with the top edge of the blanket. **B,** Take the left side of the blanket and bring it over the baby's chest. Tuck his or her right arm inside. Tuck the blanket under the baby. **C,** Take the bottom of the blanket and fold it up on top of the baby's body. Bring the right side of the blanket around the baby, making sure the arm is at the baby's side. Tuck the end of the blanket under the baby. **Source:** Hockenberry, M.J., Wilson, D., Winkelstein, M.L., & Kline, N.E. (2003). *Wong's nursing care of infants and children* (7th ed., p. 1139). St. Louis: Mosby.

Comforting the Crying Infant

Infants cry to communicate a number of things, including when they are wet, hungry, hot, cold, tired, uncomfortable, in pain, overstimulated, or lonely. You should respond to the baby's crying immediately, which helps babies feel safe and secure. ***An infant cannot be spoiled with too much attention and comfort.***

Some babies cry a lot and the parents have to figure out what comforts them. Ask the mother how she soothes her baby. You may have to try different things to find out what works for you. Follow the guidelines in Box 38–4. Tell your supervisor if the baby cannot be comforted.

Laying the Infant Down to Sleep

Safety precautions must be taken when laying the baby down to sleep, in order to lower the risk of **sudden infant death syndrome (SIDS)**—the sudden, unexplained death of an apparently healthy infant under 1 year of age, which usually occurs while the infant is sleeping.

When laying the baby down to sleep, remember the following:

- ***Always lay babies on their backs for sleep.*** Babies who sleep on their stomachs or sides have an increased risk for SIDS. Some babies have medical conditions that require them to sleep on their stomachs. Check with your supervisor and the care plan. Babies can lie on their stomachs when they are awake and being supervised.
- ***Do not lay the baby on soft bedding products.*** These include fluffy, plush products, such as sheepskin pillows, quilts, comforters, memory foam mattresses or mattress pads, or soft toys. Remove these items from the crib. Soft products might cause large amounts of carbon dioxide to pool around the baby's head, which may result in SIDS. The soft bedding also can cover the baby's nose and mouth and cause suffocation.
- ***Make sure the baby is warm but never hot.*** Overheating is thought to increase the risk of SIDS. Do not overdress the baby at bedtime. If the room temperature feels comfortable for you, it is also right for the baby. Use a lightweight blanket that you can add or remove depending on room temperature. To check if the baby is too hot, place your hand on the back of his or her neck. If the neck is sweaty, the baby is too warm.

Box 38–4 Guidelines for Soothing a Crying Infant

- Ensure all physical needs are met. Determine if the baby needs a diaper change or is hungry, hot, cold, tired, or in pain.
- Use gentle motions, such as rocking, swinging, or walking back and forth with the baby.
- Hold the baby close to your chest so that he or she can hear your heartbeat.
- Rub the baby's back or stomach.
- Swaddle the baby.

Cradle Cap, Diaper Rash, and Thrush

Many babies get cradle cap or diaper rash. Neither are life-threatening but may cause discomfort to the baby.

Cradle Cap. *Cradle cap* (seborrheic dermatitis) is a skin condition in which yellowish, scaly, or crusty patches, made up largely of oil and dead skin cells, appear on the scalp. The condition is most common in infants, but it may be seen occasionally in children up to the age of 5. These patches appear most often appear on the scalp and may even extend onto the forehead. They may also appear in the skin fold behind the baby's ears, on the ears, and in the diaper area. The most typical location is over the soft spot (anterior fontanelle) on the top of the baby's head.

Cradle cap is quite common and not difficult to treat. Mild cases usually clear up when the baby is shampooed daily with regular baby soap applied on a wet, rough facecloth wrapped around your hand. Remember to always rinse the soap completely from the baby's skin. Check the baby's care plan or with your supervisor for details on how to provide care for cradle cap on an infant. One common treatment is to soften the crusts first by massaging a small amount of baby oil into the baby's scalp and letting it remain there overnight.

Diaper rash. *Diaper rash* is a very common condition that most babies will develop at one time or another. Diaper rashes may be caused by medications (such as antibiotics), moisture, urine, or irritating chemicals in diapers (cloth or disposable). When you observe a rash on the baby you are caring for, make a note of its appearance, location, and other typical symptoms (see Box 38–5).

There are different types of rashes that are caused by different problems. Always remember to practise proper hand hygiene before and after changing the baby. If it is stated in the baby's care plan, you may have to wear gloves for changing the baby's diaper. ***Always report a rash that is new, a rash that seems to be spreading in spite of treatment, or one that is present for longer than a day.*** Common types of rashes include:

- ***Simple diaper rash.*** Simple diaper rashes are red, slightly rough, and scaly and may appear over the whole area touched by the diaper. The skin may be irritated by chemicals used in laundering cloth diapers—detergent, bleach, whitener, water softener, or soap. Plastic or rubber pants worn over cloth diapers sometimes affect the skin. The skin may also react to the chemicals used in the manufacture of disposable diapers as well as in commercial baby wipes.
- ***Ammonia rash.*** Ammonia rash is a form of diaper rash caused by urine itself. The skin is literally burned by the ammonia that is formed when urine is decomposed by normal bacteria on the skin. Not surprisingly, ammonia rash is worse after the baby has been asleep for a long period of time without a diaper change. You can identify it by the ammonia smell noticeable when you change the diaper. The baby's skin should be washed with mild soap and warm water and then dried thoroughly. Be sure to dry in between the baby's skin folds.

Box 38–5 Treating Simple Diaper Rash or Ammonia Rash

Always practise proper hand hygiene (see Chapter 20).

Keep the baby as dry as possible; change diapers frequently, even if they are only slightly wet; and avoid any airtight coverings.

If using cloth diapers, use double diapers during the daytime and triple diapers at night.

Wash the diaper area with plain water each time you change the baby. Be sure to remove any old creams that might be remaining on the baby's skin. Dry the baby's skin thoroughly, taking care to dry the baby's skin folds well. If instructed in the baby's care plan, apply a protective cream or ointment (such as zinc oxide, petroleum jelly, or an ointment combining zinc oxide, cod liver oil, petrolatum, and lanolin). Use only one type of ointment at a time unless the client's care plan has instructed you to use more than one.

Do not dust the baby's skin with cornstarch, a practice that was once commonly recommended; it has been found that it encourages the growth of fungi.

Try a different brand of laundry soap on cloth diapers. Do not use fabric softener with every wash because the baby may be sensitive to a buildup of it.

Give cloth diapers a try if you have been using disposables, or switch brands. Try disposables if you have been using cloth diapers.

Cut down on the use of commercial baby wipes, powders, and oils for the baby, and ensure that whatever products you use are mild and nonallergenic.

If you have been using coloured toilet tissue to clean the baby's genital area, switch to plain white.

To further promote healing, place a pad under the baby and let him or her lie undiapered, whenever possible, to expose the baby's skin to air.

Source: The College of Family Physicians of Canada. (2007) *Diaper rash: Tips on how to prevent and treat diaper rash.* Retrieved October 27, 2007, from http://www.cfpc.ca/English/cfpc/programs/patient%20education/diaper%20rash/default.asp?s=1. Reprinted with permission.

- ***Other causes.*** Besides these two basic types of diaper rashes, a variety of other rashes may appear in the diaper area, including those caused by an allergy to a food or a drug, a skin infection, or a contagious disease, such as chicken pox or measles.

Thrush. Thrush is a common yeast infection which resembles cottage cheese or milk curds on the sides, roof, and sometimes the tongue of a baby's mouth (Figure 38–3). Unlike milk residue, which just leaves a white coating on the baby's tongue that easily comes off, the white patches associated with thrush do not come off easily. If one of these patches is accidentally scraped away, you will find a raw, red area underneath that may bleed. Thrush is not life-threatening, but it can be very sore and would prevent the baby from eating, which would lead to dehydration.

You may first suspect thrush if the baby starts crying while breastfeeding or sucking on a pacifier or a bottle. It is most common in babies 2 months and younger but can appear in older babies, too. ***If the baby develops a fever, your supervisor should be notified immediately, as the baby may have another type of infection.***

Cause of Thrush: Yeast is present in the human body as the normal flora of the digestive system, but when their balance is disturbed, an infection sets in. Sometimes, hormonal changes or the use of antibiotics (either in a breastfeeding mother or in a baby) can cause this imbalance.

Some babies, such as low birth-weight babies, premature babies, babies born to diabetic mothers, or babies with some type of **congenital** (present at birth) problem, are more susceptible to infections than are others. Some babies are infected by their mothers during delivery through the birth canal.

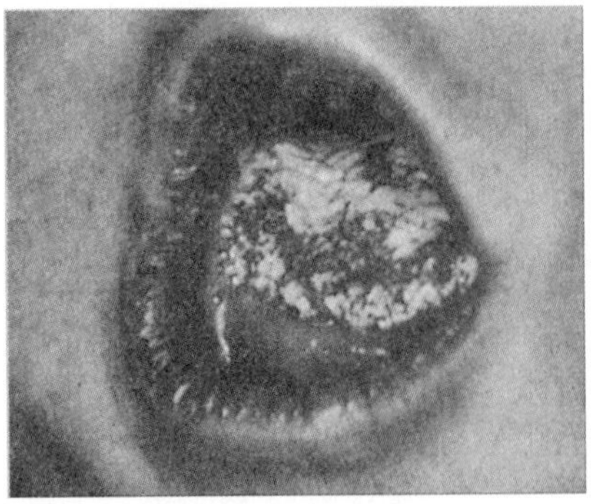

Figure 38–3 Thrush. **Source:** Seidel, H.M., Ball, J.W., Dains, J.E., & Benedict, G.W. (2003). *Mosby's guide to physical examination* (5th ed., p. 343). St. Louis: Mosby.

Treatment: If you suspect the baby has thrush, you should immediately report this to your supervisor. Some doctors may prescribe drops that the mother must place in her baby's mouth before feeding. If she is breastfeeding the baby, she may be prescribed an antifungal cream to be applied on her nipples so that she and her baby will not reinfect each other. It may take a week for the thrush to clear up after medication has been started. It is important that everyone who has contact with the baby practise proper hand hygiene methods.

Signs and Symptoms of Potentially Serious Illness

Infants can become ill quickly. Signs and symptoms may be sudden, so you must be very alert to note them. Your observations are important for the infant's safety and well-being. Tell your supervisor when the sign or symptom began. If the infant has any of the signs or symptoms listed in Box 38–6, tell your supervisor immediately. Your supervisor will tell you which care method to use.

You may need to take an infant's or child's temperature and respirations (see Chapter 41). Axillary temperatures are taken on infants, and tympanic or axillary temperatures are taken on children younger than 5 years. Apical pulses are taken on both infants and young children.

Helping Mothers Breastfeed

Many mothers breastfeed their babies, and usually both mothers and babies learn the process in a very short time. However, some mothers and babies can have difficulties in the first few weeks. This may be a stressful time for the mother. Provide a calm, supportive, and positive atmosphere. Tell your supervisor if the mother is having problems breastfeeding, as she may require additional support.

Breastfed newborns usually nurse every 2 to 3 hours throughout the day and night. Babies are fed on demand—that is, they are fed whenever they are hungry, not on a schedule. When babies want to

Box 38–6 Signs and Symptoms of Possible Serious Illness in Infants

- **Jaundice**—a yellowish colour to the skin and whites of the eyes
- Redness or drainage around the cord stump or circumcision (see pages 728 and 729)
- High temperature
- Limpness; slow response
- Screaming or crying for a long time
- Flushed or pale skin
- Heavy perspiration
- Rash
- Noisy, rapid, difficult, or slow respirations
- Coughing or sneezing
- Reddened or irritated eyes
- Turning the head to one side or putting a hand to one ear (signs of an ear infection)
- Not feeding
- Vomiting most of the feeding or between feedings
- Hard, formed stools
- Frequent watery, green, mucous, or foul-smelling stools
- Signs of dehydration:
  - Fewer than six wet diapers a day
  - Dark yellow urine
  - Decreased saliva and tears
  - Dry lips
  - Dry, wrinkled skin
  - Sunken eyes and top of head
- Stiff neck; head not pulling forward toward the chest

eat, they often become restless, suck on their fists, and cry.

At first, babies breastfeed for a short time—maybe only 5 minutes at each breast. Eventually, total nursing time may take between 20 and 30 minutes. Mothers might need help getting ready to breastfeed. Assist, as needed. If you leave the room while the mother is breastfeeding, stay within hearing distance in case she needs help. Some mothers want privacy while breastfeeding, while some others may want you to stay with them. Ask the mother what her preference is. Box 38–7 describes how you can help with breastfeeding.

Figure 38–4 A mother breastfeeding in the side-lying position.

Box 38–7 Guidelines for Helping With Breastfeeding

- Perform proper hand hygiene, and remind the mother to also do it, as it is necessary before she handles her breasts.
- Help the mother to a comfortable position. She may want to breastfeed sitting up in bed or in a chair, or she may prefer the side-lying position (Figure 38–4). If the mother is recovering from a Cesarean section or has a sore perineum after an episiotomy, she may prefer the side-lying position.
- Change the baby's diaper, if necessary. Bring the baby to the mother.
- Mothers often appreciate help getting ready for breastfeeding. Assist her, as needed. For example, bring supportive pillows and make her comfortable; provide a drink (many women get thirsty while breastfeeding), a quiet room, or a comfortable chair.
- Offer the mother a blanket to cover the baby and her breast to promote privacy during the feeding. Some women may find that using a blanket makes nursing difficult. Follow the mother's preferences.
- Help the mother burp the baby, if necessary. The baby is burped after nursing at each breast.
- Change the baby's diaper after the feeding, if necessary.
- Lay the baby in the crib if he or she has fallen asleep. ***Remember, lay the baby on the back. Do not lay the baby on the stomach or side unless the care plan instructs you to do so.***
- Record what time the baby nursed and how long on each side. Report any problems or concerns.

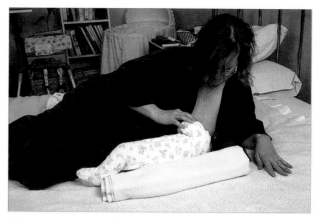

Helping Mothers Bottlefeed

Formula milk is given to infants who are not breastfed. It provides the essential nutrients needed by the infant. Formula comes in three forms: The *ready-to-feed* formula is poured directly from the can into the baby bottle (Figure 38–5). Water is added to *powdered* and *concentrated* formula. Container directions tell how much formula to use and how much water to add.

Infants must be protected from infection, so use preboiled, cooled tap water to mix the formula for infants under 4 months of age. Boiling the tap water for at least 2 minutes destroys microbes. Use tap water from the cold tap. Do not use hot tap water, well water, bottled water, or water that has been filtered or treated. Follow the care plan, and contact your supervisor if you have any questions.

Bottles are prepared one at a time or in batches for the whole day. Extra bottles are capped (Figure 38–6) and stored in the refrigerator. The prepared bottles should be used within 24 hours. After 24 hours, the formula must be discarded.

Cleaning the Equipment. Baby bottles, caps, and nipples must be thoroughly cleaned. Reusable bottlefeeding equipment is carefully washed in hot,

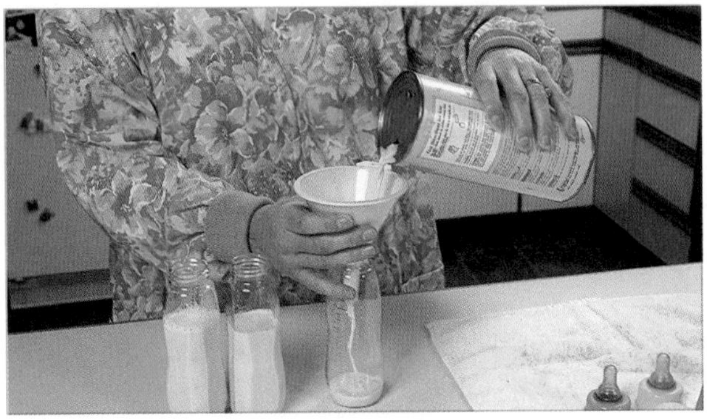

Figure 38–5 Ready-to-feed formula is poured from the can into the bottle. Use a clean funnel to avoid spilling.

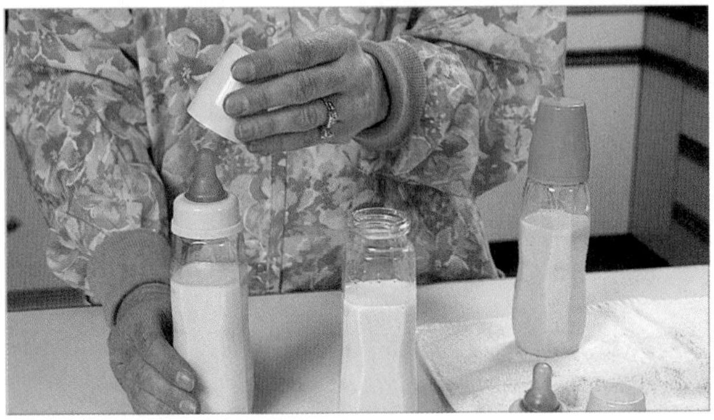

Figure 38–6 Bottles are capped for storage in the refrigerator.

1 2 3 BOTTLEFEEDING EQUIPMENT

Pre-Procedure

1 Practise proper hand hygiene.
2 Collect the following:
- Bottles, nipples, and caps
- Funnel
- Can opener
- Bottle brush
- Dishwashing soap
- Other items needed to prepare formula
- Clean dishtowel

Procedure

3 Wash the bottles, nipples, caps, funnel, and can opener in hot, soapy water. Wash other items used to prepare formula.
4 Clean inside of baby bottles with the bottle brush (Figure 38–7).
5 Squeeze hot, soapy water through the nipples (Figure 38–8) to remove all traces of the formula from them.
6 Rinse all items thoroughly in hot water.
7 Lay a clean towel on the countertop.
8 Stand the bottles upside down to drain. Place the nipples, caps, and other items on the towel. Allow the items to dry completely.

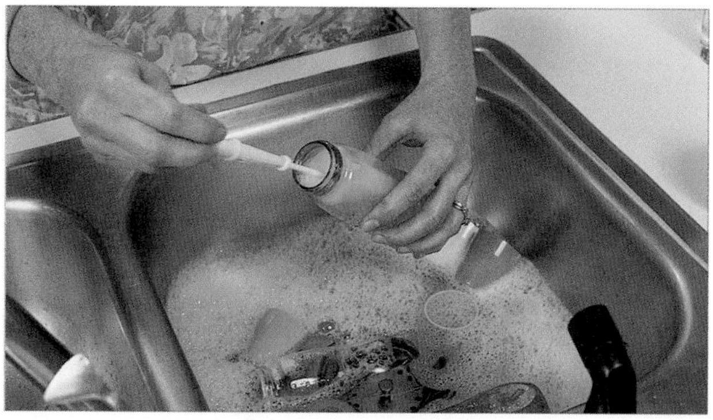

Figure 38–7 A bottle brush is used to clean the inside of the bottle.

soapy water or in a dishwasher. Complete rinsing is needed to remove all soap. Some mothers use plastic nursers, which require plastic liners that are used once and then discarded.

Bottlefeeding the Infant. Bottlefed babies usually want to be fed every 3 to 4 hours. The care plan or the mother tells you how much formula a baby needs at each feeding. Babies usually take as much formula as they need. The baby stops sucking and turns away from the bottle when he or she is full.

Babies should not be given cold formula out of the refrigerator. The bottle must be warmed in a bowl of warm water before the feeding. The formula should feel warm to touch. Test the temperature by sprinkling a few drops on the inside of your wrist (Figure 38–9). Do not set the bottle out for the formula to get to room temperature. This takes too long and allows the growth of microbes. Do not heat formula in microwave ovens. The formula can heat unevenly and burn the baby's mouth, and the microwave process will break down the nutrients in the formula.

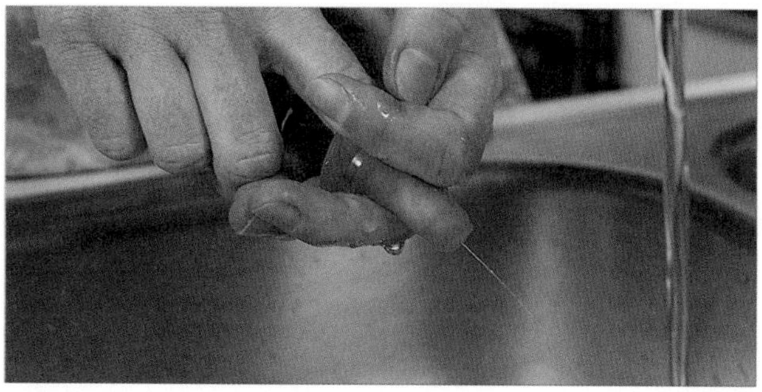

Figure 38–8 Water is squeezed through the nipples during cleaning.

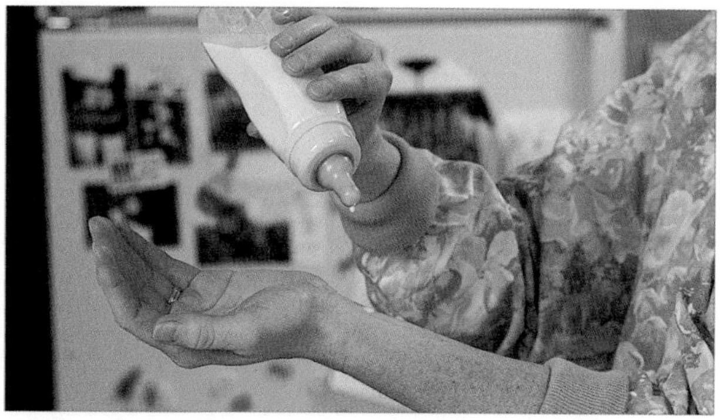

Figure 38–9 Formula should feel warm on the wrist.

The guidelines in Box 38–8 will help you bottlefeed babies.

Box 38–8 Guidelines for Bottlefeeding Infants

- Practise proper hand hygiene.
- Place the bottle in a bowl of warm water until the formula feels warm on your wrist.
- Tilt the bottle to check the flow of formula dripping out of the nipple. Two or three drops should drip out per second. Too few drops dripping indicates that the hole in the nipple is too small, and too many drops dripping indicates that the hole is too large. Change the nipple if the hole is not right, and test again.
- Assume a comfortable position for the feeding.
- Hold the baby close to you. Relax, and snuggle the baby.
- Tilt the bottle so that the neck of the bottle and the nipple are always filled (Figure 38–10). Otherwise some air might remain in the neck or nipple. If the baby swallows air, the he or she may later feel discomfort and cramping.
- ***Do not lay the baby down and prop the bottle for the feeding*** (Figure 38–11). This puts the baby at risk for choking.
- Burp the baby when he or she has taken about half the formula and at the end of the feeding.
- Do not expect the baby to always finish all of the formula. The feeding is over when the baby stops sucking and turns the head away from the bottle.
- Discard the remaining formula.
- Wash the bottle, cap, and nipple after the feeding (see *Bottlefeeding Equipment* on page 725).

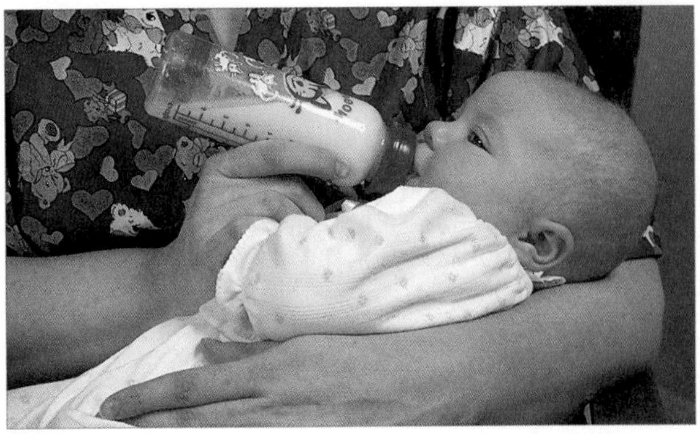

Figure 38–10 Tilt the bottle so that formula fills the bottle neck and nipple.

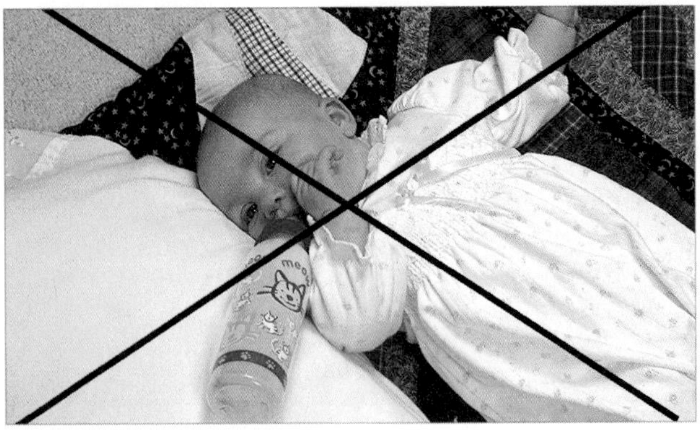

Figure 38–11 Do not prop the bottle to feed the baby.

Burping the Infant

Babies swallow some air when they are fed. Bottlefed babies swallow more air than do breastfed babies. Air in the stomach and intestines will cause the baby discomfort and cramping, which can lead to fussiness and vomiting. Burping helps get rid of the swallowed air. Most babies need to be burped after they have finished half the formula, after which they may want to continue feeding. They should be burped again after they finish the feeding.

There are three ways to position the baby for burping (Figure 38–12). One way is to hold the baby over your shoulder. First, place a clean diaper or towel over your shoulder to protect your clothing if the baby "spits up." The second way is to support the baby in a sitting position on your lap. If the baby is younger than 3 months, support the head and neck by cupping your hand under the baby's chin. Hold a towel or diaper in front of the baby. Gently pat the baby's back or rub it in circular motions until the baby burps. It may take up to 2 to 5 minutes. The third way is to lay the baby on the stomach and pat the back.

Diapering

Babies usually urinate several times a day. A baby who is only breastfed usually has stools that are bright yellow, are sweet-smelling, and have the consistency of scrambled eggs. Breastfed babies usually have bowel movements after feedings. If you introduce anything other than breast milk into a baby's diet, for example formula or solids, then the stools will change, usually to become more like an adult's

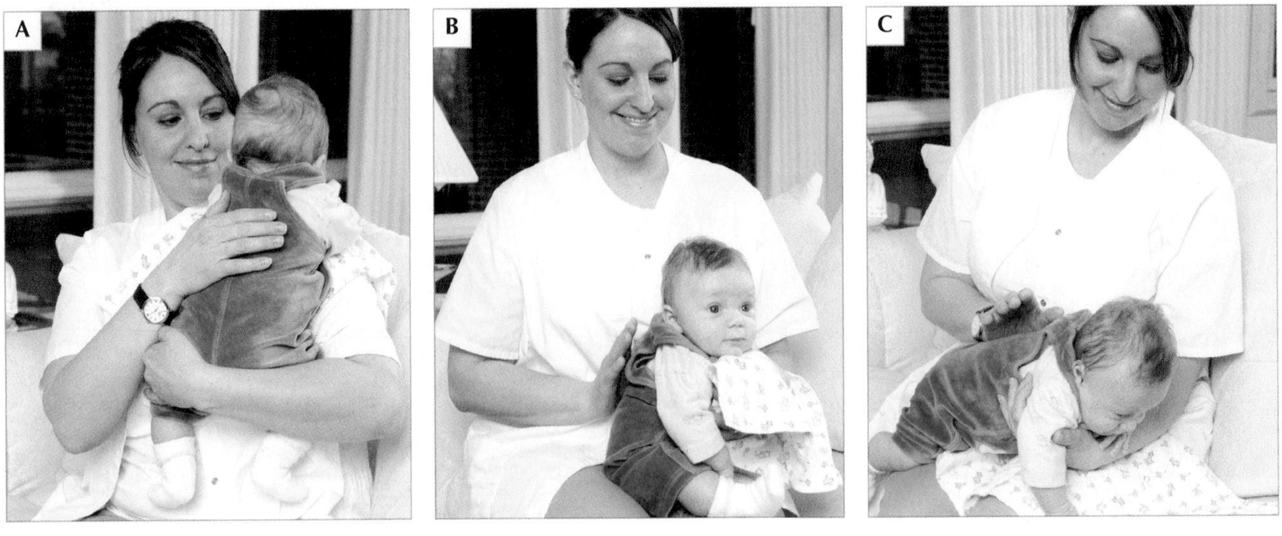

Figure 37–12 Burping a baby. **A,** The baby is held over the shoulder for burping. **B,** The baby is supported in the sitting position for burping. **C,** The baby is laid on the stomach.

(more brown, solid, and foul smelling). Until they are fed solid foods, babies usually have stools that are soft and unformed. Bottlefed babies may have three bowel movements a day.

Hard, formed stools indicate that the baby is constipated, and watery stools indicate diarrhea, which is very serious in babies, as their fluid balance can be upset quickly (see Chapter 27). Inform your supervisor immediately if you suspect a baby has constipation or diarrhea.

Diapers should be changed when they get wet or soiled, usually after a feeding. Parents may use cloth or disposable diapers. Cloth diapers may be fastened with diaper pins or Velcro strips. They are covered with plastic pants to protect against leaks. When changing a soiled cloth diaper, empty the stool into the toilet, if possible. Place used diapers and plastic pants in the diaper pail to be laundered later. They are washed in hot water with a laundry detergent made especially for baby clothes. Putting them through the wash cycle a second time without detergent helps remove all soap. They should be dried thoroughly and folded for reuse.

Disposable diapers help keep the baby dry because they absorb moisture. However, they still need to be changed whenever they become wet or soiled. When changing a soiled disposable diaper, empty the stool into the toilet, if possible. Place the diaper in the garbage. Do not flush disposable diapers or wipes down the toilet.

Changing diapers whenever they become wet helps prevent diaper rash. Moisture, stool, and urine irritate the baby's skin. If a diaper rash develops, tell your supervisor and the mother immediately. Make sure the baby is clean and dry before you apply a clean diaper. Health Canada advises that gloves are not necessary for routine diaper changes if you can avoid touching the stool or urine with your hands.[4] Check your employer's policy for the use of gloves when diapering. Always wash your hands before and after changing diapers.

To prevent falls, never turn your back on the baby when changing diapers. Gather all supplies before starting the procedure. Arrange them in an easy-to-reach place. If the baby is on a change table, keep one hand on the baby at all times.

1 2 3 DIAPERING THE BABY

Pre-Procedure

1 Practise proper hand hygiene.
2 Collect the following:
- Clean diaper
- Waterproof changing pad
- Disposable wipes, wash cloth, or cotton balls
- Basin of warm water
- Baby soap
- Baby lotion or cream, if necessary

Procedure

3 Place the baby on the changing pad.
4 Unfasten the dirty diaper. Place diaper pins out of the baby's reach.
5 Wipe the genital area with the front of the diaper, if the diaper is dry enough (Figure 38–13). Wipe from the front to the back.
6 Fold the diaper so that urine and stool are well inside. Set the diaper aside.
7 Clean the genital area from the front to back using a wet wash cloth, disposable wipes, or cotton balls. Wash with mild soap and warm (not hot) water if there is a lot of stool or if the baby has a rash. Rinse thoroughly, and pat the area dry.
8 Give cord care (page 728) and circumcision care (page 729).
9 Apply cream or lotion to the genital area and buttocks, if specified in the care plan. Do not use too much, as caking can occur.
10 Raise the baby's legs. Slide a clean diaper under the buttocks.
11 For boys, fold a cloth diaper so that the extra thickness is in the front (Figure 38–14, *A*. For girls, fold the diaper so that the extra thickness is in the back (see Figure 38–14, *B*).
12 Bring the diaper between the baby's legs.

(continued on page 728)

1 2 3 DIAPERING THE BABY

Procedure (cont'd)

13 Make sure the diaper is snug around the hips and abdomen. It should be loose near the penis if the circumcision has not healed. The diaper should be below the cord stump.

14 Secure the diaper in place. Use the tabs on disposable diapers (Figure 38–15, *A*), and make sure the tabs stick in place. Use diaper pins or Velcro strips for cloth diapers. Pins should point away from the abdomen (see Figure 38–15, *B*).

15 Apply plastic pants if cloth diapers are used. Do not use plastic pants with disposable diapers, which already have waterproof protection.

16 Put the baby in the crib, infant seat, or other safe location.

Post-Procedure

17 Rinse the stool from the cloth diaper in the toilet. Empty stool from the disposable diaper into the toilet, if possible.

18 Store used cloth diapers in a covered pail or plastic bag. Roll the disposable diaper into a ball and secure it with its tabs. Take the disposable diaper to the garbage.

19 Clean the changing pad.

20 Practise proper hand hygiene.

21 Report and record your actions and observations, according to employer policy.

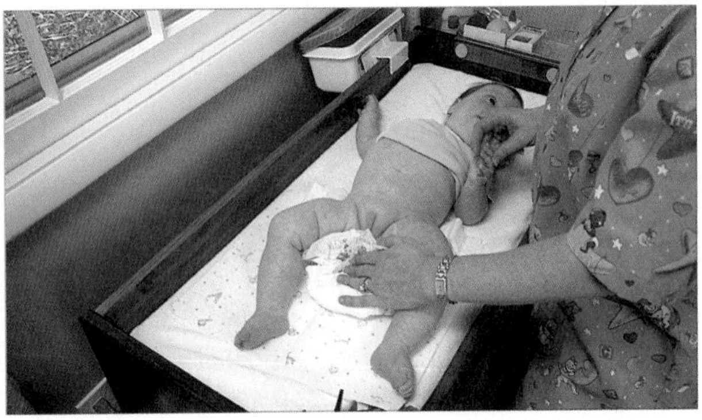

Figure 38–13 Clean the genital area with the front of the diaper.

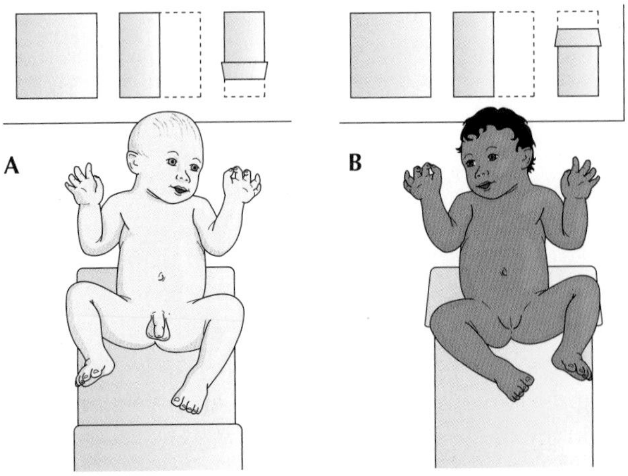

Figure 38–14 **A,** Fold a cloth diaper in the front for boys. **B,** Fold the diaper in the back for girls.

A

B

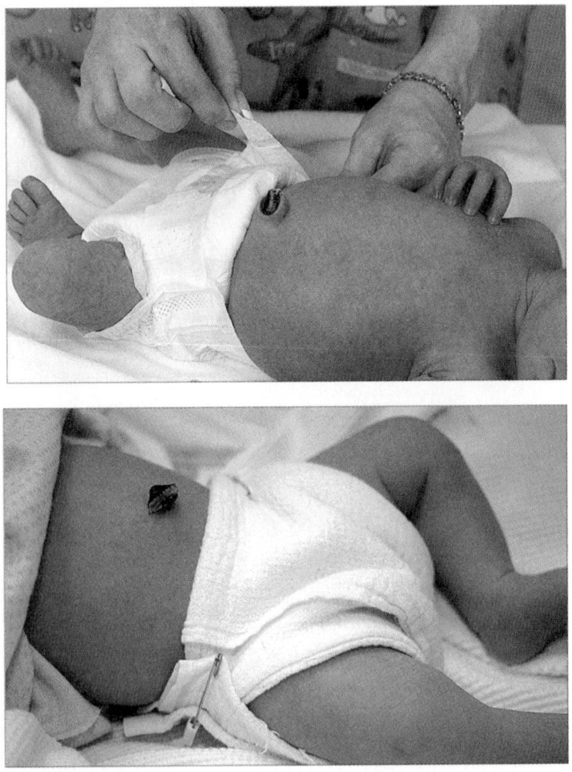

Figure 38–15 Securing a diaper. **A,** Secure disposable diaper in place with tabs. **B,** Diaper pins are sometimes used to secure cloth diapers. Point pins away from the abdomen.

Care of the Umbilical Cord

The **umbilical cord** connects the mother and the fetus (unborn baby) and carries blood, oxygen, and nutrients from the mother to the fetus (Figure 38–16). The umbilical cord is not needed after birth, so shortly after delivery, the physician or midwife clamps and cuts the cord. A stump of cord that is left on the baby dries up and falls off in 7 to 10 days. Slight bleeding may occur when the cord comes off. Do not pull the cord off—even if it looks ready to fall off.

The cord stump provides an area for the growth of microbes, so you need to ensure that it is clean and dry at all times. Cord care is done at each diaper change and is continued for 1 to 2 days after the cord comes off. The care plan and your supervisor will advise you on cord care, which usually consists of the following:

- Keeping the cord dry
- Washing your hands before and after contact with the umbilical area
- Keeping the cord clean. Gently wipe around the base of the cord with a cotton ball moistened with warm water (Figure 38–17). (Alcohol swabs are not recommended.)
- Keeping the top of the diaper below the cord to prevent the diaper from irritating the cord and to prevent the cord from being contaminated by urine.

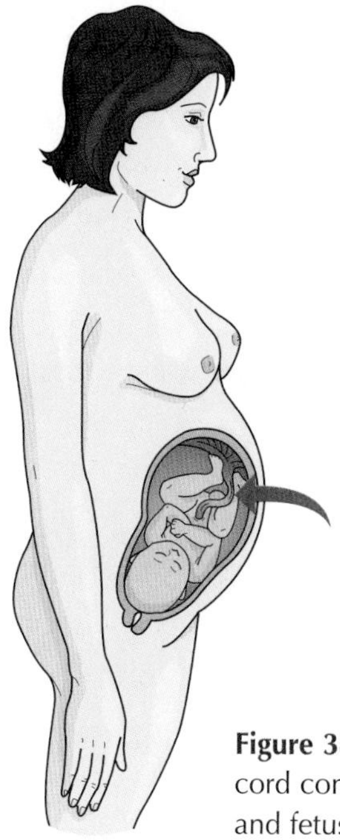

Figure 38–16 The umbilical cord connects the mother and fetus.

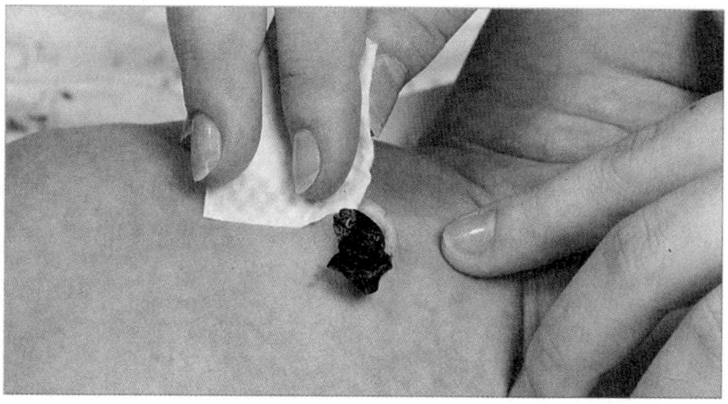

Figure 38–17 Wipe the cord stump at the base with a gauze pad moistened with warm water.

- Reporting any signs of infection, such as redness, odour, or drainage from the cord.
- Giving sponge baths to the baby until the cord falls off, after which the baby can be given a tub bath.

Caring for the Circumcised Baby

Circumcision is the surgical removal of foreskin from the penis. Not all male infants are circumcised, as the parents decide whether or not they want the procedure. The procedure promotes good hygiene and is thought to prevent certain cancers. Circumcision is usually done in the hospital before the baby goes home. In the Jewish faith, the procedure is a mandatory requirement and is conducted as a religious ceremony by a rabbi (the Jewish priest).

After a hospital circumcision, a gauze square may be applied on the penis. You should not pull this gauze off, as this can cause bleeding and scarring. Allow the gauze square to fall off on its own. The penis will look red, swollen, and sore for the first couple of days after the surgery, but the circumcision does not interfere with urination. The area should be completely healed in 10 to 14 days. Report observations of bleeding, odour, or drainage.

The penis should be thoroughly cleaned at each diaper change, especially after the baby has a bowel movement. Use mild soap and water or commercial wipes. Apply the diaper loosely to prevent the diaper from irritating the penis. Some physicians advise applying a teaspoonful of petroleum jelly to the penis to protect the penis from urine and stool. It also prevents the penis from sticking to the diaper. Use a cotton swab to apply the petroleum jelly

(Figure 38–18). Your supervisor will tell you if other measures are needed.

Bathing the Infant

Baths are very important not only to maintain cleanliness and hygiene but also to comfort and relax babies. They provide a wonderful time to hold, touch, and communicate with babies. Bath time should be part of the baby's daily routine. Some mothers like to bathe their babies in the morning and some in the evening. Follow the family's routine.

Planning and preparation are an important part of the bath routine. You cannot leave the baby alone because you forgot something and have to go and get it. Gather all necessary equipment, supplies, and the baby's clothes *before* you start the bath and place everything you need within your reach.

When bathing the baby, you should pay particular attention to the folds in the baby's skin, such as in the neck area and on the arms and legs. These folds can trap moisture, sweat, and lint from fabrics. The neck folds can also trap breast milk or formula. When skin is not cleaned thoroughly and dried, it can become excoriated (red and irritated).

The following safety measures are very important:

- Never leave the baby alone on a table or in the bathtub.
- Hold the baby securely throughout the bath. Babies are very slippery when they are wet. A wet, squirming baby can be hard to hold, so pay close attention to what you are doing.
- Room temperature for the bath should be 24°C to 27°C (75°F to 80°F). Turn up the thermostat, and close windows and doors for about 20 minutes before the bath, even if the room temperature is uncomfortable for you. In that case, remove your sweater or roll up your sleeves before starting the baby's bath.
- Pay special attention to water temperature. Babies have delicate skin that is easily burned. Bath water temperature should be 37.8°C to 40.6°C (100°F to 105°F). Bath water temperature is measured with a bath thermometer. If one is not available, test the water temperature with the inside of your wrist (Figure 38–19). The water should feel warm and comfortable on your wrist.
- Although the baby's bath should not be rushed, it is important that you are well-prepared to bathe the baby to avoid wasting time, since babies can get chilled very easily during bathing.

Two bath procedures are used for babies: (1) Sponge baths are given until the baby is about 2 weeks old or until the cord stump has fallen off and the cord site and circumcision have healed. ***The cord site must not get wet.*** (2) Tub baths (Figure 38–20) are given after the cord site and circumcision have healed.

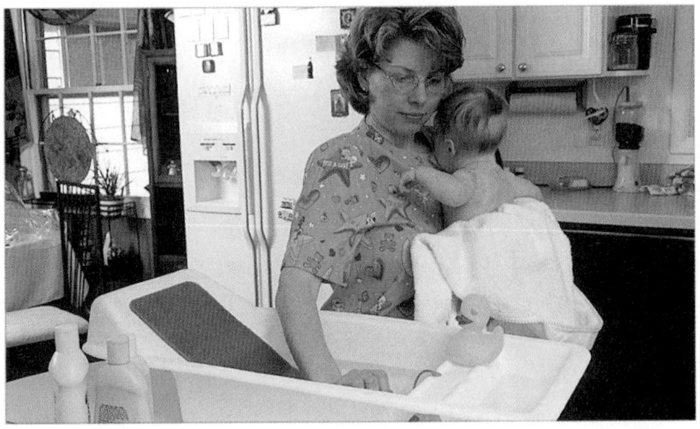

Figure 38–19 Use the inside of your wrist to test the temperature of the bathwater.

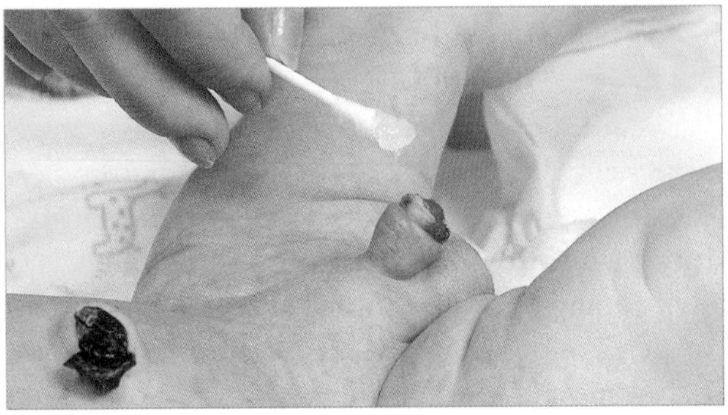

Figure 38–18 Use a cotton swab to apply petroleum jelly to the circumcised penis.

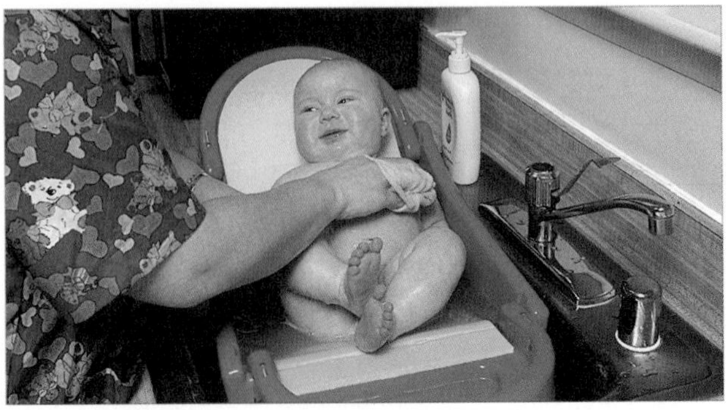

Figure 38–20 The baby is given a tub bath.

1 2 3 GIVING THE BABY A SPONGE BATH

Pre-Procedure

1 Practise proper hand hygiene.
2 Place the following items in your work area:
- Bath basin
- Bath thermometer
- Bath towel
- Two hand towels
- Receiving blanket
- Wash cloth
- Clean diaper
- Clean baby clothing
- Cotton balls
- Baby soap
- Baby shampoo
- Baby lotion

3 Fill the bath basin with warm water. Water temperature should be 37.8°C to 40.6°C (100°F to 105°F). Check the water temperature with the bath thermometer, or use the inside of your wrist. The water should feel warm and comfortable on your wrist.

Procedure

4 Undress the baby. Leave the baby's undershirt and diaper on.
5 Wash the baby's eyelids (Figure 38–21):
 a Dip a cotton ball into the water.
 b Squeeze out excess water.
 c Wash one eyelid from the inner part to the outer part.
 d Dry gently with a towel.
 e Repeat this step for the other eye with a new cotton ball.
6 Moisten the wash cloth. Clean the outside of the ear and then behind the ear. Dry with the towel. Repeat this step for the other ear. Be gentle.
7 Rinse and squeeze the wash cloth. Make a mitt with the wash cloth (Figure 38–22).
8 Wash the baby's face (see Figure 38–22). Wipe around the mouth and nose and then the cheeks and forehead. ***Do not use cotton swabs to clean inside the ears or nostrils.*** Pat the face dry.
9 Wipe under the baby's chin and in the neck creases. Dry well.
10 Pick up the baby. Hold the baby over the bath basin using the football hold. Support the baby's head and neck with one wrist and hand, while using the wash cloth in your opposite hand to wash the baby.
11 Wash the baby's head (Figure 38–23):
 a Squeeze a small amount of water from the wash cloth onto the baby's head.
 b Apply a small amount of baby shampoo to the head.
 c Wash the head using circular motions.
 d Rinse the head by squeezing water from a wash cloth over the baby's head. Be sure to rinse thoroughly. Avoid getting soap in the baby's eyes.
 e Use a small hand towel to dry the head.
12 Lay the baby on the table.
13 Remove the undershirt and diaper.
14 Wash the front of the body. Use a soapy wash cloth. You may also apply soap to your hands and wash the baby with your hands. Do not get the cord wet. Rinse thoroughly. Pat the skin dry, being sure to wash and dry all creases and skin folds.
15 Wash and dry baby's hands, feet, and between the fingers and toes.
16 Place the baby in the prone position. Wash the back and buttocks using a soapy wash cloth or your hands. Rinse thoroughly. Pat dry.
17 Give cord care (page 728) and circumcision care (page 729).
18 Apply baby lotion to the baby's body, as directed by the care plan.
19 Put a clean diaper and clean clothes on the baby.
20 Wrap the baby in the receiving blanket. Put the baby in the crib or other safe location.

Post-Procedure

21 Clean and return equipment and supplies to their proper places. Do this step when the baby is settled.
22 Practise proper hand hygiene.
23 Report and record your actions and observations, according to employer policy.

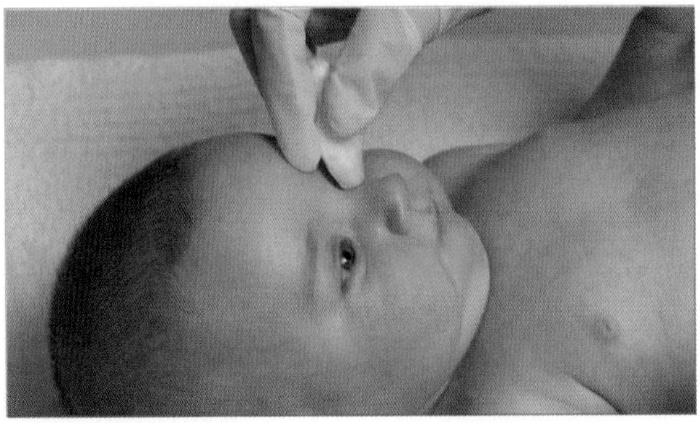

Figure 38–21 Wash the baby's eyelids with cotton balls. Clean the eyelid from the inner part to the outer part. Use a fresh cotton ball for each eye.

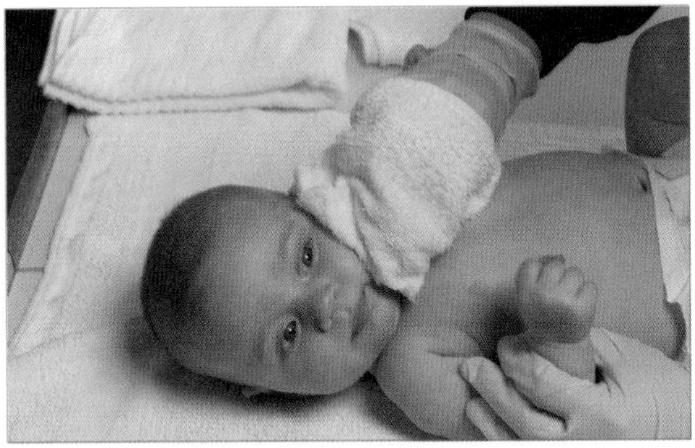

Figure 38–22 Wash the baby's face with a mitted wash cloth.

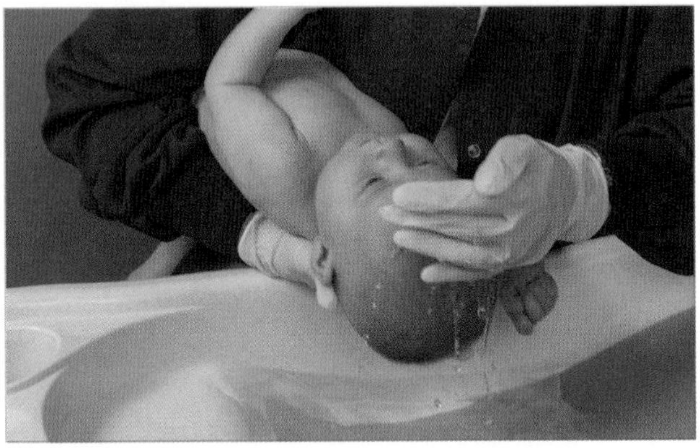

Figure 38–23 Wash the baby's head over the basin.

1 2 3 GIVING THE BABY A TUB BATH

Procedure

1 Follow steps 1 through 13 in *Giving the Baby a Sponge Bath* on page 731.

2 Hold the baby as in Figure 38–24:

- **a** Place your right hand* under the baby's shoulders. Your thumb should be over the baby's right shoulder. Your fingers should be under the right arm.
- **b** Use your left hand to support the baby's buttocks. Slide your left hand under the thighs. Hold the right thigh with your left hand.

3 Lower the baby into the water, feet first.

4 Wash the front of the baby's body. Be sure to wash all skin folds and creases. Rinse thoroughly.

5 Reverse your hold. Use your left hand to hold the baby.

6 Wash the baby's back. Rinse thoroughly.

7 Reverse your hold again. Use your right hand to hold the baby.

8 Wash the genital area.

9 Lift the baby out of the water and onto a towel.

10 Wrap the baby in the towel, taking care to cover the baby's head.

11 Pat the baby dry. Be sure to dry all skin folds and creases.

12 Follow steps 18 to 23 of the *Sponge Bath* procedure.

*This procedure was written for right-handed people. Reverse the hand positions if you are left-handed.

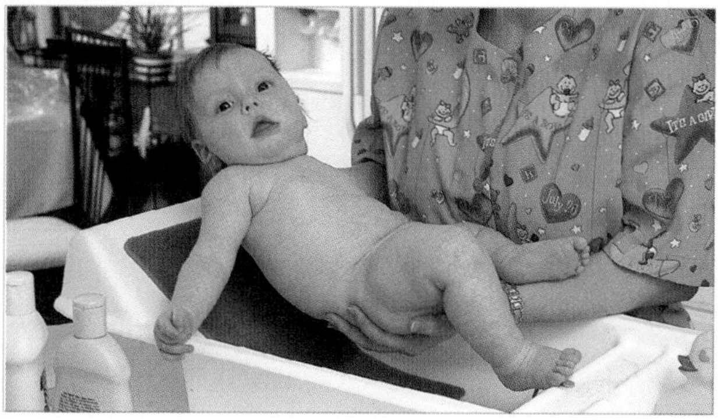

Figure 38–24 The baby is held for a tub bath.

Nail Care

The baby's fingernails and toenails should be kept short, as otherwise the baby could scratch himself or herself and others. However, you should take extreme care not to cut the baby's nails too short, as the nail tips are highly vascular and could bleed a lot if accidentally cut. Some doctors suggest gently tearing or ripping the nails to keep them short! In some cultures, mothers are taught to bite off their baby's nails to shorten them. If you do choose to cut them, nails are best cut when the baby is sleeping so that the baby does not squirm or fuss during the procedure. Use nail clippers or file nails with an emery board. If using nail clippers, clip nails straight across as for an adult (see Figure 30–10 on page 564).

Weighing Infants

Infants are weighed at birth, since the birth weight is the baseline for measuring the infant's growth. Your supervisor tells you when to weigh the baby. While you are weighing the baby, you must meet the baby's safety needs. Protect the baby from chills, by keeping the room warm and free of drafts. Also, protect the baby from falling by always keeping a hand over the baby when measuring the weight, especially if you need to look away.

1 2 3 WEIGHING THE BABY

Pre-Procedure

1 Practise proper hand hygiene.
2 Collect the following:
- Baby scale
- Paper for the scale
- Items for diaper changing (see *Diapering the Baby* on page 727)

Procedure

3 Place the paper on the scale. Adjust the scale to zero (0).
4 Undress the baby and remove the diaper. Clean the genital area.
5 Lay the baby on the scale. Keep one hand over the baby to prevent falling.
6 Read the digital display (Figure 38–25), or move the pointer until the scale is balanced.
7 Diaper and dress the baby. Lay the baby in the crib.

Post-Procedure

8 Return the scale to its proper place.
9 Practise proper hand hygiene.
10 Report and record the weight and your observations, according to employer policy.

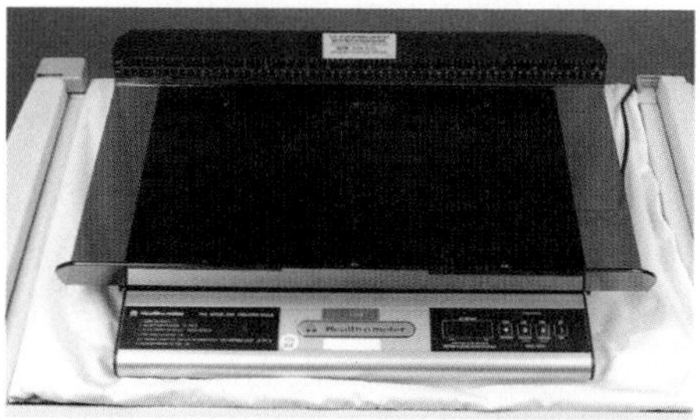

Figure 38–25 Digital infant scale.

REVIEW

Answers to these questions are at the bottom of the page.

Circle the **BEST** answer.

1. **A new mother has a red discharge evident on her pad the first few days after childbirth. This is:**
   A. Lochia
   B. Menstrual flow
   C. From her rectum
   D. Very rare

2. **A Cesarean delivery involves:**
   A. A vaginal incision
   B. A perineal incision
   C. An abdominal incision
   D. A normal delivery through the vagina

3. **A symptom of mastitis is:**
   A. Engorgement
   B. Postpartum blues
   C. Thirst while breastfeeding
   D. Pain and redness in a breast

4. **Zach is a newborn. Which of the following should be reported?**
   A. Zach looks flushed and is perspiring
   B. Zach has a soft spot on the top of his head
   C. Zach spits up a small amount when burped
   D. Zach has soft, unformed stools several times a day

5. **When holding Zach, you should:**
   A. Support his head
   B. Tell him to stop crying
   C. Let his arms and legs dangle
   D. Bounce him up and down vigorously

6. **When laying down Sarah, who is an infant, for her sleep, you should:**
   A. Lay her on her back
   B. Place pillows under her head
   C. Place her on her stomach with her head turned to the side
   D. Place stuffed animals in her bed to give her something to look at

7. **A breastfed baby is burped:**
   A. Every 5 minutes
   B. After the feeding
   C. After nursing from both breasts
   D. After feeding from one breast and then again after feeding from the other

8. **You are required to warm a baby bottle. Which of the following is *true*?**
   A. The formula should feel warm on your wrist
   B. The formula should be left out to get to room temperature
   C. The bottle is warmed for 3 minutes in the microwave
   D. The formula is warmed on the stovetop for 5 minutes

9. **When bottlefeeding, you should:**
   A. Burp the baby every 5 minutes
   B. Save remaining formula for the next feeding
   C. Lay the baby down with the bottle propped on a pillow
   D. Tilt the bottle so that formula fills the neck of the bottle and the nipple

10. **When the umbilical cord stump has not yet healed, the diaper should be:**
    A. Disposable
    B. Below the stump
    C. Snug over the stump
    D. Loose over the stump

11. **Cord and circumcision care are given:**
    A. Once a day
    B. Three times a day
    C. At every diaper change
    D. Whenever the baby has had a bowel movement

12. **When bathing babies, you should:**
    A. Keep the room temperature slightly cool
    B. Gather supplies before beginning the bath
    C. Not use soap until the cord and circumcision have healed
    D. Have the water temperature between 38.8°C and 43.3°C (102°F to 110°F).

Answers: 1.A, 2.C, 3.D, 4.A, 5.A, 6.A, 7.D, 8.A, 9.D, 10.B, 11.C, 12.B

CHAPTER 39

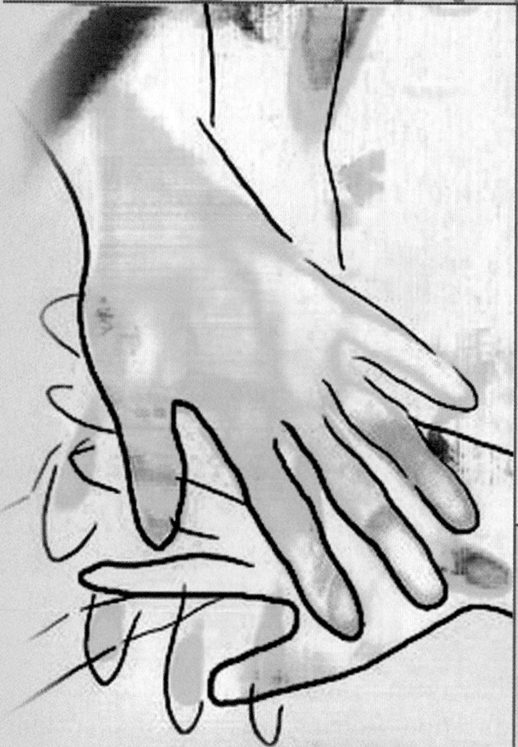

Developmental Disabilities

OBJECTIVES

- Define the key terms listed in this chapter.
- Identify the areas of functioning limited by a developmental disability.
- Explain how a developmental disability can affect the client and the family across the life span.
- Explain when developmental disabilities occur and their causes.
- Explain how various developmental disabilities affect functioning.

key terms

autism A brain disorder that impairs communication, social skills, and behaviour.

cerebral palsy (CP) A disorder affecting muscle control (*palsy*); caused by an injury or abnormality in the motor region of the brain (*cerebral*).

cognitive disability Impaired ability to learn. Also known as **intellectual disability**.

congenital Present at birth.

convulsion Violent and sudden contractions or tremors of muscle groups.

developmental disability A disability that occurs before birth, at birth, or during childhood or adolescence; impairs the child's development.

diplegia Loss of ability to move (*plegia*) corresponding parts on both (*di*) sides of the body; both arms or both legs are affected.

Down syndrome (DS) A congenital disorder caused by an extra chromosome; results in varying degrees of intellectual disability.

epilepsy A condition characterized by recurrent seizures.

Fetal alcohol effect (FAE) A milder form of FAS; the same symptoms may occur but to a lesser degree.

Fetal alcohol syndrome (FAS) A group of physical and mental abnormalities in a child as a result of alcohol consumption by the mother during pregnancy.

Fragile X syndrome The most common form among inherited developmental disorders.

intellectual disability See **cognitive disability**.

seizure Brief disturbance in the brain's normal electrical function; affects awareness, movement, and sensation.

spastic Uncontrolled contractions of skeletal muscles.

spina bifida A congenital disorder involving improper closing of the spine before birth; *spina* means backbone and *bifida* means split in two parts.

tonic-clonic seizure A seizure involving convulsions.

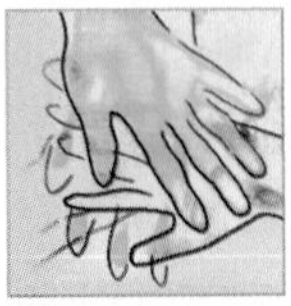

A *disability* is any loss of physical or mental function (see Chapter 4). Many disabilities begin in adulthood due to diseases, medical conditions, and injuries, or disabilities may begin before adulthood.

A **developmental disability** is a disability that occurs before birth, at birth, or during childhood or adolescence and impairs a child's development. It is often severe and is always permanent. Although the disability begins before adulthood, it remains throughout the person's life. Thus, people of all ages can have developmental disabilities.

Developmental disabilities can affect physical function, mental function, or both, limiting the person's ability to function in at least three of the following life activities:

- Self-care (eating, dressing, hygiene)
- Understanding and expressing speech and language
- Learning
- Mobility (getting around independently)
- Self-direction (solving problems and making choices and decisions)
- Independent living
- Economic self-sufficiency (earning enough income to support oneself financially)

Most clients with developmental disabilities need lifelong assistance, support, and special services, which are provided by the health care team involved in the client's care.

DEVELOPMENTAL DISABILITIES AND THE FAMILY

Families of children with developmental disabilities may face many challenges. As the support worker, be sensitive to the family's situation. Some families you work with may be adjusting to a recent diagnosis of their child's disability. They may still be figuring out the new roles and routines for all family members, so they may be under great stress. Some families may have already established their roles and routines. Remember, every family situation is different.

Most children with disabilities live with their families at home. Being a primary caregiver for a child with disabilities can be an all-consuming task, as it often takes great amounts of time, energy, and work. Many caregivers have to balance caregiving with other responsibilities, including full-time jobs and caring for other children. Parents may not leave the child with disability to spend time alone with each other because they do not want to impose on family or friends to care for the child. They may not be able to spend as much time with their other children as they would like. Parental caregivers often worry about the stigma associated with their child's disability and may feel that their child is considered as being "different" by society. They may encounter discrimination and other barriers. The constant stress and work of caregiving can lead to burnout (see Chapter 9), and the caregiver can become physically and emotionally exhausted. There can be economic and financial burdens as well, as special equipment and adaptive and assistive devices are expensive and may not be covered under the family health plan.

Home care and other community agencies often provide needed support and services. The types of community agencies available vary among the provinces and territories. Families in large cities will more likely have more support groups and agencies available than do families in small towns and rural communities. As more and more families use the Internet, they will have more access to information and group support.

As a support worker, you will be working closely with the family caregivers. You may take on some household tasks so that the parents can spend more time with the child with the disability and with their other children. You may provide respite care so that the parents can have a break from caregiving. You also may directly assist the child, according to the care plan. For example, you might help with the child's rehabilitation activities under the supervision of a physical or occupational therapist. You may accompany the child to and from school (Figure 39–1) or work with children with disabilities in schools. Children with severe disabilities may need long-term care in special facilities.

As the child and parents grow older, caring for the adolescent or adult child often becomes physically difficult. Parents may not be able to lift or move the adolescent or adult child. Parents themselves may become ill, injured, or disabled, and a parent may die. Through all these situations, the client with the developmental disability continues to need care.

Some adolescents and adults with developmental disabilities live in community and residential settings, in their own homes, or in group homes. Some may live in specially licensed long-term care facilities. Support workers in these facilities require special training to meet the needs of clients with developmental disabilities. Often the client's family continues to be involved in the care. Remember that family members have cared for the client for most of his or her life, so they understand the client's condition and needs very well. Include family members, whenever appropriate, when you provide care and services.

TYPES OF DEVELOPMENTAL DISABILITIES

There are many kinds of developmental disabilities. Generally, they are caused by conditions, illnesses, or accidents that injure the brain or body

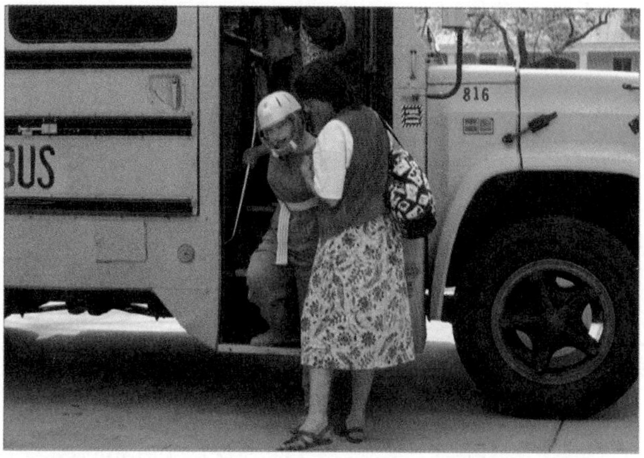

Figure 39–1 You may accompany a child with disabilities to and from school. **Source:** © Robin Sachs/Photo Edit.

before birth, during birth, or during childhood or adolescence. These include, but are not limited to, the following:

- Intellectual disabilities
- Down syndrome
- Cerebral palsy
- Autism
- Epilepsy
- Spina bifida
- Fetal alcohol syndrome

A number of children and adults have more than one condition that causes a disability. Table 39–1 lists other conditions that cause developmental disabilities.

Table 39–1	Some Conditions Causing Developmental Disabilities
Acquired brain injury	*Damage to brain tissue caused by disease, medical condition, accident, drug overdose, or violence.* As violence increases in our society, there will be more clients who will suffer brain damage. Some accidents and diseases reduce or cut off oxygen to the brain, which can destroy brain cells and cause brain injury. For example, conditions during birth, near drowning, choking, suffocation, and stroke can all cause brain injury. Certain infections (meningitis, encephalitis) or chemicals (mercury and lead poisoning) also destroy brain tissue. Unfortunately, those using street drugs risk ingesting toxic substances and overdosing. Blows to the head can batter the brain and cause brain injury, as in motor vehicle accidents, falls, sport injuries, and child abuse (including shaking). Acquired brain injuries can be permanent and severe, causing personality changes, vision problems, speech problems, muscle control problems, and intellectual disability.
Congenital heart disease	*Abnormalities in the structure or function of the heart that are present before birth.* If the affected babies survive, they may tire easily or experience delayed growth. Most congenital heart conditions must be corrected by surgery.
Fragile X syndrome	*The most common inherited cause of mental impairment and the most common known cause of autism.* It is a genetic condition caused by changes in the X chromosome, which prevents the chromosome from making the protein that it normally does. Some individuals are carriers who have a small defect in the gene and show no symptoms (called permutation). One in 259 women carry the fragile X (permutation) gene, and there is a 50% chance of her passing it on to her children; about 1 in 800 men carry the fragile X (permutation) gene and pass this gene on to all of their daughters but not to their sons. The fragile X (permutation) gene can be passed unnoticed down through generations before a child is affected with full mutation. Boys and girls can both be affected, but boys are usually affected more severely. Most males with full mutation will have developmental disabilities. Only one third to one half of girls have significant intellectual impairment. There is ongoing research into the causes for males being more affected, and recent reports suggest that since girls have two X chromosomes, even if affected, they still have one strong X chromosome, while males have only the one X chromosome that is damaged and causes full mutation. Common symptoms of Fragile X syndrome are: Mental impairment, ranging from learning disabilities to developmental disorders Attention deficit and hyperactivity Anxiety and unstable mood Autistic behaviour Long face, large ears, flat feet Hyperextension of joints, especially fingers Seizures, which affect about 25% of clients with fragile X

(continued on page 739)

Table 39–1	Some Conditions Causing Developmental Disabilities (cont'd)
Hydrocephalus	*A condition in which fluid collects in the brain* (*hydro* means water, and *cephalo* means head). Left untreated, it causes the head to enlarge and increases pressure on the brain. If the child survives, intellectual disability and neurological damage may result. To treat hydrocephalus, a shunt (a long, flexible tube) is placed in the brain and connected to a body cavity, usually the abdomen or a heart chamber. The shunt is completely enclosed inside the body. Fluid drains from the brain through the tube into the body cavity. Shunts usually stay in place for the remainder of the person's life.
Phenylketonuria (PKU)	*An inherited condition in which the body lacks an enzyme necessary to process a certain amino acid (phenylalanine).* When this amino acid builds up in the blood, it injures brain tissue. Left untreated, PKU causes intellectual disability and neurological problems. PKU can be detected with a blood test in the first few days of life. With proper treatment, brain injury can be avoided. Treatment involves maintaining a strict diet throughout life.
Shaken baby syndrome	*A term for the physical and cognitive impairments caused by shaking a baby or young child violently.* Babies and young children have weak neck muscles, and shaking them violently causes the head to swing back and forth with great force. As a result, the brain bangs against the skull wall, causing bleeding behind the eyes and in the brain. Permanent brain injury, seizures, partial or total blindness, paralysis, intellectual disability, or death can occur. Less violent but frequent shaking of a young child can also cause long-term

Intellectual Disabilities

An **intellectual disability (cognitive disability)**—an impaired ability to learn—results in below-average intelligence and limitations in the ability to function in certain areas of daily life. (*Intelligence* relates to learning, thinking, and reasoning.) The client can learn new skills but at a slower rate than normal. A client with an intellectual disability often has difficulties with communication, self-care, and social interaction. In the past, intellectual disability was called "mental retardation." In Canada, this old term is no longer considered acceptable.

An intellectual disability can be caused by any genetic abnormality, injury, or disease that impairs the development of the brain. The cause is largely unknown at this time. Some common causes of intellectual disabilities are listed in Box 39–1. People with an intellectual disability often have other disabilities as well.

Intellectual disabilities range from mild to severe. Tests that measure intelligence are called IQ tests. An average person without an intellectual disability has an IQ of about 90 to 100. People with IQ scores between 70 and 55 are considered *mildly intellectually disabled*. They may be slow to learn but are able to attend regular schools. As adults, they can function in society with some support. They can work and live in the community and need only occasional support. People who have IQ scores below 55 are considered *moderately intellectually disabled* and need daily support at home and at work. People with IQ scores below 25 are considered *severely intellectually disabled* and need constant support in all areas.

The Canadian Association for Community Living is a national association dedicated to serving people with intellectual disabilities as well as their families. The association's goal is to ensure that people with intellectual disabilities have opportunities to live meaningful, dignified lives. The association's philosophy is that people with intellectual disabilities can and should be allowed to participate in all aspects of community living. Children should live in families and be integrated into regular schools, whenever possible, and interact with other children with or without disabilities. Adults with intellectual disabilities have the right to control their lives to the fullest extent possible—that is,

Box 39–1 Causes of Intellectual Disability

Genetic Conditions

- Abnormal genes inherited from one or both parents—Fragile X syndrome and phenylketonuria (PKU) are genetic disorders that cause intellectual disability
- Missing or extra chromosomes—Down syndrome is a chromosome disorder that causes intellectual disability

Problems During Pregnancy

- Alcohol or drug use
- Poor nutrition
- Exposure to certain environmental hazards, such as X-rays or certain chemicals
- Illnesses, such as rubella (German measles) or syphilis
- Uncontrolled medical conditions, such as diabetes or human immunodeficiency virus (HIV) infection

Problems at Birth

- Premature birth
- Low birthweight
- Lack of oxygen to the baby's brain during birth

Problems After Birth

- Childhood diseases, such as whooping cough, chickenpox, and measles
- Infections, such as meningitis and encephalitis
- Acquired brain injury caused by accidents, disease, or abuse
- Severe malnutrition or neglect

they should make choices and decisions about their care and how they live. They should have friends, work at jobs, enjoy adult activities, and contribute to their communities.

People with intellectual disabilities have sexual, emotional, and social needs and desires, just like everyone else. They have the right to privacy and to love and be loved. Remember, intellectual disabilities vary from mild to severe. Some adults with intellectual disabilities have life partners; some marry and have children.

Most people with intellectual disabilities are able to control their sexual urges, but a few are not. The type of their sexual responses and where they display them may be inappropriate (see Chapter 21 for a discussion on how to deal with sexually aggressive clients). Children and adults with intellectual disabilities are vulnerable to sexual abuse. Report signs of sexual abuse immediately (see Chapter 21). Children with intellectual disabilities need to be educated about sexual abuse, safe sex, and other sexuality issues.

Down Syndrome

Down syndrome (DS) is a disorder caused by an extra chromosome. At fertilization, normally, a male sex cell (sperm) and a female sex cell (ovum), each containing 23 chromosomes, unite to form 46 chromosomes. With DS, an extra chromosome is present, so there are 47 chromosomes in the affected person. Thus, DS occurs due to an error at fertilization and is a **congenital** (present at birth) condition.

In Canada, DS is the one of the most common congenital chromosomal disorders. For every 10,000 births, 14 babies are born with DS.[1]

DS causes varying degrees of intellectual disability—usually moderate to severe. The child also has certain physical features caused by the extra chromosome (Figure 39–2):

- Small head
- Oval-shaped eyes that slant upward
- Flat face
- Short, wide neck
- Large tongue
- Wide, flat nose
- Small ears
- Short stature
- Short, wide hands with stubby fingers
- Weak muscle tone

Many children with DS have congenital heart defects and tend to have vision and hearing problems as well. They are at risk for ear infections, respiratory infections, and thyroid gland problems. Those with DS may start to show symptoms of dementia after age 35, and Alzheimer's disease is commonly diagnosed in their 40s. Genetic

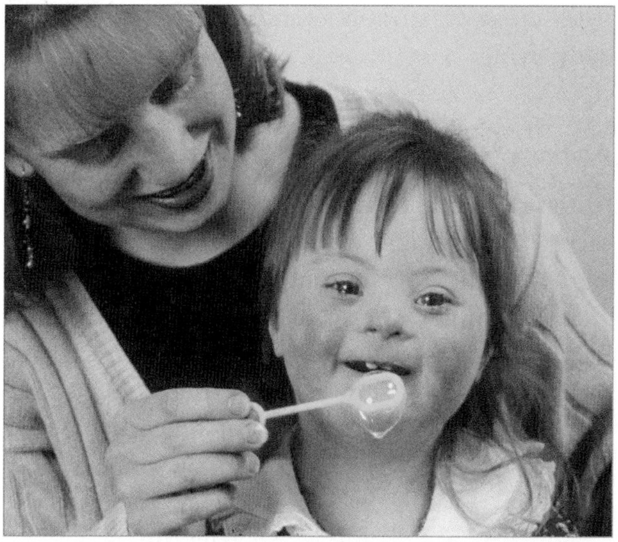

Figure 39–2 A child with Down syndrome. **Source:** Hattie Young/Science Photo Library/Publiphoto.

counsellors relate this prevalence to the effect of the extra gene.

Clients with DS need speech, language, physical, and occupational therapies, training for self-care skills, and health and sex education. Weight gain and constipation are frequent problems in these clients, so they need a well-balanced diet and regular exercise.

Cerebral Palsy

Cerebral palsy (CP), a disorder affecting muscle control (*palsy*), is caused by an injury or abnormality in the motor region of the brain (*cerebral*). Depending on which areas of the brain have been injured, one or more of the following may occur:

- Involuntary movements
- Poor coordination and posture
- Muscle weakness
- Difficulty or inability to walk
- Difficulty or inability to speak

CP may occur before, during, or shortly after birth. Lack of oxygen to the fetal or newborn brain is the usual cause. Infants at risk include those who:

- Are premature
- Have a low birthweight
- Do not cry in the first 5 minutes after birth
- Need mechanical ventilation
- Have bleeding in the brain
- Have heart, kidney, or spinal cord abnormalities
- Have blood problems
- Have seizures

Acquired brain injury in infancy and early childhood also can result in CP (see Table 39–1 on pages 738–739).

Body movements and body parts are affected. The following types of CP are the most common:

- ***Spastic cerebral palsy*—spastic** means uncontrolled contractions of skeletal muscles (*spastic* comes from the Greek *spastikos,* meaning to draw in). Muscles contract or shorten and are stiff and unable to relax. One or both sides of the body may be involved, so posture and balance are affected, and movement is stiff and jerky. The client's arms may be affected, so he or she may have difficulty eating, writing, dressing, and doing other activities of daily living. If the client's legs are affected, he or she may have difficulty walking or moving. This is the most common type of CP (about 50% of all cases of CP).
- ***Athetoid cerebral palsy***—the client cannot control movements (*athetoid* comes from the Greek *athetos*, meaning not fixed). The client has involuntary, constant, slow weaving or writhing motions that occur in the trunk, arms, hands, legs, and feet. The client might have difficulty reaching for and grasping objects and remaining upright for sitting or standing. Sometimes the tongue, face, and neck muscles may be involved, causing the client to drool or grimace.
- ***Ataxic cerebral palsy***—the client has weak muscle tone and difficulty coordinating movements (absence of [*a*] arrangement or order [*taxis*]), so he or she appears very unsteady and shaky when walking and has trouble maintaining the balance.

The following terms are used to describe the body parts affected by CP (see Chapter 18):

- ***Hemiplegia*—*hemi*** means half; *plegia* means complete or partial loss of ability to move. CP affects one side of the body—the right arm and leg or the left arm and leg. The other side functions normally. The client may be able to walk but might look a little awkward.

- ***Diplegia***—*di* means two. With **diplegia,** there is loss of ability to move (*plegia*) corresponding parts on both (*di*) sides of the body. In most cases of diplegia caused by CP, both legs are affected. The client has difficulty walking, but the upper body is not affected. (In extremely rare cases, both arms are affected, but not the legs.)
- ***Quadriplegia***—*quad* means four. CP affects all four limbs (both arms and both legs). The client cannot walk or use the arms. Usually the client also has difficulty with movement of the facial muscles and the trunk. Talking and eating may be difficult, and the client needs a wheelchair to get around.

Some clients with CP are only mildly affected. Their movements are awkward, but they can walk independently and they are not intellectually disabled. However, other clients with CP are severely affected. They can also have many other impairments and problems, including:

- Intellectual disability
- Learning disability
- Hearing impairment
- Speech impairment
- Vision impairment
- Drooling because of difficulty swallowing saliva
- Bladder and bowel control problems
- Seizures
- Difficulty swallowing
- Attention deficit hyperactivity disorder (short attention span, poor concentration, and increased activity)
- Breathing problems due to poor posture
- Pressure ulcers from immobility

Care depends on the severity of CP and the needs of the client. The goal is for the client to be as independent as possible. Physical, occupational, and speech therapy, the use of eyeglasses or hearing aids, and surgery and medications for muscle problems can all be helpful. As a support worker, you may be required to assist the client with CP with range-of-motion exercises and activities of daily living.

Autism

Autism is a brain disorder that impairs communication, social skills, and behaviour. The client has extreme difficulties relating to others. *Autos* means self; with autism, the client withdraws into the self. It may seem as if clients with autism are in their own world and uninterested in others. For example, they may not notice when someone enters a room or prefer to play alone. Some avoid physical contact and become very upset when touched.

Both verbal and nonverbal communication are affected. Many clients with autism do not develop speech. They often avoid eye contact or refuse to interact. Some are unable to understand the facial expressions on others.

Autism begins in early childhood—between the ages of 18 months and 3 years. In Canada, about 1 child in 200 is diagnosed with autism. It is one of the most common brain disorders affecting children; boys are affected more often than girls.[2]

Autism affects each client differently—mildly to severely. The following symptoms are common:

- Developing language skills slowly, if at all
- Repeating words or phrases
- Not starting or maintaining conversations
- Repeating body movements (hand flapping, finger flicking, rocking)
- Short attention span
- Spending time alone
- Showing little reaction to pain
- Overreacting to noise and touch
- Dislike of cuddling
- Frequent tantrums for no apparent reason
- Strong attachment to a single item, idea, activity, or person
- Need for routines; dislike of change
- Lack of fear
- Lack of response to others
- Being too active or too quiet
- Display of aggressive or violent behaviour
- Tendency to injure self

There is no cure for autism, but with therapy, the client may learn to change or control behaviours. Many therapies may be used:

- Behaviour modification—rewarding positive behaviours and correcting negative behaviours
- Speech and language therapy
- Music, auditory, recreation, and sensory therapies
- Occupational therapy
- Medication therapy
- Diet therapy

The client needs to develop social and work skills. Some adults with autism work and live independently, while some need support and help from family and community services. Some may live in group homes or residential care facilities.

Clients with autism may have other disorders, such as intellectual disability and epilepsy.

As a support worker caring for children or adults with autism, remember that strict routines are usually important. The client may become very upset if his or her routine is disrupted. Follow the client's routine, whenever possible. Warn the client if the routine must be changed. Children require careful supervision. Do not leave the child unattended for even a moment. The care plan provides directions on how to interact with the client with autism.

Epilepsy

Epilepsy is a condition characterized by recurrent seizures (*epilepsia*, meaning seizure). Recurrent means occurring repeatedly from time to time. A **seizure** is a brief disturbance in the brain's normal electrical function, which affects awareness, movement, and sensation.

Seizures that affect only one part of the brain are called *partial seizures*. Seizures that affect the whole brain are called *generalized seizures*. The area of the brain affected by the seizure temporarily loses its ability to function normally, so seizures may cause different reactions depending on the part of the brain affected. For example, some seizures cause the person to briefly stare and appear unresponsive; others involve convulsions (as in **tonic-clonic seizures**). A **convulsion** is a violent and sudden contraction or tremor of muscle groups. The person loses consciousness and falls to the floor. All muscle groups contract and relax, causing jerking and twitching movements of the body. Urinary and bowel incontinence may occur. A tonic-clonic seizure usually lasts for 1 to 7 minutes.

A single seizure does not mean the person has epilepsy, since a number of factors can cause a single seizure. For a diagnosis of epilepsy, the person has to have recurring seizures. The electrical system in the brain is permanently damaged, making it susceptible to seizures.

Often, the cause of epilepsy in a particular person is not known. Some of the known causes of epilepsy include acquired brain injuries (see Table 39–1 on pages 738–739), brain tumours, genetic conditions, and problems with brain development before birth.

Children and young adults are commonly affected, but epilepsy can develop at any time during a person's life. It can occur due to any problem affecting the brain, for example, cerebral palsy, intellectual disability, autism, Alzheimer's disease, stroke, tumours, and acquired brain injury.

There is no cure for epilepsy, but medications are prescribed by a physician to prevent seizures. These medications may control seizures in many people but may not work in others, and they may need brain surgery to reduce the frequency of the seizures.

When controlled, epilepsy usually does not affect learning and activities of daily living. In severe cases, people may be limited in their activities. For example, a person who has frequent seizures may not be allowed to drive, which may limit job choices and opportunities. For these clients, safety measures are needed at home, in the workplace, and for transportation and recreation.

Clients with epilepsy have an increased risk of death. They have higher rates of suicide and sudden, unexplained death, and accidental death, especially drowning.

As a support worker, it is very important for you to observe and report pre-seizure activity, what occurred during the seizure, and postseizure activity.

Spina Bifida

Spina bifida is a congenital disorder involving improper closing of the spine before birth (*spina* means backbone, and *bifida* means split in two parts). Spina bifida is one of the *neural tube defects (NTDs)* that involve the incomplete development of the brain, spinal cord, and protective coverings for these organs. Neural tube defects occur during the first months of pregnancy. Consuming sufficient folic acid before conception and during early pregnancy greatly reduces the risk of having a baby with neural tube defects (see Chapter 27).

Bones of the spinal column (vertebrae) protect the spinal cord. With spina bifida, the vertebrae do not close properly, leaving the spinal cord unprotected. The spinal cord contains nerves that send messages to and from the brain, and because the spinal cord is unprotected in spina bifida, nerve damage occurs. Affected body parts do not function properly, and partial or complete paralysis and loss of bowel and bladder control may result. Infection of the exposed spinal cord is a risk.

Spina bifida can occur anywhere in the spine. The lower back is the most common site. Types of spina bifida include:

- ***Spina bifida occulta***—(*occult* means hidden)—is the mildest form of spina bifida. A slight deficiency occurs in the vertebrae closure. However, the spinal cord and the membranes (*meninges*) that cover it remain in place. Skin usually covers the defect. In other words, the defect is hidden. The person may have a dimple or tuft of hair on the back (Figure 39–3). The spinal cord and nerves are normal. It rarely causes disability. Often there are no symptoms. Foot weakness and bowel and bladder problems may occur.
- ***Spina bifida cystica***—(*cystica* means cyst or sac)—part of the spinal column is in a pouch or sac that protrudes from the opening in the spine. A membrane or a thin layer of skin covers the sac, which looks like a large blister. Because the pouch is easily injured, infection is a risk. There are two types of spina bifida cystica (Figure 39–4):
  - *Meningocele*—(*menigo* comes from *meninx*, meaning membrane; *cele* means hernia or swelling). Meninges are the connective membranes that cover and protect the brain and spinal cord. Cerebrospinal fluid also protects the brain and spinal cord. With this type of spina bifida, a sac containing meninges and cerebrospinal fluid protrudes from the spine (see Figure 39–4 *A*, and Figure 39–5). The sac does not contain nerve tissue. The spinal cord and nerves are usually unaffected, and nerve damage usually does not occur. This defect can be corrected by surgery.
  - *Myelomeningocele* (or *meningomyelocele*)—(*myelo* means spinal cord). With this type of spina bifida, a sac containing nerves, a part of the spinal cord, meninges, and cerebrospinal fluid protrudes from the spine (see Figure 39–4 *B*). This is the most common

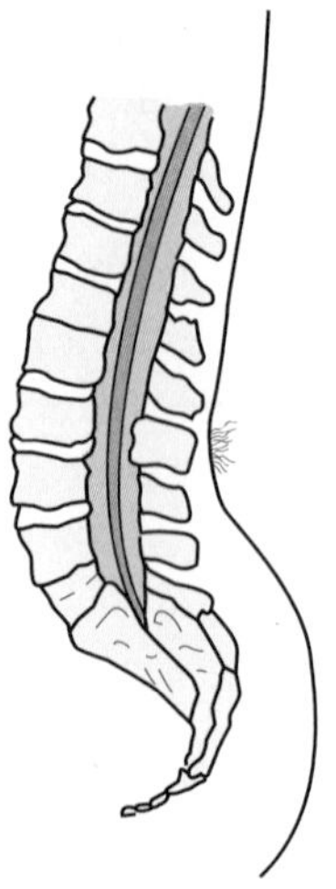

Figure 39–3 Spina bifida occulta.

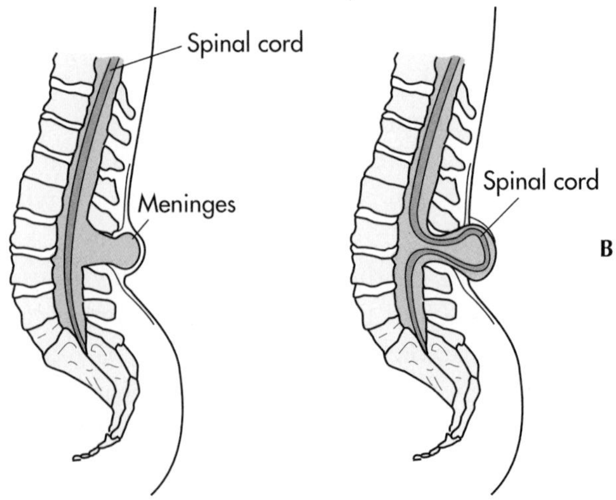

Figure 39–4 Spina bifida. **A,** Meningocele. **B,** Myelomeningocele.

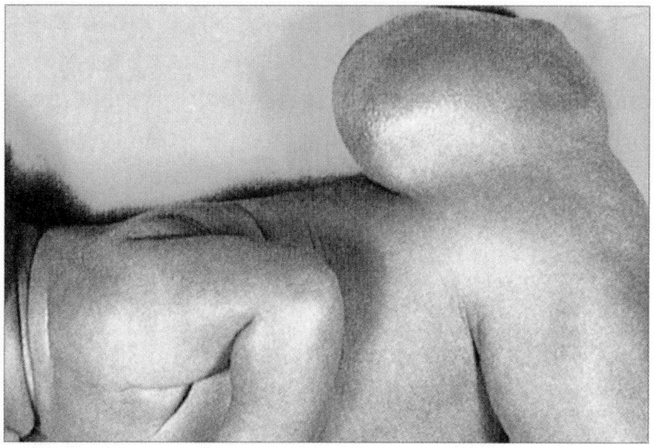

Figure 39–5 Meningocele. Surgery is performed to close the infant's back shortly after birth. **Source:** Zitelli, B.J., & Davis, H.W. (1987). *Atlas of pediatric physical diagnosis.* St. Louis: Gower Medical Publishing.

and most serious form of spina bifida, where there is severe nerve damage. The spinal cord is damaged or not properly developed. Loss of function occurs below the level of damage. Leg paralysis, lack of sensation, and lack of bowel and bladder control are common problems. The baby's back is closed with surgery, usually soon after birth. Some children and adults walk with braces or crutches, while some others will need wheelchairs.

Clients with spina bifida may have other problems or conditions, for example, learning problems, and problems with attention, language, reading, and math. They are at risk for obesity, gastrointestinal disorders, and mobility problems. Skin breakdown, depression, and social, emotional, and sexual issues are other risks. Hydrocephalus often occurs with certain types of spina bifida (see Table 39–1 on pages 738–739).

Fetal Alcohol Syndrome

Fetal alcohol syndrome (FAS) is a group of physical and mental abnormalities in a child as a result of alcohol consumption by the mother during pregnancy. In Canada, one child is born with FAS every day. It is the most common preventable developmental disability.

Physical problems include low birth weight, weak muscle tone, and poor weight gain. Heart problems, hearing loss, and abnormalities of the spine and joints may also occur. The client may have characteristic facial features, including an abnormally small head, small eye openings, thin upper lip, and a small chin.

Usually the client with FAS has an intellectual disability and often has many behavioural, learning, and emotional problems, including poor attention span, hyperactivity, poor motor skills, and slow language development. Older children and adults with FAS often have memory problems, poor judgement, difficulties with daily living skills, inability to manage anger, poor social skills, and mental health problems. Many adolescents with FAS drop out of school and get into trouble with the law. Many adults with FAS are unable to work or live independently. They require ongoing support. Women with FAS can have a normal baby as long as they do not consume alcohol during pregnancy.

Fetal alcohol effect (FAE) is a milder form of FAS, in which the same symptoms as FAS may occur, but to a lesser degree. Children with FAE are not usually intellectually disabled.

CARING FOR CLIENTS WITH DEVELOPMENTAL DISABILITIES

Clients with developmental disabilities often have complex care needs, especially if the disability is severe. You must be familiar with special equipment and self-help devices needed for each client. Follow the care plan, and consult with your supervisor if you have questions. For example, Gordon, 10, has severe cerebral palsy. He cannot walk and has limited use of his hands. He tends to slide down in his wheelchair, so a postural support is used to help keep him in good body alignment. He must be repositioned frequently to prevent pressure ulcers. Gordon also has a hearing impairment; he wears hearing aids in both ears and uses a computer to communicate. Gordon has splints on his ankles to prevent contractures. He uses a special spoon strapped to his wrist to help him eat.

When working with children and adults with developmental disabilities, remember to consider the client before the disability. For example, Frank is an intelligent, sensitive 10-year-old, who enjoys reading, going on outings, and visiting with his support worker. He also happens to have severe cerebral palsy and uses a wheelchair.

Clients with developmental disabilities have the same rights and needs as everyone else. Each client is unique. The effects of the disability vary depending on the client. Your supervisor and the care plan will tell you how to best meet each client's needs. As always, your priority when caring for these clients is to promote their dignity, independence, preferences, privacy, and safety (see the *Providing Compassionate Care: Caring for Clients With Developmental Disabilities* box.)

PROVIDING COMPASSIONATE CARE

Caring for Clients With Developmental Disabilities

- **Dignity.** Adults and children with developmental disabilities deserve to be treated with respect and in a manner that promotes their dignity. Remember to consider the client before the disability. The words you use are an important way to show respect. For example, say "clients with disabilities." Do not refer to them as "handicapped," "disabled," or "crippled." Also, do not identify the client by his or her disability. For example, it is correct to say "Mr. Joshi has autism." Do not say "Mr. Joshi is autistic." Say "Susan has an intellectual disability," not "Susan is retarded."

  Have empathy, not pity. Remember, empathy is understanding the experiences and feelings of others; pity is feeling sorry for others, which implies that you are superior to the person.

  Also, promote dignity through your actions. Extend the same courtesies and consideration that you show all clients. Be friendly, and talk with the client. Be a good listener, and show interest in their lives. Children with disabilities are like all children and need attention and love. They also need to play and have fun. Adults with disabilities are like all adults and need support and encouragement. Treat them like adults. Shake hands when introduced. Offer to shake hands even if the client has an artificial limb, has limited function in the hand, or has to shake with the left hand. Speak directly to the client in a normal tone of voice. Address adults by their title and last name, unless they tell you otherwise.
- **Independence.** The goal for clients with disabilities is to be as independent as possible. Do not make assumptions about what the client can and cannot do. Follow the care plan. Encourage the client to use self-help devices, whenever possible. Be patient, and do not rush the client.
- **Preferences.** Clients with disabilities have the right to personal choices. Provide opportunities for the client to make choices and decisions. Ask first if the client wants help and how you can provide help. Clients with disabilities must consent to procedures before you start. If the client does not want you to continue, stop. Contact your supervisor. Also, adapt your work to allow for the family's choices and preferences (unless directed otherwise in the care plan).
- **Privacy.** Medical and personal information about the client is confidential. Talk about the client only with members of the health care team who need to know. Do not expose the client. Provide privacy when performing procedures. Drape the client so as to not expose the client's body. Remember that adults with disabilities have sexual needs. Many have partners or are married. Allow for privacy for sexual practices.
- **Safety.** Most developmental disabilities create safety hazards for the client. Check with your supervisor and the care plan to determine how to ensure the client's safety. Practise the safety measures described in Chapter 19. Also, be alert to note signs of abuse. Report these to your supervisor immediately. Remember, you also must report child abuse directly to a public authority (see Chapter 21).

REVIEW

Answers to these questions are at the bottom of the page.

Circle the **BEST** answer.

1. **All developmental disabilities occur:**
   - A. During adulthood
   - B. From trauma
   - C. During pregnancy
   - D. Before birth, at birth, or during childhood or adolescence
2. **These statements are about developmental disabilities. Which one is *true*?**
   - A. Self-care, learning, and mobility are always affected
   - B. The disability is permanent
   - C. Physical and intellectual impairment always occur together
   - D. The person cannot hold a job
3. **All people with intellectual disabilities:**
   - A. Cannot learn new skills
   - B. Have IQ scores over 90
   - C. Require care in a special setting
   - D. Have an impaired ability to learn
4. **An intellectual disability:**
   - A. Is always severe
   - B. Is an inability to learn
   - C. Causes fluid to collect in the brain
   - D. Affects the motor region in the brain
5. **Down syndrome occurs:**
   - A. At fertilization
   - B. During the first month of pregnancy
   - C. Any time before, during, or after birth
   - D. From trauma
6. **A person with Down syndrome always has some degree of:**
   - A. Cerebral palsy
   - B. Autism
   - C. Impaired mobility
   - D. Intellectual disability
7. **Cerebral palsy is usually caused by:**
   - A. An extra chromosome
   - B. A high fever
   - C. Lack of oxygen to the brain
   - D. Infection during pregnancy
8. **A person with the spastic type of cerebral palsy has problems with:**
   - A. Learning
   - B. Drooling
   - C. Posture, balance, and movement
   - D. Weaving motions of the trunk, arms, and legs
9. **Symptoms of autism appear:**
   - A. At fertilization
   - B. During pregnancy
   - C. At birth
   - D. In early childhood
10. **A person with autism has:**
    - A. Impaired movement
    - B. Problems relating to people
    - C. Diplegia
    - D. A buildup of an amino acid in the blood
11. **A person with epilepsy always has:**
    - A. Seizures
    - B. Diplegia
    - C. Weak muscle tone
    - D. Low IQ
12. **Which of the following is used to control epilepsy?**
    - A. Physical therapy
    - B. Occupational therapy
    - C. Medications
    - D. A shunt
13. **Spina bifida involves:**
    - A. Improper closing of the spine
    - B. Seizures
    - C. Abnormalities in the structure of the heart
    - D. Changes in the X chromosome
14. **Which of the following is common with spina bifida?**
    - A. Short attention span
    - B. Hearing and vision problems
    - C. Seizures
    - D. Bowel and bladder problems
15. **Fetal alcohol syndrome is caused by:**
    - A. Acquired brain injury
    - B. Shaking an infant
    - C. The mother drinking alcohol during pregnancy
    - D. Abnormal chromosomes

Answers: 1.D, 2.B, 3.D, 4.B, 5.A, 6.D, 7.C, 8.C, 9.D, 10.B, 11.A, 12.C, 13.A, 14.D, 15.C

CHAPTER 40

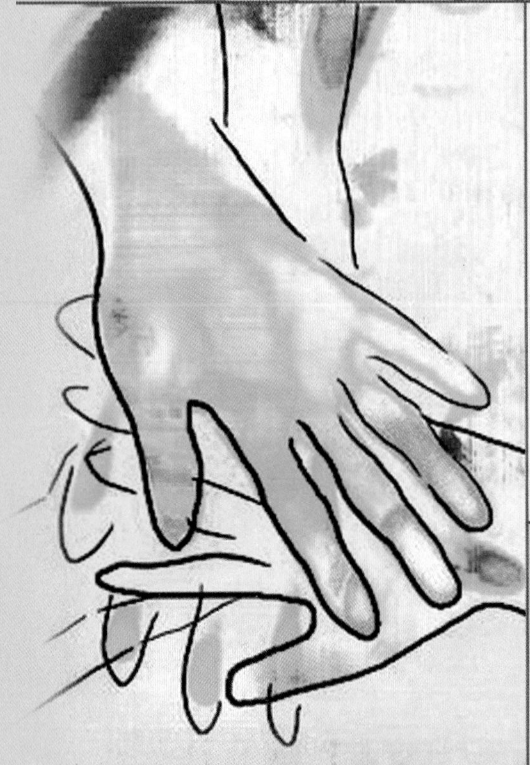

Assisting With Medications

OBJECTIVES

- Define the key terms listed in this chapter.
- Identify your role in assisting with medications.
- Summarize how drugs work in the body.
- List factors affecting drug action.
- List the different forms of medications.
- Differentiate between *assisting* with medications and *administering* medications.
- Identify guidelines to follow when assisting with medications.
- List the eight "rights" of assisting with medications.
- Summarize what you would do if you made a medication error.
- Outline your main responsibilities when assisting with medications.
- Apply the procedures described in this chapter.

key terms

absorption The passage of a drug from the site of administration into the bloodstream.

adverse effect An undesireable, posssibly harmful drug side effect.

alternative remedies Herbal or other "natural" products that do not require a physician's prescription; not considered part of conventional medicine.

anaphylaxis A life-threatening sensitivity to a substance (antigen).

antigen A substance, usually a protein, that the body recognizes as foreign and that can evoke an immune response.

blister pack A transparent moulded piece of plastic with multiple compartments, sealed to a sheet of cardboard with a foil backing, used to package individual-dose medications. Also known as *bubble pack*.

distribution The path the drug takes from the bloodstream to the body tissues of the intended site of action.

dosette, pill box Containers that store medications in separate compartments arranged by day or hour (see Figure 40–2).

drug antagonism An unusually weak drug effect that occurs when taking two or more drugs at the same time.

drug synergism An unusually strong drug effect that occurs when taking two or more drugs at the same time.

excretion The way the drug exits the body; excreted through the stool, urine, or skin.

generic name of drug The name given to a drug approved by Health Canada. It is also known as the "official name" of a drug.

medication A drug or other substance used to prevent or treat disease or illness.

metabolization Chemical reactions that take place to convert a drug from smaller molecules into waste products before it can exit the body. Most drugs are metabolized in the liver.

metered dose inhaler (MDI) A pressurized canister of medication, surrounded by a plastic case that has a mouthpiece. Pressing the MDI releases a single dose of medication as a mist.

over-the-counter (OTC) medication A medication that can be bought without a physician's prescription.

prescription (Rx) medication A medication that is prescribed by a physician and dispensed by a pharmacist.

route How a medication enters and is absorbed in the body.

scope of practice The legal limits of a health care role.

side effect A response to a medication that occurs in addition to the intended or main response.

therapeutic Causing a desired, positive effect in the body.

trade name of drug The name given to a drug by the manufacturer. Also known as *proprietary name.*

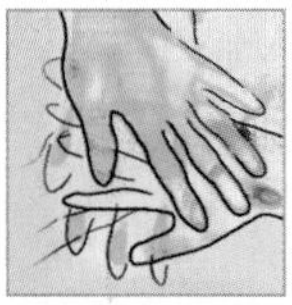

Medications are drugs and other substances used to prevent or treat diseases or illnesses. Many clients living in community settings take their medications independently. This is called *self-directed medication management*. This chapter discusses how support workers assist clients with medications.

As a support worker, you may be responsible for assisting a client with his or her medication in many different situations and settings. For example, if you work in a retirement home or group home, this may be one of your duties. Some clients need assistance when taking medications when they are not able to reach the medicines or get them out of the container.

This chapter is adapted from: Birchenall, J., & Streight, E. (1997). *Mosby's textbook for the home care aide*. St. Louis: Mosby; Lilley, L. L., Harrington, S., Snyder, J. S., & Swart, B. (2007). *Pharmacology and the nursing process in Canada*. Toronto: Mosby Elsevier. The author acknowledges the contributions of the authors of these textbooks.

Some clients may have difficulty reading the labels on the medication containers or may be too shaky to take the medications themselves. ***Remember that assisting with medications must be specifically part of your job description and within your scope of practice in your province. You must also be taught how to do this for each client by either a Registered Nurse, a Licensed/Registered Practical Nurse or a Registered Psychiatric Nurse, depending on your province.*** (See Box 40–1.)

SCOPE OF PRACTICE: YOUR ROLE

Your role in assisting with medications depends on your provincial or territorial legislation, employer policy, and your training and education. Refer to Chapter 11 to read more about the laws that govern support workers across Canada. You may be required to assist a client with medications if you work in a client's home or in community settings (e.g., retirement homes or group homes). Ensure that you are clear about what your duties include and that you have been taught how to perform each of the tasks that you are expected to do.

Your role may involve *one or more* of the following:

- Reminding the client to take a medication
- Bringing medication containers to the client
- Bringing pre-poured medications, prefilled syringes, blister packs, or dosettes (pill boxes) to the client
- Reading the prescription label to the client
- Loosening or removing container lids or opening blister packs
- Checking the dosage against the medication label
- Providing water or other fluids, as needed
- Supervising the client as he or she places the medication into the hand, measuring spoon, or cup
- Steadying the client's hand while he or she places medications or administers eye drops, nasal sprays, and so on.
- Documenting the medications that you gave in the client's medication administration record (MAR), according to your agency's policy.

You are *not* responsible for monitoring the outcome of the drug therapy. The physician, RN, or case manager is responsible for this. However, you

Box 40–1 "Assisting" Versus "Administering" Medications

Assisting with medications and *administering* medications are two very different functions. Assist means *to help*; administer means *to give*.

Assisting with medications involves helping clients to self-medicate. For example, you hand them their medications, or you open the bottles or packages for them. This is strictly a *mechanical* function, that is, you perform the functions the client would normally perform with his or her hands/feet in order to obtain the medication.

Administering medications involves measuring medications or getting them into the person's body, and it requires special judgement and knowledge. Clients and residents in facilities usually have medications administered to them, and some home care clients also need health care workers to administer their medications. Administering medications is beyond your **scope of practice**. In some provinces, ***in some special circumstances,*** you may be asked by your supervisor to perform a controlled act, such as giving an insulin injection. Some provinces and territories allow support workers to administer some forms of medications under certain conditions. ***Never assume this responsibility, as this is beyond your usual scope of practice. If you are asked to administer medication, it is your employer's responsibility to ensure that you are formally trained, supervised, and monitored by a registered staff member. It is then your responsibility to ask questions for clarification and to safely follow those instructions. This function must be in your job description, as part of your employment agreement.***

A small mistake when assisting with or administering medications can cause serious harm. Follow employer policies and provincial/territorial laws to protect your clients, your employer, and yourself. When assisting with medications, follow the guidelines in Box 40–2. Check the care plan to see how much assistance is required.

Box 40–2 Guidelines for Assisting Clients With Medications

- Always follow employer policy.
- Always wash your hands, and work in a well-lit environment, away from avoidable distractions.
- Review the care plan with your supervisor before assisting the client with medications. Follow the eight "rights" of assisting with medications (see Box 40–3 on p. 761).
- Bring the right medication containers to the client. Read the labels carefully. Compare container labels with the care plan and the medication administration record (MAR).
- Know the correct dose of each medication. Check the care plan and the MAR.
- Give a glass of water (or other liquid) with oral medications, as ordered.
- Store medications:
  - In a special place just for the client's medications; the client's medications should be stored separately from those of others
  - In a cool but dry place (not in the bathroom medicine cabinet)
  - Out of reach of children and of adults with dementia
  - In the original labelled container
  - With lids tightly closed
  - According to any special storage directions, for example, "Store in the refrigerator"
- Do not leave medications at the client's bedside. Do not assume that the client will take them correctly. Remain with the client until he or she has finished taking the medications.
- Do not remove labels from the containers.
- Never use medication in a container that is unlabelled or that has an unreadable label.
- Do not use discolored or deteriorated medications. Check the expiry date on the labels before giving medications to the client. Notify your supervisor of expired or deteriorated medications.
- If you notice that the medications are running low, tell the client or family and your supervisor.
- Check with your supervisor before discarding any unused medications.
- Listen to the client. If he or she questions something about a medication, STOP—do not assist with self-medication. Call your supervisor immediately.
- Report to your supervisor if the client:
  - Does not take medications correctly
  - Does not understand why the medication should be taken and does not know the dosage or the schedule
  - Refuses to take the medication or forgets or omits a dose; the client should not take a double dose if one is omitted
  - Shows any side effects (for example, vomiting, rash, breathing difficulty, itching, or diarrhea)
  - Wants to take medications (including OTC medications or alternative remedies) that are not listed on the MAR and care plan
- Record your actions, according to employer policy. When applicable, the client records on the MAR. Assist, as directed.
- Report and record if a medication is not taken or is omitted. Explain why.

must observe for and report any changes in the client's condition or behaviour.

The nurse or pharmacist teaches the client about the medications he or she is taking. After this, clients should be able to take medications accurately and know the medication's desired effect, when and how to take the medication, any side effects to watch for, and foods or other medications to avoid or omit. If your client does not have this information, notify your supervisor.

Many clients receive their medications in a **blister pack**, or bubble pack, (Figure 40–1). Blister packs are supplied by the client's pharmacy with the client's medications for that day or time grouped together, plastic heat-sealed to a cardboard card. Clients would then open the appropriate blister pack (or direct you to do it for them) and take their medications.

Clients often store medications in a **dosette**, which is also known as a **pill box** (Figure 40–2). Dosettes have compartments that organize the medications by day or by hour. They help clients remember what they have taken and what medications remain to be taken each day. If the client is

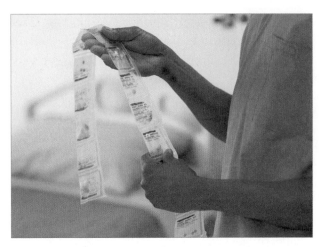

Figure 40–1 Blister (bubble) packs are supplied by the client's pharmacy and contain the medications the client has to take at that time. **Source:** Brian Hillier.

unable to fill the dosette, a nurse or family member may do so. This is *not* your responsibility.

When you assist a client with medications in the client's home or in community settings such as retirement homes or group homes, ensure that you are clear about what your duties include. Check with your employer or supervisor should you have any questions. Remember that medication errors can easily occur and that they are always avoidable!

Always check to find out if the client is allergic to the medication you are about to give. Allergies should be listed on the MAR. Clients may be wearing Medic Alert bracelets that indicate any drug allergies (Figure 40–3).

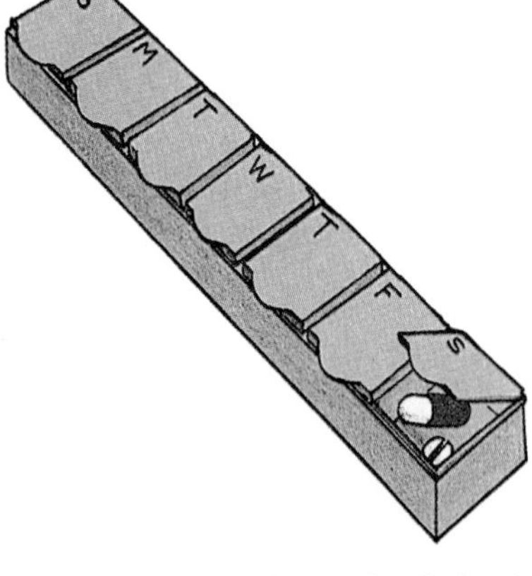

Figure 40–2 Dosettes are pill boxes that help clients keep track of their daily medications. **Source:** Birchenall, J., & Streight, E. (2003). *Mosby's textbook for the home care aide* (2nd ed., p. 348). St. Louis: Mosby.

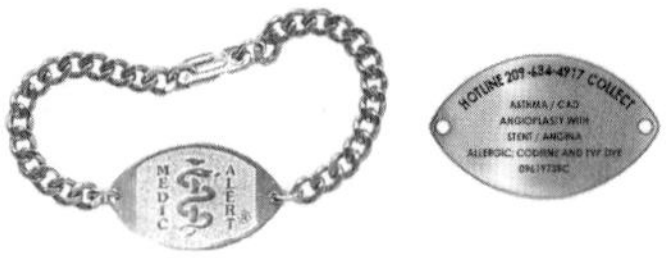

Figure 40–3 A MedicAlert bracelet has the client's emergency medical information, including drug allergies, engraved on the back. **Source:** Potter, P.A., Perry, A.G., Ross-Kerr, J.C., & Wood, M.J. (2006). *Canadian fundamentals of nursing* (3rd ed., p. 839). Toronto: Elsevier.

HOW MEDICATIONS WORK IN THE BODY

Purpose of Medications

Medications (drugs) are chemical substances that cause a specific effect on the body and are prescribed and taken by people to obtain various desired results in the body. Some medications might *treat illness* or pain—for example, aspirin to reduce the pain of a headache. Other medications *promote health*—for example, a stool softener to help reduce discomfort during bowel movement. And some medications *prevent illness*—for example, an antibiotic to prevent possible development of an infection after surgery.

Drug Action

Medications enter the body in a variety of ways. *How* the medication enters the body (in order for it to start working) is known as the **route.** The medications listed in Table 40–1 refer to some types of medications and their routes. Some other types of medication such as injections and intravenous medications are not included in the table because you will not be responsible for assisting with or administering them.

Depending on the route, the body must *absorb* and *distribute* the drug in order for it to work and *metabolize* the drug to prepare to rid the remaining materials (molecules of the drug the body no longer needs) from the body, that is, *excrete* them from the body. For example, the blood pressure pill that a client swallows must enter the stomach, be broken down into small molecules, enter the bloodstream (**absorption**), and travel throughout the body to reach its intended tissues (**distribution**) so that it can cause the intended effect. After the drug has done what it was intended to do in the body, it must be then broken down into smaller waste particles and sometimes converted into other substances the body can then use (i.e, **metabolization**, which usually takes place in the liver), and then be removed from the body, usually in the stool or in the urine **(excretion).**

Table 40–1 Types of Medications and Their Routes

Route	Form	Description	
Oral: Solids or semi-solids	Capsules	Small gelatin containers that hold medications	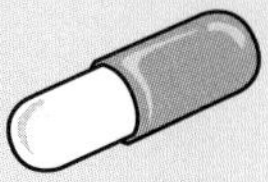
	Lozenges	Flat discs containing medication in a flavoured base. Lozenges are held in the mouth, where they dissolve and slowly release medication	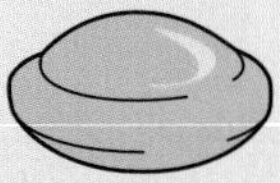
	Tablets	Dry, powdered medications that have been formed into hard disks or cylinders	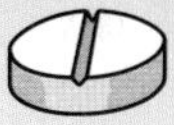
Oral: Liquids	Elixirs	Medication dissolved in liquid containing alcohol or water and flavourings	
	Suspensions	Medication suspended in a liquid and usually labelled "Shake before use"	
	Syrups	Medication dissolved in a concentrated sugar solution	
Topical	Ointments or creams	Semi-solid material containing medication; applied externally	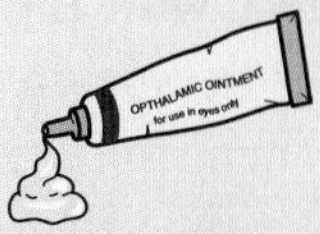
	Transdermal discs or patches	Medication on a small disc or patch that is applied to unbroken skin; absorbed through the skin over a 24-hour period	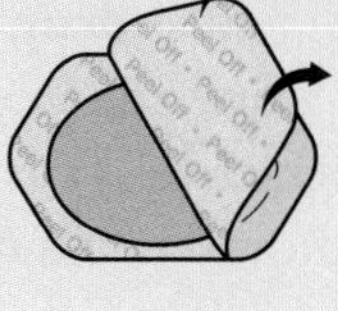
Eye, Ear	Drops	Liquid form of medication in a special container that allows one drop at a time to be administered; usually eye drops, ear drops, and nose drops	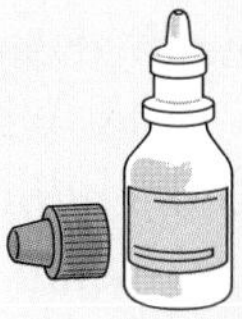
Parenteral	Liquid for injection	Liquid form of medication that is injected using a *syringe* (a device consisting of a plastic tube filled with medication, a plunger, and an attached needle)	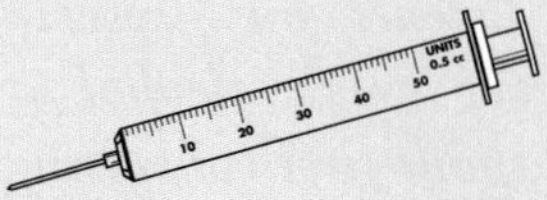

(continued on page 754)

Table 40–1 Types of Medications and Their Routes (cont'd)

Route	Solids	Description
Inhalation	Aerosols	Medication particles suspended in air or gas that are inhaled into the lungs; administered through a **metered dose inhaler (MDI).** An MDI ("puffer" or "inhaler") is a small cylinder used with a special delivery system. Many people use the MDI with holding chambers, especially if they are very young, old, or frail. The client uses it to inhale the medication through the mouth in specifically measured (metered) doses. 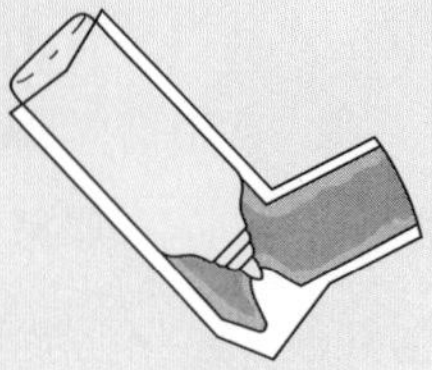
Suppositories	Rectal or vaginal	Solid form of medication for insertion into the rectum or vagina. Body temperature causes the suppository to dissolve and the medication is released and absorbed by the mucous membranes in this area 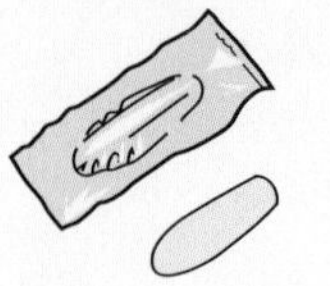

Source: Birchenall, J., & Streight, E. (2003). *Mosby's textbook for the home care aide* (2nd ed., p. 345). St. Louis: Mosby.

Drug Interactions

The way that medications interact with other drugs or substances in the body (e.g., alcohol) is also important, as mixing these substances may cause an undesirable effect on the client. For example, a client might take an **OTC (over-the-counter)** medication, and depending on its nature, it might interact with the prescription medication that his or her doctor prescribed.

When the combined effect of two drugs is greater than the effect of either drug given alone, it is known as **drug synergism.** This combined effect can cause the client to become extremely drowsy, hyperactive, or nauseated. When combined, some medications can even affect that client's heart function or blood pressure.

Some medications will counteract the actions of other drugs when combined. For example, an antacid might prevent an antibiotic or birth control pill from being absorbed in the stomach. This is called **drug antagonism.**

Clients on prescribed medications should never drink alcohol or take OTC medications without first consulting a doctor, pharmacist, or nurse, as serious harm may result from combining medications and other drugs or alcohol.

TYPES OF MEDICATIONS

Medications come in many forms. Table 40–1 lists some of the most common types.

Clients may take:

- ***Over-the-counter (OTC) medications***—medications that can be bought without a physician's prescription, for example, acetaminophen (brand name Tylenol) and cough syrup.
- ***Alternative remedies***—herbal or other "natural" products that do not require a physician's prescription, for example, ginseng and shark cartilage. Alternative remedies are usually not considered part of conventional medicine.
- ***Prescription (Rx) medications***—medications that require a physician's prescription and are dispensed by a pharmacist, for example, antibiotics and blood pressure medications.

You assist *only* with medications that are listed in the care plan. If a client requests your help with medications that are not in the care plan (including OTC medications and alternative remedies), notify your supervisor.

Clients might ask support workers to purchase or obtain OTC medications or alternative remedies for them. Refuse to do this respectfully, but firmly. Inform your supervisor about the client's request.

Drug Effects and Classifications

Medications can have *topical*, *local*, or *systemic* effects, according to *where* in the body the medication works. A cream that you rub on your skin might have a *topical* effect, that is, the cream only works on the skin surface. An eye drop medication might cause a *localized* effect, that is, it only works in the eye in which you put it. The pill that you take for your headache might have a *systemic* effect, that is, it might also help relieve pain elsewhere in your body.

Drugs are classified according to how they work—for example, an antibiotic works by eliminating or reducing harmful bacteria in the body. We can generalize that most antibiotics share some common side effects, so there will be common observations or responsibilities for you to keep in mind when assisting a client with taking them. You should know that in some clients, most drugs might cause nausea or vomiting.

Table 40–2 lists common responsibilities for you when giving medications under certain classifications, with an example of a common drug (both its generic and trade names) in each classification. The **generic name** of a drug refers to its chemical name, while the **trade name** refers to its trademarked, packaged name given by the manufacturer. ***While this list includes many of the main drug classifications and the observations or responsibilities that you might encounter in your support work, it does NOT address more complex issues, such as drug interactions, and does not discuss all of the necessary observations or responsibilities for each classification of drugs. These are only guidelines. You MUST check with your supervisor to find out if there are any specific observations that must be made for a particular client.***

Factors Affecting Drug Action

Drugs should be stored in a dry, safe place so that they do not undergo any chemical change. Most drugs should never be stored in direct sunlight, and some drugs need to be stored in the refrigerator in order to remain chemically stable. You must read the label on the drug container and follow the instructions carefully.

The same drug can affect two people very differently because one person's body cells differ from those of another person, according to age, body size, sex, genetic factors, emotional state, and physical condition. Table 40–3 briefly describes how each of these factors effect drug actions.

Side Effects

Most medications have side effects. A **side effect** is another response to a medication that occurs along with the intended response. For example, some blood pressure pills will cause a client's heart rate to slow down; or a person taking pain medication may experience pain relief as well as drowsiness, nausea, and constipation. Many side effects are predictable and harmless, but some can be so serious or harmful (these are called **adverse effects**) that the physician may order the medication to be stopped.

Drug Allergy

A drug allergy is an abnormal response to a drug caused by the body fighting or attacking the drug (which is then called an **antigen**) by releasing chemicals called *antibodies*. Antibodies attack the antigen and can cause symptoms ranging from mild (skin rashes, swelling, puffiness, nasal drainage, itchy eyes), to moderate (fever, wheezing, extreme weakness, nausea, and vomiting), to severe (anaphylactic shock, severe low blood pressure, cardiac arrest).

Anaphylaxis—from the Greek *ana* (without) and *phylaxis* (protection)—is life-threatening sensitivity to an antigen. In severe cases, anaphylactic shock can occur within seconds. Signs and symptoms include:

- Sweating
- Shortness of breath

- Low blood pressure
- Irregular pulse
- Respiratory congestion
- Swelling of the larynx (laryngeal edema)
- Hoarseness
- Dyspnea

Anaphylactic shock is an emergency, and the emergency medical service (EMS) system must be activated immediately. The client needs special medications, such as an Epinephrine Auto Injector, to reverse the allergic reaction. Until emergency help arrives, keep the client lying down, ensuring

Table 40–2 Drug Classifications and Your Responsibilities

Drug Classification	Drug Action	Example (generic and trade names)	Observations and Responsibilities
Alzheimer's medications	Treat mild to moderate symptoms of Alzheimer's disease	donepezil HCL (Aricept)	Report any nausea, diarrhea, vomiting, and muscle cramps. Client may be fatigued easily
Analgesics (non-narcotic)	Relieve mild to moderate pain	acetaminophen (Tylenol)	Might cause stomachache, so is often instructed to be taken with food
Analgesics (narcotic)	Relieve severe pain	acetaminophen 325 mg; caffeine & codeine 30 mg (Tylenol #3)	Report excessive drowsiness, constipation
Antacids	Relieve heartburn	calcium carbonate (TUMS)	Should not be taken within 2 hours of another medicine, as it might interfere with that drug's absorption
Anti-anginals	Relieve anginal chest pain	nitroglycerin (Nitrostat)	May cause dizziness in client. Wear gloves while handling some of these drugs to avoid a bad headache
Anti-anxiety medications	Reduce anxiety	lorazepam (Ativan)	Might cause drowsiness and sleepiness; client should be careful when driving
Antibiotics	Eliminate or reduce harmful bacteria	ampicillin (Novo-Ampicillin)	Check for diarrhea, vomiting. Some clients may experience a bitter aftertaste. Ensure clients finish the entire course prescribed, unless told not to by the doctor or pharmacist
Anticoagulants	Reduce blood clotting	dalteparin sodium (Fragmin)	May make clients more prone to bruising and bleeding; they must use care when brushing teeth or shaving. Report bruises on body, blood in urine
Anticonvulsants	Reduce seizures	phenytoin sodium (Dilantin)	Make sure that mouth care is done often. Thickening of the gingiva may cause tenderness when brushing teeth
Anti-emetics	Reduce nausea, motion sickness	Scopolamine (Transderm-V)	Make sure the client has good mouth care to eliminate mouth sores and bad taste in mouth

(continued on page 757)

Table 40–2 Drug Classifications and Your Responsibilities (cont'd)

Drug Classification	Drug Action	Example (generic and trade names)	Observations and Responsibilities
Antihypertensives	Reduce blood pressure	ramipril (Altace)	Client should get up slowly to avoid dizziness or lightheadedness
Anti-parkinsonian agents	Reduce symptoms of Parkinson's disease	levodopa-carbidopa (Sinemet)	Report dizziness, pain, drowsiness, or irritability
Anti-psychotics	Reduce psychosis, severe agitation, severe vomiting, or hiccups	haloperidol (Haldol)	Watch for hand tremors and dizziness. Notify the nurse if you see any grimacing
Anti-tussives	Liquefy phlegm, making it easier to cough	dextromethorphan (Robitussin DM)	Should be taken *after* taking other drugs; clients must not drink fluids for 10 to 15 minutes to give chance for drug to be absorbed into throat tissues
Anti-virals	Reduce virus reproduction	acyclovir (Zovirax)	Headache, nausea
Bronchodilators	Reduce spasm in breathing passages	salbutamol (Ventolin)	Watch for dry mouth. May cause shakiness and tremors in hands and increased heart rate in clients
Decongestants	Reduce nasal congestion	pseudoephedrine (Sudafed)	May cause dry mucous membranes and rebound congestion (congestion gets worse after drug wears off)
Diuretics	Lower blood pressure and body swelling by increasing urinary output	furosemide (Lasix)	Depending on drug, some clients must eat more potassium-rich foods (bananas, baked white potatoes); more frequent urination
Hypoglycemic agents	Improve insulin production in body	glyberide (Diabeta)	Report any nausea, vomiting, diarrhea, dizziness, or weakness
Insulin	Makes up for lack of natural insulin	insulin regular, human biosynthetic (Humulin-R)	Report any blurred vision, dry mouth, extreme hunger, or chest palpitations
Laxatives	Help with bowel movements	bisacodyl (Dulcolax)	May cause diarrhea; encourage plenty of fluids and high-fibre diet to reduce need for laxatives
Nonsteroidal anti-inflammatory drugs (NSAIDs)	Reduce pain that comes with swelling	ibuprofen (Motrin)	May cause upset stomach, so should never be taken on an empty stomach
Thyroid replacements	Make up for lack of natural thyroid	levothyroxine sodium (Eltroxin)	Report menstrual irregularities, nausea, or vomiting

Table 40–3 Factors Affecting Drug Actions in the Body

Factor Affecting Drug Action in the Body	Description
Age	Young children and older adults may absorb, distribute, metabolize, and excrete drugs very differently from the way young adults do because their digestive organs may not be efficient enough.
Body size	A dose of medication that would be **therapeutic** in a large, overweight adult might be an overdose in a small, thin adult of the same age because the drug level would be more concentrated in the small person. Note that some drugs are stored in the adipose tissue, and this could lead to a buildup of that drug in the body over time.
Sex	Drugs affect men and women differently, depending on their body sizes, hormones, and other factors such as muscle mass.
Genetic factors	Some people have an inherited tendency to react to certain medications—for example, if Mr. Jones had a very unusual reaction to an anaesthetic, doctors may choose not to give the same anaesthetic to his daughter.
Emotional state	A severe emotional state will usually cause a person's heart rate and blood pressure to change, which may, in turn, change the way a drug is absorbed, metabolized, and excreted.
Physical condition	Certain diseases will affect how well a drug is absorbed, distributed, metabolized, or excreted—for example, clients with kidney disease may not be able to excrete certain drugs through their urine as a person with healthy kidneys can.

that the airways are open. If cardiac arrest occurs, you must initiate CPR (cardio-pulmonary resuscitation) at once.

DOCUMENTATION

The client's medication needs and your responsibilities are detailed in the care plan as well as on the client's *medication administration record (MAR)*, which also serves as a record for actions taken. The exact form of the MAR varies by setting and employer. It always contains at least the following:

- The client's name
- The name, dose, and administration instructions for each medication
- A place to sign or initial after administering the medication

The MAR may also contain extra information, such as the client's allergies, expected side effects, and special instructions (Figure 40–4).

In facilities, a nurse is responsible for signing or initialling the MAR, and in some, an MAR is printed out daily for each client.

In community settings, an MAR is kept only when it is necessary to track specific medications and dosages. Clients who administer their own medications may not need an MAR, but when one is required, it is kept in the client's home. If a nurse administers the medications, the nurse signs the MAR. If the client self-medicates, the client signs the MAR as taught by the nurse. Observe as the client records the information on the MAR after the medication has been taken. Some clients may not be able to write because of physical disability or vision problems, and you may then need to do the recording for these clients.

MEDICATION ADMINISTRATION RECORD

Name:	Delbert Sullivan	Allergies:			Doctor's Name: J. Smith			
Day		SUN	MON	TUE	WED	THUR	FRI	SAT
Date		7/11	7/12	7/13	7/14	7/15	7/16	7/17
Drug Name	Lasix (water pill)							
Dose	1 tablet							
Action	Increases urination							
Time	One (1) daily	8 a.m.	8 a.m.	8 a.m.	8 a.m.	8 a.m.	8 a.m.	8 a.m.
		JKS						
Special Instructions	Daily weight at 8 a.m.							
	Drink plenty of fluids.							
	Watch for and report any weight gain or swelling.							
	Do not omit or increase dosage.							
	Call doctor if unable to take medication.							
Immediately Report								

Day		SUN	MON	TUE	WED	THUR	FRI	SAT
Date		7/11	7/12	7/13	7/14	7/15	7/16	7/17
Drug Name	Ferrous Sulfate (iron pill)							
Dose	1 tablet							
Action	Replaces iron in blood							
Time	Three (3) times daily	9 a.m.	9 a.m.	9 a.m.	9 a.m.	9 a.m.	9 a.m.	9 a.m.
		1 p.m.	1 p.m.	1 p.m.	1 p.m.	1 p.m.	1 p.m.	1 p.m.
		5 p.m.	5 p.m.	5 p.m.	5 p.m.	5 p.m.	5 p.m.	5 p.m.
		JKS						
		JKS						
		JKS						
Special Instructions	Take between meals.							
	Take with full glass of water.							
	Do not take with milk or antacids.							
	Will change colour of stool to black.							
	Do not crush tablet.							
	May cause constipation.							
Immediately Report	Nausea, vomiting, and diarrhea							
	Abdominal pain							

Figure 40–4 A sample medication administration record (MAR). **Source:** Birchenall, J., & Streight, E. (2003). *Mosby's textbook for the home care aide* (2nd ed., p. 347). St. Louis: Mosby.

Follow your employer's policies and procedures for recording. Ask your supervisor for help, if needed.

Understanding Abbreviations

An abbreviation is a shortened form of a word or phrase. The list on the inside back cover of this textbook gives the more common abbreviations used in health care settings. Physicians, nurses, and pharmacists use many abbreviations when ordering and managing medications. The care plan and MAR should present information as clearly as possible. However, sometimes abbreviations are used in these documents. Check with your supervisor about abbreviations used by your employer, especially when you are unsure about the meaning of an abbreviation. Never guess about the meaning of an abbreviation, as this can cause serious harm to the client.

THE EIGHT "RIGHTS" OF ASSISTING WITH MEDICATIONS

To help clients take medications accurately and safely, know and follow the eight "rights" of assisting with medications (see Box 40–3):

1. ***The right medication.*** Be sure you are assisting the client to take the right medication. The name of the medication is printed on the prescription label on the medication container (Figure 40–5). Read the label carefully, and make sure it is the same medication listed in the care plan and the MAR. Check twice.
2. ***The right person.*** Be sure the medication is for your client. Check the prescription label on the medication container, and make sure it has the client's name (both first and last names). In some homes and facilities, two clients may have the same name. Make sure you are assisting the right client. Identify the client following employer policy.
3. ***The right dose.*** The dose is listed on the prescription label, the care plan, and the MAR—for example, "Take one tablet daily" or "Apply ointment to left elbow twice a day." The correct amount of medication must be taken. For example, when Mrs. Jong removes two tablets from the container, whereas the prescription label and her care plan say that she has to take only one tablet at a time, you must point that out to her.

When the medication is in liquid form, the dose measurements may be in imperial (ounces), household (teaspoons or table-

Box 40–3 The Eight "Rights" of Assisting With Medications

1. ***Right medication.*** Read the container label. Check against the MAR and care plan.
2. ***Right person.*** Read the container label. Be sure the medication is for the client. Identify the client, according to employer policies.
3. ***Right dose.*** Be sure you know how much medication the client should be taking.
4. ***Right route.*** Be sure you know the correct route and form of the medication.
5. ***Right time.*** Bring medication to the client at correct time, or remind the client to take medications.
6. ***Right day.*** Ensure the medication is meant for that specific day.
7. ***Right expiry date.*** Always check that the medication has not expired.
8. ***Right documentation.*** Be sure to document the medication correctly, according to your agency policy.

If you have any questions or problems with any of these eight "rights," notify your supervisor.

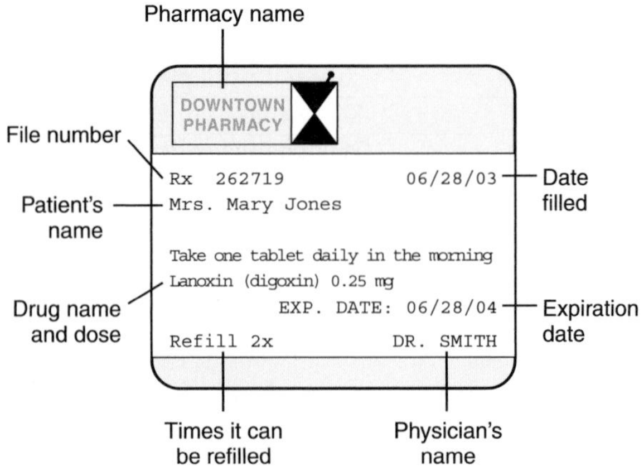

Figure 40–5 Read the prescription label before the client takes any medications. **Source:** Birchenall, J., & Streight, E. (2003). *Mosby's textbook for the home care aide* (2nd ed., p. 349). St. Louis: Mosby.

spoons), or metric (millilitres) units. Be sure the client does not measure in teaspoons when the prescription calls for millilitres. Make sure the client uses measuring spoons and measuring cups—not household spoons or cups—to measure doses.

4. ***The right route.*** The method in which the medication is taken is called the route. The prescription label, care plan, and MAR list the route. The routes are as follows:
   - *Oral*—taken by mouth and swallowed. Cough syrup is an example.
   - *Sublingual*—placed under the tongue. These are pills, tablets, or sprays that are dissolved or absorbed into the body.
   - *Topical*—applied to the skin or mucous membranes. Some topical medications are contained within the area where they are applied, for example, ointments, eye drops, and nose drops. Some are absorbed into the bloodstream and travel throughout the body, for example, transdermal discs or patches. Suppositories and medicated enemas are also topical medications because they are applied to the mucous membranes (in the rectum or vagina).
   - *Inhalant*—breathed in through the mouth or nose. Medication must be in a gas or aerosol form, for example, oxygen and medications delivered by MDIs.
   - *Parenteral*—injected by a needle into the muscle (intramuscular), a vein (intravenous), or under the skin (subcutaneous). Insulin and IV drips are examples.

   In some provinces, in some special circumstances, you may be asked by your supervisor to perform a controlled act, such as giving an insulin injection. Some provinces and territories allow support workers to administer some forms of medications under certain conditions. Never assume this responsibility, as this is beyond your usual scope of practice!

5. ***The right time.*** In order to work properly, medications must be taken at the correct time. Medications may have to be taken once a day or two, three, or four times a day, which is stated on the prescription label. For example, Mrs. Jong's prescription label states that the medication must be taken three times a day. The care plan and MAR state the exact times that the client needs to take the medication. For example, Mrs. Jong's care plan and MAR state that she should take her medication at 0600h, 1400h, and 2200h. Ensure that medications are given at the specified times. Taking medications at the wrong time of the day or taking them too close to or too far from meals and other medications can reduce their effectiveness and can even cause serious side effects.

   Some medications have to be taken when the stomach is empty—that is, 1 hour before or 2 hours after a meal. Other medications need to be taken at mealtime to reduce stomach irritation and promote absorption. The prescription labels for these medications will say "Take on empty stomach" or "Take with food or milk." Sometimes clients must avoid certain foods or beverages when taking medications. Often it is strongly recommended that alcohol and tobacco be avoided. Follow the warning labels on the prescription containers and the care plan.

   Sometimes clients are confused about when to take their medications. A client may say, "I can never remember. Do I take two tablets at 3 o'clock, or three tablets at 2 o'clock?" Tell your supervisor if this happens. The client may need a "refresher" course on taking medications properly.

   Assist the client to take all medications at the right time. If you go on an outing with the client, bring along the medications that must be taken at that time.

6. ***The right day.*** Not all medications are taken daily; some are taken every second or third day. You need to check the MAR to ensure that the medication the client is taking is meant for *that* day.

7. ***The right expiry date.*** Just like foods, medications also have expiry dates and should *never* be taken beyond their expiry date. In time, some medications either lose their potency (strength) or may even change chemically and become toxic for that client. If you ever have doubts about the expiry date, you should always check with your supervisor *before* assisting with that medication.

8. ***The right documentation.*** Any medication that is given must be documented properly, according to your agency policy. Medications are usually documented in the MAR. It is your responsibility to document any medication that you have assisted the client to take. If you have any questions about this, you need to ask your supervisor (this should be a nurse) to clarify it for you.

MEDICATION ERRORS

If you believe that you have made a drug error (or you notice a drug error that might have been committed by someone else), you need to report this to your supervisor immediately! It is the supervisor's responsibility to assess the situation and to determine the next course of action. ***Deliberate failure to report a medication error is possible grounds for immediate dismissal (losing your job) or civil action (being charged in a court of law with an offence).*** You are required to report the error, even if you think it might get you into trouble! ***You can be in more trouble if you fail to report the error than from making the error itself!***

Some errors are caused by problems in technique (such as dropping a pill down the sink by accident), by omission (such as forgetting to give a medication), by incorrectly documenting a medication, or by failing to follow any of the eight "rights." ***A drug error can cause severe harm to the client, so errors should always be reported!***

Usually, an incident report must be filled out by you and your supervisor and a copy kept with the client's chart. Incident report statistics can also identify if there is a problem that is something beyond your control (such as how the medication is labelled by the pharmacy), so it is important to include as many details as possible in the incident report. See Figure 19–29 for a sample of an incident report.

1 2 3 ASSISTING WITH ORAL MEDICATIONS

Remember to promote:

• **D**ignity • **I**ndependence • **P**references • **P**rivacy • **S**afety

Pre-Procedure

1 Identify the client, according to employer policy.
2 Explain the procedure to the client.
3 Practise hand hygiene.
4 Assist the client with hand washing.
5 Collect the following:
- Oral medications
- Standard measuring spoon, cup, or other measuring device
- Glass of water or other cool liquid
- Straw (optional)

6 Provide for privacy.

Procedure

For Medications From a Prescription Container:

7 Check label on each container (see Figure 40–5 on page 760) or on each pre-poured medication for: right medication, right person, right dose, right route, right time, right day, and right expiry date. Compare label with the MAR and care plan.
8 Loosen lid(s) on container(s), if the client cannot do so. Tell the client the name of each medication (read from the label).
9 Place the container where the client can reach it, or, hand the container to the client. Let the client read the name of the medication to you. Be sure the client wears eyeglasses, if needed.

For Medications From a Blister Pack:

7 Check blister pack label and check for: right medication, right person, right dose, right route, right time, right day, and right expiry date. Compare label with MAR and care plan.
8 Instruct the client to open the blister pack by pushing the soft plastic "bubble" and pushing the pills into a dish or saucer.

(continued on page 763)

1 2 3 ASSISTING WITH ORAL MEDICATIONS

Procedure (cont'd)

9 If the client cannot manually push open the blister pack, you can do this for the client.

For All Medications:

10 Help the client to pour the correct amount of liquid or to count the correct number of pills. Assist the client with oral medications:

- **a** If the medication is to be swallowed:
  - i. Give a sip of water to moisten the mouth
  - ii. Support the client's hand, as necessary, to pour medication
  - iii. Give a full glass of water or other cool liquid after the client puts the medication in the mouth
  - iv. Remind the client to lower the chin while swallowing
- **b** If the medication is to dissolve under the person's tongue:
  - i. Ask the client to put the medication under the tongue
  - ii. Ask the client to close the mouth and let the medication dissolve
  - iii. Remind the client not to chew or swallow the medication
  - iv. Do not give food or fluids while the medication is dissolving

11 Close the containers after use.

Post-Procedure

12 Have the client record the medications taken correctly, when applicable, or record for the client, if specified in the care plan.

13 Store materials in their proper locations.

14 Remove privacy measures.

15 Practise hand hygiene.

16 Report and record your actions and observations, according to employer policy.

1 2 3 ASSISTING WITH RECTAL SUPPOSITORIES OR ENEMAS

Remember to promote:

• **D**ignity • **I**ndependence • **P**references • **P**rivacy • **S**afety

Pre-Procedure

1 Identify the client, according to employer policy.

2 Explain the procedure to the client.

3 Practise hand hygiene.

4 Assist the client with hand washing.

5 Collect the following:

- Suppository
- Water-soluble lubricant
- Disposable gloves
- Toilet tissue

6 Provide for privacy.

Procedure

For Suppositories:

7 Check the label on the suppository for: right medication, right person, right dose, right route, right time, right day, and the right expiry date. Compare label with the MAR and care plan.

8 Assist the client into bed and into the Sims' position on the *left side.*

9 Help the client to lower or remove clothing to expose the anal area.

10 Unwrap the suppository.

11 Apply water-soluble lubricant to suppository. Do not use petroleum jelly, as it is not water soluble.

12 Give a glove to the client and see that it is put on.

(continued on page 764)

1 2 3 ASSISTING WITH RECTAL SUPPOSITORIES OR ENEMAS

Procedure (cont'd)

13 Hand to the client the suppository to be inserted into the rectum. Guide the client's hand, if necessary. (Wear a glove.)
14 Observe as the client inserts the suppository and wipes the anus with toilet tissue.
15 Have the client remove and discard the glove into the waste container.
16 Remind the client to remain on his or her side for 15 to 20 minutes to allow the suppository to dissolve and for the medication to be absorbed.

For Enemas:

This should only be performed if it is within your scope of practice for your province and you have been properly taught the correct procedure by a nurse.

10 Perform steps 7 to 9 as above. Remove enema device from its packaging and remove the cap covering the insertion tip.
11 Lubricate the insertion tip with water-soluble jelly.
12 Insert the tip into the client's rectum, up to the end of the tip. (Remember to follow the manufacturer's instructions.)
13 Gently squeeze the contents of the enema into the client. Ask the client to take slow, deep breaths while you are doing this.
14 Frequently check on the client to see of he or she is comfortable throughout the procedure. If the client develops cramping, ***stop immediately,*** and consult your supervisor.
15 Remove the enema, and wipe the client's rectal area with toilet tissue. Discard the tissue into a garbage container.
16 If the enema was intended to assist in bowel evacuation, assist the client onto the toilet, a commode chair, or a bedpan, according to his or her level of mobility. Ensure that the client is sitting as upright as possible. Provide toilet tissue.

Post-Procedure

17 Discard used materials in a waste container.
18 Assist the client with hand washing.
19 Provide the appropriate amount of privacy, and allow the client to defecate.
20 Have the client record medications taken correctly, when applicable. If specified in the care plan, record for the client.
21 Store materials in their proper location.
22 Remove privacy measures.
23 Practise hand hygiene.
24 Report and record your actions and observations, according to employer policy.

1 2 3 ASSISTING WITH EYE MEDICATIONS OR OINTMENTS

Remember to promote:

• Dignity • Independence • Preferences • Privacy • Safety

Pre-Procedure

1 Identify the client, according to employer policy.
2 Explain the procedure to the client.
3 Practise hand hygiene.
4 Assist the client with hand washing.
5 Collect the following:
- Eye medication or ointment
- Tissues or cotton balls
- Small hand mirror
- Disposable gloves (if necessary)

6 Provide for privacy.

(continued on page 765)

1 2 3 ASSISTING WITH EYE MEDICATIONS OR OINTMENTS

Procedure (cont'd)

7 Check the label on the prescription container for: right medication (be certain the preparation is for use in the eyes), right person, right dose (be certain the strength of the solution/ointment in the container is correct), right route (be certain about which eye or both eyes), right time, right day, and the right expiry date. Compare label with the MAR and care plan.

8 Loosen lid on container, if the client cannot do so.

9 Place the container within the client's reach, or hand it to him or her. Be sure the client wears eyeglasses, if needed.

10 Hold a mirror to help the client self-administer the eye medication.

11 Remove the client's eyeglasses, if worn.

12 Assist the client with:

a *Eye medication*: (Figure 40–6)

i. Guide the client's hand to grasp the lower eyelid.

ii. Observe whether the client looks up and releases drops into the lower lid.

iii. Observe whether the client closes the eye to distribute the medication.

iv. Make sure that dropper does not touch the client's eye.

b *Ointment*: (Figure 40–7)

i. Guide the client's hand to grasp the lower eyelid.

ii. Observe whether the client looks up and squeezes a small ribbon of ointment into the lower lid from inner corner of eye to outer corner of eye. (Figure 40–8)

iii. Observe that the client closes the eye to allow medication to dissolve and be distributed.

iv. Make sure that tip of tube does not touch eye surface.

Post-Procedure

13 Reseal the container.

14 Assist the client with hand hygiene.

15 Have the client record medications taken correctly, if applicable, or record for the client if specified in the care plan.

16 Store materials in their proper location.

17 Remove privacy measures.

18 Practise hand hygiene.

19 Report and record your actions and observations, according to employer policy.

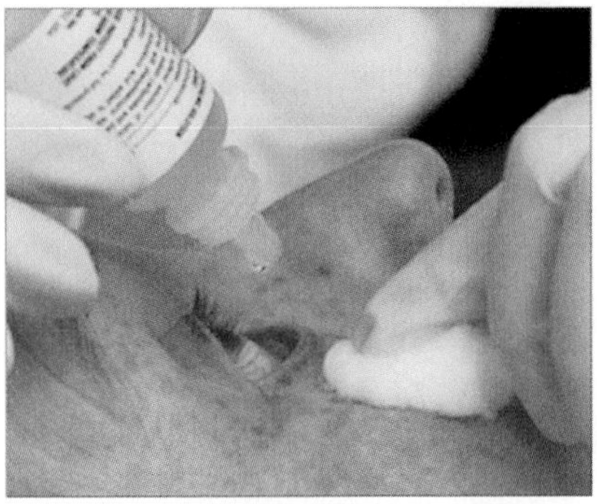

Figure 40–6 Insert the eye drop into the inside lower eye lid by holding it open with your gloved hand. **Source:** Lilley, L.L., Harrington, S., Snyder, J.S., & Swart, B. (2007). *Pharmacology and the nursing process in Canada* (p. 128). Toronto: Elsevier/Mosby.

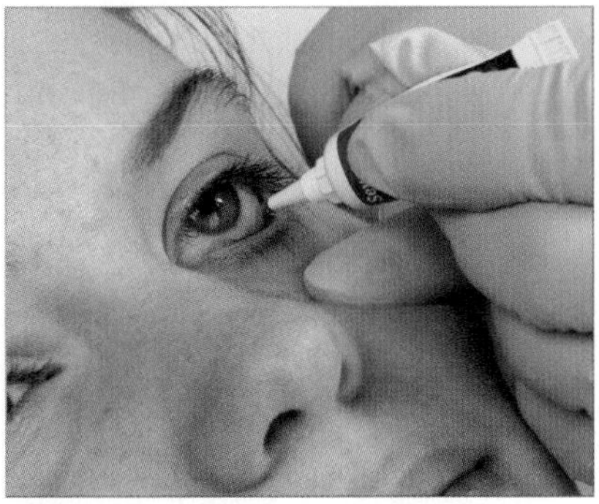

Figure 40–7 Applying eye ointment. **Source:** Lilley, L.L., Harrington, S., Snyder, J.S., & Swart, B. (2007). *Pharmacology and the nursing process in Canada* (p. 129). Toronto: Elsevier/Mosby.

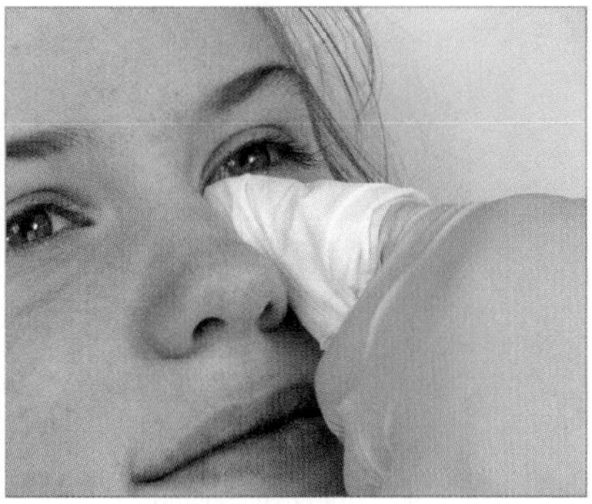

Figure 40–8 Apply gentle pressure to the inner corner of the eye for a few seconds after giving eye medications to ensure that they have time to be absorbed. **Source:** Lilley, L.L., Harrington, S., Snyder, J.S., & Swart, B. (2007). *Pharmacology and the nursing process in Canada* (p. 129). Toronto: Elsevier/Mosby.

1 2 3 ASSISTING WITH EAR DROPS

Remember to promote:

• Dignity • Independence • Preferences • Privacy • Safety

Pre-Procedure

1 Identify the client, according to employer policy.
2 Explain the procedure to the client.
3 Practise hand hygiene.
4 Assist the client with hand washing.
5 Collect the following:
- Ear drop medication
- Tissues or cotton balls
- Small hand mirror
- Disposable gloves (if necessary)

6 Provide for privacy.

Procedure

7 Check label on the prescription container for: right medication (be certain the preparation is for use in the ears), right person, right dose (be certain the strength of the solution/ointment in the container is correct), right route (be certain about which ear or both ears), right time, right day, and the right expiry date. Compare label with the MAR and care plan.
8 Loosen lid on container, if the client cannot do so.
9 Place container within the client's reach or hand it to him or her. Be sure the client wears eyeglasses, if needed.
10 Assist the client to lie on the side exposing the ear that is to receive the drop.
11 Hold the mirror so the client can self-administer the ear medication. If the client cannot manoeuvre the ear dropper, you should assist, with permission (Figure 40–9). Ensure the tip of the dropper does not touch the ear.
12 Ensure the drop(s) go into the ear canal. Gently massage the outside of the ear (the tragus), in order to allow the medication to go as far into the ear canal as possible. Place a piece of cotton ball in the ear to hold the medication in place.
13 Repeat steps 10 to 12 to assist the client with inserting drop(s) into the other ear.

Post-Procedure

13 Reseal container.
14 Assist the client with hand hygiene.
15 Have the client record medications taken correctly, when applicable, or record for the client if specified in the care plan.
16 Store materials in their proper location.
17 Remove privacy measures.
18 Wash your hands.
19 Report and record your actions and observations, according to employer policy.

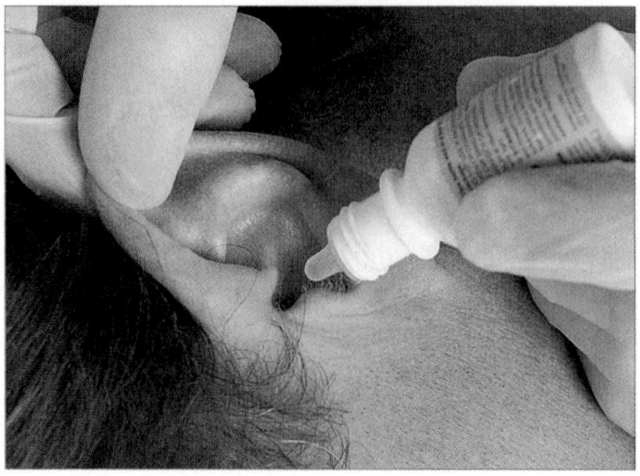

Figure 40–9 For adults, the external ear should be gently pulled upward and outward. If the client is an infant or child under 3 years of age, pull the external ear down and back. **Source:** Potter, P.A., Perry, A.G., Ross-Kerr, J.C., & Wood, M.J. (2006). *Canadian fundamentals of nursing* (3rd ed., p. 872). Toronto: Elsevier.

1 2 3 ASSISTING WITH TRANSDERMAL DISCS

Remember to promote:

• **D**ignity • **I**ndependence • **P**references • **P**rivacy • **S**afety

Pre-Procedure

1 Identify the client, according to employer policy.
2 Explain the procedure to the client.
3 Practise hand hygiene.
4 Assist the client with hand hygiene.
5 Collect the following:
- Medicated transdermal disc
- Disposable gloves
- Small garbage bag

6 Provide for privacy.

Procedure

7 Check the label on the disc container for: right medication, right person, right dose, right route, right time, right day, and the right expiry date. Compare label with the MAR and care plan.
8 Put on gloves. Give the client a glove to put on.
9 Have the client remove and discard the old disc into a waste container. Wash the skin that had been covered by the old disc.
10 Ask the client to select a new site for the new disc (any area without hair). Usually the chest or upper arm area is used.
11 Observe or help the client to apply the new disc to the skin surface. Be sure that the medicated surface of the disc is not touched by ungloved fingers. (Your skin may absorb some of the drug.) (Figure 40–10)
12 Write the date and time on the disc, making sure that it does not smudge. (*Note*: Some agencies require that you write on the disc *after* it is applied on the client, while some suggest that this should be done *before* applying it on the client. As with all steps, ensure that you follow your agency's policies.)

Post-Procedure

13 Discard disc wrapper and other used materials into a garbage bag, and tie the bag. Dispose of the bag into a lidded garbage container.
14 Remove gloves. Practise hand hygiene.
15 Have the client remove the glove, and discard it as well. Assist with hand hygiene.
16 Have the client record medications taken correctly, when applicable, or record for the person if specified in the care plan.
17 Store materials in their proper location.
18 Remove privacy measures.
19 Practise hand hygiene.
20 Report and record your actions and observations, according to employer policy.

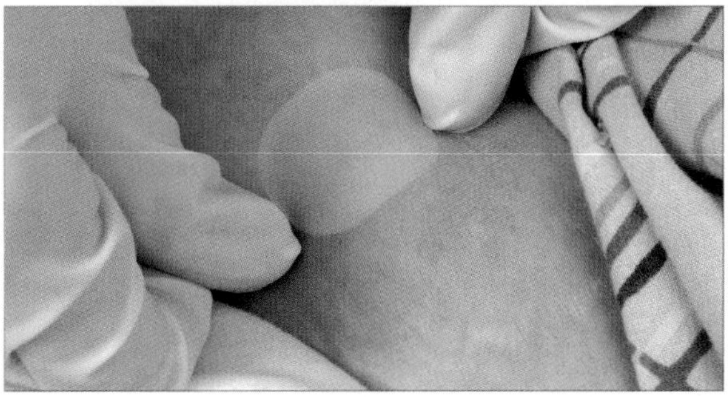

Figure 40–10 Ensure that the edges of the transdermal disc are secure after it has been applied on the client. Write the time and the date with a pen on the patch either before or after applying it, according to your agency's policy. **Source:** Lilley, L.L., Harrington, S., Snyder, J.S., & Swart, B. (2007). *Pharmacology and the nursing process in Canada* (p. 139). Toronto: Elsevier/Mosby.

1 2 3 ASSISTING WITH METERED DOSE INHALERS

Remember to promote:

• **D**ignity • **I**ndependence • **P**references • **P**rivacy • **S**afety

Pre-Procedure

1 Identify the client, according to employer policy.
2 Explain the procedure to the client.
3 Practise hand hygiene.
4 Help the client with hand washing.
5 Collect the following:
- MDI container of prescription medication
- Holding chamber (if necessary)
- Disposable gloves (if necessary)

6 Provide for privacy.

Procedure

7 Check the label on the container for: right medication, right person, right dose, right route, right time, right day, and the right expiry date. Compare label with the MAR and care plan.
8 Assist the client to shake the inhaler container vigorously.
9 Hand the MDI to the client so that he or she can use it to inhale the medication (Figure 40–11).

Post-Procedure

10 Have the client record medications taken correctly, when applicable, or record for the client if specified in the care plan.
11 Clean the MDI, according to the manufacturer's instructions, and store it in its proper location.
12 Remove privacy measures.
13 Practise hand hygiene.
14 Report and record your actions and observations, according to employer policy.

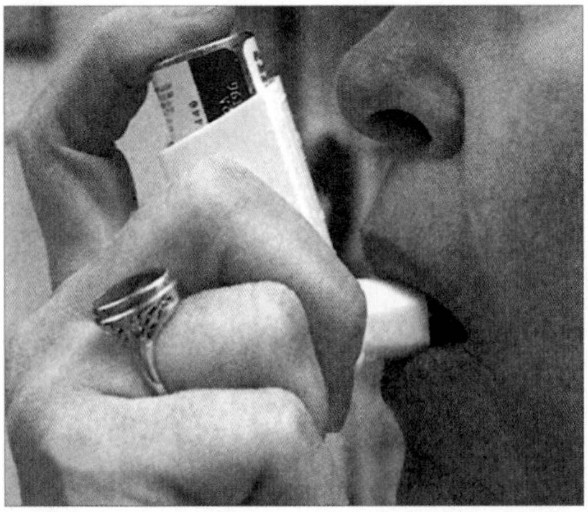

Figure 40–11 A client self-administering medication with a metered dose inhaler (MDI). **Source:** Birchenall, J., & Streight, E. (2003). *Mosby's textbook for the home care aide* (2nd ed., p. 354). St. Louis: Mosby.

1 2 3 ASSISTING WITH METERED DOSE INHALERS WITH A HOLDING CHAMBER

Remember to promote:

• **D**ignity • **I**ndependence • **P**references • **P**rivacy • **S**afety

Pre-Procedure

1 Identify the client, according to employer policy.
2 Explain the procedure to the client.
3 Practise hand hygiene.
4 Help the client with hand washing.
5 Collect the following:
- MDI container (s) of prescription medication
- Holding chamber
- Disposable gloves (if necessary)

6 Provide for privacy.

Procedure

Always double check, with either the client or your supervisor, which MDI the client should take first, especially if the client is taking two asthma medications, as the order of taking these medications is very important.

7 Check the label on the container for: right medication, right person, right dose, right route, right time, right day, and the right expiry date. Compare label with the MAR and care plan.
8 Assist the client to shake the inhaler container vigorously.
9 Assist the client to remove the from the MDI container and insert it into the holding chamber.
10 Hand the MDI and the attached holding chamber to the client, who then uses it to inhale the medication (Figure 40–12). The client should breathe normally for at least six breaths.
11 Repeat steps 8 to 10 again with the second MDI.
12 Have the client rinse the mouth with water and spit out. Instruct the client to ***not*** swallow the water.

Post-Procedure

11 Have the client record medications taken correctly, when applicable, or record for the client if specified in the care plan.
12 Clean the MDI, according to the manufacturer's instructions. Store the MDI in its proper location.
13 Remove privacy measures.
14 Practise hand hygiene.
15 Report and record your actions and observations, according to employer policy.

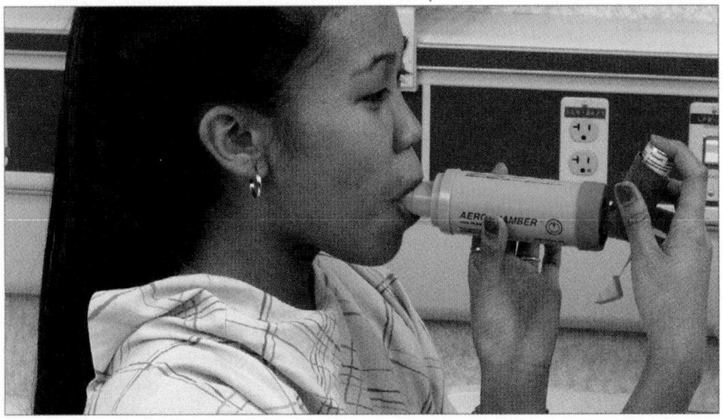

Figure 40–12 A holding chamber is often used when the client is unable to breathe deeply. It allows the client to inhale the medication while breathing normally into it. **Source:** Lilley, L.L., Harrington, S., Snyder, J.S., & Swart, B. (2007). *Pharmacology and the nursing process in Canada* (p. 135). Toronto: Elsevier/Mosby.

REVIEW

Answers to these questions are at the bottom of the page.

Circle T if the answer is true or circle F if the answer is false.

1. T F **Support workers routinely administer medications.**
2. T F **A lozenge is a type of medication.**
3. T F **Over-the-counter medications require a prescription.**
4. T F **You can purchase OTC medications for a client.**
5. T F **The physician, RN, and case manager are responsible for monitoring the outcome of the drug therapy.**
6. T F **Side effects do not need to be reported.**
7. T F **You are responsible for filling pill boxes.**
8. T F **Any person giving medications must record on the MAR, according to agency policy.**
9. T F **Medications can be taken at any time, as long as the correct dose is given.**
10. T F **When assisting with medications, you must check that the client is taking the right medication.**
11. T F **Medications should always be stored in the kitchen cabinet above the stove.**

Circle the BEST answer.

12. **Mrs. Stein has sore, swollen joints in her hands. You assist with her medications. Which of the following is *your* responsibility?**
    - A. Loosening and removing container lids
    - B. Phoning the pharmacy to order more medication
    - C. Pouring the medication for her and administering it to her
    - D. Changing the times to take her medication
13. **Which of the following is not one of the eight "rights" of assisting with medications?**
    - A. The right medication
    - B. The right colour
    - C. The right person
    - D. The right time
14. **Mrs. Smith is asking for a headache pill that is not listed on her MAR. What should you do?**
    - A. Phone her family doctor
    - B. Give it to her
    - C. Ask her daughter to give it to her
    - D. Check with your supervisor
15. **A medication should be kept:**
    - A. At the bedside, with the container open
    - B. In a warm, humid area
    - C. Along with other family members' or residents' medications
    - D. In its original labelled container
16. **Which of the following should be reported to your supervisor? The client:**
    - A. Refuses to take the medication
    - B. Needs to use a metered dose inhaler as specified on the MAR.
    - C. Says that she does not like the taste of her medication but takes it anyway
    - D. Knows what to ask her doctor about her pills on her next appointment

Answers: 1.F, 2.T, 3.F, 4.F, 5.T, 6.F, 7.F, 8.T, 9.F, 10.T, 11.F, 12.A, 13.B, 14.D, 15.D, 16.A

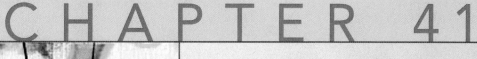

CHAPTER 41

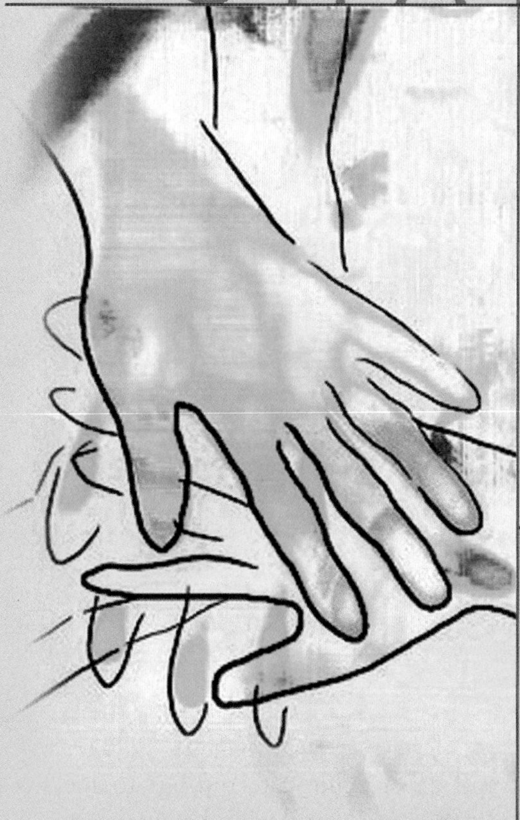

Measuring Height, Weight, and Vital Signs

OBJECTIVES

- Define the key terms listed in this chapter.
- Explain how to measure height and weight.
- Explain why vital signs are measured.
- List factors that affect vital signs.
- Identify the normal ranges for temperature sites.
- Know when to use each temperature site.
- Identify the sites for taking a pulse.
- Describe normal respirations.
- Describe factors that affect blood pressure.
- Describe the practices to follow when measuring blood pressure.
- Know the vital sign ranges for different age groups.
- Perform the procedures described in this chapter.

key terms

blood pressure The amount of force exerted by the blood against the walls of an artery.

body temperature The amount of heat in the body that is a balance between the amount of heat produced and the amount lost by the body.

bradycardia A slow (*brady*) heart rate (*cardia*); a rate less than 60 beats per minute.

diastole The period of heart muscle relaxation.

diastolic pressure The pressure in the arteries when the heart is at rest.

dysrhythmia An irregular rhythm of the pulse; beats may be unevenly spaced or skipped.

hypertension Persistent blood pressure measurements above the normal systolic (140 mm Hg) or diastolic (90 mm Hg) pressures.

hypotension A condition in which the systolic blood pressure is below 90 mm Hg and the diastolic pressure is below 60 mm Hg.

pulse The beat of the heart felt at an artery as a wave of blood passes through the artery.

pulse rate The number of heartbeats or pulses felt in 1 minute.

respiration The act of breathing air into (inhalation) and out of (exhalation) the lungs.

sphygmomanometer The instrument used to measure blood pressure.

stethoscope An instrument used to listen to the sounds produced by the heart, lungs, and other body organs.

systole The period of heart muscle contraction.

systolic pressure The amount of force it takes to pump blood out of the heart and into the arterial circulation.

tachycardia A rapid (*tachy*) heart rate (*cardia*); a rate over 100 beats per minute.

vital signs Temperature, pulse, respirations, and blood pressure.

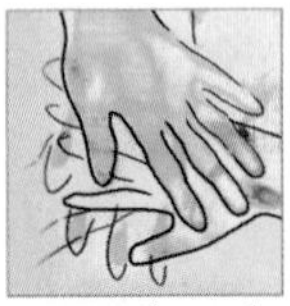

The four **vital signs** of body function are temperature, pulse, respirations, and blood pressure. Oxygen saturation (SPO_2) monitoring is considered a part of measuring vital signs in some agencies. Vital signs reflect the function of three body processes essential for life: (1) regulation of body temperature, (2) breathing, and (3) heart function. Measuring and recording vital signs, as well as height and weight, provide important information for the care planning process.

Measuring and recording height and weight are skills you need to have in all your workplace settings. Measuring and recording temperature, pulse, and respirations (TPR) are skills you need to have when working in long-term care and community settings. Measuring and recording blood pressure are additional skills required by some employers. Some provinces and territories allow support workers in hospitals and other acute care settings to measure and record temperature, pulse, and respirations, but some do not. Know your employer's policies.

MEASURING HEIGHT AND WEIGHT

Height and weight are measured when a client is admitted to a facility, and some clients may be weighed daily, weekly, or monthly. Clients may be weighed daily when there is concern about fluid retention (e.g., in congestive heart failure) and to monitor weight gain or loss. Weigh the client at the same time of day for daily, weekly, or monthly measurements. Before breakfast is the best time, as food and fluids add weight.

The client should wear only a gown or pyjamas when being weighed, as clothes add weight. Shoes or slippers add to the weight and the height. Also, have the client void (urinate) before he or she is weighed, as a full bladder affects the weight measurement. If a urine specimen is needed, collect it at this time.

There are balance beam scales, chair scales, lift scales, and wheelchair weigh scales (Figure 41–1). The most common weigh scale used in facilities is the weigh scale in the bathtub lift chair. Balance beam scales are used for clients who are able to stand, and chair and lift scales are used for those who are unable to. Wheelchair scales are used for clients confined to a wheelchair. Follow the manufacturer's instructions and employer policy when using scales.

Mechanical and digital scales are used to measure the weight of clients as well. Mechanical scales use a system of weights, in which the weights are moved to zero first and then are adjusted until the pointer is centred (Figure 41–2). Digital scales have LED displays that show the weight. Make sure the LED reads zero before weighing the client (see the *Focus on Children: Measuring Height and Weight* box.)

In the community, clients may have scales that still have imperial units (pounds). To convert to metric units, divide the pounds by 2.3 to get the weight in kilograms (e.g., 10 lb = 4.5 kg, 160 lb = 72.6 kg).

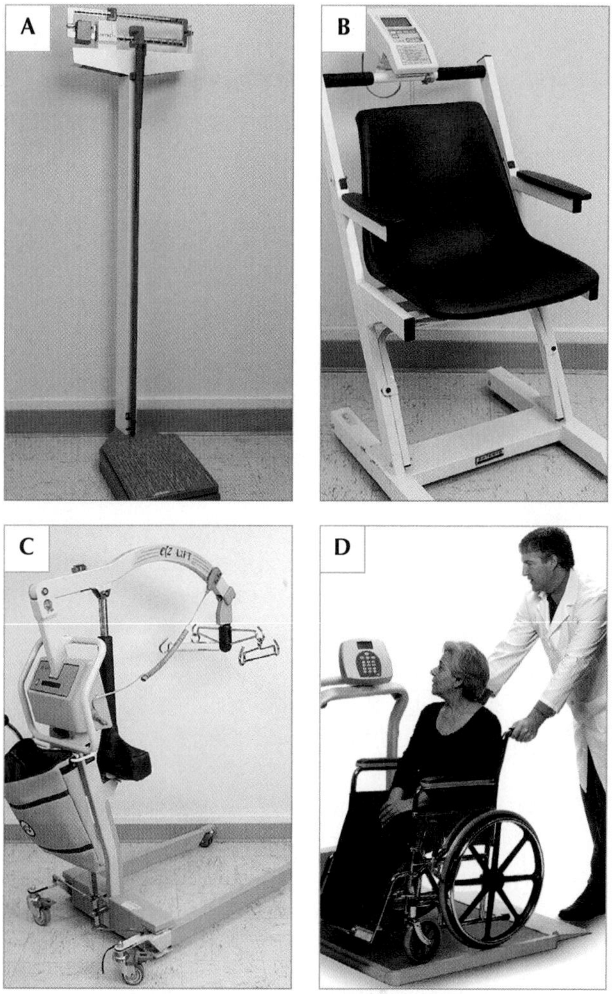

Figure 41–1 Types of scales. **A,** Balance beam scale. **B,** Chair scale. **C,** Lift scale. **D,** Wheelchair weigh scale. **Courtesy (for D):** Pelstar LLC/Health o meter Professional Scales, Alsip, IL.

focus on ›› CHILDREN

Measuring Height and Weight

Birthweight serves as the baseline for measuring an infant's growth (see Chapter 38).

In children younger than 2 years, length is measured, not height. The child is laid down on a measuring board or on a sheet of paper. Two people hold the child still, one holding the head and the other the legs. The measurement is taken from the top of the head to the heels. If using paper, mark the paper at the head and heels, and measure the distance between the two points.

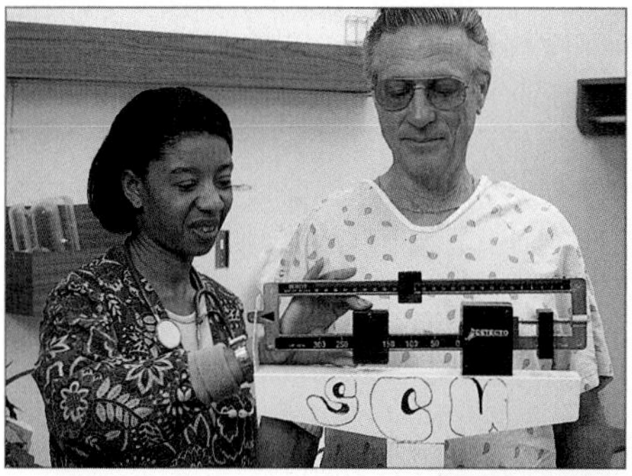

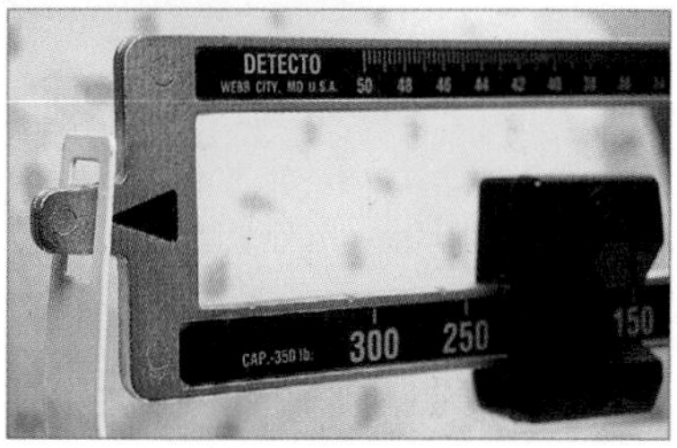

Figure 41–2 Using a mechanical scale. **A,** Adjust the weights. **B,** Read the weight when the balance pointer is in the middle.

1 2 3 MEASURING HEIGHT AND WEIGHT

Remember to promote:

• **D**ignity • **I**ndependence • **P**references • **P**rivacy • **S**afety

Pre-Procedure

1 Identify the client, according to employer policy.
2 Explain the procedure to the client.
3 Ask the client to void (see Chapter 31).
4 Perform hand hygiene.
5 Bring the scale and paper towels to the client's room.
6 Provide for privacy.

Procedure

7 *Balance beam scale (mechanical):*
  a Disinfect the scale platform, according to employer policy. Dry it with paper towels.
  b Raise the height rod.
  c Move the weights to zero (0). The pointer should be in the middle.
  d Have the client remove the robe and footwear. Assist, as needed.
  e Help the client stand on the scale platform. Arms should be at the sides.
  f Move the weights until the balance pointer is in the middle (see Figure 41–2).
  g Record the weight on your notepad or assignment sheet.
  h Ask the client to stand very straight.
  i Lower the height rod until it rests on the client's head (Figure 41–3).
  j Record the height on your notepad or assignment sheet.
  k Disinfect the scale platform after use, according to employer policy.
8 *Chair scale (mechanical):*
  a Help the client transfer from the wheelchair to the chair scale (see the *Transferring the Client to a Chair or Wheelchair* box on page 416).
  b Place the client's feet on the foot platform.
  c Move the weights until the balance pointer is in the middle.
  d Record the weight on your notepad or assignment sheet.
9 *Lift scale (mechanical):*
  a Attach the sling to the lift.
  b Place both weights on zero.
  c Level and balance the scale. Follow the manufacturer's instructions.
  d Remove the sling from the scale.
  e Place the client on the sling, and attach the sling to the lift. Raise the client about 10 cm (4 in.) off the bed (see the *Using a Mechanical Lift to Move the Client* box on page 423).
  f Move the weights until the balance pointer is in the middle.
  g Record the weight on your notepad or assignment sheet.
  h Lower the client to the bed.
  i Remove the sling.
10 Help the client dress if he or she will be up, or help the client back to bed.

Post-Procedure

11 Provide for safety and comfort.
12 Place the call bell within reach.*
13 If the client stays in bed, follow the care plan for bed rail use.*
14 Remove privacy measures.
15 Return the scale to its proper place.
16 Perform hand hygiene.
17 Report and record the measurements and your observations, according to employer policy.

*Steps marked with an asterisk may not apply in community settings.

1 2 3 MEASURING HEIGHT: THE CLIENT IN BED

Remember to promote:

• Dignity • Independence • Preferences • Privacy • Safety

Pre-Procedure

1 Identify the client, according to employer policy.
2 Explain the procedure to the client.
3 Perform hand hygiene.
4 Collect a measuring tape and ruler.
5 Ask for assistance.
6 Provide for privacy.

Procedure

7 Position the client supine, if this position is allowed.
8 Have your helper hold the end of the measuring tape at the client's heel.
9 Pull the measuring tape alongside the client's body until it extends past the head (Figure 41–4).
10 Place the ruler flat across the top of the client's head. It should extend from the client's head to the measuring tape. Make sure the ruler is level.
11 Record the height on your notepad or assignment sheet.
12 Help the client out of bed, if appropriate.

Post-Procedure

13 Provide for safety and comfort.
14 Place the call bell within reach.*
15 If the client stays in bed, follow the care plan for bed rail use.*
16 Remove privacy measures.
17 Return equipment to its proper location.
18 Perform hand hygiene.
19 Report and record the height and your observations, according to employer policy.

*Steps marked with an asterisk may not apply in community settings.

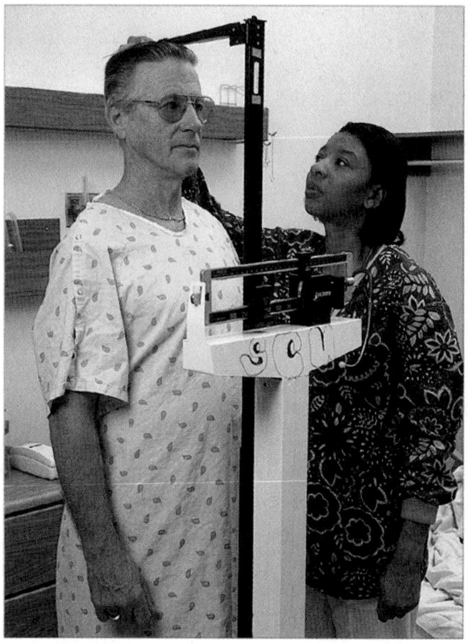

Figure 41–3 Measuring height.

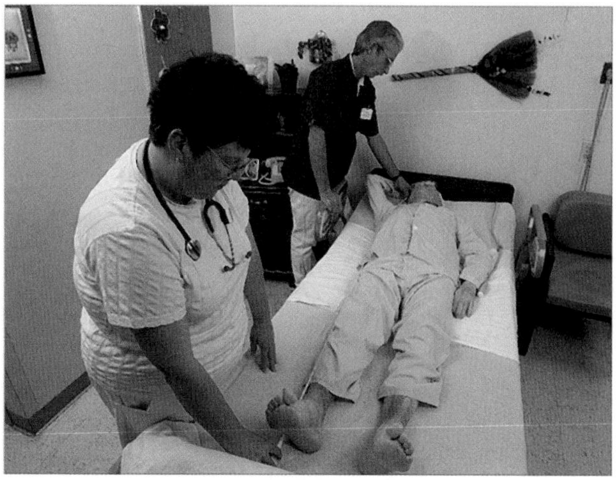

Figure 41–4 Measuring a client in bed. Extend the tape measure from the top of the client's head to the heel. Make sure the ruler is flat across the top of the client's head.

MEASURING AND REPORTING VITAL SIGNS

A person's vital signs can vary within certain limits, and they can be affected by medications, pain, illness, activity, exercise, sleep, foods, fluids, smoking, and emotions (e.g., excitement, anger, fear, and anxiety).

Vital signs are measured to detect changes in normal body function. They can indicate response to treatment and signal life-threatening events. Vital signs are part of the assessment process and are measured:

- During physical examinations
- When a client is admitted to a facility
- Several times a day for hospital clients and clients in subacute care units
- Before and after surgery
- Before and after complex procedures or diagnostic tests
- After certain care measures, such as ambulation
- After a fall or other injury
- When medications that affect the respiratory or circulatory system are taken
- Whenever the client complains of pain, dizziness, lightheadedness, shortness of breath, rapid heart rate, or not feeling well
- As often as dictated by the client's condition
- As ordered or requested by the doctor
- As stated on the care plan (usually daily or weekly)
- As instructed after the client has been given medication to relieve a fever

Vital signs reveal even minor changes in a client's condition. Accuracy is essential when you measure, record, and report vital signs. If you are unsure of the accuracy of your measurements, promptly ask your supervisor to take them again. Unless otherwise ordered, take vital signs with the client at rest, when he or she is lying down or sitting. You should always compare any readings to the client's baseline reading. Immediately report:

- Any vital sign that is changed from a previous measurement
- Vital signs above the normal range
- Vital signs below the normal range

Employers have their own methods of recording vital signs. Some use graphic flow sheets where the vital signs are graphed in red and blue ink. Some use books with pages divided into columns where the information is recorded. Whatever system your employer uses, the following information must be clearly and accurately recorded:

- Client's name
- Date
- Time the vital sign was measured
- Vital sign measurement

Some employers require that changed or abnormal vital signs be circled in red or highlighted in some way. The nurse or physician compares current and previous measurements.

BODY TEMPERATURE

Body temperature is the amount of heat in the body. It is a balance between the amount of heat produced and the amount lost by the body. It remains within a normal, safe range when a person is healthy. Temperature normally changes slightly throughout the day and in response to different factors, such as age, weather, exercise, pregnancy, the menstrual cycle, emotions, and stress. It is lower in the morning and higher in the afternoon and evening.

Illness also affects body temperature, and temperatures above or below the normal range signal illness or health problems.

Temperature Sites

Temperature is measured using the Centigrade/Celsius (C). Common sites for measuring temperature are as follows:

- Mouth (oral temperature)
- Ear (tympanic temperature)
- Underarm (axillary temperature—*axilla* means underarm)

Body temperature can also be measured in the rectum (rectal temperature), but this site is rarely used. If a rectal temperature is required, a nurse or other regulated health care provider performs the procedure. Since taking a rectal temperature involves inserting an instrument into a body cavity, *support workers are not authorized to take rectal temperatures.* If you are delegated the procedure, you need to be properly trained and supervised.

Each body site has a normal range of temperature (Table 41–1), so check with your supervisor and the care plan to find out which site to use.

Older adults have lower body temperatures than do younger people. A certain temperature may indicate fever in an older adult but may be normal body temperature in a younger person. Always report temperatures that are not within the client's normal range.

Taking Oral Temperature. Oral temperature is *not* taken if the client:

- Is unconscious
- Has had surgery or an injury to the face, neck, nose, or mouth
- Has a nasogastric tube
- Is delirious, restless, confused, or disoriented
- Is paralyzed on one side of the body
- Has a sore mouth
- Has a convulsive disorder
- Is receiving oxygen therapy

The following activities may temporarily affect oral temperature reading:

- Eating hot or cold foods
- Drinking hot or cold fluids
- Smoking
- Chewing gum

Before taking oral temperature, make sure the client has not done any of these activities within the previous 20 minutes.

Place the thermometer under the client's tongue (Figure 41–5). The tip of the thermometer should be at the base of the tongue. Ask the client to close his or her lips around the thermometer to hold it in place. The mouth must remain closed. Remind the client not to bite down on the thermometer or talk while it is in place.

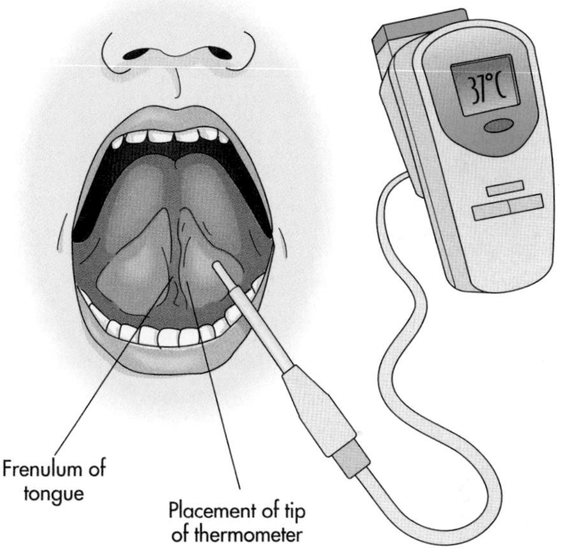

Figure 41–5 Place the thermometer at the base of the tongue.

Table 41–1 Normal Body Temperature

Site	Average Temperature	Normal Range
Mouth (oral temperature)	37.0°C (98.6°F)	35.5°C to 37.5°C (95.9°F to 99.5°F)
Ear (tympanic temperature)	37.4°C (99.3°F)	35.8°C to 38.0°C (96.4°F to 100.4°F)
Underarm (axillary temperature)	36.5°C (97.8°F)	34.7°C to 37.3°C (94.5°F to 99.1°F)
Rectal	37.5°C (99.6°F)	35.5°C to 38°C (96.6°F to 100°F)

Taking Tympanic Temperature. If oral temperature cannot be taken, tympanic temperature is usually the next choice. Special thermometers are used for the ear (Figure 41–6).

Gently pull the client's ear up and back (Figure 41–7) and insert the probe (the end of the thermometer that is temperature-sensitive) into the ear canal. The temperature is measured in 1 to 3 seconds (see the *Focus on Children: Taking Tympanic Temperature* box.)

Because temperature can be measured quickly and easily, tympanic temperature is often ordered for children and for clients with dementia. Tympanic temperature is not taken if there is any drainage from the ear.

Taking Axillary Temperature. Axillary temperature is less reliable than temperature taken at the other sites, so it is taken only when the other sites cannot be used. Axillary temperature is often taken on infants and very young children.

The axilla (underarm) must be dry. Do not use this site when the client has just had a bath. Point the thermometer tip upward and well into the client's underarm. Make sure the tip is in contact with the client's skin. The thermometer should be held in place to maintain proper position. Bring the client's arm down close against the body, and ensure that the client's forearm rests against the chest (Figure 41–8). With children, it may be helpful to hold the child while taking the temperature. This keeps the thermometer in place and comforts the child.

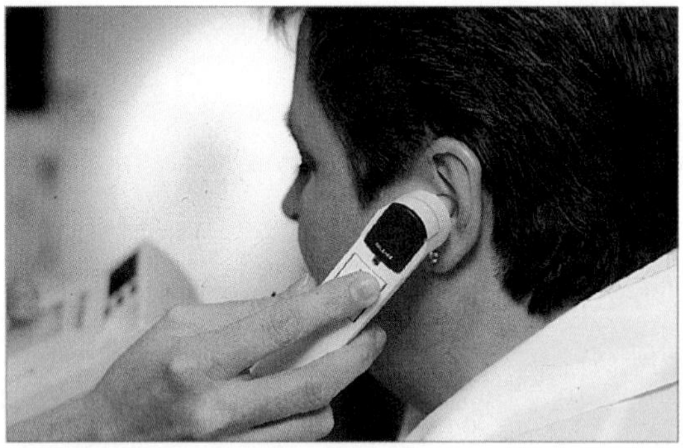

Figure 41–6 A tympanic thermometer.

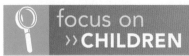

focus on
›› CHILDREN

Taking Tympanic Temperature

The shape of a child's ear canal is different from an adult's. When taking tympanic temperature on a child, gently pull the child's ear down and forward and insert the probe.

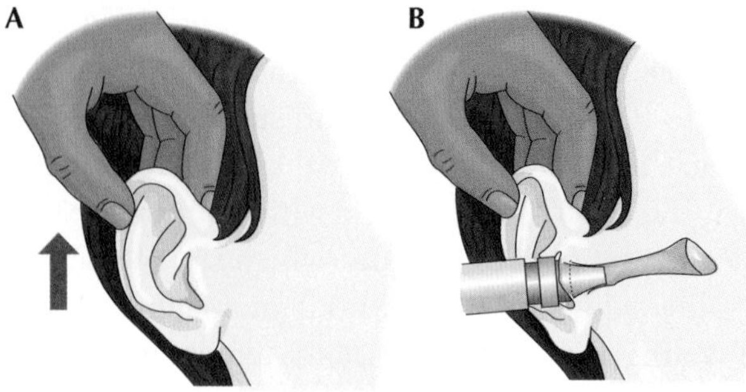

Figure 41–7 Taking an adult's tympanic temperature. **A,** Pull the ear up and back. **B,** Gently insert the probe into the ear canal.

Thermometers

A variety of thermometers are available on the market. Most facilities and agencies use electronic thermometers as well as disposable ones. Dot matrix thermometers and temperature-sensitive tape are also used. Glass thermometers are considered safety hazards and are now rarely used in any setting.

Thermometers can spread microbes, so protective disposable plastic covers are usually applied over the thermometer before use (Figure 41–9). Thermometers must always be cleaned, wiped dry, and stored, according to employer policy and the manufacturer's recommendations. Some employers

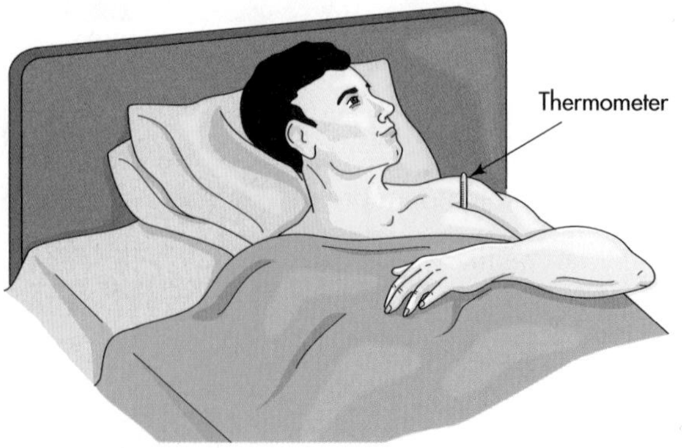

Figure 41–8 Hold the thermometer in place in the axilla by bringing the client's arm over the chest.

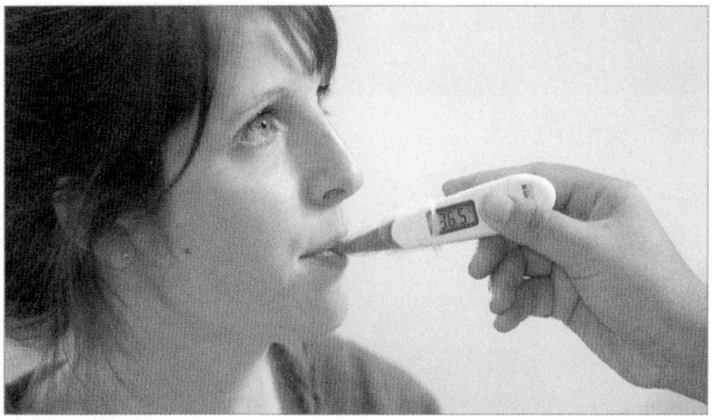

Figure 41–9 The thermometer probe is inserted into a disposable plastic cover, which helps prevent the spread of microbes. A fresh cover must be used for each client. **Courtesy:** Brian Hillier.

require that thermometers be cleaned with a disinfectant such as alcohol before and after use. Always follow medical asepsis and Standard Practices when using thermometers.

Electronic Thermometers. Electronic thermometers are battery-operated. They measure temperature within 20 to 50 seconds and display a digital readout of the temperature. Some electronic thermometers consist of a hand-held unit and a probe that is inserted into the unit (Figure 41–10). The hand-held unit is kept in a battery charger when not in use.

An electronic thermometer that has a low battery charge will not record temperature accurately. After using an electronic thermometer, replace it securely in the battery charging unit. Make sure the battery charging unit is plugged into an electrical outlet.

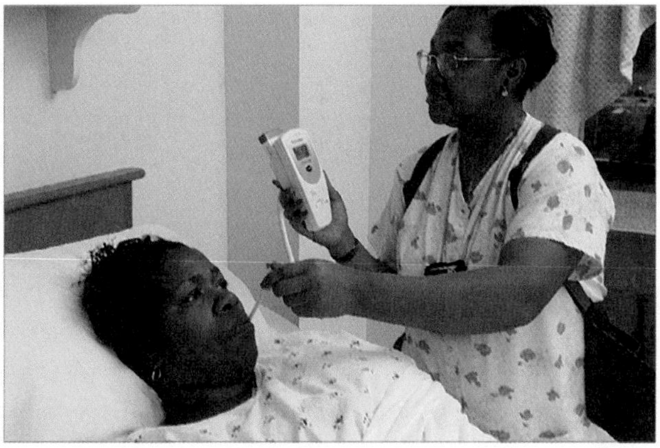

Figure 41–10 An electronic thermometer with a hand-held unit and probe.

Electronic thermometers with probes can be used for any site, and the probes may be changed depending on the site. Tympanic thermometers are electronic thermometers with probes made to fit in the ear canal (see Figure 41–6 on page 778).

A disposable protective plastic cover is slid onto the probe until it snaps in place. Electronic thermometers emit a tone or flashing light when the temperature reading is complete.

Electronic thermometers that are one-piece devices (Figure 41–11) are called digital thermometers. They have a temperature-sensitive tip on one end and an on/off button on the other end. They display a digital readout of the temperature. Some have a memory mechanism that recalls the last temperature reading. The battery is not rechargeable, but the device shuts off after about 10 minutes. These thermometers may be used to take oral or axillary temperature. They are inserted into covers before use (see Figure 41–9). Digital thermometers are used more in home care settings than in facilities (see the *Focus on Children: Special Thermometers* box.)

Dot Matrix Thermometers. Dot matrix thermometers are thin plastic strips with small chemical dots on one end (Figure 41–12). The dots change colour when heated by the body. Each dot must be heated to a certain temperature before it changes colour. These thermometers are useful to measure oral and axillary temperature and are not for use in the ear. They must be left in place for about 3 minutes before an accurate temperature can be read. They must be discarded after one use.

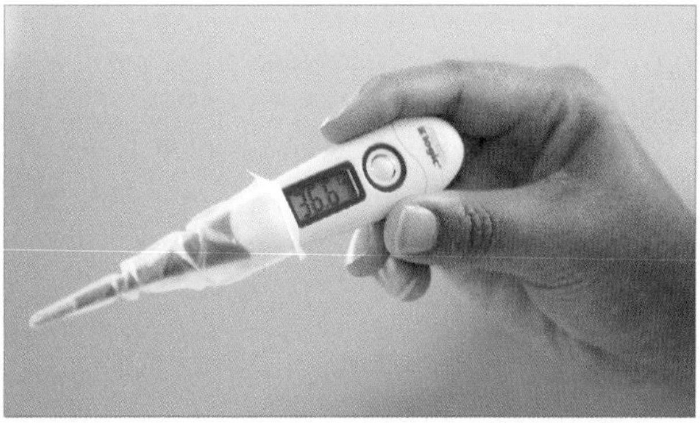

Figure 41–11 A digital thermometer. **Courtesy:** Brian Hillier.

1 2 3 TAKING TEMPERATURE WITH AN ELECTRONIC THERMOMETER

Remember to promote:

• Dignity • Independence • Preferences • Privacy • Safety

Pre-Procedure

1 Identify the client, according to employer policy.
2 Explain the procedure to the client. The client is instructed not to eat, drink, smoke, or chew gum for at least 20 minutes before the procedure.
3 Perform hand hygiene.
4 Collect the following:
- Electronic or digital thermometer
- Probe, if used. Make sure you use the correct probe for the site.
- Disposable plastic cover for thermometer or probe
- Tissues
- Towel (for axillary temperature)

5 Plug the probe into the thermometer, if used.
6 Provide for privacy.

Procedure

7 Position the client for oral, axillary, or tympanic temperature.
8 Insert the probe or thermometer tip into a disposable cover.
9 *For oral temperature:*
- **a** Ask the client to open the mouth and raise the tongue.
- **b** Place the tip of the thermometer or probe at the base of the tongue (see Figure 41–5 on page 778).
- **c** Ask the client to lower the tongue and close the mouth. Remind the client not to talk or bite down on the thermometer or probe.

10 *For tympanic temperature:*
- **a** Ask the client to turn his or her head so that the ear is in front of you.
- **b** Pull the ear up and back to straighten the ear canal (see Figure 41–7 on page 778). (In the case of children, pull the ear down and forward.)
- **c** Insert the probe gently. The probe should seal the ear canal.

11 *For axillary temperature:*
- **a** Help the client remove his or her arm from the sleeve. Do not expose the client.
- **b** Dry the axilla with the towel.
- **c** Place the tip of the thermometer or probe in the centre of the axilla, pointing upward. Make sure the tip of the probe is in contact with the client's skin.
- **d** Ask the client to place the arm over the chest to hold the thermometer or probe in place (see Figure 41–8 on page 778). Hold the arm in place if he or she cannot do it.

12 Turn on the thermometer.
13 Keep the probe or thermometer in place until you hear a tone or see a flashing or steady light.
14 Remove the probe or thermometer.
15 Read the temperature on the display.
16 Help the client put his or her arm back into the sleeve (for axillary temperature).
17 Record the client's name and temperature on your notepad or assignment sheet. Note the temperature site.
18 Use tissue to remove the plastic cover from the thermometer, or press the eject button to remove the plastic probe cover.
19 Discard tissue and plastic cover.
20 Perform hand hygiene.

Post-Procedure

21 Provide for safety and comfort.
22 Place the call bell within reach.*
23 Follow the care plan for bed rail use.*
24 Remove privacy measures.
25 Clean and store the equipment, according to employer policy. Return electronic thermometer back to the battery charging unit.
26 Perform hand hygiene.
27 Report and record your actions and observations, according to employer policy. Include the following:
- Temperature
- Site (A for axillary, T for tympanic, O for oral)
- Abnormal temperature (report at once)

*Steps marked with an asterisk may not apply in community settings.

focus on ››CHILDREN

Special Thermometers

Pacifier thermometers are a type of electronic thermometer used on infants and toddlers. They are available in stores for home use. The pacifier thermometer has four parts: (1) a storage cover, (2) a nipple with a sensor, (3) a digital display, and (4) an on/off switch. Temperature is measured in about 5 minutes.

To use the thermometer:

- Remove it from the storage case.
- Check the pacifier for cracks or holes. These can occur if the child bites or chews on the thermometer. Do not use the thermometer if it is damaged.
- Turn it on by pressing the switch.
- Place the pacifier in the child's mouth. Hold and cuddle the child.
- Read the digital display on the front of the pacifier when the thermometer beeps.
- Clean the thermometer, according to employer policy. Do not use boiling water, the dishwasher, or a sterilizer to clean the thermometer.
- Wipe the thermometer dry.
- Return it to the storage case.

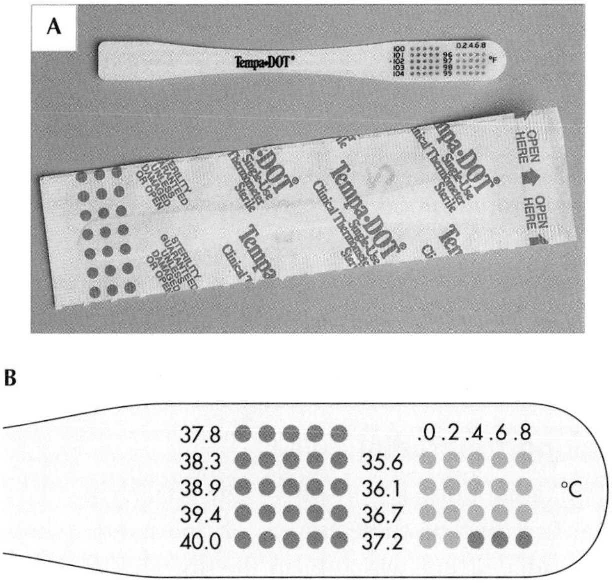

Figure 41–12 **A,** Single-use dot matrix thermometer with chemical dots. **B,** The dots change colour when the temperature is taken.

Temperature-Sensitive Tape. The temperature-sensitive tape changes colour in response to body heat (Figure 41–13). When the tape is applied to the forehead or abdomen, it shows if the temperature is normal or above normal, but exact body temperature is not measured. The colour change takes about 15 seconds. The tape is discarded after one use.

In the community setting, you may find that some clients have thermometers that show the temperature in Fahrenheit. To convert Fahrenheit to Celsius, subtract 32 from the Fahrenheit reading and then divide by 1.8 (e.g., 97.2°F = 36.2°C). To convert Celsius to Fahrenheit, multiply the Celsius reading by 1.8 and then add 32.

PULSE

Pulse is the beat of the heart felt at an artery as a wave of blood passes through the artery. The pulse is felt every time the heart beats (see Chapter 14 to review the structure and function of the heart and blood vessels.)

Sites for Taking the Pulse

You can feel the pulse by placing your fingertips over certain sites on the body. The temporal, carotid, brachial, femoral, popliteal, and dorsalis pedis (pedal) pulses are on both sides of the body (Figure 41–14). The pulse is easy to feel at these sites because the arteries are close to the body's surface and lie over a bone.

To take the pulse, support workers often use the radial site because it is easy to reach and find and the pulse can be taken without disturbing or

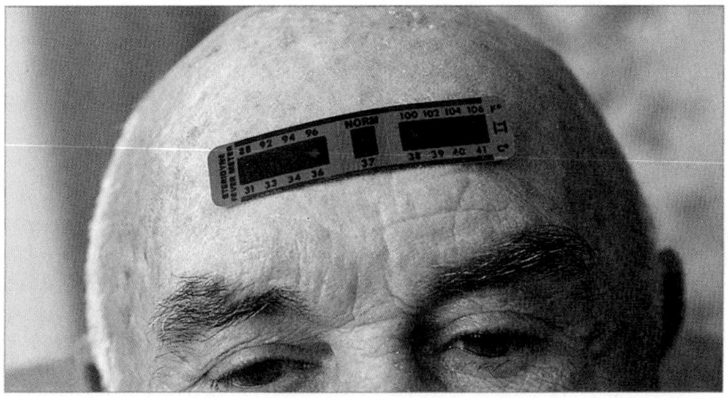

Figure 41–13 Temperature-sensitive tape.

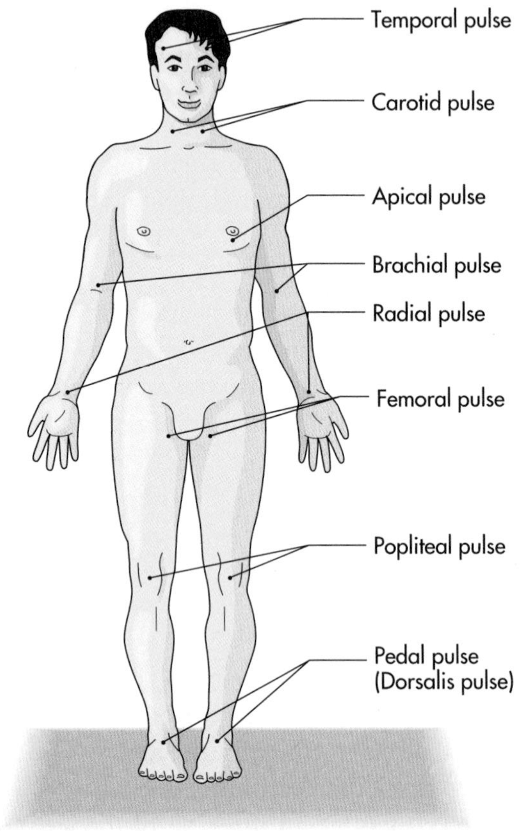

Figure 41–14 The pulse sites.

exposing the client. The carotid pulse (in adults and children) and the brachial pulse (in infants) are taken during emergencies.

Pulse Rate

Pulse rate is the number of heartbeats or pulses felt in 1 minute. The rate varies for each age group (Table 41–2) and is affected by many factors, including the following:

- Elevated body temperature (caused by fever or exposure to hot environments)
- Exercise
- Pain
- Position change (pulse rate temporarily increases when a client sits or stands after lying down)
- Caffeine
- Emotions (excitement, fear, anger, anxiety)
- Medications (can increase or slow down the pulse)

The adult pulse rate is between 60 and 100 beats per minute. A rate of less than 60 or more than 100 is not normal. Report abnormal rates at once:

Table 41–2 Pulse Ranges for Different Ages

Age	Pulse Rate (beats per minute)
Birth to 1 year	80–190
1 to 2 years	80–160
2 to 6 years	80–120
6 to 12 years	70–110
12 years and older	60–100

- **Tachycardia** is a rapid (*tachy*) heart rate (*cardia*). The heart rate is over 100 beats per minute.
- **Bradycardia** is a slow (*brady*) heart rate (*cardia*). The heart rate is less than 60 beats per minute.

You need to know the client's normal pulse range. Immediately report pulse rates that are higher or lower than normal for that client.

Rhythm and Force of the Pulse

The rhythm of the pulse should be regular, that is, the pulse should be felt in a pattern, and the same interval should be felt between beats. An irregular pulse occurs when the beats are unevenly spaced or beats are skipped. An abnormal rhythm—called **dysrhythmia**—must be reported at once.

The force of the pulse relates to its strength. A forceful pulse is easy to feel and is described as strong, full, or bounding. The hard-to-feel pulse is described as weak, thready, or feeble.

Electronic blood pressure equipment (see page 787) can also count the beats and shows the pulse rate along with blood pressure. However, it does not give information about pulse rhythm and force, which can be determined only by feeling the pulse.

Taking the Radial Pulse

The radial pulse is part of routine vital signs. Place the first two or three fingers of one hand against the radial artery, which is on the thumb side of the wrist (Figure 41–15). Do not use your thumb to take the pulse because the thumb also has a pulse, and you could mistake the pulse in your thumb for the client's pulse.

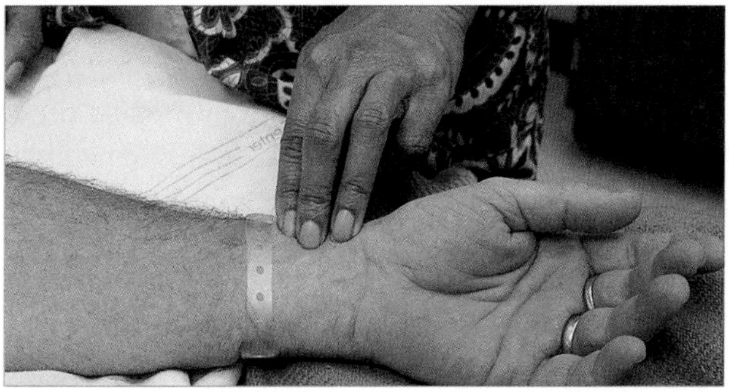

Figure 41–15 Use the middle two or three fingers to take the radial pulse.

You need a watch or clock with a second hand. If the pulse is irregular, count the beats for 1 minute. If it is regular, count the beats for 30 seconds. When you multiply the obtained number by 2, you will get the number of beats per minute.

Some employers require that the radial pulse be taken for 1 minute in all cases. Follow your employer's policy.

Report and record the following after taking the radial pulse:

- Pulse rate—beats per minute
- Pulse force—strong, full, bounding, weak, thready, or feeble
- Pulse rhythm—regular or irregular
- **Report immediately:**
  - A pulse rate less than 60 or more than 100 beats per minute
  - A pulse rate that is higher or lower than normal for the client

RESPIRATIONS

Respiration is the act of breathing air into (inhalation) and out of (exhalation) the lungs. Oxygen enters the lungs during inhalation, and carbon dioxide leaves the lungs during exhalation. Each respiration involves one inhalation and one exhalation. The chest rises during inhalation and falls

1 2 3 TAKING THE RADIAL PULSE

Remember to promote:

• Dignity • Independence • Preferences • Privacy • Safety

Pre-Procedure

1 Identify the client, according to employer policy.
2 Explain the procedure to the client.
3 Perform hand hygiene.
4 Provide for privacy.

Procedure

5 Have the client sit or lie down.
6 Locate the radial pulse. Use your first two or three middle fingers (see Figure 41–15).
7 Note if the pulse is strong or weak, and regular or irregular.
8 Count the beats for 30 seconds. Multiply the number obtained by 2. Or count the beats for 1 minute, if required by employer policy.
9 Count the beats for 1 minute, if it is irregular.
10 Record the client's name and pulse rate on your notepad or assignment sheet. Note the strength of the pulse. Note if it was regular or irregular.

Post-Procedure

11 Provide for safety and comfort.
12 Place the call bell within reach.*
13 Remove privacy measures.
14 Perform hand hygiene.
15 Report and record the pulse rate, the time you took the pulse, and your observations, according to employer policy.

*Steps marked with an asterisk may not apply in community settings.

during exhalation (see Chapter 14 for a review of the respiratory system).

The healthy adult has 12 to 20 respirations per minute. The respiratory rate is also affected by the same factors that affect temperature and pulse. Infections, heart disease, and respiratory diseases usually increase the respiratory rate.

Respirations are normally quiet, effortless, and regular. Both sides of the chest rise and fall in a uniform manner. If the chest barely moves during respiration, the breathing is described as shallow. Deep breathing occurs when the chest rises and falls significantly with every breath (see Chapter 44 for a description of abnormal respiratory patterns).

Count respirations when the client is at rest. Position the client so that you can see the chest rise and fall. To a certain extent, a client can control the depth and rate of breathing. Clients tend to change breathing patterns when they know their respirations are being counted, so try to count respirations without making the client aware of what you are doing.

Respirations are counted right after taking the pulse. Keep your fingers over the pulse site and maintain the pressure so that the client believes you are still taking the pulse. To count respirations, watch the chest rise and fall. Count how many times the chest rises and falls in 30 seconds. Remember, the rise *and* fall of the chest together is counted as 1 respiration. Multiply the number by 2 for the number of respirations in 1 minute. If an abnormal pattern is noted, count the respirations for 1 minute.

Respiratory rates vary according to age (Table 41–3). Infants and children have higher respiratory rates than do adults. Count an infant's respiratory rate for 1 minute.

Report and record the following observations after counting respirations:

- Respiratory rate
- Uniformity and depth of respirations (shallow, normal, or deep)
- Respiratory rhythm— regular or irregular
- Pain or difficulty breathing
- Any respiratory noises
- Any abnormal respiratory patterns (see Chapter 44)

1 2 3 COUNTING RESPIRATIONS

Remember to promote:

• Dignity • Independence • Preferences • Privacy • Safety

Procedure

1 Continue to hold the client's wrist after taking the radial pulse.

2 Do not tell the client you are counting respirations.

3 Begin each count when the chest rises and end when the chest falls. Count each rise and fall of the chest as 1 respiration.

4 Note the following:
- If respirations are regular
- If both sides of the chest rise uniformly
- The depth of the respirations
- If the client has pain or difficulty breathing

5 Count the respirations for 30 seconds. Multiply the number by 2.

6 Count respirations for 1 minute if they are abnormal or irregular.

7 Record respiratory rate and other observations on your notepad or assignment sheet.

Post-Procedure

8 Provide for safety and comfort.

9 Place the call bell within reach.*

10 Perform hand hygiene.

11 Report and record your actions, the time you took the respirations, and your observations according to employer policy.

*Steps marked with an asterisk may not apply in community settings.

Table 41–3 Normal Respiratory Rates by Age

Age	Respirations per minute
Newborn	30–60
Infant	30–50
Toddler	25–32
Child	20–30
Adolescent	16–19
Adult	12–20

Source: Ross-Kerr, J.C., Wood, M.J., Perry, A.G., & Potter, P.A. (2001). *Canadian fundamentals of nursing* (2nd ed., p. 699). Toronto: Harcourt Canada.

BLOOD PRESSURE

Blood pressure is the amount of force exerted by the blood against the walls of an artery. Blood pressure is controlled by:

- The force of heart contractions
- The amount of blood pumped with each heartbeat
- How easily the blood flows through the blood vessels

The period of heart muscle contraction is called **systole,** and the period of heart muscle relaxation is called **diastole.**

Both the systolic and diastolic pressures are measured. The **systolic pressure**, which is the higher pressure, represents the amount of force needed to pump blood out of the heart into the arterial circulation. The **diastolic pressure**, which is the lower pressure, reflects the pressure in the arteries when the heart is at rest.

Blood pressure is measured in millimetres (mm) of mercury (Hg). The systolic pressure is recorded over the diastolic pressure. The average adult has a systolic pressure of 120 mm Hg and a diastolic pressure of 80 mm Hg. This is written as 120/80 mm Hg.

The role of the support worker in taking blood pressure can vary from employer to employer and province to province. Ensure you are aware of your employer's policy.

Factors Affecting Blood Pressure

Blood pressure can change from minute to minute and can be affected by a number of factors (see Box 41–1). Because blood pressure can vary so easily, normal blood pressure has been assigned a range of values:

- ***Systolic pressure***—normal range is between 100 and 140 mm Hg
- ***Diastolic pressure***—normal range is between 60 and 90 mm Hg

Persistent measurements above the normal ranges of systolic and diastolic pressures are considered abnormal, and the condition is referred to as **hypertension** (see Chapter 41). In young and middle-aged adults, report any systolic pressure above 140 mm Hg at once. Also, report if the diastolic pressure is above 90 mm Hg. Likewise, systolic pressure below 90 mm Hg and diastolic pressure below 60 mm Hg must be reported, as this can be a condition referred to as **hypotension.** Low blood pressure may be normal in some clients, but hypotension may be a sign of a life-threatening problem (see the *Focus on Children: Blood Pressure* and *Focus on Older Adults: Blood Pressure* boxes.)

Equipment

A sphygmomanometer and stethoscope are used to measure blood pressure. Before using any equipment, make sure you have been properly trained to use it. Follow the manufacturer's instructions and employer policy.

Sphygmomanometer. A **sphygmomanometer** is an instrument used to measure blood pressure. It consists of a blood pressure cuff and a measuring device (*manometer*). In some provinces and territories,

Box 41–1 Factors Affecting Blood Pressure

- ***Age***—blood pressure increases with age. It is lowest in infancy and childhood and highest in adulthood.
- ***Gender (male or female)***—women usually have lower blood pressures than do men, but blood pressures tend to rise in women after menopause.
- ***Blood volume***—the amount of blood in the system. Severe bleeding lowers the blood volume and thus the blood pressure. Giving IV fluids rapidly increases the blood volume, raising the blood pressure as a result.
- ***Stress***—includes anxiety, fear, and other emotions. Blood pressure increases as the body responds to stress.
- ***Pain***—generally increases blood pressure. However, severe pain can cause shock, and blood pressure can be seriously lowered (see Chapter 47).
- ***Exercise***—increases blood pressure. Blood pressure should not be measured immediately after exercise.
- ***Weight***—blood pressure is higher in overweight people and is lowered with weight loss.
- ***Ethnicity***—blood pressure tends to be higher among Canadians of South Asian, Aboriginal, and African descents.
- ***Diet***—a high-sodium diet increases the amount of water in the body, and the extra fluid volume increases blood pressure.
- ***Medications***—can be given to raise or lower blood pressure. Other medications can cause high or low blood pressure as a side effect.
- ***Position***—blood pressure is lower when lying down and higher when standing. Sudden position changes can cause sudden changes in blood pressure (orthostatic hypotension). When standing suddenly, a rapid drop in blood pressure can occur, causing dizziness and fainting (see Chapter 24).
- ***Smoking***—increases blood pressure. The nicotine in cigarettes causes blood vessels to narrow, making the heart work harder to pump blood through narrowed vessels.
- ***Alcohol***—excessive alcohol intake can raise blood pressure.

support workers are only allowed to use digital electronic blood pressure machines. There are three types of manometers:

- ***Aneroid manometer***—has a round dial and a needle that points to the calibrations (Figure 41–16, *A*). These may be used in all settings.
- ***Mercury manometer***—has a column of mercury within a calibrated tube (Figure 41–16, *B*). Many hospitals have wall-mounted mercury manometers in patient rooms. Remember,

focus on ›› CHILDREN

Blood Pressure

As in the case of the other vital signs, in blood pressure, infants and children normally have lower values than adults do. A newborn's blood pressure is usually about 70/55 mm Hg. By 1 year of age, blood pressure increases to 90/55 mm Hg and continues to increase as the child grows older. Adult levels are reached between 14 and 18 years of age.

Taking an infant's or child's blood pressure is a complex task, as it usually involves special equipment. Measuring blood pressure in infants and children is therefore beyond a support worker's scope of practice, and the task should be the responsibility of a nurse.

focus on ›› OLDER ADULTS

Blood Pressure

With aging, arteries narrow and lose their elasticity, so the heart has to work harder to pump blood through the vessels. As a result, both the systolic and diastolic pressures are higher in older adults—a blood pressure of 160/90 mm Hg is considered normal for many older adults. It should be noted that older adults are at risk for orthostatic hypotension (see Chapter 24).

A C B D

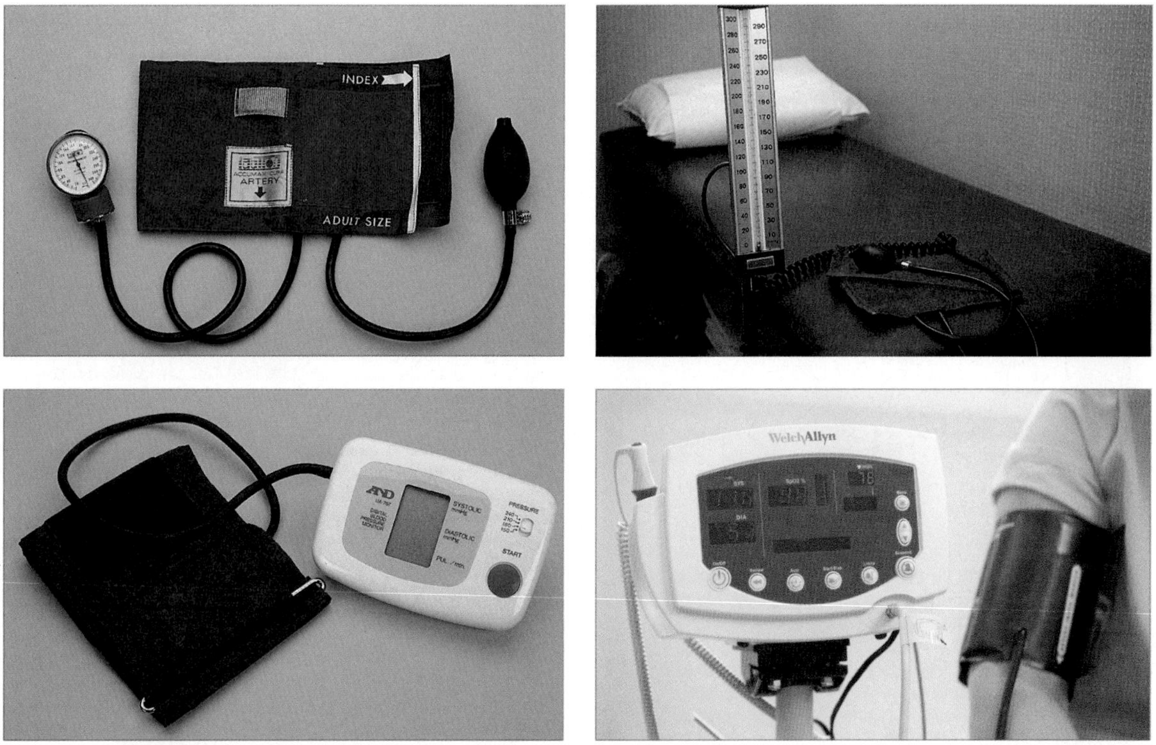

Figure 41–16 Sphygmomanometers. **A,** Aneroid manometer and cuff. **B,** Mercury manometer and cuff. **C,** Electronic manometer and cuff. **D,** Blood pressure machine on wheels. **Courtesy (for D):** Brian Hillier.

mercury is a hazardous substance. If a mercury manometer breaks, call for your supervisor at once. Do not touch the mercury, and do not let the client touch it. If possible, move the client from the area. The facility or agency must follow special procedures for handling all hazardous materials (see Chapter 19).

- ***Electronic manometer***—automatically displays the blood pressure measurement on the front of the device (Figure 41–16, *C*). The pulse rate is usually also displayed. The cuff automatically inflates and deflates on some models; some only have automatic deflation. Electronic manometers are common in facilities, and they are also available for home use. (Figure 41–16, D shows a blood pressure machine on wheels.)

The blood pressure cuff is wrapped around the upper arm of the client. Tubing connects the cuff to the manometer, and another tube connects the cuff to a small hand-held bulb. A valve on the bulb is turned so that the cuff inflates as the bulb is squeezed. The inflated cuff causes pressure over the brachial artery. The valve is turned the other way for cuff deflation, and blood pressure is measured as the cuff is deflated.

The right cuff size is important for accuracy. Children and clients with very small arms may need pediatric blood pressure cuffs, and those with very large arms may need extra-large cuffs.

Stethoscope. A **stethoscope**—an instrument used to listen to the sounds produced by the heart, lungs, and other body organs (Figure 41–17)—amplifies the sounds for easy hearing.

One of the uses of the stethoscope is to measure blood pressure. Sounds are produced as blood flows through the arteries, and the stethoscope is used to listen to these sounds in the brachial artery as the cuff is deflated. Stethoscopes are not needed with electronic sphygmomanometers.

Stethoscopes come in contact with the skin of many clients and health care team members during use, so infection control is important. The earpieces and diaphragm must be cleaned before and after each use to prevent the spread of microbes.

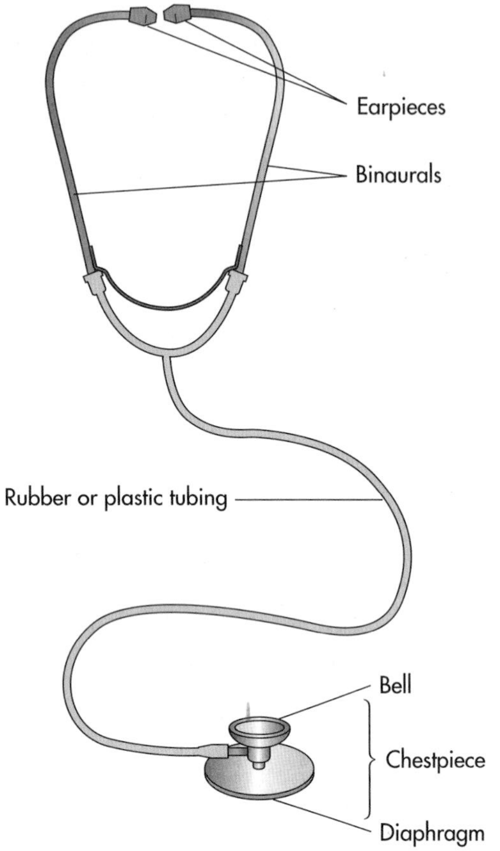

Figure 41–17 Parts of a stethoscope.

Follow these measures when using a stethoscope to measure blood pressure:

- Wipe the earpieces and diaphragm with antiseptic wipes before and after each use.
- Warm the diaphragm in your hand before touching the client with it (Figure 41–18).
- Place the earpiece tips in your ears. The bend of the tips should point forward. Earpieces should fit snugly to block out external noises. They should not cause pain or discomfort.
- Place the diaphragm over the client's brachial artery, and hold it in place (Figure 41–19).
- Prevent noise. Do not let anything touch the tubing. Ask the client to be silent.

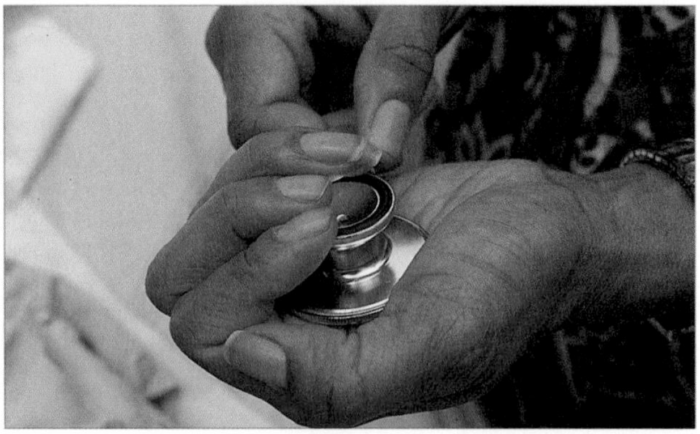

Figure 41–18 Warm the diaphragm of the stethoscope in the palm of your hand.

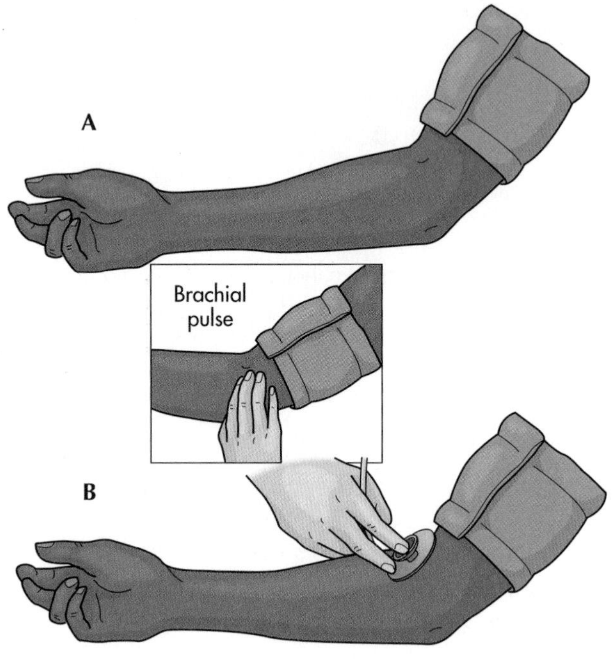

Figure 41–19 Measuring blood pressure. **A,** Apply the cuff over the brachial artery. **B,** Place the diaphragm of the stethoscope over the brachial artery.

Measuring Blood Pressure

Whenever you are asked to measure a client's blood pressure, it is very important to be accurate, as errors in measurement could cause harm to the client. Many employers do not allow support workers to measure and record blood pressure; however, if you are asked to measure blood pressure, make sure that:

- Your employer allows you to perform this procedure
- The procedure is in your job description
- You have received special training
- You have reviewed the procedure with a nurse
- A nurse is available to answer questions and to supervise you

As mentioned earlier, blood pressure is normally measured in the brachial artery. Box 41–2 lists the guidelines for measuring blood pressure.

Box 41–2 Guidelines for Measuring Blood Pressure

- Do not take blood pressure on an arm with an IV infusion, a cast, or a dialysis access site. If a client has had breast surgery, do not take blood pressure on that side. Avoid taking blood pressure on an injured arm.
- Let the client rest for 10 to 20 minutes before measuring blood pressure.
- Measure blood pressure with the client sitting or lying down. Sometimes the physician may order blood pressure to be measured in the standing position.
- Use the correct-sized blood pressure cuff for each client. For example, use a pediatric cuff for a very small arm.
- Apply the cuff to the bare upper arm. Remove any clothing that can affect the measurement.
- Make sure the cuff is snug, as loose cuffs can cause inaccurate readings.
- Place the diaphragm of the stethoscope firmly over the artery. The entire diaphragm must be in contact with the skin.
- Make sure the room is quiet. Talking, TV, radio, and sounds from the hallway can affect an accurate measurement.
- Have the manometer clearly visible.
- Measure the systolic and diastolic pressures. Expect to hear the first blood pressure sound at the point where you last felt the radial or brachial pulse. The first sound is the systolic pressure, and the point where the sound disappears is the diastolic pressure.
- Take the blood pressure again if you are not sure of an accurate measurement. Wait 30 to 60 seconds before repeating the measurement.
- Notify your supervisor at once if you cannot "hear" the blood pressure.
- Know the normal blood pressure ranges for the client. Immediately report any blood pressure measurement above or below the client's normal range.

1 2 3 MEASURING BLOOD PRESSURE

Remember to promote:

• **D**ignity • **I**ndependence • **P**references • **P**rivacy • **S**afety

Pre-Procedure

1 Identify the client, according to employer policy.
2 Explain the procedure to the client.
3 Perform hand hygiene.
4 Collect the following:
- Sphygmomanometer (blood pressure cuff)
- Stethoscope
- Antiseptic wipes

5 Provide for privacy.

Procedure

6 Clean the stethoscope earpieces and diaphragm with antiseptic wipes.
7 Have the client sit or lie down. Make sure the room is quiet and relaxing. Ask the client not to speak while you measure the blood pressure.
8 Position the client's arm level with the heart. The palm should face up.
9 Stand no more than 1 m (3 ft) away from the manometer. A mercury model must be vertical, on a flat surface, and at eye level. The aneroid type must be directly in front of you.
10 Expose the upper arm.
11 Squeeze the cuff to expel any remaining air. Close the valve on the bulb.
12 Find the brachial artery at the inner aspect of the elbow.
13 Place the arrow on the cuff over the brachial artery (see Figure 41–19, *A*). Wrap the cuff around the upper arm at least 2.5 cm (1 in.) above the elbow. It should be even and snug.
14 *Method 1:*
- **a** Place the stethoscope earpieces in your ears.
- **b** Locate the radial or brachial pulse.
- **c** Inflate the cuff until you can no longer feel the pulse. Note this point.
- **d** Inflate the cuff 30 mm Hg beyond the point where you last felt the pulse.

15 *Method 2:*
- **a** Locate the radial or brachial pulse.
- **b** Inflate the cuff until you can no longer feel the pulse. Note this point.
- **c** Inflate the cuff 30 mm Hg beyond the point where you last felt the pulse.
- **d** Deflate the cuff slowly. Note the point when you feel the pulse.
- **e** Wait 30 seconds.
- **f** Place the stethoscope earpieces in your ears.
- **g** Inflate the cuff 30 mm Hg beyond the point where you felt the pulse return.

16 Place the diaphragm over the brachial artery (see Figure 41–19, *B*). Do not place it under the cuff.
17 Deflate the cuff at an even rate of 2 to 4 mm per second. Turn the valve counterclockwise to deflate the cuff.
18 Note the point where you hear the first sound. This is the systolic reading. It should be near the point where the radial pulse disappeared.
19 Continue to deflate the cuff. Note the point where the sound disappears. This is the diastolic reading.
20 Deflate the cuff completely. Remove it from the client's arm. Remove the stethoscope.
21 Record the client's name and blood pressure on your notepad or assignment sheet.
22 Return the cuff to the case or wall holder.

Post-Procedure

23 Provide for safety and comfort.
24 Place the call bell within reach.*
25 Remove privacy measures.
26 Clean the earpieces and diaphragm with the wipes.
27 Return the equipment to its proper place.
28 Perform hand hygiene.
29 Report and record the blood pressure, the time you took the blood pressure, and your observations, according to employer policy.

*Steps marked with an asterisk may not apply in community settings.

REVIEW

Answers to these questions are at the bottom of the page.

Circle the BEST answer.

1. **The following statements are about measuring weight. Which one is *true*?**
   A. Before lunch is the best time to weigh the client.
   B. Chair and lift scales are used to weigh clients who cannot stand.
   C. A digital scale should read "12" before the client is weighed.
   D. A full bladder does not affect weight measurement.

2. **Which of the following statements is *true*?**
   A. The vital signs are temperature, pulse, respirations, and blood pressure.
   B. Vital signs cannot indicate changes in body function.
   C. Vital signs change only during illness.
   D. Sleep, exercise, medications, emotions, and noise do not affect vital signs.

3. **Which of the following should you report at once?**
   A. An oral temperature of 37.4°C
   B. A tympanic temperature of 38.2°C
   C. An axillary temperature of 36.1°C
   D. An oral temperature of 36.6°C

4. **You must take an infant's temperature. The care plan will likely tell you to take:**
   A. An oral temperature with a glass thermometer
   B. A rectal temperature
   C. An oral temperature with a tympanic thermometer
   D. An axillary temperature

5. **Which thermometer is rarely used in health care settings?**
   A. Digital
   B. Glass
   C. Electronic
   D. Dot matrix

6. **Which method is usually used to take a pulse?**
   A. The radial pulse
   B. The apical-radial pulse
   C. The apical pulse
   D. The brachial pulse

7. **Which of the following must be reported to your supervisor at once?**
   A. An adult has a pulse rate of 120 beats per minute.
   B. An infant has a pulse rate of 130 beats per minute.
   C. An adult has a pulse rate of 80 beats per minute.
   D. An adult has a pulse rate of 64 beats per minute.

8. **The following describe normal adult respirations. Which one is *true*?**
   A. There are between 8 and 12 per minute.
   B. They are quiet and effortless.
   C. They are irregular with both sides of the chest rising and falling uniformly.
   D. Noises occur on inhalation.

9. **Respirations are usually counted:**
   A. After taking the temperature
   B. After taking the pulse
   C. Before taking the pulse
   D. After taking the blood pressure

10. **Which blood pressure is normal for an adult?**
    A. 88/54 mm Hg
    B. 210/100 mm Hg
    C. 130/82 mm Hg
    D. 152/90 mm Hg

11. **When taking the blood pressure, you should:**
    A. Take the blood pressure in the arm with an IV infusion
    B. Apply the cuff to a bare upper arm
    C. Turn on the TV and radio
    D. Locate the aortic artery

12. **Which is the systolic blood pressure?**
    A. The point at which the pulse is no longer felt
    B. The point where the first sound is heard
    C. The point where the last sound is heard
    D. The point 30 mm Hg above where the pulse was felt

Answers: 1.B, 2.A, 3.B, 4.D, 5.B, 6.A, 7.A, 8.B, 9.B, 10.C, 11.B, 12.B

CHAPTER 42

Wound Care

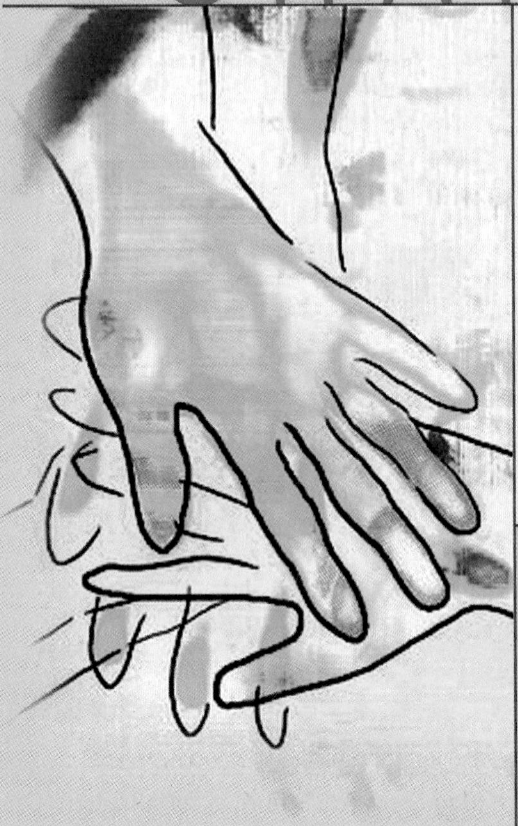

OBJECTIVES

- Define the key terms listed in this chapter.
- List clients at risk for skin tears and pressure ulcers.
- Describe the causes of skin tears and how to prevent them.
- Describe the signs, symptoms, and causes of pressure ulcers and ways to prevent them.
- Identify the pressure points in the basic bed positions and sitting positions.
- Describe the causes of leg and foot ulcers and ways to prevent them.
- Describe the process, types, and complications of wound healing.
- Describe what to observe about wounds and wound drainage.
- Explain how to secure dressings.
- Explain the guidelines for applying dressings.
- Explain the purpose of binders and the guidelines for applying them.
- Describe how to meet the basic needs of clients who have wounds.
- Apply in your practice the procedures described in this chapter.

key terms

abrasion A partial-thickness wound caused by the scraping away or rubbing of the skin.

arterial ulcer An open wound on the lower legs and feet caused by poor arterial blood flow.

bedsore See **pressure ulcer**.

bony prominence An area on the body where the underlying bone seems to "stick out." The shoulder blades, elbows, hip bones, sacrum (the bone in the lower part of the spine), knees, ankle bones, heels, and toes are all bony prominences.

bruise See **contusion**.

chronic wound A wound that does not heal easily.

circulatory ulcer An open wound on the lower legs and feet caused by decreased blood flow through arteries or veins. Also known as **vascular ulcer**.

clean wound A wound that is not infected; microbes have not entered the wound.

clean-contaminated wound A wound occurring from the surgical portal of entry into the urinary, reproductive, or digestive system.

closed wound A wound in which tissues are injured but the skin is not broken.

contaminated wound A wound with high risk of infection; pathogens have entered the wound.

contusion A closed wound caused by a blow to the body. Also known as **bruise**.

decubitus ulcer See **pressure ulcer**.

dehiscence The separation of wound layers.

dirty wound See **infected wound**.

edema Swelling in the tissues caused by an accumulation of fluid.

evisceration Separation of the wound accompanied by protrusion of abdominal organs.

full-thickness wound A wound in which the dermis, epidermis, and subcutaneous tissue are penetrated; muscle and bone may be involved.

gangrene A condition in which there is tissue death.

hematoma The collection of blood under the skin and tissues.

hemorrhage The excessive loss of blood in a short period of time.

incision An open wound with clean, straight edges; usually intentionally created with a sharp instrument.

infected wound A wound containing large amounts of bacteria and showing signs of infection. Also known as **dirty wound**.

intentional wound A wound created for treatment.

laceration An open wound with torn tissues and jagged edges.

necrotic tissue Localized tissue death as a result of disease or injury.

open wound A wound in which the skin or mucous membrane is broken.

partial-thickness wound A wound in which the dermis and epidermis of the skin are broken.

penetrating wound An open wound in which the skin and underlying tissues are pierced.

peri-wash A type of soap that is used to wash the skin. It is used primarily as a cleanser and deodorizer of the perineal area soiled by urine and feces. It also emulsifies (breaks up) feces to aid gentle, easy cleaning. Because it is pH balanced to the acid mantle (covering) of the skin, it does not have to be rinsed off like other harsher soaps.

picture-frame dressing A type of dressing in which the tape is applied to all four edges to reduce the likelihood of the dressing wrinkling or falling off.

pitting edema A type of edema that is evident by (a) first compressing your fingers into the swollen tissues, (b) then removing your fingers, (c) observing an impression of your fingers left in the skin.

pressure points Bony prominences that bear the weight of the body in certain positions, which may lead to **pressure ulcers**.

pressure sore See **pressure ulcer**.

pressure ulcer Any injury caused by unrelieved pressure. Also known as **decubitus ulcer**, **bedsore**, or **pressure sore**.

puncture wound An open wound made by a sharp object; entry of the skin and underlying tissues may be intentional or unintentional.

purulent drainage Thick drainage from a wound or body orifice that is yellow, green, or brown in colour that could indicate an infection.

shock The condition that results when there is not enough blood supply to organs and tissues.

skin tear A break or rip in the skin; the epidermis separates from the underlying tissue.

key terms

stasis ulcer See **venous ulcer**.

steri-strip A type of adhesive bandage in which thin strips are applied across a skin tear; the dressing will bring the skin edges together and hold them together while the wound heals.

tissue A group of cells that perform a similar function together.

trauma An accident or violent act that injures the skin, mucous membranes, bones, or internal organs (physical trauma) or causes an emotionally painful, distressful, or shocking result (emotional trauma) that often leads to lasting mental and physical effects (psychological trauma).

unintentional wound A wound resulting from trauma.

vascular ulcer See **circulatory ulcer**.

venous ulcer Open wounds on the lower legs and feet caused by poor blood return through the veins. Also known as **stasis ulcer**.

wound A break in the skin or mucous membrane.

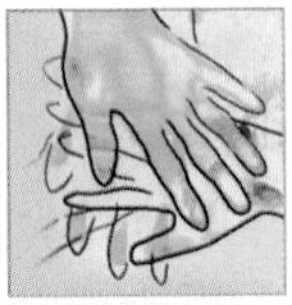

Skin is the body's first line of defence, protecting the body from microbes that cause infection and disease. As a support worker, you have to consider providing good skin care to your clients as one of your most important tasks. Infants, older adults, and clients who are disabled are at greater risk for skin breakdown because their skin can be easily injured due to limited mobility and certain health conditions that make their skin more susceptible to injury. It should be noted, however, that the skin of infants and the skin of older adults are quite different (see Chapter 14). Box 42–1 lists the common causes of skin breakdown.

A **wound** is a break in the skin or mucous membrane and becomes a portal of entry for microbes. Wounds result from many causes. A surgical incision leaves a wound, and often, wounds result from **trauma**—an accident or violent act that injures the skin, mucous membranes, bones, or internal organs. Trauma may be caused by falls, vehicle accidents, gun shots, stabbings, and other violent acts. Pressure ulcers are wounds that occur due to poor skin care and immobility. Circulatory ulcers are caused by decreased blood flow through the arteries and veins to that area of **tissue** (a group of cells that perform a similar function together).

The support worker's role in wound care depends on provincial or territorial laws, job description, and the client's condition. Whatever your role, you need to know the types of wounds, how wounds heal, and how to promote wound healing. You must prevent skin injury and give good skin care. When injury *does* occur, infection is a major threat, so wound care is important for preventing infection and further injury to the wound and nearby tissues.

Box 42–1 Common Causes of Skin Breakdown

- Age-related changes in the skin
- Skin dryness
- Fragile and weak capillaries
- General thinning of the skin
- Loss of fatty layer under the skin
- Decreased sensation to touch, heat, and cold
- Decreased mobility
- Sitting in a chair or lying in bed most or all of the day
- Chronic diseases (e.g., diabetes, high blood pressure)
- Diseases that decrease circulation
- Poor nutrition
- Poor hydration
- Incontinence
- Moisture in the dark areas of the body (skin folds, under breasts, between toes, and perineal areas)
- Pressure on bony parts (Figure 42–1)
- Poor care of fingernails or toenails
- Friction and shearing

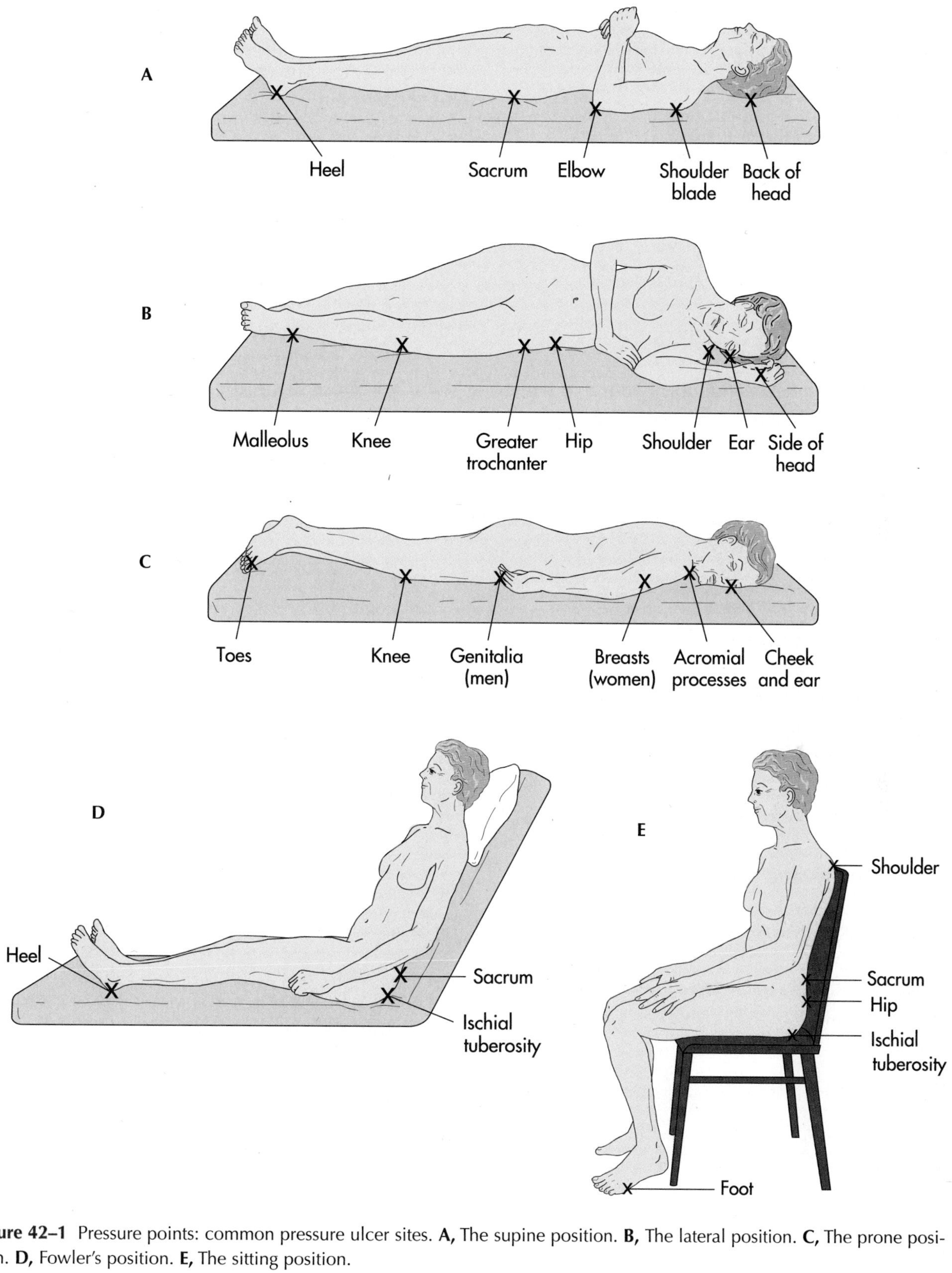

Figure 42–1 Pressure points: common pressure ulcer sites. **A,** The supine position. **B,** The lateral position. **C,** The prone position. **D,** Fowler's position. **E,** The sitting position.

TYPES OF WOUNDS

Wounds are described in many ways (see Box 42–2), including the following:

- ***Abrasion***—a partial-thickness wound caused by the scraping away or rubbing of the skin
- ***Contusion***—a closed wound caused by a blow to the body (a **bruise**)
- ***Incision***—an open wound with clean, straight edges; usually intentionally created with a sharp instrument
- ***Laceration***—an open wound with torn tissues and jagged edges
- ***Penetrating wound***—an open wound in which the skin and underlying tissues are pierced
- ***Puncture wound***—an open wound made by a sharp object; entry of the skin and underlying tissues may be intentional or unintentional

SKIN TEARS

A **skin tear** is a break or rip in the skin. The epidermis (top skin layer) separates from the underlying tissue (see Figure 23–4). The hands, arms, and lower legs are common sites for skin tears. Many older adults have very thin and fragile skin, and even slight pressure can cause a skin tear. Clients who are most likely to have skin tears are those with very dry and paper-thin skin.

Box 42–2 Types of Wounds

Intentional Wound and Unintentional Wound

- **Intentional wound**—is created for treatment; for example, surgical incisions, as well as venipunctures for starting IV therapy or for collecting blood specimens
- **Unintentional wound**—results from trauma (falls, vehicle accidents, gun shots, stabbings, and other violent acts)

Open Wound and Closed Wound

- **Open wound**—occurs when the skin or mucous membrane is broken; intentional and most unintentional wounds are open
- **Closed wound**—occurs when tissues are injured but the skin is not broken (bruises, twists, and sprains)

Clean Wound and Contaminated Wound

- **Clean wound**—is not infected. Microbes have not entered the wound; closed wounds and intentional wounds created under surgically aseptic conditions are usually clean; because the urinary, respiratory, and digestive systems are not entered, there is a reduced risk of infection
- **Clean-contaminated wound**—occurs from the surgical (sterile technique used) entry of the urinary, reproductive, or digestive system; because these systems are not sterile and contain normal flora, the risk of infection is greater than with a sterile wound
- **Contaminated wound**—has a high risk of infection; unintentional wounds (such as a stabbing) are wounds that are not created under sterile conditions and are generally contaminated; wound contamination also occurs from breaks in surgical asepsis and from the spillage of intestinal contents. Tissues may show signs of inflammation
- **Infected wound (dirty wound)**—contains large amounts of bacteria and shows signs of infection; for example, old wounds, surgical incisions into infected areas (such as a ruptured appendix), and traumatic injuries that rupture the bowel
- **Chronic wound**—does not heal easily, such as pressure ulcers and circulatory ulcers; any wound that is continually exposed to friction, pressure, or moisture can become chronic

Partial- and Full-Thickness Wounds (Described by Wound Depth)

- **Partial-thickness wound**—the dermis and epidermis of the skin are broken
- **Full-thickness wound**—the dermis, epidermis, and subcutaneous tissue are penetrated; muscle and bone may be involved.

Causes of Skin Tears

Skin tears occur due to friction, shearing (see Chapter 23), pulling, or direct pressure on the skin. Skin tears are commonly caused by:

- Bumping a hand, arm, or leg on any hard surface, such as a bed, bed rail, chair, wheelchair footrest, or table
- Holding on to a client's arm or leg too tightly
- Repositioning, moving, or transferring a client without a transfer sheet or any nonfriction surface, which can cause the client's skin to rub against the surface and even tear
- Bathing, dressing, and other tasks
- Pulling buttons or zippers across fragile skin

It is always your responsibility to be careful when moving, repositioning, or transferring clients. Skin tears are painful, and they can become portals of entry for pathogens. Tell your supervisor at once if you cause or find a skin tear, bruise, bump, or scrape (see *Supporting Mrs. Nippeskaya*).

Clients at Risk for Skin Tears

Clients at risk for skin tears include those who:

- Require moderate to complete help in moving
- Have poor nutrition or are very thin
- Are poorly hydrated
- Have altered mental awareness; for example, clients with dementia may resist care and move quickly and without warning, which can cause skin tears
- Are older

Prevention and Treatment of Skin Tears

Giving careful and safe care helps prevent skin tears and further injury. Follow the guidelines in Box 42–3.

The physician and the nurse direct skin care treatment and may order dressings. Elastic wraps protect the skin from injury and help the healing process. Follow the care plan and your supervisor's instructions.

supporting MRS. NIPPESKAYA

You are the support worker assigned to care for Olga Nippeskaya, 56, a widow with ovarian cancer currently living at the long-term care facility where you are employed. Her daughter is trying to make arrangements to move her mother to the town where she lives. Because of Mrs. Nippeskaya's illness and her treatments, she has lost approximately 50 kg (120 pounds) over the past year.

Mrs. Nippeskaya has been very weak and dizzy for several months now, and while at home, she frequently fell or bumped into the corner of her bed and dresser. She has been advised to ask for assistance to go to the washroom since being admitted to your facility. Yesterday, however, she did *not* ask for assistance, and when she stood up on her own, she lost her balance and fell to the floor hitting the side of her bed.

The nursing staff heard Mrs. Nippeskaya fall and came to her side immediately. Upon examination, they observed a 3.75-cm (1.5-in.) tear on her right buttock and a 2.5-cm (1-in.) tear on her right forearm around her elbow. She also had several bruises and scrapes on her right arm and had difficulty moving her leg. Mrs. Nippeskaya was taken by ambulance to the local hospital, where she was examined, her leg was X-rayed, and her skin tears were **steri-stripped.** Back at the facility, she agreed to be lifted with a mechanical lift (see Chapter 23) for toileting.

Today, you and your co-worker apply the mechanical lift sling carefully and properly under Mrs. Nippeskaya's hips, according to your agency's policy. However, while raising her up, you notice that there is blood on her pants over her buttock area. You carefully lower her and remove her pants to find the source of the blood.

You discover that her buttock skin tear has reopened due to friction of the mechanical lift sling on her skin. While your co-worker stays with Mrs. Nippeskaya, you summon assistance from the nurse. You are instructed to document everything you have observed and to switch to another mechanical device that does not require placing a sling around the client's buttocks. The nurse then reapplies clean steri-strips to Mrs. Nippeskaya's skin tear and fills out an incident report (see Chapter 19).

Box 42-3 Guidelines for Preventing Skin Tears

- Follow the care plan for moving, lifting, repositioning, transferring, dressing, and bathing the client.
- Keep the skin moisturized. Follow the care plan.
- Offer fluids. Follow the care plan.
- Dress and undress the client carefully.
- Dress the client in soft clothing with long sleeves and long pants. Allow the client to make choices.
- Keep your fingernails short and filed smooth.
- Keep the client's fingernails short and filed smooth. Report client's long and rough toenails to your supervisor.
- Do not wear rings with large or raised stones.
- Follow safety guidelines when transferring or lifting the client to and from a bed and wheelchair (see Chapter 23).
- Prevent friction and shearing during lifting, moving, transferring, and repositioning.
- Use a turning sheet to move and turn the client in bed.
- Use pillows to support arms and legs. Follow the care plan.
- Be patient and calm when the client is confused or agitated or resists care.
- Ensure that bed rails and wheelchair arms, footrests, and leg supports are padded. Follow the care plan.
- Provide good lighting to prevent the client from bumping into furniture, walls, and equipment.

PRESSURE ULCERS

A **pressure ulcer (decubitus ulcer, bedsore, pressure sore)** is any injury caused by unrelieved pressure that usually occurs over a **bony prominence**—an area where the bone seems to "stick out" and is compressed under the client or between the client's skin folds. The shoulder blades, elbows, hip bones, sacrum (the bone in the lower part of the spine), knees, ankle bones, heels, and toes are all bony prominences.

These bony prominences are called **pressure points** because they bear the weight of the body in certain positions (see Figure 42–1). Pressure from body weight can reduce blood supply to the area, which results in a pressure ulcer. Pressure points that are moist with perspiration or body excretions are especially prone to developing a pressure ulcer as well as bacterial infections that are very difficult to treat once they set in.

Causes of Pressure Ulcers

Pressure, friction, and shearing are common causes of skin breakdown and pressure ulcers. Other factors include breaks in the skin, poor circulation to an area, moisture (such as perspiration or urine), dry, flaky skin, and irritation from urine and stool. Pressure occurs when the skin over a bony prominence is squeezed between hard surfaces. In obese people, pressure ulcers can develop in areas where friction is caused by skin-to-skin contact.

Pressure ulcers can also occur in thin people when two bony areas are in direct contact with each other (such as knees or ankles rubbing together). The bone itself is one of the hard surfaces, while the other is usually the mattress or chair seat. This squeezing or pressure interferes with blood flow to the skin and underlying tissues, preventing oxygen and nutrients from reaching the cells (see *Supporting Mr. Hansen*) and causing the death of the involved skin and tissues (Figure 42–2).

Friction scrapes the skin, and the resulting wound creates a portal of entry for microbes. For the scraped area to heal, a good blood supply to the area and prevention of infection are necessary. A

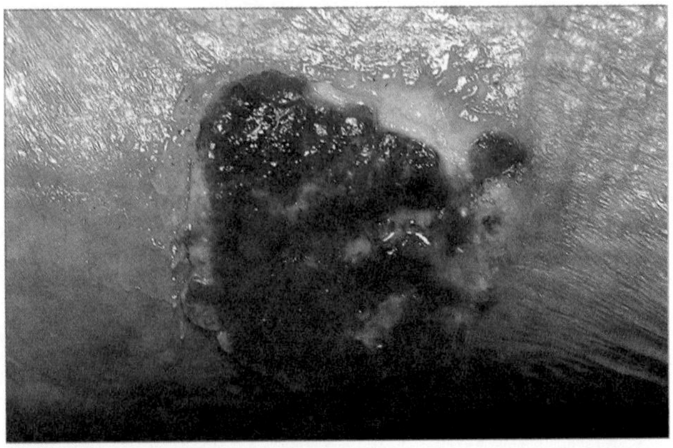

Figure 42–2 A pressure ulcer.

poor blood supply or an infection can lead to a pressure ulcer.

Other High Risk Areas. Skin fold areas—under the breasts, between the abdominal folds, on the legs and buttocks, and between toes—are also at risk for infection (which can lead to the formation of pressure sores). These areas, often missed during a bed bath, are frequently warm and moist because of perspiration and infrequent exposure to air. In addition, some clients use body lotions that tend to add moisture to the skin in these areas, increasing the risk for infection. As a support worker, it is your responsibility to wash these body areas well, ensure they are dried thoroughly, and report any signs of redness or skin irritation to your supervisor. A small piece of cloth or gauze inserted under a large breast can help prevent moisture and friction—and thus skin redness and breakdown—whenever a bra is not worn.

supporting
MR. HANSEN

Otto Hansen, a 75-year-old man, has been cared for by his wife (a retired nurse) at home since his stroke 5 years ago. He has limited use of his left side; however, being right-handed, he is able to write and to assist his wife with his care in a number of ways. His wife was admitted recently to the hospital for pneumonia, so your agency has been hired to provide respite personal care and support to him while she is recovering.

Today, while you are washing Mr. Hansen's feet, you notice a large doughnut-shaped blister on his left heel. When you ask him about the blister, Mr. Hansen tells you that when a pressure ulcer developed on his heel, his wife made something to prevent his heel from getting any worse. When he shows it to you, you see that it is a doughnut-shaped object made by wrapping a gauze strip around a circular object. The blistered area seems to be the same size and shape as the "doughnut."

Uncertain about what to do about this, you call your supervisor, who says that Mr. Hansen should discard the "doughnut." She explains that although it might prevent the heel from getting a blister, that circular surface will suffer from increased pressure when Mr. Hansen is lying in bed with his heel resting flat on the bed and this will cause a pressure ulcer to develop! You convey to Mr. Hansen what your supervisor has said. After thinking about this, he then asks you how he can prevent getting blisters (or pressure sores) on his heel in the future. How will you advise him?

Shearing. Shearing, which also exerts pressure on the skin, is caused when the skin sticks to a surface (usually the bed or chair) and deeper tissues move downward, exerting pressure on the skin (see Chapter 23). Shearing occurs when the client slides down in the bed or chair. Blood vessels and tissues are damaged, which reduces blood flow to the area and increases the risk of a pressure ulcer.

Clients at Risk for Pressure Ulcers

Clients at risk for pressure ulcers are those who:

- Are confined to bed or a chair
- Require moderate to complete help in moving
- Have loss of bowel or bladder control
- Have poor nutrition
- Have altered mental awareness
- Have problems sensing pain or pressure
- Have circulatory problems
- Are older
- Are obese or very thin

Signs of Pressure Ulcers

The first sign of a pressure ulcer is pale skin or a warm, reddened area. Colour changes in the skin may be hard to notice in dark-skinned clients, so if the client is complaining of pain, burning, itching, or tingling in the area (common signs and symptoms of poor blood flow to the area), you should report this to your supervisor. However, some clients may not feel anything unusual, so it is important that you observe your client and look for other signs of poor blood flow to the area. Box 42–4 describes pressure ulcer development. It is your responsibility to check your client's skin every time you provide personal care. You should

Box 42–4 Stages of Pressure Ulcers

Stage 1 The skin is red. The colour does not return to normal when the skin is relieved of pressure (Figure 42–3, *A*).

Stage 2 The skin cracks, blisters, or peels (Figure 42–3, *B*). There may be a shallow crater.

Stage 3 The skin is gone, and the underlying tissues are exposed and damaged (Figure 42–3, *C*). There may be drainage from the area.

Stage 4 Muscle and bone are exposed and damaged (Figure 42–3, *D*). Drainage is likely.

also immediately notify your supervisor if you observe any signs of a pressure ulcer.

Prevention and Treatment of Pressure Ulcers

Pressure ulcers develop over time. The longer that pressure is exerted on the skin, the greater is the risk that a pressure ulcer will develop.

Preventing pressure ulcers is much easier than healing them. Good support care, (which includes frequent position changes and ensuring a proper diet with lots of fluid), cleanliness, and skin care are essential. Box 42–5 lists guidelines for preventing skin breakdown and pressure ulcers. As always, it is important that you also follow your client's care plan and adhere to the preventative measures described on it.

Any client at risk for pressure ulcers is placed on a surface that reduces or relieves pressure—for example, foam, air, alternating air, gel, or water mattresses. The health care team decides on the best surface for the client.

A physician orders specific pressure ulcer treatment—wound care products, medications, treatments, and special equipment—for each client. Your supervisor and the care plan tell you what to do. The following protective devices are often ordered to prevent and treat pressure ulcers and other types of skin breakdown.

Special Beds. Some beds may have air flowing through the mattress (Figure 42–5), may be made out of a gel-like substance, or may be made out of a special foam material that conforms to the body. On these mattresses, the client seems to *float*, which allows body weight to be evenly distributed and reduces pressure on bony parts.

Another type of bed allows repositioning clients without having to move them. Depending on the bed, the client is turned to the prone or supine position, or the bed is tilted to various degrees. Body alignment does not change, but pressure

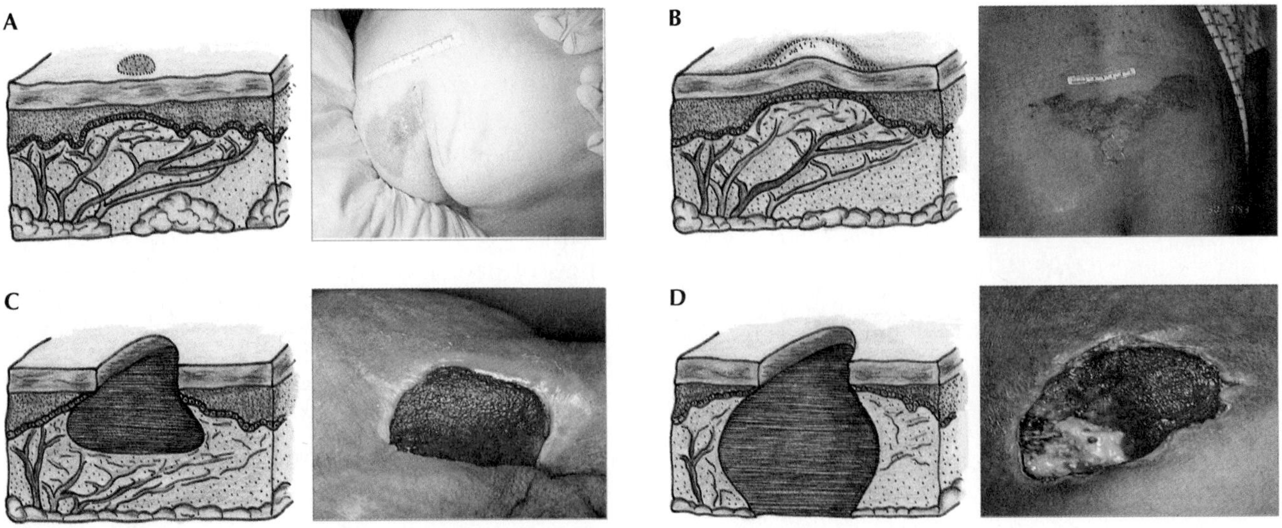

Figure 42–3 Stages of pressure ulcers. **A,** Stage 1. **B,** Stage 2. **C,** Stage 3. **D,** Stage 4. **Courtesy:** Laurel Wiersema-Bryant, RN, MSN, Clinical Nurse Specialist, Barnes-Jewish Hospital, St. Louis, MO.

Box 42–5 Guidelines for Preventing Pressure Ulcers

- Follow the repositioning schedule in the care plan. Some clients have to be repositioned at least every 2 hours and some every 15 minutes. Each client's care plan should have specific instructions with regard to that client.
- Position the client as specified in the care plan. Use pillows for support, as instructed by your supervisor. The 30-degree lateral position is recommended (Figure 42–4).
- Use proper lifting, positioning, and transferring procedures to prevent friction and shearing (see Chapter 23).
- To reduce the likelihood of shearing, do not raise the head of the bed to more than 30 degrees. Always follow your client's care plan.
- Provide good skin care. The skin must be clean and dry after bathing and kept free of moisture from urine, stool, perspiration, and wound drainage.
- Minimize exposure of skin to moisture. Check incontinent clients (those with loss of bowel or bladder control) frequently. Also check clients who perspire heavily and those with wound drainage. Change linens and clothing, as needed. Give good skin care.
- Check with your supervisor before using soap on a client. Soap can dry and irritate the skin.
- Apply a moisturizer on dry areas—hands, elbows, legs, ankles, and heels—but not on the areas under the breasts, between skin folds, and between toes. Your supervisor will tell you what to use and where to apply it. As a very wise nurse once stated, ***"Never grease a crease!"***
- Give a back massage after repositioning the client. Do not massage bony areas.
- Keep linens clean, dry, and wrinkle-free.
- Do not irritate the skin. Avoid scrubbing or rubbing when bathing or drying the client.
- Do not massage pressure points. ***Never rub or massage reddened areas, but massage the skin around the reddened area. Be careful to never scratch or irritate the skin.***
- Use pillows and blankets to prevent skin-to-skin contact and to reduce moisture and friction.
- Keep the client's heels off the bed. Use pillows or other devices, as directed. Place the pillows or devices under the lower legs from midcalf to the ankles.
- Use protective devices, as instructed by your supervisor and the care plan.
- Remind clients sitting in chairs to shift their positions every 15 minutes to decrease pressure on bony points. Assist, if requested.
- Report any signs of skin breakdown or pressure ulcers at once. Record your observations, according to employer policy.
- Remember that areas that had pressure ulcers in the past (but are now healed) are always at risk of re-developing the ulcers. Pay particular attention to these areas, and follow the above guidelines.

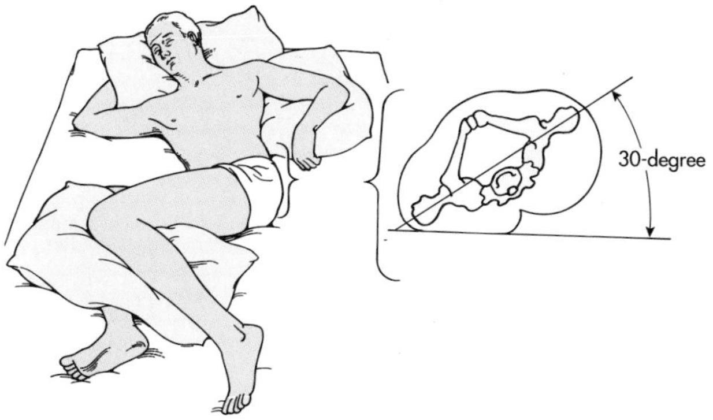

Figure 42–4 The 30-degree lateral position. Pillows are placed under the head, shoulder, and leg. This position inclines (lifts up) the hip to avoid pressure on the hip. The client does not lie on the hip as in the side-lying position. **Source:** Bryant, R.A. et al. (1992). Pressure ulcer. In R.A. Bryant, ed. *Acute and chronic wounds: Nursing management.* St. Louis: Mosby.

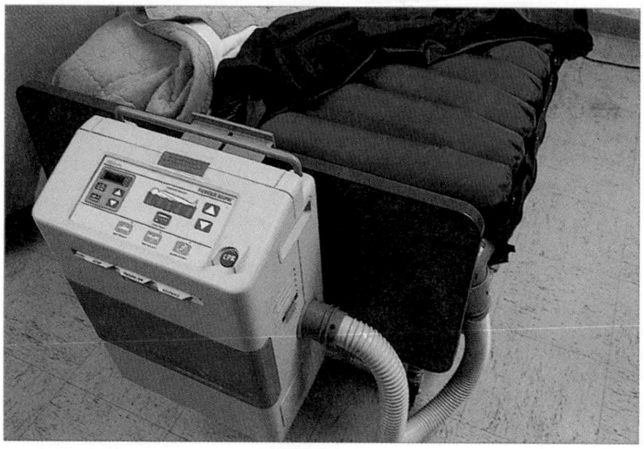

Figure 42–5 Air flotation bed.

points change as the position changes, and there is little friction. Some beds continually rotate from side to side and are useful for clients with spinal cord injuries.

Bed Cradle. A bed cradle (Anderson frame) is a metal frame placed on the bed and over the client. Top linens are brought over the cradle to prevent pressure of linens on the legs and feet (Figure 42–6). Top linens are either folded back to expose the feet if the client is too warm or may be tucked in at the bottom of the mattress and mitred, if the client prefers it. They are also tucked under both sides of the mattress to protect the client from air drafts and chilling (see the *Focus on Home Care: Bed Cradles* box.)

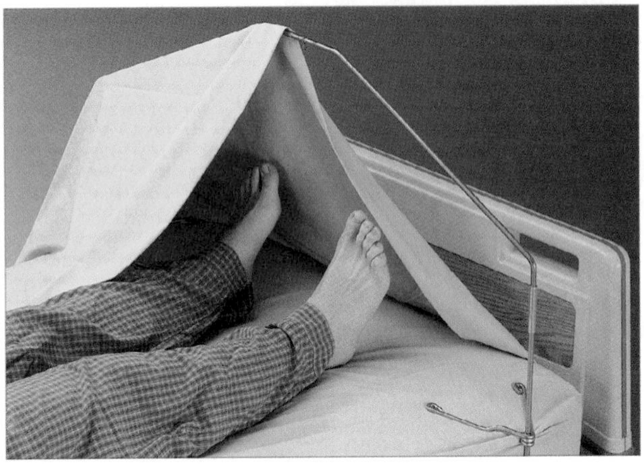

Figure 42–6 A bed cradle is placed on top of the bed. Linens are brought over the top of the cradle. **Courtesy:** J.T. Posey Company, Arcadia, California.

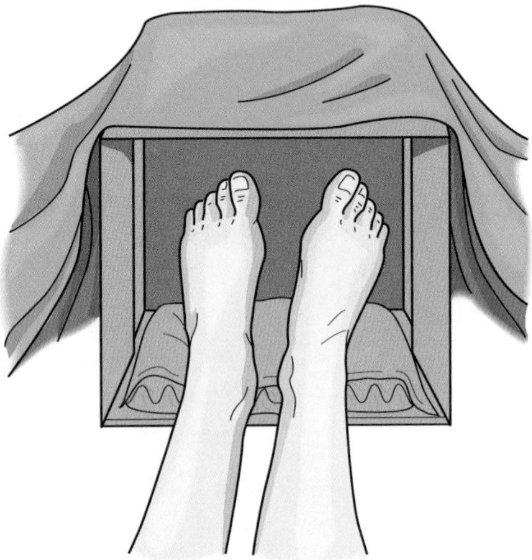

Figure 42–7 A cardboard box serves as a bed cradle. It keeps top linens off the client's feet.

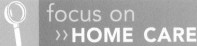

focus on
»HOME CARE

Bed Cradles

A cardboard box can be used as a bed cradle (Figure 42–7). Your supervisor would tell you how to line the box to prevent pressure on the heels.

Elbow Protectors. These devices, made of foam rubber or sheepskin, prevent friction between the bed and the elbow. They fit the shape of the elbow (Figure 42–8); some have straps to secure them in place.

Heel Elevators. Pillows or special cushions raise the heels off the bed (Figure 42–9). Special braces and splints also keep pressure off the heels.

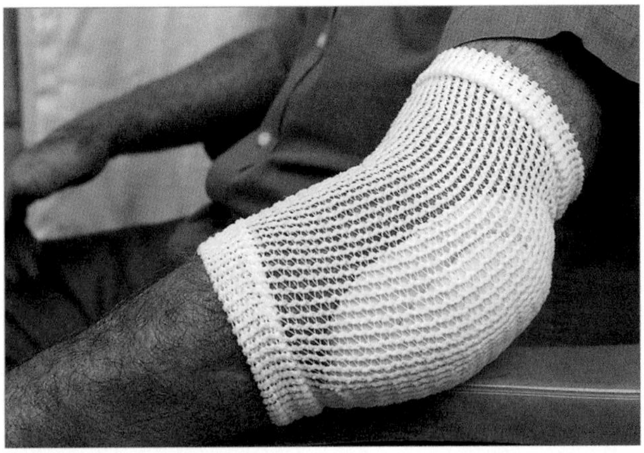

Figure 42–8 Elbow protector.

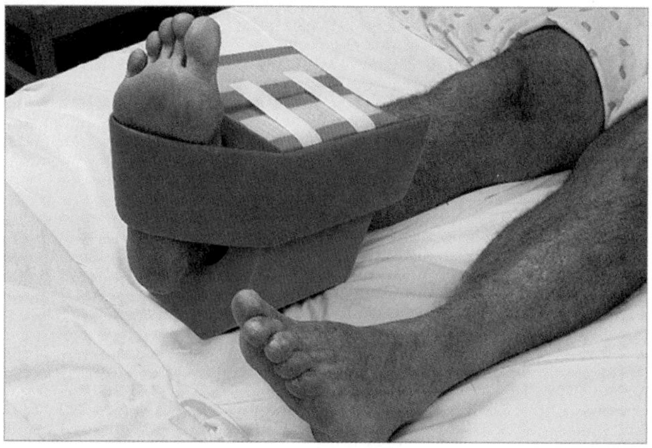

Figure 42–9 Heel elevator.

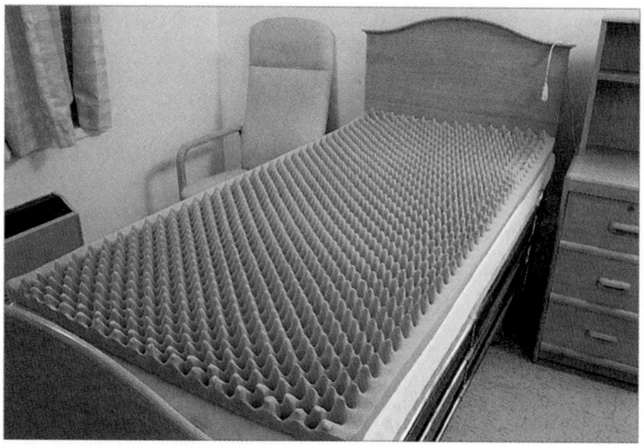

Figure 42–11 Eggcrate-like mattress on the bed.

Flotation Pads. Flotation pads or cushions (Figure 42–10) are like water beds, but they are made of a gel-like substance with an outer case of heavy plastic. The pads can be placed in chairs and wheelchairs, which allows the client to sit comfortably without the risk of developing pressure ulcers. The pad is placed in a pillowcase or special cover to prevent the plastic from coming in contact with the client's skin.

Eggcrate-like Mattress. This is a foam pad that looks like an egg carton (Figure 42–11), with peaks that distribute the client's weight more evenly. This mattress is placed on top of the regular mattress. The eggcrate-like mattress is placed in a special cover that protects it against moisture and soiling. Only a bottom sheet covers the mattress. There is some concern that this type of mattress may create pressure points, so they are not commonly used. They are, however, inexpensive and commercially available, and some family physicians still recommend them to their clients.

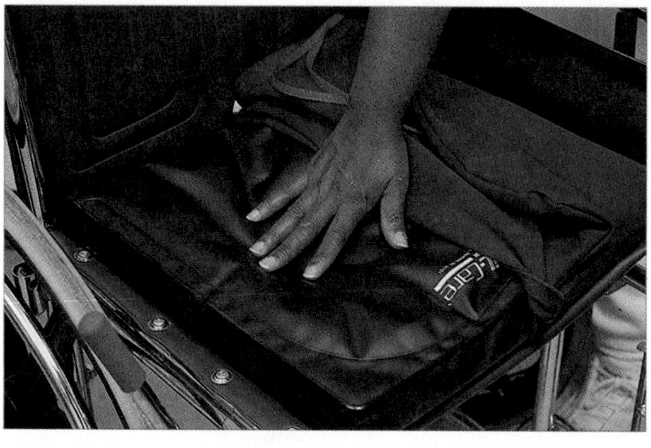

Figure 42–10 Flotation pad.

Other Equipment. Trochanter rolls and footboards are also used to prevent pressure ulcers (see Chapter 26).

LEG AND FOOT ULCERS

Some diseases may affect blood flow to and from the legs and feet, which can cause pain, open wounds, and **edema** (swelling caused by fluid collecting in tissues). Infection and gangrene can result from the open wound and poor circulation. **Gangrene** is a condition in which there is death of tissue (see Chapter 18).

The client needs special skin care, as directed by a physician. The nurse uses the care planning process to prevent skin breakdown on the legs and feet.

Circulatory Ulcers

Circulatory ulcers (vascular ulcers) are open wounds on the lower legs and feet caused by decreased blood flow through arteries or veins. People with diseases affecting the blood vessels are at risk for these ulcers on the legs and feet, which can be painful and hard to heal.

Venous Ulcers

Venous ulcers (stasis ulcers) are open wounds on the lower legs and feet caused by poor blood return through the veins (Figure 42–12 *A*). Blood travelling from the feet to return to the heart must defy gravity. Usually people who are active use their leg muscles to assist the valves in their leg veins to pump the blood upward.

Unfortunately, in some clients who are not active, are extremely obese, or have circulatory problems, blood will pool in the leg veins or the valves will not close well. As a result, blood will not be pumped back to the heart normally, and blood and fluid will collect in their legs and feet. This will result in edema (swelling in the tissues caused by an accumulation of fluid) in their legs and feet. If you compress your fingers into the swollen, edematous tissues and then take away your fingers, you will notice that your fingers have left an impression in the skin, which is called **pitting edema**.

Appearance. Edema in tissues will give them a swollen appearance. If the edema is fairly recent, the skin can also appear shiny and stretched. Edema and venous ulcers are painful and make walking difficult. Venous ulcers may weep fluid. Healing is slow, and infection is a great risk. If the edema lasts for a long period, the skin will change in appearance and texture. Small veins in the skin can rupture, allowing the hemoglobin in the blood (which gives blood its red colour) to enter the tissues, which causes the skin to turn brown in colour and become dry, leathery, and hard. Itching is common.

Causes. Heels and inner sides of the ankles are common sites for venous ulcers because these areas can be easily injured. Scratching is also a common cause of venous ulcers. Some ulcers occur spontaneously, without any specific cause.

Prevention. It is important to prevent skin breakdown caused by poor circulation which leads to stasis ulcers, which are hard to heal. Box 42–6 lists guidelines that help prevent venous ulcers. These guidelines may be part of the client's care plan.

The physician may order elastic stockings or elastic bandages (see Chapter 30), which promote comfort and circulation by providing support and pressure to the veins. Foot care by a professional with specialized training in foot care, as well as medications or wound care products, may be ordered by the client's physician or nurse practitioner.

Arterial Ulcers

Arterial ulcers are open wounds on the lower legs and feet caused by poor arterial blood flow.

Causes. These ulcers are caused by diseases or injuries that decrease arterial blood flow to the legs and feet—such as high blood pressure, diabetes, as well as narrowed arteries from aging. Smoking is a significant risk factor for vascular disease.

Appearance. The affected leg and foot may feel cold and look blue or shiny (Figure 42–12 *B*). The ulcer is often painful during rest and is usually worse at night. Arterial ulcers are found between

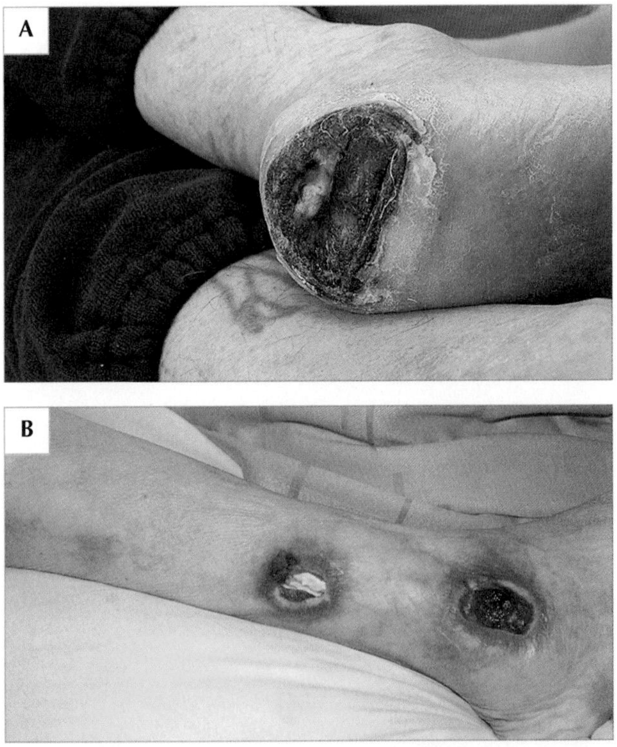

Figure 42–12 A, Venous ulcer. **B,** Arterial ulcer. Compare their appearances and how they differ from each other. **Source (for B):** Black, J.M., & Hawks, J.H. (2005). *Medical-surgical nursing: Clinical management for positive outcomes* (7th ed.). St. Louis: W.B. Saunders.

Box 42–6 Guidelines for Preventing Venous Ulcers

- Apply elastic stockings or elastic wraps, according to the care plan and if you are allowed to do so (see Chapter 30).
- Remind the client not to sit with legs crossed.
- Do not use elastic or rubber-band type garters to hold socks or hose in place.
- Provide good skin care daily. Clean and dry between the toes.
- Avoid injury to client's legs and feet.
- Keep linens clean, dry, and wrinkle-free.
- Follow the care plan for walking and exercise, as they increase venous blood flow.
- Reposition the client at least every 2 hours. Follow the care plan.
- Elevate the client's legs, according to the care plan.
- Have the client wear comfortable socks and shoes.
- Do not do anything that may irritate the skin. Avoid scrubbing or rubbing when bathing or drying the client.
- Avoid massaging over the pressure point. ***Never rub or massage reddened areas.***
- Keep the heels off the bed. Use pillows or other devices, as instructed by your supervisor. Place the pillows or devices under the lower legs from midcalf to the ankles.
- Use protective devices, as directed by your supervisor and the care plan.
- Report signs of skin breakdown, stasis ulcers, or pressure ulcers at once.

the toes, on the tops of the toes, and on the outer sides of the ankles. The heels are common sites for people on bed rest. Arterial ulcers can also occur in pressure sites from shoes that fit poorly.

Treatment and Prevention. The physician directs the client's care by treating the disease that caused the ulcer and ordering medications, wound care, and a walking program. *Very important:* You should never provide foot care unless it is specified in the client's care plan to prevent further injury. Box 42–7 lists guidelines for preventing arterial ulcers.

Box 42–7 Guidelines for Preventing Arterial Ulcers

- Urge the client to quit smoking.
- Remind clients not to sit with legs crossed.
- Avoid exposing the client to cold.
- Do not use elastic or rubber-band type garters to hold socks and hose in place.
- Make sure the client's shoes fit well.
- Keep feet clean and dry.
- Keep pressure off heels and other bony points.
- Avoid pressure under the knees.
- Check the client's legs and feet daily. Report changes in skin colour or breaks in the skin to your supervisor.
- Avoid massaging over pressure points. ***Never rub or massage reddened areas.***
- Use protective devices, as directed by your supervisor and the care plan.

WOUND HEALING

The healing process has three phases:

- ***Inflammatory phase*** (3 days). Bleeding stops, and a scab forms over the wound, which prevents microbes from entering the wound. Blood supply to the wound increases, and the blood brings nutrients and healing substances. Because blood supply increases, signs and symptoms of inflammation—redness, swelling, heat or warmth, and pain—may appear and there may be some loss of function.
- ***Proliferative phase*** (day 3 to day 21). *Proliferate* means to multiply rapidly. Tissue cells multiply to repair the wound.
- ***Maturation phase*** (day 21 to 1 or 2 years). The scar tissue gains strength and appears red and raised but eventually becomes thin and pale.

Types of Wound Healing

The healing process occurs through primary intention, secondary intention, or tertiary intention. With *primary intention* (*first intention, primary closure*), the wound is closed, and sutures (stitches), staples, clips, or adhesive strips are applied to hold the wound edges together.

Secondary intention (*second intention*) is used in contaminated and infected wounds. Wounds are cleaned and dead tissue removed. Wound edges are not brought together, and the wound is left gaping. Healing occurs naturally but takes longer, and a larger scar is formed. The threat of infection is great.

Tertiary intention (*third intention, delayed intention*) involves leaving a wound open and then closing it later. Thus tertiary intention combines secondary and primary intentions. Infection and poor circulation are common reasons for choosing tertiary intention.

Complications of Wounds

Many factors affect healing and could increase the risk of complications—for example, the client's age, general health, nutritional status and lifestyle, and the type and location of the wound. The client might be elderly, might have a medical condition (such as circulatory disease or diabetes), or have a lifestyle factor (such as smoking or poor diet) that might slow down the healing process. Other clients may be on certain medications (such as Coumadin or heparin) that will prolong bleeding and possibly delay healing.

Wound healing is dependant on good circulation to the wound and good nutrition, with a diet rich in fluids (needed for tissue hydration) as well as protein and vitamin C (needed for tissue growth and repair). The wound must be protected from infection. Sometimes, the client's doctor may prescribe antibiotics to prevent an infection from developing.

Hemorrhage. **Hemorrhage** is excessive loss of blood in a short period of time. If bleeding is not stopped, death results. Hemorrhage may be internal or external. Internal hemorrhage cannot be seen, when bleeding occurs into tissues and body cavities. A **hematoma,** which is a collection of blood under the skin and tissues, forms and the area appears swollen and has a reddish-blue colour. Shock, vomiting blood, coughing up blood, and loss of consciousness are signs of internal hemorrhage. External bleeding is visible as bloody drainage or in dressings soaked with blood. As with internal hemorrhage, shock can occur.

Shock results when there is not enough blood supply to organs and tissues. Signs and symptoms include low or falling blood pressure, rapid and weak pulse, rapid respirations, and cold, moist, and pale skin. The client is restless and may complain of thirst. Confusion and loss of consciousness eventually occur.

Hemorrhage and shock are emergencies, so notify your supervisor immediately, and assist, as requested. Remember to follow Standard Practices when in contact with blood. Gloves should always be worn, and gowns, masks, and eye protection are necessary when blood splashes and splatters are likely.

Infection. Wound contamination can occur at any time during or after an injury or surgery. Trauma often causes contaminated wounds, and surgical wounds can be contaminated during or after surgery. An infected wound has drainage and is painful and tender to touch. The client may have a fever (see Box 42–8).

Dehiscence. **Dehiscence** is the separation of the wound layers (Figure 42–13). Separation may involve the skin layer or underlying tissues, usually seen in abdominal wounds. Coughing, vomiting, and abdominal distention place stress on the wound. The client often describes the sensation of the wound popping open.

Evisceration. **Evisceration** is the separation of the wound accompanied by protrusion of abdominal organs (Figure 42–14). Causes are the same as for dehiscence.

Dehiscence and evisceration are surgical emergencies. Tell your supervisor at once if you see them. A nurse will cover the wound with large sterile dressing saturated with sterile saline, and the client will need emergency medical care.

Wound Appearance

During the healing process, physicians and nurses routinely observe the wound and its drainage for healing and complications. You need to make certain observations when assisting with wound care. You should report your observations to your supervisor and record them, according to employer policy.

Box 42–8 Wound Observations

Wound Location

- Where is the wound located on the body? Is there more than one wound? (Multiple wounds may exist from surgery or trauma.)

Wound Appearance

- Is the wound red and swollen?
- Is the area around the wound warm to touch?
- Are sutures, staples, or clips intact or broken?
- Are wound edges closed or separated? Did the wound break open?

Drainage

- Is there drainage?
- What is the amount of drainage?
- Is the damage:
  - Clear
  - Bloody
  - Watery and blood-tinged
  - Thick and green, yellow, or brown

Odour

- Does the wound or drainage have an odour?

Surrounding Skin

- Is surrounding skin intact?
- What is the colour of the surrounding skin?
- Are the surrounding tissues swollen?

Box 42–8 lists questions to consider when observing wounds.

Wound Drainage

During injury and during the inflammatory phase of wound healing, fluid and cells escape from the tissues. The amount of drainage may be small or large, depending on wound size and location and the presence of bleeding or infection. Although the nurse is responsible for changing dressings, you need to observe and report to the nurse any type of wound drainage. You may also be shown how to measure drainage tubes and to document the amount of drainage, depending on your scope of practice in your province or your employing agency.

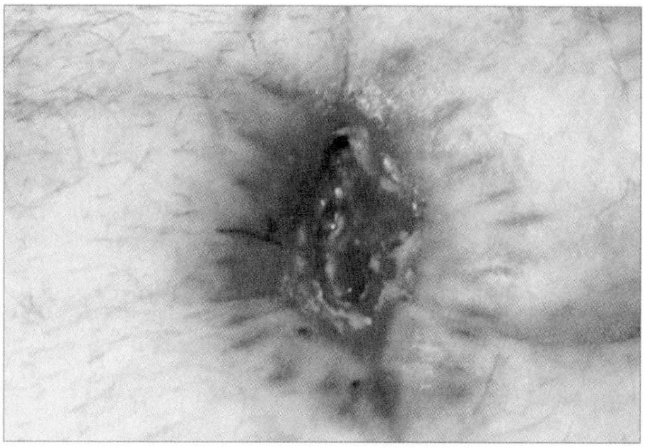

Figure 42–13 Wound dehiscence. **Source:** Morison, M. (1992). *A colour guide to the nursing management of wounds.* London: Wolfe Medical Publishers.

Major types of wound drainage are as follows:

- ***Serous drainage***—clear, watery fluid (Figure 42–15, *A*). The fluid in a blister is serous (from the Latin word *serum,* meaning clear, thin, fluid portion of blood). Serum does not contain blood cells or platelets.
- ***Sanguineous drainage***—bloody drainage (Figure 42–15, *B*). The amount and colour of sanguineous (from the Latin word *sanguis,* which means blood) drainage are important. Hemorrhage is suspected when large amounts are present. Bright red drainage means fresh bleeding, whereas older bleeding is darker.
- ***Serosanguineous drainage***—thin, watery drainage (*sero*) that is blood-tinged (*sanguineous*) (Figure 42–15, *C*).
- ***Purulent drainage***—thick drainage that is green, yellow, or brown (Figure 42–15, *D*).

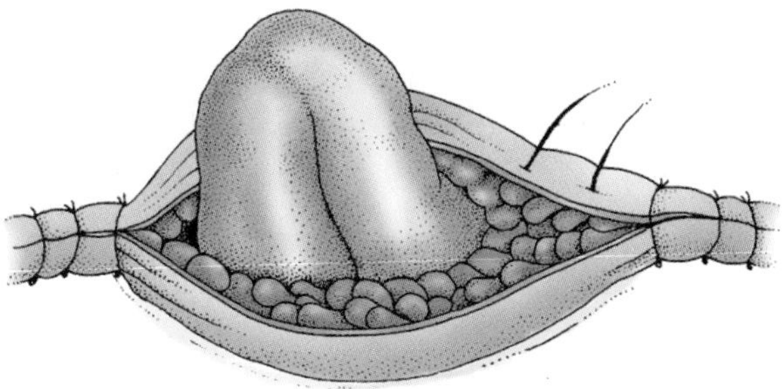

Figure 42–14 Wound evisceration. **Source:** Ignatavicius, D.D., & Workman, M.L. (2002). *Medical-surgical nursing: Critical thinking for collaborative care* (4th ed.). Philadelphia: Saunders.

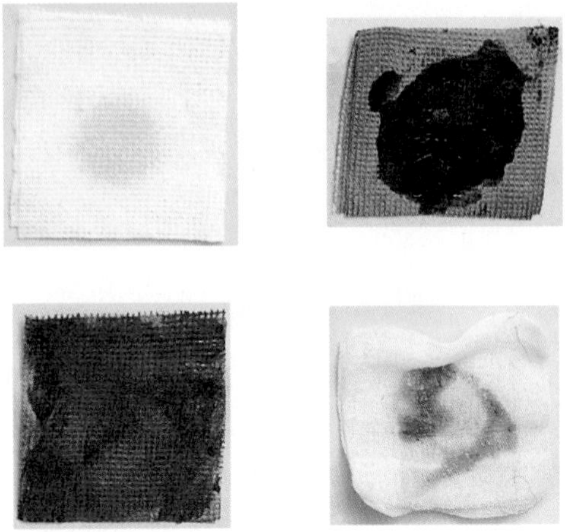

Figure 42–15 Wound drainage. **A,** Serous drainage. **B,** Sanguineous drainage. **C,** Serosanguineous drainage. **D,** Purulent drainage. **Source:** Ross-Kerr, J.C., Wood, M.J., Perry, A.G., & Potter, P.A. (2006). *Canadian fundamentals of nursing* (3rd ed., p. 1507). Toronto: Elsevier.

Drainage must leave the wound for healing to occur. If drainage is trapped inside the wound, underlying tissues swell. The wound may heal at the skin level, but underlying tissues do not close, and infection and other complications can occur. When large amounts of drainage are expected, the physician will insert a drain. A Penrose drain is a rubber tube that drains onto a dressing (Figure 42–16). Because it is an open drain, it can act as a portal of entry for microbes.

Closed drainage systems prevent microbes from entering the wound. A drain is placed in the wound and attached to suction—for example, the Hemovac (Figure 42–17) and Jackson-Pratt (Figure 42–18) systems. Depending on the wound type, size, and location, other systems may be used.

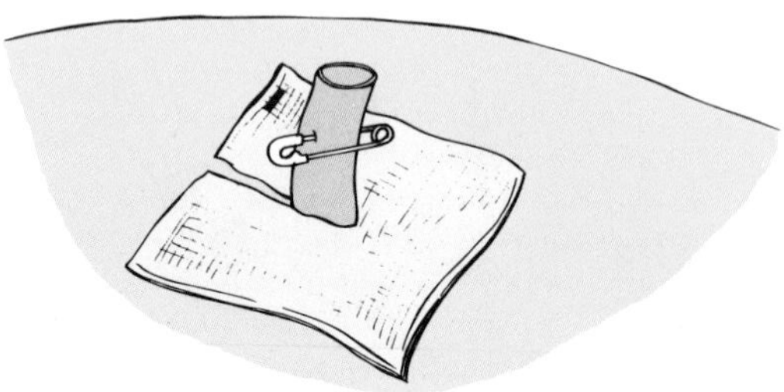

Figure 42–16 A Penrose drain. The safety pin prevents the drain from slipping into the wound. **Source:** Ross-Kerr, J.C., Wood, M.J., Perry, A.G., & Potter, P.A. (2006). *Canadian fundamentals of nursing* (3rd ed., p. 1520). Toronto: Elsevier.

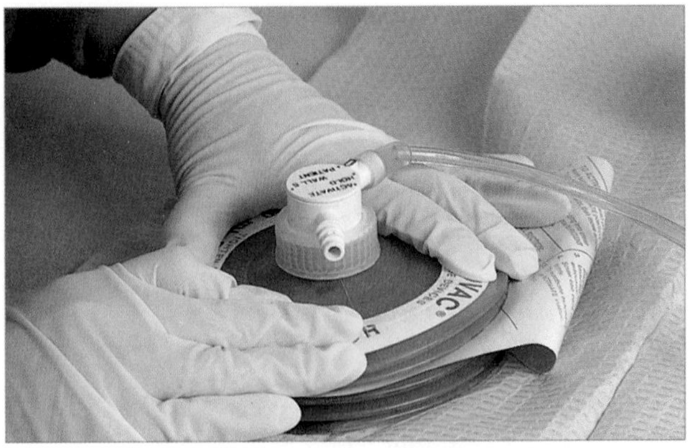

Figure 42–17 Hemovac. Drains are sutured to the wound and connected to the reservoir. **Source:** Ross-Kerr, J.C., Wood, M.J., Perry, A.G., & Potter, P.A. (2006). *Canadian fundamentals of nursing* (3rd ed., p. 1554). Toronto: Elsevier.

A nurse measures drainage in two ways:

- ***Noting the number and size of dressings with drainage***—The amount and kind of drainage are described. Are dressings saturated? Is drainage on just part of the dressing? If so, which part? Is drainage through some or all layers?
- ***Measuring the amount of drainage in the collecting receptacle***—if closed drainage is used.

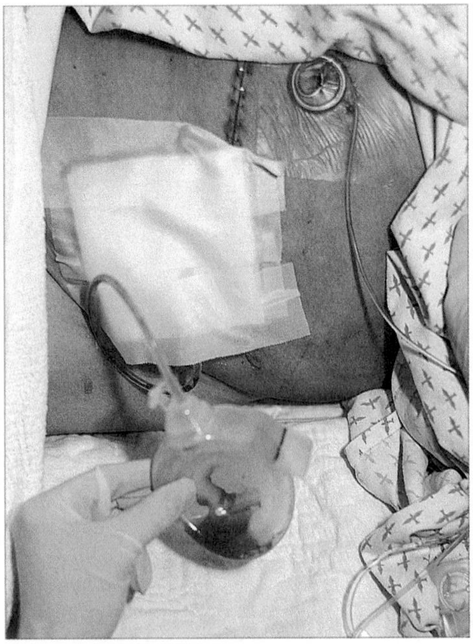

Figure 42–18 Jackson-Pratt drainage system. **Source:** Ross-Kerr, J.C., Wood, M.J., Perry, A.G., & Potter, P.A. (2006). *Canadian fundamentals of nursing* (3rd ed., p. 1520). Toronto: Elsevier.

DRESSINGS

Wound dressings have many functions:

- They protect wounds from injury and microbes.
- They absorb drainage.
- They remove dead tissue.
- They promote comfort.
- They cover unsightly wounds.
- They provide a moist environment for wound healing.
- When bleeding is a problem, pressure dressings help control bleeding.

Sterile Dressings

The type and size of dressing used depend on many factors—(a) the type of wound, (b) its size and location, (c) the amount of drainage, (d) the presence or absence of infection, (e) the dressing's function, and (f) the frequency of dressing changes. The physician and nurse choose the best type of dressing for each wound. ***Because there is such a wide range of sterile dressing types and indications for their use, and because it is beyond your scope of practice to decide on the type of dressing, this chapter will instead focus on your responsibilities with regard to a client's dressing.*** You may be asked to assist in the application of a sterile dressing (see Chapter 20).

Although you are not responsible for sterile dressing changes or for skin assessment (this is the responsibility of the nurse), you should function as the "eyes and ears" of the client, reporting important details about the dressings to the nurse (see Box 42–9).

Types of Dressings

Dressings are described by the material used and application method. Many products are available for dressing wounds. They may be dry, moist, or hydrocolloid dressings. The following are common dressings:

- ***Gauze***—comes in squares, rectangles, pads, and rolls (Figure 42–19). Gauze dressings absorb moisture.
- ***Nonadherent gauze***—is a gauze dressing with a nonstick surface. It does not stick to the wound and removes easily without injuring the tissue.

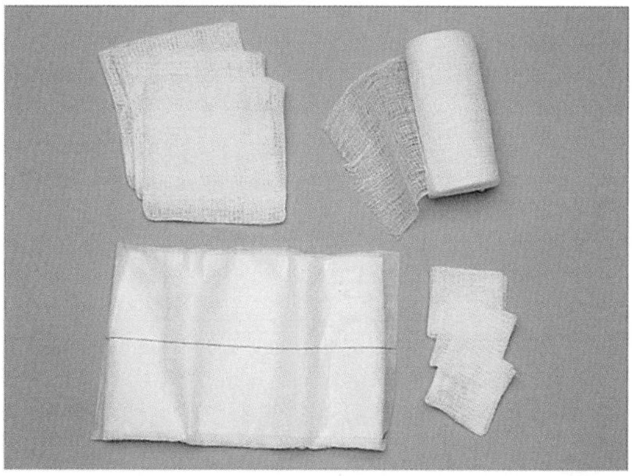

Figure 42–19 Gauze dressings. **A,** 10 x 10 cm (4 x 4 inch). **B,** Gauze roll. **C,** Abdominal pad. **D,** 5 x 5 cm (2 x 2 inch).

- ***Vapour-permeable transparent adhesive film***—air can reach the wound but fluid and microbes cannot. The wound is kept moist. Drainage is not absorbed. The transparent film allows wound observation.

Some dressings contain special agents to promote wound healing. If you assist with a dressing change, your supervisor will explain the use of the dressing to you. Dressing application methods involve a number of dressing types, depending on the client's particular type of wound. Your supervisor or the nurse will direct you with regard to the particulars of dressing change and care for each client.

Securing Dressings

Dressings must be secure over wounds, as microbes may enter the wound and drainage may escape if the dressing is dislodged (see the *Focus on Children: Dressings* and *Focus on Older Adults: Dressings* boxes on page 813).

Tape. Adhesive, paper, plastic, and elastic tapes are common. Adhesive tape sticks well to the skin, but removing the remaining adhesive can be difficult, and the adhesive can irritate the skin. Sometimes some skin may come off with the tape, causing an abrasion. When clients are allergic to adhesive tape, paper and plastic tapes are used, as these do not usually cause allergic reactions. Elastic tape allows easier movement of the body part.

Box 42–9 The Support Worker's Responsibilities to Clients With Wounds

Specific Areas	Your Responsibilities
1. Overall	• Follow the client's care plan. • Report and document any observations you have made about your client in any of the areas noted below. • Document all wound care or observations that you have made.
2. Prevention of Pressure Sores It is important that you observe your client's skin, especially over the bony prominences and report any reddened areas. Remember that these can quickly become pressure sores!	• Remove any restrictive clothing, such as socks that are too tight. These can prevent blood circulation, which will lead to skin breakdown. • Ensure the client is repositioned at least every 2 hours (***or more frequently if specified by the client's care plan!***). • Inspect bony prominences that have been compressed by any type of surface. • If the client is confined to a wheelchair, sitting on a gel pad may reduce pressure areas. • Keep bony prominences and skin folds clean and dry. Wash skin area after each soiling, and then rinse and pat dry. • Avoid oily soaps that trap bacteria, or drying, anti-perspirant soaps that can cause the skin to dry and crack. If possible, use **peri-wash**, as it does not leave a residue on the client's skin. • Massage ***around*** reddened areas only, never directly on the area, as this would only remove more skin cells. • If the client is diabetic, ***never*** perform nail care. This should be done only by a professional with specialized training in foot care. Always report reddened areas or ingrown toenails so that these can be treated as soon as possible. • Report and record your findings, according to your agency's policies.
3. Pain and Comfort A client in pain will probably not eat or participate in care. Pain may affect your client's breathing and moving, turning, repositioning, and walking. In addition, pain is exhausting and can make the client depressed or irritable. It is important that the client be made as comfortable as possible.	• Observe to find out if the client is in pain (look for grimacing, holding a body part for a long period, or tensing up during repositioning). If you find the client to be in pain, determine where, the amount, the intensity, aggravating factors and the cause so that you can report this and record it appropriately. • Handle the client gently. • Report the client's pain and details to the appropriate nurse who can give the client pain medication, if it is ordered and appropriate. • Allow pain medications to take effect before giving care (at least 1 hour). • Assist the client into a comfortable position, and frequently turn the client (according to the care plan) to avoid placing pressure on compromised areas. • If specified in the client's care plan, massage the client's bony prominences. Assist the client into a proper body alignment, and position him or her with pillows. • If the client is in bed, ensure that he or she is lying on a wrinkle-free foundation.

(continued on page 811)

Box 42–9 The Support Worker's Responsibilities to Clients With Wounds (cont'd)

Specific Areas	Your Responsibilities
4. Movement and Ambulation Movement is important for everyone because it encourages deeper respirations and better blood circulation, reduces the risk of pressure ulcers developing, increases the body's metabolism, promotes peristalsis, and improves digestion. Clients with painful wounds are often reluctant to move or to ambulate, and those with wounds that are foul-smelling may be self-conscious about leaving their rooms, even if they can.	• Encourage the client to move in bed, take deep breaths, and to turn independently as much as possible. • Following the client's care plan, assist the client into a chair (or wheelchair) or to ambulate as often as stated. If he or she is unable to ambulate, turn the client frequently, as indicated in their care plan. • Time activities around the time the client receives pain medication (at least 1 hour after), so that the client is as comfortable as possible before attempting to ambulate. • Have another worker to help, in case the client feels light-headed or faint. • Encourage the client to rise slowly and to take a few deep breaths before standing up. This might eliminate the feeling of lightheadedness.
5. Dressings Depending on the type of dressing that is ordered for your client, the appearance, care, and maintenance of the dressing may vary. Regardless of type, all dressings should be kept clean.	• Observe if the client's dressing is clean and free from bodily fluids (such as urine or feces). Report pertinent information. • If required, assist the nurse with the client's dressing change. If the wound is particularly unsightly, be careful not to let your facial expressions frighten the client.
6. Nutrition and Hydration The client's wound cannot heal with a diet that is poor in protein or vitamin C. In addition, the client must have adequate fluid to replace any lost in wound drainage. The client who is anemic will not have enough hemoglobin to bind with oxygen, so he or she must also eat an iron-rich diet.	• Take the client's care plan, dietary needs, and preferences into account, and prepare tasty treats that are high in protein and vitamin C. • If the client is diabetic, ensure that he or she does not exceed caloric restrictions.
7. Oxygenation Oxygen is a requirement for healing. On a cellular level, oxygen must bind itself to hemoglobin (part of a red blood cell) and be transported throughout the body.	• Help the client to maintain positions that will maximize lung expansion. • Gently remind the client to take several deep breaths at least every hour.

(continued on page 812)

Box 42–9 The Support Worker's Responsibilities to Clients With Wounds (cont'd)

Specific Areas	Your Responsibilities
8. Odour Some wounds (especially **necrotic**, infected ones) may be very foul smelling, and this can embarrass the client and ruin his or her appetite.	• Keep drainage containers out of the client's sight. • Open windows, whenever possible, to allow fresh air to enter the client's room. • Ensure that dressing materials are removed promptly and placed in a plastic bag that is tied to contain the odour (see Chapter 20). • Discretely use room air fresheners to mask any odour. • If possible, move the client into another room for meals.
9. Temperature Fever is the body's way of fighting infection by increasing white blood cells and blood flow to the area. ***Not all clients who have an infection will have a fever when you take the temperature.*** Some clients (like older adults or clients with immune challenges) may not have a fever, even if they have an infection.	• Often, fever is a sign of infection. Take the client's temperature, according to their care plan (see Chapter 41) and report it if there is a fever. • If the client does not have a fever, ***there may be other signs that indicate an infection*** (such as redness or swelling around the wound, tenderness, and warmth to the touch). Report any abnormal findings at once.
10. Skin Care Clean, dry skin is less likely to harbour pathogens than moist, soiled skin. Pathogens can cause skin infections, which, in turn, can lead to skin ulceration and breakdown.	• Keep the client's skin clean and dry. Avoid the use of powders, which may dry out the skin too much and may irritate the client's airway. • After washing the client's skin, rinse it thoroughly and pat it dry. Do not towel dry roughly, as this can actually tear the skin on some frail clients. • Report and record any observations of edema, bruising, swelling, or any other abnormal feature.
11. Maintaining Skin Integrity Intact skin is the body's first line of defence against pathogens. It is important that skin is kept intact, as it is easier to prevent a skin infection than it is to cure one.	• Gently transfer or position the client. Use equipment properly. Use friction-reducing equipment, such as sliding boards (see Chapter 23). • Never apply straps or boards directly on the skin, as this can increase the client's chance of getting scratched or bruised. • Ensure that the client's skin remains clean and dry at all times. Follow all of the above steps to ensure the client's skin is not damaged at any time. • Avoid tight, restrictive clothing.
12. Complications and Concerns The client may have many fears. He or she may fear scarring, disfigurement, delayed healing, and infection. Fears about the wound "popping open" are common.	• Delayed healing is a risk for clients who are older or obese or who have poor nutrition. Poor circulation and diabetes also affect healing. These conditions are risk factors for infection. • Victims of violence have many other concerns. Fear of future attacks, concerns about finding and convicting the attacker, and fear for family members are common. Victims of abuse often hide the true source of their injuries.

(continued on page 813)

Box 42–9 The Support Worker's Responsibilities to Clients With Wounds (cont'd)

Specific Areas	Your Responsibilities
The wound may be large or small. It may be visible to others—on the face, arms, or legs—or hidden by clothing. If the client had surgery, anesthesia and pain medication can affect eating and elimination.	• The wound may be disfiguring. It may affect sexual performance or the client's sense of being sexually attractive. • Amputation of a finger, hand, arm, toes, foot, or leg can affect the client's function, daily activities, and job. Eye injuries can affect vision. • Whatever the wound's location or size, the client's body image and self-esteem are often affected. Many clients with serious and disfiguring wounds have an increased need for love and acceptance. • You must be empathetic to the client's feelings. The client may be sad and tearful or angry and hostile. Adjustments may be hard and rehabilitation necessary. Be gentle and kind; give compassionate care; and practise good communication. • Other health care team members—social workers, psychiatrists, therapists, and spiritual advisers—may be involved in the client's care.

Tape is applied to secure the top, middle, and bottom of the dressing (Figure 42–20). The tape extends several centimetres beyond each side of the dressing. ***The tape must not circle the entire body part. If swelling occurs, circulation to the part would be impaired.***

If the client can tolerate it, a **picture frame dressing**—where the tape is applied to all four edges—can be used, as it is less likely to wrinkle or fall off.

Applying Dressings

Your supervisor may ask you to assist with dressing changes. Some employers let support workers apply simple, dry, nonsterile dressings to simple wounds. Box 42–10 lists guidelines for applying nonsterile

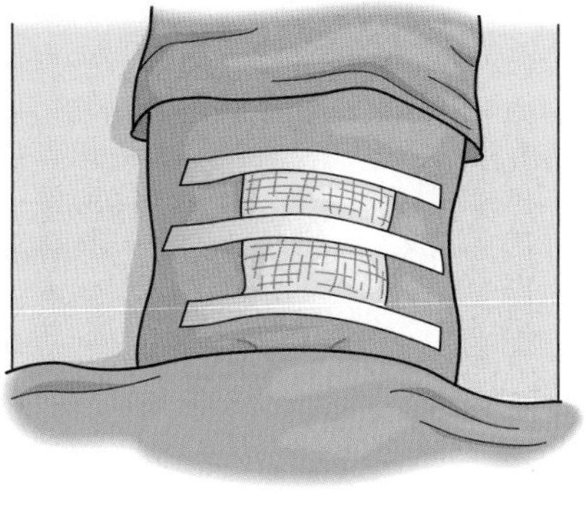

Figure 42–20 Tape is applied at the top, middle, and bottom of the dressing. Note that the tape extends several centimetres beyond both sides of the dressing.

focus on »CHILDREN

Dressings

Children are often afraid of dressing changes. Tape removal is often painful for them, and the wound's appearance can be frightening. It is important to ensure that the child is calm and cooperative, or the sterile field could become contaminated. A parent or caregiver should hold the child so that the wound can be reached with ease. Holding or playing with a favourite toy is often comforting to the child. The child may be asked to apply a dressing to a doll (and remove it), which may decrease the child's fear and apprehension about dressings.

focus on »OLDER ADULTS

Dressings

Older adults have thin, fragile skin, so it is important to prevent skin tears in them. Extreme care is therefore necessary when removing tape. One way that many nurses suggest is to "peel" the tape off by folding the edge of the tape over and dragging it back. This avoids lifting the skin which can be uncomfortable to the client and can injure the client's skin.

Box 42–10 Guidelines for Applying Nonsterile Dressings

- Make sure your province or territory allows you to perform the procedure.
- Make sure the procedure is in your job description.
- Apply dressings only under a nurse's direction and supervision.
- Review the procedure with the nurse.
- Allow time for pain medications to take effect, as the client may experience discomfort during the dressing change. The nurse will give the medication and tell you how long to wait.
- Provide for the client's fluid and elimination needs before starting the procedure.
- Collect needed equipment and supplies before you begin.
- Be aware of your nonverbal communication. Wound odours, appearance, and drainage may be unpleasant, but take care not to communicate your thoughts and reactions to the client.
- Follow Standard Practices. Wear personal protective equipment, as necessary. Never touch a wound with ungloved hands.
- Remove dressings in a way that the client cannot see the soiled side. The drainage and its odour may upset the client.
- Do not force the client to look at the wound, as the appearance of the wound can affect body image and self-esteem. The nurse will address the client's concerns about the wound.
- Remove the tape by pulling it toward the wound. You can ensure that the tape does not stick to the skin by, again, folding it back on itself.
- Remove the dressing gently. If the dressing sticks to the wound and surrounding skin, ask your supervisor if the wound can be dampened (for example, by applying sterile normal saline) to prevent the dressing sticking to the wound.
- Observe the wound, and report and record your observations, according to employer policy (see Box 42–8 on page 807).

dressings (see the *Focus on Home Care: Changing Dressings* box.)

Binders

Binders are applied to the abdomen, chest, or perineal areas to promote healing because they:

- Support wounds
- Hold dressings in place
- Reduce or prevent swelling by promoting circulation
- Promote comfort
- Prevent injury

Usually a nurse applies binders. You may provide care for clients with the following types of binders:

Straight Abdominal Binder. This type provides abdominal support and holds dressings in place (Figure 42–21). It is applied with the client supine. The top part is at the client's waist, and the lower part is over the hips. The binder is secured with pins, hooks, or Velcro.

focus on ››HOME CARE

Changing Dressings

Your supervisor may ask you to telephone him or her after removing the client's old dressing. During this telephone call, you should report your observations, and your supervisor will give you instructions on how to proceed further. Follow your employer policy for disposing of dressings. Usually employers require you to:

- Place the used dressing in a plastic bag
- Fasten the bag securely
- Dispose of the bag with the household garbage

1 2 3 APPLYING DRY NONSTERILE DRESSING

Remember to promote:

• Dignity • Independence • Preferences • Privacy • Safety

Pre-Procedure

1 Review the procedure with your supervisor.
2 Identify the client, according to employer policy.
3 Explain the procedure to the client.
4 Allow time for pain medication to take effect (at least 1 hour).
5 Provide for the client's fluid and elimination needs.
6 Practise proper hand hygiene.
7 Collect the following:
- Gloves
- Personal protective equipment, as needed
- Tape
- Dressing, as directed by the care plan
- Adhesive remover
- Scissors
- Leakproof plastic bag
- Bath blanket

8 Provide for privacy.
9 Arrange items on your work area.
10 Raise the bed to a comfortable working height. Follow the care plan for bed rail use.*

Procedure

11 Lower the bed rail near you, if it is up.
12 Help the client to a comfortable position.
13 Cover the client with a bath blanket. Fanfold the client's top linens to the foot of the bed.
14 Expose the affected body part.
15 Make a cuff on the plastic bag. Place it within reach.
16 Wear a gown and mask, if needed.
17 Put on gloves.
18 Remove tape by holding the skin down and gently pulling the tape toward the wound.
19 Remove adhesive from the skin. Wet a 10 x 10 cm (4 x 4 in.) gauze dressing with the adhesive remover. Clean away from the wound.
20 Remove the gauze dressing. Start with the top dressing. Keep the soiled side of the dressing out of the client's sight. Place the dressing in the bag. They must not touch the outside of the bag.
21 Remove the dressing directly over the wound very gently. It may stick to the wound.
22 Observe the wound and drainage (see Box 42–8 on page 807).
23 Remove gloves. Put them in the bag. Practise proper hand hygiene. (If used, raise the bed rail before leaving the bedside. Lower it when you return.)
24 Put on clean gloves.
25 Open the dressing.
26 Cut the length of tape needed.
27 Apply dressing, as directed by the care plan.
28 Secure the dressing in place. Use tape.
29 Remove your gloves. Put them in the bag. Practise proper hand hygiene.

Post-Procedure

30 Provide for safety and comfort.
31 Cover the client and remove the bath blanket.
32 Place the call bell within reach.*
33 Return the bed to its lowest position. Follow the care plan for bed rail use.*
34 Remove privacy measures.
35 Discard supplies into the bag. Tie the bag closed. Dispose of the bag, according to employer policy.
36 Clean your work surface, according to employer policy.
37 Practise proper hand hygiene.
38 Report and record your actions and observations, according to employer policy.

*Steps marked with an asterisk may not apply in community settings.

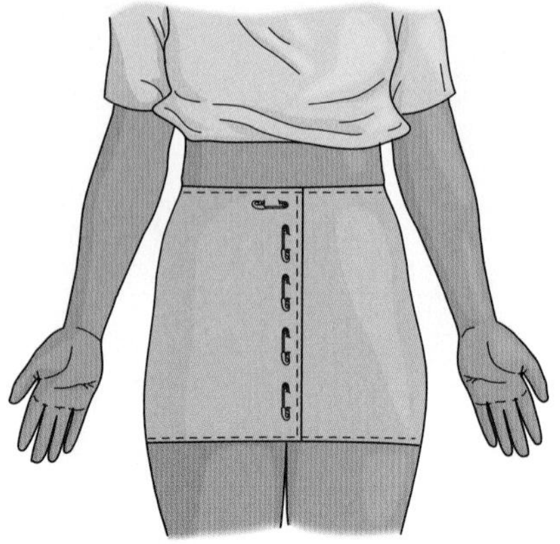

Figure 42–21 Straight abdominal binder.

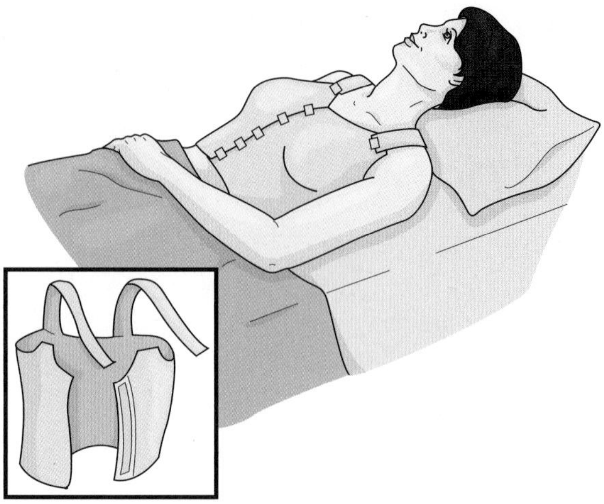

Figure 42–22 Breast binder.

Breast Binder. This type supports the breast after breast surgery (Figure 42–22). The female client is placed in the supine position when it is applied. It is pulled snugly across the chest and secured in place.

T binder. It secures dressings in place after rectal and perineal surgeries. The single T binder is used for women (Figure 42–23, *A*) and the double T binder for male clients (Figure 42–23, *B*). If perineal dressings are large in some female clients, double T binders may be needed. The waistbands are brought around the waist and pinned at the front. The tails are taken between the legs, up to the waistband, and pinned in place at the waistband.

Some employers allow support workers to apply binders. You will receive training and supervision for this task. Apply a binder so that there is firm, even pressure over the area. It should be snug without affecting breathing or circulation. Point away from the wound. Reapply the binder if it is loose, wrinkled, or out of position or if it causes discomfort. Also, change binders when they become wet or soiled.

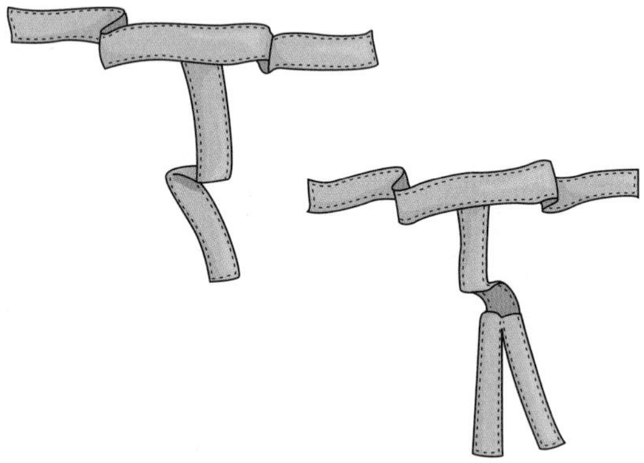

Figure 42–23 **A,** Single T binder. **B,** Double T binder.

HEAT AND COLD APPLICATIONS

Heat and cold applications are often ordered for wound care (see Chapter 43) by physicians and nurses to promote healing and comfort and to reduce tissue swelling.

REVIEW

Answers to these questions are at the bottom of page 818.

Circle T if the answer is true or circle F if the answer is false.

1. T F **Good nutrition and hydration can help prevent skin breakdown.**
2. T F **White or reddened skin is the first sign of a pressure ulcer.**
3. T F **Pressure ulcers do not usually occur over a bony area.**
4. T F **Pressure ulcers can develop from failing to reposition the client often enough.**
5. T F **Shearing and friction can cause pressure ulcers.**

Circle the BEST answer.

6. **A child fell off her bike. She has a laceration on her right leg. She has a(n):**
   A. Closed wound
   B. Infected wound
   C. Contaminated wound
   D. Intentional wound
7. **Mrs. Katz had rectal surgery. What type of wound does she have?**
   A. A clean wound
   B. A dirty wound
   C. A clean-contaminated wound
   D. A contaminated wound
8. **When skin and underlying tissues are pierced, this is called a(n):**
   A. penetrating wound
   B. incision
   C. contusion
   D. abrasion
9. **Which of the following can cause skin tears?**
   A. Keeping your nails trimmed and filed smooth
   B. Dressing clients in clothing with long sleeves and long pants
   C. Hurrying when lifting and transferring clients
   D. Padding wheelchair footrests
10. **Which of the following causes pressure ulcers?**
    A. Repositioning the client every 2 hours
    B. Scrubbing and rubbing the skin
    C. Applying lotion to dry areas
    D. Keeping linens clean, dry, and wrinkle-free
11. **Which of the following are used to treat or prevent pressure ulcers?**
    A. Hospital beds
    B. Waterbeds and flotation pads
    C. Plastic drawsheets and waterproof pads
    D. Heel "doughnuts"
12. **You can help prevent stasis ulcers by:**
    A. Using elastic rubber-band type garters to hold socks in place
    B. Keeping the client in bed as much as possible
    C. Encouraging the client to sit with legs crossed
    D. Avoiding injury to the legs and feet when giving care
13. **Which of the following areas is a common site for arterial ulcers?**
    A. On the scalp
    B. On top of the nose
    C. On the outer side of the ankle
    D. Behind the knee
14. **A wound appears red and swollen. The area around it is warm to the touch. These signs occur during:**
    A. The inflammatory phase of wound healing
    B. The proliferative phase of wound healing
    C. Healing by primary intention
    D. Healing by secondary intention
15. **A wound is healing by primary intention. While assisting with a dressing change, you note that the wound is separating. This is called:**
    A. Dehiscence
    B. Tertiary intention
    C. Evisceration
    D. Hematoma

REVIEW

Answers to these questions are at the bottom of the page.

16. **You see clear, watery drainage from a wound. This drainage is called:**
    - A. Purulent drainage
    - B. Serous drainage
    - C. Seropurulent drainage
    - D. Serosanguineous drainage

17. **Which of the following does a dressing do?**
    - A. Protects the wound from injury
    - B. Reduces swelling
    - C. Prevents healing too fast
    - D. Prevents oxygen from entering the wound

18. **You are securing a dressing with tape. Tape is applied:**
    - A. Around the entire body part
    - B. To the top and bottom of the dressing
    - C. To the top, middle, and bottom of the dressing
    - D. As the client prefers

19. **Mr. Heron has an abdominal binder. The binder is used to:**
    - A. Prevent blood clots
    - B. Prevent wound infection
    - C. Provide support and hold dressings in place
    - D. Encourage peristalsis

Answers: 1.T, 2.T, 3.F, 4.T, 5.T, 6.C, 7.C, 8.A, 9.C, 10.B, 11.B, 12.D, 13.C, 14.A, 15.A, 16.B, 17.A, 18.C, 19.C

CHAPTER 43

Heat and Cold Applications

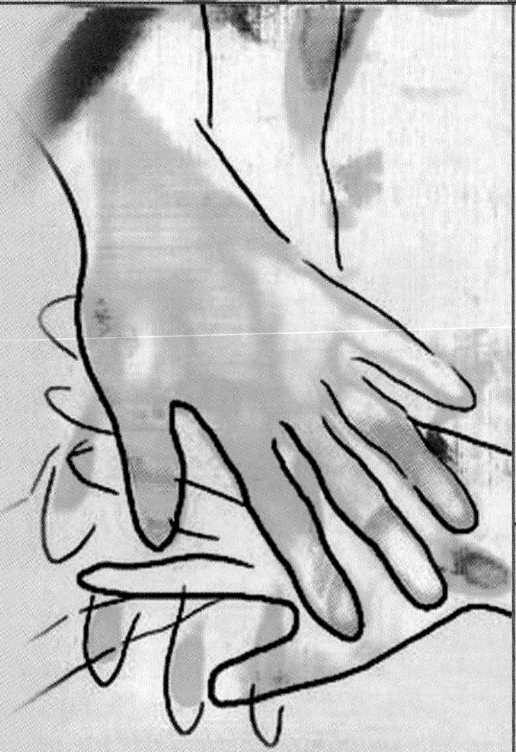

OBJECTIVES

- Define the key terms listed in this chapter.
- Identify the purposes, effects, and complications of heat and cold applications.
- List clients at risk for complications from heat and cold applications.
- List the guidelines for application of heat and cold.
- Perform the procedures described in this chapter in a safe manner.

key terms

cold pack A treatment that involves wrapping a body part with a cold—moist or dry—application.

compress A soft pad that is moistened and applied over a body area.

compression bandage A bandage designed to provide pressure to a particular area, for example, on a bleeding wound, or to limit swelling in body parts, such as ankles, by wrapping the bandage around. Also known as a *tensor bandage.*

constrict To squeeze or make narrow.

cyanosis Bluish skin colour caused by a lack of oxygenated blood in the visible tissues.

dilate To expand or open wider.

frost bite A medical condition in which damage is caused to skin and other tissues by extreme cold. Signs of **frost bite** include blisters, pale, white, or grey skin, cyanosis, shivering, numbness, pain, and burning.

gel pack A commercially produced hot-and-cold pack designed to keep its temperature over a period of time.

RICE An acronym for "**R**est, **I**ce, **C**ompression, and **E**levate" as a method of treating recent injuries.

sitz bath A special shallow plastic bathtub, filled with warm water, designed to keep the buttocks and hips immersed while in a sitting position. Sitz baths are used to soothe the discomfort from pain and swelling and reduce the chance of infection by cleansing around the perineum.

wheat/bean bags A type of heating bag that provides dry heat. It needs to be heated in a microwave. Because the beans may heat unevenly, the bag should be shaken to thoroughly mix the beans and then covered with a cloth before applying to the client's skin.

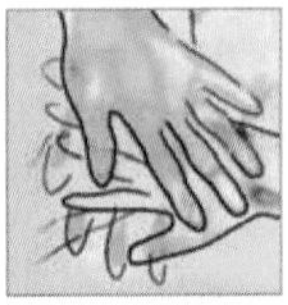

Physicians, nurses, and physical therapists use heat and cold applications to reduce tissue swelling and promote healing and comfort. Heat and cold have opposite effects on body functions. Heat increases blood flow by *dilating* blood vessels in the area being heated (Figure 43–1 *B*). Cold slows blood flow by *constricting* blood vessels in the area being cooled (Figure 43–1 *C*). Both effects can be helpful, but there are risks associated with heat and cold applications, such as severe injuries and a decrease in the ability of that body part to function well. Because of this, they should never be used unless they are in the client's care plan, and then only if this duty has been ***delegated*** to you by a nurse.

Any client receiving a heat or cold application should be frequently checked for any signs of problems related to their use (Table 43–1). ***Inspect the skin beneath the application frequently, according to the care plan. It is usually good to check the skin every 5 minutes for the first two checks, and at least every 15 minutes after that. Because not every client may report having any discomfort, you should be particularly aware of signs such as restlessness, agitation, or other changes in behaviour.***

Both heat and cold applications can be either moist or dry and produce different effects. You must thoroughly understand the purposes, effects, and complications of both heat and cold applications.

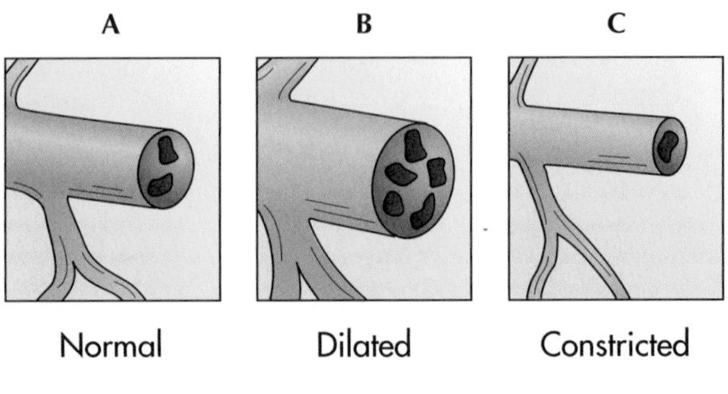

Figure 43–1 A, Blood vessel under normal conditions. **B,** Dilated blood vessel. **C,** Constricted blood vessel.

Table 43–1 Comparison of Heat and Cold Applications

	Heat	Cold
Purposes	*For chronic pain*: - Reduces pain of muscle cramps - Reduces pain related to arthritis - Promotes healing - Reduces joint stiffness	*For recent injury*: - Reduces swelling - Reduces pain - Slows bruising - Reduces insect bite itching
How it works	Expands blood vessels and assists in increasing circulation to the area	Constricts blood vessels in order to reduce swelling and pain to the area
Examples	*Moist*: - Hot/warm compress - Hot/warm soak - Sitz bath *Dry*: - Bean/wheat bags - Heating pads - Heat rubs	*Moist*: - Cold/cool water compress - Cold/cool water soak *Dry*: - Cold pack, gel pack - Ice packs, bags, and collars - Cold rubs
Length of time for application*	Do not apply longer than 15 minutes at a time Check the skin every 5 minutes	Do not apply longer than 15 minutes at a time Check the skin every 5 minutes Cold applications are usually applied at 15-minute intervals (i.e., 15 minutes on followed by 15 minutes off)
Signs of problems: Stop application and report at once	Excessive skin redness in the area Excessive facial redness Blisters Complaints of discomfort, pain, or burning (or changes in the client's behaviour) Signs of skin irritation (such as redness, rash, itching, or burning)	Pale, white, or grey skin **Cyanosis** (bluish skin colour) Shivering Complaints of discomfort, pain, numbness, or burning (or changes in the client's behaviour) Signs of skin irritation (such as redness, rash, itching, or burning)
Complications from misuse	Burns Tissue death Circulatory shock	Frost bite Tissue death Circulatory shock

These times were suggested by the Fowler-Kennedy Sports Medicine Clinic of the University of Western Ontario. Your supervisor may have more specific times, as they pertain to each individual client. You should always follow the client's care plan and the policies of your employing agency.

Source: Fowler-Kennedy Sports Medicine Clinic, University of Western Ontario.

Because of the risks involved, some employers allow only nurses to do heat and cold applications, while some others may permit support workers to do them as well. You must be certain that this is within your scope of practice.

Before you perform these procedures, it is ***your responsibility*** to make sure of the following:

- Your provincial or territorial laws and employer's policies allow you to perform the procedure.
- The procedure is in your job description.
- You have the necessary training.
- You are familiar with the equipment.
- You have reviewed the procedure with a nurse.
- A nurse is available to answer questions and to supervise you.

HEAT APPLICATIONS

Heat applications can be applied to almost any body part. They are often used for musculoskeletal injuries or problems—for example, strains, low back pain, and arthritis (see Table 43–1 on page 821).

When heat is applied to the skin, blood vessels in the area **dilate** (i.e., they expand or open wider) (Figure 43–1, *B*), and more blood flows through them. This extra blood brings more oxygen and nutrients for healing to the tissues and removes excess fluid and wastes from the area faster. The extra blood causes the overlying skin to become red and warm to the touch. When heat is used correctly, muscles in that area relax, and painful swelling is reduced.

Complications

Burns are caused when heat is applied either for too long or at too high temperatures. Pain, excessive redness, and blisters are danger signs of burns. If you observe any of these, you should remove the application and report these signs immediately. If not immediately treated, burns can lead to serious, life-threatening problems.

Some clients are at greater risk than others for burns and other complications from heat applications (Box 43–1). It is your responsibility to observe these clients closely and to protect them from injury. Follow the guidelines listed in Box 43–2 when performing heat and cold applications.

Moist and Dry Heat Applications

Moist heat application involves water coming in contact with the skin. Moist heat has certain advantages, including the following:

- Water conducts heat, so moist heat has a greater and faster effect than dry heat.
- Heat penetrates deeper with moist applications, so they have lower (cooler) temperature

Box 43–1 Clients at High Risk for Complications From Heat or Cold Applications

- ***Clients with thin, delicate, or fragile skin.*** They include infants, young children, older adults, and fair-skinned people.
- ***Clients who have decreased sensations.*** Clients who have difficulty sensing heat, cold, or pain may not realize if the application is too hot or cold and damaging their skin. Examples of situations that may reduce a person's ability to feel pain include:
  - Loss of consciousness
  - Scarring of the skin
  - Use of some medications
  - Spinal cord injuries
  - Stroke
  - Diabetes
  - Aging, which can cause decreased sensations due to changes in body function
- ***Clients with dementia or confusion.*** These clients may not recognize pain, or they may not be able to communicate that they are in pain. You need to look for changes in the client's behaviour, which can signal pain.
- ***Clients with metal implants.*** Metal conducts heat and cold, so deep tissues can be burned. Pacemakers and joint replacements are made of metal. Do not apply heat in the area of the implant.

Box 43–2 General Guidelines for Applying Heat and Cold

These guidelines apply to application of heat or cold:

- Apply only when ordered by a professional, allowed by your employer, and assigned to do so.
- Know how to use the equipment.
- Measure the temperature of moist applications before applying, according to your employer policy.
- Follow employer policies for safe temperature ranges. See Table 43–2 for heat and cold temperature ranges.
- Do not apply hot applications above 41.1°C (106°F) because tissue damage can occur. ***Only a nurse can apply a very hot application.***
- Ask your supervisor what the temperature of the application should be (see Box 43–1).
  - Heat—are used for clients at risk, cooler temperatures.
  - Cold—for clients at risk, warmer temperatures are used.
- Know the precise site of the application. Ask your supervisor to show you the site.
- Cover dry heat or cold applications with cloth before applying them. Use a flannel or terrycloth cover, towel, or pillowcase, according to your employer policy.
- Do not leave clients at risk unattended.
- Observe the skin, at least every 5 minutes, for signs of complications (see Table 43–1 on page 821).
- Observe for changes in the client's behaviour, which may indicate the client is in pain.
- Remind the client not to change the temperature of the application.
- Prevent chills. When moist heat is applied, the increased blood flow to the affected area may cause reduced blood flow to other body parts, and the client may feel chilled. Cover the client with a blanket or robe. Eliminate room drafts.
- Ask your supervisor how long to leave the application in place. Carefully watch the time. Heat and cold are applied for no longer than 15-minute periods.
- Provide for privacy. Properly drape and screen the client. Expose only the body part on which you will apply heat or cold.
- If it is safe to leave, place the call bell within the client's reach, or remain within easy hearing distance.
- Follow Standard Practices. Wear gloves if you or the client has nonintact skin.

settings than dry heat applications to prevent injury to the client.

In *dry heat applications,* water does not come in contact with the skin. The advantages of dry heat are as follows:

- The application stays at the desired temperature longer.
- Dry heat does not penetrate as deeply as moist heat. Because water is not used, dry heat needs higher (hotter) temperatures to achieve the desired effect.

With both these applications, the client is at risk for burns. It is very important, therefore, to continually check on the client and inspect the skin under the application every 5 minutes. The applications should never be left on the skin longer than 15 minutes (see the *Focus on Home Care: Dry Heat Applications* box on page 824).

Warm Compresses

Warm compresses are moist heat applications. A **compress** is a soft pad that is moistened and applied over a body area. (Compresses can be hot or cold.)

Table 43–2 Heat and Cold Temperature Ranges

Temperature	Centigrade Range	Fahrenheit Range
Very hot	41.1°C to 46.1°C	106°F to 115°F
Hot	36.6°C to 41.1°C	98°F to 106°F
Warm	33.8°C to 36.6°C	93°F to 98°F
Tepid	26.6°C to 33.8°C	80°F to 93°F
Cool	18.3°C to 26.6°C	65°F to 80°F
Cold	10.0°C to 18.3°C	50°F to 65°F

focus on ››HOME CARE

Dry Heat Applications

Wheat or Bean Bags

The use of **wheat or bean bags** has become very popular because they are easy to use and inexpensive. They can even be made at home. These bags are warmed in the microwave, but the length of warming time depends on size, components, and the heating power of the client's microwave. If the client's care plan instructs you to apply them, you should ***always do the following***:

- ***Heat the bag in the microwave only for the length of time specified in the client's care plan.***
- ***Never leave the bean bag unattended while it is heating in the microwave.*** The contents can spark or even catch on fire (similar to microwave popcorn)! Always remove the bag immediately if you begin to smell something burning.
- ***After heating, shake the bag in order to mix the beans inside***, as they usually heat unevenly.
- ***Never place these bags directly on the skin.*** They should always be wrapped in a pad or towel, to avoid injuring the client. Check with your supervisor if you are unsure of the type of cover you should use.

Heating Pads, Electric Blankets, and Hot-Water Bottles

Some of your home care clients may have electric heating pads or hot-water bottles that apply dry heat. These can create serious fire and burn risks, ***so support workers are usually not permitted to apply electric heating pads or hot-water bottles.*** If a client asks you to apply an electric heating pad or hot-water bottle, explain that your employer's policy does not allow you to do this. Find another way to provide warmth to the client—such as giving them a blanket or a sweater—and tell your supervisor about the client's request. If the client still insists on using a heating pad or hot-water bottle, he or she may need to sign a legal waiver (sometimes called a "Negotiated Risk Agreement") with your supervisor before you can apply it.

A compress is usually made of cloth—for example, a wash cloth, small towel, or gauze dressing.

Your supervisor will tell you how long to leave the application in place. The length of time should never exceed 15 minutes. Check the skin every 5 minutes. To maintain the temperature, change the compress frequently. A layer of plastic wrap and a dry towel can be used to cover the compress and retain the heat.

Sometimes commercial compresses may be ordered in the care plan. These are premoistened and packaged in foil, and before unwrapping them, they are heated under an infrared lamp, as instructed by the manufacturer. Then they are unwrapped and applied in the same manner as regular hot compresses. Commercial compresses are used once and then discarded.

1 2 3 APPLYING WARM COMPRESSES

Remember to promote:

• **D**ignity • **I**ndependence • **P**references • **P**rivacy • **S**afety

Pre-Procedure

1 Identify the client, according to employer policy. Explain the procedure to the client.
3 Practise proper hand hygiene.
4 Collect the following:
- Basin
- Bath thermometer
- Small towel, wash cloth, or gauze squares
- Plastic wrap
- Ties, tape, or rolled gauze
- Bath towel
- Waterproof pad

5 Provide for privacy.

(continued on page 825)

1 2 3 APPLYING WARM COMPRESSES (cont'd)

Procedure

6 Place the waterproof pad under the body part to be treated.
7 Fill the basin one half to two thirds full with hot water, as directed by your supervisor. Measure the water temperature.
8 Place the compress in the water.
9 Wring out the compress
10 Apply the compress to the area. Note the time.
11 Ask the client if the compress feels comfortable. If the client is comfortable, cover the compress quickly with plastic wrap. Cover the plastic wrap with a bath towel (Figure 43–2). Secure the towel in place with ties, tape, or rolled gauze.
12 Place the call bell within reach. Follow the care plan for bed rail use.*
13 Check the area every 5 minutes. The compress should never be applied longer than 15 minutes. Check for redness and complaints of pain, discomfort, or numbness. Remove the compress if any of these signs occur, and tell your supervisor immediately.
14 Change the compress if it cools down.
15 Remove the compress after 15 minutes or sooner, as directed by your supervisor. Pat the area dry with a towel.

Post-Procedure

16 Provide for safety and comfort.
17 Place the call bell within reach. Follow the care plan for bed rail use.*
18 Remove privacy measures.
19 Clean the equipment. Discard disposable items. Wear gloves for this step.
20 Follow employer policy for soiled linen.
21 Practise proper hand hygiene.
22 Report and record your actions and observations, according to employer policy.

*Steps marked with an asterisk may not apply in community settings.

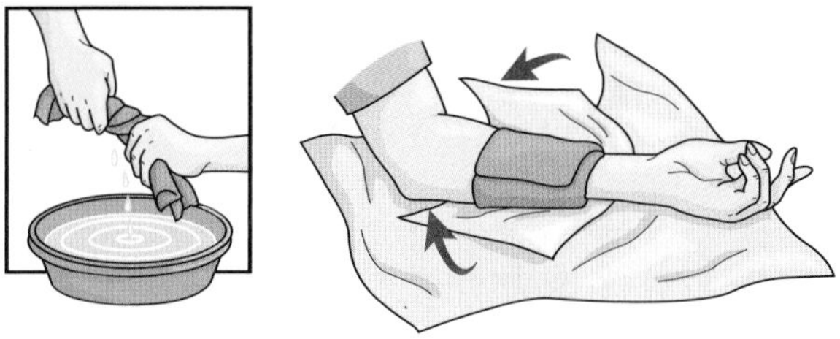

Figure 43–2 Cover a warm compress with plastic and a bath towel to prevent the compress from cooling down too quickly.

Warm Soaks

A warm soak is a warm, moist application that involves immersing a body part into heated water. This promotes circulation and muscle relaxation. Hot soaks are usually used for smaller body parts, such as a hand, lower arm, foot, or lower leg (Figure 43–3). A tub is used to soak larger parts (arm, leg, or torso). The soak lasts 15 minutes. Maintain the client's comfort and body alignment during the warm soak.

Remember to check the water temperature before soaking the body part. If the water is too hot, the skin can be burned as soon as it touches the water. If a water thermometer is not available, test the water by dipping your inner wrist in the water. If the water feels too warm, add some cold water and mix it in well.

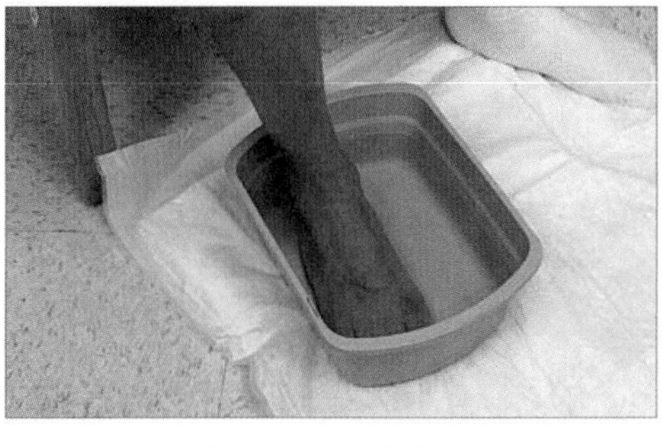

Figure 43–3 The warm soak.

1 2 3 THE WARM SOAK

Remember to promote:

• Dignity • Independence • Preferences • Privacy • Safety

Pre-Procedure

1 Identify the client, according to employer policy.
2 Explain the procedure to the client.
3 Practise proper hand hygiene.
4 Collect the following:
- Water basin or an arm or foot bath
- Bath thermometer
- Bath blanket
- Waterproof pads

5 Provide for privacy.

Procedure

6 Position the client for treatment.
7 Place the call bell within reach.*
8 Place a waterproof pad under the area to be treated.
9 Fill the water basin half full with hot water, as directed by your supervisor. Measure the water temperature. If a water thermometer is not available, test the water by dipping your inner wrist in the water. If the water feels too warm, add some cold water and mix it in well.
10 Place the body part into the water. Pad the edge of the basin with a towel. Note the time.
11 Cover the client with a bath blanket for extra warmth.
12 Check the area every 5 minutes. Check for redness and complaints of pain, discomfort, or numbness. Discontinue the soak if any of these signs are noticed. Wrap the body part in a towel, and inform your supervisor at once.
13 Check water temperature every 5 minutes. Change the water, as necessary. Wrap the body part in a towel while changing the water.
14 Remove the body part from the water in 15 minutes. Pat dry.

Post-Procedure

15 Follow steps 16 through 22 in *Applying Warm Compresses* on page 825.

*Steps marked with an asterisk may not apply in community settings.

Change the water, as necessary, to correct the temperature. Never add hot water while the body part is in the basin because you can burn the client. Instead, have the client remove the body part from the basin, assisting as necessary. Then you can safely add more hot water. Test the temperature again before assisting the client to put the body part back into the soak.

The Sitz Bath

The **sitz bath**—also considered to be a warm, moist application—involves immersing the perineal and rectal areas in warm or hot water (*sitz* from German means *seat*). Sitz baths, usually lasting for about 15 minutes, are commonly used after rectal surgery, female pelvic surgery, childbirth, and as treatment for hemorrhoids. They are used to:

- Clean perineal or anal wounds
- Promote healing
- Relieve pain and soreness
- Increase circulation
- Stimulate voiding

The disposable plastic sitz bath fits onto the toilet seat (Figure 43–4). Plastic tubing runs from the bowl of the sitz bath to a water bag, and a plastic clamp closes the tubing. The sitz bath is filled with water at an appropriate temperature. (Check with your supervisor to determine a safe temperature.) The water bag is filled with warmer water. As the water in the sitz bath cools, the tubing is

1 2 3 ASSISTING THE CLIENT TO TAKE A SITZ BATH

Remember to promote:

• Dignity • Independence • Preferences • Privacy • Safety

Pre-Procedure

1 Identify the client, according to employer policy.
2 Explain the procedure to the client.
3 Practise proper hand hygiene.
4 Collect the following:
- Disposable sitz bath, if used.
- Wheelchair, if the built-in sitz tub is used
- Bath thermometer
- Large water container
- Two bath blankets, bath towels, and clean garments
- Footstool, if the client is short
- Disinfectant solution
- Utility gloves

5 Provide for privacy.

Procedure

6 Assist the client to the bathroom or commode. Encourage the client to eliminate before the procedure.
7 *If using a disposable sitz bath:*
- **a** Place the disposable sitz bath on the toilet seat.
- **b** Fill the sitz bath two thirds full with water. Your supervisor will tell you water temperature to use. Measure the water temperature. If a water thermometer is not available, test the water by dipping your inner wrist in the water. If the water feels too warm, add some cold water and mix it in well.
- **c** Close the clamp on the tubing.
- **d** Fill the water bag with warmer water than that in the bowl. Your supervisor will tell you what water temperature to use. Measure the water temperature.
- **e** Hang the bag on a towel bar or from the top of the toilet tank. The bag must be at a higher level than the toilet seat.

8 *If using a built-in sitz tub:*
- **a** Transport the client by wheelchair to the room with the sitz bath.
- **b** Fill the sitz bath two thirds full with water. Your supervisor will tell you what water temperature to use. Measure the water temperature with a thermometer or your inner wrist.
- **c** Pad the metal part of the sitz tub with towels. Pad the part that will be in contact with the client.

9 Assist the client to remove or lower clothing below the waist, or raise the client's gown above the waist.
10 Assist the client to sit in the sitz bath.
11 Place a bath blanket around the shoulders. Place another over the legs for warmth.
12 Provide a footstool if the edge of the sitz bath causes pressure under the knees.
13 Show the client how to open the clamp to let warmer water from the bag flow into the sitz bath (with disposable sitz baths). Assist, as necessary.
14 Place the call bell within reach.*
15 Stay with a client who is weak or unsteady.
16 Check the client every 5 minutes for complaints/signs of weakness, faintness, and drowsiness. Check for a rapid pulse. If any occur, get assistance to help the client back to bed.
17 Assist the client out of the sitz bath after 15 minutes or as directed by your supervisor.
18 Assist the client to dry off and with dressing.
19 Assist the client back to his or her room.

Post-Procedure

20 Provide for safety and comfort.
21 Place the call bell within reach. Follow the care plan for bed rail use.*
22 Remove privacy measures.
23 Clean the sitz bath with disinfectant solution. Wear utility gloves.
24 Clean and return reusable items to their proper places. Follow employer policy for soiled linen. Wear gloves for this step.
25 Practise proper hand hygiene.
26 Report and record your actions and observations, according to employer policy.

*Steps marked with an asterisk may not apply in community settings.

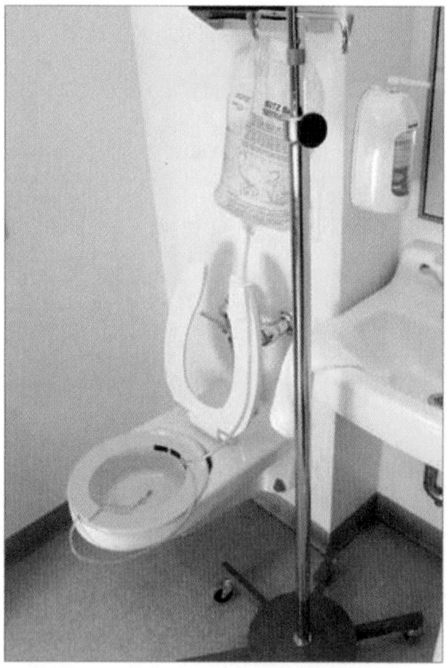

Figure 43–4 The disposable sitz bath with water bag, tubing, and clamp.

unclamped to allow the warmer water from the bag to flow into the sitz bath.

A *sitz tub* is a built-in fixture with a deep seat. The client sits in a seat filled with water (Figure 43–5), with his or her feet resting flat on the floor. Do not use an ordinary bathtub for a sitz bath. Immersing the legs and feet decreases the effectiveness of the procedure.

When using a sitz bath, blood flow to the perineal and rectal area increases. As blood flow to other body parts is reduced, the client may feel chilled. Cover the client's shoulders and knees for warmth. Reduced blood flow may also make the client feel faint, dizzy, weak, or drowsy. Check the client every 5 minutes for these signs. Stay in the room if it is not safe to leave the client alone. Allow as much privacy as possible. If it is safe to leave, place the call bell within the client's reach, or remain within easy hearing distance.

Warm Packs

A *pack* is a treatment that involves wrapping a body part with a wet or dry application. The application can be either warm or cold. Single-use (disposable) or reusable commercial packs are available. Some can be used alternatively for heat or cold, such as some commercial **gel packs**. The manufacturer's instructions will tell you how to activate the heat or cold (Figure 43–6 and Figure 43–7). Some warm

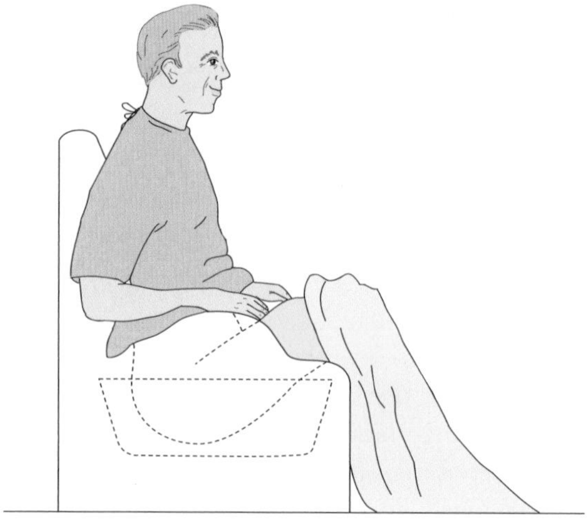

Figure 43–5 The built-in sitz tub.

packs are put in boiling water for a few minutes or warmed in a microwave oven. Other types of packs require kneading or squeezing in order to activate them to heat up. Some packs can be either warmed in hot water (to heat) or placed in the freezer (to cool). Always read warning labels, and follow the manufacturer's safety instructions.

Reusable packs should never be placed directly on the skin but should be covered with a clean, dry cloth, such as a dishcloth or towel. Follow employer policy and the manufacturer's instructions regarding how to cover the packs for use and how to clean them after use—by wiping with alcohol or washing with soap and water.

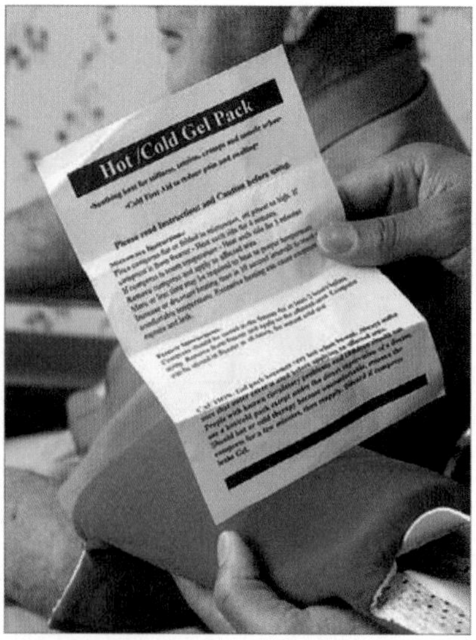

Figure 43–6 Commercial warm pack. The manufacturer's instructions explain how to activate the heat.

1 2 3 APPLYING A WARM PACK

Remember to promote:

• Dignity • Independence • Preferences • Privacy • Safety

Pre-Procedure

1 Identify the client, according to employer policy.
2 Explain the procedure to the client.
3 Practise proper hand hygiene.
4 Collect the following:
- Commercial pack
- Towel
- Pack cover
- Ties, tape, or rolled gauze (if needed)
- Waterproof pad

5 Heat the pack. Follow the manufacturer's instructions.
6 Put the pack in the cover.
7 Provide for privacy.

Procedure

8 Place the pad under the body part.
9 Apply the pack quickly. Note the time.
10 Secure the pack in place with ties, tape, or rolled gauze. Some packs are secured with Velcro straps (Figure 43–8).
11 Place the call bell within reach. Follow the care plan for bed rail use.*
12 Check the area every 5 minutes. Check for redness and complaints of pain, discomfort, or numbness. Remove the pack if any occur. Tell your supervisor at once.
13 Change the pack if it cools down.
14 Remove the pack after 15 minutes or sooner, as directed by your supervisor. Pat the area dry with the towel.

Post-Procedure

15 Follow steps 16 through 22 in *Applying Warm Compresses* on page 825.
16 Clean a reusable pack, according to employer policy and the manufacturer's instructions.

*Steps marked with an asterisk may not apply in community settings.

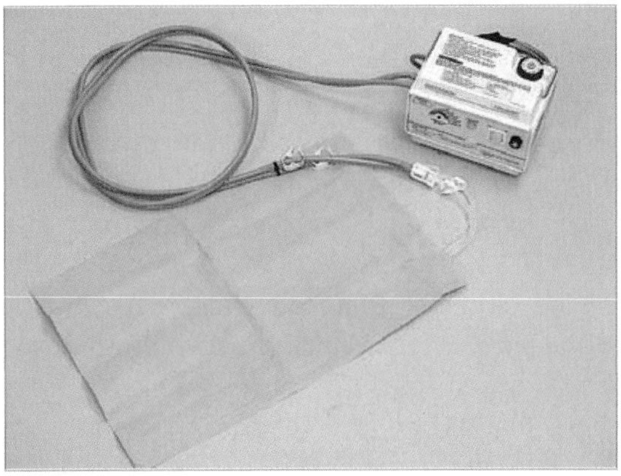

Figure 43–7 An Aquathermia pad. **Source:** Potter, P.A., & Perry, A.G. (2005). *Fundamentals of nursing* (6th ed., p. 1559). St. Louis: Mosby.

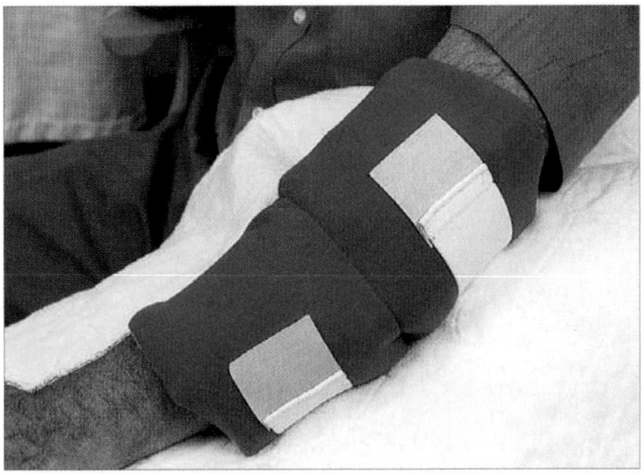

Figure 43–8 Warm pack secured with Velcro.

COLD APPLICATIONS

Cold applications are often used to treat sprains, fractures, and fever. They reduce pain, prevent swelling, and decrease circulation and bleeding. Cold applications also cool the body when fever is present.

Cold has the opposite effect of heat on body functions. When cold is applied to the skin, blood vessels **constrict** (see Figure 43–1*C* on page 820), resulting in decreased blood flow to the area and less oxygen and nutrients being carried to the tissues. Cold applications are useful immediately after an injury. The decreased circulation reduces the amount of bleeding, bruising, and swelling, and cold has a numbing effect on the skin, which helps reduce or relieve pain in the part.

Complications

Cold applications should never be used on old injuries, as they can actually cause tissue damage, called **frost bite**—the medical condition in which damage is caused to skin and other tissues due to extreme cold. Signs of frost bite include blisters; pale, white, or grey skin; cyanosis; and shivering, numbness, pain, and burning.

Complications of cold applications include pain, burns, blisters, and cyanosis. Burns and blisters tend to occur due to intense cold and when dry cold applications are in direct contact with the skin.

It is your responsibility to frequently check clients who are at high risk for complications (see Box 43–1 on page 823) and to follow the guidelines listed in Box 43–2 on page 823 in order to prevent injuries from cold applications. You should peek under the application to inspect the skin every 5 minutes for signs of complications of cold applications.

In general, cold applications should be applied and removed in 15-minute intervals (15 minutes on and 15 minutes off). Timely removal of the cold application helps prevent tissue damage resulting from overconstricted blood vessels.

Moist and Dry Cold Applications

Cold applications can be moist or dry.

- Dry cold—ice bag, ice collar, and ice glove
- Moist cold—cold compress
- Moist or dry—cold packs

Moist cold applications penetrate deeper than dry moist ones, so temperatures of moist applications should not be as low as in dry applications. You should check the skin frequently (at least every 5 minutes, or more often, as directed by your supervisor).

Ice Bags, Ice Collars, Ice Gloves, and Dry Cold Packs

Ice bags, ice collars, and ice gloves are dry cold applications. The devices are filled with crushed ice.

Reusable as well as single-use (disposable) **cold packs** are available commercially. To activate the cold, follow the manufacturer's instructions. You may need to strike, knead, or squeeze the pack. Reusable cold packs are kept in the freezer after they are cleaned after use.

Some devices have an outer covering and can be placed directly on the skin. If the device comes without a cover, it should be placed in a cover. When the cover becomes moist, remove it and apply a dry one (see the *Focus on Home Care: Ice Packs* box.)

Cold Compresses

The cold compress is a moist application that should not be left in place longer than 15 minutes. The skin under the cold compress should be checked every 5 minutes for signs of blistering, increased pain, or frost bite.

focus on ›› HOME CARE

Ice Packs

Disposable ice packs are commonly used in home settings. They are kept in the freezer until needed. A bag of frozen vegetables can be used as a makeshift ice pack. Also, plastic bags can be filled with ice, closed securely to prevent leaks, wrapped in a clean towel, dish cloth, or pillowcase and used as an ice pack. If you use a bag of frozen vegetables as an ice pack, ***make sure the vegetables are not eaten later. Remember to only apply an ice pack if your supervisor assigns this task to you and if it is within your scope of practice in your province!***

1 2 3 APPLYING AN ICE BAG, ICE COLLAR, OR DRY COLD PACK

Remember to promote:

• Dignity • Independence • Preferences • Privacy • Safety

Pre-Procedure

1 Identify the client, according to employer policy.
2 Explain the procedure to the client.
3 Practise proper hand hygiene.
4 Collect a cold pack or the following:
- Ice bag, collar, or glove
- Crushed ice
- Flannel cover, towel, or pillowcase
- Paper towels

5 *Applying an ice bag, collar, or glove:*
  a Fill it with water and place the stopper. Turn the device upside down to check for leaks.
  b Empty the device.
  c Fill the device one half to two thirds full with crushed ice or ice chips (Figure 43-9).
  d Remove excess air. Bend, twist, or squeeze the device, or press it against a firm surface.
  e Place the cap or stopper on securely.
  f Dry the device with the paper towels.
  g Place the device in the cover.

6 *Applying a cold pack:*
  a Squeeze, knead, or strike the disposable cold pack, as directed by the manufacturer. This activates the cold.
  b Place the device in the cover.

7 Provide for privacy.
8 *Applying an electric cooling pad (Figure 43–10):*
  a Cover the pad with a washable cover, such as a flannelette cover or a towel.
  b Plug in the cord in a three-prong (grounded) plug.

Procedure

9 Apply the device to the appropriate body part, as stated in the client's care plan. Secure it in place with ties, tape, or rolled gauze. Note the time.
10 Place the call bell within reach. Follow the care plan for bed rail use.*
11 Check the skin every 5 minutes. Check for signs of frost bite, including blisters, pale, white, or grey skin, cyanosis, shivering, numbness, pain, and burning. Remove the device if any occur. Tell your supervisor at once.
12 Remove the device after 15 minutes or as directed by your supervisor.

Post-Procedure

13 Provide for safety and comfort.
14 Replace the call bell within reach. Follow the care plan for bed rail use.*
15 Remove privacy measures.
16 Clean equipment. Discard disposable items. Wear gloves for this step.
17 Follow employer policy for disposing of soiled linen.
18 Practise proper hand hygiene.
19 Report and record your actions and observations, according to employer policy.
20 Clean the reusable cold pack, according to employer policy and the manufacturer's instructions.

*Steps marked with an asterisk may not apply in community settings.

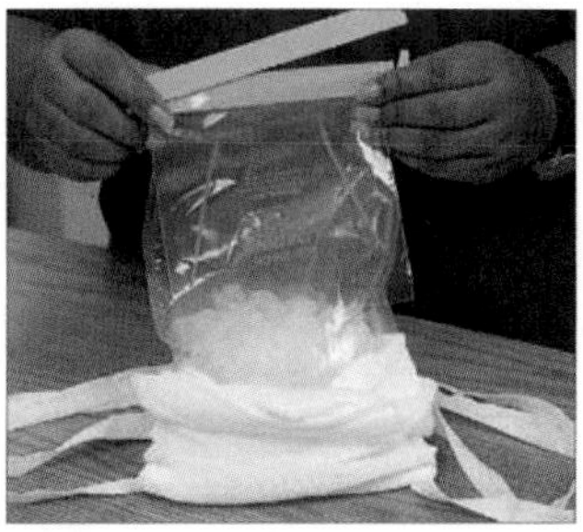

Figure 43–9 Fill the ice bag one half to two thirds full with ice. Remember to cover it before placing it on the client's skin.

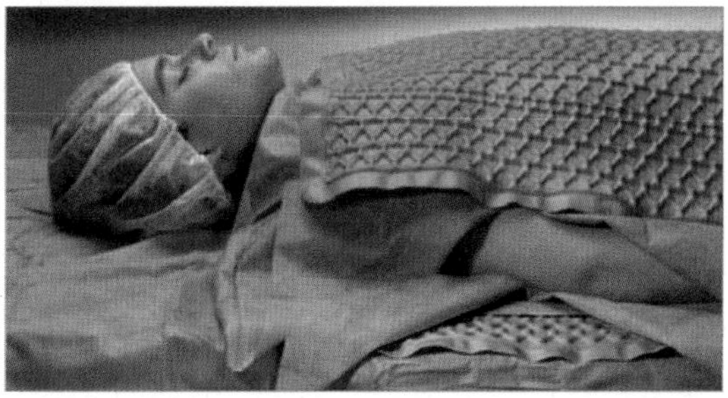

Figure 43–10 An electric cooling device. **Source:** Perry, A.G., & Potter, P.A. (2006). *Clinical nursing skills & techniques* (6th ed., p. 1324). St. Louis: Mosby.

focus on ›› FIRST AID

Remember "RICE" for Recent Injuries

If someone you know or are caring for has suffered a recent injury, you should remember the acronym that you probably learned in your first-aid class: "RICE."

R **Rest** the limb. Do not try to use it.

I **Ice.** Apply ice packs to reduce swelling and decrease pain.

C **Compression.** Wrap a **compression bandage** (also known as a **tensor bandage)** around the affected part, ensuring that it is not too tight. Signs that it is too tight include tingling and numbness, followed by increased pain and poor circulation (loss of colour) of the skin in the extremities of the affected body part.

E **Elevate** the limb to reduce possible swelling.

Remember that the client should be assessed by a health care professional, as soon as possible, in order to determine if a fracture has occurred!

1 2 3 APPLYING COLD COMPRESSES

Remember to promote:

• Dignity • Independence • Preferences • Privacy • Safety

Pre-Procedure

1 Identify the client, according to employer policy.
2 Explain the procedure to the client.
3 Practise proper hand hygiene.
4 Collect the following:
- Large basin with ice
- Small basin with cold water
- Gauze squares, wash cloths, or small towels
- Waterproof pad
- Bath towel

5 Provide for privacy.

Procedure

6 Place the small basin with cold water into the large basin with ice.
7 Place the compresses into the cold water.
8 Place the pad under the body part.
9 Wring out a compress.
10 Apply the compress to the part. Note the time.
11 Place the call bell within reach. Follow the care plan for bed rail use.*
12 Check the area every 5 minutes. Check for signs of frost bite, which includes blisters, pale, white, or grey skin, cyanosis, shivering, numbness, pain, and burning. Remove the compress if any occur. Tell your supervisor at once.
13 Change the compress when it warms up. Usually compresses are changed every 5 minutes.
14 Remove the compress after 15 minutes or sooner, as directed by your supervisor.
15 Pat the area dry.

Post-Procedure

16 Follow steps 13 through 20 in *Applying an Ice Bag, Ice Collar or Dry Cold Pack* on page 831.

*Steps marked with an asterisk may not apply in community settings.

REVIEW

Answers to these questions are at the bottom of the page.

Circle the BEST answer.

1. **Which of the following is *true* about the area of heat application?**
   - A. It will decrease the blood flow
   - B. It will cause an increase in muscle spasm
   - C. It will treat recent sprains
   - D. It can reduce joint stiffness
2. **Which of the following is the greatest threat from heat applications?**
   - A. Infection
   - B. Burns
   - C. Chilling
   - D. Pressure ulcers
3. **Who has the greatest risk of complications from a heat application?**
   - A. A 10-year-old boy
   - B. A teenager
   - C. A 40-year-old woman
   - D. An older adult with diabetes
4. **When checking the area of skin under a heat application, which of the following should you report?**
   - A. Rash
   - B. Warm skin
   - C. Relaxed muscles
   - D. Client sleeping
5. **The temperature of a hot application is usually between:**
   - A. 26.6°C and 33.8°C
   - B. 33.8°C and 36.6°C
   - C. 36.6°C and 41.1°C
   - D. 41.1°C and 46.1°C
6. **Which of these statements about moist heat applications is *true*?**
   - A. Water is never in contact with the skin
   - B. Moist heat has a greater and faster effect than dry heat
   - C. Dry heat penetrates deeper than moist heat
   - D. Heat applications are more dangerous than cold applications
7. **A client has a warm compress. Which of the following is *true*?**
   - A. The warm compress is a dry heat application
   - B. The compress is applied no longer than 5 minutes
   - C. The area is checked every 5 minutes
   - D. The compress should never be covered
8. **Which of these statements about sitz baths is true?**
   - A. The foot and leg areas are immersed in warm or hot water for 15 to 20 minutes
   - B. Weakness and fainting can occur
   - C. Sitz baths should never be used on men
   - D. The sitz bath lasts 1 to 2 hours
9. **Cold applications:**
   - A. Reduce pain, prevent swelling, and decrease circulation
   - B. Dilate blood vessels
   - C. Prevent the spread of microbes
   - D. Are warmed in a microwave oven
10. **Which of the following is a complication of a cold application?**
    - A. Fever
    - B. Excessive thirst
    - C. Infection
    - D. Cyanosis
11. **Before applying an ice bag:**
    - A. Place the bag in a freezer
    - B. Measure the temperature of the bag
    - C. Place the bag in a cover
    - D. Ask the client to void
12. **Moist cold compresses are left in place no longer than:**
    - A. 15 minutes
    - B. 30 minutes
    - C. 45 minutes
    - D. 60 minutes

Answers: 1.D, 2.B, 3.D, 4.A, 5.C, 6.B, 7.C, 8.B, 9.A, 10.D, 11.C, 12.A

CHAPTER 44

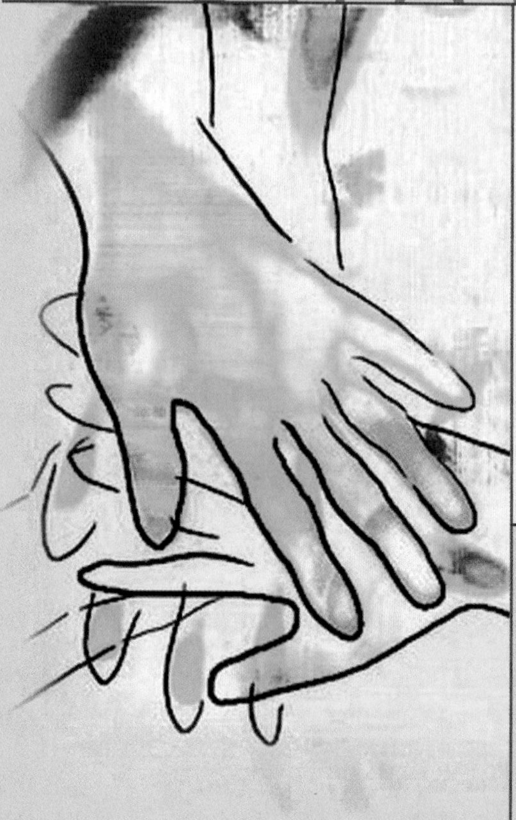

Oxygen Needs

OBJECTIVES

- Define the key terms listed in this chapter.
- Describe factors that affect oxygen needs.
- Identify the signs and symptoms of hypoxia and altered respiratory function.
- Describe tests used to diagnose respiratory problems.
- Explain measures that promote oxygenation.
- Describe devices used to administer oxygen.
- Explain how to safely assist a client with oxygen therapy.
- Describe the safety measures for suctioning.
- Explain how to assist in the care of clients with artificial airways, on mechanical ventilation, and with chest tubes.
- Apply the procedures described in this chapter to your clinical practice properly.

key terms

allergy A sensitivity to a substance that causes the body to react with signs and symptoms, such as a runny nose, wheezing, or congestion, or difficulty breathing. As part of the allergic reaction, a client's upper airway mucous membranes may swell.

apnea The lack or absence (*a*) of breathing (*pnea*).

bradypnea Slow (*brady*) breathing (*pnea*); respirations are fewer than 10 per minute.

chest tube A hollow plastic tube, surgically inserted into the chest cavity, between the inner lining and the outer lining of the lung (pleural space). The tube allows for the removal of trapped air (pneumothorax) and the drainage of blood or fluid (pleural effusion). The tube can go to an airtight drainage container or can be attached to a suction machine.

Cheyne-Stokes Respirations gradually increasing in rate and depth and then becoming shallow and slow; breathing may stop (*apnea*) for 10 to 20 seconds. This type of respiration is common when death is near.

distilled water Sterile and pure water that has been boiled and allowed to cool and condense.

dyspnea Difficult, laboured, or painful (*dys*) breathing (*pnea*).

eupnea The term for normal breathing.

face mask A device used to deliver oxygen to a client who needs extra oxygen; consists of a mask that covers the client's nose and mouth, with a plastic tube at the bottom that delivers the oxygen. The mask also has holes on either side to allow for the exhaled carbon dioxide to escape. Face masks deliver more oxygen than can nasal cannulas.

flowmeter A device that connects to an oxygen tank, a portable oxygen generator, or to a wall connection in a hospital. It regulates the flow of oxygen to the nasal cannula or face mask.

hemoptysis Bloody (*hemo*) sputum (*ptysis*, meaning "to spit").

humidified oxygen Oxygen forced through distilled water and collected into the tubing; the oxygen now contains water vapour and is less irritating to delicate mucous membranes than is plain oxygen.

hyperventilation Respirations that are more rapid (*hyper*) and shallower than normal. Sometimes, respirations may be more rapid and deeper than normal.

hypoventilation Respirations that are slow (*hypo*), shallow, and sometimes irregular.

hypoxia A deficiency (*hypo*) of oxygen in the cells (*oxia*).

intubation The process of inserting an artificial airway.

mechanical ventilation The use of a machine to move air into and out of the lungs.

nasal cannula A device used to deliver oxygen to a client who needs extra oxygen; consists of a plastic tube that fits behind the ears and a set of two prongs that are placed in the nares of the nose, and oxygen flows from these prongs. Nasal cannulas deliver less oxygen than face masks.

orthopnea Breathing (*pnea*) deeply and comfortably only while sitting or standing (*ortho*).

orthopneic position Sitting up (*ortho*) and leaning over a table to breathe.

oxygen-conserving devices Devices that help reduce oxygen wastage so that the client's oxygen supply lasts longer and he or she can go for longer outings.

pollutant A harmful chemical or substance in air or water. Air pollutants (e.g., dust, fumes, toxins, asbestos, coal dust, and sawdust) damage the lungs, and exposure can occur anywhere.

pulse oximeter A device that measures (*meter*) oxygen (*oxi*) concentration in the arterial blood; consists of a computerized monitor and a sensor (probe).

respiratory arrest Stoppage of breathing.

respiratory depression Slow, weak respirations at a rate of fewer than 12 per minute; respirations are not deep enough to bring enough air into the lungs.

SOB Acronym for "short of breath."

SpO_2 The short form for the oxygen concentration value (S = saturation, p = pulse, O_2 = oxygen).

sputum Mucus from the respiratory system that is expectorated (expelled) through the mouth.

stoma A surgically created opening into the body.

suctioning The process of withdrawing or sucking up fluid (secretions).

tachypnea Rapid (*tachy*) breathing (*pnea*); respirations are 24 or more per minute.

tracheostomy A surgically created opening (*ostomy*) through the neck into the trachea (*tracheo*).

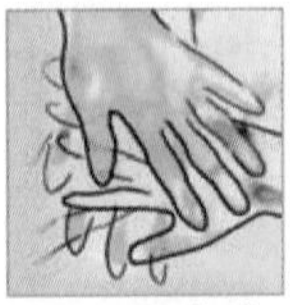

Oxygen (O_2) is a gas that is part of the air we breathe every day. It has no taste, odour, or colour. Oxygen is the most important basic need required for life, and without it, death will occur within minutes. Breathing is something that we take for granted until we experience difficulty breathing. People who have certain illnesses or are in stressful situations might experience difficulty breathing, which can affect the amount of oxygen in their blood cells.

As a support worker, you will often work with clients who have difficulty breathing or absorbing enough oxygen into their bodies. In order to survive, they require oxygen, which is supplied to them through a nasal tube or mask. It is your responsibility to know how to provide safe and effective care to these clients (see Figure 44–1, and Chapter 14 for a description of the respiratory system).

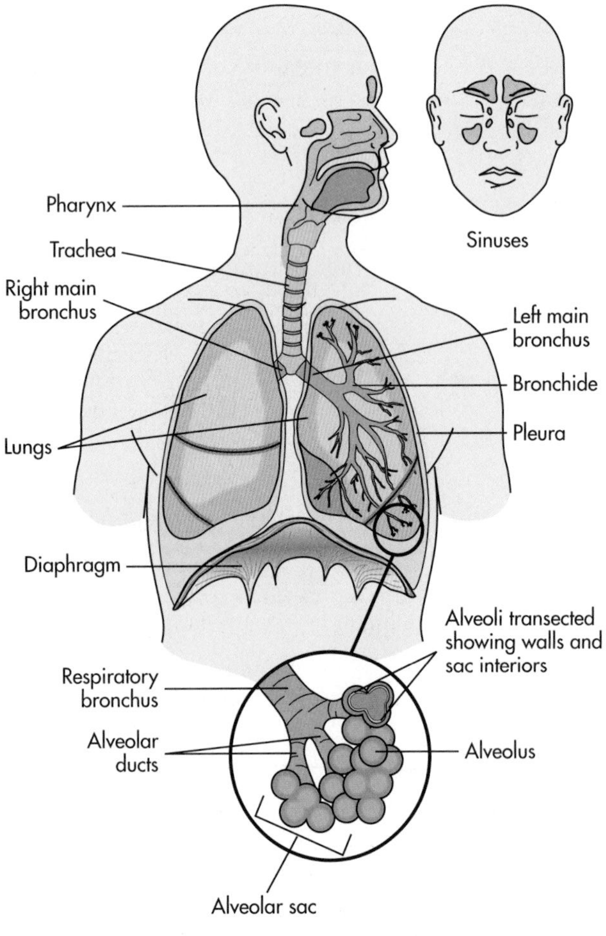

Figure 44–1 The respiratory system.

As with any task, before giving or assisting with any care described in this chapter, you should make sure of the following:

- Your province or territory allows you to perform the task.
- The task is in your job description at your agency.
- You have the necessary training.
- You know how to use the equipment.
- You have reviewed the task with a nurse.
- A nurse or respiratory technician will supervise you.

FACTORS AFFECTING OXYGEN NEEDS

For cells to get enough oxygen, the respiratory and cardiovascular systems must function properly. Any disease, injury, or surgery involving these systems can affect the body's ability to absorb oxygen from the air and deliver it to the cells. Body systems depend on each other, so altered function of any system (nervous, musculo-skeletal, or urinary) can affect oxygen absorption and delivery. Major factors affecting oxygen absorption and delivery are:

- ***Respiratory system function***—structures of the respiratory system must be intact and functioning. The airway must be open (patent), and there must be an adequate number of *alveoli* (single-celled air sacs in the lungs) to effectively absorb oxygen (O_2) and excrete carbon dioxide (CO_2), which is a waste product.
- ***Cardiovascular system function***—blood must flow normally to and from the heart to all bodily cells. When blood vessels are narrowed by disease or other causes, blood flow will be affected. Capillaries and cells must exchange O_2 and CO_2 efficiently. Oxygen is required by all cells to produce energy to carry out their proper functions.
- ***Red blood cell count***—blood must have enough red blood cells (RBCs), which contain hemoglobin. Hemoglobin is made up of iron, and it picks up oxygen in the lungs and carries it to the cells. The bone marrow produces RBCs, but health challenges (such as chemotherapy and

leukemia) can affect bone marrow function and therefore the production of RBCs, and poor diet, iron-deficiency anemia, and blood loss will also reduce the number of RBCs in blood.

- ***Nervous system function***—nervous system diseases and injuries can affect respiratory muscles, making breathing difficult or impossible. Brain injury as well as use of narcotics and depressant drugs can affect the respiratory rate, rhythm, and depth.

  Brain function is affected by O_2 and CO_2 levels in the blood. When CO_2 levels increase, the body tries to get rid of the excess CO_2 and bring in more oxygen by increasing the respiration rate.
- ***Aging***—respiratory muscles weaken and lung tissue becomes less elastic with advancing age, making coughing more difficult. If the person cannot cough to remove secretions from the upper airway, pneumonia (infection of the lungs) can develop. Older adults are at risk for respiratory complications after surgery for this reason.
- ***Exercise***—the body requires more O_2 when it is exercised, in order to supply energy needed by cells. This is usually accomplished by increasing the respiratory rate and depth (in the lungs), at a pace that keeps up with the O_2 demand throughout the body.

  Clients with heart and respiratory disease may have enough O_2 while they are at rest, but with even a slight increase in activity, their bodies may not be able to bring in enough O_2 and deliver it to the cells for energy. This stresses the heart and lungs, which (like all tissues) require oxygen to perform their necessary tasks.
- ***Fever***—when fever is present, O_2 needs increase because the body is working hard to fight the infection that is causing the fever. In order to keep up with the body's O_2 needs, the respiratory rate and depth must increase.
- ***Pain***—pain increases the need for O_2, so the body responds by increasing the respiration rate and depth. Clients with chest and abdominal injuries or surgeries are unwilling or unable to take deep breaths because it is painful to breathe in and out, which further increases their need for O_2. The extra O_2 they need is therefore supplied to them by way of a mask or tube until they can take deep breaths on their own.
- ***Drugs***—some drugs depress the respiratory centre in the brain. **Respiratory depression** involves slow, weak respirations at a rate of fewer than 12 per minute and too shallow to bring enough O_2 into the lungs. **Respiratory arrest** occurs when breathing stops. Narcotics such as morphine, Demerol, and others can slow or even stop respirations (*narcotic* comes from the Greek word *narkoun* meaning stupor or numbness). In safe amounts, when prescribed by a physician, these drugs help relieve pain. Substance abusers are at risk for respiratory depression and respiratory arrest from overdoses of these drugs.
- ***Smoking***—those who smoke inhale air that is mixed with harmful substances that can damage the lung tissue and have been proven to cause lung cancer and chronic obstructive pulmonary disease (COPD). Smoking is also a risk factor for coronary artery disease.
- ***Allergies***—an **allergy** is a sensitivity to a substance—for example, pollen, dust, foods, drugs, and smoke—that causes the body to react with signs and symptoms such as a runny nose, wheezing, or congestion. As part of the allergic reaction, the upper airway mucous membranes may swell. With severe swelling, the airway closes, resulting in shock and death. People with allergies are at risk for chronic bronchitis and asthma.
- ***Pollutant exposure***—a **pollutant** is a harmful chemical or substance in air or water. Air pollutants, for example, dust, fumes, toxins, asbestos, coal dust, and sawdust, damage the lungs. Exposure to allergens can occur at home, in the workplace, or in the community.
- ***Nutrition***—good nutrition that includes iron and vitamins (vitamin B_{12}, vitamin C, and folic acid) is necessary to produce RBCs, without which the body cannot transport O_2 to cells.
- ***Alcohol***—alcohol depresses the brain. Excessive amounts reduce the cough reflex and increase the risk of aspiration, which can cause obstructed airway and pneumonia.
- ***Drug (narcotic or barbiturate) overdose***—in normal circumstances and when used as prescribed, the proper amount of a drug will control

moderate to severe pain (narcotics) or provide sedation (barbiturates). When a narcotic or barbiturate is taken for "recreational" purposes or over the safe dosage, the breathing centre in the hypothalamus of the brain is affected, and respirations are suppressed. The brain cannot tell the person to take deep breaths, which can result in loss of consciousness or death.

ALTERED RESPIRATORY FUNCTION

The function of the respiratory system involves three processes that must work together, and respiratory function is altered if even one of these processes is affected:

1. Air moves into and out of the lungs.
2. O_2 and CO_2 are exchanged at the alveoli.
3. The blood transports O_2 to the cells and removes CO_2 from them.

Signs and Symptoms. The client who is short of breath (**SOB**) has altered respiratory function, that is, something is preventing him or her from breathing easily. Altered respiratory function may be an acute or chronic problem. When unable to breathe easily, a client may feel very anxious or may panic. He or she is uncomfortable and usually visibly struggling to breathe. The client often wants to sit up in the bed or in a chair, as he or she may have more difficulty breathing when lying flat (*orthopnea*) (see Box 44–1).

Struggling to breathe is both exhausting and dangerous for the client, as he or she usually uses more energy (and therefore more oxygen) doing so. Report your observations to your supervisor promptly and accurately so that quick action may be taken to correct the problem and prevent it from getting worse. However, you should be aware that if the client is already on oxygen, ***you should never turn up the oxygen level if you have not been directed to do so in the client's care plan. In certain circumstances, turning up the oxygen could cause extreme harm to the client and can make the client even more short of breath (SOB)!***

Box 44–1 Signs and Symptoms of Altered Respiratory Function

- Signs and symptoms of hypoxia (see Box 44–2 on page 840)
- Any abnormal breathing pattern
- Complaints of shortness of breath or being "winded" or "short-winded"
- Cough (note frequency and time of day)
  - Dry and hacking
  - Harsh and barking
  - Productive (produces sputum) or nonproductive
- Sputum
  - Colour—clear, white, yellow, green, brown, or red
  - Odour—none or foul
  - Consistency—thick, watery, or frothy (with bubbles or foam)
  - **Hemoptysis**—bloody (*hemo*) sputum (*ptysis*, meaning "to spit"); note if the sputum is bright red, dark red, blood tinged, or streaked with blood
- Noisy respirations
  - Wheezing
  - Wet-sounding respirations
  - Crowing sounds
- Chest pain
  - Location
  - Constant or intermittent (comes and goes)
  - Client's description (stabbing, knife-like, aching)
  - What makes it worse (movement, coughing, yawning, sneezing, sighing, deep breathing)
- Cyanosis
  - Skin
  - Mucous membranes
  - Lips
  - Nail beds
- Changes in vital signs
- Body position
  - Sitting upright
  - Leaning forward or hunched over a table

Abnormal Respiratory Patterns

The normal respiration rate for adults is 12 to 20 per minute. Infants and children have faster rates (see Table 41–3 on page 784). Normal respirations are quiet, effortless, and regular, and both sides of the chest should rise and fall in a uniform manner. The medical term for normal respirations is **eupnea**.

The following respiratory patterns are abnormal (Figure 44–2):

- ***Tachypnea***—rapid (*tachy*) breathing (*pnea*). Respirations are 24 or more per minute. Fever, exercise, pain, airway obstruction, and hypoxemia are common causes.
- ***Bradypnea***—slow (*brady*) breathing (*pnea*). Respirations are fewer than 12 per minute. Drug overdoses and nervous system disorders are common causes.
- ***Apnea***—the lack or absence (*a*) of breathing (*pnea*). It occurs in cardiac arrest and respiratory arrest. Sleep apnea and periodic apnea of newborns are other types of apnea.
- ***Kussmaul respirations***—deep and rapid respirations.
- ***Hypoventilation***—respirations are slow (*hypo*), shallow, and sometimes irregular. Common causes include lung disorders (such as pneumonia) that affect the alveoli. Other causes include obesity, airway obstruction, side effects of drugs, and nervous system and musculo-skeletal disorders affecting the respiratory muscles.
- ***Hyperventilation***—respirations are rapid (*hyper*) and deeper than normal. Its many causes include asthma, emphysema, infection, fever, nervous system disorders, hypoxia, anxiety, pain, and some drugs.
- ***Dyspnea***—difficult, laboured, or painful (*dys*) breathing (*pnea*). Heart disease, exercise, and anxiety are common causes.
- ***Cheyne-Stokes***—respirations gradually increase in rate and depth and then become shallow and slow. Breathing may stop (apnea) for 10 to 20 seconds. Drug overdose, heart failure, renal failure, and brain disorders are common causes. Cheyne-Stokes respirations are common when death is near.
- ***Orthopnea***—breathing (*pnea*) deeply and comfortably only in the sitting or standing (*ortho*) positions. Common causes include emphysema, asthma, pneumonia, angina pectoris, and other heart and respiratory disorders.

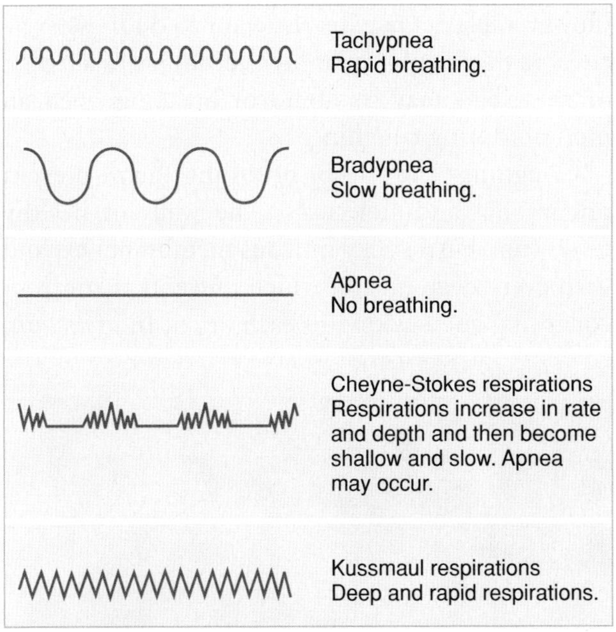

Figure 44–2 Some respiratory patterns. **Adapted from:** Phipps, W.J., et al. (2003). *Medical-surgical nursing: Health and illness perspectives* (7th ed.). St. Louis: Mosby.

Hypoxia

Hypoxia—a deficiency (*hypo*) of oxygen in the cells (*oxia*)—is one of the end results of abnormal respiratory functioning, and it is caused by any illness, disease, injury, or surgery that affects respiratory function. Hypoxia is a life-threatening condition because without enough oxygen to function, cells will be damaged or die.

The brain is very sensitive to an inadequate supply of oxygen. Restlessness, dizziness, and disorientation are early signs of hypoxia. It is important that you report signs and symptoms of hypoxia (see Box 44–2) immediately. The sooner hypoxia is diagnosed, the sooner oxygen can be given and the cause of the hypoxia treated.

Box 44–2 Signs and Symptoms of Hypoxia

- Restlessness
- Dizziness
- Disorientation
- Confusion
- Behaviour and personality changes
- Difficulty concentrating and difficulty following directions
- Apprehension
- Anxiety
- Fatigue
- Agitation
- Increased pulse rate
- Increased rate and depth of respirations
- Sitting position, often leaning forward
- Cyanosis (bluish colour in the skin, lips, mucous membranes, and nail beds)
- Dyspnea

PROMOTING OXYGENATION

For the body to get enough oxygen, air must move deeply into the lungs and reach the alveoli, where O_2 and CO_2 are exchanged. Disease and injury can prevent air from reaching the alveoli. Pain, immobility, and narcotics interfere with deep breathing and with coughing up secretions, allowing the secretions to collect in the airway and lungs, which will interfere with air movement and lung function. Secretions also provide an environment for microbes to grow and multiply, which can lead to a life-threatening infection.

To completely meet the client's oxygen needs, the care plan will list measures to promote oxygenation. Some of the measures require the administration of oxygen or other activities, for example, a short walk, that simply involve movement to expand the client's lungs. Some other measures that are commonly listed in care plans are given below.

Positioning and Providing Rest Periods

For clients confined to bed, breathing is usually easier in the semi-Fowler's or Fowler's position. Client who have alterations in respiratory functioning often prefer to sit up and lean over a table. When breathing comfortably is possible only when sitting upright, it is called *orthopnea*, and this position is called the **orthopneic position** (*ortho* means sitting or standing; *pnea* means breathing).

You can increase the client's comfort by placing a pillow on the overbed table (Figure 44–3). Make sure that the client has sufficient rest periods between activities so that he or she can breathe easier without struggling for oxygen (see Box 44–3).

When a client is confined to bed for long periods of time, it is important that he or she changes positions frequently, at least every 2 hours. If not, the lung cannot expand on one side, and secretions could pool (collect) at the bottom of the lung. Unless the physician has placed restrictions on positioning, the client should never lie on one side for a long time. You should always follow your client's care plan.

Coughing and Deep Breathing

Coughing removes mucus from the lungs, and deep breathing moves air into most parts of the lungs. Therefore, coughing and deep breathing exercises help clients with respiratory disorders and are done after surgery and during bed rest. However, clients may be reluctant to do these exercises, as they may be painful after injury or surgery, or the client may be afraid of breaking open an incision during coughing.

Coughing and deep breathing help prevent pneumonia and atelectasis. The walls of healthy lungs (lined in a sticky mucous membrane) expand with every deep breath, which prevents them from collapsing and sticking to each other. In *atelectasis,*

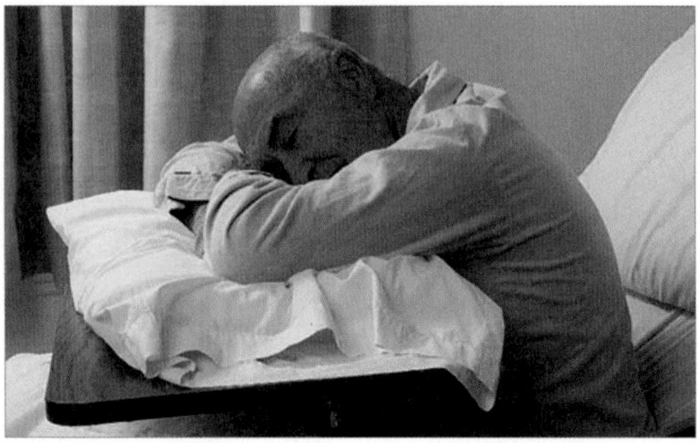

Figure 44–3 The client is in the orthopneic position. Note that a pillow has been placed on the overbed table for the client's comfort.

Box 44–3 Caring for a Client Who Has Altered Respiratory Function

When caring for the client who has altered respiratory function, whether at home or in a facility, it is important to provide care that will relax the client and reduce his or her need for more oxygen. You can do this in the following ways:

- Provide care at a time that the client is as well-rested and comfortable as possible.
- Be organized. Arrange to do all of your care in the shortest, least strenuous way possible.
- Allow for frequent rest periods.
- Assist the client into the sitting position, as it makes breathing easier. Assist the client into a semi- or high-Fowler's position, whenever possible. Clients who are sitting up can expand their lungs much more easily than those who are lying down. Place several pillows behind the client's back or use a large foam wedge if the client has one.
- Place a reclining chair for the client's naps or sleeping. A reclining chair can allow the client to sleep in a partially upright position, which gives the lungs more room to breathe.
- If the client is in a hospital bed, mechanically elevate the head of the bed to reduce the client's need to move in bed by himself or herself.
- Assist the client with moving and turning to reduce his or her oxygen need as much as possible.
- Avoid wearing perfumes that can trigger an allergic reaction, which would only make breathing more difficult for the client.
- Never wear powders or apply powders on the client, as they can irritate the airway and cause the client to have difficulty breathing.
- Be friendly and professional at all times, but try not to engage the client too much in conversation. Ask the client questions that require short or one-word answers only.
- Make sure the client is as comfortable as possible. Discomfort can cause a client to become more anxious, which, in turn, will increase their need for oxygen. Smooth out the sheets on the bed, and turn the pillow over to the smoother, cooler side. Make sure that the client does not have any restrictive clothing on.
- Encourage relaxation. Feelings of tension can contribute to breathlessness, and muscle tension can make the act of breathing harder. You can help reduce the client's tension level by promoting pleasant activities as well as relaxation exercises.
- Make sure that the bedside and the surrounding area are clean and dust-free. Wipe down all surfaces with a damp cloth (do not use disinfectants around the client, as this can trigger an allergic reaction). Remove any clutter from the room, as clutter can trap dust.
- If you must make the client's bed, make sure that the sheets are never shaken in the air (see Chapter 26).
- Open a window or use a fan to get air moving in the room, which will help the client to feel less short of breath.
- Make sure the client is well-hydrated. Most clients who are short of breath tend to breathe through the mouth, which can dry the lips, oral mucous membranes, and the throat. Apply water-soluble jelly to the lips (***never use petroleum jelly, as it is combustible and may create a risk of fire***). Have the client drink fresh water frequently, at least once every hour. Avoid the use of straws, as drinking from a straw would increase the breathing effort, which would require more energy.
- Oxygen supports combustion, so you should keep combustible items (clothing, towels, and sheets that are static-charged) away from the source of the oxygen in order to reduce the risk of a fire.
- In the winter, use a humidifier or place pans of water near radiators to moisten the room air that is breathed in, which will help loosen mucus and moisten the dry throat and nasal passages. If the phlegm in the lungs is thick, a humidifier can help loosen up that phlegm so that it is coughed up easily. Wash the humidifier or pans daily to prevent bacteria from colonizing in this warm, moist setting.
- If it is allowed on the client's care plan, offer throat lozenges or hard candy to help moisten the dry throat. Sucking on lozenges or candy often helps because it increases the production of saliva, which moistens the throat as it is swallowed.
- If the client requires oxygen therapy, make sure that there is always enough oxygen in the tank and that the oxygen tubing is not kinked. Remember to follow agency policy at all times.
- Make sure that the client is not lying on oxygen tubing, as this could (a) prevent oxygen flow through the tubing, and (b) cause pressure sores.
- Make sure that appropriate and clearly visible signs that indicate the client is receiving oxygen are posted on the door of the room where the client is receiving oxygen.

a portion of the lung collapses after mucus collects in a section of the airway, preventing air from entering into that part of the lung.

Clients who do not perform deep breathing and coughing exercises risk developing atelectasis because mucus is then allowed to collect in their lungs, increasing the chance of the sticky, mucus-lined lungs not expanding. The mucus that collects in their lungs and the mucus on the walls are attracted to each other, causing that portion of the lung to collapse. The postsurgical period, bed rest, lung disease, and paralysis are risk factors for atelectasis.

The frequency of coughing and deep breathing varies among clients, so physicians may order the exercises every 1 to 2 hours or four times a day while the client is awake. Your supervisor and the care plan will tell you which clients are suitable candidates for the exercises and when the exercises should be done. You will also be told the required number of deep breaths and coughs for the client. Follow the care plan.

Report and record the following observations after assisting the client with coughing and deep breathing:

- The number of times the client coughed and took deep breaths
- How the client tolerated the procedure

1 2 3 ASSISTING WITH COUGHING AND DEEP BREATHING EXERCISES

Remember to promote:

• **D**ignity • **I**ndependence • **P**references • **P**rivacy • **S**afety

Pre-Procedure

1 Identify the client, according to employer policy.
2 Explain the procedure to the client.
3 Practise proper hand hygiene.
4 Provide for privacy.

Procedure

5 Help the client to a comfortable sitting position—dangling, semi-Fowler's, or Fowler's.
6 Have the client take deep breaths:
- **a** Have the client place his or her hands over the rib cage (Figure 44–4).
- **b** Ask the client to exhale. Explain that the ribs should move as far down as possible.
- **c** Have the client take a breath as deep as possible. Remind the client to inhale through the nose.
- **d** Ask the client to hold the breath for 3 seconds.
- **e** Ask the client to exhale slowly through pursed lips (Figure 44–5). The client should exhale until the ribs move as far down as possible.
- **f** Repeat steps "a" through "e" four more times.

7 Ask the client to cough:
- **a** Have the client interlace his or her fingers over the incision (Figure 44–6, *A*). The client can also hold a pillow or folded towel over the incision (Figure 44–6, *B*).
- **b** Have the client take in a deep breath as in step 6.
- **c** Ask the client to cough strongly twice with the mouth open.

Post-Procedure

8 Provide for safety and comfort.
9 Place the call bell within reach.*
10 Follow the care plan for bed rail use.*
11 Remove privacy measures.
12 Practise proper hand hygiene.
13 Report and record your actions and observations, according to employer policy.

*Steps marked with an asterisk may not apply in community settings.

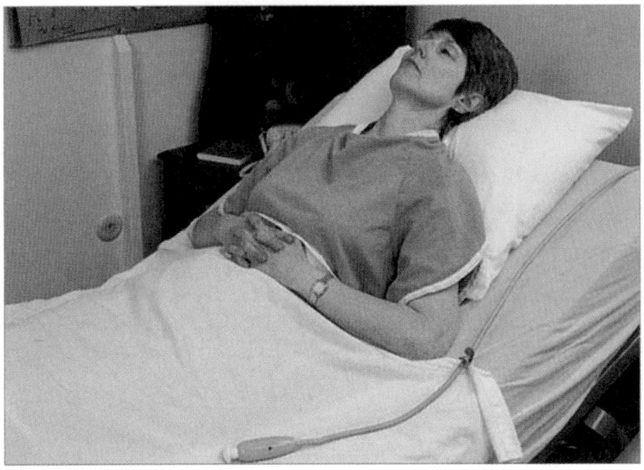

Figure 44–4 The hands are over the rib cage for deep breathing.

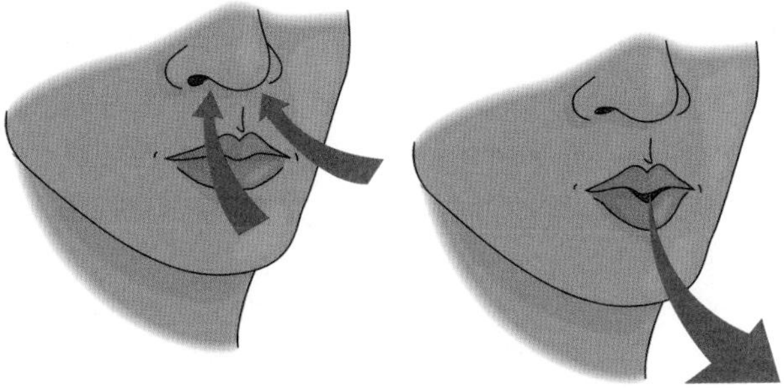

Figure 44–5 The client inhales through the nose and exhales through pursed lips during the deep-breathing exercise.

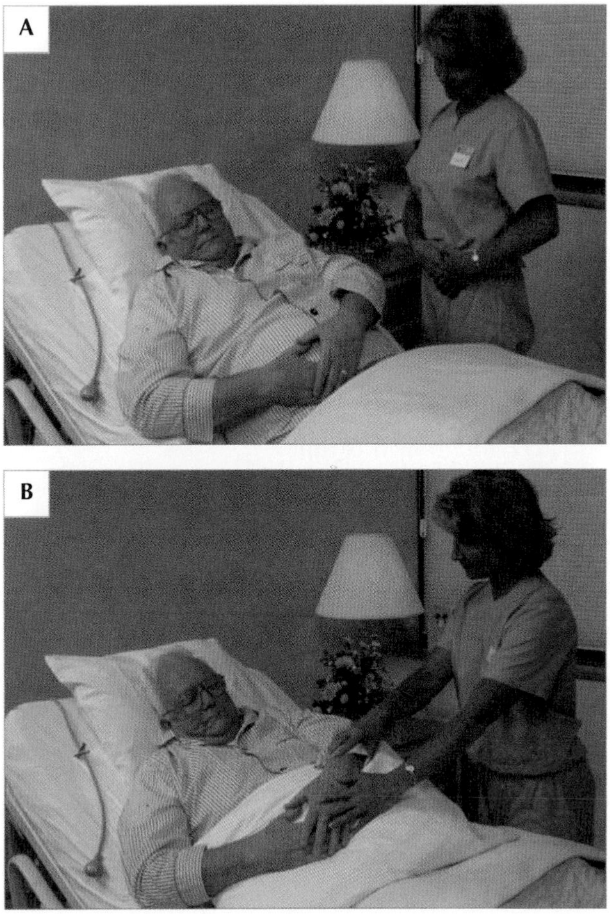

Figure 44–6 The client supports an incision for the coughing exercise. **A,** Hnads are placed over the incision for support. **B,** A pillow is held over the incision.

Incentive Spirometry

An *incentive* means encouragement. A *spirometer* is a machine that measures the amount (volume) of air inhaled. Balls or bars in the machine allow the client to see air movement during inhalation (Figure 44–7), so the client is encouraged to inhale until a preset volume of air is reached. The client inhales as deeply as possible and holds that breath for a certain time, usually for at least 3 seconds. Incentive spirometry is also called *sustained maximal inspiration (SMI)* (*sustained* means constant; *maximal* means the most or the greatest; and *inspiration* relates to breathing in).

The goal of using a spirometer is to improve lung function and prevent respiratory complications. They may be given to some clients to be used at home and to those who have had surgeries in hospitals, but they can be used by anybody the doctor thinks would benefit. By taking long, slow, and deep breaths, the client moves air deep into the lungs; secretions become loose; and O_2–CO_2 exchange occurs between the alveoli and capillaries.

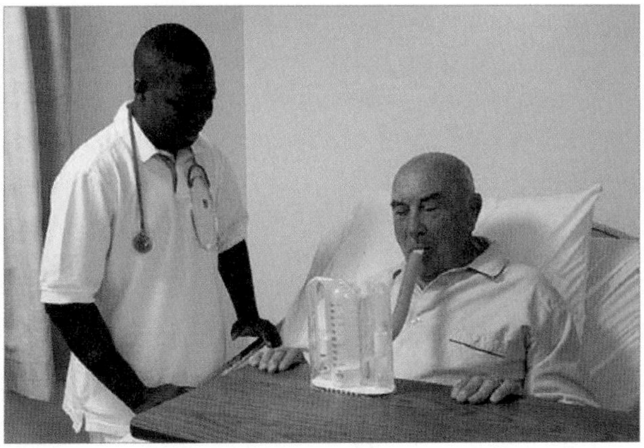

Figure 44–7 A client using a spirometer.

The device is used as follows:

- The spirometer is placed upright.
- The client exhales normally.
- The client seals his or her lips around the mouthpiece of the device.
- The client takes a slow, deep breath until the balls rise to the desired height.
- The client holds the breath for 3 to 6 seconds to keep the balls floating.
- Then the client removes his or her mouth from the mouthpiece and exhales slowly. The client may cough at this time.
- After taking some normal breaths, the client uses the device again.

Your supervisor and the care plan will tell you the following:

- How often the client needs to use incentive spirometry
- How many breaths the client needs to take
- The desired height of the floating balls

Follow employer policy for cleaning and replacing the mouthpiece.

ASSISTING WITH OXYGEN THERAPY

Disease, injury, and surgery can all interfere with a client's ability to breath easily, either directly (e.g., if the client has asthma) or indirectly (e.g., if the client has just had abdominal surgery and it hurts too much to take a deep breath). The level of O_2 in the blood is lower than normal (hypoxemia), so the physician orders oxygen therapy.

Oxygen therapy is handled in the same way as any medication. The physician prescribes the amount of oxygen, the device to use, and the times for therapy. Some clients may need oxygen constantly, while others may need it for relief of symptoms such as chest pain (in those with heart disease) or shortness of breath (in clients with respiratory diseases who may have enough oxygen while at rest but become short of breath with mild activity).

Your Role in Oxygen Therapy. As a support worker, ***you do not "give" oxygen***. In many provinces, support workers are trained to perform oral suctioning, to transfill oxygen from a liquid source tank to a portable tank (often called a *stroller unit*), and to ensure the client's oxygen unit is functioning well. The nurse and respiratory therapist, however, are responsible for starting and maintaining a client's oxygen therapy. You assist in providing safe care to clients receiving oxygen (see Box 44–3 on page 841 for a list of your duties and responsibilities).

Oxygen Sources

Whether the client is at home or in a continuing care facility, oxygen is supplied by three main delivery systems. The length of time each of these three systems lasts depends on the amount of oxygen a client uses.

Oxygen Concentrator. This machine makes oxygen by taking in room air and filtering out the oxygen (Figure 44–8). It must be plugged into a grounded electrical outlet. Because the oxygen concentrator "makes" the oxygen, it does not need to be replaced or refilled regularly. Ambulatory clients may use portable oxygen cylinders along with their concentrators to help them to be mobile and also to be prepared for a power failure. Oxygen concentrators are used in facilities and community settings, while cylinders are used by the client while on outings

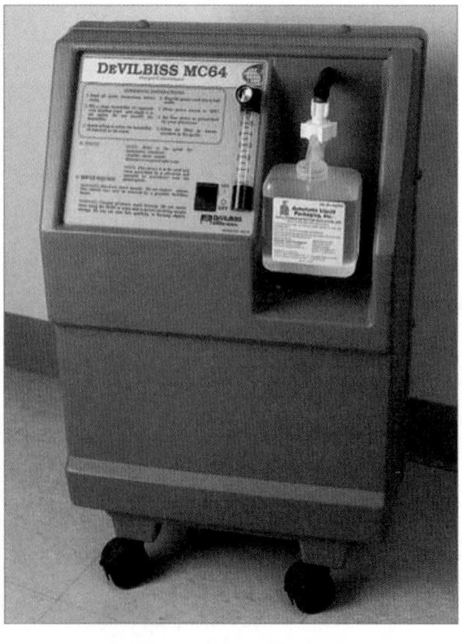

Figure 44–8 Oxygen concentrator.

from home. Some suppliers offer lightweight aluminum cylinders for easier handling.

Oxygen Cylinder. This is a tank of compressed oxygen. Large tanks are used inside the home, and small tanks are used for outings or travel. Some clients may be ambulatory but still need continuous oxygen therapy as they go about their daily lives, so they use portable oxygen cylinders (tanks) carried in a shoulder bag or wheeled in a cart (Figure 44–9). Large cylinders are often used for babies who need special breathing equipment.

The length of time cylinders last will depend on the amount of oxygen the client uses. A gauge on the cylinder shows how much oxygen is left in it (Figure 44–10). Check the gauge often, and tell your supervisor if the oxygen in the cylinder is low. Oxygen cylinders are used for clients in facility or community settings.

In hospitals and some continuing care facilities, oxygen is piped directly to each client's unit by way of a *wall oxygen outlet* (Figure 44–11) from a centrally located oxygen supply.

Liquid Oxygen System. This system stores oxygen in its liquid form. The liquid is kept in large stationary containers called reservoirs. The portable unit that can be worn over the shoulder is filled from a stationary unit (Figure 44–12) and has enough oxygen for about 8 hours of use. The liquid turns into gas before it leaves the container and is breathed in by the client.

A gauge shows the amount of oxygen in the unit. Tell your supervisor if the amount is low. Liquid oxygen is very cold, and if touched, it can freeze the skin. Follow employer procedures and the manufacturer's instructions when working with liquid oxygen. Liquid oxygen systems are used for clients in facility or community settings.

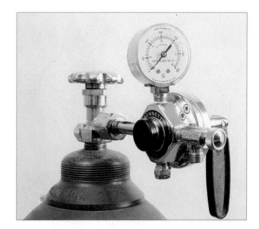

Figure 44–10 The gauge shows the amount of oxygen remaining in the tank.

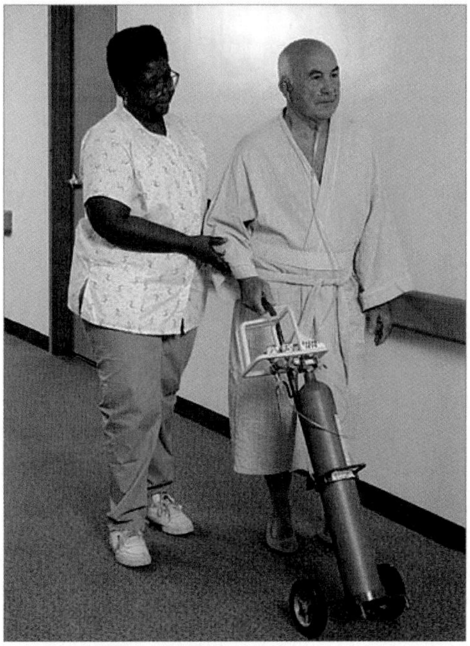

Figure 44–9 A client is using a portable oxygen tank while walking.

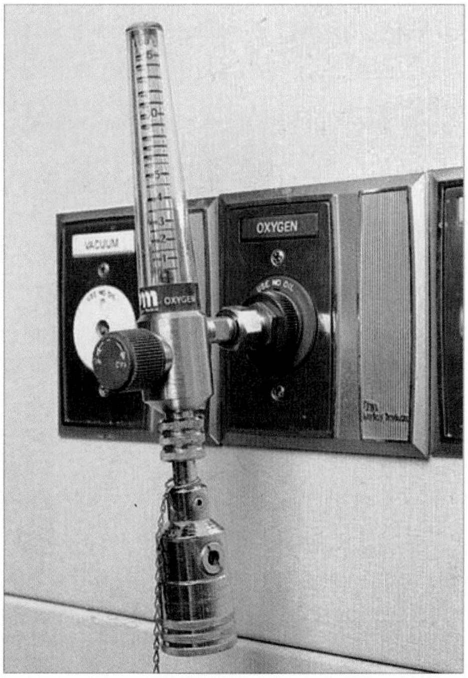

Figure 44–11 Wall oxygen outlet.

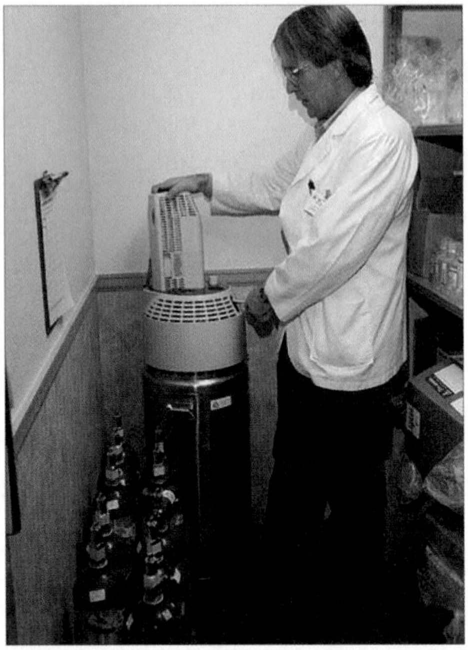

Figure 44–12 Liquid oxygen system.

With the oxygen systems described above, oxygen is delivered continuously while the client inhales and exhales. However, a lot of the oxygen is wasted when the client exhales. **Oxygen-conserving devices** help reduce this wastage so that the client's oxygen supply lasts longer and he or she can go for longer outings. Conserving devices also cut down on the number of oxygen cylinders that have to be delivered to the client.

Oxygen Therapy and Safety

Remember, you ***assist*** with oxygen therapy; you do ***not*** administer oxygen. However, It is your responsibility to provide safe care to clients receiving oxygen. Follow the safety guidelines in Box 44–4, as well as the fire safety guidelines in Box 44–5 on page 847.

Oxygen and Fire Safety

Oxygen is flammable, so the client is at risk for burns. In addition, the fire caused by an accident with oxygen devices may get out of control and cause significant damage to property and loss of life. It is very important to keep the oxygen source away from heat and open flame. Follow employer policies and the fire safety guidelines in Box 44–5.

The physician, nurse, or respiratory therapist is responsible for teaching the client and family members about oxygen safety. However, people sometimes forget or disregard safety rules (see *Supporting*

Box 44–4 Safety Guidelines for Oxygen Therapy

- Never remove the device (cannula, mask) used to administer oxygen.
- Report to your supervisor if the client removes the device.
- Make sure the device is secure but not tight.
- Check for signs of skin irritation caused by the device. Check behind the ears, under the nose (cannula), and around the face (mask). Also check the cheekbones.
- Keep the client's face clean and dry when a mask is used.
- Never shut off oxygen flow.
- Do not adjust the flow rate unless allowed by your scope of practice limitations and your employer's policy.
- Tell your supervisor immediately if the flow rate is too high or too low.
- Tell your supervisor immediately if the humidifier is not bubbling.
- Secure connecting tubing in place. Tape or pin it to the client's garment, according employer policy.
- Make sure there are no kinks in the tubing.
- Make sure the client does not lie on any part of the tubing.
- Report signs and symptoms of hypoxia, respiratory distress, or abnormal breathing patterns to your supervisor immediately (see Figure 44–2 on page 839, Box 44–1 on page 838, and Box 44–2 on page 840).
- Provide oral hygiene, as directed. Follow the care plan.
- Make sure the device is clean and free of mucus.
- Maintain an adequate water level in the humidifier.

Box 44–5 Oxygen and Fire Safety Guidelines

- Place "No Smoking" signs in the room and on the room door.
- Remove smoking materials from the room (cigarettes, cigars, pipes, matches, lighters).
- Remove materials from the room that ignite easily (alcohol, nail polish remover, oils, petroleum jelly, greases).
- Keep the oxygen source and tubing away from heat sources and open flames (e.g., direct sunlight, lit cigarettes, candles, lamps, stoves, heating ducts, radiators, heating pipes, space heaters, kerosene heaters).
- Turn off electrical items before unplugging them.
- Use electrical equipment (e.g., razor, radio, TV) only if it is in good repair.
- Use only electrical equipment that has a three-prong plug.
- Do not use materials that cause static electricity (wool and synthetic fabrics).
- Know the location of fire extinguishers and how to use them (see Chapter 19).
- If a fire occurs, turn off the oxygen. Then move the client to safety.
- Remind the client about oxygen safety. Report safety hazards immediately.

supporting MR. KALUWA

Joe Kaluwa, 88, is a retired farmer who lives in his home with his wife, Lily. Mr. Kaluwa started smoking at the age of 13, and now, after a lifetime of smoking, he has advanced emphysema and chronic obstructive pulmonary disease (COPD).

Mr. Kaluwa has been repeatedly instructed to quit smoking, but he continues to smoke a pack of cigarettes a day. Mrs. Kaluwa has forbidden smoking inside the house, so he goes outside to smoke—in the backyard during summer and in the garage in winter.

Mr. Kaluwa was hospitalized recently for his COPD and was discharged yesterday. He was sent home with a nasal cannula through which oxygen is administered to him, and he was instructed to use it all 24 hours of the day. While in the hospital, he had been warned not to allow anyone to smoke around his oxygen because of the risk for fires.

A respiratory therapist set up his oxygen tank and tubing at his home. You have been assigned to provide support care and to ensure that he maintains his oxygen therapy. This is your first visit with Mr. Kaluwa.

Today, upon your arrival, you find Mr. Kaluwa sitting in his backyard calmly smoking a cigarette. He is still connected to his oxygen tubing, with the nasal cannula in place in his nose and around his ears and the portable tank next to him. You take a quick look at his oxygen meter and find that the device is on. Mr. Kaluwa notices that you look surprised, and he tells you that he "turned down his oxygen" to be able to smoke safely. You are shocked at his behaviour and nervous about approaching him and do not know what to do.

Mr. Kaluwa). You may observe a client, visitor, or family member creating a safety hazard—for example, a home care client attempting to light a gas stove while using oxygen or a family member wanting to smoke while the oxygen device is on. These are very dangerous situations, so warn the concerned individuals of the dangers and the safety hazards. Also, call your supervisor immediately and report the situation.

Oxygen Administration Devices

The physician orders the device used to administer oxygen. The following devices are commonly ordered:

Nasal Cannula. The **nasal cannula** (Figure 44–13) is used at home or in a hospital setting to deliver oxygen to a client in need of extra oxygen. It consists of a set of two prongs that are placed in the client's nostrils and a plastic tube that fits behind the ears. The prongs, from which oxygen flows into the client, curve downward to prevent drying of the sinuses.

The nasal cannula is connected to an oxygen tank, a portable oxygen generator, or to a wall connection in a hospital through a **flowmeter**. The client can eat and talk with the cannula in place. If the prongs are placed too tightly, nasal irritation or

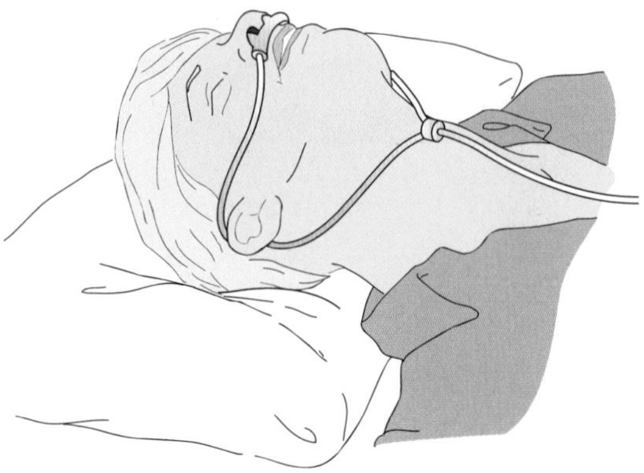

Figure 44–13 Nasal cannula.

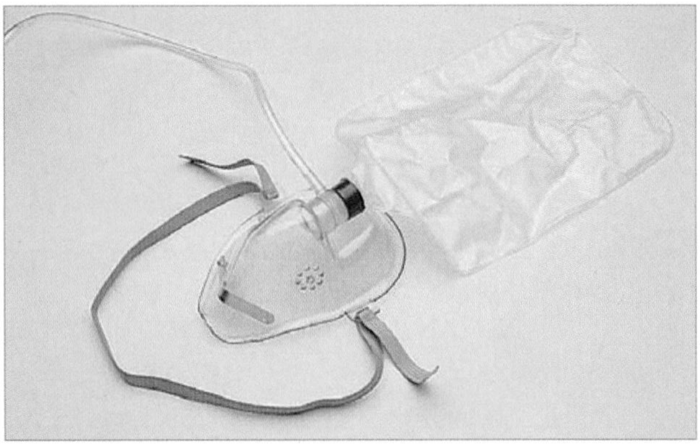

Figure 44–15 Partial-rebreather mask.

pressure on the ears and cheekbones may occur. You should always report signs or complaints of skin irritation or soreness.

Simple Face Mask. The simple **face mask** (Figure 44–14) covers the nose and mouth and is connected to an oxygen source. The mask has small holes on the sides through which room air enters during inhalation and CO_2 escapes during exhalation.

Partial-Rebreather Mask. In the partial-rebreather mask (Figure 44–15), a bag is added to the simple face mask to collect exhaled air. When breathing in, the client inhales oxygen as well as some exhaled air and some room air. The bag should not totally deflate during inhalation.

Nonrebreather Mask. This type of mask (Figure 44–16) prevents exhaled air and room air from entering the bag and, instead, allows the exhaled air to leave through holes in the mask. The bag fills up with oxygen from the oxygen source, and only oxygen from the bag is inhaled. The bag must not totally deflate during exhalation.

Venturi Mask. The venturi mask (Figure 44-17) allows precise amounts of oxygen to be given. Special colour-coded plastic adaptors that fit into the mask are connected to the source of oxygen. Each colour is coded to show what amount of oxygen the mask delivers.

Special care is needed when masks are used. Masks make talking difficult, so listen carefully when the client is trying to say something. Moisture can build up under the mask. Keep the client's face clean and dry to help prevent irritation from the mask. Report any signs of skin irritation. Masks are removed for eating, and usually oxygen is administered by nasal cannula during that time.

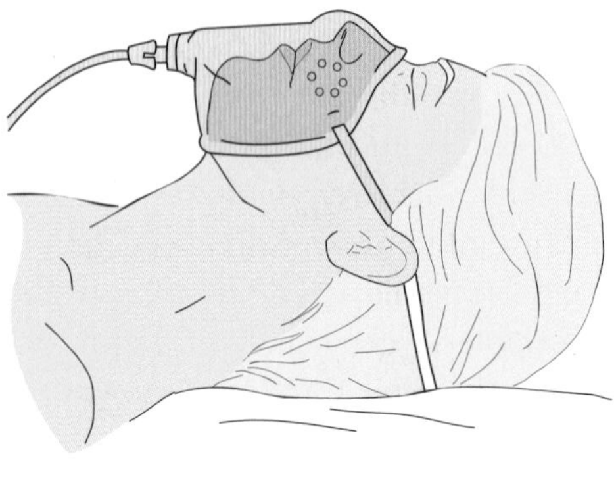

Figure 44–14 Simple face mask.

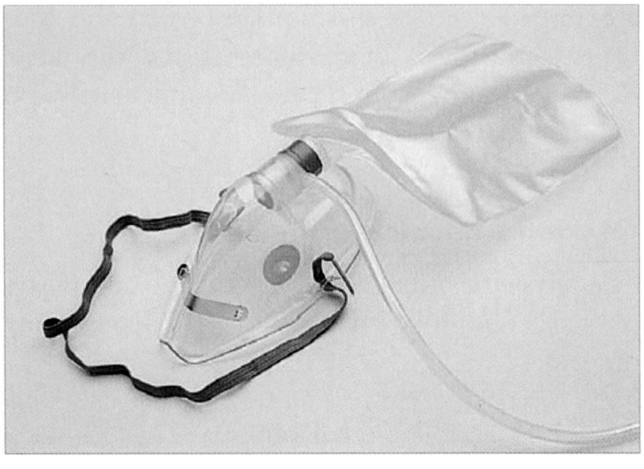

Figure 44–16 Nonrebreather mask.

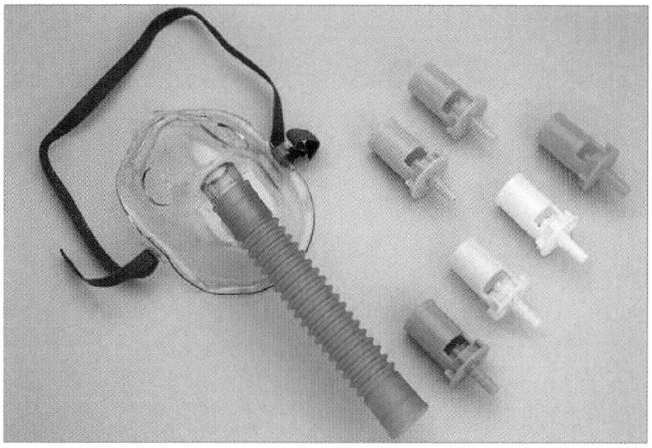

Figure 44–17 Venturi mask.

Oxygen Flow Rates

The amount of oxygen ordered by the physician and administered to the client is called the **flow rate.** The flow rate is measured in litres per minute (L/min), and the oxygen flow rate can range from 2 to 15 L/min. A nurse or respiratory therapist sets the flow rate (Figure 44–18).

Your supervisor and the care plan will specify the client's flow rate. While giving care to your clients who are receiving oxygen, always check the flow rate. Tell your supervisor immediately if the flow rate is too high or too low. A nurse or respiratory therapist will then adjust the flow rate. Some employers may allow support workers to adjust oxygen flow rates. If you are allowed to adjust the flow rate, follow employer policies and procedures.

Preparing for Oxygen Administration

Humidified Oxygen. Oxygen is a dry gas. If it is not humidified (made moist), it can dry the mucous membranes of the airways. A *humidifier* (Figure 44–19) is a system by which oxygen is forced through distilled water, allowing it to bubble up and be collected in the tubing for the client to breathe. This oxygen is now **humidified**, that is, it now contains water vapour in it. This oxygen mixed with water vapour is less drying and irritating to delicate mucous membranes than plain oxygen is.

The humidifier is filled with **distilled water,** which is pure, sterile water that has been boiled and allowed to cool and condense. Tap water is not used, as it contains impurities that can irritate the mucous membranes and damage the equipment. The humidifier is then attached to the oxygen administration system (wall outlet, oxygen tank, or oxygen concentrator).

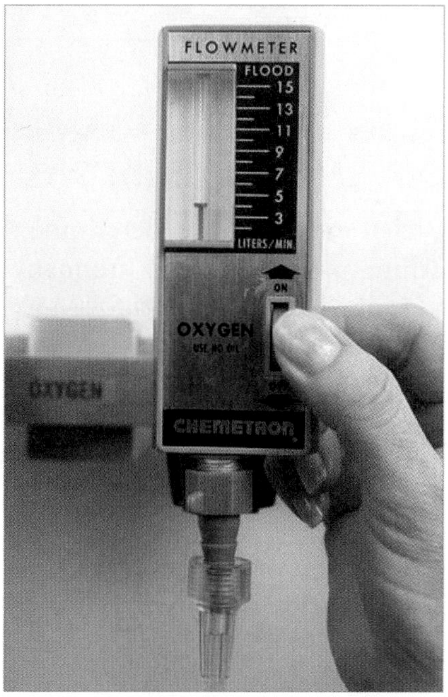

Figure 44–18 The flowmeter is used to set the oxygen flow rate.

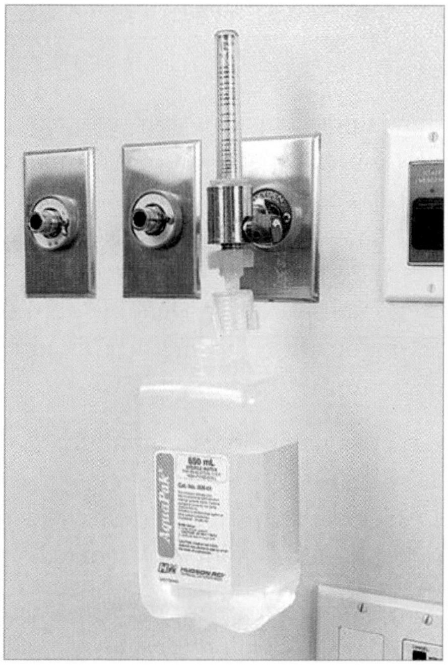

Figure 44–19 Oxygen administration system with humidifier.

1 2 3 SETTING UP FOR OXYGEN ADMINISTRATION

Remember to promote:

• Dignity • Independence • Preferences • Privacy • Safety

Pre-Procedure

1 Identify the client, according to employer policy.
2 Explain the procedure to the client.
3 Practise proper hand hygiene.
4 Collect the following:
- Oxygen administration device with connecting tubing
- Flowmeter
- Humidifier (if ordered)
- Distilled water (if using a humidifier)

Procedure

5 Make sure the flowmeter is in the OFF position.
6 Attach the flowmeter to the wall outlet or to the tank.
7 Fill the humidifier with distilled water.
8 Attach the humidifier to the bottom of the flowmeter.
9 Attach the oxygen administration device and connecting tubing to the humidifier. ***Do not set the flowmeter. Do not apply the oxygen administration device on the client.***

Post-Procedure

10 Provide for safety and comfort.
11 Place the call bell within reach.*
12 Discard packaging.
13 Make sure the cap on the distilled water bottle is secure. Store it, according to employer policy.
14 Practise proper hand hygiene.
15 Tell your supervisor when you are finished. A nurse will:
- Turn on the oxygen and set the flow rate
- Apply the oxygen administration device on the client

*Steps marked with an asterisk may not apply in community settings.

Low flow rates (1 to 2 L/min) by nasal cannula usually do not need humidification. You may be responsible for checking the water level in the humidifier and cleaning and refilling it. Follow employer procedures and your supervisor's directions.

You do not administer oxygen, but your supervisor may ask you to set up the oxygen administration system. You are told the following:

- The client's name and room and bed number (in facilities)
- The oxygen administration device ordered
- Whether humidification was ordered

Tell your supervisor when you finish setting up the oxygen administration system. A nurse will turn the oxygen on, set the flow rate, and apply the administration device.

ASSISTING WITH ASSESSMENT AND DIAGNOSTIC TESTING

The physician orders tests to determine the cause of a breathing problem. There are many respiratory tests available (see Box 44–6). Most of these tests are done at hospitals or clinics, and some are done in continuing care facilities. They are done by a physician or a specially trained nurse, respiratory therapist, or laboratory technician. You may assist the client before and after a test, as directed by your supervisor, the care plan, and assignment sheet.

You are likely to assist with pulse oximetry and to collect sputum specimens. Both procedures may provide the physician with information about the state of the client's respiratory system.

Box 44–6 Common Respiratory Tests

- ***Chest X-ray (CXR)***—an X-ray of the chest is taken to evaluate changes in the lungs.
- ***Lung scan***—the lungs are scanned to see which areas are not getting air or blood. The client inhales radioactive (*radioactive* means to give off radiation) gas and is injected with a radioisotope (a *radioisotope* is a substance that gives off radiation). Lung tissue getting air and blood "take up" the radioactive substances, and a scanner then senses the areas with radioactive substances.
- ***Bronchoscopy***—a scope (*scopy*) is passed into the trachea and bronchi (*broncho*). Airway structures are checked for bleeding and tumours. Tissue samples (biopsy) are taken, or mucous plugs and foreign objects are removed. After the procedure, the client is NPO and watched carefully until the gag and swallow reflexes return, usually in about 2 hours.
- ***Thoracentesis***—the pleura (*thora*) is punctured, and air or fluid is removed (*centesis*) from it. The physician inserts a needle through the chest wall into the pleural sac when injury or disease causes it to fill with air, blood, or fluid and affects respiratory function.

  Sometimes fluid is removed for laboratory study, and sometimes anticancer medications are injected into the pleural sac. After the procedure, which takes only a few minutes, the client is checked frequently for shortness of breath, dyspnea, cough, sputum, chest pain, cyanosis, vital sign changes, and other respiratory signs and symptoms.
- ***Pulmonary function tests***—tests that measure the amount of air moving into and out of the lungs (volume) and how much air the lungs can hold (capacity). The client takes as deep a breath as possible and, using a mouthpiece, blows into a machine. The tests are used to evaluate clients at risk for lung diseases or postoperative lung complications and to measure the progress of lung disease and its treatment.
- ***Arterial blood gases (ABGs)***—A radial or femoral artery is punctured to obtain arterial blood, and laboratory tests measure the amount of oxygen in it. Hemorrhage from the artery must be prevented, so pressure is applied to the artery for at least 5 minutes after the procedure and longer if the client has blood clotting problems.

Pulse Oximetry

A **pulse oximeter** is a device used to measure (*metry*) oxygen (*oxi*) concentration in arterial blood as well as for measuring pulse rate. *Oxygen concentration* is the amount (percent) of hemoglobin that contains oxygen. The normal range is 95 to 100%. For example, if 97% of all the hemoglobin carries O_2, tissues get enough oxygen. If only 90% of the hemoglobin contains O_2, tissues do not get enough oxygen to function. The pulse oximeter can detect low oxygen levels before any signs or symptoms appear, and the measurements are used to prevent and treat hypoxia.

A pulse oximeter, which consists of a computerized monitor and a sensor (probe), is a very delicate and expensive piece of equipment that should always be handed gently. ***Never drop or handle a pulse oximeter roughly, as this can affect the delicate sensors within it.*** Many employers now consider pulse oximetry as a regular part of taking a client's vital signs, so the support worker should be aware of the correct method of attaching it and reading it.

The sensor is attached to the client's finger, toe, nose, earlobe, or forehead (Figure 44–20). Two light beams on one side of the sensor pass through the tissues. A detector on the other side measures the amount of light passing through the tissues. Using this information, the oximeter measures the O_2 concentration, and the value and pulse rate are displayed on the monitor. Oximeters have alarms, which sound if O_2 concentration is low, the pulse is too fast or slow, or other problems occur.

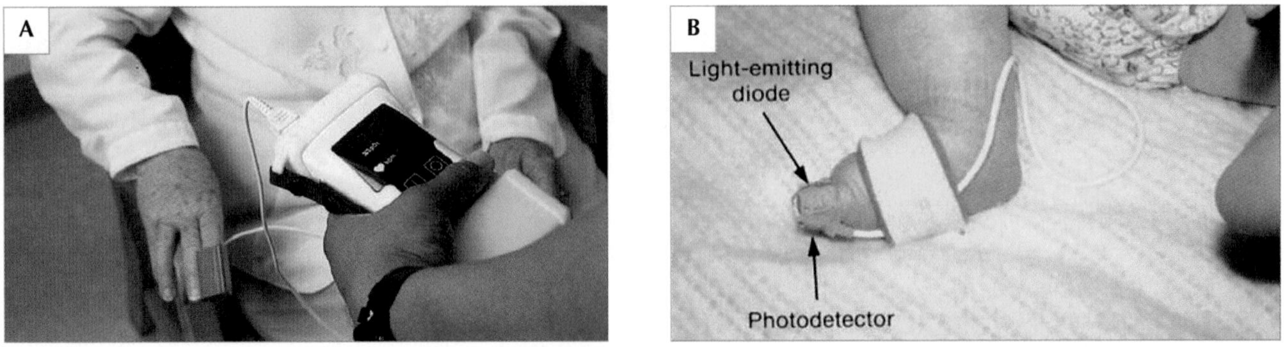

Figure 44–20 **A,** A pulse oximeter sensor is attached to a finger. **B,** The sensor is attached to an infant's toe. **Source (for B):** Wong, D.L. (1999). *Whaley and Wong's nursing care of infants and children* (6th ed.). St. Louis: Mosby.

1 2 3 USING A PULSE OXIMETER

Remember to promote:

• **D**ignity • **I**ndependence • **P**references • **P**rivacy • **S**afety

Pre-Procedure

1 Identify the client, according to employer policy.
2 Review the procedure with your supervisor.
3 Find out what site to use.
4 Explain the procedure to the client.
5 Practise proper hand hygiene.
6 Collect the following:
- Pulse oximeter and sensor
- Nail polish remover and cotton balls (if needed)
- SpO_2 flow sheet
- Tape (if needed)
- Towel

7 Provide for privacy.

Procedure

8 Provide for comfort.
9 Remove any nail polish if a finger or toe site is used. Use nail polish remover and a cotton ball. ***Do not use nail polish remover if the client is receiving oxygen therapy. Nail polish remover is flammable and dangerous near oxygen.***
10 Dry the site with a towel.
11 Clip or tape the sensor to the site.
12 Attach the sensor cables to the oximeter.
13 Turn on the oximeter.
14 Set the high and low alarm limits for SpO_2 and pulse rate. Turn on audio and visual alarms.
15 Check the client's radial pulse with the pulse on the display. The pulses should be equal. Tell your supervisor if the pulses are not equal.
16 Read the SpO_2 and the pulse rate on the display. Note the values on the flow sheet and assignment sheet.
17 Leave the sensor in place for continuous monitoring. Otherwise, turn off the device and remove the sensor.

Post-Procedure

18 Provide for safety and comfort.
19 Place the call bell within reach.*
20 Follow the care plan for bed rail use.*
21 Remove privacy measures.
22 Return the pulse oximeter to its proper place unless monitoring is continuous.
23 Practise proper hand hygiene.
24 Report and record the SpO_2, pulse rate, and other observations. Follow employer policy.

*Steps marked with an asterisk may not apply in community settings.

Small, hand-held oximeter units are available for home use. Usually the client's oxygen concentration and vital signs are measured simultaneously. Because the device is portable and used for many clients, you must make sure that it is accurate. After applying the sensor, check the client's radial pulse and compare it with the displayed pulse. The pulse rates should be the same.

A good sensor site on the client is important. Your supervisor will tell you which site to use based on the client's condition. Swollen sites and sites with skin breaks should be avoided. Because aging and vascular disease often cause poor circulation, sometimes blood flow to the fingers or toes is poor. If this is the case, the earlobe, nose, or forehead sites are used.

Bright light, nail polish, artificial nails, and movements can affect measurement accuracy. To prevent inaccurate readings, place a towel over the sensor to block out bright light. Remove nail polish on the client, or use another site. Do not use a finger site if the client wears artificial nails. Movements from shivering, seizures, or tremors affect finger sensors. The earlobe is a better site if a client has these problems. Blood pressure cuffs affect blood flow, so if using a finger site, do not measure blood pressure on that side.

Report and record measurements accurately. Use the abbreviation **SpO_2** when recording the oxygen concentration value (S = saturation, p = pulse, O_2 = oxygen). Also, report and record the following:

- The date and time
- What the client was doing at the time of measurement
- Oxygen flow rate and the device used
- Reason for the measurement (routine or change in the client's condition)
- Other observations, such as the client's cooperation with wearing the pulse oximeter

Pulse oximetry does not replace good observations. The client's condition can change rapidly. Observe for signs and symptoms of hypoxia—such as a ***change*** in the client's behaviour or ability to comprehend instructions—which can signal a drop in the client's SpO_2 level.

Collecting Sputum Specimens

Respiratory disorders cause the lungs, bronchi, and trachea to secrete mucus. Mucus from the respiratory system is called **sputum** when expectorated (expelled) through the mouth. Note that sputum is *not* saliva (spit), which is a thin, clear liquid produced by the salivary glands in the mouth.

Sputum specimens can be collected from clients in the community, in continuing care facilities, and in the hospital. Sputum specimens are studied for blood, microbes, and abnormal cells. For this test, the client must cough up sputum from the bronchi and trachea (not saliva from the mouth!); this can often be painful and hard to do. Specimens should be collected in the morning when secretions are more easily coughed up upon awakening.

The client should rinse the mouth only with water to decrease saliva and remove food particles. Instruct the client ***not*** to use mouthwash before the procedure because it can destroy some of the microbes in the mouth and give a false reading.

Ensure that the client has privacy for this procedure. The procedure can be embarrassing for the client, as the sputum is unpleasant to look at, and the coughing and expectorating sounds may disturb others nearby. If possible, collect the specimen when the roommate or family members are out of the room. Cover the specimen container, and place it in a bag, in order to keep the contents out of sight. Always follow Standard Practices (see Chapter 20) when collecting a sputum specimen.

Postural Drainage. Some clients do not have the strength to cough up sputum, so they are placed by the nurse or respiratory therapist in a certain position to allow secretions to drain by gravity (gravity causes fluids to flow downward). Coughing is then made easier for them after postural drainage. The client is positioned in such a way that a lung part is at a higher level than the airway (Figure 44–21). Positioning depends on the lung part that needs draining.

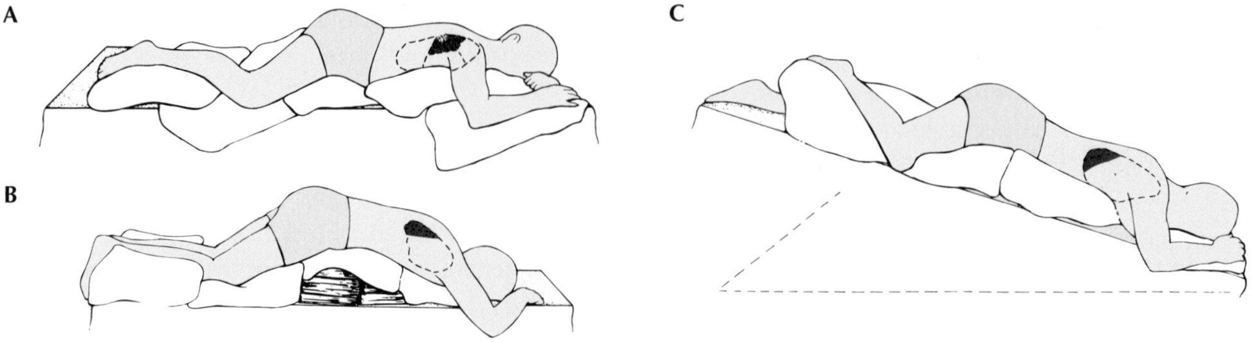

Figure 44–21 Some positions used for postural drainage. (*Note:* A nurse or respiratory therapist is responsible for postural drainage.) ***Do not place the client in these positions without supervision.*** **A,** Draining the right upper lobe. **B,** Draining the right middle lobe. **C,** Draining the right lower lobe. **Source:** Potter, P.A., & Perry, A.G. (2001). *Fundamentals of nursing: Concepts, process, and practice* (5th ed.). St. Louis: Mosby.

1 2 3 COLLECTING A SPUTUM SPECIMEN

Remember to promote:

• **D**ignity • **I**ndependence • **P**references • **P**rivacy • **S**afety

Pre-Procedure

1 Identify the client, according to employer policy.
2 Explain the procedure to the client.
3 Practise proper hand hygiene.
4 Collect the following:
- Sputum specimen container and label
- Laboratory requisition
- Disposable bag
- Gloves
- Mask (if needed)
- Tissues
- Cup of water
- Kidney basin

5 Label the specimen container.
6 Provide for privacy. If able, the client can go into the bathroom for the procedure.

Procedure

7 Put on gloves. Put on a mask.
8 Ask the client to rinse the mouth out with clear water. If the client is in bed, offer a glass of water and allow the client to spit into the kidney basin.
9 Have the client hold the container. Only the outside can be touched.
10 Ask the client to cover the mouth and nose with tissues when coughing.
11 Ask the client to take two or three deep breaths and cough up the sputum.
12 Have the client expectorate directly into the specimen container (Figure 44–22). Sputum should not touch the outside.
13 Collect 15 to 30 mL (1 to 2 tablespoons) of sputum unless told to collect more.
14 Put the lid on the container. Do not touch the inside of the lid.
15 Place the container in the bag. Attach the requisition to the bag.
16 Remove your gloves. Remove your mask.
17 Practise proper hand hygiene.

Post-Procedure

18 Provide for safety and comfort.
19 Place the call bell within reach.*
20 Remove privacy measures.
21 Practise proper hand hygiene.
22 Take the bag to the appropriate area.
23 Practise proper hand hygiene.
24 Report and record your actions and observations, according to employer policy.

*Steps marked with an asterisk may not apply in community settings.

If it is within your scope of practice for your province or your agency, you may have to assist with postural drainage. Do not attempt to position the client without supervision (see the *Focus on Children: Assisting With Treatments* box.)

Report and record the following observations after collecting a sputum specimen (Figure 44–22):

- The time the specimen was collected
- The amount of sputum collected
- How easily the client coughed up the sputum
- The consistency of the sputum

focus on
>> CHILDREN

Assisting With Treatments

Breathing treatments and suctioning are often needed to obtain sputum specimens from infants and small children. The nurse or respiratory therapist gives the breathing treatment. The nurse suctions the trachea for the sputum specimen. The infant or child is likely to be uncooperative during suctioning. You can assist by comforting the child. You might be asked to hold the child's head and arms still.

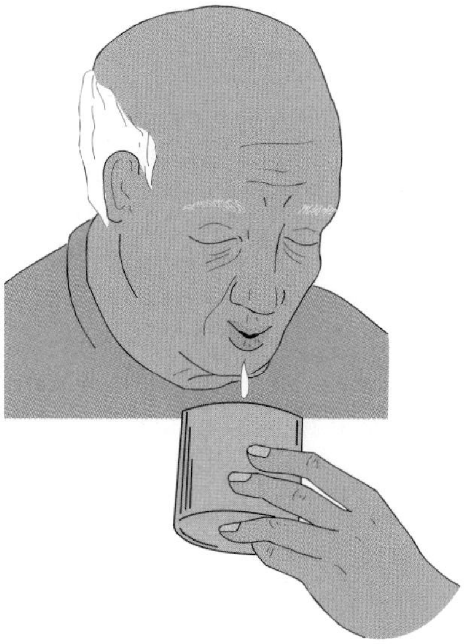

Figure 44–22 The client expectorates into the centre of the specimen container.

ARTIFICIAL AIRWAYS

Artificial airways keep the airway patent (open) and are used when:

- The airway is obstructed from disease, injury, secretions, or aspiration
- The client is semi-conscious or unconscious
- The client is recovering from anaesthesia
- The client needs mechanical ventilation

Types. **Intubation** is the process of inserting an artificial airway. Airways are usually plastic and disposable and come in adult, pediatric, and infant sizes. The following airways are commonly used:

- ***Oro-pharyngeal airway***—inserted through the mouth and into the pharynx (Figure 44–23, *A*). A nurse, paramedic, or respiratory therapist inserts the airway, usually in a hospital or in an emergency situation, on the way to a hospital.
- ***Nasopharyngeal airway***—inserted through a nostril and into the pharynx (Figure 44–23, *B*). A nurse, paramedic, or respiratory therapist inserts the airway usually in a hospital or in an emergency situation, on the way to a hospital.
- ***Endo-tracheal (ET) tube***—inserted through the mouth or nose and into the trachea (Figure 44–23, *C*) usually in a hospital or in an emergency situation, on the way to a hospital. A physician, an RN with special training, or a paramedic with special training inserts it using a lighted scope. A balloon (called a *cuff*) at the end of the tube is inflated to keep the airway in place.
- ***Tracheostomy tube***—inserted through a surgical incision (*ostomy*) into the trachea (*tracheo*) (Figure 44–23, *D*). Some tubes have cuffs; the cuff is inflated to keep the tube in place. The tracheostomy is done by a physician. *Tracheostomies* are performed in both emergency and non-emergency situations and can be both temporary and permanent.

Care of a Client With an Artificial Airway. If you are assisting with caring for a client with an artificial airway, it is normally in a hospital setting, and you are given directions by a nurse. The client's vital signs need to be checked often, and the client must

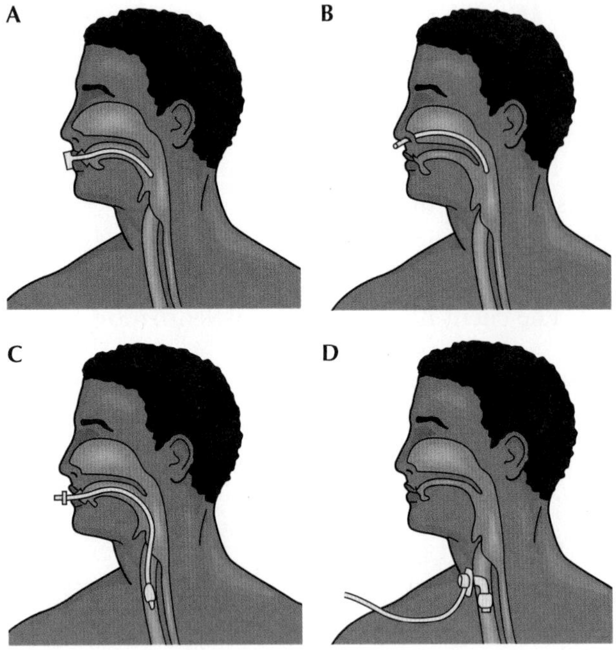

Figure 44–23 Artificial airways. **A,** Oro-pharyngeal airway. **B,** Nasopharyngeal airway. **C,** Endo-tracheal tube. **D,** Tracheostomy tube.

be observed for hypoxia and other respiratory signs and symptoms. The client needs frequent oral hygiene, as the oral mucous membranes may become dried and cracked. Your supervisor and the care plan will tell you when and how to perform oral hygiene. If an airway comes out or is dislodged, you need to tell your supervisor immediately.

Talking is hard with oro-pharyngeal and nasopharyngeal airways. Clients with endo-tracheal tubes cannot speak, but some tracheostomy tubes allow clients to speak. Paper and pencils, magic slates, communication boards, and hand signals can all be used to communicate. Follow the care plan.

Gagging and choking sensations are common with artificial airways. Comfort and reassure the client. Remind the client that the airway helps breathing. Use touch to show you care.

Tracheostomies

A **tracheostomy** is a surgically created opening (*ostomy*) through the neck into the trachea (*tracheo*). A tracheostomy tube is usually inserted through this opening, and the client breathes through the tracheostomy tube. A humidifier attachment may be needed for about 1 month after tracheostomy surgery because the trachea is now exposed to drier air.

Types. Tracheostomies can be temporary or permanent, depending on the client's circumstances. In temporary situations, tracheostomies may have been inserted because of a severe breathing crisis or blockage. In permanent cases, airway structures have been surgically removed, along with the client's larynx and epiglottis. Clients who have head and neck cancers, severe airway trauma, or brain injury may require permanent tracheostomies. Generally, a surgeon will consider a tracheostomy only when there is no other option (see the *Focus on Children: Congenital Conditions* box.) Certain groups—for example, babies, smokers, and older adults—are more vulnerable to complications following a tracheostomy.

The long-term care of clients depends on whether the tracheostomy tube is temporary or permanent. If it is temporary, it will be removed when no longer needed and the incision will be allowed to heal closed, leaving a small scar in the neck area. If the tracheostomy is permanent, the hole (**stoma**) will stay open. However, the opening tends to narrow with time, and further surgery may be needed to widen the opening. The outer tracheostomy tube needs to be changed every few months, and the site is inspected at each change. The client may be referred to a speech therapist for voice training.

Supporting the Client With a Tracheostomy. A tracheostomy tube is made of plastic or metal and has three parts (Figure 44–24):

- *Obturator*—has a round end; it is used to insert the outer cannula and then removed. (The obturator is placed within easy reach in case the tracheostomy tube falls out and needs to be reinserted. It is taped to the wall or to the bedside stand.)
- *Inner cannula*—an inner tube; it requires cleaning whenever it gets blocked with secretions, which can occur once to several times every day. It is removed for cleaning and mucus removal and then reinserted and locked in place. This keeps the airway patent. Some plastic tracheostomy tubes do not have inner cannulas.
- *Outer cannula*—is secured in place with ties around the neck or a Velcro collar. The outer cannula is not removed.

focus on
›› CHILDREN

Congenital Conditions

Some children are born with congenital (*congenital* from a Latin word that means present at birth) conditions, and some of these conditions affecting the neck and airway require tracheostomies. Some infections and foreign body aspiration cause airway structures to swell or be blocked and obstruct airflow, which necessitates emergency tracheostomies.

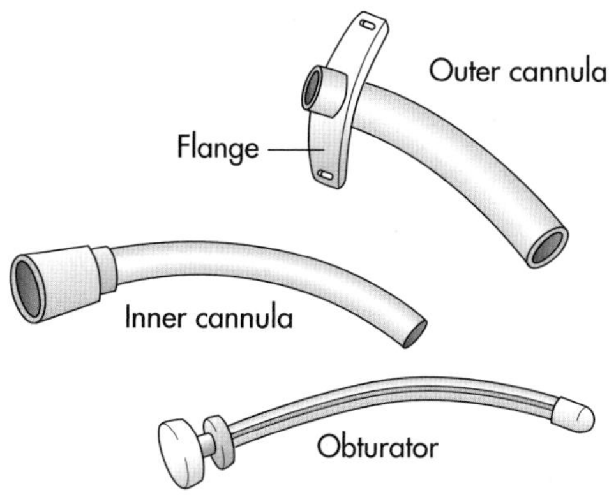

Figure 44–24 Parts of a tracheostomy tube.

The cuffed tracheostomy tube provides a seal between the cannula and the trachea (see Figure 44–23, *D*). This type is used with mechanical ventilation. The cuff prevents air from leaking around the tube and also prevents aspiration. A nurse or respiratory therapist inflates and deflates the cuff.

The tube must not come out (extubation). If it is not secured properly, it could come out with coughing or if pulled on. Damage to the airway is possible if the tube is loose and moves up and down in the trachea.

The tube must remain patent (open) at all times, in order for the client to breathe. Some clients can cough secretions up and out of the tracheostomy; some clients may require suctioning. ***Call your supervisor if the client shows signs and symptoms of hypoxia or respiratory distress. Also, call your supervisor if the outer cannula comes out.***

The client with a permanent tracheostomy may not be able to speak or may speak with great difficulty. Assist the client to communicate with you by writing. Also, look at the picture of a communication board shown in Figure 36–1. When the client tries to speak, you must remember to be patient and supportive (see Chapter 36). It might be very difficult and frustrating for the client, especially if you have difficulty understanding what he or she is trying to tell you.

Safety Measures. Nothing (such as dust, food, or water) should ever enter the stoma, as the client can aspirate on them. The following safety measures are important:

- Dressings should never have loose gauze or lint, or anything that the client can inhale.
- The stoma or tube should always be covered when the client goes outside. The client should cover the stoma with a scarf, or shirt or blouse that buttons at the neck to prevent dust, insects, and other small particles from entering the stoma.
- The stoma should never be covered with plastic, leather, or similar materials. These materials prevent air from entering the stoma, making it difficult for the client to breathe.
- The client should take tub baths, instead of showers. If showers are taken, a shower guard should be worn, and the client should hold a hand-held nozzle to direct water away from the stoma.
- Assist the client with shampooing. Remember that water should never enter the stoma.
- The stoma should be covered when the client has a shave.
- The client must not be allowed to swim, as water will enter the tube or stoma.
- Medic Alert jewellery should always be worn, and clients should also carry a Medic Alert ID card whenever they leave their homes.

Tracheostomy Care. Clients require care to their tracheostomy stoma site when there are excess secretions, when the ties or collar holding their tracheostomy in place become soiled, or when the dressing around their tracheostomy becomes soiled or moist. Such care is usually provided every 8 to 12 hours, or according to the client's care plan. Remember to follow Standard Practices (see Chapter 20) when assisting with tracheostomy care. Tracheostomy care involves:

- ***Cleaning the inner cannula***—removes mucus and keeps the airway patent. Cleaning is not necessary with inner cannulas that are disposable.
- ***Cleaning the stoma***—prevents infection and skin breakdown.
- ***Applying clean ties or a Velcro collar***—prevents infection. Remember when the ties are removed, you need to hold the outer cannula in place. The ties or collar must be secure but not tight, and you should be able to slide a finger under the ties or collar (Figure 44–25, *A*). (See the *Focus on Children: Tracheostomy Care* box.)

A

B

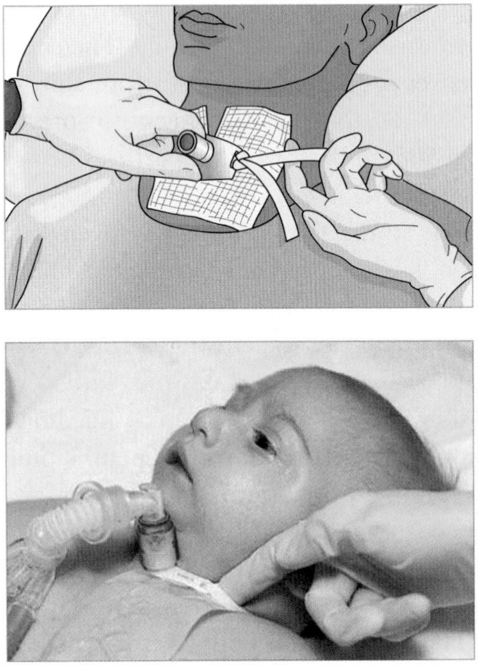

Figure 44–25 A, A finger is inserted under the ties. **B,** For children, only a fingertip is inserted under the ties. **Source (for B):** Hockenberry, M.J., & Wilson, D. (2007). *Wong's nursing care of infants and children* (8th ed.). St. Louis: Mosby.

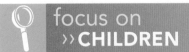

focus on ›› CHILDREN

Tracheostomy Care

As with adults, in children also the ties must be secure but not tight. You should be able to slide only a fingertip under the ties (Figure 44–25, *B*). Ties are too loose if you can slide your whole finger under them. When assisting with tracheostomy care, you must hold the child still. Position the child's head so that the neck is slightly extended.

SUCTIONING AN AIRWAY

Injury and illness often cause secretions to collect in the upper airway resulting in the following problems:

- They obstruct air flow in and out of the airway.
- They provide an environment for microbes.
- They interfere with O_2 and CO_2 exchange.
- Hypoxia can occur.

Usually coughing removes secretions, but some clients are not able to cough, or the cough is too weak to remove secretions. Some clients cannot expectorate or swallow secretions after coughing. These clients need suctioning to remove secretions.

Suctioning is the process of withdrawing or sucking up fluid (secretions). A tube connects to a suction source (wall outlet or suction machine) at one end and to a suction catheter at the other end. The catheter is inserted into the airway, and secretions are withdrawn through the catheter.

Suctioning Sites

The upper airway (nose, mouth, and pharynx) and the lower airway (trachea and bronchi) are suctioned.

- ***Oro-pharyngeal route***—the mouth (*oro*) and pharynx (*pharyngeal*) are suctioned. A suction catheter is passed through the mouth and into the pharynx.
- ***Nasopharyngeal route***—the nose (*naso*) and pharynx (*pharyngeal*) are suctioned. The suction catheter is passed through the nose and into the pharynx.
- ***Lower airway suctioning***—is done through an endo-tracheal (ET) tube or through a tracheostomy tube.

Safety Measures Related to Suctioning

If not done correctly, suctioning can cause serious harm to the client. As suctioning removes oxygen from the airway, the client may be unable to breathe during suctioning, and hypoxia and life-threatening complications can arise. The respiratory, cardiovascular, and nervous systems can be affected, and cardiac arrest, infection, and airway injury are possible. ***It is your responsibility to ensure that suctioning is within your scope of practice for your province or your agency.***

The client's lungs are hyperventilated—given extra (*hyper*) breaths (*ventilate*)—before suctioning from an ET tube or tracheostomy. An Ambu bag (Figure 44–26) is attached to an oxygen source; then the oxygen delivery device is removed from the ET or tracheostomy tube, and the Ambu bag is attached to the ET or tracheostomy tube. To give a breath, the bag is squeezed with both hands. A nurse or respiratory therapist gives 3 to 5 breaths.

Remember, oxygen is considered a medication and you do not administer medications. Therefore you need to check if your province or territory and employer allow you to operate an Ambu bag attached to an oxygen source.

Some employers limit suctioning to 10 seconds, and some allow 10 to 15 seconds for the suction cycle:

- Insert the catheter
- Apply suction
- Remove the catheter

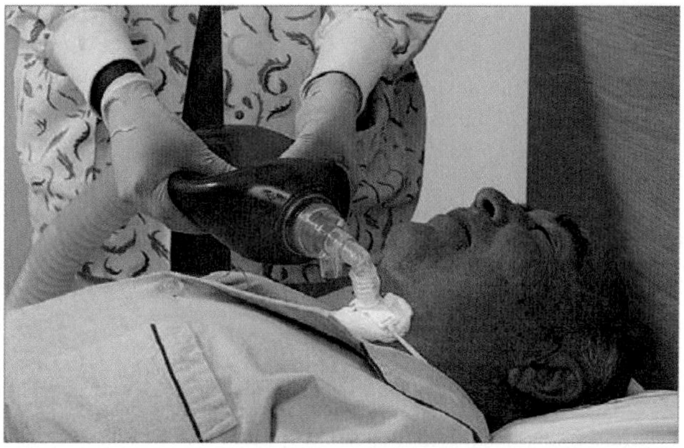

Figure 44–26 The Ambu bag. A nurse compresses it with two hands.

For infants and children, suction is applied for no longer than 5 seconds.

You might be asked to assist a nurse with suctioning. You need to understand the principles and safety measures involved in safe suctioning (see Box 44–7).

Box 44–7 Principles and Safety Measures for Suctioning

- If suctioning is within the scope of practice for your province and your agency, you should be taught the correct way to do it by a nurse or a respiratory technologist.
- Review the procedure with your supervisor (a nurse). Know what is expected of you.
- Suctioning is done as needed (*prn*). Coughing and signs and symptoms of respiratory distress signal the need for suctioning. Your supervisor tells you what signs to look for.
- Standard Practices should be followed. Secretions can contain blood and are potentially infectious.
- Sterile technique must be used (see Chapter 20).
- Your supervisor tells you the size and type of catheter to collect (Figure 44–27). Airway injury can occur if the catheter is too large.
- Needed suction equipment and supplies should be kept at the bedside so that they are readily available when the client needs suctioning.
- When suction is applied, air is sucked out of the airway, so suction should not be applied while inserting the catheter.
- The catheter is cleared with water or saline after removal.
- The catheter should be inserted smoothly to prevent injury to the mucous membranes.
- The suction catheter should be passed (inserted) no more than three times. The risk of injury increases each time the catheter is passed.
- When suctioning, ***you should not suction any deeper than the client's oral cavity. This means that the catheter should not go past the back of the client's teeth (or the gum area).*** Suctioning near the client's epiglottis can trigger a strong gag reaction. This is allowed in deep suctioning, which usually falls only within the scope of practice for nurses or respiratory technicians.
- Check the client's pulse, respirations, and pulse oximeter before, during, and after the procedure. Also observe the level of consciousness. Tell your supervisor immediately if any of the following occur:
  - A drop in pulse rate, or a pulse rate less than 60 beats per minute
  - Irregular cardiac rhythms
  - A drop or rise in blood pressure
  - Respiratory distress
  - A drop in the SpO_2 (see page 853)

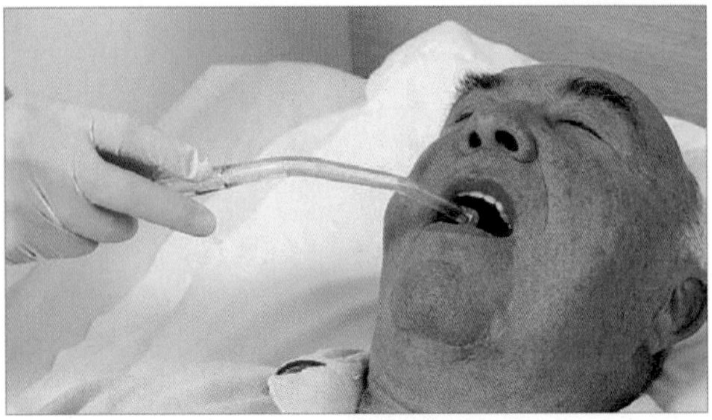

Figure 44–27 The Yankauer suction catheter is often used when there are large amounts of thick secretions.

MECHANICAL VENTILATION

With some severe problems, the client cannot breathe, or normal blood oxygen levels are not maintained. These include: (a) hypoxia caused by weak muscle effort, airway obstruction, and damaged lung tissue; (b) nervous system diseases and injuries that can affect the respiratory centre in the brain when nerve damage interferes with messages between the lungs and the brain; and (c) drug overdoses that can depresses the brain's hypothalamus breathing centre. In these situations, mechanical ventilation may be needed to save the client's life. **Mechanical ventilation** is the use of a machine to move air into and out of the lungs (Figure 44–28), allowing oxygen to enter the lungs and carbon dioxide to leave them. ***It is your responsibility to ensure that assisting with mechanical ventilation is within your scope of practice for your province or your agency.***

Mechanical ventilation is always initiated in a hospital. Some people need it for a few hours or days, while some need it longer. Clients who are on mechanical ventilation will have a **ventilator** attached to some form of artificial airway, such as an endo-tracheal tube (ET tube) or a tracheostomy tube.

Ventilators have alarms that sound when something is wrong. An alarm sounds when the client gets disconnected from the ventilator. Your supervisor (in this case, a nurse) would have to show you how to connect the ET or tracheostomy tube to the ventilator. When any alarm sounds, ***first check to see if the client's tube is attached to the ventilator. If not, attach it to the ventilator. The client can die if not connected to the ventilator.*** Then tell your supervisor at once about the alarm. ***You should never reset alarms.***

Clients needing mechanical ventilation are very ill or have other problems and injuries. Some are confused, disoriented, or cannot think clearly. Many are frightened by the machine and by thoughts of dying. Some feel relieved to get enough oxygen. Many fear the prospect of needing the machine for life. Mechanical ventilation can be painful for those with chest injuries or chest surgery. Tubes and hoses restrict movement and can cause more discomfort.

You may be asked to assist with the care of a client on mechanical ventilation. Follow the guidelines in Box 44–8.

Weaning from the ventilator is often needed. That is, the client gradually needs to breathe without the ventilator. Weaning can take many weeks. A physician, respiratory therapist, and nurse plan the weaning process. (See *Focus on Home Care: Mechanical Ventilation* box.)

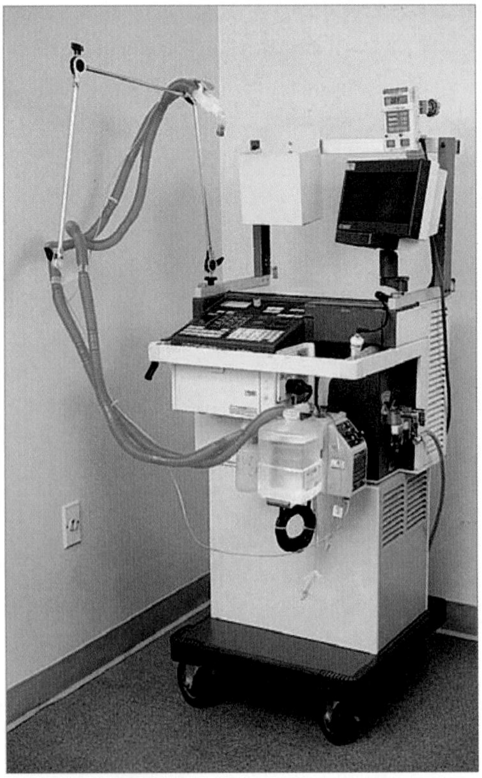

Figure 44–28 A mechanical ventilator.

focus on »HOME CARE

Mechanical Ventilation

Home care is often arranged for clients receiving mechanical ventilation. Portable ventilators are used in home care. An RN will teach you how to care for each client. Family members are taught how to assist with the client's care. Always make sure that an RN is available by phone when you are in the client's home.

CHEST TUBES

Air, blood, or fluid can collect in the pleural space (sac or cavity) when the chest has been penetrated because of injury or surgery:

- ***Pneumothorax*** is air (*pneumo*) in the pleural space (*thorax*).
- ***Hemothorax*** is blood (*hemo*) in the pleural space (*thorax*).
- ***Pleural effusion*** is the escape and collection of fluid (*effusion*) in the pleural space (*pleural*).

Pressure occurs when air, blood, or fluid collects in the pleural sac, and this pressure makes the lungs collapse. Therefore, air does not reach affected alveoli, and O_2 and CO_2 are not exchanged, which will result in respiratory distress and hypoxia. Sometimes there is so much accumulated pressure that the heart's ability to pump blood is threatened, and the situation becomes life threatening.

Hospital care is required in these cases. A physician inserts the **chest tube** to remove the air, fluid, or blood (Figure 44–29). After the client's condition has been stabilized, he or she may need rehabilitation or subacute care.

Chest tubes attach to a drainage system (Figure 44–30) that must be airtight to prevent air from entering the pleural space. This is done as follows:

- A chest tube attaches to connecting tubing.
- Connecting tubing attaches to a tube in the drainage container.

Sometimes suction is applied to the drainage system. You may be asked to assist a nurse with the client's care. Follow the guidelines in Box 44–9.

Box 44–8 Guidelines for Caring for Clients Receiving Mechanical Ventilation

- Keep the call bell within reach (in facilities).
- Make sure hoses and connecting tubing have slack. They must not pull on the artificial airway.
- Answer call bells promptly. The client is in a situation in which he or she must depend on others for basic needs.
- Explain who you are and what you are going to do. Do this whenever you enter the room.
- Give the day, date, and time every time you give care.
- Report signs of respiratory distress or discomfort at once.
- Do not change settings on the machine or reset alarms.
- Follow the care plan for communication. Since the client cannot talk, use agreed-upon hand or eye signals for "yes" and "no." All health care team members must use the same signals, or confusion, not communication, may occur. Some clients may be able to use paper and pencils, magic slates, communication boards, and hand signals to communicate. Follow the care plan.
- Ask questions that have simple answers. It may be hard to write long responses.
- Watch what you say and do, whether you are near or away from the client and family. They pay close attention to your verbal and nonverbal communication. Do not say anything that could upset them.
- Comfort and reassure the client by talking to him or her. It is also comforting when you talk about seemingly "light" topics, such as the weather, pleasant news events, gifts, and cards.
- Meet the client's basic needs. Follow the care plan.
- Use touch to reassure and comfort the client.
- Tell the client when you are leaving the room and when you will return.

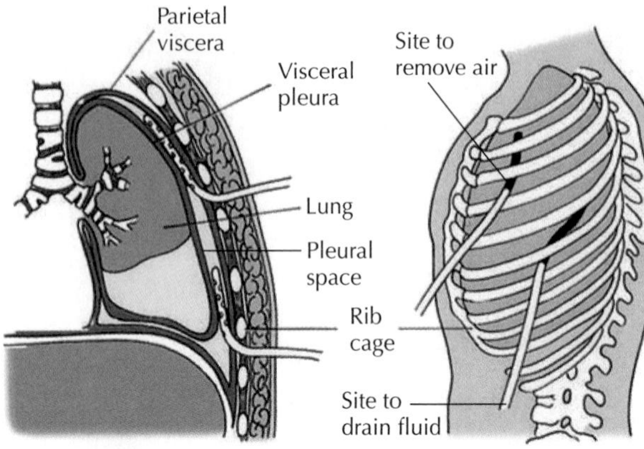

Figure 44–29 Chest tubes inserted into the pleural space. **Source:** Elkin, M.K., Perry, A.G., & Potter, P.A. (2000). *Nursing interventions and clinical skills* (2nd ed.). St. Louis: Mosby.

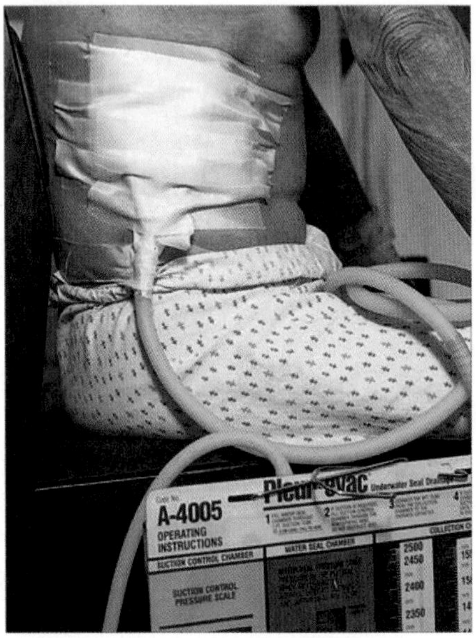

Figure 44-30 Chest tubes attached to a disposable water-seal drainage system. **Source:** Elkin, M.K., Perry, A.G., & Potter, P.A. (2000). *Nursing interventions and clinical skills* (2nd ed.). St. Louis: Mosby.

Box 44–9 Guidelines for Caring for Clients With Chest Tubes

- Keep the drainage system below the level of the client's chest.
- Check vital signs, as directed. Report vital sign changes at once.
- Report signs and symptoms of hypoxia, complaints of pain, difficulty breathing, and respiratory distress at once.
- Keep connecting tubing coiled on the bed. Allow enough slack so the chest tubes are not dislodged when the client moves. If tubing hangs in loops, drainage collects in the loop.
- Prevent tubing kinks, which can obstruct the chest tube, causing air, blood, or fluid to collect in the pleural space.
- Observe chest drainage. Report any change in chest drainage at once. This includes increases in drainage or the appearance of bright red drainage.
- Record chest drainage, according to employer policy.
- Turn and reposition the client, as directed. Be careful and gentle to prevent chest tubes from dislodging.
- Assist the client with coughing and deep breathing exercises, as directed.
- Assist with incentive spirometry, as directed.
- Note bubbling in the drainage system. Tell your supervisor at once if bubbling increases, decreases, or stops.
- Tell your supervisor at once if any part of the system is loose or disconnected.
- Keep sterile petrolatum gauze at the bedside. It is needed if a chest tube comes out.
- Call for help at once if a chest tube comes out. Cover the insertion site with sterile petrolatum gauze. Stay with the client. Then follow the nurse's directions.

REVIEW

Answers to these questions are at the bottom of page 864.

Circle the BEST answer.

1. **Alcohol and narcotics affect oxygen needs because they:**
   A. Depress the breathing centre in the brain
   B. Are pollutants
   C. Cause allergies
   D. Cause a pneumothorax

2. **Hypoxia is:**
   A. The lack of oxygen
   B. Not enough oxygen in the cells
   C. Not enough oxygen in the blood
   D. The amount of hemoglobin that contains oxygen

3. **An early sign of hypoxia is:**
   A. Dyspnea
   B. Cyanosis
   C. Restlessness
   D. Increased pulse and respiratory rates

4. **A client can breathe deeply and comfortably only while sitting. This is called:**
   A. Bradypnea
   B. Orthopnea
   C. Biot's respirations
   D. Kussmaul's respirations

5. **Which of the following is a sign of altered respiratory function?**
   A. Joint pain
   B. Nausea and vomiting
   C. Severe abdominal pain
   D. Wheezing or crowing sounds

6. **A client's SpO_2 is 98%. Which of the following is *true*?**
   A. The client needs suctioning
   B. The pulse oximeter is wrong
   C. The client's pulse is 98 beats per minute
   D. The measurement is within normal range

7. **Which of the following is a site for a pulse oximetry sensor?**
   A. Wrist
   B. Finger
   C. Upper arm
   D. The tragus of the ear

8. **The best time to collect sputum is:**
   A. On awakening
   B. After meals
   C. At bedtime
   D. After suctioning

9. **A sputum specimen is needed. You should ask the client to:**
   A. Use mouthwash
   B. Brush the teeth
   C. Apply lubricant to the lips
   D. Rinse the mouth with clear water

10. **You are assisting a client with coughing and deep breathing. Which of the following is *true*?**
    A. The client exhales through pursed lips
    B. The client should do this just after eating
    C. The client exhales deeply through the nose
    D. The client needs to be in a comfortable lying position

11. **Which of the following is useful for deep breathing?**
    A. Chest tubes
    B. Pulse oximeter
    C. Incentive spirometer
    D. Partial-rebreather mask

12. **You are assisting with oxygen therapy. You can:**
    A. Start the oxygen
    B. Decide what device to use
    C. Turn the oxygen on and off
    D. Keep the connecting tubing secure and free of kinks

13. **A client has a tracheostomy. Which of the following is *true*?**
    A. The outer cannula is removed for cleaning
    B. The obturator is inserted after the outer cannula
    C. The outer cannula must be secured in place
    D. The client is rarely at risk for aspiration

14. **A client has a tracheostomy. He or she can do the following:**
    A. Sing
    B. Shave
    C. Shower
    D. Swim

REVIEW

Answers to these questions are at the bottom of the page.

15. **A client has a tracheostomy. For the client's safety, the old ties are removed after:**
    - A. The stoma is cleaned
    - B. The dressing is removed
    - C. The inner cannula is removed
    - D. The outer cannula is held in place

16. **These statements are about suctioning. Which one is *true*?**
    - A. You can perform the procedure without wearing gloves
    - B. Suctioning is done every 2 hours
    - C. Suction is applied while inserting the catheter
    - D. A suction cycle is no more than 10 to 15 seconds

17. **Suctioning requires:**
    - A. Chest tubes
    - B. Sterile technique
    - C. An artificial airway
    - D. Mechanical ventilation

18. **Which of the following is used to hyperventilate the lungs?**
    - A. Ambu bag
    - B. Pulse oximeter
    - C. Incentive spirometer
    - D. Partial-rebreather mask

19. **Mr. Long requires mechanical ventilation. Which of the following is *true*?**
    - A. He cannot move
    - B. His call bell is useless right now
    - C. You can reset alarms on the ventilator
    - D. He has an ET tube or a tracheostomy tube

20. **An alarm sounds on Mr. Long's ventilator. What should you do first?**
    - A. Reset the alarm
    - B. Ask him what is wrong
    - C. Call your supervisor immediately
    - D. Check to see if his airway is attached to the ventilator

21. **A client has a pneumothorax. This is the collection of:**
    - A. Air in the pleural space
    - B. Blood in the pleural space
    - C. Fluid in the pleural space
    - D. Respiratory secretions in the pleural space

22. **Chest tubes are attached to a disposable water-seal drainage system. You should do the following:**
    - A. Encourage the client to stay in bed
    - B. Hang the tubing in as straight a line as possible
    - C. Keep the drainage system below the client's chest
    - D. Reinsert the tubing if it is accidentally disconnected

Answers: 1.A, 2.B, 3.C, 4.B, 5.D, 6.D, 7.B, 8.A, 9.D, 10.A, 11.C, 12.D, 13.C, 14.B, 15.D, 16.D, 17.B, 18.A, 19.D, 20.D, 21.A, 22.C

CHAPTER 45

Assisting With the Physical Examination

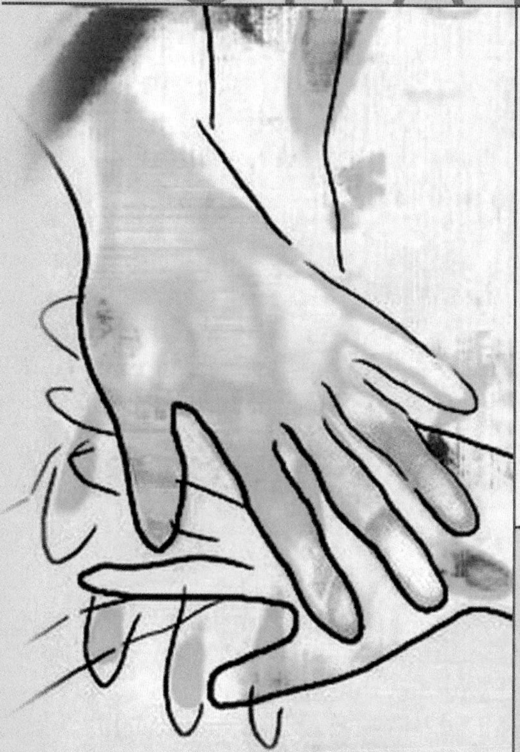

OBJECTIVES

- Define the key terms listed in this chapter.
- Explain what to do before, during, and after a physical examination.
- Identify the equipment used during a physical examination.
- Describe how to prepare a client for an examination.
- Describe the four examination positions and how to drape the client for each position.
- Explain guidelines for assisting with a physical examination.
- Perform the procedures described in this chapter.

key terms

dorsal recumbent position See **supine position**.

horizontal position See **supine position**.

knee-chest position An examination position in which the client kneels and rests the body on the knees and chest; the head is turned to one side, the arms are above the head or flexed at the elbows, the back is straight, and the body is flexed about 90 degrees at the hips.

laryngeal mirror An instrument used to examine the mouth, teeth, and throat.

lithotomy position A back-lying position in which the hips are brought down to the edge of the examination table, the knees are flexed, the hips are externally rotated, and the feet are supported in stirrups.

nasal speculum An instrument used to examine the inside of the nose.

ophthalmoscope A lighted instrument used to examine the internal structures of the eye.

otoscope A lighted instrument used to examine the external ear and the eardrum (tympanic membrane).

percussion hammer An instrument used to tap body parts to test reflexes. Also known as **reflex hammer**.

reflex hammer See **percussion hammer**.

Sims' position A left side-lying position; the right leg is sharply flexed so it is not on the left leg, and the left arm is positioned along the client's back

supine position A back-lying position; the legs are together; Also known as **dorsal recumbent position** and **horizontal position**.

tuning fork An instrument used to test hearing.

vaginal speculum An instrument used to open the vagina so that it and the cervix can be examined.

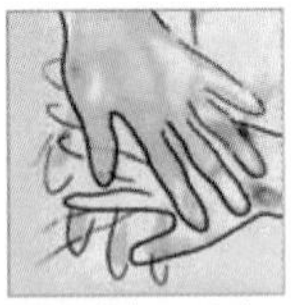

Physicians and nurses perform physical examinations (exams) for many reasons: (1) Routine health examinations are done to promote health. (2) Pre-employment physicals are done to determine fitness for work. (3) Physical examinations are also used to diagnose and treat diseases. (4) Some long-term care facilities require new clients to have a physical exam when they arrive; some require clients to have physical exams at least once a year. As a support worker in a facility, you may be asked to assist the physician or the nurse with a physical exam. In the community, you may possibly assist physicians in some aspects of a physical exam, since some physicians do still make house calls.

YOUR RESPONSIBILITIES

Your responsibilities depend on your employer's policies and procedures, as well as the examiner's preferences. You may do some or all of the following:

- Collect linens for draping the client for the procedure
- Collect examination equipment
- Prepare the room for the examination
- Transport the client to and from the exam room
- Assist with lighting
- Measure vital signs, height, and weight
- Position and drape the client
- Hand equipment and instruments to the examiner
- Stay with the client before or during the exam to provide emotional support and to prevent falls
- Label specimen containers
- Dispose of soiled linen and discard supplies
- Clean equipment
- Assist the client with putting the clothes back on and help him or her assume a comfortable position after the examination

EQUIPMENT

Instruments needed for a physical examination include, but are not limited to, the following (Figure 45–1):

- ***Ophthalmoscope***—a lighted instrument used to examine the internal structures of the eye

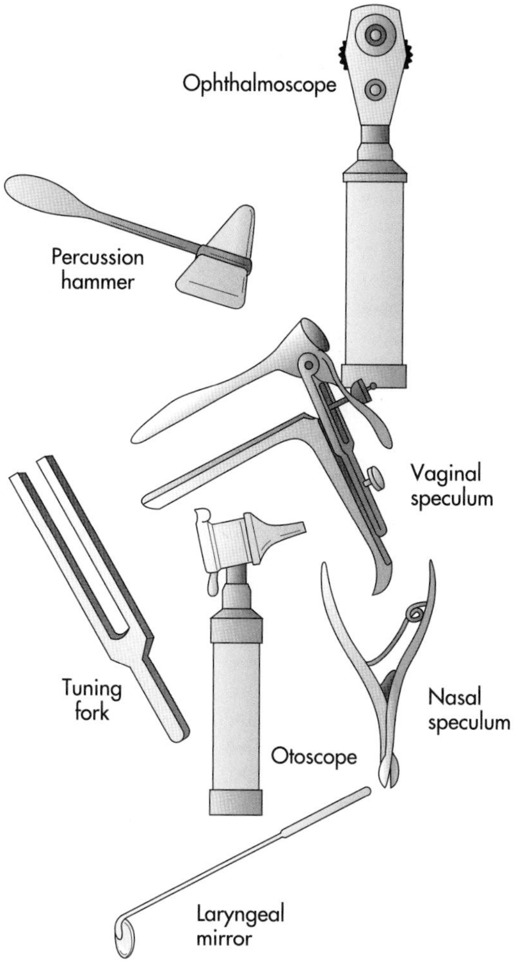

Figure 45–1 Some of the many instruments used for a physical examination.

- ***Otoscope***—a lighted instrument used to examine the external ear and the eardrum (tympanic membrane). Some scopes have parts for examining eyes and ears. They are changed into an ophthalmoscope or otoscope.
- ***Percussion hammer***—used to tap body parts to test reflexes. It is also called a **reflex hammer**.
- ***Vaginal speculum***—used to open the vagina so it and the cervix can be examined
- ***Nasal speculum***—used to examine the inside of the nose
- ***Tuning fork***—an instrument used to test hearing
- ***Laryngeal mirror***—used to examine the mouth, teeth, and throat

Many facilities have examination trays in the supply department. If one is not available, collect the items listed in *Preparing the Client for an Examination* (see page 870), and arrange them on a tray or table for the examiner.

PREPARING THE CLIENT

Many clients worry about having a physical examination because of possible findings or because of confusion or fear about what the examiner will do. Feeling discomfort and embarrassment, fearing exposure, and not knowing what the procedure involves all cause anxiety. As a support worker, you need to be sensitive to the client's feelings and concerns and prepare the client physically and psychologically for the examination.

The client has the right to know who will do the exam, why it is done, and what to expect, and this information is given to the client by the physician or nurse. If a client asks you questions about an examination, say that you will ask your supervisor to speak to him or her.

The client has the right to personal choice. The physician or nurse must inform the client about the exam and the reasons for it. The client is told who will do the exam, when it will be done, and what the procedure involves. The exam is done only if the client gives consent. The client may want a different examiner or may want a family member to be present at the exam. Some clients want to have family members with them when exam results are explained to them.

The client's right to privacy also should be protected. The examining area is screened and the room door closed. The client has to remove all clothes for a complete examination, and he or she is usually asked to wear a hospital gown, which reduces the feeling of nakedness and the fear of exposure. The client is also covered with a paper drape, bath blanket, sheet, or drawsheet. Explain to the client that only the body part being examined is exposed and that only minimum exposure will occur (see the *Focus on Children: Promoting Privacy* box).

The client is asked to void before the examination, as an empty bladder allows the examiner to feel the abdominal organs easily. A full bladder can change the normal position and shape of organs and can also cause discomfort, especially when the examiner is palpating (feeling) the abdominal organs. If a urine specimen is needed, ask the client to collect it when voiding before the exam. Explain how to collect the specimen (see Chapter 31), and when the client hands it to you, label the container.

Maintaining warmth during the examination is important, so ensure that the client—especially an ill client, older client, or a child—is protected from chilling. Keep an extra bath blanket at hand, and take measures to prevent drafts.

1 2 3 PREPARING THE CLIENT FOR AN EXAMINATION

Remember to promote:

• Dignity • Independence • Preferences • Privacy • Safety

Pre-Procedure

1 Identify the client, according to employer policy.
2 Explain the procedure to the client.
3 Perform hand hygiene.
4 Collect instruments and supplies, as requested by the examiner. These may include some or all of the following:
- Flashlight
- Blood pressure cuff
- Stethoscope
- Thermometer
- Tongue depressors (blades)
- Laryngeal mirror
- Ophthalmoscope
- Otoscope
- Nasal speculum
- Percussion (reflex) hammer
- Tuning fork
- Tape measure
- Gloves
- Water-soluble lubricant
- Vaginal speculum
- Cotton-tipped applicators
- Specimen containers and labels
- Disposable bag
- Kidney basin
- Towel
- Bath blanket
- Tissues
- Drape (sheet, bath blanket, drawsheet, or disposable drape)
- Paper towels
- Cotton balls
- Waterproof bed protector
- Eye chart (Snellen chart)
- Slides
- Gown
- Alcohol wipes
- Wastebasket
- Container for soiled instruments
- Marking pencils or pens

5 Provide for privacy.

Procedure

6 Instruct the client to remove all clothes and put on the gown provided. Assist, as necessary.
7 Ask the client to void. Offer the bedpan, commode, or urinal, if necessary. Provide for privacy.
8 Transport the client to the exam room.
9 Weigh and measure the client (see Chapter 41).
10 Help the client get on the examination table. Provide a footstool, if necessary. (Omit this step if the exam is done in the client's room.)
11 Raise the bed to its highest level. Raise the far bed rail, if used. (This step is done for an exam in the client's room.)
12 Position the client, as directed.
13 Drape the client.
14 Place a bed protector under the client's buttocks.
15 Raise the bed rail near you, if used.
16 Ensure adequate lighting.
17 Press the call bell for the nurse or examiner. Do not leave the client unattended.

focus on »CHILDREN

Promoting Privacy

Toddlers, preschool children, and school-age children are allowed to keep their underpants on during the examination. The underpants may be lowered or removed, as necessary, during the procedure.

The examiner may want height, weight, and vital signs measured, so obtain these before the examination starts and record the information on the examination form. The client is then positioned and draped for the examination. Take care to protect the client from falls and injury. Do not leave the client unattended.

POSITIONING AND DRAPING

For some examinations, special positions may be needed, and some of them may be uncomfortable and embarrassing for the client. The examiner will tell you how to position the client. Before helping the client assume and maintain the position, explain the following:

- Why the position is needed
- How to assume the position
- How the body is draped for warmth and privacy
- How long the client can expect to stay in the position

The **supine position** (**dorsal recumbent position** or **horizontal position**) is used to examine the abdomen, anterior chest, and breasts. The client lies flat on his or her back keeping the legs together. If the perineal area is to be examined, the knees are flexed and the hips externally rotated (Figure 45–2, *A*). The drape is extended over the client's body from the shoulders to the feet.

The **lithotomy position** (Figure 45–2, *B*) is used to examine the vagina. The client lies on her back, and her hips are brought to the edge of the examination table. The knees are flexed, the hips externally rotated, and the feet supported in stirrups. The client is draped as for perineal care (see Figure 29–26). Some facilities provide socks to cover the client's feet and calves. If a client finds it difficult to assume this position, the examiner will tell you how to position the client.

The **knee-chest position** (Figure 45–2, *C*) is used to examine the rectum and sometimes the vagina. The client kneels and rests the chest on the knees, with the head turned to one side. The arms are kept above the head or flexed at the elbows. The back is kept straight, and the body is flexed about 90 degrees at the hips. The client wears a gown and sometimes socks, and the drape is applied in a diamond shape to cover the back, buttocks, and thighs. This position is rarely used for older adults; they usually assume the side-lying position for rectal exams.

The **Sims' position** (Figure 45–2, *D*) is sometimes used to examine the rectum or the vagina. The client lies on the left side. The right leg is sharply flexed so it is not on the left leg. The left arm is positioned along the client's back. The drape is applied over the client in a diamond shape. The corner near the examiner is folded back to expose the rectum or the vagina.

ASSISTING WITH THE EXAMINATION

You may be asked to prepare, position, and drape the client and also to assist the physician or the nurse during the exam. When assisting with an examination, follow the guidelines in Box 45–1 (also see *Focus on Children: Providing Comfort During a Physical Exam* box).

Clients with dementia may resist the examiner and may be agitated and physically aggressive because of confusion and fear. The client who refuses or actively resists an examination must not be restrained or forced to have the procedure. The client may react better at another time, or having a family member present may calm the client. The client's rights should always be respected.

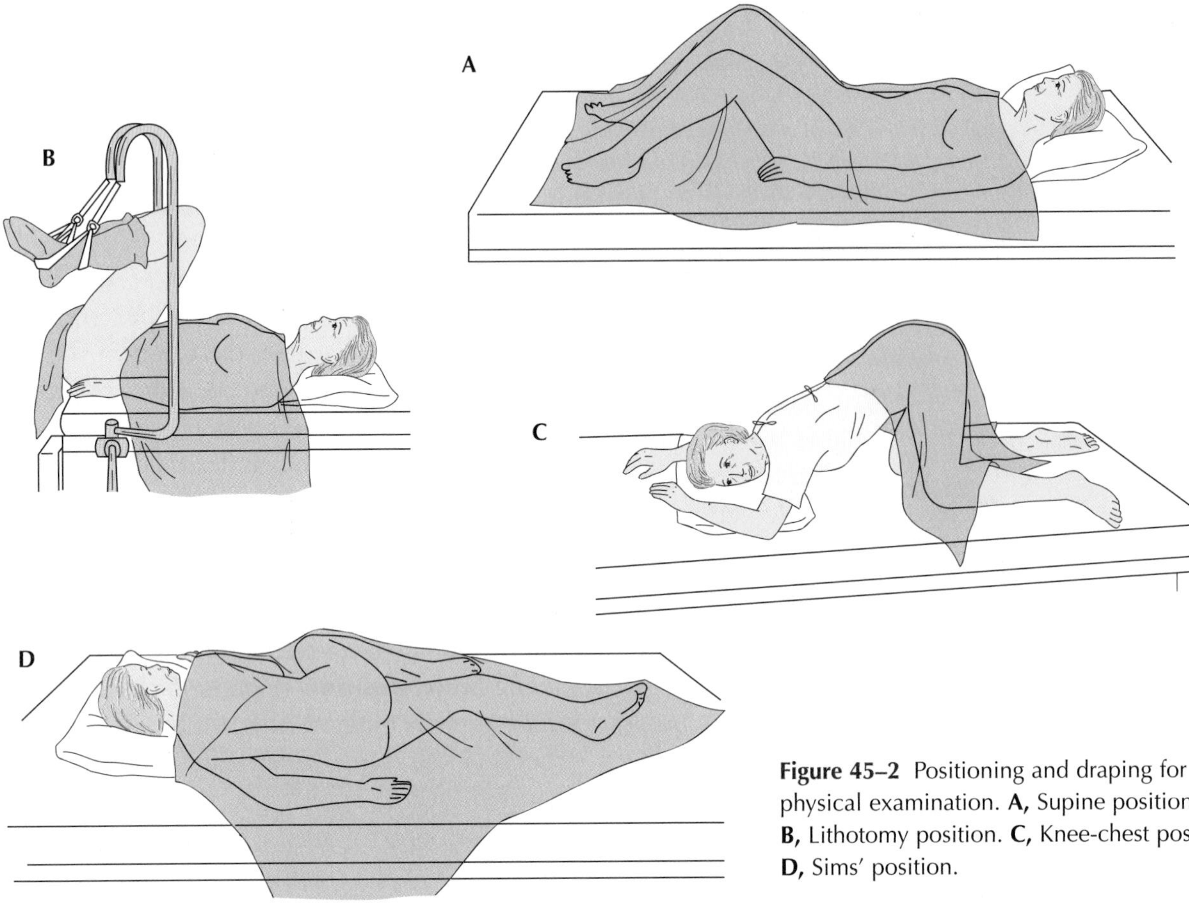

Figure 45–2 Positioning and draping for the physical examination. **A,** Supine position. **B,** Lithotomy position. **C,** Knee-chest position. **D,** Sims' position.

Box 45–1 Guidelines for Assisting With a Physical Examination

- Perform hand hygiene before and after the examination.
- Provide for privacy by screening, closing doors, and draping. Expose only the body part being examined.
- Assist with positioning, as directed by the examiner.
- Place instruments and equipment near the examiner.
- Stay in the room when a female client is examined (only if you are also a female). When a male examiner examines a female, it is required that another female be present in the room for the legal protection of both the female client and the male examiner. The presence of a female attendant also provides psychological comfort to the client. Similarly, a female examiner may want a male attendant present when she examines a male client, again for the legal protection of both parties.
- Protect the client from falling.
- Anticipate the examiner's need for equipment and supplies. When passing instruments during the physical exam, you should hand the instruments to the examiner with the handles toward the examiner. In order to keep the instrument sterile (if appropriate) or as clean as possible, you should only handle the instrument by holding it in the middle.
- Place a paper sheet or paper towel on the floor if the client is asked to stand.
- Practise medical asepsis, and follow Standard Practices.

focus on
>> CHILDREN

Providing Comfort During a Physical Exam

The examination of an infant or child is similar to an adult examination. However, a parent or other adult caregiver is required to be present. The parent or caregiver may need to hold the infant or child still during some parts of the procedure if he or she is uncooperative, which may be frightening. The child or infant may also have separation anxiety or fear of physical harm during the examination. Your calm, comforting attitude will help not only the child but also the parent or caregiver who may be feeling anxious, too.

Most of the equipment is the same as for the adult examination; however, with children, toys are sometimes used to assess development, and vaginal speculums are never used.

ASSISTING AFTER THE EXAMINATION

After the examination has been completed, the client dresses and returns to his or her room. Assist, as needed. If a lubricant has been used for vaginal or rectal examination, wipe or clean the area before the client dresses or returns to the room.

You may also be asked to do the following:

- Discard disposable items.
- Replenish supplies for the next exam.
- Clean reusable items (such as otoscope and ophthalmoscope tips, speculum, and stethoscope), according to employer policy. Return them to the tray or storage place.
- Remove the used drawsheet or paper from the examination table. Cover the examination table with a clean drawsheet or paper.
- Label specimens. Take them to the designated area, according to employer policy.
- Clean and tidy up the client's unit or examination room. Follow employer policy for disposing of soiled linens.

Remember the client's right to privacy. The results of the examination are confidential. Only members of the health care team involved in the client's care need to know the reason for the exam and its results. If the client consents, the physician may provide the result to family members. The client may share the information with others if he or she wants to. You should never disclose the results of the exam to the family or others.

REVIEW

Answers to these questions are at the bottom of the page.

Circle the **BEST** answer.

1. **The otoscope is used to:**
   A. Examine the internal structures of the eye
   B. Examine the external ear and the eardrum
   C. Test reflexes
   D. Open the vagina

2. **You are preparing Mrs. Janz for an exam. You should do the following:**
   A. Do not tell her any details of the exam, as it is not part of your role
   B. Ask her to undress
   C. Take her vital signs
   D. Leave her alone while you go to tell the nurse that Mrs. Janz is ready

3. **Which part of Mrs. Janz's exam can you do?**
   A. Test her reflexes
   B. Inspect her mouth, teeth, and throat
   C. Position and drape her
   D. Observe her perineum and rectum

4. **Mrs. Janz is in the supine position. Her hips are flexed and externally rotated. Her feet are supported in stirrups. She is in the:**
   A. Supine position
   B. Lithotomy position
   C. Knee-chest position
   D. Sims' position

5. **You will be assisting with Mrs. Janz's exam. Which of the following is true?**
   A. Hand hygiene is done before and after the examination
   B. Draping is not necessary if the door is closed
   C. You leave the room when Mrs. Janz is examined
   D. The examiner will position the client

6. **Which of the following statements is *true*?**
   A. You cannot explain the reason for the exam to the client
   B. You must keep the client safe from injury during the exam
   C. You can tell the family the results of the exam
   D. You explain what the examiner will do

Answers: 1.B, 2.B, 3.C, 4.B, 5.A, 6.B

CHAPTER 46

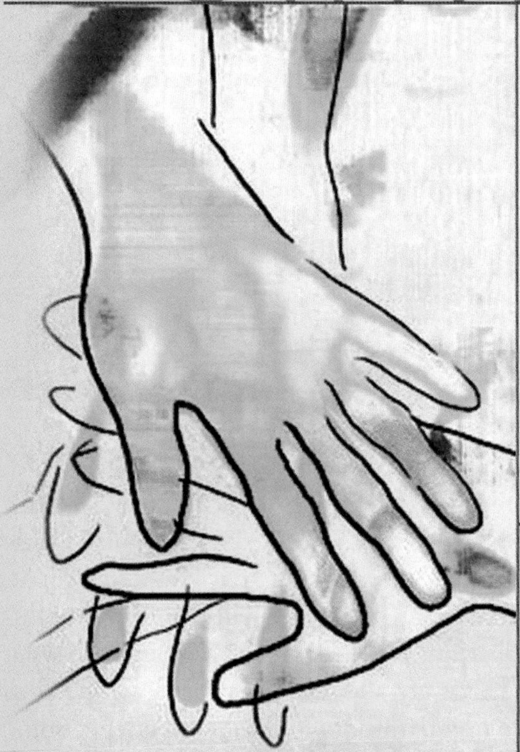

The Client Having Surgery

OBJECTIVES

- Define the key terms listed in this chapter.
- Describe the common fears and concerns of surgical clients.
- Explain how clients are physically and psychologically prepared for surgery.
- Describe how to prepare a room for the postoperative client.
- List the postoperative signs and symptoms to report to the nurse.
- Explain how circulation is stimulated after surgery.
- Describe how to meet the client's hygiene, nutrition, fluid, and elimination needs after surgery.
- Perform the procedures described in this chapter.

key terms

anesthesia The loss of feeling or sensation produced by a medication that blocks the pain impulses to the brain; usually causes loss of consciousness.

elective surgery Surgery that is scheduled but nonurgent; delaying the surgery does not result in permanent damage, disability, or death.

embolus A blood clot, an air bubble, or a fat clot (a **thrombus**) that travels through the vascular system and finally lodges in a distant blood vessel.

emergency surgery Surgery that must be done immediately to save a client's life or prevent permanent disability.

general anesthesia Unconsciousness and the loss of feeling or sensation produced by a medication

local anesthesia The loss of sensation in a small area, produced by a medication injected at the specific site.

postoperative After surgery.

preoperative Before surgery.

regional anesthesia The loss of sensation or feeling in a large area of the body, produced by the injection of a medication; the client does not lose consciousness.

thrombus A blood clot, an air bubble, or a fat clot.

urgent surgery Surgery that must be done soon to prevent further damage, disability, or disease.

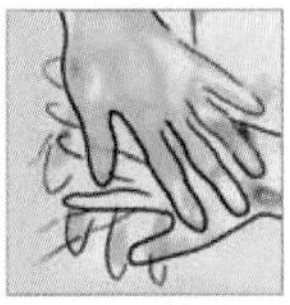

Surgery is performed on clients for many reasons, including removal of a diseased organ or body part, removal of a tumour, or repair of injured tissue. Surgery may also be done to diagnose a disease, improve appearance, and relieve symptoms. A specially trained physician, called a *surgeon*, performs the surgery.

A large number of surgeries require hospital stays; the client is admitted to the hospital before the surgery and stays for a few or several days after the surgery, for example, repair of a hip fracture. However, outpatient surgery (also called *ambulatory surgery*, *one-day surgery*, *same-day surgery*) that does not require an overnight hospital stay is also done quite frequently. The client is in the hospital for less than 24 hours. Many outpatient surgeries are done in clinics or surgical centres that are part of hospitals or physicians' offices.

Some outpatient procedures (day surgeries)—for example, a colonoscopy—will require *home preparation*. The client must take medication, as prescribed by the doctor, the day before the procedure to clear the colon of all fecal matter. Different kinds of medication are prescribed for preoperative preparation, and your supervisor will tell you the procedure to follow when assisting a client with these medications. These medications may cause diarrhea and therefore dehydration in the client. You need to ensure that the client drinks lots of fluids. Instructions from the doctor will include what types of fluids are allowed. The client will need to stay close to a bathroom and may experience some cramping. The area around the anus can become quite sore with frequent defecation. You can assist the client with the use of adult unscented wet wipes, a water spray, or a barrier cream. Home preparation for surgery can be tiring for older clients. Ensure safety if they become weak.

Surgeries may be elective, urgent, or emergency:

- ***Elective surgery***—is surgery that is scheduled but nonurgent. Delaying the surgery does not result in permanent damage, disability, or death. The surgery may be scheduled 1 day to months in advance. Often, clients are placed on waiting lists for elective surgery, for example, surgery for hip replacement.
- ***Urgent surgery***—must be done soon to prevent further damage, disability, or disease. Examples include cancer surgery and coronary artery surgery.

- ***Emergency surgery***—is surgery that must be done immediately to save a client's life or prevent disability. Clients who have been in accidents often require emergency surgery.

The client is prepared by nurses and physicians for what happens before, during, and after surgery. Clients need both physical and psychological preparation before surgery.

In hospitals, as a support worker, you will come in contact with clients before and after surgery. You may care for many clients in long-term care facilities who are recovering from surgery or provide postoperative care to clients in their homes.

PSYCHOLOGICAL CARE

Illness or injury causes many fears and concerns (see Box 46–1), and if surgery is needed, it increases these fears. Your clients may express their deepest fears about surgeries. Imagine you were in an accident, and when you woke up hours later, you were told that your right leg had been surgically amputated. How would you feel? Or if you were told you needed surgery the very next day, would you have fear of pain or death? Would you worry about who would care for your children and your home and who would earn money for your family while you were in the hospital?

Feelings are influenced by past experiences. Some clients may have had surgery before and some may not have had that experience at all. Family and friends may share experiences of their own surgeries with the client, which also can affect the client. Clients may have heard tragic stories related to surgeries—surgery on the wrong client, surgery on the wrong body part, instruments left in the body, death during surgery, and so on. Before surgery, some clients may not talk about their fears and concerns but just cry or be quiet and withdrawn; some may constantly talk about other things; some may pace restlessly; and some may act overly cheerful.

Psychological preparation before surgery is very important. As a support worker, you must respect your client's fears and concerns. The entire health care team must communicate warmth, sensitivity, and caring to the client. It must be remembered that clients may be extremely fearful of the pain that they may have to endure after surgery.

Box 46–1 Common Fears and Concerns of Surgical Clients

Fears

- Disfigurement and scarring
- Disability
- Pain during and after surgery
- Dying during surgery
- Anesthesia and its effects
- Exposure
- Severe pain or discomfort after surgery
- Tubes, needles, and other equipment used for care
- Complications
- Prolonged recovery
- More surgery or treatments
- Separation from family and friends
- Nausea and vomiting

Concerns

- Caring for children and other family members
- Taking care of pets, the house, lawn, and garden
- Payment of monthly bills, loans, mortgage or rent
- Insurance coverage for loss of earnings
- Loss of control
- Restrictions on lifestyle

Client Information

The physician explains the need for surgery and about the surgical procedure, risks, and possible complications to the client and family. Options other than surgery as well as the risks from not having surgery are also explained. The physician gives information about when the surgery is scheduled, who will perform it, and how long it will take. The physician will answer all the questions and doubts the client and family may have about the surgery and what to expect and gives instructions about pre- and postoperative care. All of this information before surgery is given by the physician or nurse. It is beyond the scope of your job to give this information.

After surgery, the physician informs the client and the family about the outcome of the surgery. The physician decides what and when to tell them. Often the health care team knows the results before the client does. Clients and families are usually anxious to know the results and may ask you, nurses, and other health care workers for information. They may ask if reports are back from the laboratory or what the reports say. While you should know what exactly the client is told, you must take care not to reveal any information about the surgery or test results to the client. If the client asks you for information, explain that you cannot give it and that you will get your supervisor to talk to him or her. Your supervisor tells you what the client and family were told and when it was told. This is confidential information, so do not repeat it to anyone.

Your Role

As a support worker, you can assist in the psychological care of the surgical client. Do the following if you are involved in preoperative and postoperative care:

- Listen to the client when he or she voices fears or concerns about surgery.
- Refer any questions about the surgery or its results to the nurse.
- Explain to the client the procedures that *you* will perform and the reasons for them.
- Communicate effectively. Use verbal and nonverbal communication (see Chapter 13).
- Report to your supervisor verbal and nonverbal signs of fear or anxiety that you have observed in the client.
- Report to your supervisor a client's request to see a spiritual adviser.

THE PREOPERATIVE PERIOD

The **preoperative** (before surgery) period may be many days or just a few minutes. If time permits, the client is prepared psychologically and physically for the effects of anesthesia and surgery. Good preoperative preparation prevents complications after surgery.

Preoperative Teaching

A nurse does the preoperative teaching and explains to the client what to expect before and after surgery. Teaching includes the following:

- ***Preoperative activities***—tests and their purposes, skin preparation, personal care, and the purposes and effects of medications.
- ***Deep-breathing, coughing, and leg exercises***—done after the surgery. These are taught by either a nurse or a physiotherapist and practised before the surgery.
- ***The recovery room***—where the client wakes up from the anesthetic (Figure 46–1). Care provided in the recovery room is explained.
- ***Food and fluids***—preoperatively clients are NPO (nothing by mouth) for several hours. Some clients receive an IV infusion after surgery. The physician orders food and oral fluids when the client's condition is stable.
- ***Turning and repositioning***—the client usually is turned and repositioned every 2 hours after surgery. The client is taught what to expect.
- ***Early ambulation***—usually the client is encouraged to walk as soon as possible after surgery.
- ***Pain***—the client is told about the type and amount of pain to expect and about medications for pain relief.
- ***Needed treatments and equipment***—the client may need a urinary catheter, nasogastric

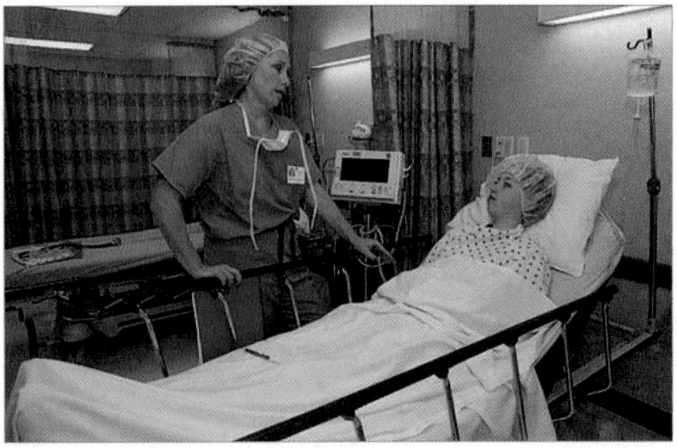

Figure 46–1 The recovery Room.

focus on
›› CHILDREN

Preparing for Surgery

The child who will be operated on as well as the parents or caregivers are psychologically prepared before the surgery. Often play is used to help the child understand what will happen. For example, dolls are used to show the anatomical site of surgery. The child and parents or caregivers are introduced to the members of the health care team who will be caring for the child. A tour of the operating room and the recovery room also is common.

tube, oxygen, wound suction, a cast, traction, or wound dressings, which are explained to the client.

- ***Position restrictions***—the patient is told if a certain position is required to be maintained after surgery—for example, after hip replacement surgery, the hip is abducted.

Special Tests

Before surgery, the physician orders tests to evaluate the client's circulatory, respiratory, and urinary systems. These tests include a chest X-ray, a complete blood count (cbc), and urinalysis. An electrocardiogram (ECG or EKG) detects any cardiac (heart) problems. To be prepared for any needed transfusions to correct anticipated blood loss, the patient's blood is tested to determine blood type (*type and crossmatch*). Other tests are done based on the client's condition and the requirements of the surgery. The client is prepared for the tests, as needed, and results are on the chart by the time of surgery.

Nutrition and Fluids

The client is usually allowed to have a light meal the day before the surgery, and then he or she has to be NPO (not allowed to eat or drink by mouth) for 6 to 8 hours before the surgery. These measures reduce the risk of vomiting and aspiration during anesthesia and after surgery. An NPO sign is placed in the client's room. Some clients may be required to take medications on the morning of surgery, for example, insulin or blood pressure medication. It is important that this is a doctor's order and that it is clearly written. Remember to remove the water pitcher and drinking glasses from the room when the patient is NPO. If the time of surgery is delayed or cancelled, your client will need nutrition during the waiting period. Check with your supervisor about the type of diet and fluids allowed.

Elimination

Abdominal surgeries usually require a preoperative enema. Cleansing enemas are common before intestinal surgeries and are ordered to clear the colon of feces so that feces do not spill into the abdominal cavity when the intestine is opened.

Enemas are also given when straining or a bowel movement could cause postoperative problems such as pain, severe bleeding (hemorrhage), or stress on the operated area. The physician specifies what enema to give and when, and usually a nurse administers the enema.

Some surgeries will necessitate urinary catheterization. For pelvic and abdominal surgeries, the bladder must be empty, as a full bladder is easily injured during surgery. Catheters also allow accurate urinary output measurements during and after surgery.

Personal Care

Personal care before surgery usually involves the following:

- ***Giving a complete bed bath, shower, or tub bath.*** A special soap or cleanser may be ordered. A bath and a shampoo help reduce the number of microbes on the body at the time of surgery.
- ***Removing makeup and nail polish.*** This is done so that the skin, lips, and nail beds can be observed for colour and circulation during and after surgery.
- ***Braiding long hair.*** All hairpins, clips, combs, and similar items as well as wigs and hairpieces are removed. Some hospitals have both male and female clients wear surgical caps to keep hair out of the face and the operative area.

- ***Giving oral hygiene to promote comfort.*** Being NPO causes thirst and a dry mouth. Ensure that the client does not swallow any water during oral hygiene (see the *Focus on Children: Preoperative Oral Hygiene* box).
- ***Removing dentures.*** Dentures are removed before preoperative medications are given, cleaned, and kept in a denture cup in a safe place. Some clients do not like being seen without their dentures, in which case allow them wear their dentures as long as possible. This promotes the client's sense of dignity and self-esteem.
- ***Removing all jewellery.*** If body piercing jewellery cannot be removed, it should be taped down.

Valuables

Valuables, such as dentures, glasses, contact lenses, hearing aids, and jewellery, are removed from clients for safekeeping. Artificial eyes and limbs also are removed, as these items are easily lost or broken during surgery. Transfers to the OR, to the recovery room, and back to the client's room also present safety risks. A note is made on the client's chart about the valuables removed and where they are kept. The client may want to continue to wear a wedding band or religious medal. If so, the item is secured in place with gauze or tape, according to hospital policy.

Skin Preparation

The skin and hair shafts contain microbes that could enter the body through the surgical incision, and a serious infection could result. The skin cannot be sterilized, but a *skin prep* can help reduce the number of microbes.

Hospital policy and the surgeon's preferences determine the area to be prepared for a specific surgery and the type of preparation to be done.

The Preoperative Checklist

A preoperative checklist (Figure 46–2) is placed at the top of the client's chart. The nurse makes sure that all items on the checklist have been completed because only when the list has been completed is the client considered to be ready for surgery. The nurse may ask you to do some things on the list, and when you complete each task, promptly report it to the nurse along with any observations. Except for positioning of bed rails, the entire checklist should be completed before preoperative medications are given.

> focus on
> ›› CHILDREN
>
> **Preoperative Oral Hygiene**
>
> A loose tooth can fall out during anesthesia and the child can aspirate the tooth. Therefore, during preoperative care, check for loose teeth when giving oral hygiene, and report any that you observe to the nurse. The nurse will note this on the preoperative checklist and inform the operating room (OR) staff.

Preoperative Medication

About 45 minutes to 1 hour before surgery, the preoperative medications are given by a physician or nurse. One medication helps the patient relax and feel drowsy, and another dries up respiratory secretions to prevent aspiration. Drowsiness, lightheadedness, thirst, and dry mouth are normal and expected (see the *Focus on Children: Preoperative Medications* box).

After the medications are given, safety measures are taken to prevent falls. Bed rails are raised, and the patient is not allowed out of bed after this, so the client must void before the medications are given. If the client needs to void after the medications are given, the bedpan or urinal is used.

The bed is kept in the lowest position or raised to the highest position, according to hospital policy. Move furniture out of the way to make room for the stretcher. Also, clear the overbed table and the bedside stand to prevent damage to equipment and valuables. Raise the bed to the highest position for transferring the client from the bed to the stretcher.

CREDIT • VALLEY

THE CREDIT VALLEY HOSPITAL

PRE-OPERATIVE CHECKLIST

Procedure: __________ **Date:** __________

____

Surgeon: __________ ☐ **SDA** ☐ **SDC**

SDC - Ride available? ☐ Yes ☐ No ☐ ICU/CCU

Allergies: __________

____

Allergy Bracelet: ☐ Yes

Infectious Disease Risk: ☐ Yes ☐ No ☐ Unknown

Yes: __________

Initial in box	YES	N/A	OR RN
Addressograph Plate			
Identification Bracelet			
Consent to Surgery			
Blood Consent			
History & Physical			
Surgical Consultation			
Pre Anaesthetic Questionnaire			
Pre-op Teaching			
Old Chart to OR			
Dentures Removed			
Capped/loose teeth/braces			
Retainers/Palate Expanders			
Contact Lenses Removed			
Hearing Aid Removed			
Prosthesis Removed			
Jewellery / Body PiercingRemoved/Taped			
Nail Polish Removed			
Undergarments removed			
Other:			
Operative Side ☐ Bil. ☐ R ☐ L ☐ N/A			
Operative Site Marked by MD			

Last void time: __________ / __________

NPO since: __________ / __________

VITAL SIGNS - Time

Temp __________ Pulse __________

Resp. __________ BP __________

Weight __________ kg SpO2 __________

Other Patient Information

Pre-operative

RN Signature/Init. __________ / __________

Date. __________

Physical & Emotional Assessment

☐ Oriented ☐ Confused

☐ Semi-Conscious ☐ Anxious

☐ Unconscious ☐ Language Barrier

Language Spoken at Home __________

IMPLANTS			**INIT.**
AV Fistula	☐ R - ARM	☐ L - ARM	______
Total Hip	☐ R	☐ L	______
Total Knee	☐ R	☐ L	______
Pacemaker	☐ Yes		______

Location: __________

Other: __________ ______

LAB RESULTS/REPORTS

☐ Hemoglobin ☐ Sickle Cell

☐ Urinalysis ☐ Cap Blood Glucose: Result: ______

☐ Sickle Cell

☐ Electrolytes ☐ Urea ☐ Creat

☐ Glucose ☐ LFTs

☐ INR/PT / PTT ☐ ECG

☐ Gr & Reserve/OB Mom ☐ CXR

☐ Crossmatch _____ units ☐ Other:

☐ Autologous _____ units

Abnormal Results:

Medication Administration	**Initial**
	/
	/
	/
	/
	/
	/

IV Solution ☐ No

IV site/cath. size

RN Signature:

Operating Room

RN Signature/Init. __________ / __________

Date. __________

5322 D HR (Sept/2005)

PRE-OPERATIVE CHECKLIST

Figure 46–2 Preoperative checklist. **Courtesy:** Credit Valley Hospital, Mississauga, ON.

focus on
» CHILDREN

Preoperative Medications

Some hospitals allow a parent or caregiver to stay with the child in the OR while anesthesia is given. The person can stay until the child loses consciousness.

Transport to the Operating Room

A nurse or an attendant brings a stretcher to the client's room, and the client is transferred onto the stretcher and covered with a bath blanket to provide warmth and prevent exposure. Falling is prevented by securing the safety straps and raising the side rails. A small pillow is sometimes placed under the client's head for comfort. Assist with all of this, as required.

After identification checks have been made, the client's chart is given to the OR staff member.

The nurse responsible for preoperative care may go with the client to the OR entrance. Often family members also are allowed to accompany the client up to this point.

ANESTHESIA

Anesthesia is the loss of feeling or sensation produced by a medication. Anesthetics are given by specially trained physicians called *anesthetists*. There are three types of anesthesia:

1. **General anesthesia**—produces unconsciousness and the loss of feeling or sensation. A medication is given intravenously or a gas is inhaled.
2. **Regional anesthesia**—produces loss of sensation or feeling in a large area of the body. The client does not lose consciousness. A medication is injected into a body part.
3. **Local anesthesia**—produces loss of sensation in a small area. A medication is injected at the specific site.

THE POSTOPERATIVE PERIOD

During the **postoperative** (after surgery) period, the client is taken to the recovery room (RR). This is often called the post-anesthesia room (PAR) or post-anesthesia care unit (PACU). In the recovery room, which is near the OR, the client recovers from the anesthetic after the surgery. This can take 1 to 2 hours, during which time the client is watched very closely. Some clients may suffer from nausea and vomiting. Vital signs are taken and observations are made frequently. The client leaves the recovery room when:

- Vital signs are stable
- The respiratory function is good
- The client can respond and is able to call for help when needed

The physician gives the transfer order, when appropriate.

Preparing the Client's Room

The room must be ready for the client's return from the recovery room. A open bed is made (see Chapter 26), and equipment and supplies needed for the client's postoperative care are brought to the room. The nurse tells you if special measures and equipment are needed. The room is prepared right after the client has been taken to the OR. Preparations include:

- Making an open bed
- Placing equipment and supplies in the room:
  - Thermometer
  - Stethoscope
  - Sphygmomanometer
  - Kidney basin
  - Tissues
  - Waterproof bed protector
  - Vital signs flowsheet
  - I&O record
  - IV pole
  - Wound dressings
  - Other items, as directed by the nurse
- Raising the bed to its highest position

- Lowering bed rails
- Moving furniture to make room for the stretcher

Return From the Recovery Room

The recovery room nurse calls the nursing unit when the client is ready for transfer, and the client is transported by the recovery room nurses. A nurse meets the client on the nursing unit, and the client is transferred from the stretcher to bed. Assist, as needed, with the transfer. Also, assist the staff with positioning the client.

Have an extra blanket ready for the client, as clients often feel cold after surgery.

Vital signs are taken by a nurse after the client has been positioned in bed. Vital signs are usually measured in the following frequencies:

- Every 15 minutes the first hour
- Every 30 minutes for 1 to 2 hours
- Every hour for 4 hours
- Every 4 hours

The nurse also observes the client and checks dressings for bleeding. Catheters, IV infusions, and other tube placements and functions are checked, and necessary care and treatments are given. Bed rails are raised, and the call bell is placed within the client's reach. When the family is allowed to see the client varies with each hospital.

Observations

The client requires careful monitoring during the postoperative period. After the client is stable, you may be asked to check the client frequently. The nurse tells you how often to check the client. This is an important function—always be alert for the signs and symptoms listed in Box 46–2, and report them to the nurse immediately.

Box 46–2 Postoperative Observations

- Choking
- A drop or rise in blood pressure
- Bright red blood from the incision, drainage tubes, or suction tubes
- A pulse rate of more than 100 or less than 60 beats per minute
- A weak or irregular pulse
- A rise or drop in body temperature
- Hypoxia (see Chapter 44)
- The need for upper airway suctioning, signalled by any of the following:
  - Tachypnea (rapid breathing)
  - Dyspnea (difficult, laboured, or painful breathing)
  - Moist-sounding respirations
  - Gurgling or gasping
  - Restlessness
  - Cyanosis (bluish colour of the skin, lips, and nails)
- Shallow, slow breathing
- Weak cough
- Complaints of thirst
- Cold, moist, clammy, or pale skin
- Increased drainage on or under dressings or on bed linens (including drawsheets, bottom sheets, and pillowcases)
- Complaints of pain or nausea
- Vomiting
- Confusion or disorientation
- Other measurements and observations, as directed by a nurse:
  - The amount, character, and time of the first voiding after surgery
  - Intake and output
  - Blood in the IV tubing
  - Redness or swelling around the IV insertion site
  - The appearance of drainage from a urinary catheter, nasogastric tube, or wound suction
  - Any other observation that can indicate a change in the client's condition

Positioning

Proper positioning after surgery promotes comfort and prevents complications. The type of surgery determines positioning and, possibly, position restrictions. The client is usually positioned for easy and comfortable breathing and to prevent stress on the incision. When the client is in the supine position, the head of the bed is usually raised slightly, and the client's head may be turned to the side, which will help prevent aspiration if vomiting occurs.

Repositioning every 1 to 2 hours helps prevent respiratory and circulatory complications. Turning may be painful for the client, so provide support, and turn the client with smooth, gentle motions. Pillows and other positioning devices are often used (see Chapters 23 and 24).

The nurse tells you when to reposition the client and the positions allowed. Usually you assist the nurse, but sometimes you will turn and reposition the client yourself when the client's condition is stable and care is simple (see the *Focus on Older Adults: Postoperative Positioning* box).

Coughing and Deep Breathing

Respiratory complications in the postsurgical period must be prevented. There are two major complications: (1) *pneumonia,* an inflammation and infection in the lung; and (2) *atelectasis*, the collapse of a portion of the lung. Coughing and deep-breathing exercises and incentive spirometry help prevent these complications (see Chapter 44) and are done every 1 to 2 hours when the client is awake. For comfort, the client should be instructed to splint their incision, if possible (see the *Focus on Older Adults: Respiratory Complications After Surgery* box).

focus on ›› OLDER ADULTS

Postoperative Positioning

Many older adults have stiff and painful joints even before surgery, and soreness of muscles, bones, and joints occurs from positioning on the operating room table. Take care to turn and reposition older adults slowly and gently.

Stimulating Circulation

After surgery, circulation must be stimulated, especially for blood flow in the legs. If blood flow is sluggish, a blood clot (**thrombus**) can form in the deep leg veins (Figure 46–3, *A*). Part of the thrombus can break loose and travel through the bloodstream. It then becomes an **embolus**—a blood clot that travels through the vascular system until it lodges in a distant vessel (Figure 46–3, *B*). An embolus from a vein can eventually lodge as far away as in the lungs (pulmonary embolus) and can cause severe respiratory problems and even death.

Leg Exercises. Leg exercises help increase venous blood flow and thus prevent the formation of a thrombus. Leg exercises are easy to do; however, provide assistance if the client is weak. If the client has had leg surgery, a physician's order is needed for the exercises. Your supervisor will tell you when the client should do the exercises. The exercises are done at least every 1 or 2 hours while the client is awake. Have the client assume the supine position and do each of the following exercises five times (see Chapter 24):

- Make circles with the toes (ankle-rotating exercises)
- Dorsiflex and plantar flex the feet (calf-pumping exercises)
- Flex and extend one knee and then the other (Figure 46–4).
- Raise and lower one leg off the bed (Figure 46–5). Repeat this exercise with the other leg.

focus on ›› OLDER ADULTS

Respiratory Complications After Surgery

Age-related changes increase the older adult's risk for respiratory complications following surgery. Since the respiratory muscles are weaker and lung tissue is less elastic, the client has less strength for coughing. Coughing, deep breathing, and incentive spirometry are, however, very important, and the client must be encouraged to do these exercises to prevent respiratory complications.

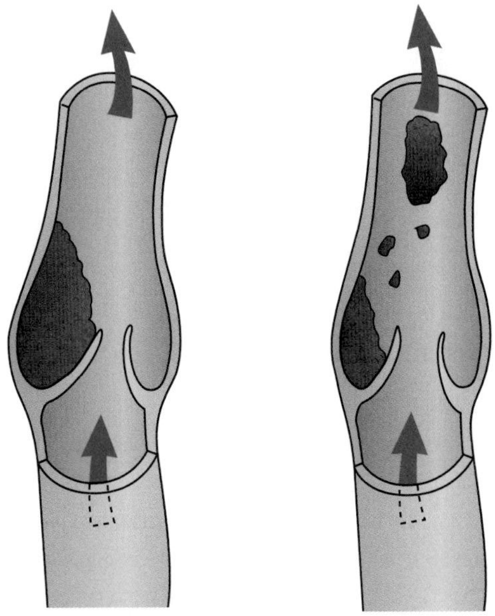

Figure 46–3 **A,** A thrombus (blood clot) is attached to the wall of a vein. The arrows show the direction of blood flow. **B,** Part of the thrombus has broken off and become an embolus. The embolus will travel in the bloodstream until it lodges in a distant vessel.

Do not place pillows under the client's calf as it may cause pooling of blood and create a risk for clot formation.

Elastic Stockings and Bandages. Elastic stockings and bandages help prevent the formation of a thrombus. The elastic exerts pressure on the veins, promoting venous blood flow to the heart. Elastic stockings or bandages are often ordered for postoperative clients and for regular use in those with heart disease and circulatory disorders.

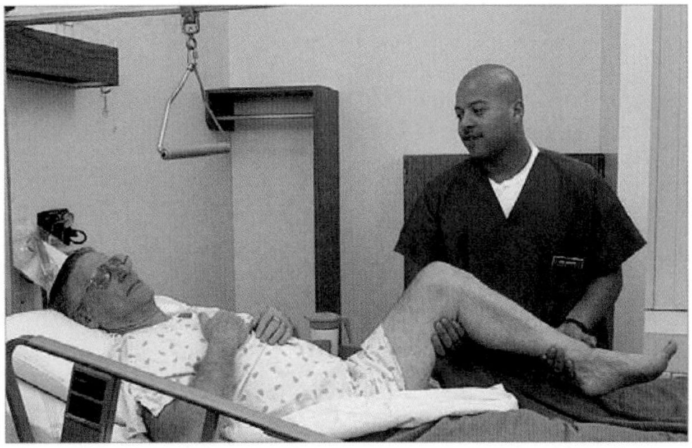

Figure 46–4 The client flexes and then extends the knee during postoperative leg exercises.

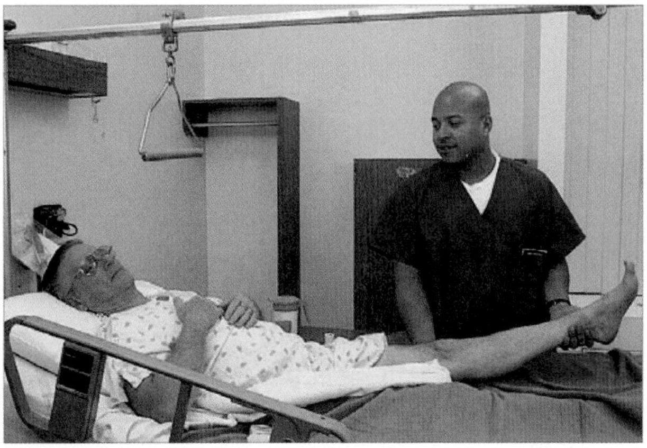

Figure 46–5 Assist the client with raising and lowering the leg.

Both elastic stockings and bandages could harm the client if applied improperly. Therefore, most hospitals allow only nurses to apply them to acute care clients. If you are assigned this task, make sure that it is in your scope of practice and that employer policy allows you to do it. Also, ensure that you have been properly trained and are closely supervised (see Chapter 30 for a discussion on the application of elastic stockings and bandages).

Early Ambulation

Early ambulation prevents postoperative circulatory complications, such as thrombus formation, pneumonia, atelectasis, constipation, and urinary tract infections. The client is usually encouraged to ambulate even on the day of surgery. The client first sits up with the legs over the edge of the bed (dangling the legs; see Chapter 23). If blood pressure and pulse are stable, the client is assisted out of bed. Usually the client does not walk very far, just a few feet in the room. Walking distance is increased as the client gains strength.

The nurse will tell you when to help the client ambulate. Usually you assist the nurse the first time the client ambulates.

Wound Healing

The surgical incision needs protection, so measures are taken to promote healing and prevent infection. Sterile dressing changes are done by a physician or a nurse. Some hospitals allow support workers to perform simple dressing care if the client is stable (see Chapter 42 for a discussion on wound healing).

Nutrition and Fluids

The client has an IV infusion upon his or her return from the OR. Continuation of the IV therapy depends on the type of surgery and the client's condition, for example, nausea and vomiting caused by anesthesia. The client's diet progresses from NPO to clear liquids, to full liquids, to a light diet, to a regular diet that is ordered by the physician. Frequent oral hygiene is important when the patient is NPO.

Some clients have nasogastric (NG) tubes (see Chapter 28) after surgery. The NG tube is attached to suction equipment to keep the stomach empty. The patient is NPO and receives IV therapy.

Elimination

Anesthesia, the surgery, and being NPO can all affect normal fecal and urinary elimination, and medications for pain relief can cause constipation. You will be asked to take measures to promote elimination, as directed by the nurse (see Chapters 31 and 32).

Fluid intake and output are measured during the postoperative period. It is important that the client urinates within 8 hours after surgery. Report the time and amount of the client's first voiding. If the client does not void within 8 hours, a catheterization is usually ordered. Some clients have catheters inserted routinely after surgery, for example, after bladder surgery (see Chapter 31 for care of the client with a catheter).

Adequate fluid intake and return to a regular diet are needed for normal bowel movement. Suppositories or enemas may be ordered if the client is constipated, and rectal tubes may be ordered for relief of flatulence (see Chapter 32).

Comfort and Rest

Pain is common after surgery. The degree of pain depends on the extent of surgery, incision site, and the presence of drainage tubes, casts, or other devices, as well as positioning during surgery that can cause muscle strains and discomfort. The physician orders medications for pain relief, and the nurse will tell you how to promote comfort and rest (see Chapter 22 for guidelines listed as part of the client's care plan).

Personal Hygiene

Personal hygiene is important for the client's physical and mental well-being. Wound drainage and skin prep solutions can irritate the skin and cause discomfort, and NPO can cause dry mouth and breath odours. Moist, clammy skin from blood pressure changes or elevated body temperatures also cause discomfort. Frequent oral hygiene, hair care, and a complete bed bath the day after the surgery help refresh and renew the client physically and psychologically. The gown should be changed whenever it becomes wet or soiled (see Chapter 29).

REVIEW

Answers to these questions are at the bottom of the page.

Circle T if the answer is true or circle F if the answer is false.

1. T F **Hair is kept out of the face for surgery by using pins, clips, or combs.**
2. T F **Nail polish is removed before surgery.**
3. T F **Women can wear makeup to surgery.**
4. T F **Clients can wear pyjamas when going to the operating room for surgery.**
5. T F **Contact lenses are removed before surgery.**
6. T F **An open bed is made before the client's return from the recovery room.**
7. T F **A drop in a patient's blood pressure is reported to the nurse immediately.**
8. T F **The client ambulates for the first time the day after the surgery.**
9. T F **Intake and output are measured after surgery.**
10. T F **A surgical client should void within 8 hours after surgery.**

Circle the BEST answer.

11. **Which of the following is *true* of elective surgery?**
    - A. The surgery is done immediately
    - B. The need for surgery is sudden and unexpected
    - C. Surgery is scheduled for a later date
    - D. General anesthesia is always used
12. **You can assist in a client's psychological preparation by explaining:**
    - A. The reason for the surgery
    - B. The procedures you will be doing
    - C. The risks and possible complications of surgery
    - D. What to expect during the preoperative and postoperative periods
13. **Preoperatively, Mr. Long is:**
    - A. NPO
    - B. Allowed only water
    - C. Given a regular breakfast
    - D. Given a tube feeding
14. **Cleansing enemas are ordered for Mr. Long preoperatively. The enemas are given:**
    - A. To clean the colon of feces
    - B. To prevent bleeding
    - C. To relieve flatus
    - D. To prevent pain
15. **Mr. Long's preoperative medication has been given to him. He:**
    - A. Must remain in bed
    - B. Is allowed to walk within his room
    - C. Can use the commode to void
    - D. Is allowed only sips of water
16. **General anesthesia:**
    - A. Is injected into a body part
    - B. Produces unconsciousness and the loss of feeling or sensation
    - C. Is a specially educated physician
    - D. Produces loss of sensation or feeling in a body part
17. **Mr. Long must do coughing and deep breathing exercises after surgery to prevent:**
    - A. Bleeding
    - B. A pulmonary embolus
    - C. Respiratory complications
    - D. Pain and discomfort
18. **Leg exercises are ordered for Mr. Long. Which of the following is *true*?**
    - A. Leg exercises stimulate circulation
    - B. Leg exercises do not prevent thrombus formation
    - C. Leg exercises are done 15 times every 1 or 2 hours
    - D. Leg exercises are done only for leg surgery
19. **Postoperatively, Mr. Long's position is changed:**
    - A. Every 2 hours
    - B. Every 3 hours
    - C. Every 4 hours
    - D. Every shift

Answers: 1.F, 2.T, 3.F, 4.F, 5.T, 6.T, 7.T, 8.F, 9.T, 10.T, 11.C, 12.B, 13.A, 14.A, 15.A, 16.B, 17.C, 18.A, 19.A

CHAPTER 47

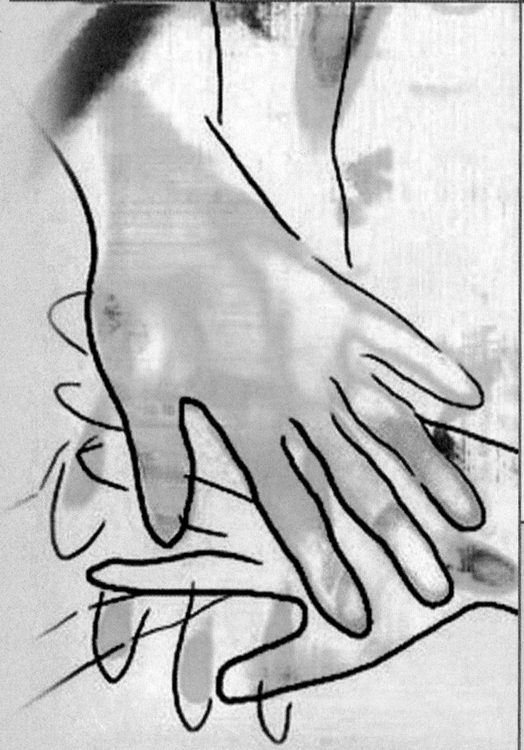

Caring for a Client Who Is Dying

OBJECTIVES

- Define the key terms listed in this chapter.
- Explain how culture, religion, and age influence attitudes toward death.
- Describe the five stages of grief.
- Explain how to help meet a dying client's needs.
- Describe the needs of the family of a dying client.
- Describe palliative care.
- Explain the importance of an advance directive.
- Identify the signs of approaching death and the signs of death.
- Describe how to assist in giving postmortem care.
- Demonstrate the procedures described in this chapter.

key terms

advance directive A legal document in which a person states his or her wishes about future health care, treatment, and personal care; the document is put into effect when the person is unable to make or express these wishes; **living will**.

anticipatory grief The sense of loss and sorrow experienced before an expected loss happens.

grief The process of moving from deep sorrow caused by loss toward healing and recovery.

living will See **advance directive**.

palliative care Services for clients (and their families) living with or dying from a progressive, life-threatening illness; these services aim to relieve suffering and improve comfort, not cure the illness.

postmortem care Care of the body after (*post*) death (*mortem*).

rigor mortis The stiffness or rigidity (*rigor*) of skeletal muscles that occurs after death (*mortis*).

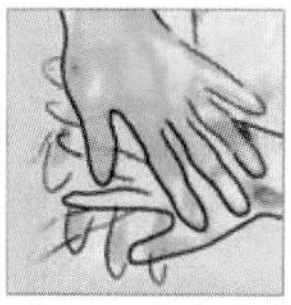

Clients who are dying are cared for in facilities or at home. Health care team members see death often, and some may be unsure of their feelings about death. They may be uncomfortable with dying clients and the subject of death. Dying clients may represent helplessness and the failure to cure and may also remind them of their own eventual death or the death of their loved ones.

As a support worker, you will be required to help meet the physical, social, emotional, intellectual, and spiritual needs of clients who are dying. Your feelings and beliefs about death and dying affect the care you give, so you need to understand both the dying process and your own attitudes toward death and dying, which will help you provide compassionate care. Before reading on, reflect on the following:

- What has been your experience with death?
- What are your feelings and beliefs about death and dying?
- How have your experiences and culture shaped your beliefs?

LIFE-THREATENING ILLNESS

Many life-threatening illnesses have no cure, and some injuries are so serious that the body cannot function. In these cases, recovery is not expected, and the illness or injury inevitably ends in death.

Health care professionals cannot predict the exact time of death. A client may have days, months, weeks, or years to live. Some clients who are expected to live for a short time live for many years, while others who are expected to live longer die much sooner than predicted. A client's hope and the will to live can influence dying and living. Some clients die sooner than expected because they lose the will to live.

ATTITUDES TOWARD DEATH

Personality, culture, religion, age, and experience influence attitudes toward death. Many people fear death; some do not believe they will die; and some accept and even look forward to death. A person's attitude toward death often changes with age and experience.

Until the beginning of the twentieth century, most Canadians died in their own homes, and families cared for loved ones who were dying. Death was considered a natural part of life. Today, however, most Canadians die in facilities. Many people have never seen a dying person or a dead body, so death is a frightening experience for them.

Culture and Religion

Practices and attitudes about death differ among cultures. Attitudes toward death are closely related to religion (see the *Respecting Diversity: Death and*

Dying Rituals box). Some believe that there is no suffering and hardship, that they will be reunited with loved ones, and that sins and misdeeds will be punished in the afterlife. Some believe there is no afterlife.

People have various religious beliefs about the body's form after death. Some believe that the body keeps its physical form, while others believe that only the spirit or soul is present in the afterlife. Some religions have the concept of *reincarnation,* which is the belief that the spirit or soul is reborn in another human body or in another life form.

Many clients experience a strengthening of their religious beliefs when they are faced with death, and religious faith often provides comfort to the dying person and the family.

Age

People's attitudes and responses to dying are highly individual. Age and stage of life are some of the major influences on people's feelings and reactions with regard to death.

Infants and toddlers have no concept of death. Between the ages of 3 and 5 years, children are curious and have some ideas about death because they know when family members or pets die, and they notice dead birds and insects. However, they may think that death is only a temporary state. Not answering their questions about death accurately and properly can cause fear and confusion. For example, children who are told "He is sleeping" may be afraid to go to sleep. Children between ages 5 and 7 know that death is final, though they may not think it will happen to them.

Adults often have more fears about death than children. They may fear pain and suffering, dying alone, separation from loved ones, and loss of dignity. They may worry about the care and support of those left behind. Some people have regrets about missed opportunities, failed relationships, or unfulfilled hopes and dreams. Some may feel that their

RESPECTING DIVERSITY

Death and Dying Rituals

Hinduism	The dying person may be laid on the floor. A priest ties a thread around the neck or wrist, and it should not be removed. After the client's death, a priest pours water in the client's mouth. The family washes the body before cremation.
Sikhism	The body of the deceased person must wear or have the five Ks: *Kesh,* uncut hair; *Kangra,* wooden comb; *Kara,* wrist band; *Kirpan,* sword; *Kach,* shorts.
Buddhism	A priest is called in before a person's death and he performs the last rites and chanting at the dying person's bedside. Burial and cremation are both acceptable.
Shinto	Jewellery is removed from the body, which is then washed and dressed in a white kimono and straw shoes.
Islam	The dying person confesses his or her sins. After death, the body is washed and wrapped in white cloth; the head is turned toward the right shoulder facing east, toward Mecca.
Judaism	The body is washed by the burial society, and someone remains with the body (Orthodox and Conservative Jews) all the time. Whenever possible, burial is to take place within 24 hours after death.
Christianity	Rituals vary greatly among groups. Many give last rites or communion to the dying person. Many groups prefer burial to cremation.

Remember, individuals may not follow every belief and practice of their culture and religion. Each client is unique. Do not judge the client by your own standards.

Source: Ross-Kerr, J.C., Wood, M.J., Potter, P.A., & Perry, A.J. (2001). *Canadian fundamentals of nursing* (2nd ed., p. 600). Toronto: Mosby.

lives did not have any meaning, but some feel that their lives did make a difference.

Older adults often have fewer fears about death, as they expect to die, and many have experienced the deaths of friends and loved ones. Some feel they have lived full and complete lives, while some have regrets. Some older adults welcome death as freedom from pain, suffering, and disability. Like younger adults, older adults often fear dying alone.

Although age and stage of life influence a person's response to dying, you cannot predict what a particular individual's response will be.

THE STAGES OF GRIEF

Grief is the process of moving from deep sorrow caused by loss toward healing and recovery. Both the client who is dying and his or her loved ones experience a range of emotions when faced with loss. Many people experience **anticipatory grief**—the sense of loss and sorrow experienced before an expected loss happens.

Dr. Elisabeth Kübler-Ross identified the following five stages of grief that a dying client and his or her family may experience:

1. ***Denial.*** During the first stage, the client refuses to believe that he or she is dying. "No, not me" is a common response. The client does not accept that the condition will end in death. He or she cannot deal with the problems or decisions related to the illness or injury. This stage can last for a few hours, days, or much longer. Some people may still be in denial when they die.
2. ***Anger.*** During this stage, the client thinks "Why me?" He or she feels anger and, sometimes, rage and may envy and resent those with life and health. Family, friends, and the health care team often become targets of anger. The client may blame him or herself or blame others and find fault with those who are loved and needed the most. If your client displays anger, remember that anger is a normal stage of grief. Do not take the anger personally, and control any urge to argue with the client.
3. ***Bargaining.*** The anger passes, and the client enters the third stage. The client now says "Yes, me, but …" Often the client bargains with God for more time, and promises are made in exchange for more time. The client may want to see a child get married, see the birth of a grandchild, have one more summer, or live for some other event. This stage may not be obvious to you, as bargaining usually is private and done on the spiritual level.
4. ***Depression.*** During the fourth stage, the client thinks "Yes, me" and is very sad. He or she mourns things that have been lost and the future loss of life. The client may cry or say little. Some clients may talk about loved ones and things that will be left behind.
5. ***Acceptance.*** This is the final stage. The client is at peace—he or she has said what needs to be said, has completed unfinished business, and accepts death. This stage may last for many months or years. Reaching acceptance of death does not mean that death is near.

All dying clients do not always go through all five stages of grieving. A client may never get beyond a certain stage. Some reach the final stage of accepting death without going through the other stages. Some move back and forth between stages. For example, a client may reach the depression stage, move back to bargaining, and then move forward to acceptance. Some clients remain in one stage until death.

The family of the dying client may also experience some or all of the five stages of grief. Often family members do not go through the stages at the same time as the client who is dying. For example, a woman may still be angry at her husband's diagnosis when her husband has reached the acceptance stage. Like dying clients, their family members also may move back and forth between stages.

Members of the health care team also experience the stages of grief. Caring for a dying client is a moving and emotional experience, and supporting a grieving family can be very difficult. As a support worker, you will grieve the loss of clients you have cared for. It is therefore important that you examine your feelings about loss and grief. Do not turn away from these feelings, and develop your own support system that includes your supervisor and co-workers. Many facilities have support groups to help team members share their grief (see Box 47–1).

Palliative Care

The idea of hospice or palliative care began as a place of comfort for weary travellers in Europe during the Middle Ages. Dr. Cecily Saunders opened the first freestanding research and teaching hospice in London, England, in 1967. In 1976, pilot projects for palliative care were started at St. Boniface Hospital in Winnipeg and the Royal Victoria Hospital in Montreal. Soon after, hospice services in Canada proliferated both in the community and hospital settings.

The terms *palliative care* and *hospice care* are often used to mean the same thing—the compassionate care of dying persons directed at comfort and pain management. **Palliative care** can be defined as the active compassionate care of the terminally ill at a time when the disease is no longer responsive to traditional treatment for cure or when prolongation of life and the control of symptoms—physical, emotional and spiritual—is the most important goal.

A hospice program provides compassionate care to dying persons. Some cities and towns have community hospice organizations, which are usually nonprofit organizations run by volunteers and sometimes working closely with home care programs.

Separate facilities called hospices also provide palliative care. Many hospices provide care in houses that once were private homes that are often located in quiet neighbourhoods in park-like settings. The goal is to provide a comfortable, peaceful setting. Some hospices provide palliative care to specific client groups, such as those dying of AIDS or cancer.

The most common facility setting is the palliative care unit within a hospital. Many long-term care facilities also provide palliative care.

The goal of hospice or palliative care is not to prolong life but to provide the best quality of life during the final days before death. The three main goals of hospice/palliative care are:

1. ***To assist in controlling the pain and symptoms of illness.*** Most terminally ill clients fear pain more than death itself. Some of a dying client's fears and anxieties can be alleviated by providing good pain control.
2. ***To ensure that death is a natural process.*** The goal of care is not to prolong life but to provide the best quality of life during the final days before death. As a result, medical interventions such as respirators and tube feedings are not used to keep clients alive.
3. ***To provide compassionate care.*** A team of professionals, nonprofessionals, and volunteers with a special interest in the field of palliative care work with sensitivity to meet the needs of the dying client and his or her family. The right to die with dignity is strongly upheld.

Because palliative care is demanding and complex, it requires the expertise of more than one health care professional and a team approach. The common goal or purpose behind all the activities is to assist the dying client and his or her family in the best way possible. Team members vary depending

Box 47–1 Case Study: Support Worker Grief

Indira works in a long-term care facility. She relates this experience about her grief following the death of a resident:

"I cared for Mrs. Giovanni on and off for 5 years. We always talked while I gave care, and I got to know her quite well. She used to tell me about her early life in Italy before she came to Canada and show me photographs of her family.

"I was with her the day before she died. She wanted me to stay with her, and I did. I didn't know her end was so near. When I heard the next day that she had died, I was really upset. I had not been this sad when other residents died. I felt sad for several weeks afterwards.

"I shared my feelings with the RN on my unit and a co-worker. It helped to talk about it. Gradually, I accepted that my feelings were a natural reaction to loss and death. Looking back, I'm glad I got to know Mrs. Giovanni so well and made time for her the day before she died."

on the situation (see Box 47–2) Some clients may choose to include a close friend as well as family members in the team, who can provide much emotional and physical care. Even in facility settings, family members and close friends are encouraged to help with the client's care, and the client himself or herself can be an active participant in his or her own care.

Although members of the team have one or more areas of expertise, their roles often overlap. For example, a client in the community may have a support worker provide assistance with personal care, but the hospice care nurse plays a similar role by bathing the client and monitoring skin condition. Another example is the nurse who assists with personal care may also provide counselling or physical therapy. Because roles overlap, it is important to ensure that the dying client receives the best care possible. Mutual respect between team members as well as communication, accurate charting, and information sharing are all essential to ensure the best care.

Caring for a Client Who Is Dying

The health care team helps meet the dying client's emotional, social, spiritual, intellectual, and physical needs, and every effort is made to promote physical and emotional comfort. The client's right to die in peace and with dignity is always kept in the forefront of these efforts (see Box 47–3 and the *Providing Compassionate Care: The Dying Client* box).

Box 47–2 Palliative/Hospice Care Team Members in the Home

Care Provider	General Responsibilities
Client and caregivers	– Caregivers may be family or friends – Participates in the decision-making process – Included in all discussions about care, whenever possible
Home care coordinator	Assesses client needs and coordinates services in the home
Support worker	– Assists the dying client with personal care and household tasks – Monitors client's situation and reports significant observations – Provides emotional support to dying client and caregivers
Hospice volunteer	Provides emotional support and information about services available to a dying client and caregivers
Spiritual adviser	Provides spiritual and emotional support to the dying client and caregivers
Occupational therapist	– Teaches caregivers and the dying client to complete activities of daily living – Provides emotional support to the dying client and caregivers
Physician	– Monitors the dying client's health status – Prescribes and monitors medications for pain and symptom management – Educates and provides emotional support to the dying client and caregivers
Physiotherapist	Teaches physical exercise and recommends assistive devices to keep the client as independent as possible
Social worker	Provides supportive counselling
Nurse	– Monitors medications and assists with pain and symptom management – Assists with personal care – Educates and provides emotional support to the dying client and caregivers

Other individuals may also assist the client and family, such as a nutritionist; a complementary therapist providing relaxation, massage, aromatherapy, acupuncture, therapeutic or healing touch, reflexology, music/art; and, of course, extended family and friends.

Emotional, Social, Intellectual, and Spiritual Needs

Clients who are dying need accurate information to make informed decisions. They may want to talk about their fears, worries, and anxieties. Some may want family and friends present, and some want to be alone. Others may want someone from the health care team to stay with them. Often clients prefer to talk at night when things are quiet and there are few distractions or because their fears and anxieties are worse at night. The following are ways you can meet a client's needs:

- ***Listening.*** If the client needs to share his or her worries and concerns with you, let the client talk. You do not need to talk or worry about saying the wrong thing or finding comforting words. Sometimes the client does not want to talk but just needs you around. Just being there and listening can be very helpful. If the client requests medical information, spiritual guidance, or counselling, immediately tell your supervisor. Remember, it is not your role to give clients information about their medical condition.
- ***Touch.*** Touch conveys caring and support when words cannot. Touch, along with silence, is a powerful and compassionate way to communicate. However, always keep in mind that some clients may not like to be touched.
- ***Respect.*** The client may share thoughts about his or her religious or spiritual beliefs with you. Be respectful as you listen to the client.

Box 47–3 The Dying Person's Bill of Rights

- I have the right to be treated as a living human being until I die.
- I have the right to maintain a sense of hopefulness, however changing its focus may be.
- I have the right to be cared for by those who can maintain a sense of hopefulness, however changing this might be.
- I have the right to express my feelings and emotions about my approaching death, in my own way.
- I have the right to participate in decisions concerning my care.
- I have the right to expect continuing medical and nursing attention even though "cure" goals must be changed to "comfort" goals.
- I have the right not to die alone.
- I have the right to be free of pain.
- I have the right to have my questions answered honestly.
- I have the right not to be deceived.
- I have the right to have help from and for my family in accepting my death.
- I have the right to die in peace and with dignity.
- I have the right to retain my individuality and not to be judged for my decisions, which may be contrary to the beliefs of others.
- I have the right to discuss and enlarge my religious and spiritual experiences, regardless of what they may mean to others.
- I have the right to expect that the sanctity of the human body will be respected after death.
- I have the right to be cared for by caring, sensitive, knowledgeable people who will attempt to understand my needs and will be able to gain some satisfaction in helping me face my death.

Adapted from: Barbus, A.J. (1975). The hospice RN: Patient's bill of rights: A dying patient's bill of last rights. *American Journal of Nursing* 75(1): 99.

Physical Needs

Dying may take a few minutes, hours, days, or weeks. Body processes slow down, the client grows weak, and changes occur in consciousness. The health care team encourages the client to do as much as possible independently during this period. As the client weakens, more help is provided with personal care. Eventually, the client may need to depend on others for all basic needs and activities of daily living.

- ***Pain relief and comfort.*** Some clients experience severe pain, and health care professionals administer medications to relieve pain. The care plan may call for other measures such as back massages and relaxation techniques. Skin care, personal hygiene, and good alignment promote comfort. Provide good mouth care, as this is comforting to the client. Follow the care plan (see Chapter 22).

PROVIDING COMPASSIONATE CARE

The Dying Client

- **Dignity.** Treat the dying client with respect, dignity, warmth, and empathy. Be sensitive to the client's wishes. Listen when the client wants to talk. Respect the client's need for quiet and silence. Do not avoid the client if you feel uncomfortable or sad. Put yourself in the client's shoes, and try to imagine how the client feels.

  Whether a client is dying at home or in a facility, the environment should be comfortable and pleasant, quiet, well lit, and well ventilated. Try to keep equipment and supplies out of view, as some clients may find equipment such as suction machines and drainage containers upsetting to look at. Display expressions of concern (such as flowers and cards) in clear view, as some clients may find these comforting.

  Be sensitive to the client's needs. Provide comfort through care and touch, if culturally appropriate for the client.

  Respect the client's religious views and practices. Do not impose your views on the client. Treat religious items and other personal possessions with care and respect.
- **Independence.** Encourage the client to do things for himself or herself without help, if he or she can. Offer to assist before actually doing something for the client. The client has the right to autonomy.
- **Preferences.** The client has the right to make choices about his or her care, treatment, and environment, so respect these choices. Ask before providing care. Respect a client's decision to refuse treatment and not prolong life. In all health care settings, the client and family should be free to arrange the room as they wish to reflect the client's choices. This shows respect and helps the client feel cared for.
- **Privacy.** The dying client has the right to privacy. Remember, do not expose the client unnecessarily during care. The client has the right not to have his or her body seen by others, so follow proper screening and privacy procedures. Provide privacy during prayer and spiritual moments. The client and family have the right to have visits in private. In facilities, privacy may need to be arranged; for example, a roommate may have to leave while the family visits. Some clients may ask to see a spiritual adviser. The client also has the right to confidentiality; protect this right before and after death. Share information about diagnosis, health, and treatment only with those involved in the client's care. Maintain confidentiality about the client's final moments and cause of death as well as statements and reactions of the family.
- **Safety.** Clients who are dying are at high risk for falls, choking, and other accidents. Know the safety measures that must be taken for each client. The dying client has the right to be free from abuse, mistreatment, and neglect. It must be ensured that family members or health care team members do not abuse or mistreat the client. Follow the safety measures described in Chapter 19.

- ***Comfort and positioning.*** Frequent position changes and supportive devices also promote comfort. You may need the help of another worker in order to turn the client slowly and gently. Semi-Fowler's position (Fowler's position with the knees slightly bent) is usually best for easing breathing problems. Ask the client what position is most comfortable.
- ***Vision and eye care.*** At the end of life, vision blurs and gradually fails, and the client may find a darkened room frightening. The room should therefore be well lit (if the client wishes), but bright lights and glares should be avoided. Since the client's vision may be failing, explain what you are doing. Secretions may collect in the corners of the client's eyes. Ease the client's discomfort by providing eye care. Follow the care plan. It may call for applying protective ointment and moist pads to the client's eyes.
- ***Hearing.*** Hearing is one of the last functions to be lost. Many clients, even unconscious ones, are able to hear until the moment of death. Always assume that the client can hear, and continue to introduce yourself and give explanations

and reassurance about the care you are giving even when the client is unconscious. Speak in a normal voice, offer words of comfort, and avoid topics that could upset the client.

- ***Speech.*** The client may have difficulty speaking, so it may be hard to understand what the client says. Some clients cannot speak at all. Anticipate clients' needs. Ask "yes" or "no" questions, and avoid asking questions that require long answers. Do not tire the client with questions, but do talk to the client.
- ***Mouth care.*** The client's mouth may feel dry, uncomfortable, or sore, and swallowing may be difficult and uncomfortable. Oral hygiene promotes comfort. Routine mouth care is given if the client can eat and drink. Frequent oral care is given as death nears and when the client has difficulty taking oral fluids. Oral hygiene is needed if mucus collects in the mouth and the client cannot swallow. Offer ice chips or small sips of fluids if the client has a dry mouth. Apply moisturizer to relieve dry, chapped lips. Follow the care plan.
- ***Nostril care.*** The client's nostrils may become crusted and irritated, usually by nasal secretions, oxygen cannulas, or nasogastric tubes. Clean the nose carefully. Apply lubricant, as directed by the care plan.
- ***Skin care.*** Circulation to the arms and legs slows as death approaches. Hands and feet may feel especially cold to the touch. Skin colour may change, and skin may appear pale or mottled (blotchy) and feel cold to the touch, but the client is usually not aware of feeling cold. The upper parts of the body may sweat as circulation to the peripheral parts fails. The body temperature may rise, and blankets may make the client feel too warm and cause restlessness, so only light bed coverings should be applied. Skin care, bathing, frequent position changes, and fresh garments and linens help keep the client comfortable. Measures must be taken to prevent pressure ulcers.
- ***Elimination.*** The dying client may have urinary or fecal incontinence. Follow the care plan for the use of incontinence products or bed protectors. Keep the client dry and clean. Give perineal care, as needed. Constipation and urinary retention are common, and the care plan may call for the use of enemas and catheter care, which may be delegated to you. Remember to follow Standard Practices.

Comforting the Family

This is a stressful time for family members, who may be very tired, sad, and tearful. Watching a loved one die and dealing with the eventual loss of that person can be very painful. If the family wants a spiritual adviser to be present with them, let your supervisor know immediately.

It may be very hard to find comforting words. Show your feelings by being respectful, empathetic, and supportive. You may need to listen to a family member who wants to talk. Do not feel the need to talk. Use touch to show your concern. In a home care setting, you can show your support in many ways. You might help by taking on household tasks while the family cares for the dying client, or you might provide respite care to give the caregivers a break. Follow the care plan.

In facilities, family members are usually allowed to stay as long as they wish, sometimes through the night. The health care team helps make them as comfortable as possible.

No matter what the setting, you need to respect the family's right to privacy while taking care not to neglect care because the family is present. Most facilities allow family members to give care. When they do, you may help them take beverage or meal breaks. Family members often hesitate to leave because they do not want to leave their loved one alone. Offering to remain with the client can be a great relief for the family and make them feel better about taking a much-needed break.

LEGAL ISSUES

A person's right to die is a much debated issue at present. Many clients do not want machines or other measures keeping them alive, so the client's informed consent is needed for any such treatment, as legally required by all provinces and territories (see Chapter 11). Clients may give or withhold consent and make their own decisions about care. Some clients, however, may be unable to do so due to confusion, dementia, or other impairments, so a substitute decision maker often makes decisions for these clients.

Advance Directive

An **advance directive** (**living will**) is a legal document in which a person states his or her wishes about future health care, treatment, and personal care. Health care includes all medical treatment: diagnostic, therapeutic, preventative, and palliative. Personal care includes shelter, hygiene, nutrition, clothing, and safety.

An advance directive is used when the person can no longer make decisions or express his or her wishes. Advance directives allow people to control their future health care. Without an advance directive, family members sometimes have to make difficult decisions on behalf of a loved one, and this can result in conflict in the family.

Every province and territory has legislation about advance directives. Most advance directives have a dual function. They allow a person to:

1. Appoint a representative (proxy) to make medical care and treatment and personal care decisions
2. Give written instructions about medical care and treatment and personal care

People often use advance directives to forbid certain types of treatment and care when there is no hope of recovery. For example, some people do not want life-sustaining measures that support or maintain life (e.g., tube feedings, ventilators, and cardio-pulmonary resuscitation [CPR]). These measures and other machines keep a person alive when death is likely. An advance directive may instruct physicians:

- Not to start measures that prolong dying
- To remove measures that prolong dying

Advance directives are known by different names and have different powers, depending on provincial or territorial legislation—in Alberta, advance directives are called *personal directives;* in Manitoba, they are called *health care directives;* and in Ontario, they are called *powers of attorney for personal care.*

Most people appoint a family member or friend to be their representative or proxy. In some cases, a lawyer may be named. The advance directive *only* comes into effect when a client can no longer make decisions about his or her own health care and personal care. When this happens, the proxy, who has been given the legal right to make decisions for the client, steps in to make decisions on behalf of the client.

In most provinces and territories, residents name a proxy to make decisions about personal care as well as medical care and treatment. However, in some parts of the country, a proxy can be used only for decisions about medical care and treatment.

Not all clients name a proxy. When no proxy is named, family members in consultation with the physician decide for the client. Some provinces, however, require a court application before any decision can be made on behalf of an incapable person.

"Do Not Resuscitate" Orders

Even when sudden and unexpected death is possible, every effort is made to save the client's life. An emergency response system is activated, and CPR is started. In facilities, nurses, physicians, and emergency staff immediately get to the client's bedside, and in the community, ambulances and paramedics rush to the scene, bringing emergency and life-saving equipment with them. CPR and other life-support measures are continued until the client is resuscitated or until a physician declares the client dead. Some facilities, however, do not offer CPR as part of their policy, so clients and new staff need to be clear about the policies and procedures of these facilities.

Physicians often write "do not resuscitate" (DNR) or "no code" orders for clients who are not expected to recover. This means that the client will not be resuscitated, and the client is allowed to die in peace and with dignity. The orders are written after consulting with the client and his or her family. The family or the proxy, in consultation with the physician, makes the decision about the DNR order if the client is not mentally able. Some people prepare an advance directive that contains DNR orders.

You may not agree with care and resuscitation decisions. However, you must follow the client's (or proxy's) wishes and the physician's orders, even if these are against your personal, religious, and cultural beliefs. If you are not comfortable with care and resuscitation decisions, discuss the matter with your supervisor.

Signs of Death

Signs that death is near may occur rapidly or slowly. These include:

- ***Loss of movement, muscle tone, and sensation***—usually begins in the feet and legs and eventually spreads to other parts. When a client's mouth muscles relax, the jaw drops, and the mouth may stay open. The client's face often looks peaceful.
- ***Slowing of peristalsis and other digestive functions***—abdominal distention, fecal/urinary incontinence, fecal impaction, nausea, and vomiting are common. The client usually refuses to eat or drink.
- ***Rise in body temperature***—the client is cool or cold to touch, looks pale, and perspires heavily.
- ***Failure of circulation***—the pulse is fast, weak, and irregular. Blood pressure begins to fall. Skin may have a mottled appearance.
- ***Failure of the respiratory system***—presence of *Cheyne-Stokes* respirations—respirations that gradually increase in rate and depth, and then become shallow, slow, and stop for up to 30 seconds. Mucus collects in the airway and causes a wet, gurgling sound as the client breathes, known as the *death rattle.*
- ***Decrease in pain and loss of consciousness***—some clients may remain conscious until the moment of death.
- ***Increased sleep***—the client may sleep a lot and not participate in conversations.
- ***Changes in eating***—the client may not be interested in eating food they once loved or have cravings for odd food.
- ***Loss of interest***—they may not watch TV or read anymore.
- ***Losing touch with reality***—the client may become removed from reality.

The physiological signs of death include absence of pulse, respirations, or blood pressure; and fixed, dilated pupils. A physician determines that death has occurred and pronounces the person dead. In some parts of Canada, RNs are allowed to pronounce death in the home when the death is expected (see the *Focus on Home Care: When Death Occurs* box).

CARE OF THE BODY AFTER DEATH

Care of the body after (*post*) death (*mortem*) is called **postmortem care,** which begins after the client is pronounced dead and when no autopsy (an examination of the body to determine the cause of death) is required. You may be asked to assist with postmortem care, and during this process, you may have contact with blood or body fluids. Follow Standard Practices.

Postmortem care is done to maintain the body's appearance by helping prevent discoloration and skin damage. Remember, the right to privacy and the right to be treated with dignity and respect should be preserved even after a client's death.

Within 2 to 3 hours after death, rigor mortis develops. **Rigor mortis** is the stiffness or rigidity (*rigor*) of skeletal muscles that occurs after death (*mortis*).

> **focus on ›› HOME CARE**
>
> **When Death Occurs**
>
> Some clients die at home, and you may be present at the time of death. Know your employer's policies and procedures. Call your supervisor, and follow his or her directions. Be supportive of the family.

1 2 3 ASSISTING WITH POSTMORTEM CARE

Remember to promote:

• **D**ignity • **I**ndependence • **P**references • **P**rivacy • **S**afety

Pre-Procedure

1 Perform hand hygiene.
2 Collect the following:
- Postmortem kit (shroud or body bag, ID tags, gauze squares, and safety pins)
- Bed protectors
- Wash basin
- Bath towels and wash cloths
- Tape
- Dressings
- Gloves
- Cotton balls
- Gown or clean garments

3 Provide for privacy.
4 Raise the bed to a comfortable working height. Make sure it is flat.*

Procedure

5 Put on gloves.
6 Bathe soiled areas with plain water. Dry thoroughly.
7 Place the body in the supine position. Straighten the arms and legs. Place a pillow under the head and shoulders (Figure 47–1).
8 Close the eyes by gently pulling the eyelids over the eyes. Apply moist cotton balls gently over the eyelids if the eyes will not stay closed.
9 Insert the dentures, if it is employer policy. If not, put them in a labelled denture container.
10 Close the mouth. If necessary, place a rolled towel under the chin to keep the mouth closed.
11 Follow employer policy about valuables, including jewellery. In many facilities, the support worker and the nurse together make a list of valuables and both sign a statement that the valuables have been placed in a sealed envelope.
12 Tape the wedding ring, if any, in place, if this is your employer's policy.
13 Follow employer policy and instructions with regard to drainage containers, tubes, and catheters.
14 Place a bed protector under the buttocks.
15 Remove soiled dressings and apply clean ones.
16 Dress the body in a clean gown, pyjamas, nightgown, or other clothes, as instructed. Position the body as in step 6.
17 Brush and comb the hair, if necessary.
18 Cover the body to the shoulders with a sheet if the family will view the body.
19 Put the client's belongings in a bag labelled with his or her name.*
20 Remove supplies, equipment, and linens. Tidy up the room. Provide soft lighting.*
21 Remove gloves. Perform hand hygiene.
22 When the family is viewing the body, leave the room, and return after the family leaves.
23 Perform hand hygiene. Put on gloves.
24 Fill out the ID tags. Tie one to an ankle or to the right big toe.*
25 Place the body in the body bag, or cover it with a sheet.* Apply the shroud as follows (Figure 47–2):
- **a** Bring the top down over the head.
- **b** Fold the bottom up over the feet.
- **c** Fold the sides over the body.
- **d** Pin or tape the shroud in place.

26 Attach the second ID tag to the shroud, sheet, or body bag.*
27 Leave the denture cup with the body.
28 Provide for privacy.
29 Remove gloves. Perform hand hygiene.

Post-Procedure

30 Strip the bed after the body has been removed. Wear gloves.*
31 Remove gloves. Perform hand hygiene.
32 Report the following to your supervisor:
- The time the body was taken by the funeral director
- What was done with jewellery, personal items, and so on
- What was done with dentures

*Steps marked with an asterisk may not apply in community settings.

Postmortem care involves positioning the body in normal alignment before rigor mortis sets in. The family may want to see the body before it is taken to the morgue or funeral home. The body should be placed in a natural position for this viewing.

In some cases, the body is prepared initially only for viewing. Postmortem care is completed later at the funeral home. If the client dies at home, the funeral home usually provides postmortem care.

Postmortem care may involve repositioning the body to clean soiled areas and to put the body in good alignment. Movement of the body can cause sounds to come from the body as air is expelled. Do not be frightened by these sounds; they are normal and expected.

As a support worker, you will not have full responsibility for postmortem care, but you may assist in the procedure.

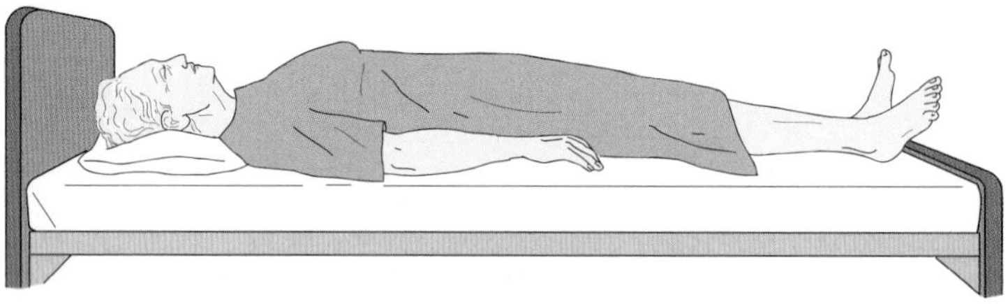

Figure 47–1 The body is in the supine position. Arms are straight at the sides. A pillow is placed under the head and shoulders.

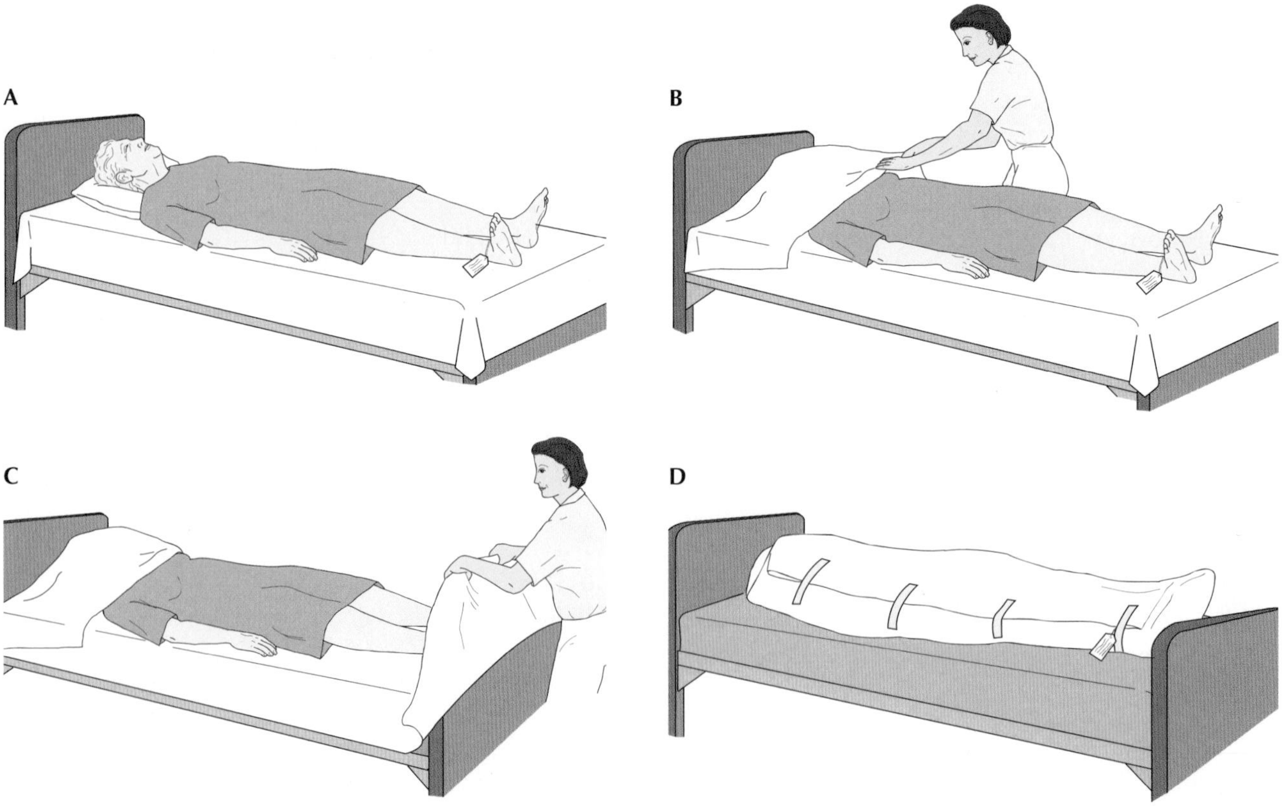

Figure 47–2 Applying a shroud. **A,** Place the body on the shroud. **B,** Bring the top of the shroud down over the head. **C,** Fold the bottom up over the feet. **D,** Fold the sides over the body. Tape or pin the sides together. Attach the ID tag.

REVIEW

Answers to these questions are at the bottom of the page.

Circle the BEST answer.

1. **Reincarnation is the belief that:**
   - A. There is no afterlife
   - B. The spirit or soul is reborn into another human body or another form of life
   - C. The body keeps its physical form in the afterlife
   - D. Only the spirit or soul is present in the afterlife

2. **Adults of all ages often fear:**
   - A. Dying alone
   - B. Reincarnation
   - C. The five stages of grief
   - D. Advance directives

3. **People in the stage of denial:**
   - A. Are angry
   - B. Make "deals" with God
   - C. Are sad or quiet
   - D. Refuse to believe they are dying

4. **Palliative care is:**
   - A. Treatment that prolongs life
   - B. Physical therapy for people with severe back pain
   - C. Massage therapy and relaxation techniques to relieve pain
   - D. Services for people with progressive and life-threatening illnesses that relieve or reduce uncomfortable symptoms

5. **When caring for a dying person, you should:**
   - A. Listen, and use touch when appropriate
   - B. Do most of the talking
   - C. Keep the room darkened
   - D. Speak in a loud voice

6. **As death approaches, the last sense to be lost is:**
   - A. Sight
   - B. Taste
   - C. Smell
   - D. Hearing

7. **Care of the dying person includes the following:**
   - A. Forcing fluids
   - B. Low sodium diet
   - C. Active range-of-motion exercises
   - D. Position changes

8. **The dying person is placed in:**
   - A. The supine position
   - B. Fowler's position
   - C. A position comfortable for the client
   - D. The dorsal recumbent position

9. **A woman is no longer able to make decisions about her own health care. Through an advance directive, she has appointed her sister as her proxy. Decisions about her health care are made by:**
   - A. Her son
   - B. Her physician
   - C. Her sister
   - D. Her lawyer

10. **A "do not resuscitate" order has been written for a client. This means:**
    - A. CPR will not be done
    - B. The person has a living will
    - C. Life-prolonging measures will be carried out
    - D. The person will be kept alive as long as possible

11. **Which of the following are signs of approaching death?**
    - A. Decreased body temperature and rapid pulse
    - B. Increased movement and muscle tone
    - C. Increased pain and blood pressure
    - D. Cheyne-Stokes respirations

12. **Postmortem care is done:**
    - A. After rigor mortis sets in
    - B. After the person is pronounced dead
    - C. When the funeral director arrives for the body
    - D. After the family has viewed the body

Answers: 1.B, 2.A, 3.D, 4.D, 5.A, 6.D, 7.D, 8.C, 9.C, 10.A, 11.D, 12.B

CHAPTER 48

Your Job Search

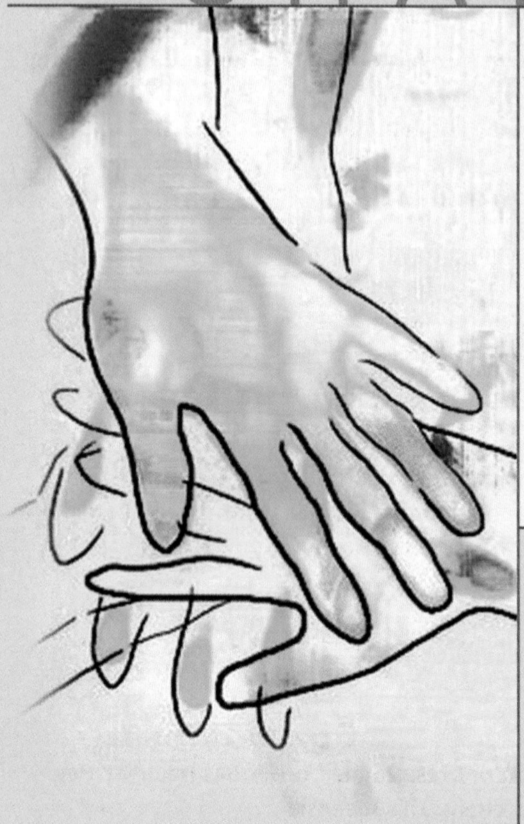

OBJECTIVES

- Summarize the key terms listed in this chapter.
- List three tools you need to organize yourself for your job search.
- Differentiate between a chronological résumé and a functional résumé.
- List three sources of advertised positions.
- Identify methods for finding out about unadvertised positions.
- List five details that are important in a letter of application.
- Summarize why you should take time completing application forms.
- List what interviewers are trying to determine during an interview.
- Summarize why the interview is a key element in the job search.
- Summarize why it is important to practise and plan before an interview.
- Name three ways to make a good impression at an interview.
- Summarize why it is important to write a thank-you note following an interview.
- Apply the techniques described in this chapter to your job application experience.

key terms

chronological résumé A résumé that highlights employment history, starting with the most current employment and working in reverse chronological order (backward) through earlier jobs.

cover letter A letter that accompanies the application; summarizes the job applied for and reasons for applying for that position.

functional résumé A résumé that highlights skills or functions and briefly lists positions held.

letter of application A letter that is included with a résumé; can be solicited or unsolicited; **cover letter**.

reference A person who can speak to a potential employer about the applicant's skills, abilities, and personal qualities.

résumé A concise one- to two-page summary of experience, education, work-related skills, and personal qualities.

solicited letter of application A letter of application that responds to an advertised position.

unsolicited letter of application A letter of application that enquires about potential openings.

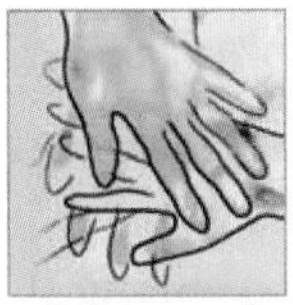

Finding a job takes discipline, focus, and hard work. For many people, the process is stressful because the end result is uncertain. However, with good preparation and a sound plan, the job search can be exciting and rewarding, as it gives you the opportunity to learn about yourself and to meet new people.

GETTING ORGANIZED

Your job search will be more successful if you get organized before you start. Choose a place in your home where you will work, and then make sure that you have the following tools in your workspace:

- ***A computer and printer***—A computer offers many benefits. It enables you to store the letters and résumés that you create and send out. It gives you Internet and e-mail access, which are important as many employers today post job openings on the Internet and correspond by e-mail. Letters and résumés prepared on the computer look more professional than handwritten letters. If you do not own a computer, you should have access to one. Most public libraries have computers available to the public, and you can obtain an e-mail account whether or not your have your own computer.
- ***A telephone with voice mail***—Prospective employers should be able to reach you by telephone. The message on your voice mail should sound professional.
- ***Office supplies***—Make sure that you have a supply of good-quality paper, notebooks, envelopes, file folders, a stapler, paper clips, Post-It notes, pens, pencils, and stamps.
- ***Resources***—Many excellent books available at the library as well as Web sites on the Internet can provide needed information to help you with your job search. Look for books and Web sites that can show you how to prepare a résumé and cover letter. Your college library or local public library should have extensive resources on the job search (see Box 48–1 for a list of useful resources).

SETTING PRIORITIES AND GOALS

Before creating your résumé, think about your priorities and goals. Determine the following:

- What type of support work do you want to pursue?

Box 48–1 Useful Resources for Your Job Search

Resource	Description
What Color Is Your Parachute?	Well-known guide on job hunting
www.jobhuntersbible.com	Web site for *What Color Is Your Parachute?*
jobfutures.ca/en/home.shtml	Web site address for Job Futures, a Canadian site that provides information on the world of work, including an overview of the labour market
www.careerbookstore.ca	Web site with a comprehensive catalogue of books on all aspects of the job search
www.resumeedge.com	Free sample résumés and cover letters
accent-resumewriting.com/tips/	Tips on résumé writing
www.job-interview.net	Sample interview questions
www.workopolis.com	Comprehensive Web site on all aspects of the job search. It posts health care positions and also allows you to post your résumé for employers to view.

- Would you prefer to work in a facility or a community setting?
- Do you want full-time or part-time work?

As discussed in Chapter 3, there are many different kinds of support work settings. If you were unsure during your course about where you would like to work, your clinical placements may have helped you make the decision. If you are still undecided, you may want to apply for work in a variety of settings.

PREPARING YOUR RÉSUMÉ

A **résumé** is a concise one- to two-page summary of your experience, education, work-related skills, and personal qualities and is the first step toward a job interview. A résumé introduces you to possible employers, so it must look and sound professional. Employers use résumés to decide which job applicants to interview, and even small errors such as spelling mistakes may negatively influence the employer's decision.

It is best to prepare your résumé well before you begin your job search. This gives you time to do it properly without rushing. As you prepare your résumé, keep the needs of prospective employers in mind. Consider what most employers look for in support workers (see Chapter 1). Remember, however, that each job is unique, so make adjustments to your résumé to fit the needs of each employer and setting. ***Keep a copy of the résumé on your hard drive as well as on a CD or external drive. Remember to update it frequently, to reflect any new courses that you have taken or work experience that you have had since the last time that you updated it.*** If you also store your résumé on a flash drive (memory stick) you have the advantage of portability when you need to print off copies of your résumé when you are away from home.

Elements of a Résumé

All résumés include information on the following:

- ***Experience***—Employers want to know what you have done that qualifies you for the position. Experience does not have to be paid work. It can come from volunteer work, field placements, special projects, and recreational activities. Stress your skills and accomplishments rather than your duties and responsibilities.
- ***Education***—Employers want to know if you have the educational qualifications required for the position. Your résumé should include the exact name of your certificate, the name of your educational institution, and the year you graduated. Also include additional training and any awards or honours you received.

The following elements are optional:

- ***Objective***—An objective on a résumé states your career goal and briefly lists relevant skills, abilities, and personal qualities. It appears at the top of the first page of your résumé, right after your name and address.
- ***Profile***—A career profile summarizes your qualifications, highlighting particular skills and experience in one brief paragraph. It usually appears on the first page of your résumé, right after your name and address. Most people include either an objective or a profile, but rarely both.
- ***Interests***—Most career consultants advise against including a separate section on interests because it takes up valuable space. Instead, they suggest incorporating accomplishments in sports or hobbies into other sections of the résumé. Include information on sports or hobbies only if it is relevant to the job. For example, mention your skills in curling if it will help to show you as an experienced team player.

Getting Started on Your Résumé

Think of the résumé as an advertisement for those experiences, skills, and qualities that you have which an employer might be seeking. Start by making a list of the skills and qualities an employer would want in a support worker; then make a list of your own skills and qualities and the experiences that helped you to develop those qualities.

If you are not able to identify your skills and qualities, start by thinking about your experiences. Ask yourself what you learned from each experience and how your experiences have influenced you.

Organizing Your Résumé

There are two basic résumé styles: (1) the chronological résumé, and (2) the functional résumé.

Chronological Résumé. A **chronological résumé** highlights employment history, starting with the most current employment and working in reverse chronological order (backward) through earlier jobs (Figure 48–1). Because of its emphasis on work history, this style of résumé is best for those with:

- ***A steady history of employment in their chosen field***
- At least 2 years' employment with one employer
- Few gaps between jobs

Functional Résumé. A **functional résumé** highlights skills or functions and briefly lists positions held (Figure 48–2). Because it emphasizes skills and abilities, rather than specific jobs, a functional résumé is best for those with:

- Little work experience in their chosen field
- ***Long periods during which they were not in the workforce***
- Frequent job changes

A functional résumé should include your employment history with dates. A résumé that excludes this information might suggest that you have something to hide.

Creating Your Résumé

You will probably need to prepare several drafts of your résumé before you are satisfied. As you prepare your drafts, ask yourself the following questions:

- ***Is the information relevant?*** You have limited space to make an impression. Mention only those experiences that say something about how well you would perform on the job.
- ***Have I been completely honest?*** Emphasize your strengths, but do not misrepresent yourself. ***It is unethical to lie.*** Do not change your qualifications, job titles, and dates of employment. Do not exaggerate your limited accomplishments if you lack experience. Remember that some employers prefer to hire inexperienced workers, who may be more motivated, flexible, and easier to train than those with experience.
- ***Have I expressed myself clearly?*** Be concise, and avoid using long words. Revise your draft to make sure it is clear. Avoid giving information in paragraphs; use bulleted points instead. Sentences should be short and direct. Start them with action words, and avoid the use of the word "I." Remember, your résumé should be only one or two pages in length.
- ***Is my résumé consistent?*** Set up the page, headings, and sentences in a consistent format. Use

bullets, bold type, italic type, or underlining in the same style throughout the document. Use the same grammatical form for each point.

- ***Have I accounted for all my time?*** Do not leave blocks of time that are unaccounted for.
- ***Is my résumé correct?*** Read over the final document several times slowly and carefully. Some people have problems proofreading their own work because they read what they think they have written rather than what is actually on the page.

Begin by reading every word out loud. Make sure that what you have written makes sense as you hear it. If you find that you cannot judge

SEAN TOOTOOSIS

16 Uptown Street, Apt. 4, Edmonton, AB T9Q 2P1, (403) 765-4321, stootoosis@elsewhere.net

PROFILE

- Experienced support worker has cared for clients with diverse needs
- Skilled at motivating clients to regain their independence
- Dedicated to creating a caring, compassionate environment
- Discreet, hard-working, and loyal

EXPERIENCE

Support Worker, Hummingbird Agency, Edmonton, AB, August 2002–Present
- Provide personal care and support to diverse client population
- Skilled at caring for clients with quadriplegia and severe physical disabilities
- Selected to assist in training new staff and writing procedures for manual
- Praised for my calm, composed, empathetic manner with clients
- Demonstrated ability to work independently under minimal supervision

Support Worker, Primrose Group Home, Edmonton, AB, June 1999–July 2002
- Assisted developmentally disabled adolescents with activities of daily living
- Developed good listening and other interpersonal skills
- Demonstrated flexibility in meeting multiple needs and finishing tasks on time
- Commended by supervisor for initiative and problem-solving skills
- Served as leader of four-person team to redesign the home's living space

Lamantia Brickworks and Patios, Edmonton, AB, March 1994–May 1999
- Demonstrated leadership skills while supervising team of four bricklayers.

EDUCATION AND TRAINING

- Certificate in Personal Support Work, Western Canadian College, Edmonton, AB, 1999
- St. John's Ambulance First Aid and CPR Level C Certification, Edmonton, AB, yearly 1999–2006

OTHER

- Spoken languages: English and Cree

Figure 48–1 Chronological résumé.

your own work impartially and objectively, ask someone to read it aloud for you.

Follow this with reading your document backward, by starting at the end of the résumé and reading each sentence backward. You are more likely to catch typos and spelling mistakes when you read this way. Do not depend on computer spell-checks to find errors. When you are satisfied with your résumé, ask at least two reliable people to proofread it.

KAYLEE SAUVÉ

105 Pine Avenue, Hamilton, ON L4W 5Y3, (905) 725-9589, ksauve@link.com

OBJECTIVE

To provide support to clients in their homes and to deliver compassionate personal care.

SKILLS AND ABILITIES

- Listening skills: composed, respectful, and empathetic
- Speaking skills: won public speaking award in secondary school
- Language skills: speak English and French fluently
- Organizational skills: ability to complete work while meeting multiple demands
- Leadership skills: strong ability to motivate others; captain of winning basketball team
- Meal preparation skills: experienced; sound knowledge of food safety and nutrition
- Mature and responsible: childcare worker for two families for six years
- Flexible: able to work in a variety of settings and adapt to different situations
- Self-reliant: confident working under minimal supervision
- Physically strong: unloaded trucks and lifted boxes at local food bank

EDUCATION

- Certificate in Personal Support Work, Ontario Institute for Applied Health Sciences, Hamilton, ON, 2006
- St. John's Ambulance First Aid and CPR Level C, Certification, Hamilton, ON, 2006
- Food Safety course, River College, Toronto, ON, 2005

EXPERIENCE

Sunset Nursing Home, Field Placement, Hamilton, ON, February 2005–April 2005
- Prepared and delivered meals for 35 residents

Ricky's Restaurant, Waitress, Hamilton, ON, Summers, May 2001–August 2005
- Greeted customers, served meals, prepared salads

Children's Caregiver, Hamilton, ON, Part-time, 1998–2004
- Cared for children ages 4 months through 9 years

Volunteer, Daily Food Bank, Hamilton, ON, January 2001–March 2004
- Unloaded trucks, stocked shelves, helped customers

Figure 48–2 Functional résumé.

Formatting and Printing

To make a good impression, your résumé must look neat and professional:

- Choose a simple, professional-looking font (typeface) such as Times New Roman or Ariel. Do not choose fancy or script-type fonts.
- Do not use more than one font.
- Keep the use of graphic devices, such as bold type, to a minimum.
- Do not crowd too much material on a page.

Most computer programs have preset résumé designs that you can use to format your résumé. Many books and Web sites also present a variety of designs that you can use. Some Web sites offer services such as formatting your résumé and posting it on the Internet. You can also have your résumé formatted by a professional. Look in the Yellow Pages under "Résumé Service" to find a centre near you. Your college may also provide this service through the career centre.

Print your résumé on good-quality white or ivory bond 8½" × 11" paper. ***Never*** use flowery designed or patterned paper. If your résumé runs to two pages, staple the pages together. ***Never*** fold the corners down together. Paper clips can be used to hold your pages together, but this is not preferred by some employers.

Note: Because résumé formats change constantly, it may be worth securing the services of professional résumé writers. Check the Yellow Pages or the Internet for names in your area.

FINDING AND FOLLOWING LEADS

The main sources for advertised positions are local newspapers, the Internet, and college career services.

- ***Employment advertisements.*** Check national, local, and community newspapers daily for advertisements.
- ***The Internet.*** Many health care facilities post job openings on their Web sites. To search the Internet, use a search engine (e.g., Google) and type in search words such as "Health Care," "Home Health Care," "Home Care," "Home Health Services," "Community Health Care," "Retirement Homes," "Nursing Homes," "Nursing Services," "Not-For-Profit Jobs/Careers," and so on. General job search Web sites such as Workopolis (see Box 48–1 on page 902) also post health care positions.
- ***College career services.*** Some colleges offer career counselling and placement services to students and members of the community. Employers post job openings on the bulletin boards at the college or on the college Web site.

Some positions are not advertised. To find out about unadvertised positions, try the following:

- ***Contact people you know.*** Friends, acquaintances, and professional contacts may help you to find work and advance your career. Make a list of people you know in the health care field, including course instructors and employers you worked for in your program placement. Ask these people if any positions are available at their workplace. They may be aware of jobs posted on bulletin boards or jobs that may become available.
- ***Check with your district home care program.*** The Web sites of your health district's home care program or community care access centre may list agencies that are used to deliver home care in the community as well as long-term care agencies.
- ***Look in the Yellow Pages.*** Look under the headings "Home Health Care," "Home Care," "Home Health Services," "Community Health Care," "Retirement Homes," "Nurses and Nurses Registries," "Nursing Homes," and "Nursing Services."
- ***Check your local library.*** Libraries often have lists of health care facilities and agencies.
- ***Attend job fairs.*** Job fairs are often held at community colleges or elsewhere in the community and may be advertised in the local newspapers, on local cable channels, or at your college.
- ***Check with your Canada Employment Centre.*** These centres often have information about local area employers and about specific job openings.

Selecting References

A **reference** is a person who can speak to a potential employer about your skills, abilities, and personal qualities. Determine who you want as references early in the job search. Do not use family members or friends as references. Previous employers are usually the best people to use as references. Other possibilities are people in positions of authority, such as teachers and camp directors. Here are some basic tips about references:

- ***Ask for the reference***—Do not use someone as a reference without asking him or her. Explain the type of work you are looking for. Do not assume the person will speak positively about you. Ask the person what he or she would say your strengths and weaknesses are. Be reasonably certain the person will speak positively about you before listing him or her as a reference. If you are applying for more than one position, be sure to ask the reference if he or she would give you a reference for *each* position.
- ***Make sure contact information is correct***—Make sure you provide accurate phone numbers or e-mail addresses to give prospective employers. Make sure that it is directed to the correct department or room, especially if you are applying to a large agency such as a hospital.
- ***Keep your references informed***—Let your references know when you are going for a job interview so that they can be prepared for a phone call from your prospective employer. They are more likely to give you a good reference if they are prepared.
- ***Follow up***—Keep your references informed about your job search. If you got the job, thank them for their help. If you did not get the job, let them know.

PREPARING A LETTER OF APPLICATION

A **letter of application**, also called a **cover letter**, is included with a résumé. There are two kinds of letters of application:

1. A **solicited letter of application** responds to an advertised position (Figure 48–3)
2. An **unsolicited letter of application** inquires about potential job openings (Figure 48–4)

A letter of application should not simply summarize the information in your résumé. It should focus on what you can *offer* by summarizing how your skills and experiences are relevant to the job you are seeking. A good letter of application is persuasive, professional, and personalized. Try to find out the specific person who is responsible for hiring you, and direct your correspondence to him or her. Most administrators do not like to receive applications or résumés from job seekers when there is a designated individual and department to deal with recruitment and hiring. A letter of application should be addressed to a prospective employer by name and be written specifically for the position you are seeking.

Determining the Employer's Needs

If a letter of application is solicited, study the advertisement carefully to determine what exactly the employer is looking for. Describe your experiences and skills that match what the employer wants. Consider if you have skills and qualities that are not listed in the advertisement but that could contribute to the position advertised. Even if you are new to support work, your course should have provided you with information about those qualities.

If you write an unsolicited letter, find out as much as you can about the employer first. As mentioned earlier in this chapter, many agencies and facilities have Web sites that contain information about their health care goals and practices. For example, a facility's Web site might emphasize respect, compassion, and innovation as important goals. In your letter, you could indicate experiences in which you have demonstrated these qualities.

Organizing a Letter of Application

Use a standard letter format to organize your letter.

Front Matter.

- ***Return address.*** Put your mailing address at the top left-hand corner of the page.

ADVERTISEMENT

Ferndale Lodge has two positions available for support workers. Reporting to the Director of Nursing Services, the successful candidates will provide personal care to residents. They must have excellent communication, problem-solving, and organizational skills. They must be able to cope with the demands of personal care service and remain calm and courteous with clients and their families at all times. They must be available to work days, evenings, nights, and weekends. Experience preferred, but not required.

Reply in confidence to: Derek Sykes, Human Resources Director, Ferndale Lodge, Box 101, Littletown, BC, V6X 2Z1.

453 Lower Town Road
Littletown, BC
V6N 4N3

September 5, 2008

Mr. Derek Sykes
Human Resources Director
Ferndale Lodge
Box 101
Littletown, BC
V6X 2Z1

Dear Mr. Sykes:

I am writing to apply for one of the support worker positions that were advertised in the September 4th issue of *The Star Daily*.

You specified that Ferndale Lodge is seeking qualified support workers with excellent communications, problem-solving, and organizational skills. I attended the support worker program at Central Vancouver College, where I developed strong organizational skills and finished in the top third of the class. Before enrolling in the support worker program, I worked as a full-time cashier while raising three children. In my position as a cashier for *Fresh Food,* I interacted with the public and treated all customers with respect, tact, and courtesy. I was promoted to the customer service desk, where I learned how to solve customers' problems efficiently and diplomatically.

I am a mature, hard-working person who enjoys working with people. I am also assertive, persuasive, and adaptable to new situations. Because I am highly motivated to begin a new career in support work, I would be a productive and enthusiastic employee. I am available to work all the times that you listed in your advertisement, including weekends.

Enclosed you will find a résumé that details my skills and experience. At your convenience, I would like to meet to discuss how I can contribute to Ferndale Lodge.

Sincerely,

Belinda Lau

Belinda Lau
(604) 345-6789
bflau@internet.ca

Enclosure

Figure 48–3 A sample advertisement and a solicited letter of application.

105 Pine Avenue Hamilton, ON L4W 5Y3	Include return address
October 15, 2008	Include today's date
Ms. Katherine Ferrero Director of Personnel Mapleview Health Care Agency 1572 Maple Road Hamilton, ON L9P 8B2	Identify the name and title of contact, and address of prospective employer
Dear Ms. Ferrero:	Include a greeting
I read in *The Sun Daily* on October 14th that Mapleview Health Care Agency is expanding its home care services. I am writing to ask you to consider me if you need support workers.	Identify the position
The article in *The Sun Daily* indicated that Mapleview Health Care Agency offers a wide range of services to people in their homes, including personal care, meal preparation, and housekeeping. While completing a support worker course at Ontario Institute for Applied Health Sciences, I acquired skills in all those areas. For my six-week field placement, I worked in the kitchen at Sunset Nursing Home, where I prepared and delivered meal trays. In this position, I learned how to balance multiple demands by delivering hot meals on time and meeting the different dietary needs of residents.	Indicate your knowledge of the facility or agency Indicate your qualifications Link your skills to the job requirements; explain what you have learned from experience
I am a mature, responsible person who works well independently and as part of a team. Because I enjoy helping people, I know you would find me a competent and enthusiastic support worker.	Highlight personal qualities and other skills relevant to the job
Please find enclosed my résumé, which outlines my skills and experience in detail. I hope to have the opportunity to meet you to discuss how I can contribute to Mapleview Health Care Agency. Next week I will call you to discuss the possibility of an interview.	Indicate that your résumé is enclosed Ask for an interview
Sincerely,	
Kaylee Sauvé	Include a signature block
Kaylee Sauvé (905) 725-9589 ksauve@link.com	
Enclosure	

Figure 48–4 An unsolicited letter of application.

- ***Today's date.*** Include today's date on the left-hand side of the letter beneath your return address.
- ***Name, title, and address of prospective employer.*** Include the contact person's name, title, and address aligned with the left-hand margin. Ensure that this information is correct. You may have to call the facility or agency to confirm it. If you are unable to find out the person's name, you may have to exclude this information.
- ***Greeting.*** Greet the person you are writing to in a professional manner. If you do not know the name, write "Dear Sir or Madam."

Body.

- ***Paragraph one.*** Identify the job, indicate how you learned about it, and explain your purpose for writing. For unsolicited letters, use this opening paragraph to ask about potential opportunities.
- ***Paragraph two.*** Explain how your qualifications, experience, and skills relate to the position you are seeking.
- ***Paragraph three.*** Describe personal qualities or additional skills that make you a suitable candidate.

Closing.

- ***Paragraph four.*** Use the concluding paragraph to ask for an interview. If the letter is unsolicited, say that you will contact the reader at a future date. Refer the reader to the enclosed résumé.
- ***Signature block.*** End the letter in a professional manner by writing "Sincerely" or "Yours Truly." Leave some space, and type your name at the end of the letter. Sign in ink above the typed name. Add your phone number and e-mail address (if you have one) after your name. Type "Enclosure" at the bottom of the page to indicate that your résumé is enclosed.

Writing Your Letter

You will probably have to write several drafts to create a convincing letter. First, concentrate on putting down your main points or an outline. As you revise the content of the letter, ask yourself the following questions:

- ***Have I emphasized relevant skills and qualities?*** Mention experiences that demonstrate the skills, qualities, and attitudes necessary to support work. For example, if you have worked as a sales clerk, emphasize your positive interactions with clients.
- ***Have I emphasized accomplishments and skills?*** Rather than simply listing the tasks performed, explain what your experience has taught you. You might say "Working as a sales clerk taught me how to interact with the public in a warm, courteous, and respectful manner."
- ***Have I used an appropriate tone?*** Your letter should be written in a respectful, capable, and professional tone. Be persuasive without being boastful. Minimize the use of the word "I" to sound more modest. If you lack experience, avoid an apologetic tone.
- ***Is my letter concise?*** Your letter should not be more than one page long. If it is longer, edit out some of the details.
- ***Does my letter sound and look professional?*** Proofread your letter carefully and have at least two reliable people also read it. Create it on a computer. Use a standard business letter format, and print out the letter on high-quality paper. Double-check that your contact information is correct. You want to be completely sure that a prospective employer can reach you.

Delivering Your Letter

Hand-deliver your letter of application and résumé, whenever possible, to make sure it arrives on time. Another method of delivery is to courier the letter to a prospective employer. Follow up with a telephone call to the appropriate person to find out if the letter reached him or her. If you respond to an advertisement, send out your letter and résumé as soon as possible. Sometimes the earliest applicants get more attention simply because their applications arrived first.

Many employers request that letters and résumés be submitted by e-mail (see Box 48–2). Because

Box 48–2 Sample of an E-mail to an Employer When Submitting a Résumé

Subject: Job Application and Résumé

Dear Sir or Madam:

I am applying for the position of Support Worker that you advertised in the *London Free Press* on July, 4, 2008, and have attached a cover letter with my résumé. As you can see, I am available for hire immediately.

Sincerely,
Mariane Blankette

software programs vary, your résumé could lose its formatting or the prospective employer may have difficulty opening your attachment. If you send your letter and résumé by e-mail, send a hard copy as well. (However, if the employer asks the applicant not to submit a hard copy, you need to abide by this request.)

Tips on Conveying Professionalism Electronically

Since many employers post job opportunities on the Internet and many apply electronically, here are a few tips to ensure that you get the best attention:

- Your e-mail background should be electronically neutral. Do not have a patterned or designed background.
- Ensure that your e-mail address is a professional one. ***Never create a childish or offensive e-mail address.***
- Never use "cyber-speak," that is, short forms or acronyms for words (such as "LOL" or "CU later"). When using the Internet for professional purposes, you should use full sentences, appropriate punctuation, and correct and appropriate spelling and grammar.
- Ensure that your résumé is in the correct format (i.e., Microsoft Word, or WordPerfect). If you are unsure, contact the agency to find out or send the résumé in both formats.
- Do not have attachments or postscripts that open automatically (that indicate that you listen to a particular radio station, for example).

COMPLETING A JOB APPLICATION FORM

For some positions, you are expected to complete a preset job application form when employers need to find out specific information about applicants. Some institutions also use forms as a way to test applicants' reading and writing skills. It is a good idea to attach your résumé to the job application form, even when one is not required.

Most application forms ask for information about the following:

- Your legal eligibility to work in Canada
- Your education
- Your work-related skills
- Your employment history
- Names and phone numbers of employers
- Reasons for leaving previous jobs
- The names and phone numbers of three references

Remember that the completed application form says something about you. It should be professional looking and have no spelling or grammar mistakes or unfilled columns. Do a thorough job of filling the form. If possible, take two copies of the form home with you. Use one as a rough copy and the other as your final copy. Ask someone reliable to read and check the final copy. If you make an error on the final copy, use eraser fluid to make the correction.

Application forms often require detailed information, such as the reason for leaving a job. You must answer every question truthfully. If you have been fired, or if you have an inconsistent work history, consider attaching a note of explanation.

Some employers require you to submit an online application form. Be just as careful with an online application as you would be with a hard copy. Ask someone reliable to read it over before you send it.

THE INTERVIEW

You will not be hired as a support worker unless someone first interviews you and decides you are the right person for the job. During the interview, a prospective employer is trying to determine the following:

- Do you have the educational qualifications for the job?
- Do you have the skills necessary to do the job, or can you learn those skills?
- Will clients and co-workers respond well to you?
- Will you be a reliable, responsible, and motivated employee?

The interview is a key factor in any job search. From the interview, prospective employers decide if you have essential personal qualities such as compassion, respect, and enthusiasm. They can also judge if you are a good listener, if you speak clearly, and if you are at ease with others.

Interviewers may ask questions to find out the following:

- Can you handle the stress of working with seriously ill people?
- Can you deal with interpersonal conflict?
- Would you respond calmly and responsibly to an emergency?
- Are you capable of being firm and assertive with clients?
- Are you flexible enough to adapt to a variety of situations?
- Can you handle multiple demands and conflicts?
- Can you work under minimal supervision?
- Do you have initiative?
- Are you an effective team player?
- Can you handle routine problems on your own?
- Are you discreet?
- Do you respect individual differences?
- Are you a quick learner?
- Are you effective at managing your time?

Many interviewers ask situational questions, which are questions that are designed to find out what you would do in certain situations. You may be asked a question about an imaginary situation, or you may be asked to describe what you did in a particular situation.

Always be well prepared for an interview. When you are nervous, it can be difficult to think and speak clearly. If you have thought about possible questions and answers, you are more likely to be at ease. To prepare for an interview, think about the following:

- ***The position.*** Make sure you understand the nature of the position. Learn about the employer's services, clients, and philosophy. This may require some research. Check information about the employer that is available to the general public, such as Web sites and brochures. Talk to friends, instructors, and acquaintances who know the agency or facility. Review the skills and qualities that are essential to support work.
- ***Your qualities, skills, and experience.*** Develop a clear understanding of yourself: your values, skills, qualities, interests, goals, strengths, and weaknesses. Write these down, along with specific experiences that illustrate each.
- ***The interviewer.*** Put yourself in the interviewer's place. Review your cover letter and résumé. Why do you think you were selected for an interview? What concerns might the interviewer have about you? For example, if you are young and inexperienced, the interviewer may be concerned about your maturity level. If you have never remained in a job for more than a year, the interviewer may be concerned about your commitment. Be prepared to address these issues.

The Group Interview

More Than One Applicant. Occasionally, an agency may want to fill several positions, especially if it is short-staffed. In order to save time and trouble for the people who are doing the interviewing, the agency may group two or more applicants together in a room and ask each applicant specific questions. After one applicant has answered the question directed at him or her, the other applicants are invited to respond. Following this group interview, the applicants may be then interviewed individually.

The benefit for you of this interview type is that you might feel less nervous to know that "you are not alone." On the other hand, however, some applicants may be intimidated to think that their answers may be compared unfavourably with the answers of the other applicants in the room.

It is important to watch your body language and your responses during this type of interview. Try to watch each of the applicants as he or she answers questions. It is important that you appear friendly and polite. Do not ever cut someone off while he or she is speaking. This type of interviewing is a good technique for the interviewers to identify a "team player" who has effective communication skills (see Chapter 13).

More Than One Interviewer. This type of interview takes place with one applicant but two or more interviewers, who will take turns asking the applicant a question. The interviewers usually read from a written list of prepared questions. Occasionally, the interviewers may ask the applicant an unscripted question for clarification of something the applicant has said.

This type of interview is usually a very thorough one, and the applicant may leave the room feeling overwhelmed. You should be aware that the interviewers are trying to determine if you can handle questions well and if you can answer them in an honest and sincere manner. They may ask you questions that test your ability to solve problems, so they might ask you questions that begin with "What would you do if…."

It is important that you make eye contact with each interviewer as he or she is asking the question (see Chapter 13). Remember to use words and body language that show that you are friendly and approachable. The interviewers also want to know how well you can apply what you have learned in your support worker education to the scenarios that they present to you. These questions can be easily practised with a friend or a classmate.

Practising for Your Job Interview

Practice will give you confidence. When practising, focus on listening skills, relaxation techniques, and responses to questions you think might be asked.

Developing Listening Skills. The ability to listen is an important skill for interviews. If you fail to listen, you will not make a good impression. Since listening is essential in support work, an employer is unlikely to hire a poor listener as a support worker. Be a good listener during the interview by avoiding the following:

- Failing to concentrate on what the interviewer is saying
- Failing to ask for clarification if the question is unclear
- Talking too much
- Responding to questions too quickly without thinking first about the answer

Practising Relaxation Techniques. You will probably listen more attentively if you feel relaxed in the interview. Deep breathing exercises and other relaxation techniques can help you relax (see Chapter 9).

Practising Your Responses. Most interviewers ask similar questions. See Box 48–3 for a list of commonly asked questions. Practise your responses to these questions in front of a mirror or with a friend.

Planning

Plan ahead so that things go smoothly on the interview day.

- Decide what you are going to wear and make sure that the clothing is cleaned and pressed. Get a haircut, if you need one.
- If the route to the venue of the interview is unfamiliar, do a "practise run" so that you will not get lost on the interview day. Leave yourself at least 30 minutes to spare in case of traffic holdups on the way to the interview.
- Prepare a portfolio with a fresh copy of your résumé, notepaper, and a pen that works. Include a list of references with their complete contact information. It is a good idea to include a list of questions to ask during the interview.

Making a Good Impression

In an interview, first impressions are crucial. Poor impressions can be difficult to change, no matter how well you do later in the interview. From the moment you meet a prospective employer, you need to present a calm and professional image. This applies even when you stop by to pick up an application form. Pay attention to your grooming, your clothing, and your conduct.

Box 48–3 Common Interview Questions

- Tell me a little about yourself.
- What are your strengths?
- What are your weaknesses?
- Tell me about your last job.
- What did you like best/least about your last job?
- Why did you leave your last job?
- Why do you want to be a support worker?
- What do you think are the three most important qualities in a support worker?
- What do you think you can bring to support work?
- What do you think is the biggest challenge in support work?
- What do you like best/least about support work?
- Describe a situation in which you have met several demands.
- Describe a typical day in your last job.
- How did you manage your time in your last job?
- What did you learn from your last job?
- Give me an example of how you have worked as part of a team.
- Tell me about a time you showed initiative on the job.
- Tell me about a problem you had in your last job. How did you handle it?
- Tell me about a conflict you had with a client or co-worker. How did you handle it?
- What would your former supervisor tell me about your strengths and weaknesses?
- I am going to give you a made-up situation. Tell me how you would handle it.

In addition, some employers may present a scenario that involves some kind of witnessed abuse by a co-worker. The employer may ask you how you would handle or deal with this type of situation, both at the time that you witnessed it and later.

Grooming.

- Make sure your hair is clean, neat, and away from your face.
- Brush and floss your teeth. If you are a heavy coffee drinker or a smoker, bring breath mints with you (but do not have them in your mouth during the interview).
- Be careful not to wear too much makeup.
- Wear minimum jewellery. Avoid large bracelets, rings, and earrings.
- Remove body ornaments such as nose rings and eyebrow studs; cover tattoos.
- Do not wear any perfume.
- Make sure your nails are trimmed. If you wear nail polish, use a neutral colour.
- If possible, wash your hands before you shake hands with the interviewer, especially if your palms perspire when you are nervous.

Clothing.

- Men should wear a business suit, or jacket and pants, and a tie. Women should wear a business suit, dress, jacket and skirt, or jacket and tailored pants. Do not wear jeans, T-shirts, or shorts. Avoid tight clothing. Your outfit should be coordinated and should fit properly. It should also be in good repair and wrinkle-free.
- Women should make sure that hosiery is in good repair. Carry an extra pair of stockings in your purse.
- Shoes should be in good repair and well polished. Avoid casual shoes, such as running shoes or sandals, and shoes with very high heels.

Conduct.

- Arrive in the lobby 5 to 10 minutes before the interview.
- Do not bring anyone with you. If someone has driven you to the place, ask the person to wait outside.
- Do not chew gum, smoke, or eat as you wait for the interviewer. Ensure that your clothing does not smell of tobacco.
- Do not ask to use the phone, talk on a cell phone, or text-message anyone.

- Do not talk with the receptionist, unless he or she starts the conversation.
- If you feel nervous, take deep breaths to calm yourself.

Interview Tips

Being adequately prepared should help you feel relaxed during the interview. If you feel calm, you are more able to focus on details that may help you get the job. Some of these are discussed below.

Use a Firm Handshake. When you meet the interviewer, shake hands and smile. Use a firm handshake. A limp, clammy handshake makes a poor impression. Make sure your hands are dry. If your palms are perspiring, wipe them on a tissue as you wait in the lobby.

Do Not Use the Interviewer's First Name. The exception is if you are asked by the interviewer to do so. However, do address the interviewer by name.

Project a Confident Image. Stand or sit straight, breathe deeply to relax, and avoid nervous habits such as picking at your fingernails or fiddling with your hair. Be aware of gestures and body language that might be perceived negatively such as crossed arms. Look the interviewer in the eye, and keep your hands folded in your lap.

Listen Carefully. If you listen carefully, you should be able to answer questions concisely and directly. Do not be afraid to ask the interviewer to repeat a question.

Take Your Time. Many people speak quickly when they are nervous. Slow down, take a deep breath, and think about the question before you answer. A question answered too quickly may sound rehearsed.

Answer Questions Honestly. You must be honest in your answers. If you do not understand a question or are unsure of an answer, say so. Do not try to hide aspects of your past that you think may disqualify you from the job. Instead, explain how you have learned from past mistakes. For example, if you were fired from your last position, explain the reason and give examples of how you have corrected the behaviour.

Speak Positively About Your Previous Job. Do not demean, ridicule, appear upset with, or speak critically about your previous employer, regardless of the circumstances. To do otherwise may suggest a negative attitude.

Use Experiences to Support Opinions. When you are asked your opinion, support your answer with examples from your experience. For instance, after saying "I think it's important for support workers to know their scope of practice," describe a situation that illustrates this point. If you are inexperienced, use an example from your course of study.

Ask the Right Questions. Most interviewers conclude by asking if you have any questions. The questions you prepared in advance may have been answered during the interview. Rather than trying to think up new questions, it is acceptable to say something like "No, I don't have any questions. You have addressed all the questions that I had during our discussion." If you do have a question, make sure that it is appropriate. Do not ask questions about the salary, benefits, hours, and vacation times. You can ask about these when you are offered the position.

Concluding the Interview. At the end of the interview, thank the interviewer for his or her time. Show confidence and enthusiasm by saying something like "I am really interested in working for your facility, and I am sure I could be a productive member of your staff." Whatever you say, it is important to be genuine.

Follow-Up

Send a brief thank-you note after an interview. Write the note as soon as possible, no later than the day following the interview. The thank-you note will indicate that you are enthusiastic and courteous, and it might set you apart from other candidates.

The note can be handwritten or prepared on a computer. If you write the note by hand, use a plain white note card. Write at least one draft before you write the final copy. Ask someone else to read the note before you send it. Mail the note rather than sending it by e-mail. It shows the employer you are prepared to make an effort.

Express your thanks for the interview and reinforce your interest in the position. Sign your name on the card (see Figure 48–5 for a sample note).

THE EMPLOYMENT OFFER

You may be offered the position at the end of the interview or within a few days following the interview. You may wait weeks before hearing anything. Instead of waiting by the phone, continue to explore other opportunities. Even if you are not offered a job, the interview experience will have been worthwhile if you learn something from it. Review the interview process by asking yourself the questions in Box 48–4.

If you are not offered the job, contact the employer to find out why. Ask if you can talk to the person who interviewed you, either in person or on the phone. Most employers are willing to talk to people who are genuinely interested in improving their skills.

Accepting an Offer

A conditional offer is often made in the form of a letter of hire, that your employer will show you at the end of the interview, during a subsequent meeting, or by mail. Signing the conditional offer (and

October 03, 2008

Dear Ms. Frye,

Thank you for the interview on Wednesday morning. I appreciated the opportunity to meet you and to discuss your needs for the support worker position at Greenacres.

As I mentioned at the end of the interview, I am very interested in the position. I am sure that my recent experience in home care would enable me to make an immediate contribution to your care team.

Once again, thank you for your time and interest. I look forward to hearing from you.

All the best,

Sumi Ramarashan
(604) 432-7376

Figure 48–5 A sample thank-you note.

Box 48–4 Learning From the Interview Experience

- Was I prepared enough? Did I practise my listening skills, relaxation techniques, and responses to potential questions?
- Did I arrive for the interview in plenty of time?
- Did I pay enough attention to my grooming, my clothing, and my conduct?
- Did I project a calm, professional, positive image?
- Did I listen attentively?
- Did I speak clearly and calmly?
- Did I answer all questions honestly?
- Did I use my experiences to support my opinions?
- Did I relate my skills and experience to the requirements of the job?
- Did I show enthusiasm for the job?
- Did I express interest in the job at the end of the interview?
- Did I send a thank-you note after the interview?

faxing or mailing it back, if necessary) indicates that you have accepted the position. Before you accept an offer of employment, find out as much as you can about the terms of your employment. Find out if the offer is conditional and if the job begins with a trial period.

Terms of Employment. At the time of the job offer, make sure that you clarify your wages, your hours of work, requirements, and expectations. If, for example, a car is required for the position, find out the employer's policy on car mileage and repairs. Many employers publish procedure manuals that should address your questions.

If the job is a contract position, find out the length of the contract, the terms of the contract, and what is and is not included in the contract prior to accepting the offer.

If you are hired directly by a client or a client's family, you must specify the terms of your employment. The client may be required to contribute to Unemployment Insurance and Canada Pension Plan. He or she may also be required to submit your taxes directly to the government. Before you accept employment directly with a client, read Revenue Canada's booklet *Employee or Self-Employed* (Catalogue Number: RC4110(E) 1219), which is available at your local Canada Customs and Revenue Agency Office.

Conditional Offer. In the health care field, an offer of employment is often conditional, meaning that you must meet certain conditions or requirements before you are hired. These usually include a health report signed by your family physician that confirms that you are in good health and a police record check that shows that you do not have a criminal record. You are responsible for providing all documents that are required. Some employers may also require that you have certain equipment necessary to perform the job. For example, in community settings, a cell phone may be essential.

Probation. Most employers hire new staff for a probationary (trial) period that lasts 3 to 6 months. During this time, both you and the employer can decide if you are the right fit for the job. Within this period, the employer can end your employment at any time and you can leave without the usual two-week notice.

Benefits. Find out what you can about an employer's benefits package. Many employers have booklets that explain their benefit plan. Benefits do not usually begin until the end of the probationary period. If you work part-time, you may not be eligible for benefits. Be especially careful to find out about benefits if you are working directly for a client in his or her home.

How to Refuse or Leave a Job Without Burning Bridges

Occasionally, you might decide that you cannot work at an agency (or decide to leave an agency). This is a difficult thing to do, as it is important that the agency has a good impression of you. Many employers spend a lot of time and effort to train their employees and are understandably not happy when they leave, especially after a short period of time. Remember, you might want to return to that agency in the future! Ask to meet with your supervisor in person, and show up for this meeting dressed professionally. Remember, this is the *last* chance that you have to make a good impression!

If you are refusing a job or leaving a job because you are going back to school, have been hired at another agency on a full-time basis (assuming it is a part-time job here), are moving to another city, or you are pregnant and have decided not to work for some time, this is easy to convey to an employer. It is important—whatever the reason—that you be honest, tactful, and pleasant to the employer.

If, however, you are leaving because you do not like the atmosphere of the workplace or you are unhappy about the agency in any way, you need to be able to state this tactfully as well! Prepare what you are going to say ahead of time. If necessary, write down your thoughts on small index cards so that you can refer to them, if necessary. Always begin by stating what you *liked* about the agency. Be as fair as possible, remembering that you wanted to work there once!

When stating what you do not like about the agency, be as specific as possible. Instead of stating, "Well, I don't like the staff," you can be more specific (and therefore more honest) if you can say, "I do not agree with the afternoon staff who put residents in bed by 6:30 pm. I think the residents should have a say as to when they are put to bed, and their families should be involved in the decision process." Remember, you must always be honest. Do not lie or exaggerate a story to win favour with the supervisor!

Your statements inform the supervisor of the issues that exist in the agency. If you are a valued employee, the supervisor might ask if you would reconsider your decision to leave. This is a choice only you can make. Regardless of whether your decision is to stay or leave, you should always be professional and pleasant when conveying it.

REVIEW

Answers to these questions are at the bottom of the page.

Circle T if the answer is true or circle F if the answer is false.

1. T F It is best to prepare your résumé before you begin your job search.
2. T F A résumé is revised for each position applied for.
3. T F Every résumé should include an objective and a career profile.
4. T F A chronological résumé is best for those with a steady work history in their chosen field.
5. T F A functional résumé should not include employment history.
6. T F Résumés should make extensive use of graphics.
7. T F It is best to ask your references what they plan to say about you.
8. T F A letter of application should summarize the information from your résumé.
9. T F A solicited letter of application inquires about potential job openings.
10. T F A letter of application should list duties held in previous positions.
11. T F Most employers overlook small mistakes on letters, résumés, and applications.
12. T F It is acceptable to wear jeans to an interview as long as they are clean.
13. T F It is unacceptable to bring a friend to an interview, even if she or he stays in the lobby.
14. T F The ability to listen is one of the most important skills for an interview.
15. T F It is a good idea to bring a prepared list of questions to an interview.
16. T F It is usually not necessary to practise answering questions before an interview.
17. T F Assume you can address the interviewer by his or her first name.
18. T F It is best not to ask about salary, benefits, and holidays during an interview.
19. T F Never admit in an interview that you have been fired from a previous position.
20. T F If an offer is conditional, it is usually firm.

Answers: 1.T, 2.T, 3.F, 4.T, 5.F, 6.F, 7.T, 8.F, 9.F, 10.F, 11.F, 12.F, 13.T, 14.T, 15.T, 16.F, 17.F, 18.T, 19.F, 20.F

APPENDIX

Support Workers From Across Canada

Province	Job Title(s)	Education	Examinations
British Columbia	Home Support Worker Community Health Worker Long-Term Care Aids Home Support Worker Resident Care Attendant Health–Care Aide Health–Care Assistant	Community colleges Private Schools	No regulatory or comprehensive exam
Alberta	Support Worker Health–Care Aide	Community colleges Private Schools	—
Saskatchewan	Home Care Aide Health-Care Aide Home Support Health–Care Worker Long-Term Care Aide Nurse's Aide Resident Care Attendant Special Needs Assistant Continuing Care Assistant	Community colleges Private Schools	
Manitoba	Home Care Aide Home Care Attendant	Community colleges Private schools Dual credit programs (in some school divisions)	No provincial exam
Ontario	Personal Support Worker Health–Care Aide Personal Care Attendant Home Support Worker Patient Services Associate	Community colleges Private Schools District School Boards	No comprehensive exam required for community college graduates Comprehensive exam required for graduates from private schools A provincial certification exam (monitored by the CESBA PSW committee) is required from graduates of most district school boards
Quebec	Nursing Assistant Home Support Worker	Community colleges Private schools Community colleges	—

Support Workers From Across Canada (cont'd)

Province	Job Title(s)	Education	Examinations
New Brunswick	Home Care Worker	Community colleges Private schools	—
Nova Scotia	Personal Care Worker Continuing Care Assistant	Community colleges	—
Prince Edward Island	Home Care and Support Provider	Community colleges Private schools	—
Newfoundland & Labrador	Home Health–Care Aide Home Health–Care Assistant	Community colleges Private schools	—
Yukon Territory	Home Support Worker/ Nursing Home Attendant	Community colleges	—
Northwest Territories	Home Support Worker	Community colleges Private schools	—
Nunavit	Home Support Worker Nursing Home Attendant	Community colleges Private schools	—

GLOSSARY

abbreviation A shortened form of a word or phrase.

abduction Movement of a body part away from the median plane.

abrasion A partial-thickness wound caused by the scraping away or rubbing of the skin.

absorption The passage of a drug from the site of administration into the bloodstream.

abuse Physical or mental harm caused by someone in a position of trust—such as a family member, partner, or caregiver.

accessibility A principle of the *Canada Health Act* that states that people must have reasonable access to insured health care services.

accountability Being willing to accept responsibility and to explain your actions, inactions, or omissions, intentions, and decisions. Accountability cannot be shared: it rests solely on an individual.

acetone A compound that appears in the urine from the rapid breakdown of fat for energy.

acquired brain injury Damage to brain tissue caused by disease, medical condition, accident, or violence.

acquired immune deficiency syndrome (AIDS) AIDS is caused by the human immunodeficiency virus (HIV). HIV damages the immune system and makes a person susceptible to opportunistic infections.

act A specific law that has passed through the required legislative steps.

active listening A nonjudgemental communication technique that focuses not only on understanding the content of what is being said but also on the underlying emotions and feelings conveyed by the sender. This technique helps develop rapport and fosters trusting relationship.

activities of daily living (ADLs) Self-care activities people perform daily to remain independent and to function in society.

acute care Health care that is provided for a relatively short time (usually days to weeks) and is intended to diagnose and treat an immediate health issue.

acute illness Illnesses (such as influenza) and disabilities (such as a broken arm) which have a sudden onset and last for a relatively short period of time.

acute pain Sudden pain due to injury, disease, trauma, or surgery; it generally lasts less than 6 months.

adduction Movement of a body part toward the median plane.

administrator The name given to the person appointed by that province's Provincial Courts to administer the estate of a client who has died without leaving a will.

admission Official entry of a client into a hospital or other health care facility.

adolescence A time of rapid growth and psychological and social maturity that occurs with puberty. Because the start of puberty varies between the genders and between individuals, the approximate age range is from 10 years old for girls and 12 years old for boys until the age of 18.

adult day care See **Community day program**.

advance directive A legal document in which a person states his or her wishes about future health care, treatment, and personal care; the document is put into effect when the person is unable to make or express these wishes; **living will**.

advanced care directive See **advanced directive**.

advanced directive Legal documents that allow people to convey their decisions about their own end-of-life care. These documents are signed ahead of time, usually when the client is admitted to a long-term care facility. They are usually done in consultation with the client, his or her next of kin (usually one with power of attorney), the client's physician, and the agency's Director of Care (usually the nurse or supervisor in charge). Also known as **advanced care directive.**

adverse effect An undesirable, possibly harmful side effect of a drug.

affect A word that describes a person's feelings, emotions and moods, and the way the person demonstrate them.

affective disorders A group of mental disorders involving feelings, emotions, and moods.

afternoon care Routine care given in a facility that occurs between lunch and evening meal.

ageism Bias and discrimination against older adults; feelings of intolerance or prejudice toward a person or group of people because of their age.

age-related macular degeneration (AMD; ARMD) The breakdown (degeneration) of the macula (the light-sensitive part of the retina).

agnosia The impaired recognition of familiar objects or people, which occurs with dementia.

allergy A sensitivity to a substance that causes the body to react with signs and symptoms, such as a runny nose, wheezing, or congestion, or difficulty breathing. As part of the allergic reaction, a client's upper airway mucous membranes may swell.

alopecia Hair loss.

alternative remedies Herbal or other "natural" products that do not require a physician's prescription; not considered part of conventional medicine.

Alzheimer's disease (AD) A progressive, degenerative disease that gradually destroys nerve cells (neurons) in most areas of the brain and causes thinking and memory to become seriously impaired; the most common form of dementia.

AM care Routine care given in a facility before lunch. AM care sometimes occurs before breakfast. Also known as **early morning care** and **morning care**.

ambulation The act of walking.

amenorrhea Absence of at least three consecutive menstrual periods as normally expected to occur.

amputation The removal of all or part of an extremity.

amyotrophic lateral sclerosis (ALS) A neurological disorder that results in the loss of all muscle control but does not affect intelligence. Also known as **Lou Gehrig's disease**.

anaphylaxis A life-threatening sensitivity to a substance (antigen).

anatomical position The body is standing erect, with face forward, arms at the sides and palms of the hands facing outward.

anesthesia The loss of feeling or sensation produced by a medication that blocks the pain impulses to the brain; usually causes loss of consciousness.

angina pectoris Chest (*pectoris*) pain (*angina*) due to ischemia, a lack of blood supply to the heart muscle that is usually caused by an obstruction or spasm of the coronary arteries because of coronary artery disease.

anterior The front surface of the body—often used to indicate the position of one structure to another; located at or toward the front of the body or body part; ventral.

anticipatory grief The sense of loss and sorrow experienced before an expected loss happens.

antigen A substance, usually a protein, that the body recognizes as foreign and that can evoke an immune response.

anxiety A vague, uneasy feeling, including a sense of impending danger or harm.

anxiety disorders A group of mental disorders in which anxiety is the main symptom.

apathy An absence or lack of emotional feeling, which appears to be indifference.

aphasia Partial or complete loss (*a*) of speech and language skills (*phasia*), caused by brain injury.

apnea The lack or absence (*a*) of breathing (*pnea*).

apraxia Impairment of skilled motor system, resulting in problems with feeding or dressing oneself.

apraxia of speech Inability (*a*) to move (*praxia*) the muscles used to speak. Apraxia is usually caused by a brain injury.

arrhythmia Abnormal (*a*) heart rhythm (*rhythmia*).

arterial ulcer An open wound on the lower legs and feet caused by poor arterial blood flow.

arteries Blood vessels that carry blood away from the heart.

arthritis Joint (*arthr*) inflammation (*itis*).

arthroplasty Surgical replacement (*plasty*) of a joint (*arthro*).

asepsis Asepsis is the practice of reducing or eliminating potential pathogens (bacteria, viruses, fungi, and parasites). There are two levels of asepsis: (a) medical asepsis, for which the goal is the exclusion of all *pathogenic micro-organisms* through medical aseptic technique, and (b) surgical asepsis, which aims to exclude *all micro-organisms and their spores* through surgical aseptic technique.

aspiration Inhaling fluid or an object into the lungs.

assault Intentionally attempting or threatening to touch a client's body to cause harm without the client's consent.

assertiveness A style of communication in which thoughts and feelings are expressed positively and directly without offending others.

assessment Collecting information about the client; a step in the care planning process.

assigning Giving responsibility for providing care.

assisted-living facility See **supportive housing facility**.

asthma Respiratory disease characterized by narrowed air passages; episodes of difficulty breathing (asthma attacks) occur.

atrophy Marked shrinkage or wastage of a specific body part or tissue.

authority The legal right to do something.

autism A brain disorder that impairs communication, social skills, and behaviour.

autonomy Having free choice to make decisions that affect one's life. Also known as **self-determination**.

ball-and-socket joint A joint that allows movement in all directions. It is made up of the rounded end of one bone and the hollow end of another bone. The rounded end of one fits into the hollow end of the other.

base of support The area on which an object rests. If the base of support is adequate, this will prevent the object from tipping.

battery The touching of a client's body without the client's consent.

bed rails The metal or plastic sides of a hospital bed that are used to prevent a client from falling out of bed.

bedsore See **pressure ulcer**.

beneficence Doing or promoting good.

benefits Types of assistance that are provided through available insurance premiums. An example of one benefit would be a medical physical examination without any additional cost to the consumer.

benign Noncancerous.

bias When one person's point of view prevents him or her from impartially judging the issues relating to the subject being considered.

binge An episode where an individual eats a much larger amount of food than most people would in a similar situation. Binging is not a response to intense hunger but is usually a response to depression, stress, or low self-esteem.

binge eating A compulsive disorder, in which an individual has periods of uncontrolled, impulsive, or continuous binging.

biofilm A thin film that sticks to the teeth; it contains saliva, microbes, and other substances.

biohazardous waste Items that may be harmful to others because they are contaminated with blood, body fluids, secretions, or excretions; *bio* means life and *hazardous* means dangerous or harmful.

bipolar affective disorder An illness characterized by periods of serious depression, followed by episodes of mania (mental hyperactivity or "highs," irritable moods, and disorganized behaviour).

blended family A couple with two or more children, and at least one of the children is the natural child of both members of the couple, and at least one child is the stepchild of either member of the couple.

blister pack A transparent moulded piece of plastic with multiple compartments, sealed to a sheet of cardboard with a foil backing, used to package individual does medications. Also known as *bubble pack*.

blood pressure The amount of force exerted by the blood against the walls of an artery.

body alignment The way in which body parts (head, trunk, arms, and legs) are positioned in relation to one another, whether lying, sitting or standing. Also known as **posture**.

body dysmorphic disorders Altered body image perceptions, which lead to disturbances in eating behaviours and an abnormal concern with body weight and shape. Also known as **eating disorders.**

body language Posture, appearance, facial expressions, body movements, eye contact, and gestures that send messages to others.

body mechanics The movement of the body. Proper body mechanics ensures the body moves in an efficient and careful way.

body temperature The amount of heat in the body that is a balance between the amount of heat produced and the amount lost by the body.

boil A skin disorder caused by the infection of a hair follicle. Also known as **furuncle.**

bony prominence An area on the body where the underlying bone seems to "stick out." The shoulder blades, elbows, hip bones, sacrum (the bone in the lower part of the spine), knees, ankle bones, heels, and toes are all bony prominences.

brace An apparatus worn to support or align weak body parts or to prevent or correct problems with the musculoskeletal system; orthosis.

bradycardia A slow (*brady*) heart rate (*cardia*); a rate less than 60 beats per minute.

bradypnea Slow (*brady*) breathing (*pnea*); respirations are fewer than 10 per minute.

Braille A writing system for the blind that uses raised dots for each letter of the alphabet.

bruise See **contusion**.

burnout A state of physical, emotional, and mental exhaustion.

C. difficile (***Clostridium difficile***) is a bacterium that causes diarrhea and colitis. It is the most common cause of infectious diarrhea in hospitalized patients in the industrialized world and one of the most common infections in hospitals and long-term care facilities.

call bell A safety device for hospital patients and long-term care residents that enables them to call for assistance.

calorie The amount of energy produced as the body burns food.

Canada Health Act (1984) Federal legislation that clarifies the types of health care services that are insured; it also outlines five principles **(comprehensiveness, universality, portability, accessibility,** and **public administration)** that must be met by provinces and territories to qualify for federal health money.

Canadian Charter of Rights and Freedoms (1982) A law which states that Canada values equality and diversity and that no one should be abused or has the right to treat others unfairly; the *Charter* is part of the Canadian Constitution and is a constitutional document. It applies at the federal level, and all other laws must be consistent with its rules. The *Charter* lists the basic rights and freedoms to which all Canadians are entitled.

cancer A group of diseases characterized by out of control cell division and growth.

capillaries Tiny blood vessels that carry blood away from the heart; food, oxygen, and other substances pass from the capillaries to the cells.

care conference A meeting that occurs on admission and on an ongoing basis, usually once or twice a year. The purpose of the meeting is to discuss a client's care. It is attended by the client (if able), family/significant others/advocate, and members of the health care team. Also known as **family conference**.

care plan A document that details the care and services the client should receive.

care planning process The method used by nurses and case managers to plan the client's care with the team. Also known as the **nursing process.**

caring Concern for clients', as well as their families', dignity, independence, preferences, privacy, and safety at all times. True *caring* means honesty, sensitivity, comforting, discretion, and respect while showing this concern.

carrier A person who is able to transfer a pathogen to others without getting an active infection himself of herself because the pathogen has become part of that person's normal flora.

cartilage Connective tissue, which cushions the joint.

case manager See **team leader**.

cataract Clouding of the eye's lens.

catheter A tube used to drain or inject fluid through a body opening.

catheterization The process of inserting a catheter.

celiac disease A disorder of the small intestine caused by a reaction to gluten protein.

cell The basic functional unit of body structure.

centre of gravity The horizontal midpoint of a person's body. Also known as **line of gravity**.

cerebral palsy (CP) A disorder affecting muscle control (*palsy*); caused by an injury or abnormality in the motor region of the brain (*cerebral*).

cerebral vascular accident (CVA) See **stroke**.

cervical mucus A viscous discharge secreted by the glands in the cervix.

Cesarean section A surgical incision into the abdominal and uterine walls; the baby is delivered through the incision.

chart A legal document that details a client's condition or illness and responses to care; record.

charting See **documentation.**

chemical restraints Medication that is ordered by a doctor and given to a client to control unsafe, undesirable, or bizarre behaviour or movement. A chemical restraint is not given to cure a person's medical condition but merely to control behavioural symptoms.

chest tube A hollow plastic tube, surgically inserted into the chest cavity, between the inner lining and the outer lining of the lung (pleural space). The tube allows for the removal of trapped air (pneumothorax) and the drainage of blood or fluid (pleural effusion). The tube can go to an airtight drainage container or can be attached to a suction machine.

Cheyne-Stokes respirations Respirations gradually increasing in rate and depth and then becoming shallow and slow; breathing may stop (*apnea*) for 10 to 20 seconds. This type of respiration is common when death is near.

Child neglect When a child's parents or other caregivers are not meeting the essential needs for emotional, psychological, and physical development.

cholecystitis Inflammation of the gallbladder.

chronic care Treatment and care given for a pre-existing or long-term illness or health problem. Also known as **long-term** or **continuing care**.

chronic illness An ongoing illness, slow or gradual in onset, that may or may not grow worse over time. Because chronic illness cannot be cured, the focus of care is on preventing complications of the illness; illnesses (such as AIDS) or disabilities (such as paraplegia) that are permanent and last throughout the person's life. Also called *long-term illnesses* in some provinces.

chronic obstructive pulmonary disease (COPD) A chronic lung disorder that obstructs (blocks) the airways; refers to chronic bronchitis and emphysemia.

chronic pain Pain that lasts longer than 6 months; it may be constant or occur off and on.

chronic wound A wound that does not heal easily.

chronological résumé A résumé that highlights employment history, starting with the most current employment and working in reverse chronological order (backward) through earlier jobs.

circulatory ulcer An open wound on the lower legs and feet caused by decreased blood flow through arteries or veins. Also known as **vascular ulcer**.

circumcision The surgical removal of foreskin from the penis.

cirrhosis Chronic liver disease characterized by normal liver cells being replaced by scar tissue.

civil law Laws that deal with relationships between people.

clean technique A method of giving care using proper hand washing and clean equipment in order to reduce the risk of spreading pathogens. Also known as **medical asepsis** or "no touch" technique**.**

clean wound A wound that is not infected; microbes have not entered the wound.

clean-contaminated wound A wound occurring from the surgical portal of entry into the urinary, reproductive, or digestive system.

client A person receiving care or support services in a community setting; a general term for all people receiving health care or support services: hospital patients, facility residents, and clients in the community.

clinical depression See **major depression.**

closed questions Questions that are structured so that the response can be restricted to one word, such as "yes" or "no," or a few words.

closed wound A wound in which tissues are injured but the skin is not broken.

cognitive disability Impaired ability to learn. Also known as **intellectual disability**.

cognitive function Brain function involving memory, thinking, reasoning, understanding, judgement, and behaviour functions of the brain.

cognitive impairment The loss of a person's ability to remember, think, reason, understand, or live independently.

cold pack A treatment that involves wrapping a body part with a cold—moist or dry—application.

colitis Inflammation of the bowel.

colonization A process during which bacteria live on or in the body and survive as part of that person's normal flora.

colostomy An artificial opening (*stomy*) between the colon (*colo*) and the abdominal wall.

combining vowel A vowel added between two roots or between a root and a suffix to make pronunciation easier.

communicable disease A disease caused by microbes that spread easily. Also known as **contagious disease.**

communicable phase The period when a person is infectious and can spread pathogens on to others.

community day program A daytime community-based program for people with physical or mental health problems or older adults who need assistance. Also known as **adult day care** and **adult day centre**.

community-based services The health care and support services provided outside of a facility setting and in a community setting.

compassion Compassion is the awareness of the misfortune and suffering of another person and the desire and actions taken to reduce or alleviate the problem.

competence Performing one's job safely and within one's scope of practice or legal limits.

complex care facility See **long-term care facility**.

complex care A term used in some provinces as a guide to describe clients who need 24-hour professional care within a residential care facility. Also known as **long-term care** or **complex continuing care.**

comprehensiveness A principle of the *Canada Health Act* that states that all necessary health services, including hospitalization and access to physicians and surgical dentists, must be insured.

compress A soft pad that is moistened and applied over a body area.

compression bandage A bandage designed to provide pressure to a particular area, for example, on a bleeding wound, or to limit swelling in body parts, such as ankles, by wrapping it around. Also known as a **tensor bandage**.

condom catheter A sheath that slides over the penis; tubing connects the catheter and drainage bag.

conduct Personal behaviour that is based on moral principles.

confidentiality Respecting, guarding, and using discretion with personal and private information about a client.

conflict A clash between opposing interests and ideas.

confusion A mental state in which the person's memory and judgement are usually impaired and the person is disoriented to person, time, or place.

congenital Present at birth.

congestive heart failure (CHF) Condition occurring when the heart cannot pump blood normally; causes a buildup (congestion) of fluid in the tissues.

conjunctivitis An inflammation of the clear membrane that covers the white part of the eye and lines the inner surface of the eyelids. The nonmedical term for this is **pink eye.**

consent Agreeing or giving approval, such as to medical treatment, health care, or personal care services.

constipation A condition in which bowel movements are less frequent than usual; the stool is hard, dry, and difficult to pass.

constrict To squeeze or make narrow.

contagious disease A disease that is very likely to spread to others.

contaminated wound A wound with high risk of infection; pathogens have entered the wound.

contamination The process of being exposed to microorganisms, including pathogens.

continuing care facility See **long-term care facility**.

continuing care Medical, nursing, and support services provided over the course of months or years to people who cannot care for themselves. Also known as **long-term care** or **chronic care**.

contracture The lack of joint mobility caused by abnormal shortening of a muscle.

contusion A closed wound caused by a blow to the body. Also known as **bruise**.

convalescent care Comprehensive, inpatient care provided to people who are recovering from surgery, injury, an acute illness, or an exacerbation of a disease process. Convalescent care provides less intensive care than acute care in a hospital but more intensive care than that provided in long-term care facilities. The duration of care in a subacute care setting is time-limited. The goal is to help the client recover to be strong enough to go back into the community. If that is not possible, the client will be transferred to a long-term care facility. Also known as **subacute care** and **transitional care.**

convulsion Violent and sudden contractions or tremors of muscle groups.

coronary artery disease (CAD) A condition in which the coronary arteries are narrowed or blocked.

cover letter A letter that accompanies the application; summarizes the job applied for and reasons for applying for that position.

crime A violation of a criminal law.

criminal law Laws concerned with offences against the public and against society in general.

Crohn's disease A chronic, inflammatory condition of the gastro-intestinal tract.

cross-contamination The spread of pathogens from one source to another.

cultural conflict This term refers to negative feelings and conduct that can result when people from one culture try to assert their own set of values and behaviours onto another culture. In individuals, feelings of cultural conflict can also be caused by living within different cultures at the same time.

culture The characteristics of a group of people—the language, values, beliefs, customs, habits, ways of life, rules of behaviour, and traditions—that are passed from one person to the next and from one generation to the next. Culture is not limited to ethnic background but can extend to any group of interacting individuals that share similar learned characteristics.

cyanosis Bluish skin colour caused by a lack of oxygenated blood in the visible tissues.

cyst An abnormal closed sac, which may contain air, fluids, or semi-solid material.

cystitis A bladder infection.

Daily Value (DV) How a serving fits into the daily diet; expressed as a percentage based on recommended daily intake.

dandruff Excessive amount of dry, white flakes on the scalp.

deconditioning The loss of muscle strength from inactivity.

decubitus ulcer See **pressure ulcer**.

deep Distant from the surface of the body.

defamation Injuring the name and reputation of a client by making false statements to a third person.

defecation The process of excreting feces from the rectum through the anus; bowel movement.

defence mechanism An unconscious reaction that blocks unpleasant or threatening feelings.

dehiscence The separation of wound layers.

dehydration A decrease in the amount of water in body tissues; excessive loss of water from tissues.

delegation A process by which an RN authorizes another health care provider to perform certain tasks.

delirium A state of temporary mental confusion that can occur suddenly.

delusion A fixed, false belief that is not based on reality.

delusions of grandeur False and exaggerated beliefs about one's importance, talent, or wealth. For example, a woman believes that she is a goddess or the prime minister.

delusions of persecution False beliefs that one is being mistreated, abused, or harassed. For example, a man believes that his neighbour wants to kill him.

dementia A general term that describes the progressive loss of brain functions, which include cognitive and social functions. It is not a single disease but a group of illnesses that involve memory, behaviour, learning, and communication.

dependence The state of relying on others for support; being unable to manage without help.

dermatitis Inflammation of the skin caused by direct contact with an irritating or allergy-causing substance.

Determinants of Health The most important factors, such as lifestyle, environment, human biology and health services, that determine health status in an individual or a population of people.

detoxification A process that involves allowing abused substances to exit the body naturally or medically removing the substance from the body. The person being detoxified may go into **drug withdrawal**.

development The maturation toward adulthood that is usually characterized by physical changes and increased ability and functionality.

developmental disability A disability that occurs before birth, at birth, or during childhood or adolescence; impairs the child's development.

developmental task An activity that must be mastered during a stage of development.

diabetes A metabolic disorder characterized by hyperglycemia (high blood sugar levels) and resulting from low levels of insulin or a resistance to insulin's effect on a cellular level.

diabetic retinopathy A disorder (*pathy*) caused by diabetes, in which the blood vessels in the retina are damaged.

diarrhea The frequent passage of liquid stools.

diastole The period of heart muscle relaxation.

diastolic pressure The pressure in the arteries when the heart is at rest.

digestion The process of physically and chemically breaking down food so that it can be absorbed for use by the cells.

dignity The state of feeling worthy, valued, and respected.

dilate To expand or open wider.

diplegia Loss of ability to move (*plegia*) corresponding parts on both (*di*) sides of the body; both arms or both legs are affected.

DIPPS This acronym stands for dignity, independence, preferences, privacy, and safety. All clients have the right to compassionate care, which includes dignity, respect for their independence, respect for their own preferences, respect for their need for privacy, and need for safety.

dirty wound See **infected wound**.

disability The loss of physical or mental function.

discharge Official departure of a client from a hospital or other health care facility.

discretion Ability to use responsible judgement in order to avoid causing distress or embarrassment to a person.

discrimination Behaviour that prejudges or treats people unfairly, based on their group membership.

disease prevention Strategies that prevent the occurrence of disease or injury.

disinfection The process of destroying pathogens.

disorientation Another name for confusion.

distal The farthest away from the trunk of the body or the point of origin; the part farthest from the centre or from the point of attachment.

distilled water Sterile and pure water that has been boiled and allowed to cool and condense.

distribution The path the drug takes from the bloodstream to the body tissues of the intended site of action.

diversity The state of different individuals and cultures coexisting together.

diverticulosis The condition (*osis*) of having small pouches in the colon that bulge outward (*diverticulum*).

documentation Recording the care you have given the client and the observations you have made during care. Documentation is a legal requirement for health care providers. Support workers working in the community or the home care setting are required to document the care provided. In facilities, support workers may or may not document care, depending on the agency's policy.

dominant progressive hearing loss The impairment of nerves used to hear.

dorsal Located at or toward the back of the body or body part; posterior.

dorsal recumbent position See **supine position**.

dorsiflexion Bending the toes and foot up at the ankle.

dosette, pill box Containers that store medications in separate compartments arranged by day or hour (see Figure 40–2).

Down syndrome (DS) A congenital disorder caused by an extra chromosome; results in varying degrees of intellectual disability.

drawsheet A small sheet placed over the middle of the bottom sheet; it helps keep the mattress and bottom linens clean and dry; can be used to turn and move the client in bed.

droplet A drop of liquid.

drug antagonism An unusually weak drug effect that occurs when taking two or more drugs at the same time.

drug synergism An unusually strong drug effect that occurs when taking two or more drugs at the same time.

drug tolerance A state in which a person abusing a substance needs larger and larger amounts of it to experience the same effect.

drug withdrawal A physical reaction that occurs when a person abusing a substance stops taking it. Signs and symptoms of withdrawal may include depression, agitation, abdominal cramps, nausea, diarrhea, and painful muscle spasms, and the symptoms can be severe.

DSM-IV (*Diagnostic and Statistical Manual of Mental Disorders, Fourth Edition*) A manual published by the American Psychiatric Association, used throughout North America to classify mental illnesses.

dysarthria Difficulty (*dys*) in speaking clearly (*arthria*), caused by weakness or paralysis in the muscles used for speech.

dysphagia Difficulty (*dys*) swallowing (*phagia*).

dyspnea Difficult, laboured, or painful (*dys*) breathing (*pnea*).

dysrhythmia An irregular rhythm of the pulse; beats may be unevenly spaced or skipped.

dysuria Painful or difficult (*dys*) urination (*uria*).

ear infection See **otitis media**.

eardrum See **tympanic membrane**.

early morning care See **AM care**.

eating disorders See **body dysmorphic disorders**.

eczema A persistent inflammatory condition of the skin that can include recurring skin rashes.

edema Swelling in the tissues caused by an accumulation of fluid.

elective surgery Surgery that is scheduled but nonurgent; delaying the surgery does not result in permanent damage, disability, or death.

electroconvulsive therapy (ECT), A procedure in which an electric current is briefly applied to the brain to produce a seizure for quick relief of severe symptoms of depression or when there is no response to other forms of treatment. It is not known exactly how ECT works, but it is believed that ECT works by altering brain chemicals, serotonin, endorphins, and adrenalin.

electronic privacy Not disseminating a client's image, words, character description, or comments about his or her reputation by electronic means, including posting or forwarding these on any Web site, chat room, or e-mail address on the Internet, by way of cell phones, electronic listening devices, spy cameras, computers, or personal messaging devices of any sort.

embolus A blood clot, an air bubble, or a fat clot (a thrombus) that travels through the vascular system and finally lodges in a distant blood vessel.

emergency surgery Surgery that must be done immediately to save a client's life or prevent permanent disability.

emotional abuse An attack on a person's self-esteem, such as constantly insulting, humiliating, or rejecting him or her, or saying that he or she is "stupid" or "bad." All of these can harm the person's sense of worth and self-confidence. People at any age could be emotionally abused.

emotional health Well-being in the emotional dimension achieved when people feel good about themselves.

emotional illness See **mental illness**.

emotional neglect Occurs when a person's need to feel loved, wanted, safe, and worthy is not met. Emotional neglect can range from the context of the abuser simply being unavailable to that in which the abuser openly rejects the person. People at any age could be emotionally neglected.

empathetic listening A nonjudgemental technique that requires the listener to be attentive to the sender's feelings.

empathy The ability to recognize, perceive, and have an understanding of another person's emotions by being able to "put oneself into his or her shoes."

end-of-life care See **palliative care**.

enema The introduction of fluid into the rectum and lower colon.

engorged breasts Breasts that are filled with milk, which makes them swollen, hard, and painful. Engorgement usually decreases once breastfeeding is established or within 1 or 2 days after breast milk dries up.

enteral nutrition Giving nutrients by way of the intestine (*enteral*).

environmental restraints Barriers, furniture, or devices that prevent a client from having free movement.

epilepsy A chronic disorder of recurring seizures.

episiotomy An incision made in the perineum to increase the size of the vaginal opening for the delivery of the baby.

equitable A fair, reasonable, and just choice.

erythrocytes Red blood cells that make up the blood; the cells that carry oxygen from the lungs to body tissues.

ethical dilemma This is a situation that will often involve an apparent conflict between opposing moral choices, and choosing one would result in going against another moral choice.

ethics The principles or values that guide us when deciding what is right and what is wrong, and what is good and what is bad.

ethnic identity The ethnic background a person considers himself or herself to be part of, based usually on similar language and customs. Ethnic identity is not the same as citizenship, as people can be a citizens of one country but consider themselves to be part of another ethnic group.

ethnicity Groups of people who share a common history, language, geography, national origin, religion, or identity.

euphoria An exaggerated or abnormal sense of physical or emotional well-being that is not based on reality or truth.

eupnea The term for normal breathing.

eustachian tube The name for the tiny drainage pipe in the middle ear.

evaluation Assessing and measuring; a step in the care planning process.

evening care HS care or **PM care.**

evisceration Separation of the wound accompanied by protrusion of abdominal organs.

excretion The way the drug exits the body; excreted through the stool, urine, or skin.

executor, executrix See **guardian of property.**

expressive aphasia Difficulty in speaking or writing.

expressive-receptive aphasia Difficulty in speaking and understanding language.

extension Straightening a body part.

external rotation Turning the joint outward.

face mask A device used to deliver oxygen to a client who needs extra oxygen; consists of a mask that covers the client's nose and mouth, with a plastic tube at the bottom that delivers the oxygen. The mask also has holes on either side to allow for the exhaled carbon dioxide to escape. Face masks deliver more oxygen than can nasal cannulas.

failure to thrive A term to describe infants, babies, or children who are below the norms for body weight, growth, or cognitive development.

false imprisonment Unlawful restraint or restrictions of a client's freedom of movement.

family A biological, legal, or social network of people who provide support for one another.

family conference See **care conference.**

fanfold A method of folding sheets, in which the sheet is folded back and forth, in a form that resembles a fan.

febrile respiratory illness (FRI) is a term used to describe a wide range of respiratory infections, such as colds, influenza, influenza-like illness (ILI) and pneumonia spread through droplets**.** People with FRI may have a fever of greater than 38°C and new or worsening cough or shortness of breath. *Note*: Some elderly people or people with immune problems may *not* have a high fever.

fecal impaction The prolonged retention and accumulation of feces in the rectum.

fecal incontinence The inability to control the passage of feces and gas through the anus. Also known as **anal incontinence.**

feces The semisolid mass of waste products in the colon.

fetal alcohol effect (FAE) A milder form of FAS; the same symptoms may occur but to a lesser degree.

fetal alcohol syndrome (FAS) A group of physical and mental abnormalities in a child as a result of alcohol consumption by the mother during pregnancy.

fibromyalgia A condition associated with aching, stiffness, and fatigue in muscles, ligaments, and tendons.

financial abuse The misuse of a person's money or property.

flatulence The excessive formation of gas in the stomach and intestines.

flatus Gas or air from the stomach or intestines passed through the anus.

flexion Bending a body part.

flow rate The volume of fluid over a prescribed period.

flowmeter A device that connects to an oxygen tank, a portable oxygen generator, or to a wall connection in a hospital. It regulates the flow of oxygen to the nasal cannula or face mask.

focusing Limiting the conversation to a certain topic.

Foley catheter See **indwelling catheter.**

fomite Any nonliving object that is capable of carrying infectious organisms and may be serve as a mode of transmission.

foodborne illness An illness transmitted by contaminated food products, which includes improperly cooked or stored foods.

footdrop The foot falls down at the ankle (permanent plantar flexion).

fracture A broken bone.

fracture pan A small thin rimmed bedpan that is about 1 cm deep at one end. It is often given to clients who cannot manoeuvre themselves onto a larger bedpan, for example, someone who has had a hip fracture. Also called a **slipper pan.**

Fragile X syndrome The most common form among inherited developmental disorders.

friction The rubbing of one surface against another.

frost bite A medical condition in which damage is caused to skin and other tissues by extreme cold. Signs of **frost bite** include blisters, pale, white, or grey skin, cyanosis, shivering, numbness, pain, and burning.

full-thickness wound A wound in which the dermis, epidermis, and subcutaneous tissue are penetrated; muscle and bone may be involved.

functional incontinence Urinary incontinence caused by physical conditions or environmental barriers that prevent the client from reaching the toilet on time.

functional résumé A résumé that highlights skills or functions and briefly lists positions held.

furuncle A skin disorder caused by the infection of a hair follicle. Also called a **boil.**

gangrene A condition in which there is tissue death.

gastroenteritis More commonly known as "stomach flu," this childhood illness causes vomiting and diarrhea and can lead to dehydration, particularly in very young children and the frail older adult.

gastro-esophageal reflux disease (GERD) A disorder of the digestive system which causes heartburn.

gastro-jejunostomy tube A tube which connects the stomach to the jejunum.

gastrostomy tube A tube inserted through an opening (*stomy*) into the stomach (*gastro*).

gavage Tube feeding.

gel pack A commercially produced hot-and-cold pack designed to keep its temperature over a period of time.

gender The condition of being male or female, such as the *sex* of a person.

general anesthesia Unconsciousness and the loss of feeling or sensation produced by a medication

generic name of drug The name given to a drug approved by Health Canada. It is also known as the "official name" of a drug.

genetic endowment This is the genetic makeup that predisposes individuals to a wide range of responses that affect health status.

geriatrics The branch of medicine that provides care for older adults.

gerontology The study of the aging process.

glaucoma An eye disease that causes pressure within the eye and vision loss.

glucosuria Sugar (*glucos*) in the urine (*uria*).

gout A painful disease caused by the accumulation of uric acid in the cartilage of a joint.

grief The process of moving from deep sorrow caused by loss toward healing and recovery.

group home A residential facility in which a small number of people with physical or mental disabilities live together and are provided with supervision, care, and support services.

growth Increase in physical size and weight. It occurs in a slow and steady manner but has marked times of acceleration that occur after birth and during puberty.

guardian of property The person chosen by the deceased client to deal with his or her possessions, as it states in the will. Also known as **executor and executrix**.

hallucination Seeing, hearing, smelling, tasting, or feeling something that is not real.

hand hygiene The process of removing soil and excess microbes from the hands. Hand hygiene may be accomplished by either **hand washing** or the use of **waterless hand rubs** that sanitize the hands. Hand hygiene should always be practised before and after client contact or when in contact with any soiled material. Wearing latex or vinyl gloves should never take the place of hand hygiene. Hand hygiene should always be performed after removing the gloves.

hand washing The process of removing soil and excess microbes from the hands, using soap and running water. It is one form of **hand hygiene**.

harassment Troubling, tormenting, offending, or worrying a client by one's behaviour or comments.

hazardous material Any substance that presents a physical hazard or a health hazard in the workplace.

health The state of well-being in all dimensions of one's life.

health care associated infection (HAI) An infection acquired while a person is a patient, client, or resident in a health care facility or while receiving care from a health care provider. This term has replaced the term "**nosocomial infection.**"

health care ethics The philosophical study of what is morally right and wrong when providing health care services.

health promotion A strategy for improving the population's health by providing the necessary information and tools so that individuals, groups, and communities can make informed decisions that promote health and wellness.

heart attack See **myocardial infarction**.

hematoma The collection of blood under the skin and tissues.

hematuria Blood (*hemat*) in the urine (*uria*).

hemiplegia Paralysis (*plegia*) of one side (*hemi*) of the body; the arm and leg, body organs, vision, the tongue, and the swallowing mechanisms on the affected side can all be compromised.

hemoglobin The substance in red blood cells that carries oxygen and gives blood its colour.

hemoptysis Bloody (*hemo*) sputum (*ptysis*, meaning "to spit").

hemorrhage The excessive loss of blood in a short period of time.

hepatitis Inflammation (*itis*) of the liver (*hepa*) caused by a viral infection.

herpes simplex virus 1 (HSV 1) This virus is the cause of the common, nonsexually transmitted, cold sore. The infection is often triggered during times of physical or psychological stress. The initial symptom is a localized tingling or itching sensation. It is soon followed by a painful raised area on the skin that will form an abscess and scab over. It usually takes 7 to 10 days to heal.

Herpes zoster This is the reactivation of the varicella zoster virus, the virus that causes chickenpox. Previous exposure to chicken pox is therefore necessary. Herpes Zoster is a neurological disease, usually occurring during times of stress and immunosuppression. It is characterized by itching, tingling, and pain and followed by skin lesions that begin as a rash that turn into blisters. Also known as **shingles.**

high Fowler's position A semi-sitting position in bed; the head of the bed is elevated 45 to 60 degrees or the person is propped up with a backrest or pillows.

hinge joint A joint that allows movement in one direction.

hirsutism Excessive and increased hair growth in women in locations where the occurrence of visible, coarse hair is normally minimal or absent (such as on the face or neck). Men who are described as being *hirsute* have an abundant (or above average) amount of body hair or have coarse, visible body hair in areas of the body where men usually do not, such as on the foreheads, noses, or backs.

HIV (human immunodeficiency virus) The virus that causes **AIDS**. HIV damages the immune system and makes a person susceptible to opportunistic infections.

hives (wheals) A common form of an allergic reaction which causes raised red skin welts.

hoarding Collecting things and putting them away in a guarded manner.

holism A concept that considers the whole person; the whole person has physical, social, emotional, intellectual, and spiritual dimensions.

home care Health care and support services provided to people in their places of residence.

home management The cleaning and organizing of a home.

homeostasis a stable internal environment in our bodies.

homophobia The irrational fear of, aversion to, discrimination and contempt against homosexuality and homosexuals.

horizontal position See **supine position**.

hormone A chemical substance secreted by specialized glands into the bloodstream.

hospice A portion of palliative care that provides home, residential or in-patient care to a patient and who has a terminal diagnosis and is no longer seeking life-prolonging care. The philosophy of hospice is to provide support for the patient's emotional, social, and spiritual needs as well as medical symptoms as part of treating the whole person. Hospice workers try to make the client's last days as painless, comfortable, and dignified as possible.

HS care Routine care given in a facility in the evening at bedtime (HS means hour of sleep). Also known as evening care or **PM care.**

humidified oxygen Oxygen forced through distilled water and collected into the tubing; the oxygen now contains water vapour and is less irritating to delicate mucous membranes than is plain oxygen.

Huntington's disease An inherited neurological disorder; causes uncontrolled movements, emotional disturbances, and cognitive losses.

hyperextension Excessive straightening of a body part.

hypertension High blood pressure; persistent blood pressure measurements above the normal systolic (140 mm Hg) or diastolic (90 mm Hg) pressures.

hyperthyroidism A disorder caused by an overactive thyroid gland.

hyperventilation Respirations that are more rapid (*hyper*) and shallower than normal. Sometimes, respirations may be more rapid and deeper than normal.

hypotension A condition in which the systolic blood pressure is below 90 mm Hg and the diastolic pressure is below 60 mm Hg.

hypothyroidism A condition caused by an underactive thyroid gland.

hypoventilation Respirations that are slow (*hypo*), shallow, and sometimes irregular.

hypoxia A deficiency (*hypo*) of oxygen in the cells (*oxia*).

ileal conduit An artificial bladder fashioned out of a section of the ileum. Urine drains from the ureters into this newly created artificial bladder and then through the client's stoma.

ileostomy An artificial opening (*stomy*) between the ileum (small intestine; *ileo*) and the abdominal wall.

illness The loss of physical or mental health.

immoral Actions conflicting with traditionally held moral principles and are often regarded as indecent or deviant.

immunity Protection against a certain disease or infection; the person with immunity will not get or be affected by the disease.

impetigo A contagious skin disorder caused by bacteria.

implementation Carrying out or performing; a step in the care planning process.

incident report A report submitted whenever an accident, error, or unexpected problem arises in the workplace. Also known as an **occurrence report.**

incision An open wound with clean, straight edges; usually intentionally created with a sharp instrument.

incubation period The time between exposure to a pathogenic organism, and when signs and symptoms first appear.

independence The state of not depending on others for control or authority.

indwelling catheter A catheter that is inserted into the bladder, through the urinary meatus and urethra, so urine drains constantly into a drainage bag. Also known as **Foley** or **retention catheter**.

infancy The first year of life that is characterized by rapid physical, psychological, and social growth and development. Also known as **newborn**.

infected wound A wound containing large amounts of bacteria and showing signs of infection. Also known as **dirty wound**.

infection A disease state resulting from the invasion and growth of microbes in the body.

infection control Policies and procedures to prevent the spread of infection within health care settings.

inferior The lower parts of the body or indicating below a superior surface.

influenza A highly contagious infection of the respiratory tract by the causative virus in airborne droplets. Symptoms include sore throat, cough, fever, muscular pains, and weakness.

influenza Respiratory tract infection; the "flu."

informal giving practices Ways of giving which are not part of a formal celebration, for example, random acts of kindness.

informed consent Legal condition whereby a client has been given the relevant information so that she or he can appreciate and understand the situation and the potential implications and still consent to an action or procedure.

ingrown hair A hair that curls into the side wall of the hair follicle or into the skin surface, which causes the skin to become inflamed. Also known as **razor bumps**.

ingrown nails Toenails that grow in at the side of the nailbed.

inpatient A patient who is assigned a bed and is admitted to stay in a facility overnight or longer.

insomnia A chronic condition in which the client cannot go to sleep or stay asleep throughout the night.

intake The amount of fluids taken in by the body.

intellectual disability See **cognitive disability**.

intellectual health Well-being in the intellectual dimension achieved through an active, creative mind.

intentional wound A wound created for treatment.

interdependence The state of depending on one another.

interdisciplinary team See **multidisciplinary team**.

internal rotation Turning the joint inward.

interpersonal communication The exchange of information between two people, usually face to face.

intervention An action or measure taken by the health care team to help the client meet a goal in the care plan.

intradisciplinary team A team of providers from the same specialty.

intravenous (IV) therapy Fluids given through a needle or catheter inserted into a vein; referred to as IV, IV therapy, and IV infusion.

intubation The process of inserting an artificial airway.

invasion of privacy Violating a client's right not to have his or her name, photograph, private affairs, health information, or any personal information exposed or made public without consent.

irritable bowel syndrome (IBS) A disorder of the bowel characterized by abdominal pain and changes in bowel habits.

isolation precautions Guidelines for preventing the spread of pathogens; includes **Standard Practices** and **Transmission-Based Precautions**.

jaundice A yellowing of the skin and the white part (conjunctiva) of the eyes.

jejunostomy tube A tube inserted into the intestines through an opening (*stomy*) into the middle part of the small intestine (*jejunum*).

justice Treating people in a fair and equal manner.

ketone body A byproduct of the metabolism of protein.

knee-chest position An examination position in which the client kneels and rests the body on the knees and chest; the head is turned to one side, the arms are above the head or flexed at the elbows, the back is straight, and the body is flexed about 90 degrees at the hips.

laceration An open wound with torn tissues and jagged edges.

lactation The process of producing and secreting milk from the breast.

laryngeal mirror An instrument used to examine the mouth, teeth, and throat.

late adulthood Occurs approximately at the age of 65 years and older. This stage is characterized by adjusting to decreased physical strength and loss of health, retirement and reduced income, coping with the death of a partner, developing new friends and relationships, and preparing for one's own death.

late childhood Occurs between leaving childhood and dependency on others and entering adolescence. The approximate age range is 9 to 12 years. It is characterized by becoming independent of adults and learning to depend on oneself, developing and keeping friendships with peers, understanding the physical, psychological, and social roles of one's gender, developing moral and ethical behaviour, developing greater muscular strength, coordination and balance, and learning how to study.

lateral position A side-lying position that uses pillows to support the back and separate the lower legs.

lateral Relating to or located at the side of the body or body part; the farthest away from the midline of the body.

laundry care symbols Symbols on garment tags that indicate how to launder or care for specific garments.

legislation A body of laws that govern the behaviour of a country's residents.

letter of application A letter that is included with a résumé; can be solicited or unsolicited; cover letter.

leukocytes White blood cells that are part of the blood; the cells are part of the immune system that fight infection.

liable Being legally responsible.

libel Making false statements that hurt the reputation of another client. Statements are in the form of a permanent record and are usually in print, writing, or through pictures or drawings.

lice Small, insect-like parasites that live on the human body, most commonly on the skin, hair, and genital area. They feed on human blood and lay their eggs on body hair and in clothing. The word "lice" is plural for the word "louse."

licensed practical nurse (LPN) See **registered practical nurse.**

lift Moving a person from one place to another, without his or her weight-bearing or assistance.

lift sheet See **turning sheet, slider sheet**.

line of gravity The line dividing the body where the collection of the person's mass and all the weight of the object can be considered to be concentrated. Also known as **centre of gravity**.

lithotomy position A back-lying position in which the hips are brought down to the edge of the examination table, the knees are flexed, the hips are externally rotated, and the feet are supported in stirrups.

living will A document that lets the reader (for example, health care professionals or family members) know one's preferences about care intended to sustain life. In most long-term care facilities, it is part of an **advance directive**. Anyone can have a living will. However, it is not legally enforceable.

local anesthesia The loss of sensation in a small area, produced by a medication injected at the specific site.

lochia Postpartum vaginal discharge that begins as a bloody discharge and changes in colour and amount.

log-rolling Turning the person as a unit, in alignment, with one motion. The client's knee may be bent, if necessary, but his or her neck and spine should be turned in one step and never twisted.

long-term care Medical, nursing, and support services provided over the course of months or years to people who cannot care for themselves. Also known as **complex care, chronic care,** or **continuing care** in other provinces.

long-term care facility A facility that provides accommodations, 24-hour nursing care, and support services to people who cannot care for themselves at home but who do not need hospital care.

Lou Gehrig's disease See **amyotrophic lateral sclerosis**.

low-Fowler's position A semi-sitting position in bed; the head of the bed is elevated 15 to 30 degrees, or the person is propped up with a backrest or pillows.

lunge (or stride) step A position whereby you place one foot in front of the other foot, keeping both feet about a shoulder length apart. This stance will enable you to keep your balance while performing the various tasks related to moving, positioning, transferring, or lifting clients.

major depression A state of mind in which a person has severe feelings of worthlessness, self-blame, sadness, disappointment, and emptiness that last for weeks and interfere with the person's ability to perform activities of daily living. Also known as **clinical depression**.

malignant Cancerous; characterized by progressive and uncontrolled growth.

manual lift Physically moving a client who cannot weight-bear without the assistance of a mechanical lift.

marginalization Preventing a person from having any power or control over his or her life or health care because of language, life circumstances, or role in society, resulting in the person being shunned from mainstream society. For example, people addicted to drugs or alcohol and sex-trade workers are often **marginalized** from society.

marginalize To exclude people who are not part of the majority culture.

mastitis An infection of the breast.

mechanical lift A device that can elevate and move the person while in a special body sling. This device reduces the risk for injury to the support worker.

mechanical ventilation The use of a machine to move air into and out of the lungs.

medial Relating to or located at or near the middle or midline of the body or body part; the closest to the midline of the body.

medical asepsis Practices that reduce the number of pathogens and prevent their spread. Also known as **clean technique.**

medical diagnosis The identification of a disease or condition by a physician.

medicare Canada's national health care insurance system; publicly funds all the cost of medically necessary health services.

medication A drug or other substance used to prevent or treat disease or illness.

melena The passage of dark, tarry stools containing decomposing blood that is usually an indication of bleeding in the upper part of the alimentary canal and especially the esophagus, stomach, and duodenum.

menarche The time when menstruation first begins.

Ménière's disease An increase of fluid in the inner ear causing pressure in the middle ear; vertigo, tinnitus, and hearing loss occur.

menopause The time when menstruation stops.

menstruation The process in which the lining of the uterus breaks up and is discharged from the body through the vagina.

mental disorder See **mental illness.**

mental health A state of mind in which a person copes with and adjusts to the stresses of everyday living in socially acceptable ways. It is influenced by three factors: inherited characteristics, childhood nurturing, and life circumstances.

mental health care services Services provided to individuals and families confronting mental illness or disorders. Also known as **psychiatric services.**

mental health disorder See **mental illness**.

mental illness A disturbance in a person's ability to cope with or adjust to stress; thinking, mood, or behaviours are affected, and functioning is impaired. Also known as **mental health disorder, emotional illness**, or **psychiatric disorder.**

metabolism The burning of food for heat and energy by the cells; the body's physical and chemical processes that create and use energy. It is also associated with the breaking down of chemicals for excretion.

metabolization Chemical reactions that take place to convert a drug from smaller molecules into waste products before it can exit the body. Most drugs are metabolized in the liver.

metastasis The spread of cancer to other parts of the body.

metered dose inhaler (MDI) A pressurized canister of medication, surrounded by a plastic case that has a mouthpiece. Pressing the MDI releases a single dose of medication as a mist.

methicillin-resistant *Staphylococcus aureus* (MRSA) A type of multidrug-resistant organism (MRO) that is resistant to the antibiotic called methicillin.

microbe See **micro-organism**.

micro-organism A form of life (*organism*) that is so small (*micro*) it can be seen only with a microscope**.** Also known as **microbe**.

micturition See **urination**.

middle adulthood Occurs approximately between 40 to 65 years of age. This stage is characterized by seeing children growing up and moving away from home, adjusting to physical changes, developing leisure activities, and relating to aging parents.

middle childhood Ages 6 to 8 years is characterized by developing the social and physical skills needed for playing games, learning to get along with peers, learning behaviours and attitudes appropriate to one's own gender, learning basic reading, writing, and arithmetic skills, developing a conscience and morals, and developing a good feeling and attitude about oneself.

mildew A microscopic, fungal parasite that is responsible for the black discoloration that is often visible over bathroom surfaces and causes a foul odour in bathrooms.

mites Small, often microscopic, invertebrates that can infest stored food and are parasitic to animals and plants.

mobility The ability to move around.

morals Actions that are founded on the fundamental principles of right and virtuous conduct, rather than legalities or customs. The opposite of moral is **immoral**.

morning care See **AM care**.

multidisciplinary team A team of health care providers from a variety of backgrounds and specialties who work together to meet the client's needs. Also known as **interdisciplinary team**.

multidrug-resistant organism (MRO) A strain of bacteria that is very difficult to treat with common antibiotics; examples are MRSA and VRE.

multiple sclerosis (MS) Progressive neurological disease, in which nerve impulses are not sent to and from the brain in a normal manner.

muscle atrophy A decrease in size or a wasting away of muscle.

myocardial infarction (MI) Death (*infarction*) of heart tissue (*myocardium*) caused by lack of oxygen to the heart. Also known as **heart attack**.

nasal cannula A device used to deliver oxygen to a client who needs extra oxygen; consists of a plastic tube that fits behind the ears and a set of two prongs that are placed in the nares of the nose, and oxygen flows from these prongs. Nasal cannulas deliver less oxygen than face masks.

nasal speculum An instrument used to examine the inside of the nose.

nasogastric (NG) tube A tube inserted through the nose (*naso*) into the stomach (*gastro*).

nasointestinal tube A tube inserted through the nose (*naso*) into the small intestine (*intestinal*)

necrosis Death of cells, tissues, or organs as a result of disease or injury.

necrotic tissue Localized tissue death as a result of disease or injury.

need (basic human) That which is necessary or desirable for maintaining life and psychosocial well-being.

negative reinforcement Encouraging a behaviour by penalizing the person when that behaviour is not demonstrated.

neglect When a child's parents or other caregivers are not meeting the essential needs for emotional, psychological and physical development.

negligence Failing to act in a careful or competent manner and thereby harming a client or damaging property.

newborn During **infancy,** a baby is called a newborn, or a *neonate*.

nocturia Frequent urination (*uria*) at night (*noct*).

"no-lift" policy Agency regulations that prohibit you from manually lifting clients over a certain weight. You need to use a mechanical lifting device instead. In some agencies, "no-lift" policies extend to include situations where the client is agitated or uncooperative.

nonmaleficence The ethical principle of doing no harm.

nonpathogen A microbe that does not usually cause infection or disease and is not harmful to humans.

nonverbal communication Messages sent without words.

normal flora The mixture of different environmental organisms usually found on the surface of the skin and mucous membranes.

Norovirus This family of viruses causes nearly 50% of all gastroenteritis (stomach pain, diarrhea, and vomiting) around the world. Formerly also known as **Norwalk Virus** and **Norwalk-like virus**.

Norwalk virus and **Norwalk-like virus** See **Norovirus.**

nosocomial infection See **health care associated infection (HAI).**

nuclear family A family consisting of a father, a mother, and children.

nursing diagnosis A statement describing a health problem that is treated by nursing measures.

nutrients Substances that are ingested, digested, absorbed, and used by the body

nutrition The many processes involved in the ingestion, digestion, absorption, and use of foods and fluids by the body.

oath of confidentiality A pledge that all health care workers must sign, which promises that the signer will respect and guard personal and private information about a client, family, or agency. Signing the document obligates you not to reveal information obtained in the course of your work.

objective data See **signs.**

observation The active process of sensing and assimilating information within the context that has been constructed from past experiences.

occurrence report See **incident report.**

OH&S (occupational health and safety) legislation Federal and provincial laws designed to protect employees from injuries and accidents in the workplace; these laws outline the rights and responsibilities of employers, supervisors, and workers.

oliguria Scant amount (*olig*) of urine (*uria*); usually less than 500 mL in 24 hours.

open wound A wound in which the skin or mucous membrane is broken.

open-ended questions Questions that invite a person to share thoughts, feelings, or ideas.

ophthalmoscope A lighted instrument used to examine the internal structures of the eye.

oral hygiene Measures performed to keep the mouth and teeth clean; mouth care.

organs Groups of tissues that work together to perform special functions.

orthopnea Breathing (*pnea*) deeply and comfortably only while sitting or standing (*ortho*).

orthopneic position Needing to sit up (*ortho*) and lean over a table to breathe.

orthosis The process of straightening or correcting a deformity.

orthostatic hypotension A drop in (*hypo*) blood pressure when the client stands up (*ortho* and *static*); postural hypotension. Also known as **postural hypotension**.

orthotic Apparatus worn for support or alignment of parts of the musculo-skeletal system and to prevent or correct problems associated with it; a brace.

osteomyelitis Inflammation or infection of the bone.

osteoporosis A bone disorder (*osteo*) in which the bone becomes porous and brittle (*poros*).

ostomy The surgical creation of an artificial opening.

otitis media Infection (*itis*) of the middle (*media*) ear (*ot*); caused by either a virus or a bacteria, that most often occurs in children under the age of 2 but is also common between the ages of 5 and 6; it is triggered by respiratory illnesses picked up in kindergarten or first grade. Also known as **ear infection.**

otosclerosis a condition (*osis*) in which there is hardening (*sclero*) of the ossicles in the middle ear (*oto*).

otoscope A lighted instrument used to examine the external ear and the eardrum (tympanic membrane).

outpatient A patient who does not stay overnight in a facility.

output The amount of fluid lost by the body.

overflow incontinence The leaking of urine when the bladder is too full.

over-the-counter (OTC) medication A medication that can be bought without a physician's prescription.

oxygen-conserving devices Devices that help reduce oxygen wastage so that the client's oxygen supply lasts longer and he or she can go for longer outings.

palliative care Services for clients (and their families) living with or dying from a progressive, life-threatening illness; these services aim to relieve suffering and improve comfort, not cure the illness; end-of-life care provided in an interdisciplinary approach to care and service provision. Also known as **end-of-life care.**

pandemic An epidemic that has spread over a large region or even worldwide.

panic An intense and sudden feeling of fear, anxiety, terror, or dread for no obvious reason.

paralysis Complete or partial loss of ability to move a limb or muscle group.

paranoia Extreme suspicion about a person or a situation.

paraphrasing Restating someone's message in one's own words.

paraplegia Paralysis (*plegia*) from the waist down.

parasite Animals that live off other animals.

Parkinson's disease Neurological disorder in which cells in certain parts of the brain are gradually destroyed; causes tremors, muscle stiffness, slow movement, and poor balance.

partial-thickness wound A wound in which the dermis and epidermis of the skin are broken.

pathogen A microbe that can cause harm, such as an infection or a disease.

patient A person receiving care in a hospital setting.

pediculosis Infestation with lice.

pediculosis capitis Infestation of the scalp (*capitis*) with lice.

pediculosis corporis Infestation of the body (*corporis*) with lice.

pediculosis pubis Infestation of the pubic (*pubis*) hair with lice.

pelvic tilt A standing position whereby your pelvis is tilted by tightening the stomach muscles and flattening out the small of the back. It is used prior to lifting an object or transferring a resident in order to reduce the risk of back injury.

penetrating wound An open wound in which the skin and underlying tissues are pierced.

percussion hammer An instrument used to tap body parts to test reflexes. Also known as **reflex hammer**.

percutaneous endoscopic gastrostomy (PEG) tube A tube inserted into the stomach (*gastro*) through a stab or puncture wound (*stomy*) made through (*per*) the skin (*cutaneous*); a lighted instrument (*scope*) allows the physician to see inside the body cavity or organ (*endo*).

perineal care (pericare) Cleansing the genital and anal areas.

peripheral Away from the centre of the body.

peristalsis Involuntary muscle contractions in the digestive system that move food through the alimentary canal; the alternating contraction and relaxation of intestinal muscles.

peri-wash A type of soap that is used to wash the skin. It is used primarily as a cleanser and deodorizer of the perineal area soiled by urine and feces. It also emulsifies (breaks up) feces to aid gentle, easy cleaning. Because it is pH balanced to the acid mantle (covering) of the skin, it does not have to be rinsed off like other harsher soaps.

personal protective equipment (PPE) Special clothing and equipment that act as a barrier between microbes and a person's hands, eyes, nose, mouth, and clothes; includes gloves, gowns, masks, and eye protection.

personal space The area immediately around one's body.

personality disorder A group of disorders involving rigid and socially unacceptable behaviours.

phantom limb pain Pain felt in a body part that is no longer there.

phlebitis An inflammation of a vein.

phototherapy A treatment for **seasonal affective disorder (SAD);** involves exposure to light directed from a box containing white fluorescent light tubes.

physical abuse Force or violence that causes pain, injury, and sometimes death; the deliberate application of force to any part of a child's body, which may result in a nonaccidental injury.

physical health Well-being in the physical dimension achieved when the body is strong, fit, and free of disease.

physical neglect This occurs when a child's needs for food, clothing, shelter, cleanliness, medical care, and protection from harm are not adequately met.

physical restraints Garments or devices used to restrict movement of the whole body or parts of the body.

picture-frame dressing A type of dressing in which the tape is applied to all four edges to reduce the likelihood of the dressing wrinkling or falling off.

pink eye See **conjunctivitis.**

pitting edema A type of edema that is evident by (a) first compressing your fingers into the swollen tissues, (b) then removing your fingers, (c) observing an impression of your fingers left in the skin.

pivot joint A joint that allows turning from side to side.

planning Establishing priorities and goals and developing measures or actions to help the client meet the goals; a step in the care planning process.

plantar flexion The foot (*plantar*) is bent (*flexion*) with the toes pointed away from the leg.

plastic drawsheet A drawsheet placed between the bottom sheet and the cotton drawsheet to keep the mattress and bottom linens clean and dry.

PM care See **HS care**.

pneumonia Infection of the lung tissue.

podiatrist A physician who specializes in the evaluation and treatment of diseases of the foot.

pollutant A harmful chemical or substance in air or water. Air pollutants (e.g., dust, fumes, toxins, asbestos, coal dust, and sawdust) damage the lungs, and exposure can occur anywhere.

polyuria The production of abnormally large amounts (*poly*) of urine (*uria*).

portability A principle of the *Canada Health Act* that states that residents continue to be entitled to coverage from their home province even when they live in a different province or territory or out of the country.

positive reinforcement Encouraging a behaviour by rewarding the desired behaviour after it is demonstrated.

posterior The back surface of the body—often used to indicate the position of one structure to another. See **dorsal.**

postmortem care Care of the body after (*post*) death (*mortem*).

postoperative After surgery.

postpartum After (*post*) childbirth (*partum*).

postpartum blues Feelings of sadness or mild depression in the mother during the first 2 weeks after childbirth; baby blues.

postpartum depression A major depression at any point during the first year after childbirth.

postpartum psychosis The most severe form of postpartum depression; the mother may experience delusions, hallucinations, and suicidal thoughts.

postural hypotension See **orthostatic hypotension.**

posture Body alignment.

preferences The right to or the act of selecting someone or something over another or others.

prefix A word element placed at the beginning of a word to change the meaning of the word.

prejudice An attitude that forms an opinion on a person based on his or her membership in a group. It is formed from the word "prejudge," which implies that value assumptions regarding a person are formed before meeting or knowing that person.

preoperative Before surgery.

presbycusis The gradual hearing (*cusis*) loss associated with aging (*presby*).

presbyopia The gradual inability to focus (*opia*) on close objects; a condition associated with aging (*presby*).

preschool Ages 3 to 5 years and is characterized by increasing ability to communicate and understand others, the ability to perform self-care activities, learning the differences between the sexes, learning right from wrong and good from bad, learning to play with others, and developing family relationships.

prescription (Rx) medication A medication that is prescribed by a physician and dispensed by a pharmacist.

pressure points Bony prominences that bear the weight of the body in certain positions, which may lead to **pressure ulcers**.

pressure sore See **pressure ulcer**.

pressure ulcer Any injury caused by unrelieved pressure. Also known as **decubitus ulcer**, **bedsore**, or **pressure sore**.

primary care nurse A primary care nurse is responsible for the ongoing management of the health of a client, which includes liaising with other heath care team members, the client/resident and her or his family. In a long-term care (complex care) environment, the primary care nurse may or may not be directly involved in providing care on a daily basis.

primary caregiver A person who is responsible for providing care to a dependent individual, regardless of the dependant's age; a person—usually a family member or close friend—who assumes the responsibilities of caring for an ill or disabled client in the home.

privacy Privacy is the state of being free from unsanctioned intrusion, as well as the degree to which an individual can determine which personal information is to be shared with whom and for what purpose. It is one of the most important and comprehensive of all human rights, and yet it is one of the hardest to protect.

professionalism An approach to work that demonstrates respect for others, commitment, competence, and appropriate behaviour.

prognosis The expected course of recovery, which may range from recovery to death, based on the usual outcome of the illness.

pronation Turning downward.

prone position A front-lying position on the abdomen, with the head turned to one side.

prostheses (singular, prosthesis) Artificial replacements for missing body parts.

proximal Nearest to the trunk of the body or the point of origin; the part nearest to the centre or to the point of origin.

proxy See **substitute decision maker**.

pseudo-dementia A word that means false (*pseudo*) dementia. Pseudo-dementia often occurs when severe depression causes cognitive changes that mimic dementia.

psoriasis A chronic skin disorder which affects the skin and joints. It commonly causes red scaly patches to appear on the skin.

psychiatric disorder See **mental illness**.

psychiatric services See **mental health care services**.

psycho-geriatrics A specialty which involves the study of the causes and treatment of dementia, behavioural disturbances, and psychiatric problems in older adults.

psychological abuse Emotional abuse.

psychosis A mental state in which perception of reality is impaired.

psychosocial health Well-being in the social, emotional, intellectual, and spiritual dimensions of one's life.

psychotherapy A form of therapy in which a client explores his or her thoughts, feelings, and behaviours with help and guidance from a mental health specialist.

puberty The period when the reproductive organs begin to function and secondary sex characteristics appear.

public administration A principle of the *Canada Health Act* that states that provincial health insurance must be administered by a public authority on a nonprofit basis.

pulse The beat of the heart felt at an artery as a wave of blood passes through the artery.

pulse deficit The difference between the apical and radial pulse rates.

pulse oximeter A device that measures (*meter*) oxygen (*oxi*) concentration in the arterial blood; consists of a computerized monitor and a sensor (probe).

pulse rate The number of heartbeats or pulses felt in 1 minute.

puncture wound An open wound made by a sharp object; entry of the skin and underlying tissues may be intentional or unintentional.

purulent drainage Thick drainage from a wound or body orifice that is yellow, green, or brown in colour that could indicate an infection.

pyelonephritis Inflammation of the pelvis or of the kidney

quadriplegia Paralysis (*plegia*) of all four (*quad*) limbs and the trunk; paralysis from the neck down.

racism Feelings of superiority over, and intolerance or prejudice toward, a person or group of people who may be different in physical appearances or cultural practices.

radiating pain Pain that is felt not just at the site of tissue damage but extends to nearby areas.

range of motion (ROM) Moving a joint to the extent possible without causing pain.

razor bumps See **ingrown hair**.

reactive depression A term that some health care professionals use to describe normal reactions, such as feelings of loss and sadness, to what a person has just experienced.

receptive aphasia Difficulty understanding language.

record See **chart**.

recording The process of documenting care provided and observations made. Also known as **charting** and **documentation**.

reference A person who can speak to a potential employer about the applicant's skills, abilities, and personal qualities.

reflex An involuntary movement in response to a stimulus.

reflex hammer See **percussion hammer**.

reflex incontinence The loss of urine at predictable intervals.

regional anesthesia The loss of sensation or feeling in a large area of the body, produced by the injection of a medication; the client does not lose consciousness.

registered nurse (RN) A health care professional who is licensed and regulated by the province or territory to maintain overall responsibility for the planning and provision of client care. RNs study for a longer period of time than do RPNs/LPNs, allowing for greater depth and breadth of foundational knowledge in the areas of clinical practice, decision making, critical thinking, leadership, research utilization, and resource management.

registered practical nurse (RPN) A health care professional, licensed and regulated by the province or territory to carry out nursing techniques and client care. Both categories of nurse (RNs and LPN/RPNs) study from the same body of nursing knowledge, although RPNs study for a shorter period of time than RNs, resulting in a more focused body of foundational knowledge. They can work both independently and as part of the health team along with an RN. Also known as a **licensed practical nurse (LPN)** in many provinces.

registered psychiatric nurse (RPN) A nurse who is educated and registered in his or her own province to provide care specifically to individuals whose primary needs relate to mental, emotional, and developmental health.

regulations Detailed rules that implement the requirements of a legislative act.

regurgitation The backward flow of food from the stomach into the mouth.

rehabilitation services Therapies and educational programs designed to restore or improve the client's independence and functional abilities.

rehabilitation The process of restoring a client to the highest level of functioning possible through the use of therapy, exercise, or other methods.

relationship The connection between two or more people, shaped by the roles, feelings, and interactions of those involved.

remission Periods when the signs and symptoms of a disease lessen or disappear.

renal calculi Kidney (*renal*) stones (*calculi*).

repression Keeping (or "burying") unpleasant or painful thoughts from the conscious mind.

reservoir The environment in which microbes live and grow; host.

resident A person living in a long-term care (also known as a **residential**) facility.

residential facility A facility that provides living accommodations and services; includes assisted-living facilities, long-term care facilities, group homes, and retirement residences.

respect Showing acceptance and regard for another person.

respiration The act of breathing air into (inhalation) and out of (exhalation) the lungs; the process of supplying the cells with oxygen and removing carbon dioxide from them.

respiratory arrest Stoppage of breathing.

respiratory depression Slow, weak respirations at a rate of fewer than 12 per minute; respirations are not deep enough to bring enough air into the lungs.

respite care Temporary care of a person who requires a high level of support, care and supervision that gives the client's caregivers a break from their duties.

restraint Any device, garment, barrier, furniture, or medication that limits or restricts freedom of movement or access to one's body.

résumé A concise one- to two-page summary of experience, education, work-related skills, and personal qualities.

retention catheter A Foley or indwelling catheter.

retinal detachment The separation of the retina from its supporting tissue.

retirement residence A facility that provides accommodation and supervision for older adults.

Reye's syndrome A rare but potentially fatal disease causing inflammation of the brain, which can occur during the recovery stage of flu or chickenpox. It has been seen in children who take aspirin.

RICE An acronym for "**R**est, **I**ce, **C**ompression, and **E**levate" as a method of treating recent injuries.

right The entitlement of a person or persons to something. For example, Canadians have a **right** to safety and security.

rigor mortis The stiffness or rigidity (*rigor*) of skeletal muscles that occurs after death (*mortis*).

root A word element containing the basic meaning of the word.

rotation Turning the joint.

route How a medication enters and is absorbed in the body.

Routine Practices See **Standard Practices**.

safety The state of being free from actual, threatened, or imagined danger, risk, or injury.

same-sex family A family in which both adults who live together in a loving, intimate relationship are of the same gender.

scabies A highly contagious skin infection caused by a mite.

schizophrenia An extremely complex mental health disorder characterized by delusions, hallucinations, disturbances in thinking, and withdrawal from social activity. The exact causes are still a mystery, but it is believed to be caused by a biochemical imbalance.

scleroderma A chronic disease caused by excessive deposits of collagen in the skin or other organs.

scope of practice The legal limits and extent of a health care worker's role. This will vary from province to province and employer to employer.

seasonal affective disorder (SAD) A type of depression that occurs each year at the same time, usually starting in fall or winter and ending in spring or early summer. It is common in colder regions, where people tend to spend a majority of their winter months indoors. Signs and symptoms may range from mild to severe, and the condition is often mistaken for major depression.

secondary prevention Prevention strategies designed to intervene when risk factors or early indicators of a health-related problem are present.

seizure Brief disturbance in the brain's normal electrical function; affects awareness, movement, and sensation.

self-actualization Experiencing one's potential.

self-awareness Understanding one's own feelings, moods, attitudes, preferences, biases, qualities, and limitations.

self-determination See **autonomy**.

self-esteem Thinking well of oneself and being well thought of by others.

serous exudate The drainage from the body of serum, the watery portion of the blood, and high concentration of protein, cells, and other solid debris.

sexism Feelings of intolerance or prejudice toward a person or group of people because of their gender.

sexual abuse Unwanted sexual activity; occurs when a child is used for sexual purposes by an adult or an adolescent; involves exposing a child to any sexual activity or behaviour.

sexual harassment Any conduct, comment, gesture, threat, or suggestion that is sexual in nature; a form of sexual abuse.

sexually transmitted infections (STIs) Diseases that are spread by sexual contact.

sharps Equipment or item that may pierce the skin; includes needles, razor blades, and broken glass.

shearing The process in which skin sticks to a surface and the muscles under the skin slide in the direction the body is moving. Shearing can result in skin tearing.

shock The condition that results when there is not enough blood supply to organs and tissues.

side effect A response to a medication that occurs in addition to the intended or main response.

signs Are objective data gained through observation and the use of other senses about a client's health. Also known as **objective data**.

Sims' position A left side-lying position; the upper leg is sharply flexed so that it is not on the lower leg, and the left arm is positioned along the client's back.

single-parent families Families in which the adult head of the household does not have a partner who shares the home.

sitz bath A special shallow plastic bathtub, filled with warm water, designed to keep your buttocks and hips immersed while in a sitting position. Sitz baths are used to soothe the discomfort from pain and swelling and reduce the chance of infection by cleansing around the perineum.

skin tear A break or rip in the skin; the epidermis separates from the underlying tissue.

slander Making false statements that hurt the reputation of another person. Statements are usually verbalized and have no permanent record.

slider board A friction-reduced board with handles, which is placed under a person, is grasped by the handles, and then slid (with the client on the board) from one bed to another.

slider sheets Sheets used to slide clients up in the bed. The slider sheet has a slippery surface to reduce friction

slipper pan See **fracture pan**.

SOB Acronym for "short of breath."

social health Well-being in the social dimension achieved when people have stable and satisfying relationships.

social integration See **social support**.

social support Equipping a person with the skills and knowledge necessary to successfully live independently outside of an institution. Also known as **social integration**.

social support system An informal group of people who help each other or others.

solicited letter of application A letter of application that responds to an advertised position.

spastic Uncontrolled contractions of skeletal muscles.

sphygmomanometer The instrument used to measure blood pressure.

spina bifida A congenital disorder involving improper closing of the spine before birth; *spina* means backbone and *bifida* means split in two parts.

spiritual health Well-being in the spiritual dimension achieved through the belief in a purpose greater than the self.

SpO_2 The short form for the oxygen concentration value (S = saturation, p = pulse, O_2 = oxygen).

spore coat The protective shell that surrounds dormant bacteria and viruses, which protects them from external harm.

spousal abuse Abuse of a partner by a partner in an intimate relationship, such as a marriage or common-law relationship. The abuse may be physical, sexual, emotional, or financial, or any combination of them.

sputum Mucus from the respiratory system that is expectorated (expelled) through the mouth.

Standard Practices Guidelines to prevent the spread of infection from blood, body fluids, secretions, excretions, nonintact skin, and mucous membranes. Also known as **Routine Practices** or **Standard Precautions**.

Standard Precautions See **Standard Practices**.

stasis ulcer See **venous ulcer**.

stereotype An overly simple or exaggerated view of a group of people; assumptions made of a certain ethnic or cultural group by assuming that they are "all alike" or by believing that everyone in that group act or behave in a certain way.

sterile Free of all microbes, both pathogens and nonpathogens as well as their spores.

sterile field A work area free of all microbes, both pathogens and nonpathogens.

sterile technique See **surgical asepsis**.

sterilization The process of destroying *all* microbes.

steri-strip A type of adhesive bandage in which thin strips are applied across a skin tear; the dressing will bring the skin edges together and hold them together while the wound heals.

stethoscope An instrument used to listen to the sounds produced by the heart, lungs, and other body organs.

stigma A characteristic that marks a person as different or flawed.

stoma A surgically created opening through which a portion of the body cavity is brought to the outside environment.

stool Excreted feces.

straight catheter A catheter that is inserted to drain the bladder and is then removed.

strep throat A throat that is infected with **streptococci**.

streptococci (singular, *streptococcus*) A type of bacteria that cause **strep throat** and other problems.

stress The emotional, behavioural, or physical response to an event or situation.

stress incontinence The leaking of urine during exercise and certain movements.

stressor An event or situation that causes stress.

stroke A stroke is the sudden death of some of the brain cells due to a lack of oxygen. A stroke occurs when blood flow to the brain is affected, by blockage or rupture of an artery to the brain, resulting in abnormal function of brain. Also known as **cerebral vascular accident (CVA)**.

subacute care See **convalescent care**.

subjective data See **symptoms**.

substance-dependence disorder (substance-abuse disorder) The deliberate misuse of medications, illegal drugs, alcohol, or other substances.

substitute decision maker for health care A person authorized to make health decisions, such as to give or withhold consent on behalf of the client if the client is unable to do so.

substitute decision maker for property This is the person who would represent the incapable client's interests regarding his or her property.

suctioning The process of withdrawing or sucking up fluid (secretions).

sudden infant death syndrome (SIDS) The sudden, unexplained death of an apparently healthy infant under 1 year of age.

suffix A word element placed at the end of a root to change the meaning of the word.

suffocation Occurs when breathing stops due to lack of oxygen.

sundowning The name given for the condition in which the signs, symptoms, and behaviours of dementia increase at bedtime or during hours of darkness.

superficial Near the surface of the body.

superior Situated above.

supination Turning upward.

supine position A back-lying position; the legs are together; Also known as **dorsal recumbent position** and **horizontal position**.

support worker Support workers provide services to people who need help with their daily needs, both in facilities and in the community.

supportive housing facility A residential facility where residents live in their own apartments and are provided support services. Assisted living facilities are increasingly providing services to young and middle-age adults, and are not limited to a majority of older adults. Also known as an **assisted-living facility**.

suppository A cone-shaped, solid medication that is inserted into a body opening; it melts at body temperature.

suprapubic catheter A catheter that is surgically inserted into the bladder through the abdomen.

surgical asepsis Practices that keep equipment and supplies free of *all* microbes. Also known as **sterile technique**.

sympathy Feeling compassion for, or commiseration with, another person.

symptoms Information reported by a client that cannot be directly observed by others. Also known as **subjective data**.

syncope A brief loss of consciousness; fainting.

systems Organs that work together to perform special functions.

systole The period of heart muscle contraction.

systolic pressure The amount of force it takes to pump blood out of the heart and into the arterial circulation.

tachycardia A rapid (*tachy*) heart rate (*cardia*); a rate over 100 beats per minute.

tachypnea Rapid (*tachy*) breathing (*pnea*); respirations are 24 or more per minute.

tartar Hardened biofilm on teeth.

task A function, procedure, or activity that you assist with or perform for the client.

team leader A health care professional who assesses, monitors, and evaluates a client's needs in a community care setting; also co-ordinates team services. In a care facility setting, a team leader, usually a nurse, is responsible for managing the care of the clients. The team leader also provides direction to support workers. Support workers report to the team leader. Also known as **case manager**.

Telehealth Medical telephone call centres where nurses give advice to callers on health issues.

therapeutic Causing a desired, positive effect in the body.

thrombus A blood clot, an air bubble, or a fat clot; forms in a blood vessel.

tinnitus Ringing in the ear.

tissue A group of cells that perform a similar function together.

toddlerhood Occurs between the age of 1 to 3 years. Characterized by tolerating separation from the primary caregiver, gaining control of bowel and bladder functions, using words to communicate, and starting to assert independence.

tonic-clonic seizure A seizure involving convulsions.

tort A wrongful act committed by an individual against another person or the person's property.

toxic shock syndrome (TSS) A rare, often life-threatening, illness that develops suddenly after an infection. TSS can quickly affect several different organ systems including the liver, lungs, and kidneys. It has been linked to the use of tampons in postpartum women.

tracheostomy A surgically created opening (*ostomy*) through the neck into the trachea (*tracheo*).

trade name of drug The name given to a drug by the manufacturer. Also known as *proprietary name*.

transfer Moving a client from one room or unit to another or to another facility; to move a client from one place to another, using the client's assistance with partial to full weight-bearing.

transfer belt A strong strap that is secured around the client's/resident's waist, to help and support the client to stand, sit, and walk. It is removed after the activity is completed.

transfer board A smooth board placed between two surfaces (for example, a chair and a wheelchair) that allows the client to slide over more easily. Transfer boards are usually used when the client cannot weight-bear but can assist by using her or his upper body.

transfer of function Is a process by which an RN authorizes another health care provider to perform certain tasks

transient ischemic attack (TIA) A temporary interruption of blood flow in the brain.

transitional care See **convalescent care**.

Transmission-Based Precautions Guidelines to contain pathogens within a certain area, usually the client's room.

trauma An accident or violent act that injures the skin, mucous membranes, bones, or internal organs (physical trauma) or causes an emotionally painful, distressful, or shocking result (emotional trauma) that often leads to lasting mental and physical effects (psychological trauma).

tuberculosis (TB) A bacterial infection, usually affecting the lungs; a chronic infection caused by the bacterium *Mycobacterium tuberculosis*, usually transmitted through airborne droplets reaching a person's respiratory system.

tumour An abnormal lump or mass caused by cells growing out of control; tumours are benign or malignant.

tuning fork An instrument used to test hearing.

turning sheets Turning sheets are used to safely move a client up in bed, and they give support workers a more secure grasp. These sheets can be made of a variety of materials of waterproofed material, or even a folded sheet. Turning sheets prevent pain, skin damage, and bone and joint damage by protecting the client's skin from friction and **shearing** when the client is moved in bed. Also known as **slider sheets**, **lift sheets**.

tympanic membrane A thin oval-shaped layer of skin at the end of the external ear canal, which transmits sound to the middle ear. Also known as the **eardrum**.

umbilical cord The structure that carries blood, oxygen, and nutrients from the mother to the fetus.

unintentional wound A wound resulting from trauma.

universality A principle of the *Canada Health Act* that states that all residents are entitled to the same basic level of health care services across the country.

unregulated care providers (UCPs) A broad term applied to staff who assist nurses and other health care professionals in giving care.

unsolicited letter of application A letter of application that enquires about potential openings.

upper respiratory infections (URIs) This is the medical term for colds and other viral illnesses that affect the throat, nose and sinuses.

ureterostomy An artificial opening (*stomy*) between the ureter (*uretero*) and the abdomen.

urge incontinence The loss of urine in response to a sudden, urgent need to void.

urgent surgery Surgery that must be done soon to prevent further damage, disability, or disease.

urinary frequency The need to urinate at frequent intervals.

urinary incontinence The inability to control the passage of urine from the bladder; the loss of bladder control.

urinary tract infection (UTI) An infection in the urinary system.

urinary urgency The need to void immediately.

urination The process of emptying urine from the bladder. Also known as **micturition** or **voiding**.

urticaria A common form of an allergic reaction which causes raised red skin welts. (wheals). Also known as **hives**.

vaginal speculum An instrument used to open the vagina so that it and the cervix can be examined.

vascular ulcer See **circulatory ulcer**.

vector An organism that spreads infection by transmitting pathogens from one host to another but is not the cause of the infection.

veins Blood vessels that carry blood back to the heart.

venous ulcer See **stasis ulcer**.

ventral See **anterior**.

verbal communication Messages sent through the spoken word.

verbal report A spoken account of care provided and observations made.

vertigo Dizziness.

vital signs Temperature, pulse, respirations, and blood pressure.

voiding See **urination**.

VRE (vancomycin-resistant *Enterococcus*) A type of multidrug-resistant organism (MRO).

waterless hand rubs (waterless antiseptic hand-wash) Hand hygiene products containing 60 to 90% alcohol that are rubbed into the hands, and then allowed to dry completely. These rubs are used before and after direct contact with a client, bedding, or any object which may be contaminated with pathogens.

wellness The achievement of the best health possible in all dimensions of one's life.

wheals Raised red skin welts.

wheat/bean bags A type of heating bag that provides dry heat. It needs to be heated in a microwave. Because the beans may heat unevenly, the bag should be shaken to thoroughly to mix the beans and then covered with a cloth before applying to the client's skin.

word element A part of a word.

Workplace Hazardous Materials Information System (WHMIS) A national system that provides safety information about hazardous materials; includes labelling, material safety data sheets (MSDSs), and employee education.

workplace violence Any physical assault or threatening behaviour that occurs in a work setting that is directed toward the client and/or members of the health care team.

wound A break in the skin or mucous membrane.

young adulthood Ages approximately 18 to 40 years and is characterized by choosing an education and an occupation, selecting and learning to live with a partner, becoming a parent and raising children, developing a satisfactory sex life.

REFERENCES

Chapter 2

1. Public Health Agency of Canada. (1999). *Appendix C: Key determinants of health.* Retrieved June 28, 2007, from http://www.phac-aspc.gc.ca/ph-sp/phdd/docs/common/appendix_c.html.
2. Health Canada. (2005). *Canada's health care system.* Retrieved January 28, 2008, from http://www.hc-sc.gc.ca/hcs-sss/pubs/system-regime/2005-hcs-sss/del-pres_e.html

Chapter 4

1. World Health Organization. (1948) *Definition of health.* Retrieved January 25, 2008, from http://www.who.int/suggestions/faq/en/
2. Centre for Addiction and Mental Health. (2007). *Low-risk drinking guidelines.* Retrieved July 2, 2007, from http://www.camh.net/About_Addiction_Mental_Health/Drug_and_Addiction_Information/low_risk_drinking_guidelines.html
3. Nuu-chah-nulth Nursing Program. (2007). Retrieved July 2, 2007, from http://www.nuuchahnulth.org/tribal-council/nursing.html
4. Lalonde, M. (1974). *Toward a healthy future: Second report on the health of Canadians.* Ottawa: Government of Canada. Retrieved January 25, 2008, from http://www.phac-aspc.gc.ca/ph-sp/phdd/pube/perintrod.htm
5. Public Health Agency of Canada. (2004). *What determines health?* Retrieved April 20, 2007, from http://www.phac-aspc.gc.ca/ph-sp/phdd/determinants/determinants.html#unhealthy

Chapter 6

Arnold E., and Underman Boggs, E. (1999). *Interpersonal relationships: Professional communication skills* (3rd ed., p. 82). Philadelphia: Saunders.

Chapter 8

Potter, P.A, Griffin A., Perry, Ross-Kerr, J.C., and Wood, M.J. *Canadian fundamentals of nursing* (2nd ed., p. 240). Toronto: Harcourt Canada, 2001.

Chapter 9

Douglas, M.E., and Douglas, D.N. (1993). *Manage your time, your work, yourself* (pp. 16–17). New York: American Management Association.

Chapter 10

ALS Society of Canada. (2008). Retrieved January 25, 2008, from http://www.als.ca/default.aspx

Chapter 11

1. Province of British Columbia. (2004). *Community care and assisted living update, order in Council No. 476/04.* Retrieved January 25, 2008, from http://www.health.gov.bc.ca/ccf/ccal/ccalaupda.html
2. Ontario's *long-term care act,* 1994, S.O. 1994, c. 26, s. 3(1). *Consolidated as of: January 1, 2005.* Retrieved January 25, 2008.
3. Carlyle Peterson Lawyers, 700 Richmond Street, Suite 216, London, Ontario N6A 5C7 Tel. (519) 432-0632, Fax. (519) 432-0634.
4. Department of Justice, Canada. (1985). *Access to information and privacy.* Retrieved October 27, 2007, from http://www.justice.gc.ca/en/ps/atip/index.html

Chapter 12

1. Sorrentino, S. (1998). *Mosby's textbook for nursing assistants* (5th ed., p. 102). St. Louis: Mosby.
2. Davidhizar, R. E., and Giger, J. N. (1998). *Canadian transcultural nursing: Assessment and intervention* (p. 115). St. Louis: Mosby.
3. Davidhizar, R. E., and Giger, J. N. (1998). *Canadian transcultural nursing: Assessment and intervention* (p. 29). St. Louis: Mosby.
4. Sorrentino, S. (1998). *Mosby's textbook for nursing assistants* (5th ed., p. 98). St. Louis: Mosby.
5. Potter, P.A., Perry, A., Ross-Kerr, J.C., and Wood, M.J. (2001). *Canadian fundamentals of nursing* (p. 119). Toronto: Harcourt Canada.
6. Davidhizar, R. E., and Giger, J. N. (1998). *Canadian transcultural nursing: Assessment and intervention* (p. 51). St. Louis: Mosby.
7. Davidhizar, R. E., and Giger, J. N. (1998). *Canadian transcultural nursing: Assessment and intervention* (p. 31). St. Louis: Mosby.
8. Davidhizar, R. E., and Giger, J. N. (1998). *Canadian transcultural nursing: Assessment and intervention* (p. 30). St. Louis: Mosby.
9. Davidhizar, R. E., and Giger, J. N. (1998). *Canadian transcultural nursing: Assessment and intervention* (p. 28). St. Louis: Mosby.

Chapter 16

1. Gillis, D.E. (1995). *Promoting health eating to children: A look at successful Canadian programs.* Published by the National Institute of Nutrition. Retrieved September 27, 2007, from http://www.cfc-efc.ca/docs/ninut/00000350.htm.

2. BC Health Guide. (2007). *Healthy eating for children.* Retrieved September 27, 2007, from http://www.bchealthguide.org/kbase/topic/special/tn9188/sec3.htm.
3. Pless, B., and Miller, W. (2000). *Unintentional injuries in childhood: Results from Canadian health surveys.* Ottawa: Minister of Public Works and Government Services. Retrieved July 10, 2007, from http://www.phac-aspc.gc.ca/dca-dea/publications/unintentional_e.html.
4. National Institute of Child Health and Human Development. (2003). Retrieved June 11, 2007 from http://www.cnn.com/HEALTH/9905/03/infant.deaths/; National Institute of Child Health and Human Development. (2003).Retrieved June 11, 2007, from http://www.nichd.nih.gov/news/releases/deaths2.cfm.
5. Body and Health Canada. (2008) *Vaccination and your child.* Retrieved January 25, 2008, from http://bodyandhealth.canada.com/channel_health_features_details.asp?channel_id=145&relation_id=16435&health_feature_id=137&article_id=406.
6. Alberta Government Children's Services. Retrieved September 27, 2007, from http://www.child.gov.ab.ca/acyi/parenting/health/illness/page.cfm?pg=index.
7. Baby Centre. (2007). Retrieved November 20, 2007, from http://www.babycenter.ca/baby/health/whentoosicknursery/?printFriendly=yes, and Healthy Ontario, retrieved November 20, 2007, from http://www.healthyontario.com/ConditionDetails.aspx?disease_id=76).

Chapter 18

1. National Cancer Institute of Canada. (2002). *Canadian cancer statistics, 2002.*
2. Laboratory Centre for Disease Control. Retrieved February 2003, from http://www.hc-sc.gc.ca/hpb/lcdc/publicat/cdic/ cdic173/cd173b_e.html
3. Arthritis Society. *Rheumatoid arthritis.* Retrieved February 2003, from http://www.arthritis.ca/types%20of%20arthritis/ra/default.asp?s=1
4. Multiple Sclerosis Society of Canada. Retrieved February 2003, from http://www.mssociety.ca/en/information/ default.htm
5. ALS Society of Canada. *The ALS Society of Canada.* Retrieved February 2003, from http://www.als.ca
6. Heart and Stroke Foundation of Canada. Retrieved February 2003, from, http://www.heartandstroke.
7. Ontario Lung Association. Retrieved February 2003, from http://www.on.lung.ca/ola/aboutus.html
8. Canadian Diabetes Association. Retrieved February 2003, from http://www.diabetes.ca/Section_About/prevalence.asp

Chapter 19

Norris, M. A., Walton, R. E., Patterson, C. J., Feightner, and the Canadian Task Force on Preventive Health Care. (2007). *Recommendation statement: Prevention of falls in long-term care facilities.* Retrieved July 11, 2007, from http://www.ctfphc.org/Full_Text/CTF_FallsPrevn_RS_Aug05.pdf

Chapter 20

1. Ministry of Health and Long Term Care (2006**).** *Provincial Infectious Diseases Advisory Committee (PIDAC) Annual Report.* Retrieved June 23, 2007, from http://www.health.gov.on.ca/english/providers/program/infectious/pidac/pidac_mn.html
2. Government of Canada (2007). *Pandemic Influenza.* Retrieved January 25, 2008, from http://www.influenza.gc.ca/index_e.html.
3. Stephen T. Abedon (November 21, 1998). *Control of Microbial Growth.* Retrieved August 13, 2007, from http://www.mansfield.osu.edu/~sabedon/biol2030.htm

Chapter 21

1. Statistics Canada (2000). *Family Violence in Canada: A Statistical Profile* (p. 11). Retrieved July 25, 2007, from http://www.statcan.ca:80/English/freepub/83-224-XIE/0000085-224-XIE.pdf
2. Wathen, C. N. & MacMillan H. L. et al. (2003). Prevention of violence against women: Recommendation statement from the Canadian task force on preventive health care. *Journal de Association Médicale Canadienne, 169*(6), 582–584.
3. Public Health Agency of Canada. *Child abuse and neglect overview paper.* Retrieved June 11, 2007, from http://www.phac-aspc.gc.ca/ncfv-cnivf/familyviolence/html/nfntsnegl_e.html
4. Public Health Agency of Canada. *What is child abuse?* Retrieved June 11, 2007, from http://www.phac-aspc.gc.ca/ncfv-cnivf/familyviolence/html/nfntsnegl_e.html
5. Hockenbury, M., Wilson, D., Winkelstein, M., and Kline, N. (2003). *Wong's nursing care of infants and children* (7th ed.). St. Louis: Mosby; Public Health Agency of Canada. *Child abuse and neglect overview paper.* Retrieved June 11, 2007, from http://www.phac-aspc.gc.ca/ncfvcnivf/familyviolence/html/nfntsnegl_e.html
6. MacDonald, P.L., Hornick, J. P., Robertson, and G. B., and Wallace, J. E. (1991). *Elder abuse and neglect in Canada* (p. 29). Toronto: Butterworths.
7. Public Health Agency of Canada. *Abuse of older adults: A fact sheet from the Department of Justice Canada.* Retrieved May 21, 2007, from http://www.justice.gc.ca/en/ps/fm/adultsfs.html#ftn34

Chapter 30

1. Dellinger, M. (2007). *Caring for your African American or biracial child's hair.* Retrieved September 4, 2007, from http://adoption.about.com/od/africanamericanhaircare/ss/blackhaircare_2.htm
2. Shavers.co.uk. (2005). *Electric shaver maintenance.* Retrieved September 5, 2007, from http://www.shavers.co.uk/shavermaintenance.php
3. Look Good Feel Better. (2004). *Wig care.* Retrieved September 29, 2007, from http://www.lookgoodfeelbetter.org/women/hair_help/wig_care.htm

Chapter 34

1. Canadian Mental Health Association. (2002). *Mental Health and Mental Illness in Canada: Facts and Figures.* Retrieved January 27, 2003, from http://www.cmha.ca/mhw2002/ facts_fig.htm.
2. *Telemental health in Canada.* Retrieved March 24, 2007, from ***http://www.hc-sc.gc.ca.***
3. Health Canada. (2002). *A Report on mental illnesses in Canada.* Ottawa: Author.
4. The Traumatic Stress Group. (2003). *What is PTSD?* Retrieved April 15, 2007, from http://dev.www.uregina.ca/traumatic/
5. Schizophrenia Society of Canada. (2005). *Understanding schizophrenia.* Retrieved July 2, 2007, from http://www.schizophrenia.ca/english/index.php
6. Claudia Black. (1989). *Anger.* Retrived February 29, 2008, from www.authorsden/visit/viewpoint.asp?id=9017
7. Health Canada. (2002). *A report on mental illness in Canada*, p. 90. © Health Canada Editorial Board Mental Illnesses in Canada, Cat. No. 0-662-32817-5. Retrieved from http://www.hc-sc.gc.ca; The Canadian Mental Health Association. (1993). *Preventing suicide.* Toronto: National Office. Retrieved from http://www.cmha.ca/english/info_centre/mh_pamphlets/mh_ pamphlet_12.htm.
8. Centre for Addiction and Mental Health. (2007). *Low-Risk Drinking Guidelines.* Retrieved July 2, 2007 from: http://www.camh.net/About_Addiction_Mental_Health/Drug_and_Addiction_Information/low_risk_drinking_guidelines.html

Chapter 35

1. *People With Alzheimer's disease and related dementias.* Retrieved April 7, 2003, from http://www.alzheimer.ca/english/disease/ stats-people.htm
2. *Alzheimer disease: The progression of Alzheimer's disease.* Retrieved January 25, 2008, from http://www.alzheimer.ca/english/disease/stats-people.htm
3. *Pick's disease.* Retrieved January 25, 2008, from http://alzheimers.about.com/od/diagnosisissues/a/picks.htm
4. *Creutzfeldt–Jakob Disease.* Retrieved January 25, 2008, from http://alzheimers.about.com/od/diagnosisissues/a/cjd.htm
5. *The progression of Alzheimer disease.* Retrieved January 25, 2008 from http://www.alzheimer.ca/english/disease/progression-3stages.htm
6. *The ABCDs of Behaviour Management.* Retrieved January 25, 2008, from http://www.bendigohealth.org.au/Regional-Dementia-Management/Library.html

Chapter 36

Joanette, Y., Lafond, D., and Lecours, A.R. (1993). *The client with aphasia. Living with aphasia: Psychosocial issues* (pp. 19–36). D. Lafond, et al., eds. San Diego: Singular Publishing Group.

Chapter 37

1. *AMD awareness: About age-related macular degeneration (AMD).* Retrieved April 30, 2003, from http://www.cnib.ca/ amd/edu/amd_info.htm
2. Lewis, S.M., Heitkemper, M.M., and Dirkson, S.R. (2000). *Medical-surgical nursing: Assessment and management of clinical problems,* 5th ed. St. Louis: Mosby.

Chapter 38

1. Health Canada. (2000). *Family-centred maternity and newborn care: National guidelines* (p. 6.19). Ottawa: Minister of Public Works and Government Services.
2. Sword, W., Busser, D., Gannon, R., and Swinton, M. (July 13, 2007). *Care of women following referral for probable postpartum depression. Strategies in Women Health Care,* symposium of the 18th International Nursing Research Congress Focusing on Evidence-Based Practice.
3. Health Canada. (2000). *Family-centred maternity and newborn care: National guidelines* (p. 6.21). Ottawa: Minister of Public Works and Government Services.
4. Health Canada. (March, 2007). *Routine practices and additional precautions for preventing the transmission of infection in health care. Canadian communicable disease report* . Toronto: Author.

Chapter 39

1. Health Canada. (2002). *Congenital anomalies in Canada: A perinatal health report* (p. 2).
2. *Geneva Centre for Autism.* Retrieved March 2003, from http://www.autism.net

INDEX

Page numbers followed by b indicate boxes, f, figures; t, tables.

PROCEDURES